Estimated Safe and Adequate Daily Dietary Intakes (ESADDIs) of Selected Vitamins and Minerals*

| Category | Age (years) | Vitamins | | Trace Elements† | | | | |
		Biotin (µg)	Pantothenic acid (mg)	Copper (mg)	Manganese (mg)	Fluoride (mg)	Chromium (µg)	Molybdenum (µg)
Infants	0-0.5	10	2	0.4-0.6	0.3-0.6	0.1-0.5	10-40	15-30
	0.5-1	15	3	0.6-0.7	0.6-1	0.2-1	20-60	20-40
Children and	1-3	20	3	0.7-1	1-1.5	0.5-1.5	20-80	25-50
adolescents	4-6	25	3-4	1-1.5	1.5-2	1-2.5	30-120	30-75
	7-10	30	4-5	1-2	2-3	1.5-2.5	50-200	50-150
	11+	30-100	4-7	1.5-2.5	2-5	1.5-2.5	50-200	75-250
Adults		30-100	4-7	1.5-3	2-5	1.5-4	50-200	75-250

*Because there is less information on which to base recommendations for allowances of minerals, these figures are not given in the main table of RDAs and are provided here in the form of ranges of recommended intakes.

†Since toxic levels for many trace elements may be reached with only several times usual intakes, the upper levels for the trace elements given in this table should not be habitually exceeded.

> "It ain't what you don't know that hurts you... Its knowin' what aint so." —Will Rogers

Estimated Minimum Sodium, Chloride, and Potassium Requirements for Healthy Persons

Age	Weight (kg)	Sodium (mg)*†	Chloride (mg)*†	Potassium (mg)‡
Months				
0-5	4.5	120	180	500
6-11	8.9	200	300	700
Years				
1	11	225	350	1000
2-5	16	300	500	1400
6-9	25	400	600	1600
10-18	50	500	750	2000
>18§	70	500	750	2000

*No allowance has been included for large, prolonged losses from the skin through sweat.

†There is no evidence that higher intakes confer any additional health benefit.

‡Desirable intakes of potassium may considerably exceed these values (~13,500 mg for adults).

§No allowance has been included for growth. Values given for people under 18 years of age assume a growth rate corresponding to the 50th percentile reported by the National Center for Health Statistics and averaged for males and females.

ESSENTIALS
of NUTRITION and
DIET THERAPY

www.mosby.com

ESSENTIALS of NUTRITION and DIET THERAPY

with 115 illustrations

seventh edition

Sue Rodwell Williams
Ph.D., M.P.H., R.D.

President, SRW Productions, Inc.
and Clinical Nutrition Consultant,
Davis, California

Mosby

St. Louis Baltimore Boston Carlsbad
Chicago Minneapolis New York Philadelphia Portland
London Milan Sydney Tokyo Toronto

Publisher: Sally Schrefer
Editor: Yvonne Alexopoulos
Associate Developmental Editor: Melissa K. Boyle
Project Manager: Dana Peick
Production Editor: Cindy Deichmann
Designer: Amy Buxton
Senior Composition Specialist: Joan Herron
Manufacturing Manager: Betty Mueller

A Note to the Reader:

The author and publisher have made every attempt to check dosages and nursing content for accuracy. Because the science of pharmacology is continually advancing, our knowledge base continues to expand. Therefore we recommend that the reader always check product information for changes in dosage or administration before administering any medication. This is particularly important with new or rarely used drugs.

Seventh Edition

Copyright © 1999 by Mosby, Inc.

Previous editions copyrighted 1974, 1978, 1982, 1986, 1990, 1994

Printed in the United States of America
Composition by Mosby Electronic Production
Lithography/color film by Top Graphics
Printing/binding by Von Hoffmann Press

Mosby, Inc.
11830 Westline Industrial Drive
St. Louis, Missouri 63146

International Standard Book Number 0-323-00398-2

99 00 01 02 03 / 9 8 7 6 5 4 3 2 1

To my students,
whose "whys" and "hows" and "so whats"
keep my feet to the fire of knowledge
and make the learning process exciting
and ever new to me

Preface

Through six previous editions, this compact "little" book has served the needs of students and teachers in the health sciences in many community colleges, as well as providing a sound but simple reference for busy practitioners. In truth, in all its editions, as its title indicates, it has captured and distilled the essence of my larger, more comprehensive college and university textbook, *Nutrition and Diet Therapy*, to lay a faithful foundation for further study and practice.

In this new seventh edition I have adhered to these same fundamental goals. But as in the previous completely reformatted edition, here I have rewritten much of the material to reflect a rapidly developing science and society. Thus its expanded current material and its organization continue to meet the more comprehensive needs of beginning students in the allied health professions today. All the while, it retains its sound, simple, substantive content, thoroughly updated and realistically applied to meet human health needs in our rapidly changing modern world.

NEW TO THIS EDITION

As indicated, this book is in essence an abridgement of my larger text. It follows a similar format and style to facilitate learning and lay a beginning foundation for sound clinical practice. To achieve these goals in this current edition, I have made a number of changes:

CHAPTER CHANGES

Instead of placing all of the discussion of stress and its effect on health in one separate chapter, I have placed its components in related chapters so that it may be more closely associated with specific diseases and health problems, thus guiding students to immediately relate stress factors with the problem at hand.

Each chapter applies the expanding science of nutrition to changing health care needs and developing technologic tools for its clinical practice and management. For example, Chapter 17, "Feeding Methods: Enteral and Parenteral Nutrition," updates and expands information about these rapidly developing means of special nutrition support; and Chapter 23, "Nutrition and AIDS," provides current coverage of the special nutritional needs of the rapidly growing number of HIV-infected and AIDS patients worldwide, especially in the developing countries.

CHAPTER ORDER AND COORDINATION

Chapters are positioned to aid learning and reflect current science and practice.

Several chapters have been repositioned or combined since previous editions to aid learning and reflect current science and practice.

Chapter 2, "Digestion, Absorption, and Metabolism," is positioned before the chapters on the macronutrients—carbohydrates, fats, and proteins—at the request of teachers and students using this beginning text, to provide basic knowledge first of the nature of the nutrients involved.

Chapter 6, "Energy Balance and Weight Management," combines two topics previously treated in separate chapters for a better understanding of their basic relationship in practice.

Chapter 13, "Nutrition for Adults: Early, Middle, and Later Years," provides a balanced and comprehensive view of the varying needs of adults at different age periods, rather than a previous limited focus mainly on the aged, to better reflect the current health care emphasis on health maintenance and disease prevention.

Chapter 18, "Gastrointestinal Diseases," has been updated to include current knowledge and changes in nutritional management of problems of the gastrointestinal tract and its accessory organs. For example, new knowledge has changed the treatment of peptic ulcer disease; discovery of the cystic fibrosis gene and its biochemical mechanism effect on pancreatic secretions has changed treatment of the resulting pancreatic insufficiency and malabsorption; and advancing knowledge of viruses causing liver disease has led to new vaccines and reinforced nutritional care of the various stages of the disease, including advanced cirrhosis and encephalopathy.

Chapter 19, "Diseases of the Heart, Blood Vessels, and Lungs," continues to reflect the coordinated functions of each component of the overall circulatory system and unique actions of system sections, such as the role of the arterial vessels' inner endothelial lining in controlling hypertension.

Chapter 25, "Nutritional Support in Disabling Disease and Rehabilitation," has been revised and expanded to include treatment and rehabilitative care in the fields of *musculoskeletal problems* such as rheumatoid arthritis and osteoarthritis; *neuromuscular injury and disease* from the growing problem of neurologic injuries or from developmental disabilities of childhood (cerebral palsy, epilepsy, spina bifida, Down syndrome); and *progressive neurologic disorders* of middle and older adulthood (Parkinson's and Huntington's diseases, Guillain-Barré syndrome, amyotrophic lateral sclerosis or Lou Gehrig disease, multiple sclerosis, myasthenia gravis, Alzheimer's disease). In each case I have focused on life-changing effects and the role of nutritional support.

ILLUSTRATIONS AND DESIGN

A number of illustrations, many two- and four-color, greatly enhance the overall design and provide learning support. These added graphs, charts, and photographs portray concepts introduced and help students grasp the clinical problems encountered in patient care.

ENHANCED READABILITY AND STUDENT INTEREST

A large amount of the text has been rewritten as indicated to incorporate new material in a writing style designed to capture student interest and present comprehensive subject matter in a sound and simple manner. Many new advances in basic and clinical science are explained and applied. Issues of student interest and public-professional controversy are discussed. The many examples used open up meaning and understanding. Topics of current relevance clarify questions and concerns.

LEARNING AIDS WITHIN THE TEXT

This new text continues to use many learning aids throughout the text.

CHAPTER OPENERS

To alert students to the topic of each chapter and draw them into its study, each chapter opens with an illustration and a couple of brief focusing paragraphs on the chapter topic.

CHAPTER OUTLINES

The major sections are listed at the beginning of each chapter and indicated by special type for ease in reading comprehension.

KEY TERMS

Key terms important to the student's understanding and application of the material in patient care are presented in three steps. They are first identified in bold-face type in the body of the text. Some are particularly pertinent to the discussion and defined on the right-hand side of each right page. And finally, all are collected in a comprehensive glossary for easy reference at the end of the book. This three-level approach to vocabulary development greatly improves the overall study and use of the text.

CHAPTER SUMMARIES

To help the student pull the chapter material together again as a whole, each chapter concludes with a summary of the key concepts presented and their significance or application. The student can then return to any part of the material for repeated study and clarification as needed.

REVIEW QUESTIONS FOR TESTING COMPREHENSION

To help the student understand key parts of the chapter or apply it to patient problems, questions are given after each chapter text for review and analysis of the material presented.

CHAPTER REFERENCES

To provide immediate access to all references cited in the chapter text, a full list of these key references is given at the end of each chapter, rather than collected at the end of the book.

FURTHER READING

In addition to referenced material in the text, an annotated list of suggestions for further reading for added interest and study is provided at the end of each chapter. These selections extend or apply the material in the text according to student needs or areas of special interest. The annotations themselves improve the student's ability to use them by identifying pertinent parts of the reference.

ISSUES AND ANSWERS

A special feature of each chapter is a concluding brief article on nutrition-related issues or controversies based on the text discussion. These interesting and motivating studies help the student to see the importance of scientific thinking and develop sound judgment and openness to different points of view.

CASE STUDIES

In many chapters, realistic case studies lead the student to apply the text material to related patient care problems. Each case is accompanied by questions for case analysis. These cases also help alert the student to applications of nutritional therapy for similar patient care needs in their own clinical assignments.

DIET GUIDES

A variety of diet guidelines are highlighted in the clinical chapters in Part Three.

APPENDIXES

The revised appendixes include a number of materials for use as reference tools and guidelines in learning and practice. Food value tables include nutrient and energy references for a variety of basic foods.

INDEX

The index extends the basic text cross-referencing and provides a quick reference to the book's content.

SUPPLEMENTARY MATERIALS

Several available supplements enhance the teaching-learning process. Information on these helpful packages may be obtained from the publisher.

INSTRUCTOR'S MANUAL AND TEST BANK

Prepared by Joanne Spaide, University of Northern Iowa, this valuable tool features chapter overviews; behavioral objectives; chapter outlines with teaching notes on controversial topics; individual/group activities; transparency masters; and an extensive test-item bank of approximately 1250 questions, prepared by

E. Ruth Yurchuck, consultant in nursing assessment and evaluation.

COMPUTERIZED TEST BANK

Qualified adopters of the text receive a computerized test bank package compatible with the IBM and Macintosh computers. This software provides a unique combination of user-friendly aids and enables the instructor to select, edit, delete, or add questions and construct and print tests and answer keys.

TRANSPARENCY ACETATES

Illustrations of important, hard-to-understand concepts are available as transparency acetates. These useful tools facilitate learning of key concepts discussed in the text and are free to adopters of the text.

SELF-STUDY GUIDE

This concise little companion continues to serve as a general learning aid during initial courses, as well as a tool for review of the text for professional examinations or for practitioners needing to update knowledge. It includes many items to support learning of each chapter's content: (1) chapter focus; (2) summary-review quiz; (3) discussion questions to stimulate thinking; (4) true-false and multiple choice test items to test comprehension; (5) numerous guides for individual and group projects that involve experiments, case studies, and situational problems that apply learning; and (6) inquiry questions that relate an "Issues and Answers" article to current health care problems.

MOSBY'S NUTRITRAC CD-ROM

Packaged in every *Essentials of Nutrition and Diet Therapy* 7th edition text, this interactive nutrient analysis CD-ROM includes a unique food list with more than 2200 items, selected activities, and food exchange lists. The program allows students to input food intake and physical activities to determine total kcalories consumed and expended over a certain period of time.

PERSONAL APPROACH

My person-centered approach in past editions remains in this new text. It is enhanced by: (1) a personal writing style that reflects my own convictions and commitments about student learning and patient care; (2) extensive use of ever-expanding personal files and materials gathered from current research, my own clinical practice, teaching, and biochemical-metabolic work; and (3) practical applications of scientific knowledge in realistic *human* terms to find personal solutions to individual problems.

ACKNOWLEDGMENTS

A textbook of this sort is never the work of one person. It develops into the planned product through the committed hands and hearts of a number of persons. It would be impossible to name all the individuals involved, but several groups deserve special recognition.

First of all, I am grateful to the reviewers who gave their valuable time and skills to strengthen the manuscript: Rhonda B. Armstrong, Mary Babcock, Kay Gilbert, Judy Hammond, Dorothy G. Herron, Karen Kirmis, Jane Kufus-Krump, and Lillie M. Nash.

Second, I am indebted to Mosby and the many persons there who had a part in this extensive project. I especially thank my editor of nutrition publications, Yvonne Alexopoulos, who supported me all the way to meet tight management requirements; and my developmental editor, Melissa Boyle, whose capable talents helped shape the book's final pages. To our marketing managers, Janet Blanner and Tom Wilhelm, and the many fine Mosby marketing representatives throughout the country, I owe a great deal for their help in guiding the result of my efforts to its ultimate users. I am also grateful for the help of Manager of Editing and Prepress Production, Peggy Fagen, and all the associated artists and photographers who participated in this project.

I also thank my own staff during the various stages of preparing the manuscript, especially to my research assistant Mary Herbert, who gathered the comprehensive materials I requested. Most of all, I owe a special debt of gratitude to my author's editor, James C. Williams, for writing assistance on many of the learning aids articles, for expert copyediting throughout, and for producing the manuscript. I also give special thanks to my many students, interns, colleagues, clients, and patients over the years, all of whom have taught me much; and to my family, who never cease to support all my efforts and who always share in whatever I am able to achieve.

Sue Rodwell Williams
Davis, California

Rhonda B. Armstrong, RN, MSN
Nursing Instructor
Department of Associate Degree
  Nursing
Hinds Community College
Jackson, Mississippi

Mary Babcock, RD, BS, MS, MS
Adjunct Professor
Wilkes University
Wilkes-Barre, Pennsylvania

Kay Gilbert, PhD, RD
Instructor
Science Department
Truckee Meadows Community
  College
Reno, Nevada;
Consultant and Owner
Gilbert and Gilbert Consultants
Reno/Sparks, Nevada

Judy Hammond, RNC, PhD
Instructor
Associate Degree Nursing
Tyler Junior College
Adjunct Faculty;
Allied Health
University of Texas at Tyler
Tyler, Texas

Dorothy G. Herron, PhD, RN, CS
Assistant Professor
School of Nursing
University of Maryland at Baltimore
Baltimore, Maryland

Karen Kirmis, MS, RD
Director of Foods and Nutrition
Human Ecology Department
Marygrove College
Detroit, Michigan

Jane Kufus-Krump, MS, LRD
Associate Professor
Science Department
North Dakota State College
  of Science
Wahpeton, North Dakota

Lillie M. Nash, MS, RN, CDN
Assistant Professor
Long Island University
Brooklyn, New York

*Mosby, Inc. extends thanks to
the reviewer of Mosby's
NutriTrac CD-ROM:*

**Sister M. Marguerite Polcyn,
  BS, MS, PhD**
Professor of Health Education
Department of Health and Wellness
Lourdes College
Sylvania, Ohio

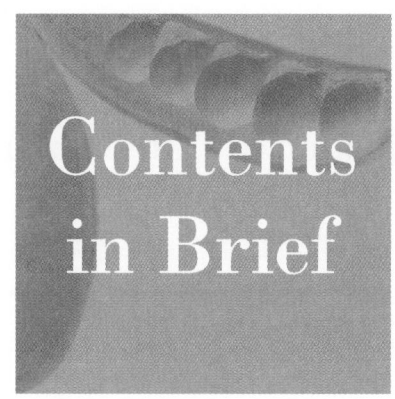

Contents in Brief

Part 3

Introduction to Clinical Nutrition

Contents

Part 1

Introduction to Human Nutrition

Part 2

Community Nutrition: The Life Cycle

Part 3

Introduction to Clinical Nutrition

ESSENTIALS
of NUTRITION and
DIET THERAPY

Introduction
to Human
Nutrition

Part 1

Chapter

1

Nutrition and Health

This chapter introduces the study of nutrition in health and health care. Whatever the basis of your present interest, a sound base of nutrition knowledge and skills is fundamental.

Current knowledge of nutrition and its basic science foundations reflects our rapidly changing world in terms of a changing food supply, expanding population, and phenomenal scientific knowledge. Nutrition is rapidly emerging as a vital component in personal health care and in our national nutrition and health policies to meet human need.

A primary means of promoting health and preventing disease rests on a wholesome food supply for all persons and the sound nutrition it provides. In this chapter we introduce a person-centered approach to nutrition and health care, an important focus throughout your study.

NUTRITION AND HUMAN HEALTH

THE SCIENCE OF NUTRITION

For the most part, knowledge about nutrition builds on two fundamental areas of science. First, the physical sciences of biochemistry and physiology help us see how nutrition relates to our physical health and well-being. Second, behavioral sciences help us better understand how nutrition is interwoven with our unique nature as human beings. Throughout our study here, you will see both of these areas of learning at work in our lives.

For example, some basic principles of biochemistry show us that, in our physical being, human organisms are marvelously complex groupings of chemical compounds constantly at work in an array of reactions designed to sustain life. Nutrients, the basic currency of nutrition, are chemical compounds or elements. The integrating work of human physiology brings the beauty of order out of a seemingly internal chaos of individually functioning cells and organs, blending them into a total functioning whole. Physiologists call this highly sensitive level of internal control **homeostasis**.

However, if we were defined only by our physical components, we would not be fully human. We learn human aspects of being and nutrition from the behavioral sciences, which are rooted in our earliest awareness of psychosocial beginnings and life experiences. Attitudes toward food and eating patterns develop throughout the lifespan from the acculturating influences of our primary family and relatives, our friends, ethnic group, community, nation, and even our world. How we perceive ourselves and our food, what we choose to eat, why we eat what we do and in what manner, all become integral parts of human nutrition.

FOOD AND NUTRIENTS

The word **nutrition** refers to nourishment that sustains life. It centers on the food people eat and how it nourishes their lives not only physically, but also socially and personally. The science and art of human nutrition both focus on nourishing human life. They do this in many ways. From the moment of conception until death, the quality of the diet throughout life enables persons to cope with environmental stress and disease.[1] We need energy to carry out vital functions such as breathing as well as to cope with environmental stress and support physical activity. We must constantly replenish these energy needs with food to sustain physical life. But food also nourishes the human spirit. We all have our particular "soul food," our comfort foods, those special "warm fuzzies" for the heart.

Nutrition is thus defined as the food people eat and how it nourishes their bodies. **Nutritional science** comprises the body of scientific knowledge governing the nutritional requirements of humans for maintenance, growth, activity, and reproduction. **Dietetics** is the health profession having primary responsibility for the practical application of nutritional science to persons and groups of persons in various conditions of health and disease. The **registered dietitian (RD)**, especially the **clinical nutrition specialist**, is the nutrition authority on the health care team. The RD, in collaboration with the physician and nurse, carries the major responsibility for nutritional care of patients and clients. The **public health nutritionist** is responsible for nutritional care of groups of people in the community, especially those high-risk groups who require assessment of need and community programs to meet these needs.

Functions of food and nutrients

The respective functions of food and nutrients in human nutrition need to be distinguished. First of all, we should dispense with the myth that any particular food or food combination is required by the body for health. The human race has subsisted for centuries with wide varieties of foods, depending on what was available to eat and what the culture designated as human food. Various foods serve as important vehicles for taking nutrients into the body and bringing human pleasure and comfort. Instead, it is these specific chemical compounds or elements—the **nutrients**—in a wide *variety* of foods that the body requires. Approximately 40 essential nutrients are known; others are probably yet to be discovered. Known essential nutrients include **macronutrients**—carbohydrates, fats, and proteins—whose constituent substances supply energy and build tissue, and **micronutrients**—vitamins and minerals—that the body uses in much smaller amounts to regulate and control body processes. Water is the overall vital nutrient sustaining all our life processes. The term **metabolism** refers to the sum of all these chemical processes in the body that sustain life and health. The first part of this text will cover your study of these important nutrients.

Nutrient interrelationships

An important nutritional metabolic fact will emerge increasingly in your study of nutrition, the fundamental principle of *nutrient interaction*. This principle states the following:

1. Individual nutrients have many specific metabolic functions, including primary and supporting roles, and
2. No nutrient ever works alone.

The human body is a fascinating whole made up of many parts and processes. Intimate metabolic relationships exist among all the basic nutrients and their **metabolites**. This key principle of nutrient interaction will be demonstrated more clearly in the following chapters. Remember, we may separate nutrients for study purposes, but they do not exist that way in the body. Nutrients are always interacting as a dynamic whole to produce and maintain the human body, providing energy, building and rebuilding tissue, and regulating metabolic processes.

ENERGY SOURCES

The energy-yielding nutrients—carbohydrates, fats, and proteins—provide primary and alternate sources of energy.

Carbohydrates

Dietary carbohydrates, starches and sugars, provide the body's primary source of fuel for heat and energy. They also maintain a stored source of energy known as *glycogen*, sometimes called "animal starch" because its structure is so similar to that of plant starch. Each gram of carbohydrate consumed yields 4 **kilocalories** (kcalories or kcal). This number is called the "fuel factor." A well-balanced diet for a healthy person supplies approximately 50% to 60% of the total kcalories from carbohydrates. The majority of these kcalories are derived from complex carbohydrate foods (starches) and a smaller amount from, simple carbohydrate foods (sugars).

Fats

Dietary fats from animal and plant sources provide the body's alternate or storage form of heat and energy. Fat is a more concentrated fuel, yielding 9 kcalories for each gram consumed. The fuel factor of fats is therefore 9. Fats should supply no more than 25% to 30% of the total kcalories of a healthy person's well-balanced diet. The majority of this amount, approximately two thirds, should consist of unsaturated fats, rather than saturated fats (see *Chapter 4*).

Proteins

The body may draw on dietary or tissue protein to obtain needed energy when the fuel supply from carbohydrates and fats is insufficient. Protein yields 4 kcalories per gram, making its fuel factor 4. Quality protein should provide approximately 15% to 20% of the total kcalories of a healthy person's well-balanced diet. Therefore although protein's primary function is tissue building, some may be available for energy as needed.

---

clinical nutrition specialist Specialty practice of a registered dietitian with an advanced degree in nutritional science and training in clinical nutrition.

dietetics Management of diet and the use of food; the science concerned with the nutritional planning and preparation of foods.

homeostasis State of relative dynamic equilibrium within the body's internal environment; a balance achieved through the operation of various interrelated physiologic mechanisms.

kilocalorie The general term *calorie* refers to a unit of heat measure and is used alone to designate the *small calorie*. The calorie used in nutritional science and the study of metabolism is the *large calorie,* 1000 calories, or kilocalorie, to be more accurate and avoid use of very large numbers in calculations.

macronutrients The three large energy-yielding nutrients: carbohydrates, fats, and proteins.

metabolism Sum of all the various biochemical and physiologic processes by which the body grows and maintains itself (anabolism) and breaks down and reshapes tissue (catabolism), transforming energy to do its work. Products of these various reactions are called *metabolites.*

metabolites Any substance produced by metabolism or by a metabolic process.

micronutrients The two classes of small non-energy-yielding elements and compounds: minerals and vitamins, essential in very small amounts for regulation and control functions in cell metabolism and for building certain body structures.

nutrients Substances in food that are essential for energy, growth, normal functioning of the body, and maintenance of life.

nutrition The sum of the processes involved in taking in food nutrients, assimilating and using them to maintain body tissue and provide energy; a foundation for life and health.

nutritional science The body of scientific knowledge, developed through controlled research, that relates to the processes involved in nutrition—national, international, community, and clinical.

public health nutritionist A professional nutritionist, accredited by academic degree course of university and special graduate study (MPH, DrPH) in schools of public health accredited by the American Association of Public Health, responsible for nutrition components of public health programs in varied community settings—county, state, national, international.

registered dietitian (RD) A professional dietitian, accredited by academic degree course of university and graduate study (MS, PhD), clinical and administration training, and having passed required registration examinations administered by the American Dietetic Association.

TISSUE BUILDING

Protein is the primary nutrient used in tissue building; minerals, vitamins, and fatty acids also play a role.

Proteins

The primary function of protein is tissue building. Dietary protein foods provide **amino acids**, the building units necessary for constructing and repairing body tissues. This is a constant, dynamic process of modeling and remodeling according to need that ensures growth and maintenance of a strong body structure and vital substances for tissue functioning.

Minerals

Various minerals have numerous functions. For example, two of the major minerals, calcium and phosphorus, help build and maintain bone tissue; the trace mineral iron helps build hemoglobin, a red blood cell's vital oxygen carrier.

Vitamins

As just one example of the role of vitamins in tissue building, vitamin C helps develop the cementing intercellular ground substance necessary for building strong tissue and preventing tissue bleeding.

METABOLIC REGULATION AND CONTROL

All of the multiple biochemical processes that comprise body metabolism, which are required for providing energy and building tissue, must be controlled in exquisite detail to maintain a smoothly running, balanced operation. Otherwise there would be chaos within the body systems and death would eventually result. Life and health result from a dynamic balance, a state of *homeostasis*, among all of the body parts and processes. Vitamins and minerals are nutrients that play a vital role in metabolic regulation and control; water provides the necessary fluid environment.

Vitamins

Many vitamins function as coenzyme factors, or components of cell enzyme systems, to govern chemical reactions in cell metabolism. This is true, for example, of most B-complex vitamins.

Minerals

Many minerals also serve as coenzyme factors in cell metabolism. An interesting structural example is that of the trace element cobalt, which is a central constituent of vitamin B_{12} (cobalamin) and thus functions as a component of this vitamin used to combat pernicious anemia.

Other nutrients

Water and dietary fiber also function as regulatory agents. In fact, water is *the* fundamental agent for life, providing the essential solution base for all metabolic processes. Dietary fiber helps regulate the passage of food through the gastrointestinal tract and influences absorption of various nutrients.

LEVELS OF NUTRITIONAL STATUS

Individual nutritional status will vary depending on a person's living situation, available food supply, and health. You will be concerned with these varying levels as you assess your own nutritional status or that of others.

Ideal nutrition

Evidence of sound positive nutrition includes a well-developed body, ideal weight for body composition (ratio of muscle mass to fat) and height, and good muscle development and tone. The skin is smooth and clear, the hair is glossy, and the eyes are clear and bright. Posture is good; the facial expression should be alert. Appetite, digestion, and elimination are normal. Detailed characteristics of good and poor states of nutrition are given in Table 1.1. Begin to think about these signs as you get into your nutrition study and look for them as you become a more skilled observer. Well-nourished persons are much more likely to be alert, both mentally and physically. They are not only meeting their day-to-day needs but also maintaining essential nutrient reserves for resisting infectious diseases and generally extending their years of normal functioning.

Borderline nutrition

As the descriptive label indicates, persons with only a borderline nutritional status may manage to meet their minimum day-to-day nutritional needs; however, they lack nutritional reserves to meet any added physiologic or metabolic demand from injury or illness, sustain fetal development during pregnancy, or attain proper growth in childhood. A state of borderline nutrition may exist in persons with poor eating habits or those who are living in stressed environments on low incomes. Dietary surveys have shown that approximately one third of the United States population is living on diets below the optimal level. This does not necessarily mean that these Americans are undernourished; some persons can maintain general health on somewhat less than the optimal amounts of various nutrients. On the average, however, persons who do not get enough of these nutrients have greater risk of physical illness than persons who are well nourished. The human body has great capacity to adapt to such lowered nutritional states, but it can only sustain a given amount of physiologic stress before signs of malnutrition appear.

Malnutrition

Signs of malnutrition appear when nutritional reserves are depleted and nutrient and energy intake is insufficient to meet day-to-day needs or added metabolic

Table

1.1   Clinical signs of nutritional status

Features	Good	Poor
General appearance	Alert, responsive	Listless, apathetic, cachexic
Hair	Shiny, lustrous, healthy scalp	Stringy, dull, brittle, dry, depigmented
Neck glands	No enlargement	Thyroid enlarged
Skin, face, neck	Smooth, slightly moist, good color, reddish pink mucous membranes	Greasy, discolored, scaly
Eyes	Bright, clear, no fatigue circles	Dryness, signs of infection, increased vascularity, glassiness, thickened conjunctivae
Lips	Good color, moist	Dry, scaly, swollen, angular lesions (stomatitis)
Tongue	Good pink color, surface papillae present, no lesions	Papillary atrophy, smooth appearance, swollen, red, beefy (glossitis)
Gums	Good pink color, no swelling or bleeding, firm	Marginal redness or swelling, receding, spongy
Teeth	Straight, no crowding, well-shaped jaw, clean, no discoloration	Unfilled cavities, absent teeth, worn surfaces, mottled, malpositioned
Skin, general	Smooth, slightly moist, good color	Rough, dry, scaly, pale, pigmented, irritated; petechiae, bruises
Abdomen	Flat	Swollen
Legs, feet	No tenderness, weakness, swelling, good color	Edema, tender calf, tingling, weakness
Skeleton	No malformations	Bowlegs, knock-knees, chest deformity at diaphragm, beaded ribs, prominent scapulas
Weight	Normal for height, age, body build	Overweight or underweight
Posture	Erect, arms and legs straight, abdomen in, chest out	Sagging shoulders, sunken chest, humped back
Muscles	Well-developed, firm	Flaccid, poor tone, undeveloped, tender
Nervous control	Good attention span for age, does not cry easily, not irritable or restless	Inattentive, irritable
Gastrointestinal function	Good appetite and digestion, normal, regular elimination	Anorexia, indigestion, constipation or diarrhea
General vitality	Endurance, energetic, sleeps well at night, vigorous	Easily fatigued, no energy, falls asleep in school, looks tired, apathetic

stress. A large number of malnourished people live in high-risk conditions of poverty. These conditions influence the health of all persons involved but especially the lives of the most vulnerable ones—infants, children, pregnant women, and elderly adults. Prenatal care for many women who are poor, young, and lack education is often inadequate or nonexistent, resulting in poor pregnancy outcomes and high infant mortality rates. One out of five United States children lives in persistent poverty and suffers stunted growth and deficiency disease such as **anemia**, as well as lowered resistance to infections, disease, impaired learning ability, apathy, and reduced activity levels. Such chronically inadequate diets in the young child prevent catch-up growth after episodes of infection and produce lasting effects on intellectual development.[2] Most stunted children become stunted, less productive adults.[3] Low socioeconomic status and malnutrition are positively related in the increasing American population of older adults.[4] Many studies also document widespread hunger and malnutrition among the poor, especially among the growing number of homeless persons.[5-7]

We also find malnutrition in our hospitals and long-term care facilities. For example, hypermetabolic disease or prolonged illness, especially among older persons with chronic conditions, places added stress. In such situations, often the person's daily nutrient and energy intake is insufficient to meet needs. Nutrition assessment procedures, fundamental to appropriate clinical care, are described in *Chapter 15.*

amino acid An acid containing the essential element nitrogen (in the chemical group -NH$_2$). Amino acids are the structural units of protein and the basic building blocks of the body.

anemia Blood condition characterized by decreased number of circulating red blood cells, hemoglobin, or both.

Overnutrition

Some persons may be in a state of overnutrition that gradually results in degrees of overweight and obesity from excess energy intake over time. In a sense, overnutrition can be viewed as another form of malnutrition, especially when excess caloric intake produces gross harmful body weight and fatness—morbid obesity. Childhood and adolescent obesity may set the stage for continuing adult obesity, increasing the risk for chronic disease. Harmful overnutrition also occurs in persons who use excessive "megadoses" of nutrient supplements that, over time, produce damaging tissue effects.

NUTRITION AND NATIONAL HEALTH PROBLEMS

DIET, NUTRITION, AND CHRONIC DISEASE

Over the past few years, a series of significant reports linking health and nutrition have continued to guide the American people and national health policy makers in relating specific dietary factors to leading United States health threats and chronic disease problems. These ongoing chronic health problems include coronary heart disease, high blood pressure, stroke, some types of cancer, diabetes, and obesity.

Nutrition and health

In 1988, *The Surgeon General's Report on Nutrition and Health* was issued in response to the increasing concerns of scientists, health professionals, and the American public about the effects of typical American dietary patterns on the incidence of chronic diseases that are leading causes of death and disability in this country.[8] Based on the weight of the evidence presented and the magnitude of the health problems involved, recommendation was made for dietary changes to reduce use of foods high in fats and salt and to increase foods high in complex carbohydrates and fiber.

Diet and health

In 1989, the Diet and Health Committee of the Food and Nutrition Board, National Research Council, issued its extensive research report, *Diet and Health: Implications for Reducing Chronic Disease Risk*.[9] On the basis of its systematic evaluation of the scientific evidence relating dietary components, foods, food groups, and dietary patterns to health maintenance and reduction of chronic disease risk, the 19-member interdisciplinary committee proposed dietary guidelines in line with those of the Surgeon General, specifically, reducing total fat intake to 30% or less of the total kcalories, with associated reductions in saturated fats and cholesterol.

Healthy people 2000

In 1990, the United States Department of Health and Human Services (USDHHS), Public Health Service, issued a report applying the recommendations indicated above in a system of specific objectives to reach these national health goals by the year 2000.[10-11] Targeted are the particularly vulnerable groups in our population who suffer from poor diets, malnutrition, and poor health: older Americans with chronic disease and disability, infants and young children (one in four lives in poverty), and the increasing numbers of homeless people.

NUTRITION GUIDES FOR HEALTH PROMOTION

During the years since the early 1900s, a number of food and nutrient guides have been developed to meet nutrition and health needs of Americans. Although not always apparent in these guides, a number of underlying assumptions about food, nutrition, and health have directed their design and reflected not only developing nutritional science but also social, political, and economic events of the times. They have addressed needs during wars and emergencies as well as in economic depressions. With our changing modern health problems, the focus of these guides has shifted from preventing primary deficiency diseases of insufficient nutritional intake to controlling chronic diseases of affluence and excess.

In general, these nutrition guides may be classed in three groups: nutrient and energy standards, food guides, and dietary guidelines, each serving different needs. They are reviewed briefly here for reference and guidance in your study.

NUTRIENT STANDARDS: THE RECOMMENDED DIETARY ALLOWANCES (RDAS)

United States standards

Most of the developed countries of the world have set up standards for intake of major nutrients by healthy persons categorized by age and sex. They serve as guidelines for maintaining healthy populations. These standards are not intended to indicate individual requirements or therapeutic needs. Rather they serve as a reference based on current scientific knowledge for intake levels of the essential nutrients judged to be adequate for meeting the known nutritional needs of most healthy population groups. In the United States these nutrient and energy standards have been called the **Recommended Dietary Allowances (RDAs)**. Such standards are similar in different countries, but may vary somewhat according to their purpose and use.

Development of the RDAs

The first RDA standards grew out of a national nutrition conference for defense held in 1941 during World War II.[11] A summary background for the nutrient and energy recommendations, based on developing nutritional science, was first published in 1943 as a guide for nutrition workers in planning and obtaining food supplies for national defense and general population needs for good nutrition. Since this first edition of the RDAs, a new edition has been published about every 4 years with revisions of the standards based on expanding scientific research. The tenth edition, issued in 1989, was the work of the 1989 dietary allowances subcommittee of the Food and Nutrition Board, National Research Council, National Academy of Sciences.[12] The Academy has numerous councils and is supported by the National Institutes of Health. (See United States RDA tables on the inside covers of this book.)

Based on expanding nutritional science and population needs, especially for the increasing number of older adults, new United States standards are currently being developed.[13] In collaboration with Canadian scientists, American nutrition experts are currently producing an expanded United States framework of age groups under the new working title of "Dietary Reference Intakes" (RDIs).[13-15] These new RDI standards will consist of three reference numbers: (1) the redefined RDA, (2) an estimated average requirement, and (3) an upper limit for safe intake. Seven nutrient-specific panels of the overall Dietary Reference Intake Committee are now at work:

1. Calcium and related nutrients
2. Folate and related nutrients
3. Antioxidants and related nutrients
4. Trace elements
5. Electrolytes and water
6. Energy and macronutrients
7. Nonnutrient food components

Other standards

Canadian and British standards are similar to the US standards. In less developed countries where such factors as quality of protein foods available must be considered, workers look to standards such as those set by the Food and Agriculture Organization (FAO) of the World Health Organization (WHO). All of these standards provide nutrient and energy guidelines to help health workers in a variety of population groups promote good health through sound nutrition.

Food group guides

To interpret and apply sound nutrient standards, health workers need practical food guides to use in nutrition education and food planning with individuals and families. Two such food guides, very different in nature and serving different needs, are the basic food groups guide and the food exchange lists.

Basic food groups guide

Probably the most familiar food group guide is the long-used but limited tool issued by the United States Department of Agriculture (USDA), reflecting in its origin agricultural commodity concerns as well as nutritional ones and initially called the Basic Four Food Groups Guide. Over the years, the USDA has issued a succession of basic food guides, each reflecting needs and concerns of the time.

In 1991, the USDA issued a new revised edition, reflecting current national goals for increasing carbohydrate intake to supply the bulk of the energy needs with the fruit, vegetable, and starch/bread groups; the revision also recommended limiting fat intake by modifying the milk, meat, and fat groups.[16] This new approach, titled *The Guide to Daily Food Choices*, is summarized in Table 1.2. A subsequent graphic form, *The Food Guide Pyramid* (Figure 1.1), followed to illustrate the relative amounts of each food group in the daily diet. This revised basic food groups guide, especially in its visual pyramid form, has proved to be a useful educational tool and continues in its modified form. It is designed to represent a total diet, not just a foundation, and to fill a need for simple guidance.[17]

The exchange lists food guide

This guide was introduced in 1950 by the American Diabetes Association and the American Dietetic Association as a meal planning tool for managing diets for persons with diabetes. Organized quite differently from the USDA guide, *The Exchange Lists Food Guide* was based on the unique concept of food exchanges, with foods grouped on the basis of equivalent food values. Soon it was apparent that this guide was also a useful short-method tool for calculating and planning any diet, such as those for weight reduction, in which control of the energy nutrients—carbohydrate, fat, and protein—as well as kcalories for both total and nutrient distribution, was the goal.

Since foods in each group in the exchange system were equal to one another in the portions indicated, group items could be freely exchanged within individual groups, thus maintaining consistent food values and kcalories. At the same time this freedom of exchange within single groups allowed a great variety of foods and food combinations to be used in planning meals and snacks. This food exchange group guide has been widely used as a nutrition tool for meal planning, education, and counseling.

---

recommended dietary allowances (RDAs) Recommended daily allowances of nutrients and energy intake for population groups according to age and sex, with defined weight and height. The RDAs are established and reviewed periodically by a representative group of nutritional scientists, in response to current research. These standards vary very little among the developed countries.

Table

1.2   The guide to daily food choices—a summary

Food group	Servings	Major contributions	Foods and serving sizes*
Bread, cereals, rice, pasta	6-11	Starch Thiamin Riboflavin† Iron Niacin Folate Magnesium‡ Fiber‡ Zinc	1 slice of bread 1 oz ready-to-eat cereal $^1/_2$-$^3/_4$ cup cooked cereal, rice, pasta
Vegetables	3-5	Vitamin A Vitamin C Folate Magnesium Fiber	$^1/_2$ cup raw or cooked vegetables 1 cup raw leafy vegetables
Fruits	2-4	Vitamin C Fiber	$^1/_4$ cup dried fruit $^1/_2$ cup cooked fruit $^3/_4$ cup juice 1 whole piece of fruit 1 melon wedge
Milk, yogurt, cheese	2 (adults§) 3 (children, teens, young adults, pregnant or lactating women)	Calcium Riboflavin Protein Potassium Zinc	1 cup milk $1^1/_2$ oz cheese 2 oz processed cheese 1 cup yogurt 2 cups cottage cheese 1 cup custard/pudding $1^1/_2$ cups ice cream
Meat, poultry, fish, dry beans, eggs, nuts	2-3	Protein Niacin Iron Vitamin B_6 Zinc Thiamin Vitamin B_{12}‖	2-3 oz cooked meat, poultry, fish 1-$1^1/_2$ cups cooked dry beans 4 tbsp peanut butter 2 eggs $^1/_2$-1 cup nuts
Fats, oils, sweets	Foods from this group should not replace any from the other groups. Amounts consumed should be determined by individual energy needs.		

From the US Department of Agriculture, revised edition of former *Basic Four Food Groups Guide*.
*May be reduced for child servings.
†If enriched.
‡Whole grains especially.
§≥25 years of age.
‖Present only in animal food choices.

In 1986, a major revision of the exchange lists was published to meet ongoing nutrition and medical research and national dietary guidelines for health promotion and reduction of chronic disease risk factors. The long-familiar basic six food groups were completely reorganized and their list order changed to emphasize use for health: (1) starch/bread, and an "other carbohydrate" group including a few sweets; (2) meat, with subgroups of lean, medium-fat, and high-fat items and tips for reducing portion size and fat; (3) vegetables; (4) fruits; (5) milk, with subgroups for reducing fat; and (6) fat, with subgroups for unsaturated and saturated food sources. Three expanded lists were added: free foods and seasonings, combination foods, and foods for occasional use. In all groups, values for dietary fiber and sodium were identified and food sources were flagged. A new edition specifically revised and designed for weight management was also issued.

Figure 1.1   Eating right pyramid. A guide to daily food choices. (Modified from the U.S. Department of Agriculture, 1992.)

The current 1995 exchange lists revisions for meal planning have been extended and rearranged in three groups for easier use (see Appendix L, Exchange Lists for Meal Planning)[18]:

1. *Carbohydrate group.* Includes the previous carbohydrate lists—starch (previously starch-bread), fruits, vegetables, milk—and a new list, other carbohydrates, such as cakes, cookies, and other sweets.
2. *Meat and meat substitutes group.* Includes the previous protein foods in the meat list (lean, medium-fat, and high-fat) with a new list, very lean, and various meat substitutes.
3. *Fat group.* The fat foods are divided into three lists: monounsaturated, polyunsaturated, and saturated fat, recognizing the health benefits of using small amounts of the unsaturated fats and reduced amounts of saturated fats.

In addition, various items have been added to the exchange lists, such as fat-modified, vegetarian, and fast-food items. Tips are included on how to purchase and prepare certain foods. A revised updated edition of Exchanges for Weight Management has also been issued.[19]

HEALTH PROMOTION GUIDELINES

In recent years, several general dietary guidelines for health promotion have been issued in the United States that reflect the growing health concerns of government, professional groups, and the public. Though not quan-

tifying food use as do the food group guides above, they call attention to proposed food habit changes to reduce chronic disease risks and enhance health. The guidelines have proved useful in nutrition education and counseling.

United States dietary guidelines

These basic health guidelines have developed from public and professional concern about chronic health problems in an aging population and a changing food environment.[20] The USDA and the USDHHS issued the current fourth edition in 1995, *Nutrition and Your Health: Dietary Guidelines for Americans*, based on extensive study by expert advisory committees and supplying supporting references for each guideline. In familiar positive terms, the statements emphasize health promotion through risk reduction and relate current scientific thinking to America's leading health problems.[21-23] They are actively supported by the American Dietetic Association and continue to serve as useful general guides for a concerned public. Although no guidelines can guarantee health or well-being, and although people differ widely in their food needs, these seven general statements can lead people to evaluate their food and exercise habits and move toward general improvements. Good food habits based on moderation and variety help build sound, healthy bodies (see *Practical Application* box, p. 20).

Shortly after the initial publication of the general United States Dietary Guidelines, two similar but more specific sets of dietary guidelines were issued, applying

Nutrition and your health: dietary guidelines for Americans

Eat a variety of foods

Foods are the preferred form of consuming nutrients. About 40 different known nutrients, and probably additional as yet unknown factors, are needed to maintain health. No single food can supply all the essential nutrients in the amounts needed. Thus the greater the variety of foods used, the less likely a person is to develop either a deficiency or an excess of any single nutrient. One way to ensure variety, and with it a balanced diet, is to select foods each day from all the major food groups.

Balance the food you eat with physical activity—maintain or improve your weight

Excessive fatness is associated with some chronic disorders such as hypertension and diabetes, which in turn relate to heart disease. A healthy body weight, however, must be determined individually, for many factors are involved, such as body composition, body metabolism, genetics and physical activity.

Choose a diet with plenty of grain products, vegetables, and fruits

Complex carbohydrate foods (starches) are better fuel sources for energy than are simple carbohydrates (sugars) and fats. Starches also contain many essential nutrients and kcalories needed for energy. With increased use of processed and refined foods, the modern American diet is relatively low in dietary fiber. Increas-ing the use of less-refined complex carbohydrates will help increase dietary fiber. Evidence exists that certain types of dietary fiber may help control chronic bowel diseases, contribute to improved blood glucose management for persons with diabetes mellitus, and bind lipids such as cholesterol. Starches, especially forms with more dietary fiber, may therefore be **substituted,** for some of the fats and sugars as energy sources.

Choose a diet low in fat, saturated fat, and cholesterol

Americans as a population have traditionally consumed a high-fat diet. In some persons, excess fat leads to high levels of blood fats and cholesterol carried in lipoprotein compounds. Elevated serum levels of these fats and cholesterol are associated with a higher risk of coronary heart disease. Thus it is wise to cut down on fats in general, using them only in moderation.

Choose a diet moderate in sugars

The major health hazard from eating too much sugar is tooth decay (dental caries). Contrary to popular opinion, however, too much sugar does not itself cause diabetes. It can only contribute to poor control of diabetes in persons who have inherited the disease. Most Americans consume a relatively large amount of sugar, much of it coming from processed food products. Again, moderation is the key.

Choose a diet moderate in salt and sodium

Excessive sodium is not healthy for anyone, especially for persons with high blood pressure. In general, since many processed food products contain considerable sodium or salt and since most Americans eat more sodium than they need, it is wise to limit the use of these products, especially "salty" ones, and reduce added salt in food preparation. These practices will lower individual salt tastes, which are learned habits and not biologic necessities. Ample sodium is found as a natural mineral in foods to meet usual needs.

If you drink alcoholic beverages, do so in moderation

Alcoholic beverages tend to be high in kcalories and low in nutrients. Limited food intake may accompany large alcohol intake. Also, heavy drinking contributes to chronic liver disease and some neurologic disorders, as well as some throat and neck cancers. Thus moderation is the key, if alcohol is used at all.

References

Kennedy E et al: The 1995 Dietary Guidelines for Americans: an overview, *J Am Diet Assoc* 96(3):234, 1996.

U.S. Departments of Agriculture and Health and Human Services: *Nutrition and your health: dietary guidelines for Americans,* ed 4, Home and Garden Bulletin No 232, Washington, D.C., 1995, U.S. Government Printing Office.

these general goals to two major United States health problems, heart disease and cancer (see Chapters 19 and 24).

Revised every 5 years since 1980, the current 1995 Dietary Guidelines for Americans is the first edition to be published under mandate of Congress.[21-23] In this issue, the USDA and the USDHHS include a statement on physical activity for the first time, along with a continuing dietary focus on the principles of variety, balance, and moderation (see *Practical Application* box, p. 12).

PERSONAL ASSESSMENT OF FOOD PATTERNS

PERSONAL PERCEPTIONS OF FOOD

Traditionally, each person develops food habits and ways of eating that are influenced by factors such as ethnic background, cultural patterns, family habits, socioeconomic status, health, available food, and personal likes and dislikes. However, today increasing ethnic diversity has influenced food patterns and brought a greater intermingling of a variety of foods and ideas about food. How persons perceive themselves in relation to food and food patterns plays an important role in developing their own attitudes toward food and personal eating behavior.

A simple way to get a basic idea of the general nutritional value of your own food habits is to examine briefly what you actually eat. First, keep a record of everything you eat and drink for a few days, noting the time, place, activity, and persons with you, if any. Sometimes these factors are a revelation because we eat by habit, usually according to where we are and what we are doing, not because of any serious thought or plan. Second, evaluate everything you had to eat or drink each day: (1) check the revised basic food groups shown in Table 1.2 to get a rough estimate of your use of representative foods in each group; (2) use the food exchange lists provided in Appendix K to determine the energy-yielding values of the macronutrients involved in your food choices (see *To Probe Further* box, below).

To Probe Further

Personal perceptions and analysis of food patterns

What are your own personal perceptions of your eating patterns? What are your food habits, attitudes, and values? To find some answers, check yourself for a few days, using some of the procedures discussed here.

First, keep a detailed record of everything you eat and drink for 3 days: 2 weekdays and 1 weekend day. Make it as complete as possible. Keep a small pocket pad with you and jot down what you eat or drink throughout the day and evening, while your memory is still clear on details. Include any factors influencing your choices: what was it, how much, how prepared or brand name, where and what time, alone or with someone, how you were feeling at the time. Just this brief recording process alone is a good start because it may tell you some things about your eating habits that you were not aware of before. Remember that you are going to analyze this record, so make it as readable, accurate, and detailed as possible.

Second, using the Food Guide Pyramid (p.11), list the foods you ate or drank under their respective food grouping as best you can by what they were. Then compare what you ate with the amounts listed and estimate how closely your choices fulfilled the recommended daily food choices and what you may be short on.

Third, go through the same process of listing each food you ate in its respective food group, this time using the new food exchange lists (Appendix K) to integrate your choices with the energy-yielding macronutrients: carbohydrates, proteins, and fats. Total the amount of each nutrient you consumed. Look particularly at your total amount of fat (g) and kcalories. How close is your total amount of fat to the recommended amount in the national diet and health objectives of 30% of the total day's kcalories? How closely do you match your RDA for kcalories?

Fourth, compare your eating patterns with the national dietary guidelines for healthy Americans (see p. 20). Are there any statements that your eating patterns do not fit? Is there anything in your food habits that you think you may change?

Now that you have thought about it, how do you see yourself as an eater? Are there any food behaviors that you may want to modify to promote health? Any with which you see you're doing a good job?

The simple approach of analyzing food records by basic food groups and food exchange lists can be helpful for increased awareness of personal food patterns. It has even been useful in larger studies of population groups to provide meaningful information about the quality of food habits.

NUTRITIONAL ANALYSIS BY NUTRIENTS AND ENERGY VALUES

A more comprehensive nutritional analysis of food intake records for a wide range of macronutrients and their subgroupings, as well as micronutrient and energy values, can easily be accomplished by using a number of computer programs. In this age of computers, colleges usually have computer equipment available in a computer laboratory or individual students may have their own. If computer equipment is not available, a limited analysis can be done by hand, using standard food value reference tables (see Appendix A). Currently there is general concern about dietary fat in relation to risk of heart disease, so an analysis that focuses on the total fat and cholesterol would prove useful in making changes in food habits.

TO SUM UP

Over the past few years, the role of nutrition in human health has been changing in response to our changing society. The scientific base of nutrition is expanding in both its physical and behavioral foundations. Health goals and objectives have become more person-centered, with a focus on health promotion.

Health status in general has a fundamental nutritional base. To meet these needs, nutritional standards (RDAs/RDIs) have been developed on the basis of current scientific research, as have a number of general and specific food guides and dietary guidelines, for the purpose of disease prevention.

QUESTIONS FOR REVIEW

1. Describe the science of nutrition in terms of its major basic science foundations. What contributions does each make toward understanding human nutrition?
2. Why is the concept of change fundamental in the science of nutrition?
3. Define the terms *nutrition* and *dietetics*. Identify personal roles of professional practitioners in the field of human nutrition.
4. Compare the four general levels of individual nutritional status and describe factors or situations that would contribute to each condition.
5. Compare the three major types of nutritional guides in terms of their nature and use. Give illustrations of each type, and describe what you see as strengths and weaknesses in each case.
6. Keep a 1-day food record of everything you eat or drink, noting nature of the food, method of preparation, and portion consumed. Analyze your food record—by computer if available—in terms of nutrient and kcalorie intake in comparison with the RDAs/RDIs. Do you see ways of improving your diet?

REFERENCES

1. Scrimshaw NS: Nutrition and health from womb to tomb, *Nutr Today* 32(2):55, 1996.
2. Brown JL, Pollitt E: Malnutrition, poverty, and intellectual development, *Sci Am* 274(2):38, 1996.
3. Scrimshaw NS: The new paradigm of public health nutrition, *Am J Public Health* 85(5):622, 1995.
4. Beyer K et al: Nutrition screening among rural older persons, *Nutr Today* 31(1):24, 1996.
5. Bassuk EL et al: Single mothers and welfare, *Sci Am* 275(4):60, 1996.
6. Bassuk EL et al: Homelessness in female-headed families: childhood and adult risk and protective factors, *Am J Public Health* 87(2):241, 1997.
7. Breakey WR: It's time for the public health community to declare war on homelessness, *Am J Public Health* 87(2):153, 1997.
8. US Department of Health and Human Services, Public Health Service: *The Surgeon General's report on nutrition and health,* PHS Pub No 88-50210, Washington, DC, 1988, US Government Printing Office.
9. Food and Nutrition Board, Committee on Diet and Health, National Academy of Sciences—National Research Council: *Diet and health: implications for reducing chronic disease risk,* Washington, DC, 1989, National Academy Press.
10. US Department of Health and Human Services, Public Health Service: *Healthy people 2000: national health promotion and disease prevention objectives,* Washington, DC, 1990, US Government Printing Office.
11. American Dietetic Association: Healthy people 2000: nutrition objectives, *J Am Diet Assoc* 91(12):1515, 1991.
12. Food and Nutrition Board, National Research Council: *Recommended dietary allowances,* ed 10, Washington, DC, 1989, National Academy Press.
13. Russell RM: New views on the RDAs for older adults, *J Am Diet Assoc* 97(5):515, 1997.
14. Monsen ER: New dietary reference intakes proposed to replace the recommended dietary allowances, *J Am Diet Assoc* 96(8):754, 1996.
15. Wu C: Nutrition guides to cover health, safety, *Sci News* 151(16):237, 1997.

16. US Department of Agriculture: *Guide to daily food choices,* Washington, DC, 1991, U.S. Government Printing Office.

17. U.S. Department of Agriculture: *Eating right food pyramid,* Washington, DC, 1992, U.S. Government Printing Office.

18. American Dietetic Association, American Diabetes Association: *Exchange lists for meal planning,* Chicago, 1995, American Dietetic Association.

19. American Dietetic Association: *Exchange lists for weight management,* Chicago, 1995, American Dietetic Association.

20. US Department of Agriculture, US Department of Health and Human Services: *Nutrition and your health: dietary guidelines for Americans,* ed 4, Home and Garden Bulletin No 232, Washington, DC, 1990, U.S. Government Printing Office.

21. Bialostosky K, St. Joer ST: The 1995 Dietary Guidelines for Americans, *Nutr Today* 31(1):6, 1996.

22. Kennedy E et al: The 1995 Dietary Guidelines for Americans: an overview, *J Am Diet Assoc* 96(3):234, 1996.

23. Kirby J: New Dietary Guidelines: new opportunity for consumer education, *J Am Diet Assoc* 96(3):228, 1996.

▄ FURTHER READING

Callaway CW: Dietary Guidelines for Americans: an historical perspective, *J Am Coll Nutr* 16(6):510, 1997.

Goldberg JP, Hellwig JP: Nutrition research in the media: the challenge facing scientists, *J Am Coll Nutr* 16(6):544, 1997.

These two articles discuss two perspectives of the Dietary Guidelines for Americans. Callaway describes the interesting history of these guidelines since their beginning in 1980. They have been published every 5 years by the USDA and USDHHS and are intended for healthy adults to reduce risks for certain diet-related chronic conditions. Goldberg and Hellwig focus on the public media as the most popular vehicle through which consumers obtain nutrition information and the need for scientists to communicate their research findings more effectively with the public.

Millen BE et al: Population nutrient intake approaches dietary recommendations: 1991 to 1995 Framingham Nutrition Studies, *J Am Diet Assoc* 97(7):742, 1997.

The population studied here are current offspring of the well-known original heart study initiated in Framingham, Massachusetts, in 1948 and conducted periodically since then in the Framingham Offspring-Spouse population studies, including ages 12 to 60 years, with current data here being the fifth study between 1991 and 1995. This ongoing work has provided valuable interesting information concerning the history of heart disease in this stable population.

Issues Answers

Positive health promotion, not negative blame

Some critics of the current health promotion/self-care movement say that it sabotages some peoples' efforts to maintain health by blaming them when they become ill. This is a misplaced accusation. It apparently started when the public and practitioners alike, alarmed by the soaring costs of health care, sought ways in which individuals could reduce their chances of becoming ill. The result is the growing field of preventive health.

Many preventive health care practitioners are sensitive, skilled professionals who have used varied methods of sharing their knowledge and skills with the public:

- Identification of risks
- Patient education regarding special illnesses
- Medical self-care
- Alternatives to traditional medical care
- Promotion of "wellness" as a state of mind or an attitude

Their task has not been easy because (1) their recommendations are often taken over and redefined or changed by business opportunists; (2) there are no guarantees that every recommendation will achieve the same results (for example, everyone who jogs 10 miles a day does not escape heart disease); (3) our culture stresses "antihealth" habits (for example, availability of high-sodium and high-fat convenience foods and heavy alcohol use and overeating promoted by the media); and (4) health activists are viewed as attempting to impose their personal value systems on others.

However, recommendations of some of these practitioners are not based on solid research and tend to yield inconsistent results. Because these "opinions" almost always involve the personal habits of the client, the "wellness" promoter is in effect telling people that it's their own fault if they're sick—they don't eat the right foods, they aren't keeping their weight down, they smoke/drink too much, they even *think* too much. In doing so, they may be confusing the issue in several cases:

- Is it really the 16-year-old's fault that he eats too much when in his lifetime he's seen over 300,000 TV commercials, most of which advertise readily available food?
- Is it the fault of the working woman that she relies on high-sodium, high-fat convenience foods to feed her family?

- Is the low-income patient with no recreation available other than meal preparation totally at fault for his obesity?
- And what about the countless patients with chronic diseases who received no preventive health information from their physicians for decades before seeing a wellness practitioner? Are they responsible for their own heart attacks or liver disease?

Physicians and other health professionals who have improved their own health because of wellness practices can contribute to the wellness of their patients without conducting a crusade against them. They can teach those same health-promoting ideas nonjudgmentally, rather than concentrating only on the "challenge" or threat of illness.

When the "victim" role is reinforced, circumstances that created vulnerability to poor health in the first place are perpetuated and legitimatized. Further attempts to help are often turned down. To avoid this type of situation, the health practitioner should:

Examine personal value systems. Is my own work designed to point a finger at the victim or truly help the client to help himself?

Consider every aspect of the client. Is it really within my client's power to control food intake at home? What social, financial, or other factors may be limiting choice of foods or choice of activities other than eating? How can these be addressed?

Be realistic. If current research is not conclusive, should I avoid presenting recommendations as being "failure proof"?

Practitioners may benefit in their health promotion activities by determining which persons may be open to such approaches and which may not. A health-promoting lifestyle profile is a helpful tool for investigating patterns of health behavior and the effects of efforts to change these behaviors. Six areas involved in these behaviors must be considered in working with each client: (1) degree of health responsibility, (2) capacity for self-fulfillment, (3) exercise capacity and amount, (4) nutritional status and problems, (5) interpersonal support, and (6) capacity for coping with stress. A checklist of positive health behaviors in each of these areas can be constructed to develop true client-centered health care. For example, items concerned with nutrition may focus on meal patterns and food choices.

Current trends in health promotion indicate that health and nutrition education efforts have increased dramatically over the past decade and resulted in behavioral change. Substantial evidence supports the fact that these health promotion activities can alter public health behaviors, preventing disease by reducing risks for health problems.

References

Hahn NI: Variety is *still* the spice of a healthful diet, *J Am Diet Assoc* 95(10):1096, 1995.

Klawitter B: Counseling and learning: child, adolescent, adult, elderly and family. In Helm KK, Klawitter B: *Nutrition therapy,* Lake Dallas, TX, 1995, Helm Seminars.

Millen BE: Population nutrient intake approaches dietary recommendations: 1991 to 1995 Framingham nutrition studies, *J Am Diet Assoc* 97(7):742, 1997.

Chapter

2

Digestion, Absorption, and Metabolism

In this chapter, we begin our story of what happens to the foods we eat and their general fate in the body. We look first at the integrated overall body systems that handle them. Once the body receives the foods we eat, unique structures and functions transform them for our use. In the following chapters of Part 1 you will discover many marvelous details of the individual nutrients and their roles in human health.

The overall physiologic and biochemical process involved has three integrated parts: digestion, absorption, and metabolism. We begin with a look at the gastrointestinal tract and then follow the path of the nutrients to the cells. We see how each part of the system makes its own special contribution to the whole integrated operation.

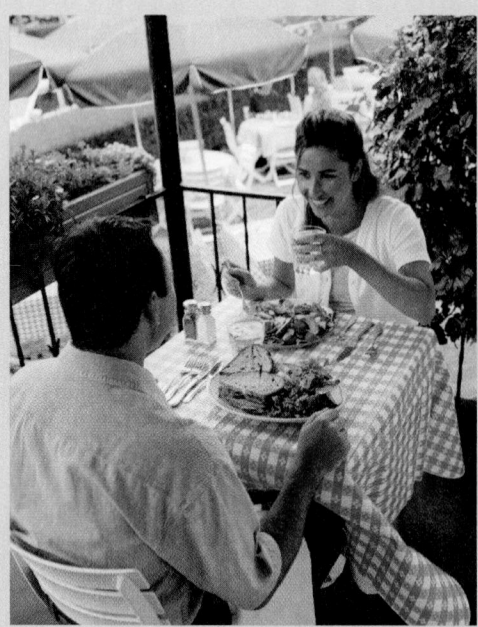

THE HUMAN BODY AS A DYNAMIC WHOLE

THE CONCEPTS OF CHANGE AND BALANCE

The foods we eat contain the necessary nutrients for our survival, but these life-sustaining nutrients must first be released and transformed into available units the body can use. Through a successive interrelated system of balanced change, the foods we eat are transformed into simpler substances and then into other, still simpler, substances that our cells can use to sustain life. All these many changes prepare food for use by the body. Together they constitute the overall digestion-absorption-metabolism process.

The overall physiologic and biochemical process involved has three integrated parts: digestion, absorption, and metabolism. We begin in this chapter with a broad view of the gastrointestinal tract. Then in following chapters we will see how each individual nutrient in our food travels this marvelous pathway and is transformed into key products to nourish and sustain our lives.

THE CONCEPT OF WHOLENESS

Body integrity

The parts of this overall process of change do not exist separately. Each is unique, but together they compose one continuous integrated *whole*. Look carefully at the respective components of the gastrointestinal tract and their relative position in this overall body system (Figure 2.1). Follow the fate of food components as they travel *together* through the successive parts of the gastrointestinal tract and into the body cells. This fundamental body system has rightly been called "the portal to nutrient utilization."[1]

Reasons for human life systems

Why is this intricate complex of activities so necessary to human life? Two reasons are apparent: (1) *Food* as it naturally occurs and as we eat it is not a single component but a mixture of chemical substances, or nutrients. If these substances are to release their stored energy and building materials for use, they must be separated into their respective components so that the body may handle each one as a separate unit. (2) *Nutrients* released from the food may still remain unavailable to the body, and some additional means of changing their forms must follow. The intermediate units must be broken down, simplified, regrouped, and rerouted. This complex chemical work must take place because the human being, whose life is developed and sustained in a dynamic internal chemical environment, is the most highly organized and intricately balanced of all organisms. This high level of internal bodily control and balance is called **homeostasis**,

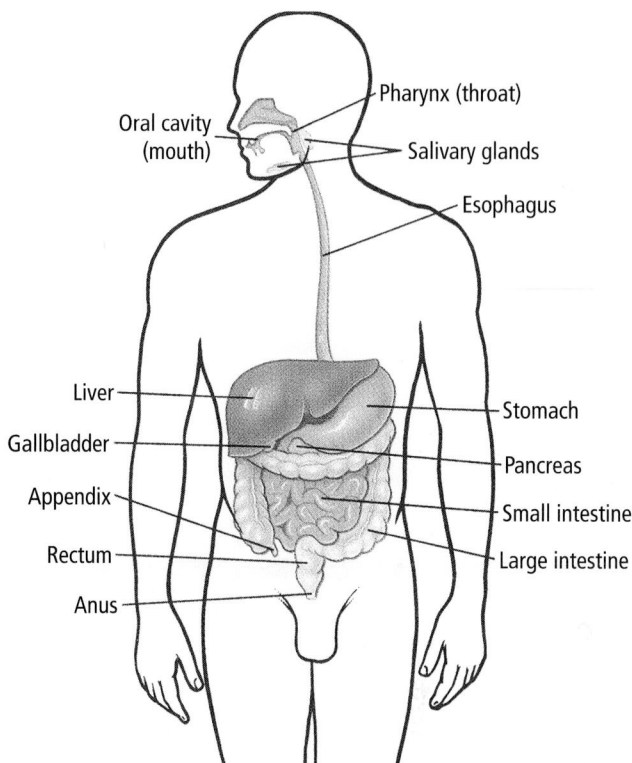

Figure 2.1   The gastrointestinal system. Through the successive parts of the system, multiple activities of digestion liberate and reform food nutrients for our use. (From Seeley RR, Stephens TD, Tate PP: *Anatomy and physiology,* ed 2, New York, 1992, McGraw-Hill.)

which is achieved through the effectiveness and beauty of the body's homeostatic mechanisms.[2] This view of the human body as an integrated physiochemical organism is basic to an understanding of human nutrition, both in health and in disease.

BASIC PRINCIPLES OF DIGESTION

Digestion initially prepares the food for the body's use. Two basic types of action are involved—muscular and chemical.

---

digestion   The process of breaking down food to release its nutrients for absorption and transport to the cells for use in body functions.

homeostasis   State of relative dynamic equilibrium within the body's internal environment; a balance achieved through the operation of various interrelated physiologic mechanisms.

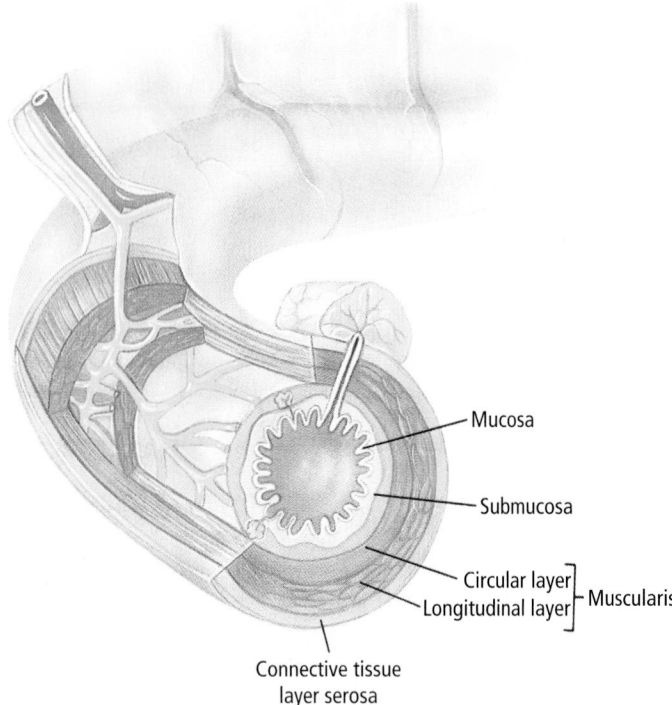

Figure 2.2   Muscle layers of the intestinal wall. (From Raven P, Johnson: *Biology,* ed 3, New York, 1992, McGraw-Hill.)

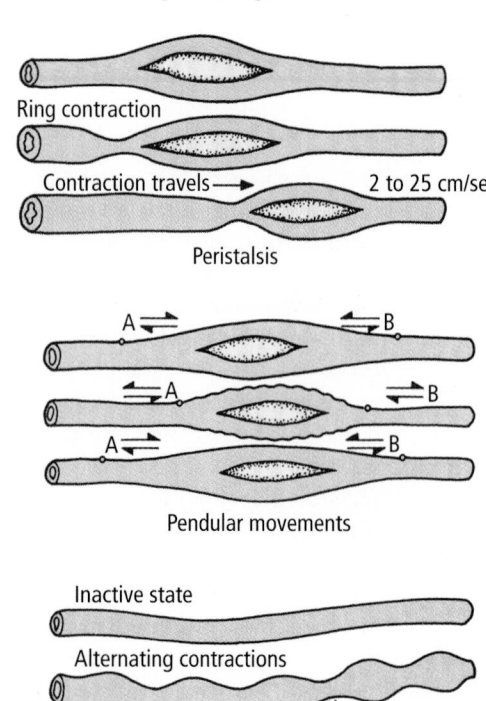

Figure 2.3   Types of movement produced by muscles of the intestine: peristaltic waves from contraction of deep circular muscle, pendular movements from small local muscles, and segmentation rings formed by alternate contraction and relaxation of circular muscle.

GASTROINTESTINAL MOTILITY: MUSCLES AND MOVEMENT

Food is prepared for chemical digestion by initial breakdown by specific enzymes, which takes place through a number of neuromuscular, self-regulating processes. These actions work together to move the food mass along the alimentary tract at the best rate for digestion and absorption of the nutrients.

Types of muscles

Organized muscle layers of the gastrointestinal wall, shown in Figure 2.2, provide the necessary motility for digestion. From the outside surface inward the layers are (1) the **serosa**, (2) a *longitudinal muscle layer*, (3) a *circular muscle layer*, (4) the *submucosa*, and (5) the **mucosa**. Also, imbedded in the deeper layers of the mucosa is a thin layer of smooth muscle fibers called the *muscularis mucosae*. The interaction of these smooth muscle layers make possible four necessary types of movement (Figure 2.3):

1. *Longitudinal muscles*. The long, smooth muscles, arranged in fiber bundles that extend lengthwise along the gastrointestinal tract, help propel the food mass along the tract.
2. *Circular contractile muscles*. In the circular muscle layer, smooth muscle fibers extend around the gut. They form rhythmic contractile rings that cause sweeping waves along the digestive tract and push

the food mass forward. These regularly occurring propulsive movements are called **peristalsis**.

3. *Sphincter muscles*. More defined circular muscles occur at strategic points to provide muscle sphincters that act as valves—pyloric, ileocecal, and anal—to prevent reflux and control movement of food mass in its forward passage.
4. *Mucosal muscles*. The imbedded thin layer of smooth muscle produces *local constrictive contractions* that occur every few centimeters. They mix and chop the food mass as it moves along the tract, effectively churning the mass and mixing it with secretions to form a semiliquid **chyme** ready for digestion and absorption.

In summary, the interaction of the gastrointestinal muscles produces two basic types of action:

- General muscle tone or tonic contraction that ensures continuous passage and valve control, and
- Periodic, rhythmic contractions that mix and propel the food mass.

As a result, these alternating muscular contractions and relaxations force the contents forward and facilitate specific digestion and absorption.

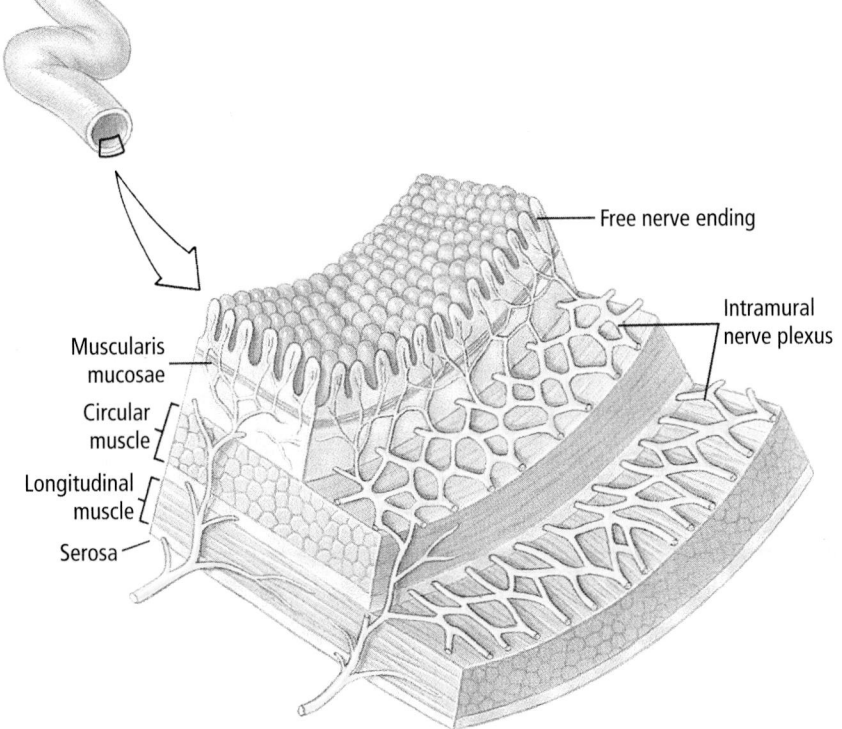

Free nerve ending

Intramural
nerve plexus

Muscularis
mucosae

Circular
muscle

Longitudinal
muscle

Serosa

Figure 2.4   Innervation of the intestine by
intramural nerve plexus. (Medical and Scientific Illustration.)

Nervous system control

Throughout the gastrointestinal tract specific nerves regulate these muscular actions. An interrelated network of
nerves within the gastrointestinal wall, called the **intramural nerve plexus** (Figure 2.4), extends from the
esophagus to the anus. This network of nerve fibers controls muscle tone of the gastrointestinal wall, regulates
the rate and intensity of muscle contractions, and coordinates the various movements.[3]

Gastrointestinal secretions

Food is digested chemically by the combined action of a
number of secretions. Generally these secretions are of
four types:
1.   *Enzymes.* Specific kind and quantity split desig-
    nated chemical bonds within the structure of
    specific nutrient compounds, freeing their com-
    ponent parts.
2.   *Hydrochloric acid and buffer ions.* These agents
    produce the necessary pH for the activity of
    given enzymes.
3.   *Mucus.* This agent lubricates and protects the
    inside wall tissues of the gastrointestinal tract
    and facilitates food mass passage.
4.   *Water and electrolytes.* These agents provide a bal-
    anced solution base in sufficient volumes to cir-
    culate the organic substances released.
Special cells in the mucosal tissue of the gastrointestinal
tract, or in adjacent accessory organs, especially the pancreas, produce these secretions. The secretory action of
these cells or glands is stimulated by the intake of food,

by the sensory nerve network, or by hormones specific for
certain nutrients.

Mouth and esophagus: preparation and delivery

Up to this point, we have generally viewed the gastrointestinal tract in terms of integrated muscular-secretory
functions that govern its operation as a whole. Here we
begin to follow this operation through its successive parts

chyme   Semifluid food mass in gastrointestinal tract following gastric digestion.

mucosa   The mucous membrane comprising the inner
surface layer of gastrointestinal tract tissues, providing
extensive nutrient absorption and transport functions.

peristalsis   A wavelike progression of alternate contraction and relaxation of the muscle fibers of the gastrointestinal tract.

serosa   Outer surface layer of the intestines interfacing
with the blood vessels of the portal system going to the
liver.

intramural nerve plexus   Network of nerves in the walls of
the intestine that make up the enteric nervous system controlling muscle action and secretions for digestion and
absorption.

to see what happens when we eat food. Actually, eating starts a remarkable physiologic event. It prepares food for entry into a complex system that radically changes its form and finally nourishes the body with its contents. Each step of the way requires motility and secretions. In this first step, highly synchronized actions prepare food in the mouth, control the intricate act of swallowing, and deliver the food to the stomach by way of the esophagus.

Mastication

Initial biting and chewing begin to break food down into smaller particles. The teeth and other oral structures are particularly suited for this function. The incisors cut; the molars grind. Tremendous force is supplied by the jaw muscles: 55 lb of muscular pressure is applied through the incisors, 200 lb through the molars. Mastication allows an enlarged surface area of food to receive constant enzyme action. Also, the fineness of the food particles eases the continued passage of material through the gastrointestinal tract.

Swallowing

The process of swallowing involves both the mouth and the pharynx. It is intricately initiated and controlled by the brainstem "swallowing center."[4] Swallowing is extremely rapid, taking less than 1 second. It can be initiated voluntarily, but once started it proceeds as an involuntary reflex. Muscles at the base of the tongue aid the process.

Esophagus

The esophagus is a muscular tube connecting the mouth or pharynx with the stomach and that serves as a channel for eating to carry the initial food mass into the body for processing and absorption. Functionally, it may be divided into three main parts[4]:

1. *Upper esophageal sphincter (UES)*. The UES controls the passage of food into the esophagus. At rest, between intakes of food, the UES muscle is closed. Within 0.2 to 0.3 seconds after a swallow of food or drink, nerve stimuli immediately open the sphincter to receive the nourishment.
2. *Esophageal body*. A mixed **bolus** of food particles passes immediately down the esophagus largely by peristaltic waves controlled by nerve reflexes. Gravity aids the movement of food down the esophagus in the upright position.
3. *Lower esophageal sphincter (LES)*. The LES controls the passage of the food mass from the esophagus into the stomach for continuing digestion. When the LES muscles maintain an excessively high degree of muscle tone, even while resting, spasms may occur and the muscles fail to open when person swallows, a condition called *achalasia*, from its unrelaxed muscle state (see Chapter 18).

Table 2.1   Comparative pH values and approximate daily volumes of gastrointestinal secretions

Secretion	pH	Daily volume (ml)
Salivary	6.0-7.4	1000
Gastric	1.0-3.5	1500
Pancreatic	8.0-8.3	1000
Small intestinal	7.5-8.0	1800
Brunner's gland	8.0-8.9	200
Bile	7.5-7.8	1000
Large intestinal	7.5-8.0	200
TOTAL		6700

Modified from Guyton AC, Hall JC: *Textbook of medical physiology,* ed 9, Philadelphia, 1996, WB Saunders.

Entry into the stomach

At the point of entry into the stomach, the *gastroesophageal constrictor muscle* relaxes to allow food to enter. Then it contracts again to prevent regurgitation or reflux of the now acidic stomach contents up into the esophagus. When regurgitation does occur, through failure of this mechanism, the person feels it as "heartburn." Two clinical problems may hinder normal food passage at this point: (1) *cardiospasm*, caused by failure of the constrictor muscle to relax properly, or (2) *hiatal hernia*, caused by protrusion of the upper part of the stomach into the thorax through an abnormal opening of the diaphragm.

CHEMICAL OR SECRETORY DIGESTION

In the mouth, three pairs of salivary glands—*parotid, submaxillary,* and *sublingual*—secrete serous material containing *salivary amylase*. This is an enzyme specific for starches. Mucus is also secreted to lubricate and bind the food particles. Stimuli such as sight, smell, taste, and touch—and even thoughts of likes and dislikes in food—greatly influence these secretions. The normal daily secretion of saliva ranges between 800 and 1500 ml, with a pH range of 6 (approximately neutral) to 7.4, as shown in Table 2.1. Food remains in the mouth only a short time, so starch digestion here is brief and is terminated by the acid medium of the stomach.

STOMACH: STORAGE AND INITIAL DIGESTIVE PROCESSES

MOTILITY

The major parts of the stomach are shown in Figure 2.5. Muscles in the stomach wall provide three basic motor functions: storage, mixing, and controlled emptying. As

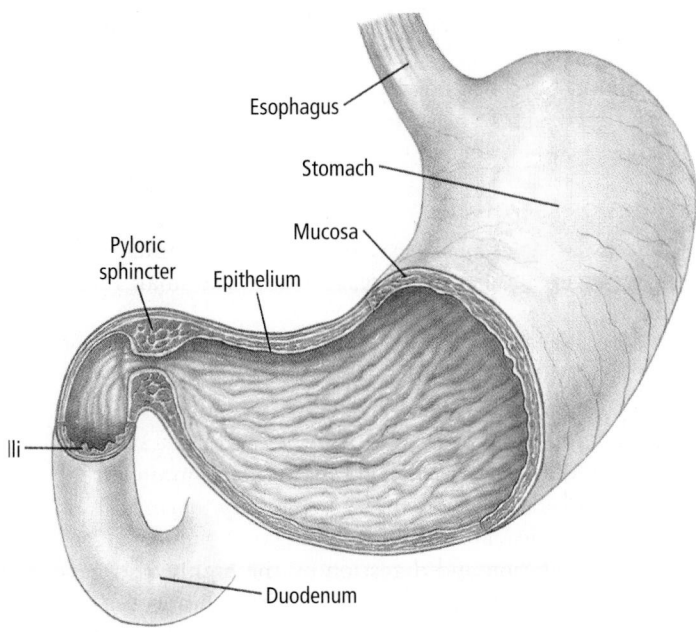

Esophagus

Stomach

Pyloric
sphincter
Mucosa
Epithelium

lli

Duodenum

Figure 2.5   Stomach (From Raven P, Johnson: *Biology,* ed 3, New York, 1992, McGraw-Hill.)

the food mass enters the stomach, it lies against the stomach walls, which can stretch outward to store as much as 1 L. Local tonic muscle waves gradually increase their kneading and mixing action as the mass of food and secretions moves on toward the pyloric valve at the distal end of the stomach. Here waves of peristaltic contractions reduce the mass to a semifluid chyme. Finally, with each wave, small amounts of chyme are forced through the pyloric valve. This sphincter muscle constricts and periodically relaxes, then constricts again to control the emptying of the stomach contents into the duodenum. This control releases the acid chyme slowly enough to be buffered by the alkaline intestinal secretions. The kilocaloric density of a meal, in addition to its particular volume and composition, influences the rate of stomach emptying.

CHEMICAL OR SECRETORY DIGESTION

Types of secretion

Stomach secretions contain three basic types of materials: acid, mucus, and enzymes.
1. *Acid.* Hydrochloric acid is produced to prepare certain enzymes and materials for digestion and absorption by creating the necessary degree of acidity for given enzymes to work. For example, the range of pH necessary for the enzyme pepsin to act on protein is 1.8 to 3.5; at a pH of 5 or above there is little or no activity.

2. *Mucus.* Special mucous secretions protect the stomach lining from the eroding effect of the acid. This **mucus** also binds and mixes the food mass and helps move it along.
3. *Enzymes.* The main enzyme in the stomach is *pepsin,* which begins the breakdown of protein. It is first secreted in the inactive form *pepsinogen,* which is then activated by the hydrochloric acid present. A small amount of *gastric lipase (tributyrinase)* is present and works on emulsified fats such as butterfat. This is a relatively minor activity, however. In childhood an enzyme called *rennin* (not to be confused with the vital lifelong renal enzyme *renin*) is also present in gastric secretions to aid in the coagulation of milk. Rennin is absent in adults.

Control of secretions

Stimuli for these gastric secretions come from two sources:
1. *Nerve stimulus* is produced in response to the senses, ingested food, and emotions. For example, anger and hostility increase secretions. Fear and depression decrease secretions, and inhibit blood flow and motility as well.
2. *Hormonal stimulus* is produced in response to the entrance of food into the stomach. Certain stimulants, especially caffeine, alcohol, and meat extracts, cause the release of a local gastrointestinal hormone **gastrin** from mucosal cells in the antrum, which in turn stimulates the secretion of more hydrochloric acid. When the pH reaches 2, a feedback mechanism stops further secretion of the hormone to prevent excess acid formation. Another local gastrointestinal hormone, **enterogastrone,** is produced by glands

bolus   Rounded mass of food formed in the mouth and ready to be swallowed.

enterogastrone   A duodenal peptide hormone that inhibits gastric hydrochloric acid secretion and motility.

gastrin   Hormone secreted by mucosal cells in the antrum of the stomach that stimulates the parietal cells to produce hydrochloric acid. Gastrin is released into the stomach in response to stimulants, especially coffee, alcohol, and meat extracts. When the gastric pH reaches 2 to 3, a feedback mechanism cuts off gastrin secretion and prevents excess acid formation.

mucus   Viscid fluid secreted by mucous membranes and glands, consisting mainly of mucin (a glycoprotein), inorganic salts, and water. Mucus serves to lubricate and protect the gastrointestinal mucosa and to help move the food mass along the digestive tract.

in the duodenal mucosa. This hormone counteracts excessive gastric activity by inhibiting hydrochloric acid secretion, pepsin secretion, and gastric motility.

Small intestine: major digestion, absorption, and transport

Motility

Intestinal muscle layers
Note the exquisite structural arrangement of the intestinal wall shown in Figure 2.2. Finely coordinated intestinal motility is achieved by the three basic layers of muscle: (1) the thin layer of smooth muscle imbedded in the mucosa, the *muscularis mucosae*, with fibers extending up into the villi; (2) the circular muscle layer; and (3) the longitudinal muscle next to the outer serosa.

Types of intestinal muscle actions
Under the control of the nerve plexus, wall-stretch pressure from food, or hormonal stimuli, these muscles produce two different types of movement to aid digestion:
1. *Propulsive movements*. Peristalsis produced by waves of contracting deep circular muscle propels the food mass slowly forward. The intensity of the wave may be increased by food intake or by the presence of irritants, causing in some cases long sweeping waves over the entire intestine. A series of local segmental contractions also aids the forward movement of the food mass.
2. *Mixing movements*. Peristalsis and local constrictive contractions that occur every few centimeters in the muscle wall mix and chop the food mass as it moves along the gastrointestinal tract. This combined action effectively churns the food mass, gradually mixing it with secretions to form the semi-liquid chyme ready for digestion and absorption.

Thus the interaction of the gastrointestinal muscles produces two basic types of action: (1) a general muscle tone or tonic contraction that insures continuous passage and valve control and (2) periodic, rhythmic contractions that mix and propel the food mass. These alternating muscular contractions and relaxations force the contents forward and facilitate appropriate digestive and absorptive processes.

Chemical or secretory digestion

Major role of small intestine
More than any other part of the entire gastrointestinal tract, the small intestine carries the major burden of chemical digestion. Thus this area secretes a large number of enzymes, each specific for some member of the macronutrients—carbohydrates, fats, and proteins. These specific enzymes are secreted from both the intestinal glands and the pancreas (Table 2.2).

Types of secretions
Four basic types of digestive secretions complete this final process of chemical breakdown in the small intestine:
1. *Enzymes*. A number of specific enzymes (see Table 2.2) act on specific nutrients to cause a final breakdown of the nutrient materials in food to forms the body can absorb and use.
2. *Mucus*. Intestinal glands located immediately inside the duodenum secrete large quantities of mucus. This secretion protects the mucosa from irritation and digestion by the highly acid gastric juices at this point. Additional mucous cells on the intestinal surface continue to secrete mucus when touched by the moving food mass. This secretion lubricates and protects the tissues.
3. *Hormone*. In response to the presence of acid in the entering food mass, mucosal cells in the upper part of the small intestine produce the local gastrointestinal peptide hormone **secretin**.[5] In turn, secretin then stimulates the pancreas to send alkaline pancreatic juices into the duodenum to buffer the entering gastric acid chyme. The unprotected intestinal mucosa alone at this point could not withstand this high degree of acidity.
4. *Bile*. Another important aid to digestion and absorption in the small intestine is bile, an emulsifying agent for fats (see *To Probe Further* box, p. 33). A large volume of bile is produced in the liver as a dilute watery solution. It is then concentrated and stored by the gallbladder (Figure 2.6). When fat enters the duodenum, the local gastrointestinal peptide hormone **cholecystokinin (CCK)** is secreted by glands in the intestinal mucosa and stimulates the gallbladder to contract and release the needed bile. The bile-conserving *enterohepatic circulation of bile* (Figure 2.6), between the liver, gallbladder, and gastrointestinal tract, serves the needs of all organs involved.[6]

Factors influencing secretions
In the small intestine, as well as in other sections of the system, many factors influence various secretions. These factors include controls by hormones and nerve plexus, stimulated by physical contact with the food materials and by emotions. These influencing factors are summarized in Figure 2.7.

Table 2.2 Summary of digestive processes			
Nutrient	**Mouth**	**Stomach**	**Small intestine**
Carbohydrate	Starch $\xrightarrow{\alpha\text{-amylase}}$ Dextrins		Pancreas
			Starch $\xrightarrow{\text{Amylase}}$ Maltose and sucrose (Disaccharides)
			Intestine
			(Monosaccharides)
			Lactose $\xrightarrow{\text{Lactase}}$ Glucose and galactose
			Sucrose $\xrightarrow{\text{Sucrase}}$ Glucose and fructose
			Maltose $\xrightarrow{\text{Maltase}}$ Glucose and glucose
Protein		Protein $\xrightarrow{\text{Pepsin HCl}}$ Polypeptides	Pancreas
			Proteins, Polypeptides $\xrightarrow{\text{Trypsin}}$ Dipeptides
			Proteins, Polypeptides $\xrightarrow{\text{Chymotrypsin}}$ Dipeptides
			Polypeptides, Dipeptides $\xrightarrow{\text{Carboxypeptidase}}$ Amino acids
			Intestine
			Polypeptides, Dipeptides $\xrightarrow{\text{Aminopeptidase}}$ Amino acids
			Dipeptides $\xrightarrow{\text{Dipeptidase}}$ Amino acids
Fat		Tributyrin (butterfat) $\xrightarrow{\text{Tributyrinase}}$ Glycerol	Pancreas
			Fatty acids Fats ^{Lipase} Glycerol
			Glycerides (di-, mono-)
			Fatty acids
			Intestine
			Fats $\xrightarrow{\text{Lipase}}$ Glycerol
			Glycerides (di-, mono-)
			Fatty acids
			Liver and gallbladder
			Fats $\xrightarrow{\text{Bile}}$ Emulsified fat

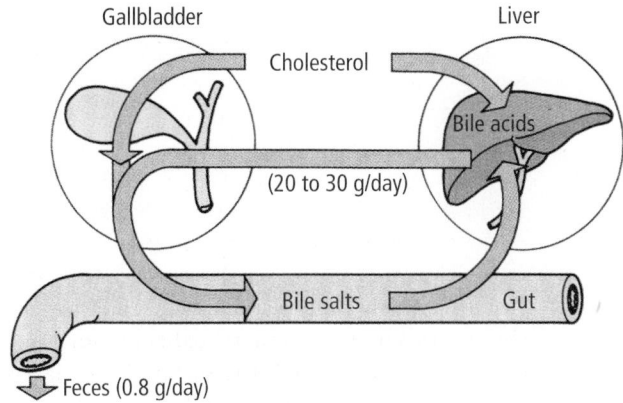

Figure 2.6   Enterohepatic circulation of bile salts.

ABSORPTION

End products of digestion

After digestion of the food nutrients is complete, the simplified end products are ready for **absorption**, aided by a number of transport mechanisms. The end products include the *monosaccharides* glucose, fructose, and galactose from carbohydrates; *fatty acids* and *glycerides* from fats; and *amino acids* from proteins. In some cases, incom-

pletely digested nutrients remain in the intestine and cause gas.[7] For example, in sensitive persons lacking lactase, lactose remains in the intestine and causes problems (see *Issues & Answers*, p. 35). Some small peptides may be absorbed intact and finally broken down to amino acids within the mucosal absorptive cells. Vitamins and minerals are also liberated. Finally, with a water base for solution and transport plus necessary electrolytes, the total fluid food mass is now prepared for absorption as part of the large gastrointestinal circulation (Table 2.3).

absorption   Transport of digested nutrients into body circulation to cells.

cholecystokinin (CCK)   A peptide hormone secreted by the mucosa of the duodenum in response to the presence of fat. The cholecystokinin causes the gallbladder to contract. This contraction propels bile into the duodenum, where it is needed to emulsify the fat. The fat is thus prepared for digestion and absorption.

secretin   Hormone produced in the mucous membrane of the duodenum in response to the entrance of the acid contents of the stomach into the duodenum. Secretin in turn stimulates the flow of pancreatic juice, providing needed enzymes and the proper alkalinity for their action.

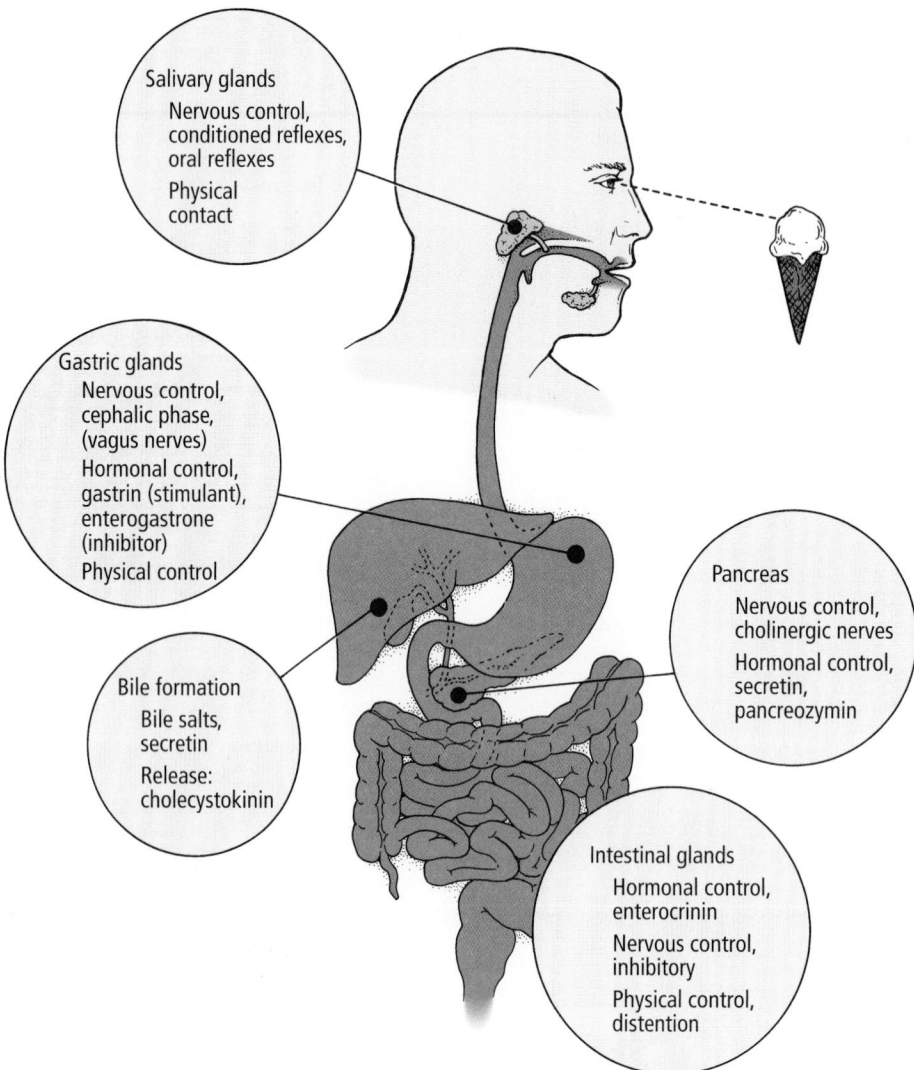

Figure 2.7   Summary of factors influencing secretions of the gastrointestinal tract.

Surface structures

Viewed from the outside, the intestine appears smooth, but the inner mucosal surface lining is quite different. Note carefully in Figure 2.8 the three types of convolutions and projections that greatly enhance the absorbing surface area:

- *Mucosal folds.* Large mucosal folds, similar to hills and valleys in a mountain range, can easily be seen by the naked eye.
- *Villi.* Fingerlike projections on these folds, called **villi**, can be seen through a simple microscope.
- *Microvilli.* Extremely small projections on each villus that can be seen only with an electron microscope. The array of **microvilli** covering the edge of each villus is called the *brush border* because it looks like bristles on a brush. Each villus has an ample network of blood capillaries, as well as a central lymph vessel called a *lacteal* for

the absorption of fat substances that have a creamy, milklike appearance at this point.

Absorbing surface area

The three structures of the small intestine—mucosal folds, villi, and microvilli—increase the inner absorbing surface area some 600 times over that of the outside serosa.[2,8] These special structures, plus the contracted length of the live organ—630 to 660 cm (21 to 22 ft)—produce a tremendously large absorbing surface. This inner surface of the small intestine, if stretched out flat, would be as large or larger than half a tennis or basketball court! All three of these mucosal structures serve as a unit for the absorption of nutrients. Although the intestine is popularly known as the lowly "gut," it is actually one of the most highly developed, exquisitely fashioned, specialized tissues in the human body.

Figure 2.8   Intestinal wall. Note the arrangement of muscle layers and the structures of the mucosa that increase the surface area for absorption—mucosal folds, villi, and microvilli. (Medical and Scientific Illustration.)

Table 2.3	Daily absorption volume in gastrointestinal system		
	Intake (L)	Intestinal absorption (L)	Elimination (L)
Food ingested	1.5		
Gastrointestinal secretions	8.5		
TOTAL	10.0		
Fluid absorbed in small intestine		9.5	
Fluid absorbed in large intestine		0.4	
TOTAL		9.9	
Feces			0.1

Mechanisms of absorption

Absorption of the finely dispersed water-based nutrient solution is accomplished through the wall of the small intestine by means of a number of transport processes, depending on the nature of the nutrient and the prevailing electrochemical fluid pressure gradient.

1. *Passive diffusion and osmosis.* When no opposing pressure exists, molecules small enough to pass through the capillary membranes diffuse easily into the capillaries of the villi in the direction of the pressure flow, in quantities that depend on their solute concentration (Figure 2.9). This varying solute concentration of electrolytes determines the electrochemical gradient based on the degree and direction of the osmotic pressure (see Chapter 8, Minerals-Water Balance).[2]

2. *Facilitated diffusion.* Even though the pressure gradient is favorably flowing from greater to lesser concentration, which characterizes the process of diffusion, some particular molecules may be too large to go through the membrane pores easily and may require assistance. In such cases, a specific integral membrane protein facilitates passage by carrying the particular nutrient molecules across the membrane.

3. *Energy-dependent active transport.* Nutrient molecules must cross the intestinal epithelial membrane to feed hungry tissue cells even when the fluid flow pressures are against them. Such

microvilli   Minute vascular structures protruding from the surface of villi covering the inner surface of the small intestine, forming a "brush border" that facilitates absorption of nutrients.

villi   Small protrusions from the surface of a membrane; fingerlike projections covering mucosal surfaces of the small intestine.

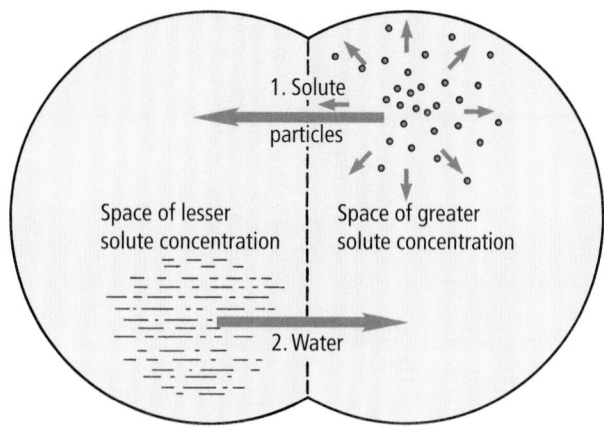

Figure 2.9   Movement of molecules, water, and solutes by osmosis and diffusion.

Figure 2.10   Pinocytosis—engulfing of large molecules by the cell.

"active" work requires extra energy supplied by the cell's metabolism and a "pumping" mechanism (see *To Probe Further* box, p. 33). A special membrane protein carrier, often coupled with the active transport of sodium, assists the process. The active sodium-coupled transport of glucose is an example of this action. A remarkable enzyme, *sodium- and potassium-dependent adenosinetriphosphatase (Na+-, K+-, ATPase)*, which is present in the cell membrane, supplies the energy for this interesting pumping action.

4. *Engulfing pinocytosis*. At times, fluid and nutrient molecules use still another means of reaching the tissue circulation outposts in the villi. In these instances, when the particular particle touches the absorbing cell membrane, the membrane dips inward around the fluid and nutrient material, surrounding it to form a *vacuole*, and then engulfs it. The materials are then conveyed through the cell cytoplasm and discharged into the circulation. Occasionally, smaller whole proteins, as well as neutral fat droplets, may be absorbed by pinocytosis (Figure 2.10).

Routes of absorption

After their absorption by these various processes, the nutrients from carbohydrates and proteins, being water soluble, enter the portal bloodstream directly and travel to the liver and other body tissues. Only fat, which is not water soluble, is unique in its route. Fats are carried in a bile complex into the cells of the intestinal wall, enzyme-processed there to human lipid compounds, converted to a complex with protein as a carrier, and packaged as lipoproteins. These packages of fat flow into the lymph; empty into the **cisterna chyli**, the major central abdominal collecting vessel of the body's lymphatic system; travel upward into the chest through the thoracic duct;

and finally flow into the venous blood at the left subclavian vein. Then these initial lipoproteins, called chylomicrons from their large fat load just absorbed, are rapidly cleared from the blood by the special fat enzyme lipoprotein lipase. Exceptions to this route of fat absorption are the medium-chain and short-chain fatty acids, which are more water soluble and hence absorbed directly into blood circulation. However, most of the fats in the human diet are made of long-chain fatty acids, are not water soluble, and must travel the lacteal lymphatic route described.

LARGE INTESTINE: FINAL ABSORPTION AND WASTE ELIMINATION

Absorption of water is the main task remaining for the large intestine. The actual capacity of the **colon** for water absorption is great; the net maximum is approximately 5 to 6 L. In daily function, however, it absorbs most of the 1 to 2 L it receives from the ileum.[1,2] Related nutrient factors, such as electrolytes, minerals, vitamins, amino acids, intestinal bacteria, and nondigestible residue, are also involved.

WATER ABSORPTION

Within a 24-hour period about 500 ml of the remaining food mass leaves the *ileum*, the last portion of the small intestine, and enters the *cecum*, the pouch at the start of the large intestine. Here the *ileocecal valve* controls passage of the semiliquid chyme. Normally the valve remains closed, but each peristaltic wave relaxes the valve and squirts a small amount of chyme into the cecum. This mechanism holds the food mass in the small intestine long enough to ensure digestion and absorption of vital nutrients.

The watery chyme continues to move slowly through the large intestine, aided by mucous secretion from mucosal glands and muscle contractions. The major portion of the water in the chyme, 350 to 400 ml, is absorbed in the first half of the colon. Only about 100 to 150 ml remains to form the feces.

This food residue mass now begins to slow its passage. A meal, having traveled the 630 to 660 cm (21 to 22 ft) of the small intestine, starts to enter the cecum about 4 hours after it is consumed. About 8 hours later it reaches the sigmoid colon, having traveled about 90 cm (3 ft) through the large intestine. In the sigmoid colon the residue descends still more slowly toward the anus, where the remainder is finally eliminated as feces. As much as 25% of a meal may remain in the rectum for up to 72 hours.

MINERAL ABSORPTION

Electrolytes, mainly sodium, are transported into the bloodstream from the colon. Intestinal absorption is a major balance control point for many of the minerals, and much of the dietary intake remains unabsorbed for elimination in the feces. For example, 20% to 70% of calcium and 80% to 85% of iron ingested are eliminated. The bioavailability of nutrients, especially minerals and vitamins, is largely reflected by their relative overall absorption from the diet during their passage through the gastrointestinal system.[2,8] This is an important aspect of nutrient balance and dietary evaluation.

VITAMIN ABSORPTION AND BACTERIAL ACTION

Intestinal absorption also serves as a balance control point for some of the vitamins, determining how much the body will keep and how much it will excrete.[8] In addition, bacteria in the colon are closely associated with a number of vitamins. For example, colon bacteria synthesize vitamin K and some of the B-complex vitamins, which are then absorbed from the colon to help meet daily needs. At birth the colon is sterile, but intestinal bacterial flora soon become well established. The adult colon contains large numbers of bacteria; the predominant species is *Escherichia coli*. Great masses of the bacteria are passed in the stool.

OTHER BACTERIAL ACTION

Intestinal bacteria also affect the color and odor of the stool. The brown color is a result of bile pigments formed by the colon bacteria from **bilirubin**. Thus in conditions that hinder bile flow, the feces may become clay colored or white. The characteristic odor results from *amines*, especially *indole* and *skatole*, which are formed by bacterial enzymes from amino acids.

Intestinal gas, or flatus, contains hydrogen sulfide or methane produced by the bacteria. Gas formation, a common complaint, is often caused not so much by specific foods as by the state of the body that receives them (see *Practical Application* box, p. 30). Many foods have been labeled "gas formers" but in reality these effects are highly variable from one person to another and such classifications have little or no scientific basis.[7]

DIETARY FIBER

Since humans have no microorganisms or enzymes to break down dietary fiber, this residue from plant carbohydrate remains after nutrient digestion and absorption (see Chapter 3). However, pectin, one of the soluble fibers, is degraded in the large intestine. Undigested fiber contributes important bulk to the diet and helps form the feces. Fully formed and ready for elimination, normal feces contain about 75% water and 25% solids. The solids include fiber, bacteria, inorganic matter such as minerals, a small amount of fat and its derivatives, some mucus, and sloughed-off mucosal cells.

Some major aspects of nutrient absorption are summarized in Table 2.4.

METABOLISM

The various absorbed nutrients, including water and electrolytes, are carried to the cells to produce many substances the body needs to sustain life. Cell metabolism encompasses the total continuous complex of chemical changes that determine the final use of the individual nutrients.

CARBOHYDRATE METABOLISM

Sources of blood glucose
Both carbohydrate and noncarbohydrate substances provide sources of blood glucose:

1. *Carbohydrate sources.* Three carbohydrate sources provide blood glucose: (1) dietary starches and

---

bilirubin A reddish bile pigment resulting from the degradation of heme by reticuleodothelial cells in the liver; a high level in the blood produces the yellow skin symptomatic of jaundice.

cisterna chyli Cistern or receptacle of the chyle; a dilated sac at the origin of the thoracic duct, which is the common trunk that receives all the lymphatic vessels. The cisterna chyli lies in the abdomen between the second lumbar vertebra and the aorta. It receives the lymph from the intestinal trunk, the right and left lumbar lymphatic trunks, and two descending lymphatic trunks. The chyle, after passing through the cisterna chyli, is carried upward into the chest through the thoracic duct and empties into the venous blood at the point where the left subclavian vein joins the left internal jugular vein.

colon The large intestine extending from the cecum to the rectum.

Digestion's sometimes embarrassing effects

A common complaint of many persons after eating a meal or certain foods is the discomfort, and sometimes embarrassment, of "gas." This gas is a normal by-product of digestion, but when it becomes painful or apparent to others it may become a physical and social problem.

The gastrointestinal tract normally holds about 3 ounces of gas, moving along with the food mass and silently absorbed into the bloodstream. Sometimes extra gas collects in the stomach or intestine, creating an embarrassing, though usually harmless, situation.

Stomach gas

Gas in the stomach results from uncomfortable air bubbles trapped there. It occurs when a person eats too fast, drinks through a straw, or otherwise takes in extra air while eating. Burping relieves it. But these tips may help to avoid this social slip:

- Avoid carbonated beverages
- Don't gulp

- Chew with your mouth closed
- Don't drink from a can or through a straw
- Don't eat when you're nervous

Intestinal gas

The passing of gas from the intestine is usually a social embarrassment. This gas is formed in the colon, where bacteria attack non-digested items, causing them to decompose and produce gas. Carbohydrates release hydrogen, carbon dioxide, and in people with certain types of bacteria in the gut, *methane*. All three of these products are odorless (though noisy) gases. Protein produces *hydrogen sulfide* and such volatile amines as *indole* and *skatole*, which add a distinctive aroma to the expelled air. However, these suggestions may help control the problem:

- Cut down on simple carbohydrates—sugars. Especially observe milk's effect to see if *lactose intolerance*, a gastrointestinal disorder

caused by lack of the necessary enzyme lactase to digest lactose, may be the real culprit. Substitute cultured forms such as yogurt or use milk treated with a lactase product such as LactAid or Lactrase.
- Eliminate all known food offenders. These vary among individuals, but beans, onions, cabbage, and high-fiber wheat are among the most common.
- Once relief is achieved, you may add more complex carbohydrates and small amounts of high-fiber foods to the diet—slowly. Once small amounts are tolerated, somewhat greater amounts can be tried. If there is still no relief, a medical examination may be needed to rule out or treat an overactive gastrointestinal tract.

References
Levine B: ...About lactose intolerance, *Nutr Today* 31(2):78, 1996.

---

sugars, (2) glycogen stored in liver and muscle tissue (the hydrolysis of glycogen to form glucose is called **glycogenolysis** or simply **glycolysis**), and (3) products of intermediary carbohydrate metabolism, such as lactic acid and pyruvic acid.

2. *Noncarbohydrate sources.* Both protein and fat provide additional indirect sources of glucose. Certain amino acids from protein are called *glucogenic amino acids* because they form glucose after they are broken down. About 58% of the protein in a mixed diet is composed of glucogenic amino acids. Thus more than half of dietary protein may ultimately be used for energy if sufficient carbo-

hydrates and fat are not available for fuel. After the breakdown of fat into fatty acids and *glycerol*, the small glycerol portion (about 10% of the fat) can be converted to glycogen in the liver and made available for glucose formation. The production of glucose from protein, fat, and intermediary carbohydrate metabolites is called **gluconeogenesis**.

Uses of blood glucose

Three uses of glucose serve to regulate the blood glucose within a normal range of 70 to 140 mg/dl (3.9 to 7.8 mmol/L). The prior cutoff point for diabetes mellitus was recently raised from 120 mg/dl (6.6 mmol/L) to the pre-

Table

2.4 Intestinal absorption of some major nutrients

Nutrient	Form	Means of absorption	Control agent or required cofactor	Route
Carbohydrate	Monosaccharides (glucose and galactose)	Competitive	—	Blood
		Selective	—	
		Active transport via sodium pump	Sodium	
Protein	Amino acids	Selective	—	Blood
	Some dipeptides	Carrier transport systems	Pyridoxine (pyridoxal phosphate)	Blood
	Whole protein (rare)	Pinocytosis	—	Blood
Fat	Fatty acids	Fatty acid–bile complex (micelles)	Bile	
	Glycerides (mono-, di-)		—	Lymph
	Few triglycerides (neutral fat)	Pinocytosis	—	Lymph
Vitamins	B_{12}	Carrier transport	Intrinsic factor (IF)	Blood
	A	Bile complex	Bile	Blood
	K	Bile complex	Bile	From large intestine to blood
Minerals	Sodium	Active transport via sodium pump	—	Blood
	Calcium	Active transport	Vitamin D	Blood
	Iron	Active transport	Ferritin mechanism	Blood (as transferritin)
Water	Water	Osmosis	—	Blood, lymph, interstitial fluid

sent normal limit of 140 mg/dl (7.8 mmol/L) by the American Diabetes Association and the American Dietetic Association.

1. *Energy production.* The primary function of glucose is to supply energy to meet the body's constant demand. A vast array of interacting metabolic pathways employing many specific successive cell enzymes accomplish this task in a highly efficient manner.
2. *Energy storage.* Two storage forms may be used for glucose: (a) *glycogen*—glucose may be converted to glycogen and stored in limited amounts in the liver and muscle tissue; only a small supply of glycogen is present at any one time, and it turns over rapidly; (b) *fat*—after energy demands have been fulfilled, any excess glucose is converted to fat and stored as adipose tissue.
3. *Glucose products.* Small amounts of glucose are used in the production of various carbohydrate compounds, which have significant roles in overall body metabolism. Examples include DNA and RNA, galactose, and certain amino acids.

These sources and uses of glucose act as checks and balances to maintain normal blood glucose levels by adding glucose to the blood or removing it as needed.

Hormonal controls

A number of hormones directly and indirectly influence the metabolism of glucose and regulate the blood glucose level.

1. *Blood glucose–lowering hormone.* Only one hormone, *insulin*, acts to lower blood glucose. It is produced by special beta cells in the pancreas. These cells are scattered in cell clusters forming "islands" in the pancreas, thus the name *islets of Langerhans*, after the scientist Paul Langerhans (1847-1888), who, as a young German medical

gluconeogenesis Production of glucose from keto acid carbon skeleton from deaminated amino acids and the glycerol portion of fatty acids.

glycogenolysis Specific term for conversion of glycogen into glucose in the liver; chemical process of enzymatic hydrolysis or breakdown by which this conversion is accomplished.

glycolysis Initial energy production enzyme pathway outside the mitochondria, by which six-carbon glucose is changed to active three-carbon fragments of acetyl CoA, the fuel ready for final energy production in the mitochondria to the high-energy phosphate bond compound adenosine triphosphate (ATP).

student, first discovered and studied them. Insulin regulates blood glucose through several actions: (1) *glycogenesis* stimulates the conversion of glucose to glycogen in the liver for constant energy reserve; (2) *lipoprotein* stimulates conversion of glucose to fat for storage in adipose tissue; and (3) *cell permeability* to glucose is increased, allowing it to pass into the cells for oxidation to supply needed energy.

2. *Blood glucose–raising hormones.* A number of hormones effectively raise blood glucose levels:

   • *Glucagon*, produced by pancreatic islet alpha cells, acts opposite to insulin, increasing breakdown of liver glycogen to glucose and maintaining blood glucose during fasting sleep hours.

   • *Somatostatin*, produced in the pancreatic delta cells and in the hypothalamus, suppresses insulin and glucagon and acts as a general modulator of related metabolic activities.

   • *Steroid hormones*, originating from the adrenal cortex, release glucose-forming carbon units from protein and act as insulin antagonists.

   • *Epinephrine*, originating from the adrenal medulla, stimulates the breakdown of liver glycogen and a quick release of immediate glucose.

   • *Growth hormone (GH)* and *adrenocorticotropic hormone (ACTH)*, released from the anterior pituitary gland, act as insulin antagonists.

   • *Thyroxine*, originating from the thyroid gland, influences the rate of insulin breakdown, increases glucose absorption from the intestine, and liberates epinephrine.

LIPID METABOLISM

Lipid synthesis and breakdown

Two organ tissues, the liver and adipose tissue, form an overall balanced axis of lipid metabolism. Both function in lipid synthesis and breakdown. The fatty acids released from lipids are used by body cells as concentrated fuel to produce energy.

Lipoproteins

These lipid-protein complexes provide the major transport form of lipids in the blood circulation. An excess amount in the blood produces a clinical condition called *hyperlipoproteinemia*. Lipoproteins are produced in the intestinal wall after initial absorption of dietary lipids and in the liver for constant recirculation to and from cells.

Hormonal controls

Since lipid and carbohydrate metabolism are closely interrelated, the same hormones are involved:

   • *GH*, *ACTH*, and *thyroid-stimulating hormone (THS)*, all from the pituitary gland, increase the release of free fatty acids from stored body lipids by imposing energy demands.

   • *Cortisone* and *hydrocortisone*, from the adrenal gland, cause release of free fatty acids.

   • *Epinephrine* and *norepinephrine* stimulate breakdown of lipids.

   • *Insulin*, from the pancreas, promotes lipid synthesis, whereas *glucagon* has the opposite effect of breaking down lipid tissues to release free fatty acids.

   • *Thyroxine*, from the thyroid gland, stimulates lipid tissue release of free fatty acids and also lowers blood cholesterol levels.

PROTEIN METABOLISM

Anabolism, or tissue building

Protein metabolism centers on the essential balance between anabolism (tissue building) and catabolism (tissue breakdown). The process of anabolism builds protein tissue through the synthesis of new protein. This build-up is specifically governed by a definite pattern—a specific "blueprint" provided by DNA in the cell nucleus—that requires specific amino acids. Specific selection and supply of amino acids are necessary. Control agents include specific cell enzymes and coenzymes. Also, specific hormones—growth hormone, gonadotropins, and thyroxine—control or stimulate the building of tissue protein.

Catabolism, or tissue breakdown

Amino acids released by tissue breakdown, if not reused in new tissue synthesis, are further broken down and used for other purposes. Two main parts of these amino acids result: the nitrogen-containing group and the remaining nonnitrogen residue.

1. *Nitrogen group.* The nitrogen portion is first split off of the amino acid, a process called **deamination**. The nitrogen is converted to ammonia and excreted in the urine or retained for use in making other nitrogen compounds.

2. *Nonnitrogen residue.* The nonnitrogen residues are called **keto acids**. They may be used to form either carbohydrates or fats. They may also be reaminated to form a new amino acid.

As in the case of tissue building, cell enzymes and coenzymes, as well as hormones, influence tissue catabolism. In health, there is a dynamic equilibrium between the two processes of anabolism and catabolism to sustain growth and maintain sound tissue.

METABOLIC INTERRELATIONSHIPS

Each of the chemical processes of body metabolism is purposeful, and all are interdependent. They are designed

To Probe Further

Absorption aids: bile circulation and pumping mechanisms

The body has a remarkable capacity for developing mechanisms to maintain its metabolic balances. Two such mechanisms are the enterohepatic circulation of bile and the pumping mechanisms for absorbing nutrients.

The enterohepatic circulation of bile

The efficiency of the enterohepatic circulation of bile salts between the small intestine and the liver demonstrates the body's amazing ability to conserve materials needed for its basic functions. Because these built-in conservation systems maintain their own balance, they are called *homeostatic mechanisms*. They are specifically designed to sustain life in a relatively stable state of equilibrium among the multitude of interdependent elements and subsystems that make up the human organism.

For example, of the 20 to 30 g of bile acids circulated daily in the body to aid in the digestion and absorption of fats, only about 0.8 g is lost in the feces. Therefore, only this small amount needs to be replaced daily by newly synthesized bile. After its tasks in digestion and absorption of fat—emulsifying and transporting—are completed, the bile is separated from its lipid complex, returned to the liver, and recirculated again and again.

Pumping mechanisms for absorbing nutrients

Various nutrients cross absorbing membranes by biologic devices called "pumps." The use of the word *pump* for this type of absorbing mechanism may be confusing at first; but it is a helpful term when you understand it.

Remember that what makes a pump function as a pump is the *threat of vacuum*, a situation that cannot exist in biologic organisms. A pump pulls material from one place to another by the exercise of negative pressure. The pump is able to "suck" material from one place to another because the new site *cannot endure the absence of material*.

It is from this characteristic of nature that biochemists and physiologists have adapted the name *pump*. The empty site's absolute necessity for something to fill its space provides the impetus to move molecules across membranes. A biochemical "pumping mechanism" is one that works by pulling a fresh molecule in to fill a place that has been emptied by the removal of a molecule that was formerly present.

References

Hofmann AF: Bile secretion and the enterohepatic circulation of bile acids. In Feldman M, Scharschmidt BF, eds: *Gastrointestinal and liver disease*, ed 6, vol 1, Philadelphia, 1998, Saunders.

---

to fill two essential needs: production of energy and growth and maintenance of healthy tissue. The controlling agents in the cells for all of these intricately balanced processes to proceed in an orderly fashion are the cell enzymes, their coenzymes (many of which involve key vitamins and minerals), and special hormones. Overall, human metabolism is an exciting biochemical process, designed to develop, sustain, and protect our most precious possession—life itself.

TO SUM UP

Nutrients are converted into usable forms via digestion and absorption. Metabolism is the means by which the body uses these nutrients to produce energy, build and rebuild body tissues, and maintain normal body functions.

Digestion consists of two basic activities: muscular and chemical. Muscular activity is responsible for food's mechanical breakdown by such means as mastication and movement of food along the gastrointestinal tract by such motions as peristalsis. Chemical activity involves enzymatic action that degrades food into smaller and smaller components for absorption.

Absorption involves the passage of food's nutrients from the gut into the bloodstream across the intestinal

---

deamination Removal of amino group (NH_2) from amino acid.

keto acid Amino acid residue after deamination. The glycogenic keto acids are used to form carbohydrates. The ketogenic keto acids are used to form fats.

wall. It occurs mainly in the small intestine via a number of efficient mechanisms.

Cell metabolism handles the absorbed nutrients. This metabolic work is accomplished by a large number of biochemical reactions that result in energy and maintain a dynamic balance between tissue breakdown and rebuilding.

▬ QUESTIONS FOR REVIEW

1. Describe five types of movement involved in the motility necessary for digestive processes.
2. Identify digestive enzymes and any cofactors secreted by the following glands or organs: salivary, mucosal, intestinal, pancreatic, liver. What activity do they perform on lipids, proteins, and carbohydrates? What stimulates their release? What inhibits their activity?
3. Describe four mechanisms of nutrient absorption from the small intestine. Describe the routes taken by the breakdown products of lipids, proteins, and carbohydrates after absorption. Why must lipids follow a different route?
4. Describe in detail two major activities that occur in the large intestine.

▬ REFERENCES

1. Greene HL, Moran JR: The gastrointestinal tract: regulator of nutrient absorption. In Shils ME, Olson JA, Shike M, eds: *Modern nutrition in health and disease,* ed 8, Philadelphia, 1994, Lea & Febiger.
2. Guyton AC, Hall JE: *Textbook of medical physiology,* ed 9, Philadelphia, 1996, Saunders.
3. Furness JB, Bornstein JC: The enteric nervous system and its extrinsic connections. In Yamada T, ed: *Textbook of gastroenterology,* vol 1, New York, 1995, Lippincott.
4. Clouse RE, Diamant NE: Motor physiology and motor disorders of the esophagus. In Feldman M, Scharschmidt BF, Sleisenger MH, eds: *Gastrointestinal and liver disease,* vol 2, ed 6, Philadelphia, 1998, Saunders.
5. Bunnett NW, Walsh JH: Gastrointestinal hormones and neurotransmitters. In Feldman M, Scharschmidt BF, Sleisenger MH, eds: *Gastrointestinal and liver disease,* ed 6, vol 1, Philadelphia, 1998, Saunders.
6. Hofmann AF: Bile secretion and the enterohepatic circulation of bile acids. In Feldman M, Scharschmidt BF, Sleisenger MH, eds: *Gastrointestinal and liver disease,* ed 6, vol 1, Philadelphia, 1998, Saunders.
7. Strocchi A, Levitt MD: Intestinal gas. In Feldman M, Scharschmidt BF, Sleisenger MH, eds: *Gastrointestinal and liver disease,* ed 6, vol 1, Philadelphia, 1998, Saunders.
8. Marsh MN, Riley SA: Digestion and absorption of nutrients and vitamins. In Feldman M, Scharschmidt BF, Sleisenger MH, eds: *Gastrointestinal and liver disease,* ed 6, vol 2, Philadelphia, 1998, Saunders.

▬ FURTHER READING

Mattes RD: Physiologic responses to sensory stimulation by food: nutritional implications, *J Am Diet Assoc* 97(4):406, 1997.

The author reviews the interesting effect sensory stimulation has on physiologic processes, such as effects of sight, smell, taste, and texture of food, that prepare the body to better absorb and use the ingested nutrients, an overall effect called the preabsorptive or cephalic phase response.

Roberfroid MB et al: Colonic microflora: nutrition and health, *Nutr Rev* 53(5):127, 1995.

This special workshop report of an International Life Sciences Institute presents an excellent summary and conclusion of the unique activities and major nutritive and protective functions of the microorganisms that form a complex ecosystem in the human colon.

Issues Answers

Lactose intolerance: common problem worldwide

Picture this: a natural disaster strikes a poor nation, leaving thousands homeless and with very little food. CARE, UNICEF, and other international organizations work quickly to collect and ship foodstuffs to the area. Yet the people find it difficult to be grateful: since the shipments began, they have found themselves not only without shelter but also in distress—gastrointestinal distress.

One of the most common foodstuffs shipped to impoverished areas is milk. And one of the most common problems throughout the world is *lactose intolerance*—a condition that results in abdominal cramps, nausea, bloating, or diarrhea when milk is consumed. The problem stems from a deficiency of *lactase*, a digestive enzyme found in the microvilli of the small intestine that hydrolyzes milk sugar (lactose) into its component monosaccharides, glucose and galactose, for absorption.

All mammals are born with sufficient amounts of lactase to accommodate the high lactose levels in "mother's milk." In animal species the amount of enzyme activity drops off significantly shortly after birth. In most humans this drop occurs after the age of 5 years.

Only a few among the human species of the world do not experience this significant childhood drop in the enzyme lactase. These are mostly Northern Europeans, a few African cattle-raisers, and residents of the northwestern sector of India who manage to digest lactose very easily throughout adulthood. The remaining majority of the world's population experience symptoms on drinking as little as a half pint of milk.

Most lactose-intolerant persons can digest well such cultured or fermented milk products as buttermilk, yogurt, or cheese and can use these as their primary source of calcium. But the problem of supplying these items in disaster areas is difficult or unacceptable. Even cheese is too expensive an item to be used frequently to satisfy calcium needs of American school children through school breakfast and lunch programs. The nutritional benefits of lactose-rich foods may become crucial in offsetting deficiency signs among those in dire need.

However, continuing study seems to cloud the calcium relationship issue further. Sensitive tests used to measure the subjects' calcium absorption and their lactase status have indicated that calcium may be absorbed better in lactase-deficient persons than in lactase-sufficient ones. Also, it seems that the presence or absence of lactose in the intestinal food mix when the calcium was taken had no effect on its absorption. So what do we tell persons who are lactase-deficient about supplementing their dietary intake of calcium? They have several options, all of which may have drawbacks for some: (1) using low-lactose milk treated with lactase products such as Lactaid or Lactrase; (2) using cultured or fermented forms of milk such as yogurt or buttermilk; (3) trying small amounts of milk at a time and only with meals; and (4) using lactose supplements in tablet form with meals.

To cloud the issue still further, there is the question about validity of persons' subjective responses and symptoms related to milk tolerance. In some studies of adults, all of whom have claimed to be lactose-intolerant, when fed whole milk only about a third of them have been proved by tests to be true lactose-intolerant individuals.

Nonetheless, the option of substituting cultured milk products or the lactase-treated milk is a possible solution. The low-lactose milks are sweeter than regular milk but have proved to be both acceptable and more effective at reducing symptoms than the alternate product, sweet acidophilus milk. Processing of the low-lactose product involves incubation with yeast lactose, which increases the cost only 2 to 3 cents per liter, keeping it inexpensive enough to be considered for mass distribution. If it continues to demonstrate its effectiveness and safety, those involved with food assistance programs may find low-lactose milk to be the means of overcoming an enzymatic barrier to optimal nutrition throughout the world.

References

Hertzler SR et al: How much lactose is low lactose? *J Am Diet Assoc* 96(3):243, 1996.

Strocchi A, Levitt MD: Intestinal gas. In Feldman M, Scharschmidt BF, Sleisenger MH, eds: *Gastrointestinal and liver disease,* ed 6, vol 1, Philadelphia, 1998, Saunders.

Chapter

3

Carbohydrates

With this chapter, we begin a three-chapter sequence on the macronutrients: carbohydrates, fats, and proteins. Among all the nutrients, these three share a unique capacity, the ability to yield energy.

Carbohydrates have long been of prime importance in the human diet as the primary source of energy for the body. They are the most important fuel source in the body. Over the ages they have nurtured cultures throughout the world, providing the major energy source to sustain work and human development.

In this chapter we look first at the nature of this major macronutrient and its function as the basic body fuel.

Figure 3.1   Photosynthesis. In the presence of sunlight and the green leaf pigment chlorophyll, green plants use the raw materials water and carbon dioxide to produce glucose and starch by capturing the sun's energy and transforming it into chemical energy in the food products stored in roots, stems, and leaves and returning oxygen to the atmosphere. (Medical and Scientific Illustration.)

THE NATURE OF CARBOHYDRATES

BASIC FUELS: STARCHES AND SUGARS

The basic fuel forms of carbohydrates are starches and sugars that occur naturally in our foods. Energy on the planet Earth comes ultimately from the sun and its tremendous reactions. In the presence of this life-giving sunlight, plants use their internal process of **photosynthesis** to transform the sun's energy into the stored plant fuel form of carbohydrates, as shown in Figure 3.1. In this important process, plants use carbon dioxide from the air and water from the soil—along with the plant pigment *chlorophyll* in their green leaves, which serves as a chemical catalyst—to manufacture starches and sugars.[1] Because the human body can rapidly break down various forms of starches and sugars to yield body energy, carbohydrates are called "quick energy" foods. They provide our major source of energy.

DIETARY IMPORTANCE

There are practical reasons for the large quantities of carbohydrates in diets all over the world. First, carbohydrates are widely available, easily grown in plants as grains, vegetables, and fruits. In some countries, carbohydrate foods make up almost the entire diet of the people. In the American diet about half of the total kcalories is in the form of carbohydrates. Second, carbohydrates are relatively low in cost. And third, they may be stored easily. Compared with other types of foods, carbohydrate

---

photosynthesis   Process by which plants containing chlorophyll are able to manufacture carbohydrate by combining CO_2 from air and water from soil. Sunlight is used as energy; chlorophyll is a catalyst.

$$6\,CO_2 + 6\,H_2O + Energy \rightarrow Chlorophyll \rightarrow C_6H_{12}O_6 + 6\,O_2$$

---

foods can be kept in dry storage for relatively long periods without spoilage. Modern processing and packaging further extend the shelf life of carbohydrate products almost indefinitely.

CLASSIFICATION OF CARBOHYDRATES

The term **carbohydrate** comes from the chemical nature of the compound. It is composed of the elements carbon, hydrogen, and oxygen, with the hydrogen/oxygen ratio usually that of water—CH_2O. Carbohydrates are classified according to the number of basic sugar, or *saccharide*, units making up their structure.

MONOSACCHARIDES

The simplest form of carbohydrate is the **monosaccharide**, often called a simple (single) sugar. The three main monosaccharides important in human nutrition are glucose, fructose, and galactose.

Glucose

A moderately sweet sugar, glucose is found naturally in only a few foods, such as corn syrup. It is mainly created in the body from starch digestion. In human metabolism, all other types of sugar are converted into glucose. Glucose, sometimes called by its older name *dextrose* in hospital intravenous solutions, is the form in which carbohydrates circulate in the bloodstream. Blood glucose levels normally range from about 3.9 to 7.8 mmol/L (70 to 140 mg/dl). The term *hyperglycemia* refers to an elevated blood glucose level. *Hypoglycemia* results from blood glucose levels below the normal range. In recent years, public controversy has developed concerning the condition of hypoglycemia (see *Practical Application* box, p. 40). Glucose is the ultimate common refined body fuel that is oxidized in the cells to give energy.

Fructose

The sweetest of the simple sugars, fructose is found in fruits and other substances, such as honey. However, honey should not be given to infants under 1 year of age because of the possibility of botulism. In the United States, fructose intake has greatly increased since it was introduced in 1970 as a high-fructose corn syrup used in food processing, especially in soft drinks. In human metabolism fructose is converted to glucose to be burned for energy. Fructose can cause gastrointestinal distress if present in the intestines in too large an amount.

Galactose

The simple sugar galactose is not found free in foods but is produced in human digestion from lactose (milk sugar)

and is then converted to glucose in the liver. This reaction is reversible, and during lactation glucose may be reconverted to galactose for use in milk production.

The general physiologic and nutritional importance of these major monosaccharides (called *hexoses* from their basic six-carbon structure) is summarized in Table 3.1.

DISACCHARIDES

The **disaccharides** are simple (double) sugars composed of two monosaccharides linked together. The three main disaccharides of physiologic importance are sucrose, lactose, and maltose. Their respective monosaccharide components follow:

$$\text{Sucrose} = \text{glucose} + \text{fructose}$$
$$\text{Lactose} = \text{glucose} + \text{galactose}$$
$$\text{Maltose} = \text{glucose} + \text{glucose}$$

Notice that glucose is a major component in each of these disaccharides.

Sucrose

Sucrose is the common "table sugar" made commercially from sugar cane and sugar beets. It is the most prevalent disaccharide. With the increasing use of processed foods, sucrose contributes some 30% to 40% of the total kcalories in the American diet (see *Issues & Answers,* p. 51). Sucrose can be found in all forms of common sugar, molasses, and in some fruits and vegetables such as pineapple and carrots.

Lactose

The sugar in milk is called *lactose* because of its source. It is formed in the body from glucose to supply the needed sugar component of milk during lactation. It is the least sweet of the disaccharides, about one sixth as sweet as sucrose. When milk sours, as in the initial stages of cheese making, the lactose changes its form and separates out in the liquid whey from the solid curd. The curd is then processed for cheese. Thus although milk has a relatively high carbohydrate content in the form of lactose, one of its main products—cheese—has very little or none. Approximately 75% of adults worldwide are lactose-intolerant, but can tolerate such lactose-free milk products as cheese.[2,3] Also, use of a commonly marketed lactase enzyme supplement with meals also prevents the discomfort of symptoms such as gas, cramping, bloating, stomach rumbling (borborygmi), altered bowel habits, and diarrhea.

Maltose

Maltose occurs in commercial malt products of starch breakdown and in germinating cereal grains. As such, it is a negligible *dietary* carbohydrate. But it is a highly significant *metabolic* carbohydrate as an intermediate product of starch digestion.

Table 3.1	Summary of physiologic and nutritional significance of selected monosaccharides	
	Source	**Significance**
Hexoses		
D-Glucose	Fruit juices; hydrolysis of starch, cane sugar, maltose, and lactose	Body "sugar"; blood and tissue fluids; cell fuel
D-Fructose	Fruit, juices, honey; hydrolysis of sucrose from cane sugar	Changed to glucose in the liver and intestine to serve as basic body fuel
D-Galactose	Hydrolysis of lactose (milk sugar)	Changed to glucose in the liver; cell fuel; synthesized in mammary gland to make lactose of milk; constituent of glycolipids and glycoproteins

Table 3.2	Summary of physiologic and nutritional significance of selected disaccharides	
	Source	**Significance**
Maltose	Starch digestion by amylase, commercial hydrolysis; malt and germinating cereals	Hydrolyzed to D-glucose; basic body fuel and metabolite; fermentable
Sucrose	Cane and beet sugar, sorghum cane, carrots, pineapple	Hydrolyzed to glucose and fructose; body fuel
Lactose	Milk	Hydrolyzed to glucose and galactose; body fuel; constituent for milk production during lactation

The general physiologic and nutritional significance of the disaccharides is summarized in Table 3.2. The United States Department of Agriculture (USDA) Nationwide Food Consumption surveys (NFCS) indicate that the percent of energy from total sugars minus lactose is about 18% in the United States and that consumers of relatively large amounts of sugars do not necessarily have poorer quality diets.[4]

POLYSACCHARIDES

Much more complex carbohydrates are called **polysaccharides** because they are made up of *many* single glucose (saccharide) units. The most important polysaccharide in human nutrition is starch. Other forms are glycogen and dextrins. The nondigestible forms of dietary fiber, cellulose and other noncellulose polysaccharides, provide important bulk in the diet.

Starch

In human nutrition, starch is by far the most significant polysaccharide. It is a relatively large complex compound made up of many coiled or branching chains of single glucose units. It yields only glucose on digestion. The cooking of starch not only improves its flavor but also softens and ruptures the starch cells, which makes digestion easier. Starch mixtures thicken when cooked because the portion that encases the starch granules has a gel-like quality that thickens the mixture the same way that pectin causes jelly to set.

Resistant starch

Until recently starch was thought to be completely digested and absorbed in the small intestine. However, studies have shown that starch from many sources, including cereals, potatoes, bananas, and legumes, is not completely broken down and passes on to the large intestine generally intact.[5,6] The extent of starch break-

---

carbohydrate Compound of carbon, hydrogen, and oxygen; starches, sugars, and dietary fiber made and stored in plants; major energy source in the human diet.

disaccharides Class of compound sugars composed of two molecules of monosaccharide. The three most common are sucrose, lactose, and maltose.

monosaccharide Simple single sugar; a carbohydrate containing a single saccharide (sugar) unit.

polysaccharides Class of complex carbohydrates composed of many monosaccharide units. Common members are starch, dextrins, dietary fiber, and glycogen.

Hypoglycemia: fact or fiction?

Recent controversy has developed concerning *hypoglycemia*, the condition of low blood sugar. Is it fact or fiction? Probably some of both. The lay public associates hypoglycemia with an excessive amount of sugar in the diet and at various times has attributed a number of symptoms to this condition ranging from hunger and headaches to depression and crime. On the other hand, members of the medical community have fueled the problem with statements about "nonhypoglycemia" or hypoglycemia as a "nondisease."

Clinically, hypoglycemia is usually defined as a blood glucose level of 2.2 mmol/L (40 mg/dl) or lower after consumption of a meal or a glucose load. Clinicians and consumers alike agree on some of the symptoms, for example, nervousness, anxiety, hunger, palpitations, and headaches. But they disagree about causes of the problem, methods of diagnosis, and treatment.

Cause

While consumers have generally named excess dietary sugar as the culprit, clinicians have specifically identified two types of hypoglycemia and their known causes:

- **Reactive hypoglycemia** occurs after a meal and most frequently affects persons who have recently had gastric surgery or who have diabetes.
- **Fasting hypoglycemia** occurs after extended periods without adequate food intake or from poor eating habits. It may also be caused by several drugs: (1) alcohol, which blocks glucose production by the liver; (2)

hypoglycemic medications used to treat diabetes; and (3) salicylate in aspirin. More serious conditions that may cause this effect include: (1) tumors of the pancreas that stimulate excessive insulin secretion, and (2) adrenal insufficiency, a rare condition that prevents the adrenal glands from responding to certain body needs, especially under stress. Unrelieved general stress, whatever the cause, increases metabolic demands on the body and can contribute to hypoglycemia.

Diagnosis

A normal blood glucose range is about 3.9 to 7.8 mmol/L (70 to 140 mg/dl); for comparison, the current cutoff point for diabetes is 7.8 mmol/L (140 ml/dl). The traditional basis for medical diagnosis of hypoglycemia has been the oral glucose tolerance test. The patient drinks a beverage containing 75 to 100 g of glucose, and the blood glucose levels are measured at half-hour intervals for up to 5 hours. But this test situation itself is unrealistic and induces the abnormal response. So, more recently, physicians have used blood tests at the time the person is experiencing the characteristic symptoms to obtain a more realistic measure.

Treatment

In general, the lay public believes that hypoglycemia should be treated with a very low-carbohydrate, high-protein diet. However, a very low-carbohydrate diet will make it difficult for the body to obtain sufficient amounts of glucose to achieve and maintain

normal blood sugar levels. It is evident now from current carbohydrate research, that a diet of frequent small meals, rich in complex carbohydrates and a good dietary fiber content, with fewer simple carbohydrates and sugars, will maintain a more stable blood sugar level while preventing periods of low blood sugar.

Sound approaches

The simple procedure for home blood glucose monitoring developed for persons with diabetes can be used by persons with hypoglycemic symptoms to test their own blood sugar levels at the time they are exhibiting symptoms. They should keep a record of results, which will provide an accurate profile of the blood glucose levels in the free home environment. This procedure can provide a therapeutic tool for use in counseling and teaching. If the record shows no documented hypoglycemic periods, a sensitive counselor can help the person gain more insight into the problem, exploring other reasons for the symptoms. On the other hand, if the record documents actual hypoglycemia, further diagnostic evaluation is required. This technique is simple, accurate, and effective for persons being evaluated for reactive or postprandial hypoglycemia.

References

Guyton AC, Hall JE: *Textbook of medical physiology,* ed 9, Philadelphia, 1996, Saunders.

Jensen RT, Norton JA: Endocrine tumors of the pancreas. In Feldman M, Scharschmidt BF, Sleisenger MH, eds: *Gastrointestinal and liver disease,* ed 6, vol 1, Philadelphia, 1998, Saunders.

down within the small intestine varies, depending on the food's physical form, so that a substantial amount of the total starch, called *resistant starch*, escapes digestion in the small intestine and enters the colon.[5] Three main types of resistant starch occur naturally in the human diet: (1) physically trapped starch, found in coarsely ground or chewed cereals; (2) ungelatinized starch granules, which are highly resistant to digestion by the starch enzyme α-amylase until gelatinized, for example, uncooked potato, green banana, and high-amylose starch; and (3) starch polymers, mainly amylose, which are produced when starch is cooled (as in cooled cooked potato) after gelatinization.[7] This undigested starch has been linked with cancer prevention, as well as control of diabetes and hyperlipidemia.[8] Finally, in the large intestine, mostly in the colon, energy is salvaged from resistant starch through bacterial fermentation.[9] The principal products of fermentation, the short-chain fatty acids, provide a valuable energy source and have important effects on the colonic epithelium, which may be a major protective factor against cancer of the large intestine.[9,10]

Starch is also by far the most important source of dietary carbohydrate worldwide. It is recognized as a significant factor in human nutrition and health. For example, standards of United States Dietary Guidelines, as outlined in Chapter 1, recommend that about 50% to 55% of the total kcalorie value of the diet come from carbohydrates, with a greater portion of that allowance coming from complex carbohydrate starch foods. In many other countries, where starch is the staple food material, it makes up an even greater portion of the diet. The major food sources of starch include cereal grains, legumes, potatoes, and other vegetables.

Glycogen

The animal storage compound comparable to starch in plants is **glycogen**. It is formed during cell metabolism and stored in relatively small amounts in the liver and muscle tissues. Liver stores help sustain normal blood glucose levels during fasting periods such as sleep hours, and muscle stores provide immediate fuel for muscle action, especially during athletic activity. Sometimes athletes practice pregame "glycogen loading" to provide added fuel stores for use during athletic events (see Chapter 14). Dietary carbohydrate is essential to maintain these needed glycogen stores and prevent the stress symptoms of low carbohydrate intake—fatigue, dehydration, and energy loss—as well as other undesirable metabolic effects such as *ketoacidosis* (see Chapter 20) and excessive protein breakdown. The US Food and Nutrition Board of the National Research Council recommends a carbohydrate intake of at least 100 g/day to prevent these symptoms. Most diets provide well over 200 g/day, with the average diet containing 300 g or more.

Dextrins

Dextrins are polysaccharide compounds formed as intermediate products in the breakdown of starch. This starch breakdown occurs constantly in the process of digestion.

Starch + water	→	soluble starch + maltose
Soluble starch + water	→	dextrins + maltose
Dextrins + water	→	maltose
Maltose + water	→	glucose + glucose

Oligosaccharides

These carbohydrates are small portions of partially digested starch, ranging in size from about 3 to 10 monosaccharides. They form either naturally through the process of digestion or commercially through acid hydrolysis. **Oligosaccharides** are irregular in form and, when digested, yield their few constituent monosaccharides. These small sugars are used extensively in special formulas for infants or persons with gastrointestinal problems because they are designed for easier digestion. These smaller sugars are also used in sports drinks—for example, Exceed (Ross)—in which they may contribute about 47.5% of the total glucose in the solution (see Chapter 14).

Some naturally occurring oligosaccharides are constructed with bonds that cannot be broken by human enzymes, so they are indigestible. For example, two of these—stachyose and **raffinose**—are found in legumes such as beans, peas, and soybeans. These small sugars provide a feast for bacterial flora in the intestines, producing a large amount of gas that can bring discomfort and embarrassment.

DIETARY FIBER

Dietary fiber may be classed into three major groups according to structure and properties, with one of these groups having five different members.

---

glycogen A polysaccharide, that is, a large compound of many saccharide (i.e., sugar) units. It is the main body storage form of carbohydrate, largely stored (with relatively rapid turnover) in the liver, with lesser amounts stored in muscle tissue.

oligosaccharides Intermediate products of polysaccharide carbohydrate breakdown that contain a small number (from 3 to 10) of single sugar units of the monosaccharide glucose.

raffinose A colorless crystalline trisaccharide component of legumes, composed of galactose and sucrose connected by bonds that human enzymes cannot break; thus it remains whole in the intestines and produces gas as bacteria attack it.

Table 3.3   Summary of dietary fiber classes

Dietary fiber class	Plant parts	Functions
Cellulose	Main cell wall constituent	Insoluble; holds water, functions as laxative, reduces elevated colonic intraluminal pressure; binds minerals
Noncellulose polysaccharides		
Hemicellulose	Secretions, cell wall material	Mostly insoluble; holds water, increases stool bulk, reduces colonic pressure; binds bile acids
Pectins	Intracellular cement material	Soluble; binds cholesterol and bile acids
Gums	Special cell secretions	Soluble; binds cholesterol and bile acids; slows gastric emptying; provides fermentable material for colonic bacteria with production of volatile fatty acids and gas
Mucilages	Cell secretions	Soluble; slows gastric emptying time; fermentable substrate for colonic bacteria; binds bile acids
Algal substances	Algae, seaweeds	Soluble; slows gastric emptying time; fermentable substrate; binds bile acids
Noncarbohydrate		
Lignin	Woody part of plants	Insoluble; antioxidant; binds bile acids and metals

Cellulose

This **dietary fiber** is the chief constituent of the framework of plants. Humans cannot digest cellulose because they lack the necessary digestive enzymes. Therefore, it remains in the digestive tract and contributes important bulk to the diet. This bulk helps move the food mass along and stimulates *peristalsis* (see Chapter 2). Cellulose makes up the principal structural material in plant cell walls and provides most of the substance formerly labeled "crude fiber," a term now obsolete (see *To Probe Further* box, p. 48). The main food sources are stems and leaves of vegetables, seed and grain coverings, skins, and hulls.

Noncellulose polysaccharides

The noncellulose fiber carbohydrates include five members: hemicellulose, pectins, gums, mucilages, and algal substances. They absorb water and slow gastric emptying time. All of them except hemicellulose are gumlike water-soluble substances that aid in binding cholesterol and controlling its absorption. They also prevent colon pressure by providing bulk for normal intestinal muscle action.

Lignin

This substance is the only noncarbohydrate type of dietary fiber. It is a large compound that forms the woody part of plants. In the intestine it combines with bile acids to form insoluble compounds, thus preventing their absorption. Lignin contributes the memorable sandy texture of pears and lima beans.

Table 3.4   Summary of soluble and insoluble fibers in total dietary fiber

Insoluble	Soluble
Cellulose	Gums
Most hemicelluloses	Mucilages
Lignin	Algal polysaccharides
	Most pectins

A summary of these dietary fiber classes is given in Table 3.3. Compare their solubility groupings in Table 3.4. Some main food sources of the various types of dietary fiber are indicated in Table 3.5. Also, in the food exchange lists (Appendix K) the high-fiber foods in each food group are indicated. Comparisons of fiber content of some selected foods are given in Table 3.6.

Physiologic effects

In general, dietary fiber produces various effects on the food mix consumed and its fate in the body. Most of these effects are caused by its physiologic properties:

- *Water absorption.* Dietary fiber's capacity to absorb water contributes to its bulk-forming laxative effect, thus influencing the transit time of the food mass through the digestive tract and the consequent absorption of the various nutrients.

Table

3.5 Selected food sources of various classes of dietary fiber

Dietary fiber class	Grains	Fruits	Vegetables
Cellulose	Bran	Apples	Beans, peas
	Whole wheat	Pears	Cabbage family
	Whole rye		Root vegetables
			Tomatoes, fresh
Noncellulose polysaccharides			
Hemicellulose	Bran		
	Cereals		
	Whole grains		
Pectins		Apples	Green beans
		Citrus fruits	Carrots
		Berries, especially strawberries	
Gums	Oatmeal	Food products thickener, stabilizer	Dried beans, other legumes
			Vegetable gums used in food processing
Mucilages		Food products thickener, stabilizer	
Algal substances		Food products thickener, stablizer	
Noncarbohydrate			
Lignins	Whole wheat	Strawberries	Mature vegetables
	Whole rye	Peaches	
		Pears	
		Plums	

- *Binding effect*. Such fibers as the noncellulose substances influence blood lipid levels through a binding effect, a capacity to bind cholesterol and bile salts and prevent their absorption. However, excessive dietary fiber can have the undesirable effect of binding such minerals as iron, zinc, or calcium, thus preventing needed absorption and creating an unbalanced diet effect.
- *Colon bacteria effect*. The colon bacteria effect on fermentation substrates for bacterial action produces volatile fatty acids and gas. A rare form of abnormal gut fermentation causing increased levels of blood ethanol has been reported.[11]

Various clinical applications have centered largely on diabetes mellitus, coronary heart disease, colon cancer, and other intestinal problems such as diverticulosis.[8,10] Some of these clinical associations between dietary fiber and various health problems are summarized in Table 3.7.

Dietary fiber recommendation

Sufficient evidence now exists to suggest that Americans should increase their intake of dietary fiber by consuming more whole grain products, fruits, and vegetables, and that fiber supplements are not appropriate for healthy persons. Recent studies indicate that the average dietary fiber intake of American adults is only 11 g/day, when a recommendation of about 20 to 35 g/day appears wise.[10,12] This goal can easily be achieved through generous use of whole grains, legumes, vegetables, fruits, seeds, and nuts. Indiscriminate use of bran is not justified.

Complex carbohydrates

The term *complex carbohydrate* refers to large molecular forms of carbohydrate such as starch and dietary fiber. These foods make up a large part of the diet, and since the 1970s they have been an important component of various dietary guidelines. As a result, there is a growing discussion and consensus among scientists and the public to add complex carbohydrates to the nutrition label on foods.[13]

---

dietary fiber Nondigestible form of carbohydrate that is of nutritional importance in gastrointestinal disease such as diverticulosis and in reducing serum lipid and glucose levels related to chronic conditions such as heart disease and diabetes.

Table 3.6 Dietary fiber and kcalorie values for selected foods

Foods	Serving	Dietary fiber (g)	Kcal	Foods	Serving	Dietary fiber (g)	Kcal
Breads and cereals				**Vegetables, cooked—cont'd**			
All Bran	1/2 cup	8.5	70	Broccoli	1/2 cup	2.2	20
Bran (100%)	1/2 cup	8.4	75	Beans, green	1/2 cup	1.6	15
Bran Buds	1/3 cup	7.9	75	Tomato, chopped	1/2 cup	1.5	17
Corn Bran	2/3 cup	5.4	100	Cabbage, red and white	1/2 cup	1.4	15
Bran Chex	2/3 cup	4.6	90	Kale	1/2 cup	1.4	20
Cracklin' Oat Bran	1/3 cup	4.3	110	Cauliflower	1/2 cup	1.1	15
Bran Flakes	3/4 cup	4.0	90	Lettuce, fresh	1 cup	0.8	7
Air-popped popcorn	1 cup	2.2	25	**Fruits**			
Oatmeal	1 cup	2.5	144				
Grapenuts	1/4 cup	1.4	100	Apple	1 medium	3.5	80
Whole-wheat bread	1 slice	1.4	60	Raisins	1/4 cup	3.1	110
				Prunes, dried	3	3.0	60
Legumes, cooked				Strawberries	1 cup	3.0	45
Kidney beans	1/2 cup	7.3	110	Orange	1 medium	2.6	60
Lima beans	1/2 cup	4.5	130	Banana	1 medium	2.4	105
				Blueberries	1/2 cup	2.0	40
Vegetables, cooked				Dates, dried	3	1.9	70
Green peas	1/2 cup	3.6	55	Peach	1 medium	1.9	35
Corn	1/2 cup	2.9	70	Apricot, fresh	3 medium	1.8	50
Parsnip	1/2 cup	2.7	50	Grapefruit	1/2 cup	1.6	40
Potato, with skin	1 medium	2.5	95	Apricot, dried	5 halves	1.4	40
Brussels sprouts	1/2 cup	2.3	30	Cherries	10	1.2	50
Carrots	1/2 cup	2.3	25	Pineapple	1/2 cup	1.1	40

Table 3.7 Relationship between fiber and various health problems

Problem	Effect of fiber	Possible mode of action	Future research needs
Diabetes mellitus	Reduces fasting blood sugar levels Reduces glycosuria Reduces insulin requirements Increases insulin sensitivity	Slows carbohydrate absorption by: Delaying gastric emptying time Forming gels with pectin or guar gum in the intestine, thus impeding carbohydrate absorption "Protecting" carbohydrates from enzymatic activity with a fibrous coat Allowing "protected" carbohydrates to escape into large colon where they are digested by bacteria	Influence of short-chain fatty acid production or metabolism of glucose and fats in the liver Exact mechanisms by which fiber influences glucose metabolism
	Inhibits postprandial (after meals) hyperglycemia	Alters gut hormones (for example, glucagon) to enhance glucose metabolism in the liver	

Continued.

Table

3.7   Relationship between fiber and various health problems—cont'd

Problem	Effect of fiber	Possible mode of action	Future research needs
Obesity	Increases satiety rate	Prolongs chewing and swallowing movements	Cause of increased satiety rate reported by subjects
	Reduces nutrient bioavailability	Increases fecal fat content	Effect of nutrient binding on nutritional status
	Reduces energy density	Inhibits absorption of carbohydrates in high-fiber foods	Studies based on food composition and kcaloric density instead of fiber content alone
		Decreases transit time	Effects of different types of fiber on gastric, small intestine, and colonic emptying time
	Alters hormonal response	Alters action of insulin, gut glucagon, and other intestinal hormones	
	Alters thermogenesis		
Coronary heart disease	Inhibits recirculation of bile acids	Alters bacterial metabolism of bile acids	Influence of fiber on cholesterol content of specific lipoprotein fractions (see Chapter 20)
		Alters bacterial flora, resulting in a change in metabolic activity	Influence on production of short-chain fatty acids
		Forms gels that bind bile acids	Role of dietary fiber as an independent variable in reducing risk of heart disease
		Alters the function of pancreatic and intestinal enzymes	
	Reduces triglyceride and cholesterol levels*	Reduces insulin levels†	Relationship between lipoprotein turnover and glucose turnover/sensitivity to insulin
		Binds cholesterol, preventing absorption	Effect of higher concentration of bile salts on colon function
		Slows fat absorption by forming gel matrices in the intestine	
Colon cancer	Reduces incidence of disease‡	Bile acids or their bacterial metabolites may affect the structure of the colon, its cell turnover rate, and function	Testing of current hypotheses regarding the effects of dietary factors on the structure of the colon and cell turnover rate
Other gastrointestinal disorders Diverticular disease Constipation Hiatal hernia Hemorrhoids	Reduces pressure from within the intestinal lumen Increases diameter of the intestinal lumen, thus allowing intestinal tract to contract more, propelling contents more rapidly and inhibiting segmentation§	Decreases transit time Increases water absorption, resulting in a larger, softer stool	

*This effect is based on epidemiologic studies, usually observed in combination with reduced fat intake.
†Insulin is required for fat synthesis.
‡Preventive effect of fiber is assumed from epidemiologic studies that associate low-fiber, high-fat diets with an increased incidence of disease.
§Segmentation increases pressure and weakness along the walls of the intestinal tract.

FUNCTIONS OF CARBOHYDRATES

ENERGY

As indicated, the primary function of carbohydrates in nutrition is to provide fuel for energy production. Fat is also a fuel, but the body needs only a small amount of dietary fat, mainly to supply the essential fatty acids. To function properly, however, the body tissues require a daily dietary supply of carbohydrates sufficient to provide a major portion, 55% to 60%, of the total kcalories.

The amount of carbohydrates in the body, though relatively small, is important to maintain energy reserves. For example, in an adult male about 300 to 350 g is "stored" in the liver and muscle tissues as glycogen, and about 10 g is present in circulating blood glucose (Table 3.8). This total amount of available glycogen and glucose provides energy sufficient for only about half a day of moderate activity. Thus carbohydrate foods must be eaten regularly and at moderately frequent intervals to meet the constant energy demands of the body.

SPECIAL FUNCTIONS OF CARBOHYDRATES IN BODY TISSUES

As part of their general function as the body's main energy source, carbohydrates serve special functions in many body tissues.

Glycogen reserves

As indicated, the liver and muscle glycogen reserves provide a constant interchange with the body's overall energy balance system. Thus these reserves protect cells from depressed metabolic function and injury.

Protein-sparing action

Carbohydrates help regulate protein metabolism. The presence of sufficient carbohydrates for energy demands of the body prevents the channeling of too much protein for this purpose. This protein-sparing action of carbohydrates allows the major portion of protein to be used for its basic structural purpose of tissue building.

Antiketogenic effect

Carbohydrates also relate to fat metabolism. The amount of carbohydrates present in the diet determines how much fat will be broken down, thus affecting the formation and disposal rates of *ketones*. Ketones are intermediate products of fat metabolism, which normally are produced at a low level during fat oxidation. However, in such extreme conditions as starvation or uncontrolled diabetes, as well as the unwise use of very low-carbohydrate diets, carbohydrates are inadequate or unavailable for energy needs, so too much fat is oxidized. Ketones accumulate, and the result is *ketoacidosis* (Chapter 20). Sufficient dietary carbohydrate, 55% to 60% of the energy nutrients, prevents this damaging excess of ketones.

Table 3.8	Postabsorptive carbohydrate storage in normal adult man (70 kg [154 lb])		
		Glycogen (g)	Glucose (g)
Liver (weight 1800 g)		72	
Muscles (mass weight 35 kg [77 lb])		245	
Extracellular fluids (10 L)			10
Component totals		317	10
TOTAL STORAGE		327	

Heart action

Heart action is a life-sustaining muscular exercise. Although fatty acids are the preferred regular fuel for the heart muscle, the glycogen reserve in cardiac muscle is an important emergency source of contractile energy. In a damaged heart, poor glycogen stores or low carbohydrate intake may cause cardiac symptoms and angina.

Central nervous system function

A constant supply of carbohydrates is necessary for the proper functioning of the central nervous system (CNS). The CNS regulatory center, the brain, contains no stored supply of glucose and is therefore especially dependent on a minute-to-minute supply of glucose from the blood. Sustained and profound hypoglycemic shock may cause irreversible brain damage. In all nerve tissue, carbohydrates are indispensable for functional integrity.

Although a more detailed and integrated discussion of digestion, absorption, and metabolism of the macronutrients is given in Chapter 2, a brief summary of these aspects for each individual macronutrient is presented at the end of each introductory macronutrient chapter, to set the scene for the larger picture that follows. Here we provide that summary outline for carbohydrates.

DIGESTION-ABSORPTION-METABOLISM SUMMARY

DIGESTION

Most carbohydrate foods, starches and sugars, cannot immediately be used by the cells to make energy available. They must first be changed into the refined fuel for which the cell is designed—*glucose*. The process by which these vital changes are made is *digestion*. The digestion of carbohydrate foods proceeds through the successive parts of the gastrointestinal tract, accomplished by two types of actions: (1) mechanical or muscle functions that render the food mass into smaller particles, and (2) chemical processes in which specific enzymes break down food nutrients into smaller usable metabolic products.[14]

MOUTH

Mastication breaks food into fine particles and mixes it with the salivary secretions. During this process, a salivary amylase (ptyalin) is secreted by the parotid gland. It acts on starch to begin its breakdown into dextrins and maltose.

STOMACH

Successive wavelike contractions of the muscle fibers of the stomach wall continue the mechanical digestive process. This action is called *peristalsis*. It further mixes food particles with gastric secretions to allow chemical digestion to take place more readily. The gastric secretion contains no specific enzyme for the breakdown of carbohydrates. The hydrochloric acid in the stomach stops the action of salivary amylase. But before the food mixes completely with the acid gastric secretion, as much as 20% to 30% of the starch may have been changed to maltose. Muscle actions continue to bring the food mass to the lower part of the stomach. Here the food mass is now a thick creamy *chyme*, ready for its controlled emptying through the *pyloric valve* into the duodenum, the first portion of the small intestine.

SMALL INTESTINE

Peristalsis continues to aid digestion in the small intestine by mixing and moving the chyme along the **lumen** in the length of the tube. Chemical digestion of carbohydrates is completed in the small intestine by specific enzymes from two sources: the pancreas and intestine.

Pancreatic secretions

Secretions from the pancreas enter the duodenum through the common bile duct. They contain a pancreatic amylase, which continues the breakdown of starch to maltose.

Intestinal secretions

Intestinal secretions contain three disaccharidases—**sucrase, lactase**, and **maltase**. These enzymes act on their respective disaccharides to render the monosaccharides—glucose, galactose, fructose—ready for absorption. These specific disaccharidases are integral proteins of the brush border of the small intestine that break down the disaccharides as absorption takes place. The digestive products, the monosaccharides, are then immediately absorbed into the portal blood circulation.

A summary of the major aspects of carbohydrate digestion through these successive parts of the gastrointestinal tract is given in Table 3.9.

ABSORPTION

The refined fuel glucose is now ready to be carried to the individual cells to be stored or "burned" to produce energy. The body rapidly absorbs glucose, the basic end product of carbohydrate digestion, and transports it to the cells throughout the body. The major glucose absorption mechanism is an active transport "pumping" system requiring sodium as a carrier substance. Of the total carbohydrates absorbed, 80% is in the form of glucose by the sodium cotransport mechanism; the remaining 20% is galactose from milk and some fructose.[14,15]

Absorbing structures

The absorbing surface area of the small intestine is uniquely enhanced by its three basic structures: mucosal folds, villi, and microvilli, which are described in detail in Chapter 2. Together, these structures provide a greatly increased absorbing surface that allows 90% of the digested food material to be absorbed in the small intestine. Only water absorption remains for the large intestine.

Route of absorption

By way of the capillaries of the villi, the simple sugars enter **portal** circulation and are transported to the liver. Here fructose and galactose are converted to glucose, which is either used immediately for fuel or converted to glycogen for brief storage. Then glycogen constantly reconverts to glucose as needed by the body.

METABOLISM

Definition

The general term **metabolism** refers to the sum of the various chemical processes in a living organism by which energy is made available for the functioning of the entire

---

lactase Enzyme that splits the disaccharide lactose into its two monosaccharides, glucose and galactose.

lumen The cavity or channel within a tube or tubular organ, such as the intestines.

maltase Enzyme that breaks down the disaccharide maltose into two units of glucose, a monosaccharide.

metabolism Sum of all the various biochemical and physiologic processes by which the body grows and maintains itself (anabolism) and breaks down and reshapes tissue (catabolism), transforming energy to do its work. Products of these various reactions are called *metabolites*.

portal An entryway, usually referring to the portal circulation of blood through the liver. Blood is brought into the liver by the portal vein and out by the hepatic vein.

sucrase Enzyme splitting the disaccharide sucrose into its two monosaccharides of glucose and fructose.

To Probe Further

The semantics of fiber: a question of definition

Much of the confusion concerning fiber in the diet has centered on semantics. No term has seemed fully acceptable to cover all the different types of fiber or the various meanings involved. The older word *roughage* and the current general term *fiber* denote a rough, abrasive material of the physical nature observed in plant cellulose, a woody type of material. However, a number of the undigestible materials in food have a soft amorphous gel-like character, more soluble in physical nature and hence having different properties and functions.

This difference in physical properties adds to the problem nutritionists and clinicians have had in determining a more precise nutritional and clinical significance for fiber in the human diet and in defining the variety of food substances involved. Further problems have surrounded methods of accurately analyzing and measuring these substances in the variety of food sources.

The general term *fiber* was initially applied to a variety of indigestible carbohydrate and noncarbohydrate substances for which specific hydrolytic enzymes are lacking in the human digestive system. Confusion resulted mainly from the erroneous interchange of the two terms *dietary fiber* and *crude fiber*.

Dietary fiber refers to the total amount of naturally occurring material in foods, mostly plants, that is not digested. This includes (1) plant dietary fiber from such foods as whole grains, legumes, vegetables, fruits, seeds, and nuts; (2) undigested animal tissue polysaccharides; (3) undigested pharmaceutical products; and (4) undigested biosynthetic polysaccharides. Refined diets in Western countries usually contain little fiber in the energy foods— starches, sugars, and fats. Diets in rural communities of other developing countries contain much more fiber. Research suggests that these higher-fiber diets protect against a wide variety of Western diseases.

Crude fiber is the material remaining after vigorous treatment of the food sources with acid and alkaline agents in the laboratory. These were the initial results given in most food value tables. These strong laboratory processes remove a good portion of the total dietary fiber that cannot withstand such treatment. Because the proportion of total dietary fiber and crude fiber varies widely among specific foods, depending on the fiber composition of a particular food, the fiber values given in earlier food value tables have had limited usefulness. However, as new laboratory procedures are developed, better information is being provided. Thus the term *crude fiber* is of little value in current usage.

The current term of choice, although not perfect, is *dietary fiber*. It refers to the indigestible residues of plant foods: (1) cellulose; (2) noncellulose polysaccharides, including hemicellulose, pectins, gums, mucilages, and algal substances; and (3) the single noncarbohydrate member, lignin, which plants produce in the process of becoming woody. All resist digestion by any human digestive enzymes, but all are valuable in nutrition and related disease.

References

Marsh MN, Riley SA: Digestion and absorption of nutrients and vitamins. In Feldman M, Scharschmidt BF, Sleisenger MH, eds: *Gastrointestinal and liver disease,* ed 6, vol 2, Philadelphia, 1998, Saunders.

Slavin JL: Whole grains and health: separating the wheat from the chaff, *Nutr Today* 29(4):6, 1994.

Staff: Special report: Complex carbohydrates: the science and the label, *Nutr Rev* 53(7):186, 1995.

organism. It includes all the processes by which basic structures are built and maintained, function, and then break down to be rebuilt. Products of specific metabolic processes are called **metabolites**.

Cell metabolism of carbohydrate products

Cells are the functional units of life in the human body. In cell nutrition the most important end product of carbohydrate digestion is glucose because the other two monosaccharides—fructose and galactose—are eventually converted to glucose. The liver is the major site of the intricate machinery that handles glucose. However, energy metabolism occurs in all cells. In these individual cells, glucose is burned to produce energy through a series of chemical reactions involving specific cell enzymes. The final energy produced is then available to the cell to do its work. Extra glucose not immediately needed for energy may also be changed to adipose tissue and stored as a reserve fuel. Review details of these interactive metabolic activities among the nutrients in Chapter 2.

	Enzyme	Action
Mouth	Salivary amylase: ptyalin	Starch → dextrins → maltose
Stomach	None	Starch hydrolysis continued briefly
Small intestine	Pancreatic amylase: amylopsin	Starch → dextrins → maltose
	Intestinal disaccharidases:	
	Sucrase	Sucrose → glucose + fructose
	Lactase	Lactose → glucose + galactose
	Maltose	Maltose → glucose + glucose

Table 3.9 Summary of carbohydrate digestion

Metabolic concept of unity

Here and in following discussions of other nutrients, a central significant scientific principle will emerge—*the unity of the human organism.* The human body is a whole made up of many parts and processes that possess unequaled specificity and flexibility. Intimate metabolic relationships exist among all the basic nutrients and metabolites. Thus it is impossible to understand any one of the body's many metabolic processes without viewing it in relationship to the whole.

Therefore, in all your study and work with patients and clients, remember this important fact: **All nutrients do their best work in partnership with other nutrients.** From this fundamental fact you can draw two practical conclusions: (1) the emphasis in health teaching and nutrition education should be on achieving an overall sound balanced nutritional basis for any dietary program, and (2) some deficiency states may be related to an illness and its medical treatment, may have their origin in a fad, or may be caused by long-term, overzealous emphasis on one particular nutrient to the exclusion of other equally essential ones.

To sum up

Carbohydrates supply most of the world's population with its primary source of energy. A product of photosynthesis, carbohydrate is widely distributed in nature and its food products are easy to store and generally low in cost.

There are two basic types of carbohydrates: simple and complex. *Simple carbohydrates* consist of single- and double-sugar units (monosaccharides and disaccharides),

which are easily digested and provide quick energy. *Complex carbohydrates*, or polysaccharides, are less easily prepared for use. Though they vary somewhat in their effect on blood sugar, generally they provide energy more slowly and prevent large fluctuations in blood glucose levels.

In addition to providing general body energy, carbohydrates maintain liver, heart, brain, and nerve tissue function. They also prevent the breakdown of both lipids and proteins for energy, which results in excessive production of toxic metabolic by-products. *Dietary fiber,* a complex carbohydrate that forms the indigestible part of plants, also affects the digestion and absorption of foods in ways that have proved beneficial to good health.

■ QUESTIONS FOR REVIEW

1. Refer to the RDA table to determine the daily caloric need of a 25-year-old woman who is 5 ft 4 inches tall and weighs 125 pounds. How many kcalories should be provided by carbohydrates in her diet? How much fiber is recommended?

2. Give a general description of the clinical effects of fiber in each of the following disease states: diverticular disease, hyperlipidemia, diabetes mellitus, and colon cancer.

3. Your client, Mr. Brown, wants desperately to lose 20 pounds before meeting his future in-laws next month. He purchased a month's worth of liquid protein and takes multivitamins daily. He seems adamant about not eating any starches or sweets. Based on your readings, how would you explain the effects of a very low-carbohydrate diet on carbohydrate functions so that he will know why carbohydrates are important even in a weight-loss program?

■ REFERENCES

1. Nevins DJ: Sugars: their photosynthesis and subsequent biological interconversions, *Am J Clin Nutr* 61(suppl 5S):996S, 1995.

2. Levine B: ...About lactose intolerance, *Nutr Today* 31(2):78, 1996.

3. Hertzler SR et al: How much lactose is low lactose? *J Am Diet Assoc* 96(3):243, 1996.

4. Gibney M et al: Consumption of sugars, *Am J Clin Nutr* 62(suppl 1S):178S, 1995.

5. Tagliabue A et al: The effect of raw potato starch on energy expenditure and substrate oxidation, *Am J Clin Nutr* 61(5):1070, 1995.

metabolite   Any substance produced by metabolism or by a metabolic process.

6. Cummings JH, Englyst HN: Gastrointestinal effects of food carbohydrate, *Am J Clin Nutr* 61(suppl 5S):938S, 1995.

7. Muir JG et al: Food processing and maize variety affects amounts of starch escaping digestion in the small intestine, *Am J Clin Nutr* 61(1):82, 1995.

8. Hylla S et al: Effects of resistant starch on the colon in healthy volunteers: possible implications for cancer prevention, *Am J Clin Nutr* 67:136, 1998.

9. Behall KM, Howe JC: Resistant starch as energy, *J Am Coll Nutr* 15(3):248, 1996.

10. Slavin JL: Whole grains and health: separating the wheat from the chaff, *Nutr Today* 29(4):6, 1994.

11. Joneja JM, Ayre EA, Paterson K: Abnormal gut fermentation: the "auto-brewery" syndrome, *J Can Diet Assoc* 58(2):97, 1997.

12. Traber PG: Carbohydrate assimilation. In Yamada T, ed: *Textbook of gastroenterology,* vol 1, New York, 1995, Lippincott.

13. Special Workshop Report: Complex carbohydrates: the science and the label, *Nutr Rev* 53(7):186, 1995.

14. Marsh MN, Riley SA: Digestion and absorption of nutrients and vitamins. In Feldman M, Scharschmidt BF, Sleisenger MH, eds: *Gastrointestinal and liver disease,* ed 6, vol 2, Philadelphia, 1998, Saunders.

15. Guyton AC, Hall JE: *Textbook of medical physiology,* ed 9, Philadelphia, 1996, Saunders.

■ FURTHER READING

Blackburn GL et al: The effect of aspartame as part of a multidisciplinary weight-control program on short- and long-term control of body weight, *Am J Clin Nutr* 65:409, 1997.

McNutt K, Sentko A: Sugar replacers, *Nutr Today* 31(6):255, 1996.

These researchers and consumer specialists describe interesting informative data and professional experience with the growing group of sweeteners in the United States, collectively called sugar replacers. These intense sweeteners provide the volume and taste of sugar but are sugar-free reduced-calorie sweeteners, used extensively in sugar-free food products.

Filer LJ Jr, Reynolds WA: Lessons in comparative physiology: lactose intolerance, *Nutr Today* 32(2):79, 1997.

Suarez L et al: Tolerance to the daily ingestion of two cups of milk by individuals claiming lactose intolerance, *Am J Clin Nutr* 65:1502, 1997.

These two articles describe interesting and unusual experiences with lactose intolerance. Filer and Reynolds tell a fascinating tale of experience with saving the lives of a pair of valuable juvenile Pandas on loan from China to the Los Angeles Zoo, when Reynolds discovered the Panda bear species was genetically intolerant to the milk being fed them. She successfully substituted a lactose-free enteral formula product, Ensure (Ross), which the Pandas readily accepted. The Pandas recovered, going on to the San Francisco Zoo and then home to China in good health. The second article reports the study of Suarez' group, which concluded that persons self-described as lactose intolerant were actually able to tolerant two cups of milk per day with no symptoms in a double-blind, randomized, crossover trial.

Issues & Answers

The sugar phobia syndrome

The Puritan ethic that "pleasure is evil" has probably done as much as has the lack of accurate nutrition information in popular media to promote Americans' general fear of sweets in their diet. But like so many other things in our lives, sugar itself is not "bad." Rather, the real problem is *excess* sugar and the health implications of overconsumption, often to the exclusion of the variety of nutrients the body needs for a healthy balanced diet. Actually, carbohydrate-rich foods have provided people with one of their primary sources of nutrients—and pleasure—since the beginning of time. Because of an inborn taste for sweets, the simpler the carbohydrate, the greater the pleasure it often provides. Nonetheless, as some persons protest and as any good Puritan can tell you, "If it's good tasting, it must be bad for you."

Although this premise is highly conjectural, it is becoming obvious that Americans have developed a fear of carbohydrates, especially in one of its simplest forms—sugar. This fear is greatly manifest in the American's obsession with weight control and the use of sugar substitutes. Popular media usually advise dieters to eliminate excess kcalories by avoiding starches, which actually provide a major source of carbohydrates for populations around the world. And especially, they say, avoid sugar. This advice is based on the belief that sugar not only contributes a large number of kcalories to the average diet, but also is responsible for such ills as heart disease, diabetes, hypoglycemia, hyperactivity in children, and dental caries. Only in the case of dental caries is the evidence indisputable. Much of the belief in other areas is based on limited evidence and requires both clarification and qualified application.

Kilocalories

Approximately 20% to 25% of the total kcaloric intake of the average American diet is provided by sugar, often through pies, cakes, ice cream, and other rich desserts high in fat. However, although USDA consumer surveys report wide use of sugars, reports indicate that consumers of relatively high amounts of sugars do not necessarily have poorer quality diets. Since fat provides more than twice the number of kcalories per serving as sugar, the dieter should be primarily concerned with reducing this nutrient. Actually, intelligent persons should be concerned with reducing the overall *excessive* kcaloric intake, mainly from fat.

Heart disease

Sucrose has been associated with elevated levels of cholesterol, low-density lipoproteins (LDL), and plasma triglycerides, especially in carbohydrate-sensitive persons. The same association has been made with fructose, a nutritive sweetener often promoted as an alternate to commonly used sugar (sucrose), because it is one-and-a-half times sweeter and therefore less is required to achieve the desired taste level. Of course, if high sugar use replaces factors in the diet, such as fiber and other nutrients that are believed to be associated with reducing heart disease risk, it may contribute significantly to an *increased* risk for heart disease.

Diabetes mellitus

Excess amounts of sugar and other simple carbohydrates can contribute to elevated blood glucose levels in persons with diabetes, but current dietary guides for diabetes management include occasional moderate choices of sweets. Contrary to popular opinion, sugar is *not* a cause of diabetes. It is only one of many variables, such as total kcaloric intake or stress, that can raise blood sugar levels.

Hypoglycemia

Sugar intake initially brings some hyperglycemia, which in turn triggers the release of insulin. The insulin output, which may exceed the need, then reduces the blood sugar level, and in some sensitive individuals these levels may become abnormally low. The popular press has often recommended a very low-carbohydrate, high-protein diet to counteract this effect, while condemning the use of sugar entirely. However, current research indicates that a diet low in simple sugars, whatever their form, and more liberal in complex carbohydrates and dietary fiber is effective in raising the blood glucose to a normal level, even in persons with diabetes.

Attention deficit hyperactivity disorder

Some practitioners have observed changes in the behavior of some children consuming high-sugar diets and noted greater activity, ease of stimulation, and other signs suggesting an association between sugar intake and an attention deficit disorder, or hyperactivity. But a number of problems have clouded the issue, including the absence of reliable methods for measuring a child's behavior, the possibility of environmental factors, such as stress, contributing to the changed behavior, and the lack of conclusive controlled studies relating sugar intake to a decreased attention span and hyperactivity.

Dental caries

Dental caries is the one health problem that has been proved to be "caused" by sugar. However, the effect of sugar has been waning because of the widespread practice of fluoridation, which together with better dental care and regular toothbrushing has greatly reduced the incidence of caries.

Despite sugar's questionable contribution to major health problems, the "fear of sugar" has led the public to increase its demand for alternative sweeteners (see Chapter 20). These agents include both nonnutritive sweeteners, such as saccharin, and nutritive sweeteners such as aspartame (made from two amino acids, phenylalanine and aspartic acid), or alternate sugars such as lactose or fructose in smaller amounts. But our history of the use of such alternate sweeteners is rather dismal. For example, although they consume enough sugar substitutes to replace 150 kcalories worth of sugar every day, Americans still have failed to make a dent either in the total amount of sugar they consume—as much as 63 kg (140 lb) per person per year—or in the average body weight of the population.

There are two possible explanations in some persons for the failure of artificial sweeteners to work as sugar substitutes:

- **Physiologic response differences**. Artificial sweeteners do not replace the desire for sugar because they do not trigger the same physiologic responses mediated by neurotransmitters in the brain and induced by sugar to produce satiety. Although for many persons the level of natural sweetness provided by vegetables, fruits, and milk often satisfies the need for a sweet taste, the average user of nonnutritive sweeteners may find that the desire for "something sweet" is even greater than that of the average sugar user. A more positive response, however, seems to be the experience of many users of some of the newer increasing number of sugar replacers on the market.
- **Increased fat intake**. Some users of artificial sweeteners try to achieve satiety by increasing their intake of fats, thereby sabotaging their weight loss efforts. To complicate matters even further, a number of studies indicate that individuals who consume average or even above average amounts of sugar tend to be thinner, not because of the sugar, but because they lead much more active lives. It has been suggested that persons use sugar as a means of satisfying short-term energy needs because of its kcaloric content and ease of digestion. For example, a group of South African sugar cane cutters who manually move up to 7 tons of cane every day and consume approximately 27% of their 6000 kcalories/day diet in the form of sugar are neither obese nor diabetic and maintain serum cholesterol levels that average 100 mg/dl *less* than those of most healthy Americans.

Even though there is growing evidence indicating that sugar may not be as "bad" as some people seem to believe, sugar eaters may benefit from a little pseudo-Puritanical advice: too much of *anything* can be harmful. The *excessive* sugar users may well consider these objective facts:

- Sugar is purely a fuel supplying energy to the body. It lacks other nutrients essential for growth and health maintenance. Thus if it replaces significant amounts of other foods in the diet, the result may be malnutrition and obesity.
- Sugar is cariogenic, and although fluoride and good dental care do reduce the incidence of dental caries, controlled intake of sugar is recommended as another preventive measure.
- Excessive sugar can elevate blood lipid levels in susceptible persons; it can contribute to serum triglyceride levels for those in whom elevated serum triglycerides is a problem. It may also contribute to elevated blood glucose levels in persons with diabetes. Also, sugar can contribute to serum triglyceride levels for those in whom elevated serum triglycerides are a problem.
- The use of artificial sweeteners may help prevent some of these health problems, but it is wise to temper their use in the light of current knowledge.

Artificial sweeteners may not fully satisfy the need for satiety or the physiologic experience of a sweet taste for all persons. In fact, in some individuals they may even increase the desire for "real" sweets.

Excessive amounts of sugar substitutes also can cause problems, such as diarrhea in the case of sorbitol. Aspartame—approved for widespread use in soft drinks—enjoys a large consumer market, but because it is made from two amino acids—phenylalanine and aspartic acid—it cannot be used freely by children with phenylketonuria (PKU).

Summing up, consumers should become aware of the benefits of *moderate* sugar use, as well as problems of *excessive* amounts of sugar and its substitutes. Then they can make intelligent decisions regarding their use.

References

Blackburn GL et al: The effect of aspartame as part of a multidisciplinary weight-control program on short- and long-term control of body weight, *Am J Clin Nutr* 65:409, 1997.

Gibney M et al: Consumption of sugars, *Am J Clin Nutr* 62(suppl 1S):178S, 1995.

McNutt K, Sentko A: Sugar replacers: a growing group of sweeteners in the United States, *Nutr Today* 31(6): 1996.

Natah SS et al: Metabolic response to lactitol and xylitol in healthy men, *Am J Clin Nutr* 65:947, 1997.

Payne ML et al: Sorbitol is a possible risk factor for diarrhea in young children, *J Am Diet Assoc* 97(5):532, 1997.

Chapter 4

Fats

Lipids, the second of our energy-yielding macronutrients, have, for the most part, had negative reporting for the past few years because of their association with a number of chronic diseases. This is especially true with heart disease. But the real culprit, as with many things, is the excess fat we eat. Fat itself is an essential nutrient.

Traditionally, fat has held a prominent place in the American diet. However, spurred by our justified health concerns, our attitudes and habits regarding lipids in general have begun to change.

Our goal here is to help achieve some balance in our food habits and our attitudes toward lipids and health. Based on the information provided about the nature of lipids and their role in nutrition, we will see why we need a moderate amount of fat for energy and overall health.

LIPIDS IN NUTRITION AND HEALTH

HEALTH NEEDS FOR LIPIDS

We need some lipids in our food and in our bodies to keep us healthy. This need is indicated by the number of functions lipids perform in nutrition, both in our diets and in our overall body metabolism.

Food lipids

The lipids in our food provide energy, essential nutrients, and satiety, as the following list explains:

- *Fuel source for energy.* Food lipids supply a basic continual source of fuel for the body to store and utilize as needed for energy. Food lipids yield 9 kcalories per gram when oxidized in the body in comparison with carbohydrates and protein, which yield 4 kcalories per gram.
- *Essential nutrient supply.* Food lipids supply the essential fatty acids, especially **linoleic acid**, and cholesterol as needed to supplement the body's endogenous supply.
- *Food satiety.* Lipids in the diet supply flavor to food and a certain mouth feel that artificial substitutes try to mimic that contributes to a feeling of satisfaction that lasts longer than does the feeling of satisfaction after eating carbohydrates and protein. Our food choices are strongly influenced by taste and texture, much of which lipids contribute, thus enhancing our eating pleasure.[1] This satiety is enhanced by the fuller texture and body that fat contributes to food mixtures and the slower gastric emptying time it brings.

Body lipids

The body stores energy as **adipose** tissue. These lipid tissue reserves serve a number of vital functions that are essential to health and life itself:

- *Energy.* A major function of lipids in nutrition is to supply an efficient fuel to all tissues, although the central nervous system and brain depend on a steady supply of glucose.
- *Thermal insulation.* The layer of lipid deposits directly underneath the skin controls body temperature within the range necessary for life.
- *Vital organ protection.* A weblike padding of adipose tissue surrounds vital organs such as the kidneys, protecting them from mechanical shock and providing a structure for support.
- *Nerve impulse transmission.* Lipid layers surrounding nerve fibers provide electrical insulation and transmit nerve impulses.
- *Tissue membrane structure.* Lipids serve as vital constituents of the cell membrane structure, helping transport nutrient materials and metabolites across cell membranes.

- *Cell metabolism.* Combinations of lipids and protein, known as lipoproteins, carry lipids in the blood to all cells.
- *Essential precursor substances.* Lipids supply necessary components, such as fatty acids and cholesterol, for the synthesis of many materials required for metabolic functions and tissue integrity.
- *Carriers of fat-soluble vitamins.* Lipids serve as essential transport for fat-soluble vitamins A, D, E, and K to the cells for vital metabolic needs.

HEALTH PROBLEMS WITH LIPIDS

From lists such as the one given previously and world health reports, it is evident that lipids make up an essential nutrient class.[2] But if lipids are as vital to human health as indicated, what is the problem with fat in the diet? As with so many things, the old maxim holds true: you need what you need, but you don't need more than you need. Specifically, health problems with lipids focus on two main issues: too much dietary fat, reflected in too much body fat, and too much of the dietary fat coming mostly from animal food sources.

Amount of fat

Too much fat in the diet provides excessive kcalories, more than required for immediate energy needs. The excess is stored as excess adipose tissue, thereby increasing body weight. How much fat is in your own diet? You might try figuring it out for a day (see *Practical Application* box, p. 56). This increased body weight—more precisely, an increased proportion of body fat making up the total body composition—has been associated with such health problems as diabetes, hypertension, and heart disease. Look for specific relationships between increased body weight and these health problems in later chapters on these topics.

Kind of lipids

Current research has shown a clear relation between a diet containing excess saturated fat and cholesterol, which come from animal sources, to *atherosclerosis*, a blood vessel disease characterized by fatty plaques on interior vessel walls that can eventually fill the vessel and cut off blood circulation (see Chapter 20). This disease process contributes to heart attacks and strokes (see *Issues & Answers,* p. 65).

THE PHYSICAL AND CHEMICAL NATURE OF LIPIDS

PHYSICAL CHARACTERISTICS

Lipids include such substances as fat, oil, and related compounds that are greasy to the touch and insoluble in water. Some basic food forms of lipids are easily seen as fat: butter, cream, exterior meat fat, bacon, oil, mayonnaise, and salad dressings. Other food forms are more hidden: egg yolk, internal tissue fat of meats, olives, avocados, nuts, and seeds.

CHEMICAL CHARACTERISTICS

The chemical class name for fats and fat-related compounds is **lipids**. By chemical definition, these are all **organic** compounds, consisting mainly of a chain of the basic element carbon as a "backbone," with attached hydrogen and oxygen atoms and other radicals. They all have in common a relation to the **fatty acids**. Thus the same basic chemical elements that make up carbohydrates—carbon, hydrogen, and oxygen—also make up the fatty acids and their related lipids. But in general the two nutrients differ in two main ways: (1) lipids are more complex in structure, with more carbon (C) and hydrogen (H) and less oxygen (O); (2) lipids' common structural units are the fatty acids, whereas carbohydrates are less complex structures largely composed of simple sugar units. Fatty acids are also refined fuel forms that some cells, such as those constituting the heart muscle, prefer over glucose. In our discussion here, we look first at the basic structural units, the fatty acids, and their unique characteristics of saturation, essentiality, and chain length. Then we focus on the nature of the basic lipids, known as triglycerides, that the fatty acids build.

BASIC LIPIDS: FATTY ACIDS AND TRIGLYCERIDES

SATURATION OF FATTY ACIDS

The state of **saturation** or unsaturation gives lipids their varying textural characteristics. Saturated lipids are harder, less saturated ones are softer, and unsaturated ones are usually liquid oils. This differing state results from the ratio of hydrogen to carbon in the structures of the respective fatty acids that make up a particular lipid. If a given fatty acid is filled with as much hydrogen as it can take, the fatty acid is said to be completely *saturated* with hydrogen. If, however, the fatty acid has less hydrogen, it is obviously less saturated. Three terms designate the varying degree of saturation:

- **Saturated**. Food lipids composed of saturated fatty acids are called *saturated fats*. The most saturated forms are found in tropical oils such as coconut and palm kernel oils (88% and 80% total fat).[1] Other sources are mainly of animal origin, for example, meats and whole milk dairy products.
- **Monounsaturated**. Food lipids composed mainly of fatty acids with one less hydrogen atom creating one double bond are called *monounsaturated fats*. These lipids are mostly from plant sources, for example, olive oil and canola oil, which is derived from a variety of rapeseed.
- **Polyunsaturated**. Food lipids composed mainly of unsaturated fatty acids with two or more places unfilled with hydrogen creating double bonds are called *polyunsaturated fats*. These lipids are from plant sources. Notable exceptions are coconut oil, palm oil, and cocoa butter, which are saturated.

ESSENTIAL FATTY ACIDS

The terms *essential* and *nonessential* are applied to nutrients according to their relative necessity in the diet. The particular nutrient is essential if the body cannot manufacture it and therefore must obtain it from the diet, since a failure to do so would result in a deficiency disease. In this case, for example, if lipids make up only 10% or less of the diet's daily kcalories, the body cannot obtain adequate amounts of the essential fatty acids. Three fatty acids—linoleic, linolenic, arachidonic—are the only ones known to be essential for the complete nutrition of humans.[3] Actually, only linoleic acid is a *true* **essential fatty acid (EFA)** because the other two may be naturally synthesized from it. These fatty acids, linoleic, linolenic, and arachidonic acids, serve important body functions:

- *Membrane structure.* Linoleic acid strengthens cell membranes, helping prevent a harmful increase in skin and membrane permeability. A linoleic

---

adipose Fat present in cells of adipose (fatty) tissue.

essential fatty acid A fatty acid required in the diet because the body cannot synthesize it.

fatty acid The structural components of fats.

linoleic acid The ultimate essential fatty acid for humans.

lipids Chemical group name for fats and fat-related compounds such as cholesterol, lipoproteins, and phospholipids; general group name for organic substances of a fatty nature, including fats, oils, waxes, and related compounds.

organic Carbon-based chemical compounds.

saturated To cause to unite with the greatest possible amount of another substance through solution, chemical combination, or the like. A saturated fat, for example, is one in which the component fatty acids are filled with hydrogen atoms. A fatty acid is said to be saturated if all available chemical bonds of its carbon chain are filled with hydrogen. If one bond remains unfilled, it is a monounsaturated fatty acid. If two or more bonds remain unfilled, it is a polyunsaturated fatty acid. Fats of animal sources are more saturated. Fats of plant sources are unsaturated.

How much fat are you eating?

Keep an accurate record of everything you eat or drink for 1 day. Be sure to estimate and add amounts of all fat or other nutrient seasonings used with your foods. (If you want a more representative picture and have a computer available with nutrient analysis software, keep a 1-week record and calculate an average of the 7 days.)

Calculate the total kilocalories (kcal) and grams of each of the energy nutrients (carbohydrate, fat, and protein) in everything you eat. Multiply the total grams of each energy nutrient by its respective fuel value:

carbohydrate ____ g × 4 =   kcal
fat ____ g × 9 = _____   kcal
protein ____ g × 4 = ____ kcal

Calculate the percentage of each energy nutrient in your total:

Fat kcal ÷ total kcal × 100 = % fat kcal in diet

Compare this figure with fat in the average American's diet (35%); with the United States dietary guidelines (25% to 30%); and with your own needs.

acid deficiency leads to a breakdown in skin integrity, resulting in characteristic eczema and skin lesions. A similar effect also occurs in other tissue membranes throughout the body.

- *Cholesterol transport.* Like other fatty acids, linoleic acid combines with cholesterol to form cholesterol esters for transport in the blood.
- *Serum cholesterol.* As do other unsaturated fatty acids, linoleic acid helps lower serum cholesterol levels. It plays a key role in both transport and metabolism of cholesterol.
- *Blood clotting.* With its closely associated metabolic products arachidonic acid and linolenic acid, linoleic acid helps prolong blood clotting time and increase fibrinolytic activity.
- *Local hormonelike effects.* Linoleic acid is a major metabolic precursor of a group of physiologically and pharmacologically active compounds known as *prostaglandins*, *prostacyclins*, *thromboxanes*, and *leukotrienes*, which are called **eicosanoids** because of their structure (see *To Probe Further* box, p. 57). These eicosanoid compounds have extensive local hormonelike effects.[4,5] They are synthesized in the body from arachidonic acid, which is derived from essential linoleic acid. The synthesis of these highly active important compounds is diagrammed in Figure 4.1, which also shows some of their significant physiologic functions and sites.

Prostaglandins

Of these groups of *eicosanoid* compounds related to the omega-3 long-chain fatty acids, perhaps the most familiar is the group of **prostaglandins** because of their exten-

sive functions. They were first discovered by Swedish investigators in their study of reproductive physiology, identified initially in human semen, and named prostaglandins because they were thought to originate in the prostate gland. They are now known to exist in virtually all body tissues, acting as local hormones to direct and coordinate important biologic functions. For example, they have been shown to be powerful modulators of vascular smooth muscle tone and platelet aggregation and hence have a significant relationship to cardiovascular disease.[4,5]

CHAIN LENGTH OF FATTY ACIDS

Another characteristic of fatty acids, important in their absorption, is the length of the carbon chain composing their structure. The long-chain fatty acids are more difficult to absorb and require a helping carrier. The short- and medium-chain fatty acids are more soluble in water and hence easier to absorb directly into the bloodstream. In intestinal malabsorption disease, when the absorbing mucosal surface is inflamed or infected, short- or medium-chain fat products are preferred. A commercial product called MCT (medium-chain triglycerides) is an oil made of short- and medium-chain fatty acids that can be used in the diet just as any ordinary vegetable oil.

TRIGLYCERIDES

Basic structure

Triglycerides are the storage form of fatty acids. The name indicates the basic chemical structure: three fatty acids attached to a **glycerol** base. Thus lipids are **glycerides** composed of glycerol and fatty acids. When glycerol is combined with one fatty acid it is called a *mono-*

To Probe Further

Omega-3 fatty acids: health or hype?

Often with new nutrition research findings come a heavy dose of hype and a new diet fad. This is especially true when the research holds promise for combating heart disease and its dreaded fatty arteries, as well as other chronic health problems. Such is the case with the *omega-3* fatty acids and their rich presence in fatty fish.

But if you can get past the commercial hype and maintain perspective, you'll find some remarkable scientific data accumulating. Scientific interest was first sparked by earlier observations among Greenland Eskimos, who eat a diet rich in fish oils but have a low incidence of heart disease. These fish oils contain high levels of the class of long-chain polyunsaturated fatty acids called *omega-3* fatty acids. ω is the last letter in the Greek alphabet, used by scientists for naming fatty acid classes by the structure of their carbon chain, counting from the end of the chain. There is an especially high level of one of these omega-3 fatty acids in fish oils, **eicosapentaenoic acid (EPA)** (from Greek *eicosa-*, twenty; *penta-*, five). The name designates its structure, abbreviated 20:5 × 3, meaning a long-chain polyunsaturated fatty acid of 20 carbons with 5 double bonds (unsaturated points), the first double bond located at carbon 3, counting from the omega end of the carbon chain.

Accumulating evidence supports the potential nutritional and clinical relevance of these omega-3 fatty acids. The National Institutes of Health (NIH) is studying both synthesis and comparative effects of these fatty acids. The human body obtains omega-3 EPA mainly from fatty fish in the diet but can synthesize it from linolenic acid. The other two essential fatty acids, linoleic and arachidonic, are omega-6 fatty acids, closely related in their metabolic pathways and functions. In fact, the two precursor essential fatty acids, linolenic (omega-3) and linoleic (omega-6) acids, compete for the same metabolic enzyme systems in the body in producing their *eicosanoid* substances. The optimal dietary balance of omega-3 and omega-6 fatty acids and their metabolic balance effects is under study. These highly active local hormone substances have highly significant physiologic effects in helping to modulate and balance cardiovascular functions, possibly affecting intestinal cancer development, as well as supporting normal growth and development.

References

Grimsgaard S et al: Highly purified eicosapentaenoic acid and docosahexaenoic acid (DHA) in humans have similar triacylglycerol-lowering effects but divergent effects on serum fatty acids, *Am J Clin Nutr* 66:649, 1997.

Levine BS: ...About DHA, *Nutr Today* 32(6):248, 1997.

Whelan J: Polyunsaturated fatty acids: signaling agents for intestinal cancer? *Nutr Today* 32(5):213, 1997.

---

eicosanoids Long-chain fatty acids composed of 20 carbon atoms.

glyceride Group name for fats; any of a group of esters obtained from glycerol by the replacement of one, two, or three hydroxyl (OH) groups with a fatty acid. Monoglycerides contain one fatty acid; diglycerides contain two fatty acids; triglycerides contain three fatty acids. Glycerides are the principal constituent of adipose tissue and are found in animal and vegetable fats and oils.

glycerol A colorless, odorless, syrupy, sweet liquid; a constituent of fats usually obtained by the hydrolysis of fats. Chemically, glycerol is an alcohol; it is esterified with fatty acids to produce fats.

prostaglandins Group of naturally occurring substances, first discovered in semen, derived from long-chain fatty acids that have multiple local hormonelike actions, including regulation of gastric acid secretion, platelet aggregation, body temperature, and tissue inflammation.

triglyceride Chemical name for fat, indicating structure; attachment of three fatty acids to a glycerol base. A neutral fat, synthesized from carbohydrate and stored in adipose tissue, it releases free fatty acids into the blood when hydrolyzed by enzymes.

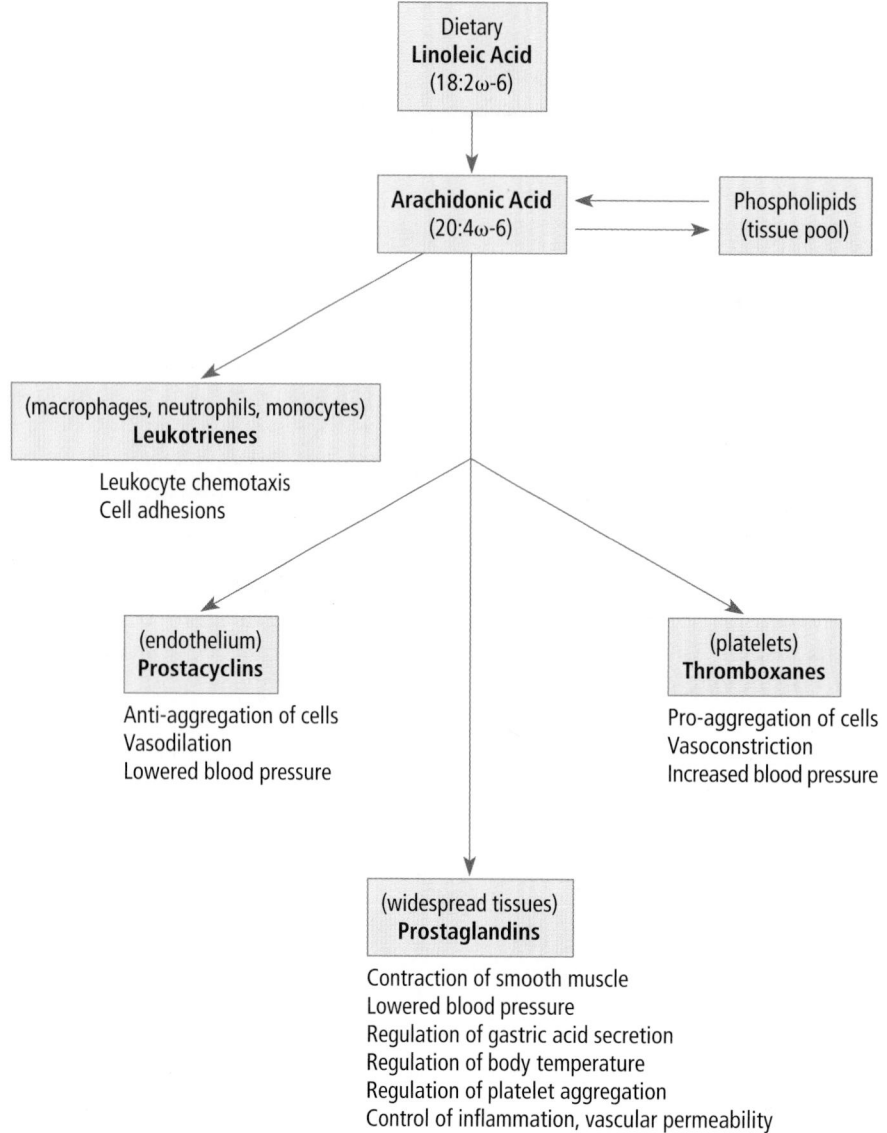

Figure 4.1   Synthesis, sites, and functions of eicosanoids.

glyceride, with two fatty acids a *diglyceride*, and with three fatty acids a *triglyceride*. Whether in food or in the body, fatty acids combine with glycerol to form glycerides. Most natural lipids, whether from animal or plant sources, are triglycerides. These lipids, the triglycerides, occur in body cells as oily droplets. They circulate in water-based blood serum encased in a covering of water-soluble protein. These lipid-protein complexes are called *lipoproteins*. They serve multiple functions throughout the body.

Nature of food lipids

Food lipids, as well as body lipids, are composed of saturated and unsaturated fatty acids. If the food lipid is made up mainly of saturated fatty acids, it is called a saturated lipid. Foods from animal sources—such as meat, milk, and eggs—contain saturated fats. Conversely, food from plant sources such as the vegetable oils are usually

unsaturated. A general saturated-unsaturated spectrum of food lipids is shown in Figure 4.2. The animal food lipids on the saturated end of the spectrum are solid; those toward the center become somewhat less saturated and are softer. The plant lipids on the unsaturated end are free-flowing oils that do not solidify even at low temperatures. Exceptions are tropical oils such as coconut oil and palm oil, which are saturated lipids. Such saturated plant fats are used extensively in commercial products because they are usually cheaper oils. Because such higher fat-processed food items have become an increasing part of the modern diet, it is important to read product labels carefully. The current food labels on processed foods indicate these distinctions in fat composition. The general distinction in saturation, as shown in Figure 4.2, as well as food labels on processed foods, may be helpful in explaining to persons on modified fat diets some wise choices of food fats.

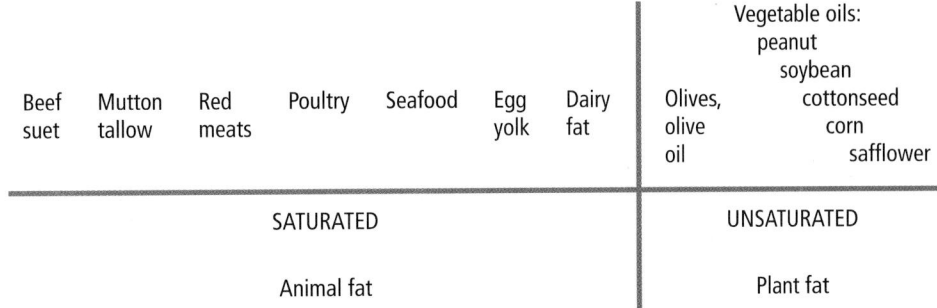

| | | | | | | | | | Vegetable oils: |
Beef suet	Mutton tallow	Red meats	Poultry	Seafood	Egg yolk	Dairy fat	Olives, olive oil		peanut soybean cottonseed corn safflower
			SATURATED					UNSATURATED	
			Animal fat					Plant fat	

Figure 4.2   Spectrum of food fats according to degree of saturation of component fatty acid.

Cis and trans unsaturated fatty acid products

The unsaturated oils can be hardened commercially into products such as margarine and shortening by injection of hydrogen gas to saturate them, a process called **hydrogenation**. Recently, health professionals have been concerned about the increasing number of hydrogenated food products being made from the *cis* and *trans* forms of unsaturated fatty acids. First, compare this difference in structure of the commonly occurring monounsaturated fatty acid, oleic acid, with its one unsaturated double bond occurring in the middle of its chain of 18 carbon atoms:

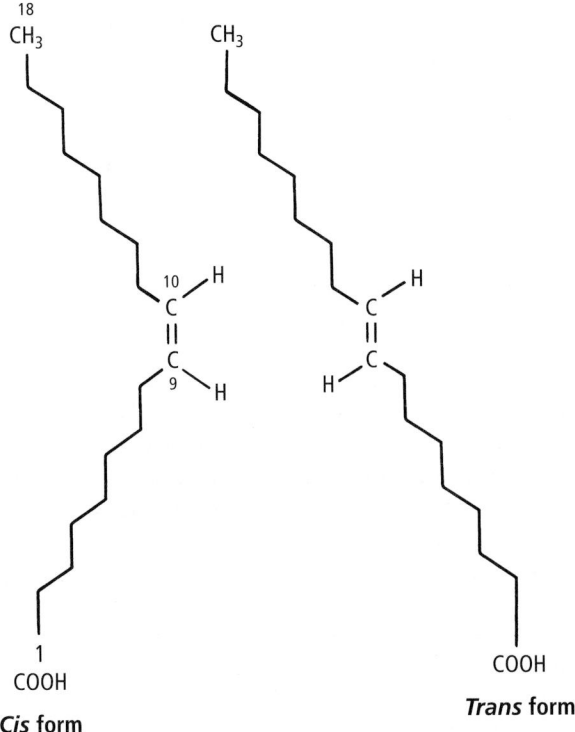

Cis form   ***Trans* form**

When double bonds occur naturally in food lipids, the fatty acid chains usually bend at those points so that the remaining parts of the structure are on the same side of the bond. In this case the form is called *cis* (same side). All fatty acids in naturally occurring lipids are in the *cis*

form. However, when vegetable oils are partially hydrogenated to make food products, the normal bend is changed so that the remaining parts are on opposite sides of the bond. In this case the form is called *trans* (opposite side). Commercially hydrogenated lipids in margarine and many other products are in the *trans* form. With the increasing use of these products, especially margarine, there is some debate about possible effects of the accumulating *trans* form in the body. Some of these observed effects include elevation of serum lipids, inhibition of essential fatty acid metabolism, and modification of membrane properties. In response to these growing health concerns, the food industry has developed solid fats low in *trans* fatty acids for the food industry to meet the current demand for nonhydrogenated solid fats.[6]

VISIBLE AND HIDDEN FOOD FAT

As indicated, food fats are sometimes called "visible" or "hidden" fats according to how obvious they are in food. In most cases the food fat is quite evident, such as in butter, margarine, oil, salad dressing, bacon, and cream, which account for about 40% of the fat in the American diet. However, less obvious hidden fats in foods such as meat, milk (unless it is a nonfat form), eggs (only in the yolk; the white is pure protein), nuts, seeds, olives, and avocados contribute more to our fat intake. A large part of this fat comes from our relatively high consumption of meats. Even when all the fat is trimmed off a cut of meat, its lean portion still contains 4% to 12% hidden fat. Higher grades of meat, both prime and choice, have considerable "marbling"—tiny fat deposits within the muscle tissue. This is especially true of beef, a major meat on the American market. Thus the meat and milk food groups together contribute about half the fat in the American diet.

---

hydrogenation   Process of hardening liquid vegetable oils by injecting hydrogen gas to produce margarines and shortenings.

Early reports of the ongoing USDA's Continuing Survey of Food Intakes by Individuals (CSFII) indicate that men consume 34% of total calories from fat and 11% from saturated fat, and that women consume 32% of total calories from fat and 11% from saturated fat.[7] The current Dietary Guidelines for Americans (see Chapter 1) recommend that all persons above age 2 choose a diet with no more than 30% of calories from total fat and less than 10% of calories from saturated fat. Yet even with increasing health concerns about their fat intake, Americans still seem ambivalent. They cut down in some areas, but at the same time purchase larger amounts of red meats with considerable nonseparable fat, such as ground beef and hamburgers. This conflicting pattern of meat fat consumption, often termed "meat fat madness," suggests that such contradictory choices are made by an ill-informed public. But the meat industry, challenged by health-conscious consumers, has been developing leaner breeds through genetic engineering and promoting leaner cuts in smaller portions for low-fat cooking. In addition, regular and fast-food restaurants have begun to develop leaner menu items.

SPECIAL LIPID-RELATED COMPOUND: CHOLESTEROL

Structure

Although **cholesterol** is often discussed in connection with dietary lipids, it is not a fat (triglyceride) itself. Many people confuse cholesterol with saturated fat. Cholesterol is a lipid-related compound that is quite different from triglycerides in structure. Generally, cholesterol travels in the bloodstream attached to long-chain fatty acids, forming cholesterol **esters**.

Functions

Cholesterol is a vital substance in human metabolism. It belongs to a family of substances called **steroids**, or sterols, and is a precursor to all steroid hormones. A cholesterol compound in the skin, *7-dehydrocholesterol*, is irradiated by sunlight's ultraviolet rays and activated in the body to produce vitamin D hormone. It is also essential in the formation of bile acids, which emulsify fats for enzymatic digestion and then serve as a carrier for fat absorption. Cholesterol is widely distributed in all cells of the body and is found in large amounts in brain and nerve tissue. It is an essential component of cell membranes. It is no wonder therefore that a constant supply of so vital a material for body processes would be made in body tissues, mainly in the liver. If a person consumed *no* cholesterol at all, the body would still synthesize a needed supply.

Food sources

Cholesterol occurs naturally in all animal foods. There is none in plant foods. Its main food sources are egg yolks and organ meats such as liver and kidneys. In fact, cholesterol occurs *only* in animal fats and tissues, *not* in plant fats or tissues. Therefore vegetable oils do not contain cholesterol. Plant oils may vary in degree of saturation, but *none* of them contain cholesterol.

Health concerns

Cholesterol has been increasingly implicated in vascular disease as a large risk factor in the development of *atherosclerosis*, the underlying pathology in coronary heart disease, in which cholesterol-containing fatty plaques build up on blood vessel walls. If this plaque forms a blood clot and narrows the major arteries serving the heart muscle, a heart attack is triggered. If this process initiates a clot that finally lodges in an artery in the brain, it causes a stroke. Current research has confirmed the association of this process with elevated serum cholesterol levels (Chapter 20). Thus government health officials and health professionals have recommended that Americans reduce their dietary cholesterol to no more than 300 mg/day. Current CSFII results reported above indicate that men consume an average of 334 mg/day, exceeding the recommended 300 mg/day; women average 212 mg/day, meeting the recommendation.[7] The various U.S. dietary guidelines (see Chapter 1) likewise recommend that Americans reduce their dietary cholesterol intake to about 300 mg/day, along with maintaining an appropriate level of physical exercise and body weight. An increase in soluble types of dietary fiber—described in the previous chapter—is also recommended because these fibers bind bile acids and dietary cholesterol, which helps in eliminating excess cholesterol from the body.

SPECIAL COMPOUND LIPIDS: LIPOPROTEINS

Function

The liver serves as the center for receiving fatty acids and cholesterol from the diet and body tissues, packaging them into lipoproteins and releasing them into the circulation.[8] The lipoproteins are important combinations of lipids with protein and other lipid-related components that are highly significant in human nutrition. Chemically they are not true compound lipids but are *complexes* (noncovalent structures) of lipids and covering protein, which—together with **apoproteins**—serve as the major vehicle for lipid transport in the bloodstream (see Chapter 20).

Lipid transport

Lipids are insoluble in water. This simple characteristic poses a problem in carrying lipids to cells in a water-based circulatory system. The body has solved this problem through the development of the **lipoproteins**, packages of lipids wrapped in water-soluble protein. These plasma lipoproteins contain fatty acids, triglycerides, cholesterol, **phospholipids**, and traces of other materials such as fat-soluble vitamins and steroid hormones. The high or low density of the lipoprotein is determined by its relative loads of lipids and protein. The higher the protein ratio, the higher the density.

Thus the lipoproteins are usually classified according to density and by relative lipid and cholesterol loads as follows[8]:

1. *Chylomicrons.* These are formed in the intestinal wall following a meal and carry the large fat load from the meal just consumed to liver cells for initial conversion to other transport lipoproteins.
2. *Very low-density lipoproteins (VLDLs).* These are formed in the liver in the fasting intervals between meals and replace chylomicrons as the major transporters of triglycerides in the continuing process of lipid transport and metabolism and deliver endogenous triglycerides to tissue cells.
3. *Intermediate low-density lipoproteins (ILDLs).* These are formed from VLDLs and continue the delivery of endogenous triglycerides to tissue cells.
4. *Low-density lipoproteins (LDLs).* These are formed from VLDLs and ILDLs and carry cholesterol to the peripheral tissue cells.
5. *High-density lipoproteins (HDLs).* These are formed in cell metabolism and carry cholesterol from the cells to the liver for breakdown and elimination from the body.

The lipoproteins are closely associated with lipid disorders and vascular disease; look for details of their structures and functions in Chapter 20.

DIGESTION-ABSORPTION-METABOLISM SUMMARY

DIGESTION

The basic lipid fuel—various animal and plant lipids (triglycerides) that naturally occur in food—is taken into the body with the food. Then the task is to change these basic fuel lipids into a refined fuel form that the cells can burn for energy. This key refined fuel is the individual *fatty acid.* The body accomplishes this task through the process of lipid digestion.

Mouth

No major chemical lipid breakdown takes place in the mouth. In this first portion of the gastrointestinal tract, the main action is mechanical as lipids are broken up into smaller particles through chewing and moistened for passage into the stomach with the general food mass.

Stomach

Little if any chemical lipid digestion takes place in the stomach. General peristalsis continues the mechanical mixing of lipids with the stomach contents. No significant amount of enzymes specific for lipids is present in the gastric secretions except a gastric **lipase** (tributyrinase), which acts on emulsified butterfat. As the main gastric enzymes act on other specific nutrients in the food mix, lipids are separated from the mix and made readily accessible to their own specific chemical breakdown in the small intestine.

Small intestine

Not until lipids reach the small intestine do the chemical changes necessary for lipid digestion occur. Digestive agents from three major sources are present: the biliary tract—consisting of the liver and gallbladder—which contributes a preparation agent, and the pancreas and the small intestine, which both release specific enzymes.

1. *Bile from the liver and gallbladder.* The presence of lipids in the duodenum stimulates the secretion

---

apoprotein A separate protein compound that attaches to its specific receptor site on a particular lipoprotein and activates certain functions, such as synthesis of a related enzyme. An example is apoprotein C II, an apoprotein of HDL and VLDL that functions to activate the enzyme lipoprotein lipase.

cholesterol A fat-related compound, a sterol ($C_{27}H_{45}OH$). It is a normal constituent of bile and a principal constituent of gallstones. In body metabolism cholesterol is important as a precursor of various steroid hormones, such as sex hormones and adrenal corticoids. Cholesterol is synthesized by the liver. It is widely distributed in nature, especially in animal tissue such as glandular meats and egg yolk.

ester A compound produced by the reaction between an acid and an alcohol with elimination of a molecule of water. This process is called esterification. For example, a triglyceride is a glycerol ester. Cholesterol esters are formed in the mucosal cells by combination with fatty acids, largely linoleic acid.

lipase Group of fat enzymes that cut the ester linkages between the fatty acids and glycerol of triglycerides (fats).

lipoprotein Noncovalent complexes of fat with protein. The lipoproteins function as major carriers of lipids in the plasma, since most of the plasma fat is associated with them. Such a combination makes possible the transport of fatty substances in a water medium such as plasma.

phospholipid Any of a class of fat-related substances that contain phosphorus, fatty acids, and a nitrogenous base. The phospholipids are essential elements in every cell.

steroids Group name for lipid-based sterols, including hormones, bile acids, and cholesterol.

Figure 4.3   Micellar complex of fats with bile salts for transport of fats into intestinal mucosa.

Table 4.1	Summary of fat digestion	
Organ	**Enzyme**	**Activity**
Mouth	None	Mechanical, mastication
Stomach	No major enzyme	Mechanical separation of fats as protein and starch digested out
	Small amount of gastric lipase tributyrinase	Tributyrin (butterfat) to fatty acids and glycerol
Small intestine	Gallbladder bile salts (emulsifier)	Emulsifies fats
	Pancreatic lipase (steapsin)	Triglycerides to diglycerides and monoglycerides in turn, then fatty acids and glycerol

of **cholecystokinin**, a local hormone from glands in the intestinal walls. In turn, cholecystokinin causes contraction of the gallbladder, relaxation of the sphincter muscle, and subsequent secretion of **bile** into the intestine via the common bile duct. The liver produces a large amount of dilute bile, then the gallbladder concentrates and stores it, ready for use with lipids as needed. The function of bile is that of an **emulsifier**. The process of *emulsification* is not a chemical digestive action itself, but it is an important first preparation step for the chemical digestion of lipids through its specific enzymes. This preparation process accomplishes two important tasks: (1) it breaks the lipids into small particles, or globules, which greatly enlarges the total surface area available for action of the enzyme, and (2) it lowers the surface tension of the finely dispersed and suspended lipid globules, which allows the enzymes to penetrate more easily. This process is similar to the wetting action of detergents. The bile also provides an alkaline medium for the action of the lipid enzyme lipase.

2. *Enzymes from the pancreas.* Pancreatic juice contains an enzyme for lipids and one for cholesterol. First, *pancreatic lipase*, a powerful lipid enzyme, breaks off one fatty acid at a time from the glycerol base of lipids. One fatty acid plus a diglyceride, then another fatty acid plus a monoglyceride, are produced in turn. Each successive step of this breakdown occurs with increasing difficulty. In fact, separation of the final fatty acid from the remaining monoglyceride is such a slow process that less than one third of the total fat present actually breaks down completely. The final products of lipid digestion to be absorbed are fatty acids, diglycerides, monoglycerides, and glycerol. Some remaining lipids may pass into the large intestine for fecal elimination. Second, the enzyme *cholesterol enterase* acts on free cholesterol to form cholesterol esters by combining free cholesterol and fatty acids in preparation for absorption.

3. *Enzyme from the small intestine.* The small intestine secretes an enzyme in the intestinal juice called *lecithinase*. As its name indicates, it acts on lecithin, a *phospholipid*, to break it down into its components for absorption.

A summary of lipid digestion in the successive parts of the gastrointestinal tract is given in Table 4.1.

ABSORPTION

The task of lipid absorption is not easy. The problem is that lipids are not soluble in water and blood is basically water. Hence lipids always require some type of solvent carrier. To accomplish this task of transporting lipids from the small intestine into the bloodstream, the body has three basic stages of operation.

Stage I: initial lipid absorption

In the small intestine, bile combines with products of lipid digestion in a **micellar bile-lipid complex**. This unique carrier system, shown in Figure 4.3, takes lipid digestion products along its initial passage into the intestinal wall.

Stage II: absorption within the intestinal wall

Once inside the wall of the small intestine, the bile separates from the lipid complex and returns in the *enterohepatic circulation* to accomplish its task over and over again. Two important actions on the lipid digestion products occur inside the intestinal wall: (1) *enteric*

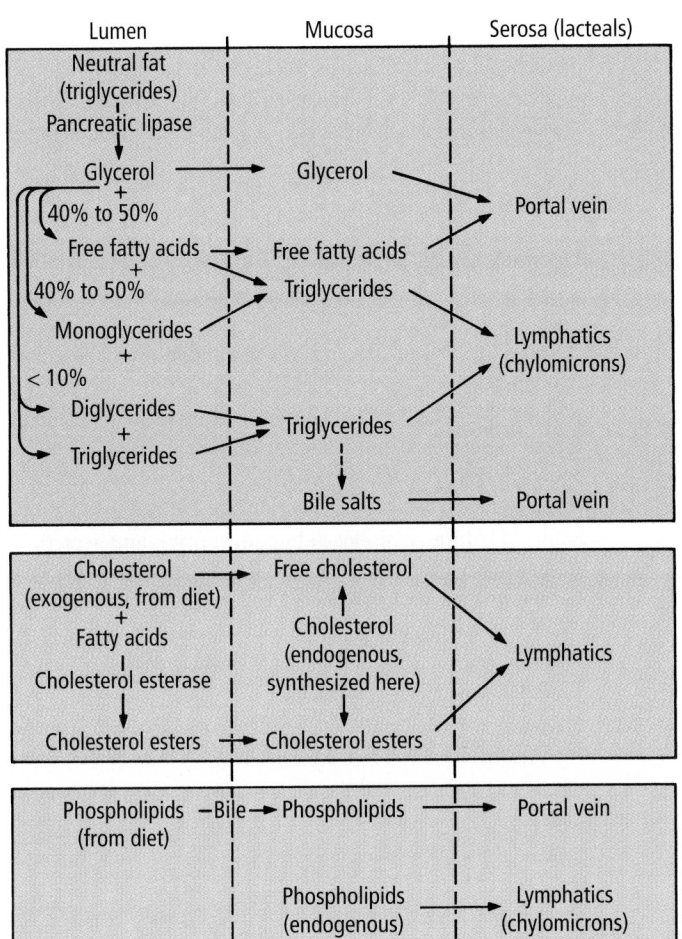

Figure 4.4   Absorption of fat, cholesterol, and phospholipids.

lipase action: an enteric lipase within the cells of the intestinal wall completes the digestion of the remaining glycerides, and (2) *triglyceride synthesis*: with the resulting fatty acids and glycerol, new human triglycerides are formed as body lipids, ready now for final absorption and circulation.

Stage III: final lipid absorption and transport

These newly formed human lipids—triglycerides—and other lipid materials present are combined with a small amount of protein covering to form lipoproteins called **chylomicrons**. These packages of lipids, in a milklike liquid called *chyle*, cross the cell membrane intact into the lymphatic system and then into the portal blood. Here a final lipid-clearing enzyme, *lipoprotein lipase*, helps clear the large meal load of dietary lipids from circulation. In the liver the lipids are converted to other lipoproteins for transport to the body cells for energy and other structural functions.

Figure 4.4 illustrates the general process of lipid absorption through its three stages.

bile   A fluid secreted by the liver and transported to the gallbladder for concentration and storage. It is released into the duodenum upon entry of fat to facilitate enzymatic fat digestion by acting as an emulsifying agent.

cholecystokinin (CCK)   A peptide hormone secreted by the duodenal mucosa in the presence of fat. The cholecystokinin causes the gallbladder to contract. This contraction propels bile into the duodenum, where it is needed to emulsify the fat. The fat is thus prepared for digestion and absorption.

chylomicrons   Initial lipoproteins, carrying a large fat load formed in the intestinal wall after a meal for absorption of the food fats into circulation.

emulsifier   An agent that breaks down large fat globules to smaller, uniformly distributed particles. This action is accomplished in the intestine chiefly by the bile acids, which lower surface tension of the fat particles. Emulsification greatly increases the surface area of fat, facilitating contact with fat-digesting enzymes.

micellar bile-lipid complex   A combination of bile and fat in which the bile emulsifies fat into very minute globules or particles that can be absorbed easily into the small intestine wall in preparation for the final stage of absorption into circulation to the cells.

METABOLISM

In the body cells, fatty acids are utilized as concentrated fuel to produce energy. These derived units of lipids have about twice the energy value of glucose products. As seen in the broad picture of metabolism discussed in Chapter 2, cell metabolism of lipids is closely interrelated with that of the other nutrients.

TO SUM UP

Lipids make up an essential nutrient class that, in addition to supplying the highest density of energy among the energy nutrients, insulates the body against low temperatures and protects vital organs from damage. Lipids also aid in the transmission of nerve impulses, production of metabolic precursors, formation of cell membrane structure, and transport of other molecules such as protein.

Lipids are composed of glycerol and attached fatty acids of varying lengths and degrees of saturation. Essential fatty acids are long-chain unsaturated fatty acids that cannot be manufactured by the body. The major one is linoleic acid. Its functions include improving skin integrity, lowering serum cholesterol levels, prolonging blood clotting time, and developing a group of special substances called *ecosanoids*—including *prostaglandins*—that are involved in many tissue activities, such as maintenance of the smooth muscle tone of blood vessels and platelet aggregations.

The type and amount of dietary lipids can affect health. Large amounts of saturated lipids and cholesterol increase the risk for cardiovascular disease and other general health problems. Too small an amount of lipids can result in a deficiency of the essential fatty acid, linoleic acid. Americans get about 35% of their total kcalories from lipids: the United States Dietary Guidelines recommend a limit of 30%. When lipids provide 10% or less of total kcalories, deficiency symptoms occur.

QUESTIONS FOR REVIEW

1. Two persons with strong family histories of cardiovascular disease are concerned about avoiding heart problems. Both reduce their cholesterol intake and avoid butter. The first person replaces butter with stick margarine made from corn oil, the second with corn oil itself. Which person might have more success with avoiding heart disease? Identify and describe two characteristics of a dietary lipid component that may affect this rate of success.

2. A woman runner concerned about her health dropped her total lipid intake to an amount supplying about 10% of her total caloric intake. What health problems would you expect her to encounter?

REFERENCES

1. Drewnowski A: Why do we like fat? *J Am Diet Assoc* 27(suppl 7): S58, 1997.
2. Staff report: Nutrition science and policy: WHO and FAO joint consultation: fats and oils in human nutrition, *Nutr Rev* 53(7):202, 1995.
3. Klein S, Jeejeebhoy KN: The malnourished patient: nutritional assessment and management. In Feldman M, Scharschmidt BF, Sleisenger MH, eds: *Gastrointestinal and liver disease,* ed 6, vol 1, Philadelphia, 1998, Saunders.
4. Sellin JH: Intestinal electrolyte absorption and secretion. In Feldman M, Scharschmidt BF, Sleisenger MH, eds: *Gastrointestinal and liver disease,* ed 6, vol 2, Philadelphia, 1998, Saunders.
5. Guyton AC, Hall JE: *Textbook of medical physiology,* ed 9, Philadelphia, 1996, Saunders.
6. Hernandez E, Lusas EW: Trends in transesterification of cottonseed oil, *Food Tech* 51(5):72, 1997.
7. Cleveland LE et al: "What we eat in America" survey, *Nutr Today* 32(1):37, 1997.
8. Stolz A: Liver physiology and metabolic function. In Feldman M, Scharschmidt BF, Sleisenger MH, eds: *Gastrointestinal and liver disease,* ed 6, vol 2, Philadelphia, 1998, Saunders.

FURTHER READING

Hahn NI: Replacing fat with food technology, *J Am Diet Assoc* 97(1):15, 1997.

McNutt K: What's bothering Olestra opponents? *Nutr Today* 32(1):41, 1997.

Jacobson MF: Letter to the editor: Olestra, *Nutr Today* 32(3):135, 1997.

These interesting articles describe the nature of fat replacers being developed in today's marketplace and the concerns raised by some users and professionals that are being explored and debated with the food industry developers.

Rolls BJ, Miller DL: Is the low-fat message giving people a license to eat more? *J Am Coll Nutr* 16(6):535, 1997.

Scarbrough FE: Some Food and Drug Administration perspectives of fat and fatty acids, *Am J Clin Nutr* 65(suppl): 1578S, 1997.

These authors, professors and administrators, provide interesting background in the ongoing debate concerning fat replacers and the broader questions raised concerning food labels to improve communication with consumers about fat and fatty acid contents of foods, the amount of fat in the American diet, and health-related problems.

Issues Answers

The dietary fat and cholesterol controversy

Over the past two decades, despite overwhelming evidence relating fat and cholesterol to heart disease, questions about the nature and extent of this relationship still seem to arise. What have we learned? Has learning led to actions? What issues remain? How are they being resolved?

Background

Controversy first arose when individual studies led to the first official concern about America's habit of consuming rich food. Justly alarmed by the increasing extent of major disease in the population, a Senate Committee on Nutrition and Health issued a plan for attacking the leading cause of death—coronary heart disease. Its approach was direct and apparently simple: it would advise millions of Americans to reduce their dietary intake of fats, saturated fats, and cholesterol. These early recommendations were based on research showing that people who eat large amounts of fat, as Americans do, tend to develop heart disease more often than people who follow leaner diets. This sounds reasonable. But it is not as simple as it sounds. Americans seem to love their fat, and a great many food industries with vested interests would like to whet these appetites.

We soon learned that getting Americans to reduce their fat intake was not easy then, nor is it any easier now, for several reasons:

1. *Taste and texture.* Fats make food more tasteful and give a pleasing texture. This is a taste cultivated over the past few years by our marketplace and is probably why some 40% to 45% of the kcalories of the American diet were then made up of fats.
2. *Prevalence in the diet.* Meat, milk, eggs, and cheese provide about half of the fat Americans consume. Because these products are so prevalent in the diet, the task of reducing animal fat components—such as saturated fats and cholesterol—is *very* challenging, to say the least.

Further, the task of making *any* dietary recommendations for Americans is always complicated by the nature of our society.

3. *Heterogenous population.* The United States population is such a heterogenous group—with wide variety of food preferences dictated by culture, religion, food availability, and personal likes and dislikes—that change is extremely difficult.

4. *Population size.* The United States population is so large—with persons who require a wide range of dietary fat, depending on individual health and energy needs—that making any standard to cover personal requirements is also difficult.

Obviously any recommendation that attempts to be specific about amounts of nutrients or types of food to eat would be difficult to make. Yet specifics were apparent in these initial guidelines:

- *Total fat.* Reduce total fat consumption to 30% of energy intake.
- *Saturated fat.* Reduce saturated fat consumption to about 10% of the total energy intake. Balance that with polyunsaturated and monounsaturated fats, which should account for about 10% of the energy intake.
- *Cholesterol.* Reduce cholesterol consumption to about 10% of the energy intake.

These initial guidelines also recommended that Americans cut their meat consumption to meet these recommendations. Obviously, this conflicted with the interests of meat-producing and meat-marketing industries.

During the following years, health officials and professional groups began to recognize that dietary guidelines must provide for a three-way balance among the following:

- The individual's *need* for fat
- The effects of *excess* dietary fat
- The public's *need* for education and guidance in preventive health

Apparently, these suggestions were taken to heart. Through two revisions our current national dietary guidelines have emerged, in essence advising Americans to eat a variety of foods, maintain an appropriate weight, and limit intake of total fat, saturated fat, and cholesterol. These early recommendations strengthened our preventive care approach to health maintenance and vascular disease. These goals are now embodied not only in the current dietary guidelines (see Chapter 1), but also in official reports, such as the National Research Council's *Diet and Health: Implications for Reducing Chronic Disease Risk* and the US Department of Health and Human Services' specific directions in *Healthy People 2000: National Health Promotion and Disease Prevention Objectives*. A part of this pattern was the establishment of the National

Cholesterol Education Program by the Heart, Lung, and Blood Institute of the National Institutes of Health, based on the strong findings of the large Lipid Clinics Coronary Primary Prevention Trials. A panel of experts brought together by the Institute, working with more than 20 health agencies, outlined for physicians important steps of cholesterol monitoring and diet as the primary attack on heart disease.

In addition, the Bogalusa Heart Study, a longitudinal study now in its twentieth year of monitoring the health and lifestyle of children growing into adulthood in the Louisiana town of Bogalusa, continues to reinforce the fact that the artery changes underlying heart disease begin early in life in genetically predisposed individuals and are enhanced by elevated serum cholesterol. This program's dedicated investigator and other cardiologists indicate that preventive cardiology should start early in life, especially with children at high risk, instilling principles of a "prudent" diet to control for excess fat, cholesterol, and energy intake, along with the value of exercise and an active life.

Current issues

The current debate focuses on four basic questions:

1. Why do the large number of studies that show a definite decline in heart disease with lowering cholesterol fail to show a similar reduction in deaths from heart disease?
2. How should we deal with children's diets in the light of the demonstrated diet-cholesterol link?
3. What do we do about the drug alternative in this age of scarce health care dollars?
4. And the most recent question raised is, how do we control the resulting increased carbohydrate intake, especially in sugars?

The question of heart disease mortality

Multifactorial disease. The question about results of the cholesterol campaign in terms of fewer deaths from heart disease appears to be part of the reality that heart disease is multifactorial, with numerous factors other than just cholesterol contributing to its development. These well-known factors include lifestyle behaviors such as lack of exercise, smoking, the consumption of excessive high-kcaloric food, and obesity; predisposing disease factors, such as hypertension and diabetes; and the important genetic factor. There is a difficulty in untangling the many intertwined factors. It also shows how difficult it is in a free-living population to know precisely what people eat and the limitations of the dietary history method. One large, ongoing study of coronary artery disease risk development in young adults reports that early data show a general difference between the recommended intakes of total fat, saturated fat, and cholesterol and the actual dietary intakes of

young adults, regardless of age and educational level. It seems that we still have a long way to go toward improving our food habits.

Data analysis. Another possible answer and resolution of the mortality issue may lie in the method used to analyze the large amount of data collected. For the most part, each of the many experimental and clinical studies has been analyzed separately. Now an Oxford University statistician indicates that the new technique of meta-analysis, or overview of all the accumulative data, would vastly add to the power of the analysis.

The question of children and cholesterol

An important question concerns what to do about screening and proposing dietary intervention for children. Longstanding studies show that fatty streaks of the artery disease process begin in childhood, as indicated by autopsies of young Americans killed in the Korean war that showed a high frequency of advanced lesions. Also, ongoing study that tracks children through adulthood has indicated a correlation between a childhood elevated blood cholesterol level and continued serum elevation in adulthood. But other investigators believe that drawbacks to childhood screening, family conflicts, the potential labeling, and as well as the cost of universal screening, exceed its benefits. Officially, the National Cholesterol Education Program has endorsed a specific cholesterol monitoring program limited to children over 2 years of age whose genetic predisposition is evidenced by parents who have premature coronary heart disease. Most families and practitioners express approval of this approach. A good plan with children's diets, expressed by one wise nutritionist, may well be a positive one of gradually reducing fat intake while maintaining a normal eating environment and avoiding strained relationships involving food. One of the easiest ways of focusing on the positive aspects of such a diet is to increase the child's intake of fruits and vegetables and low-fat whole-grain products—such as cereals and breads—in snacks and at meals, as well as to moderate the amounts of low-fat meats and nonfat milk.

The question of drug alternatives

A final question involves the alternative to failure of diet therapy—the use of drugs. Several drugs have proved useful in clinical studies for their cholesterol-lowering effect. But the magnitude of the cost involved for a significant number of our population would be enormous. Estimates for such drug therapy have ranged from $329 to $1744 per patient per year depending on the drug chosen and its dose. These figures are based on wholesale drug costs. It is clear that future recommendations for these drugs must include a careful assessment of their cost-effectiveness.

The question of high carbohydrate intake, especially sugars

This final question relates to the increased intake of carbohydrates resulting from control of fat intake. The relationship between a low-fat, high-carbohydrate diet and elevated fasting plasma triglyceride level has been known for some years. However, the effect of such a diet on plasma high-density lipoprotein (HDL) concentration has been somewhat ignored. Currently, evidence is accumulating from controlled trials that when carbohydrate replaces saturated fat in the diet there is a decrease in the level of plasma HDL. This effect is strongest with dietary sugars. However, it is also observed with diets high in complex carbohydrates such as starches. Also, large epidemiologic studies now show that populations consuming low-fat, high-carbohydrate diets have low plasma HDL concentrations. Katan and other researchers are now recommending that dietary saturated fats be replaced with monounsaturated and polyunsaturated fats instead of carbohydrates.

As you can see there are no easy answers. But there are real proposals that are bringing some solutions. In the meantime, perhaps more of us can examine our own lifestyles and turn our basic food habits in the lower fat direction.

References

Howell WH: Diet and blood lipids, *Nutr Today* 32(3):110, 1997.

Hu FB et al: Dietary fat intake and the risk of coronary heart disease in women, *N Engl J Med* 337(21):1491, 1997.

Katan MB: Effect of low-fat diets on plasma high-density lipoprotein concentrations, *Am J Clin Nutr* 67(suppl):573S, 1998.

Nicklas TA et al: Impact of meat consumption on nutritional quality and cardiovascular risk factors in young adults: the Bogalusa Heart Study, *J Am Diet Assoc* 95(8):887, 1995.

Olson RE: The folly of restricting fat in the diet of children, *Nutr Today* 30(6):234, 1995.

Schaefer EJ: Effects of dietary fatty acids on lipoproteins and cardiovascular disease risk: summary, *Am J Clin Nutr* 65(suppl):1655S, 1997.

Stevens VJ et al: Dietary Intervention Study in Children (DISC): intervention design and participation, *J Nutr Ed* 27(3):1995.

Tsetsonis NV et al: Acute effects of exercise on postprandial lipemia: a comparative study in trained and untrained middle-aged women, *Am J Clin Nutr* 65:525, 1997

Chapter

5

Proteins

In this chapter, which completes our introductory sequence on the macronutrients, we look at protein. It is quite different from its partners, carbohydrates and fats. Although protein also yields energy as needed, its main job is building and rebuilding body tissue. It is the body's major provider of nitrogen, the essential element for all living beings.

Here, then, we focus primarily on the body's builder. We see how protein accomplishes this unique task through its marvelous building units, the amino acids.

PHYSICAL AND CHEMICAL NATURE OF PROTEINS

GENERAL DEFINITION

When Dutch chemist Johann Mulder (1802-1880) first classified protein in 1838 as a prime substance of all life forms, he could scarcely guess how far-reaching his work would become. From Mulder's early grasp of what he was seeing, protein has become recognized as the essential life-substance of all living matter.[1] Today we know as fact his early insight.

In many ways, proteins act to shape our lives. They act as structural units to build our bodies. As enzymes, they change our food into nutrients our cells can use. As antibodies, they shield us from disease. As peptide hormones, they send messages that coordinate continuous body activity. Proteins do much more: they guide our growth during childhood and then maintain our bodies throughout adulthood. They ensure our nutritional well-being. They make us the unique individuals that we are.

CHEMICAL NATURE

The proteins we eat do none of this wonderful work as proteins. Their specific structural chemical units—*amino acids* released at initial digestion—provide the living, working currency of our body cells. These unique units are composed of the basic elements carbon, hydrogen, and oxygen and the special element of all living matter—nitrogen. It is with these basic units of life-substance that we begin this chapter.

THE NATURE OF AMINO ACIDS

The story of protein must begin with its unique building materials, the **amino acids**. A major life-sustaining task of the human body is the constant building and rebuilding of all its body tissues. The name of these building units, the amino acids, indicates that they have a dual nature. The word *amino* refers to base (alkaline) substance, so we at once confront a paradox. How can a chemical material be both a base and an acid at the same time and why is this important here? Consider the significance of this fact as you first examine the structure of amino acids.

GENERAL PATTERN AND SPECIFIC STRUCTURE

A common baseline pattern holds for all amino acids. First, look carefully at the characteristic common core pattern built around a central *alpha*-carbon:

Amino group — NH_2 — C — COOH — Carboxyl group; H (α-carbon atom); R (Side-chain group)

Now note here the significant parts of the amino acid structure:

1. *Amino (base, NH$_2$) group.* This part of the molecule carries the essential nitrogen and, in its ionic form, the positive charge.
2. *Carboxyl (acid, COOH) group.* This part of the molecule is the characteristic acid group in all acids and, in the amino acid ionic form, it carries the negative charge.
3. *Varying attached radical.* The R stands for *radical*, a general term for parts of a chemical compound. In the common core pattern figure it stands for the varying attached side chains on amino acids, each one different, thus making each amino acid specific.[2] Note the structure of the two simplest amino acids glycine and alanine based on the core amino acid pattern:

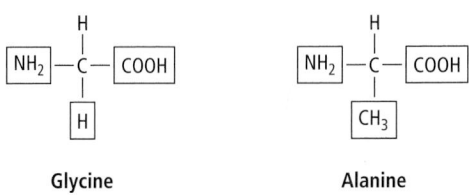

Glycine   Alanine

Also, compare a larger size amino acid, for example, the newest named essential amino acid *arginine* (see p. 70), which has an extended carbon chain and three additional nitrogen radicals.

Thus it is the unique side group radical (R) attached to the common baseline pattern that makes each of the amino acids that constitute protein unique. Amino acids are made of the same three elements—carbon, hydrogen, and oxygen—that make up carbohydrates and fats. But amino acids and their proteins have an additional important element—*nitrogen*—as the base (alkaline—NH$_2$) portion of their structure. There are 22 amino acids, all of which are important in the body's metabolism. They all have the same basic core pattern, but each is unique because it has a specific different side group attached.

ESSENTIAL AMINO ACIDS

All amino acids are necessary for building our various body tissue proteins. However, 10 of these 22 amino

---

amino acid An acid containing the essential element nitrogen (in the chemical group —NH$_2$). Amino acids are the structural units of protein and are the basic building blocks of the body.

acids are designated as **essential amino acids** because the body cannot synthesize them in sufficient quantity or at all. The most recently (1992) declared essential amino acid is arginine, based on its sufficient, though limited, quantity produced by the body, and discovery of its therapeutic properties, for which scientists declared it "molecule of the year."[3,4]

$$NH_2 - \underset{\underset{\displaystyle CH_2}{\overset{\displaystyle |}{\underset{\displaystyle CH_2}{\overset{\displaystyle |}{\underset{\displaystyle CH_2}{\overset{\displaystyle |}{\underset{\displaystyle NH}{\overset{\displaystyle |}{\underset{\displaystyle C=NH}{\overset{\displaystyle |}{\underset{\displaystyle NH_2}{\overset{\displaystyle |}{}}}}}}}}}}{\overset{\displaystyle H}{\overset{\displaystyle |}{C}}} - COOH$$

Arginine

Arginine modulates the bioavailability of nitrous oxide (NO), a powerful vasodilator in the blood vessels that inhibits atherogenesis (see Chapter 19). Increasingly, the biochemical mystique and complexity of the NO molecule is extending to the amino acid arginine from which it is derived.[5] The 10 essential amino acids are listed in Table 5.1. The remaining amino acids—12 of them, which we can synthesize in our own bodies—are then labeled "nonessential" amino acids. Actually this is a poor choice of label in the sense that all 22 of the amino acids are necessary for building the various body tissue proteins. However, the concept of *dietary* essentiality for

Table 5.1	Amino acids required in human nutrition, grouped according to nutritional dietary essentiality
Essential amino acids	**Nonessential amino acids**
Arginine	Alanine
Histidine	Aspargine
Isoleucine	Aspartic acid
Leucine	Cystine (cysteine)
Lysine	Glutamic acid
Methionine	Glutamine
Phenylalanine	Glycine
Threonine	Hydroxylysine
Trypotophan	Hydroxyproline
Valine	Proline
	Serine
	Tyrosine

From Williams SR: *Nutrition and diet therapy,* ed 8, St Louis, 1997, Mosby.

these so-designated 10 amino acids is important to remember in assessing protein quality.

This dual chemical structure of amino acids, combining both acid (**carboxyl** group—COOH) and base (amino—NH₂) factors, gives them a unique **amphoteric** nature. As a result, an amino acid in solution can behave either as an acid or a base, depending on the pH of the solution. This means that amino acids have a **buffer** capacity, which is an important clinical characteristic.

THE BUILDING OF PROTEINS

The building units, amino acids, are used by the body to construct specific tissue proteins. This process is made possible by the nature of amino acids, which enables them to form peptide linkages and arrange themselves into peptide chains.

TISSUE PROTEIN STRUCTURE

Peptide bond

The dual chemical nature of amino acids—the presence of a base (amino—NH₂) group containing nitrogen on one end and an acid (carboxyl—COOH) group on the other—enables them to join in the characteristic chain structure of proteins. The end amino group of one amino acid joins the end carboxyl group of another amino acid beside it. This characteristic joining of specific amino acids in a specific sequence to make a specific protein is called a **peptide bond**. Long chains of amino acids linked in this manner form proteins and are called *polypeptides*. These peptides may vary in chain length from relatively short chains of 3 to 15 amino acids, called *oligopeptides*, to medium-sized polypeptides, such as insulin, with chains of either 21 or 30 amino acids.

Large complex proteins

Larger still are complex proteins of several hundred amino acids that require special techniques to study, such as x-ray crystallography. Scientists now can view polypeptides in the exciting four-dimensional technique of nuclear magnetic resonance (NMR) spectroscopy, allowing them to examine closely much bigger complex proteins. This new view enables researchers to learn how long protein chains fold and twist in space.[6,7] This knowledge helps them understand how enzymes and other proteins work, as well as aiding them in new drug design.

To make a compact structure, the long polypeptide chains coil or fold back on themselves in a spiral shape called a **helix** or in a "pleated sheet" arrangement. They are held together in some instances by additional strengthening cross-links of sulfur and hydrogen bonds.

TYPES OF PROTEINS

The proteins illustrate a huge diversity of compounds produced by specific amino acid linkages. As a result, according to their varied specific structures, tissue proteins perform many vital roles in body structure and metabolism. Consider several examples here.

Myosin

This fibrous type of protein in muscle fiber, shown in Figure 5.1, is composed of 153 amino acid long chains that coil and unfold on contraction and relaxation. Shaped into long rods, these fibers end in two-headed bundles so that they can change their shape and bend, making it possible to tighten and contract muscles and then relax them.

Collagen

This structural protein, shown in Figure 5.2, is made up of three separate polypeptide chains wound around each other to produce a triple helix. Thus strengthened, the collagen is shaped into long rods and bundled into stiff fibers because its job is to strengthen bone, cartilage, skin, and other body structures to maintain their form.

Hemoglobin

This globular-type protein, shown in Figure 5.3, is made up of four globin polypeptide chains in a molecule of hemoglobin. Each chain has several hundred amino acids, conjugated with the nonprotein portion—an oxygen-carrying pigment *heme*—which attaches to iron. The globin, in a compact globular shape, wraps around the heme and forms protective pockets to secure the iron and facilitate its exposure to oxygen as it travels in circulating red blood cells.

Albumin

This major plasma protein is made up of similar compact globular shaping. It consists of a single polypeptide chain of 584 amino acids, twisted and coiled into helixes held together by 17 disulfide bridges.[8,9]

Other examples of tissue proteins shaped for special structural or metabolic roles in the body include antibodies of the immune system, such as gamma globulin; the blood protein fibrinogen; some regulating hormones, such as insulin, thyroxin, and the gastrointestinal peptides; and all of the enzymes.

COMPLETE AND INCOMPLETE FOOD PROTEINS

A common way of designating the quality of protein foods is whether they are complete or incomplete in terms of the amounts of essential amino acids that they contain.

Complete protein foods

Foods called complete protein foods are those that contain all the essential amino acids in sufficient quantity and ratio to meet the body's needs. These proteins are of animal origin: eggs, milk, cheese, and meat, including

---

amphoteric Having opposite characteristics; capable of acting either as an acid or a base, combining with both acids and bases.

buffer Mixture of acidic and alkaline components that, when added to a solution, is able to protect the solution against wide variations in its pH, even when strong acids and bases are added to it. If an acid is added, the alkaline partner reacts to counteract the acidic effect. If a base is added, the acid partner reacts to counteract the alkalizing effect. A solution to which a buffer has been added is called a buffered solution.

carboxyl (COOH) The monovalent radical, -COOH, occurring in those organic acids termed carboxylic acids.

essential amino acid Any one of ten amino acids that the body cannot synthesize at all or in sufficient amounts to meet body needs, so it must be supplied by the diet and is hence a *dietary* essential. These ten specific amino acids are arginine, histidine, isoleucine, leucine, lysine, methionine, phenylalanine, threonine, tryptophan, and valine.

helix A coiled structure as found in protein. Some are simple chain coils; others are made of several coils, as in a triple helix.

peptide bond The characteristic joining of amino acids to form proteins. Such a chain of amino acids is termed a peptide. Depending on its size, it may be a dipeptide fragment of protein or a large polypeptide.

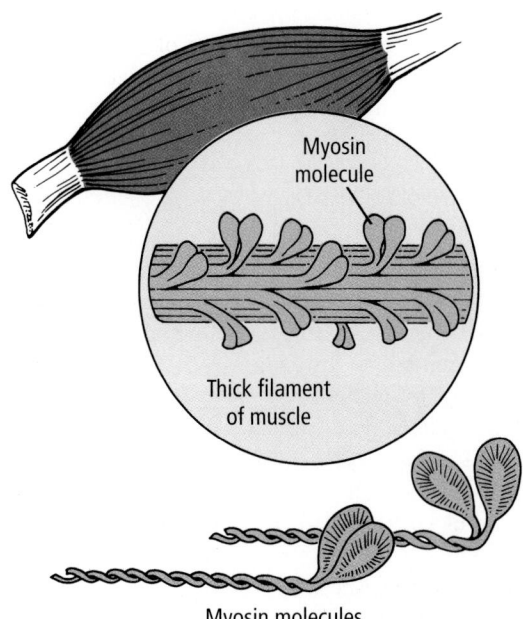

Myosin molecule

Thick filament of muscle

Myosin molecules

Figure 5.1   Myosin is a globulin in muscle that, in combination with actin, forms actomyosin, the fundamental contractile unit of muscle active with ATP.

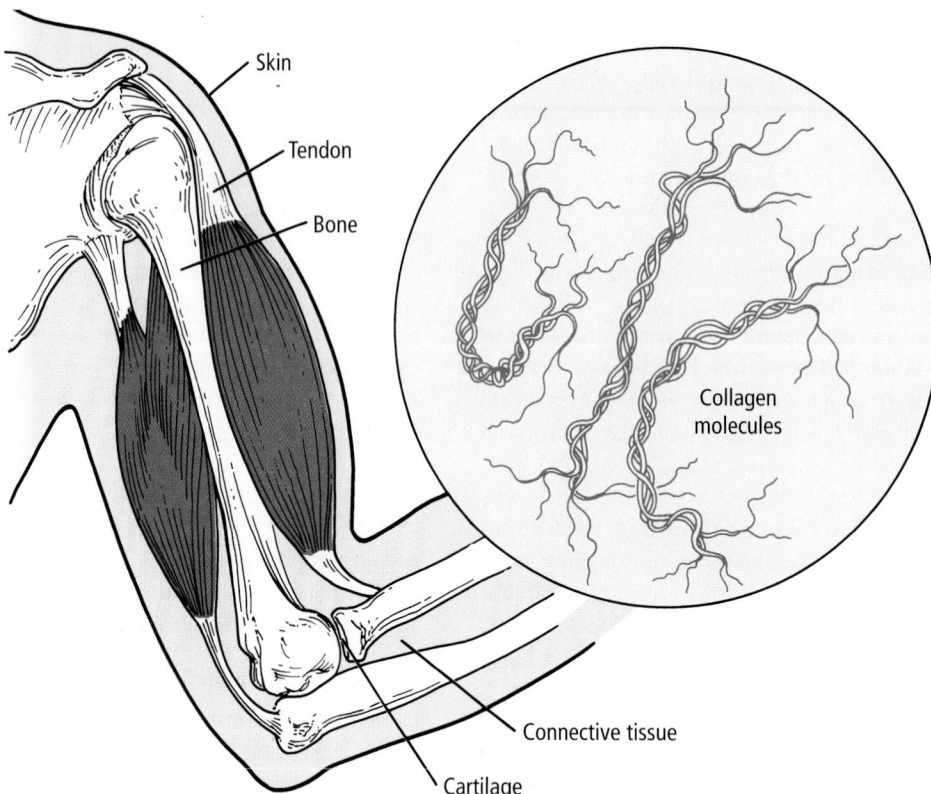

Figure 5.2   Tissues that contain collagen, the basic structural material forming connective tissue throughout the body.

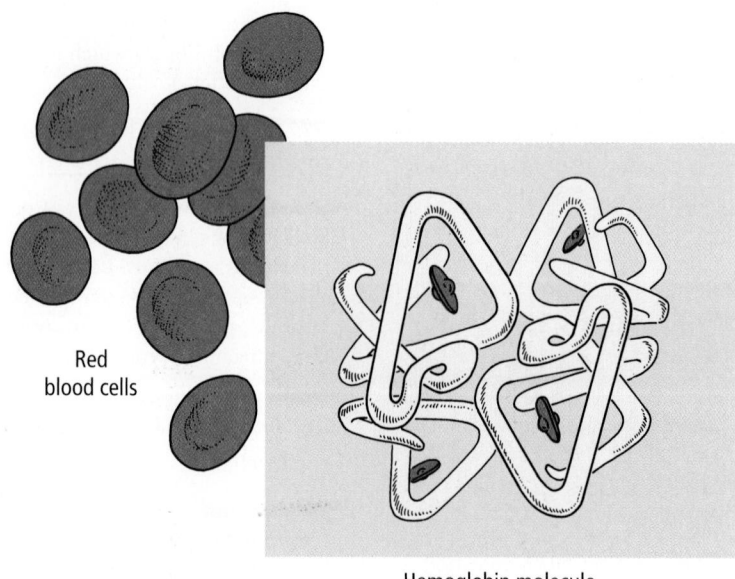

Figure 5.3   Hemoglobin is an oxygen-carrying protein of red blood cells.

poultry and fish. Another protein of animal origin, gelatin, does not qualify because it lacks three essential amino acids—tryptophan, valine, and isoleucine and has only small amounts of leucine.

Incomplete protein foods

Foods called **incomplete protein foods** are those deficient in one or more of the essential amino acids. These proteins are mostly of plant origin: grains, legumes, nuts, and seeds. In a mixed diet, however, animal and plant proteins complement one another. Even a mixture of plant proteins alone can provide adequate amounts of amino acids when our basic use of various grains is expanded to include soy protein and other dried legume (beans and peas) storage proteins.[10-12] The value of *variety* in the diet is therefore evident.

In the final analysis, the most significant measure of the protein quality of the diet depends on use of a variety of foods in the total food mix consumed, so that the amino acid patterns of the various diet components, both complete and incomplete food proteins, complement one another and the total protein intake is sufficient to meet the body's total need. A sound diet is the best way to obtain needed protein, eliminating any need for amino acid supplements (see *Practical Application* box, p. 74).

FUNCTIONS OF PROTEIN

GROWTH AND TISSUE-BUILDING MAINTENANCE

The primary function of dietary protein is to supply building material for growth and maintenance of body tissue. It does this by furnishing amino acids in appropriate amounts and types for efficient synthesis of specific cellular tissue proteins. Nitrogen, in its key position in amino acids and hence in building body tissues, is *the* vital element in our body's structure. Without it, we—and life as we know it on our planet—would not exist. Unlike carbohydrates and fats, which contain no nitrogen, protein is about 16% nitrogen. Protein also supplies amino acids for other essential nitrogen-containing substances such as enzymes and hormones.

SPECIFIC PHYSIOLOGIC ROLES

All amino acids supplied by dietary protein participate in growth and tissue maintenance. But some also perform other important physiologic and metabolic roles. For example, *methionine* is an agent in the formation of choline, which is a precursor of acetylcholine, one of the major neurotransmitters in the brain. In addition, methionine is the precursor not only of the nonessential amino acid cystine, but also of the lesser known ones **carnitine** and **taurine**, which are now known to have widespread metabolic functions (see *To Probe Further* box,

p. 80). *Tryptophan* is the precursor of the B vitamin niacin and of the neurotransmitter serotonin. *Phenylalanine* is the precursor of the nonessential amino acid tyrosine, leading to formation of the hormones thyroxine and epinephrine. In addition, protein antibodies provide essential components of the body's immune system, and plasma proteins guard water balance. In the extreme metabolic stress of malnutrition in children, kwashiorkor and marasmus, for example, decreased rates of whole-body protein synthesis and breakdown give stark evidence to these constant protein needs for normal growth and development.[13,14]

AVAILABLE ENERGY

Protein also contributes to the body's overall energy metabolism. This occurs as needed in the fasting state or during extended physical effort, such as marathon running, but not in the fed state. After the removal of the nitrogen-containing portion of the constituent amino acid, the amino acid residue—its carbon "skeleton" is called a *keto*-acid—may be converted either to glucose or to fat. On the average, 58% of the total dietary protein may become available when needed to be burned for energy. Thus sufficient amounts of nonprotein kcalories from carbohydrates are always needed to spare protein for its primary building purpose and to prevent unnecessary protein breakdown in the process of providing energy.

DIGESTION-ABSORPTION-METABOLISM SUMMARY

After the source of basic body building materials—the food protein—is secured, it must be changed into the needed ready-to-use building units—the amino acids. This work is done through the successive parts of the gastrointestinal tract by the mechanical and chemical processes of digestion.

---

carnitine A naturally occurring amino acid ($C_{17}H_{15}NO_3$) formed from methionine and lysine, required for transport of long-chain fatty acids across the mitochondrial membrane, where they are oxidized as fuel substrate for metabolic energy.

incomplete protein food A protein food having a ratio of amino acids different from that of the average body protein and therefore less valuable for nutrition than complete protein food.

taurine A sulfur-containing amino acid, $NH_2(CH_2)_2$ SO_2OH, formed from the essential amino acid methionine. It is found in various body tissues, such as lungs and muscles, and in bile and breast milk.

Amino acids on the grocery shelf

Have you seen persons shopping for amino acids and taking them singly or as multiple supplements for a number of supposed improvements in health and fitness or as remedies for health problems? Such persons buy tryptophan for insomnia, lysine and arginine for herpes, even glutamine for gluttony, and multiple combinations for athletic prowess or chronic illness. But these and other such health claims have repeatedly been refuted.

Two groups of persons most vulnerable to such claims are athletes and elderly persons. In the first group, athletes and their coaches are always searching for that "competitive edge" and often turn to various substances to advance it. The belief that protein is a major energy source and builds muscle strength leads to the use of amino acid supplements in an effort to attain this result. But carbohydrates and fats—not proteins—are fuel substrates in muscle tissue, and excess protein only places excess metabolic burden on the body. It is exercise, not protein, that increases and strengthens muscles. In the second group, older adults seek to avoid health problems or relieve the pain and stress of chronic illnesses of aging. The belief that amino acids will provide such magic elixirs is ill advised. They are both an expensive burden for

many older adults on fixed incomes and an ineffective source of needed protein, the latter of which is better found in an improved diet containing all the nutrients that work best together.

In the case of one essential amino acid—tryptophan—touted among food faddists as a "natural" agent to relieve depression and insomnia, the megadose toxic levels of use—about 3000 mg every night—had severe, even deadly, consequences for a number of persons. When a significant number of such cases were reported, including 19 deaths, the Food and Drug Administration recalled all products containing tryptophan nationwide. The products may now be off the shelves of health food stores and pharmacies, but the lesson of such abuses remains.

This health fad of "amino acid shopping" is probably only partially based on research redefining our ideas about "essential" and "nonessential" amino acids. More likely, it is taking advantage of the public's ignorance regarding the function of amino acids. Even if each individual amino acid is found to have a specific physiologic effect, they must *all* be present in specific amounts to build and maintain body proteins.

Thus persons concerned about their amino acid intake and seeking some supplement to enhance it should be cautioned as follows:

- They probably already get at least twice as much protein as they need, including all the essential amino acids, if their diet is based on typical American fare.
- Research on the effect of each amino acid refutes claims in most cases and warns of possible severe effects, even death, of toxic megadose abuse, as was the case with tryptophan.
- They can get all the currently known essential amino acids from a diet that includes even small amounts of animal products such as eggs and/or milk with a wide mix of vegetables.
- In the final analysis, such individuals need to be reminded, as researchers and practitioners alike state: "Sound diet is still the best way to maintain health."

References

Hertzman PA et al: Association of the eosinophilia-myalgia syndrome with the ingestion of tryptophan, *N Engl J Med* 322:869, 1990.

Kessler DA: The Food and Drug Administration and its problems, *N Engl J Med* 326:70, 1992.

Philen RM et al: Survey of advertising for nutritional supplements in health and bodybuilding magazines, *JAMA* 268(8):1009, 1992.

Mouth

In the mouth, only mechanical breaking up of the protein foods by chewing occurs. Here the food particles are mixed with saliva and passed on as a semisolid mass into the stomach.

Stomach

Because proteins are such large complex structures, a series of enzymes is necessary to finally break them down to produce the amino acids. These chemical changes, through a system of enzymes, begin in the stomach. In fact, the stomach's chief digestive function in relation to all foods is the initial partial enzymatic breakdown of protein. Three agents in the gastric secretions help with this task: pepsin, hydrochloric acid, and rennin.

1. **Pepsin.** The main gastric enzyme, specific for proteins, is **pepsin**. It is first produced as an inactive **proenzyme (zymogen)**, *pepsinogen*, by a single layer of cells (the chief cells) in the mucosa of the stomach wall. Pepsinogen then requires hydrochloric acid to be transformed into the enzyme pepsin. The active pepsin then begins splitting the peptide linkages between the protein's amino acids, changing the large polypeptides into successively smaller peptides. If the protein were held in the stomach longer, pepsin could continue the breakdown until individual amino acids resulted. However, with normal gastric emptying time, only the beginning stage is completed by the action of pepsin.

2. **Hydrochloric acid.** Gastric hydrochloride is an important catalyst in gastric protein digestion. It provides the acid medium necessary to convert pepsinogen to pepsin. Clinical problems result from lack of the normal secretion of hydrochloric acid.

3. **Rennin.** This gastric enzyme (not to be confused with the renal enzyme *renin*) is present only in infancy and childhood and disappears in adulthood. It is especially important in the infant's digestion of milk. Rennin and calcium act on the casein of milk to produce a curd. By coagulating milk, rennin prevents too rapid a passage of the food from the child's stomach.

Small intestine

Protein digestion begins in the acid medium of the stomach and is completed in the alkaline medium of the small intestine. A number of enzymes, from secretions of both the pancreas and the intestine, take part in protein digestion:

1. **Pancreatic secretions.** Three enzymes produced by the pancreas continue breaking down proteins to simpler and simpler substances:
   - **Trypsin** is secreted first as inactive trypsinogen and is then activated by the hormone enterokinase, which is produced by glands in the duodenal wall. The active enzyme trypsin then acts on protein and large polypeptide fragments carried over from the stomach, producing smaller polypeptides and dipeptides.
   - **Chymotrypsin** is produced by special cells in the pancreas as inactive chymotrypsinogen and then activated by the trypsin already present. Chymotrypsin continues the same protein-splitting action of trypsin.

- **Carboxypeptidase**, as its name indicates, attacks the carboxyl end (acid—COOH) of the peptide chain. It in turn produces smaller peptides and some free amino acids.

2. **Intestinal secretions.** Glands in the intestinal wall produce two more protein-splitting enzymes in the peptidase group:
   - **Aminopeptidase** releases amino acids one at a time from the nitrogen-containing amino end (base—NH_2) of the peptide chain. Through this cleavage, it produces smaller short-chain peptides and free amino acids.
   - **Dipeptidase**, the final enzyme in this protein-splitting system, breaks the remaining dipeptides into their two, now free, amino acids.

Through this total system of protein-splitting enzymes, the large complex proteins are broken down into progressively smaller peptide chains and finally into free amino acids, now ready for absorption by the intestinal mucosa. A summary of these steps in protein digestion is given in Table 5.2.

ABSORPTION

The construction sites in the body for building necessary specific tissue proteins are in the *cells*. Each cell, depending on its particular nature and function, has a

---

aminopeptidase Protein-splitting enzyme that cuts the peptide bond (linkage) at the amino end of amino acids, splitting off the amino group $-NH_2$.

carboxypeptidase A protein enzyme that splits off the chemical group *carboxyl* (-COOH) at the end of peptide chains, acting on the peptide bond of the terminal amino acid having a free-end carboxyl group.

chymotrypsin One of the protein-splitting and milk-curdling pancreatic enzymes, activated in the intestine from precursor chymotrypsinogen. It breaks peptide linkages of the amino acids phenylalanine and tyrosine.

dipeptidase Final enzyme in the protein-splitting series that cleaves the one remaining amino acid bond in dipeptides.

pepsin The main gastric enzyme specific for proteins. Pepsin begins breaking large protein molecules into shorter chain polypeptides, proteoses, and peptones. Gastric hydrochloric acid is necessary to activate pepsin.

proenzyme An inactive precursor converted to the active enzyme by the action of an acid, another enzyme, or other means. Also called zymogen.

trypsin A protein-splitting enzyme formed in the intestine by action of enterokinase on the inactive precursor trypsinogen.

Table 5.2   Summary of protein digestion

| Organ | Enzyme | | | Digestive action |
	Inactive precursor	Activator	Active enzyme	
Mouth			None	Mechanical only
Stomach (acidic)	Pepsinogen	Hydrochloric acid	Pepsin	Protein $\rightarrow$ polypeptides
			Rennin (infants) (calcium necessary for activity)	Casein $\rightarrow$ coagulated curd
Intestine (alkaline)				
Pancreas	Trypsinogen	Enterokinase	Trypsin	Protein, polypeptides $\rightarrow$ polypeptides, dipeptides
	Chymotrypsinogen	Active trypsin	Chymotrypsin	Protein, polypeptides $\rightarrow$ polypeptides, dipeptides
			Carboxypeptidase	Polypeptides $\rightarrow$ simpler peptides, dipeptides, amino acids
Intestine			Aminopeptidase	Polypeptides $\rightarrow$ peptides, dipeptides, amino acids
			Dipetidase	Dipeptides $\rightarrow$ amino acids

specific job to do. Thus its proteins must be specifically structured.

Absorption of amino acids

The end products of protein digestion are the amino acids. They are water soluble, so their absorption directly into the water-based bloodstream poses no problem. These building units are rapidly absorbed from the small intestine into the portal blood system through the fine network of villus capillaries, by means of competitive active transport.

1. *Active transport system.* Most of the amino acid absorption takes place in the first section of the small intestine, the duodenum. An energy-dependent active transport, using pyridoxine (vitamin B_6) as a carrier, absorbs the amino acids into the blood circulation, delivering them into the cells for eventual metabolism.

2. *Competition for absorption.* When we eat a mixed diet containing a variety of different amino acids, the amino acids compete with each other for absorption. The amino acid present in the largest quantity retards the absorption of the others. In plasma, circulating amino acids also compete for entry receptor sites for transport across cell membranes into the cell.

Absorption of peptides and whole proteins

A few larger fragments of short-chain peptides or smaller intact proteins are absorbed as such and then by **hydrolysis** within the absorbing cells yield their amino acids. These whole protein molecules may play a part in the development of immunity and sensitivity. For example, antibodies in the mother's colostrum, the premilk breast secretion, are passed on to her nursing infant.

METABOLISM

In human nutrition the amino acids are the "metabolic currency" of protein. It is with the fate of these vital compounds that the metabolism of protein is ultimately concerned. Protein's fascinating array of complex metabolic activities are intricately interwoven with those of carbohydrates and fats. Here we will look briefly at the fundamental metabolic concept of protein and nitrogen balance. This will provide a base for relating the tissue-building processes of **anabolism** with those of the breaking-down processes of **catabolism** to maintain these important protein balances.

The concept of balance

Many interdependent checks and balances exist throughout the body to keep it in working order. There is a constant ebb and flow of materials, a building up and breaking down of parts, and a depositing and taking up of components. The body has built-in controls that operate as finely tuned coordinated responses to meet any situation that disturbs its normal condition or function. This resulting state of dynamic equilibrium is called **homeostasis**, and the various mechanisms designed to preserve it are called *homeostatic mechanisms*. This highly sensitive balance between body parts and functions is life-sustaining. As more and more is learned about human nutrition and physiology, older ideas of a rigid body structure are giving way to this important concept of *dynamic equilibrium*—balance amid constant change. All body constituents are in a constant state of flux, although some tissues are more actively engaged than others. This dynamic concept can be seen in all metabolism. It is especially striking in protein metabolism.

Protein balance

Overall protein balance involves concepts of protein turnover, compartments, amino acid pool, and nitrogen balance.

1. *Protein turnover.* For a number of years the use of radioactive isotopes has clearly demonstrated that the body's protein tissues are continuously being broken down into amino acids and then resynthesized into tissue proteins. When "labeled" amino acids are fed, they can be traced—that is, rapidly incorporated into various body tissue proteins.   The rate of this protein turnover varies in different tissues. It is highest in the intestinal mucosa, liver, pancreas, kidney, and plasma. It is lower in muscle, brain, and skin. It is much slower in structural tissues such as collagen and bone.

2. *Protein compartments.* Body protein exists in a balance between two compartments—tissue protein and plasma protein. These stores are further balanced with dietary protein intake. Protein from one compartment may be drawn to supply need in the other. For example, during fasting, resources from the body protein stores may be used for tissue synthesis. But even when the intake of protein and other nutrients is adequate, the tissue proteins are still being constantly broken down, reshaped, and reformed according to body need. Such a dynamic state is necessary to life and growth because the body is an open system. It must sustain a dynamic balance not only within its own internal environment but also with its larger and extended external environment.

   The body's state of stability then is the result of tissue **protein balance** between the rates of protein breakdown (catabolism) and protein synthesis (anabolism). In periods of growth the synthesis rate is higher so that new tissue can be formed. In conditions of starvation, wasting disease, and more gradually as aging continues in elderly persons, tissue breakdown exceeds that of synthesis, and the body gradually deteriorates.

3. *Metabolic amino acid pool.* Amino acids derived from tissue breakdown and amino acids from dietary protein digestion and absorption both contribute to a common collective metabolic "pool" of amino acids throughout the body that are available for use (Figure 5.4). A balance of amino acids is thus maintained to supply the body's constant needs. Shifts in balances between tissue breakdown and dietary protein intake ensure a balanced mixture of amino acids. From this reserve pool, specific amino acids are supplied to synthesize specific body proteins.

4. *Nitrogen balance.* Another useful reference for indicating a person's state of protein balance is **nitrogen balance**. Total nitrogen balance involves all sources of nitrogen in the body—protein nitrogen as well as nonprotein nitrogen present in other compounds, such as urea, uric acid, ammonia, and other body tissues and fluids. It is the net result of nitrogen gains and losses in all the body protein. A person is in a harmful state of negative nitrogen balance when the loss of body protein exceeds the input of food protein. Such a state exists in conditions such as long-term illness, a hypermetabolic wasting disease, or starvation.

PROTEIN REQUIREMENTS

It is clear that protein is an essential nutrient. But just how much and what kind do we actually need? We know that some people get far less than they need. On a worldwide basis, protein-energy malnutrition is a major health concern, especially in underdeveloped

anabolism Metabolic process by which body tissues are built.

catabolism The breaking-down phase of metabolism, the opposite of anabolism. Catabolism includes all the processes in which complex substances are progressively broken down into simpler ones. Catabolism usually involves the release of energy. Together, anabolism and catabolism constitute metabolism, which is the coordinated operation of anabolic and catabolic processes into a dynamic balance of energy and substance.

homeostasis State of relative dynamic equilbrium within the body's internal environment; a balance achieved through the operation of various interrelated physiologic mechanisms.

hydrolysis Process by which a chemical compound is split into other simpler compounds by taking up the elements of water, as in the manufacture of infant formulas to produce easier-to-digest derivatives of the main protein casein, the cow's milk base. This process occurs naturally in digestion.

nitrogen balance The metabolic balance between nitrogen intake in dietary protein and output in urinary nitrogen compounds such as urea and creatinine. For every 6.25 g dietary protein consumed, 1 g nitrogen is excreted.

protein balance Body tissue protein balance between building up tissue (anabolism) and breaking down tissue (catabolism) to maintain healthy body growth and maintenance.

countries. In contrast, however, protein deficiency is not a problem in America and most other Western societies. Actually, most persons in America eat two or three times as much protein as they really need, largely as a result of the extensive role of meat and dairy products in cultural food habits. For example, United States surveys have indicated that foods of animal origin contribute about two thirds of the daily protein intake, with some 48% from meat, including poultry and fish; 17% from dairy products; and 4% from eggs.[15] But such excess protein intake often creates other problems. First, excessive intake of animal protein foods—which carry animal fat—can contribute to obesity and vascular health problems. Second, the excessive nitrogen load can place accumulative burden on the kidneys for nitrogen excretion. Clinicians have begun to raise questions about the long-term effects of habitual excess protein intake on the human kidney, designed in earlier ages to handle a different supply of protein.

FACTORS INFLUENCING PROTEIN REQUIREMENTS

Tissue growth

The primary purpose of protein in the diet is to supply amino acids in the quantity and quality necessary for growth and maintenance of tissue. Thus any period of growth increases the need for protein. Growth-related factors include age, body size, and general physical state. Also, special periods of rapid growth—such as the growth of the fetus and maternal tissue during pregnancy—require added protein.

Diet

Other factors include the nature of the protein in the diet and its ratio or pattern of amino acids. There must be sufficient nonprotein foods in the diet to have a protein-sparing effect, so that the total amount of protein will not be diminished for energy requirements. Also, the digestibility and absorption of the protein is affected by the cooking of the food, and time intervals between eating protein foods lowers the competition for absorption sites and enzymes.

Illness or disease

Any illness or disease will usually increase the requirement for protein. Diseases accompanied by fever usually increase the need for protein because of the increase in basal metabolic rate and the general breaking down of tissue. Traumatic injury requires extensive tissue rebuilding. Postsurgical states require protein for wound healing and to replenish losses. Extensive tissue destruction, as occurs with burns, requires considerable increase in protein intake for the healing process (see Chapter 22).

MEASUREMENT OF PROTEIN REQUIREMENTS

It is evident, then, that two basic measures of protein requirement must be considered: quantity and quality.

Protein quantity

The quantity of protein needed is the basis for establishing the total protein requirement. Actually, the human body *requires* somewhat less than the nutrient standards state because the standard *allows* for a safety margin to cover the variety of needs in a given population. Thus the United States standards are stated in terms of recommended dietary *allowances*, not as set *requirements*. The current RDA standard for adults has been generally set at 0.8 g/kg (2.2 lb) of body weight.[15] This amounts to about 63 g/day for a man aged 25 to 50 weighing 79 kg (174 lb) and 50 g/day for a woman of the same age weighing 63 kg (138 lb). Increased protein is indicated

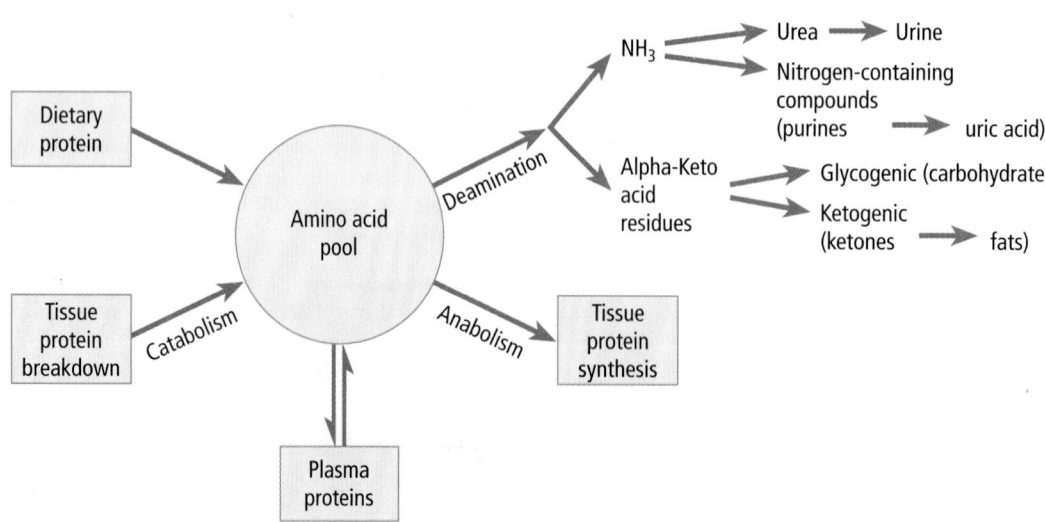

Figure 5.4   Balance between protein compartments and amino acid pool.

during pregnancy and lactation. The needs of infants and children vary according to age and growth patterns.

Protein quality

Because the value of a protein depends on its content of essential amino acids, in the final analysis the measure of protein need must be based on its amino acid quality. Guidelines for protein needs, based on nitrogen balance studies determining specific amino acid requirements, have been developed (Table 5.3).

Comparative quality of food proteins

The nutritive value of a food protein is often expressed in terms of its *chemical score*, a value derived from its amino acid composition. Using the amino acid pattern of a high-quality protein food—such as egg—and giving it a value of 100, other foods are compared according to their ratios of essential amino acids. Of these necessary amino acids, the one showing the greatest dietary deficit is called the **limiting amino acid** because when it is used up in making a specific protein, it limits the ability of the body to make more of that protein.

Other measures also determine aspects of protein quality:

1. *Biologic value (BV)* based on nitrogen balance.
2. *Net protein utilization (NPU)* based on biologic value and degree of digestibility.
3. *Protein efficiency ratio (PER)* based on weight gain of a growing test animal divided by its protein intake.

A comparison of the scores of various protein foods with their nutritive values based on these measures is shown in Table 5.4. A sound diet is the best way to obtain needed protein. There is no need for amino acid supplements. They are both costly and inefficient (see *Practical Application* box, p. 74).

VEGETARIAN DIETS

There are three main types of vegetarian diets: (1) ovolactovegetarian (including dairy foods and eggs), (2) lactovegetarian (including dairy foods), and (3) pure vegan (no animal protein). These main types, as well as others involving further deletions and combinations, are planned as any diet to secure needed nutrients and sufficient energy kcalories (see *Issues & Answers,* p. 83). The American Dietetic Association's current position paper on vegetarian diets indicates that the former conscious combining of complementary plant proteins within a given meal is unnecessary.[16] Interesting recipes for preparing nutritionally sound vegetarian meals are now widely available as a result of increased public interest. In general, in relation to animal protein sources, larger amounts of vegetable protein foods must be consumed to obtain comparable amounts of complete protein.

limiting amino acid The amino acid in foods occurring in the smallest amount, thus limiting its availability for tissue structure.

Table 5.3 Estimates of amino acid requirements

Amino acid	Infants, age 3-4 mo	Children, age 2 ~ yr	Children, age 10-12 yr	Adults
Histidine	28	?	?	8-12
Isoleucine	70	31	28	10
Leucine	161	73	42	14
Lysine	103	64	44	12
Methionine plus cystine	58	27	22	13
Phenylalanine plus tyrosine	125	69	22	14
Threonine	87	37	28	7
Tryptophan	17	12.5	3.3	3.5
Valine	93	38	25	10
Total without histidine	714	352	214	84

Requirements, mg/kg per day, by age group

From the Food and Nutrition Board, National Academy of Sciences—National Research Council: *Recommended dietary allowances,* ed 10, Washington, DC, 1989, National Academy Press.

Table 5.4 Comparative protein quality of selected foods according to chemical (amino acid) score, biologic value (BV), net protein utilization (NPU), and protein efficiency ratio (PER)

Food	Chemical score	BV	NPU	PER
Egg	100	100	94	3.92
Cow's milk	95	93	82	3.09
Fish	71	76	—	3.55
Beef	69	74	67	2.30
Unpolished rice	67	86	59	—
Peanuts	65	55	55	1.65
Oats	57	65	—	2.19
Polished rice	57	64	57	2.18
Whole wheat	53	65	49	1.53
Corn	49	72	36	—
Soybeans	47	73	61	2.32
Sesame seeds	42	62	53	1.77
Peas	37	64	55	1.57

Data adapted from Food and Nutrition Board, National Academy of Sciences—National Research Council: *Recommended dietary allowances,* ed 10, Washington, DC, 1989, National Academy Press.

To Probe Further

Recently rediscovered amino acids

Sometimes little known nutrients that have really been around for some time spark renewed interest and are "rediscovered" as their metabolic and clinical importance becomes more evident. Such is the case with two more recently rediscovered nutrients usually classed as amino acids—taurine and carnitine. Taurine was first isolated in 1872 and carnitine in 1905, but only now are their extensive metabolic activities and nutritional needs being recognized by modern research.

Taurine

Taurine is a sulfur-containing amino acid [NH_2 $(CH_2)_2SO_3H$] formed from methionine and cysteine metabolism. The interest in taurine stemmed largely from increased awareness of its need in infant formulas to make them nutritionally similar to human milk. It is one of the most abundant free amino acids in human milk and was first added to infant formulas in 1984 to meet the body's need for amino acids. Taurine is also the most abundant free amino acid in the body's total intracellular fluid. It plays a vital role in many of the body's physiologic events through its antioxidant ability as well as antimicrobial function in leukocytes.

Dietary sources of taurine are largely animal protein foods, the intake generally less than 200 mg/day. It is virtually absent in plant foods and hence in strict vegetarian diets. Its now known list of wide metabolic credits is receiving well-deserved attention, and extensive research is ongoing. Its functions, for example, relate to bile acid synthesis, regulation of heart beat, control of brain neurons and central nervous system activity, maintenance of membrane stability, and integrity of retinal and vision function. Perhaps its key functional word is *stability*.

Carnitine

Carnitine (C_7H_{15}-NO_3) is formed from methionine and lysine, with vitamins C and B_6, niacin, and iron acting as necessary nutrient cofactors with the cell enzymes in its synthesis. Thus the nutritional status of the individual greatly influences the capacity of the liver and kidney, major synthesis sites, to make carnitine.

Renewed research and clinical interest in carnitine have increased with the advent of total parenteral nutrition (TPN) technology and advanced knowledge of genetic disease. Carnitine deficiencies have been observed in persons with related genetic metabolic disorders and hypermetabolic disease and trauma patients receiving TPN. These deficiencies have been corrected by carnitine supplementation. Its major metabolic role is associated with the transport of long-chain fatty acids across the mitochondrial membranes, thus stimulating the oxidation of these fuel substrates for metabolic energy. Continuing research is revealing broader functions in forming complex esters with many of the *acyl compounds*, metabolic intermediary products from fats and carbohydrates. An accumulation of such metabolites in cells can inhibit cell enzyme functions and become toxic, creating a secondary carnitine deficiency. Carnitine supplements have been effective, for example, in such conditions as ischemic heart disease, drug reactions, and a number of inborn errors of metabolism, including organic acidemias. Carnitine converts many of the acyl compounds to less toxic forms and removes them from the cell.

As with taurine, dietary sources of carnitine are largely limited to animal protein foods. It is absent from plant proteins, hence from strict vegetarian diets. Actually, the only carnitine in such vegan diets would be from the soy-based Indonesian food *tempeh* and only then from the mold used in the fermentation process. Infants receiving soy formula, then, would need a supplement, so carnitine has been added to such products. Studies indicate that oral carnitine is about 55% to 85% bioavailable from normal Western diets.

As a result of carnitine's metabolic functions, it has become an important metabolic tool in conditions often requiring carnitine supplementation: (1) diseases of the liver and kidney, the major sites of carnitine synthesis; (2) major chronic illnesses or extensive injuries complicated by malnutrition and requiring TPN; (3) genetic metabolic disease affecting fatty acid metabolism and producing organic acidemias; and (4) deficiencies in premature infants with immature enzyme systems. Its clinical nutrition and medical attention are obviously well-deserved.

References

Broquist HP: Carnitine. In Shils ME, Olson, JA, Shike M, eds: *Modern nutrition in health and disease,* vol 1, ed 8, Philadelphia, 1994, Lea & Febiger.

Guyton AC, Hall JE: *Textbook of medical physiology,* ed 9, Philadelphia, 1996, Saunders.

Hayes KC, Troutwein EA: Taurine. In Shils ME, Olson JA, Shils M, eds: *Modern nutrition in health and disease,* vol 2, ed 8, Philadelphia, 1994, Lea & Febiger.

O'Flaherty L et al: Intestinal taurine transport: a review, *Eur J Clin Invest* 27:873, 1997.

Stapleton PP et al: Host defense—a role for the amino acid taurine? *J Parenter Enter Nutr* 22(1):42, 1998.

TO SUM UP

Proteins build tissue, perform various physiologic roles, and provide energy. Amino acids are the structural components of proteins. There are 22 in total, 10 of which the body cannot synthesize at all or in adequate amounts. These 10 are called essential amino acids (EAAs). Food proteins are considered "complete" when they contain all 10 EAAs in appropriate amounts. Animal proteins are complete. Vegetable proteins are incomplete but can be mixed with complete proteins or with each other to provide all 10 EAAs for the day.

Amino acids participate in protein building (anabolism) or breakdown (catabolism). Both processes are dictated by genetic information and hormonal influences. *Anabolism* occurs when specific amino acids required for each protein are present. If one is missing, the protein is not formed—the law of "all or none." *Catabolism* occurs when the body tissues are broken down. The amino acid splits into its nitrogen group, which helps to form amino acids or other nitrogen compounds, and its nonnitrogen residue, which can form carbohydrates for energy or fat storage. In the unfed state, proteins are broken down for energy. Thus dietary carbohydrates have a protein-sparing effect.

Protein requirements are influenced by growth needs and rate of protein synthesis, food protein quality, and dietary carbohydrate and fat levels. Clinical factors affecting protein needs include fever, disease, surgery, or other trauma to body tissues.

■ QUESTIONS FOR REVIEW

1. What is the difference between essential and nonessential amino acids? List the names of the essential amino acids.
2. Explain the term "protein-sparing effect." Which nutrients have this effect?
3. List and describe factors that affect dietary protein needs.
4. Calculate your own protein intake for a day and compare it with your general need according to the RDA allowances.
5. A vegetarian couple decides to raise their 2-year-old daughter on a strict vegan diet. As expected, the child does not often finish meals and snacks on fruits and whole grain biscuits. Eventually, they notice that she is falling behind in her growth rate and becoming thin. What food patterns would you expect in this family? What dietary factor may be involved in the child's poor growth? What advice would you offer these parents to improve their child's nutritional status? Plan one day's meals for this family, indicating amounts for the child that would meet her dietary protein need, while still adhering to a typical vegan meal pattern.

■ REFERENCES

1. Munro HN: Historical introduction: the origin and growth of our present concepts of protein metabolism. In Munro HN, Allison JB, eds: *Mammalian protein metabolism,* vol 1, New York, 1964, Academic Press.
2. Williams SR: *Nutrition and diet therapy,* ed 8, St Louis, 1997, Mosby.
3. Koshland DE: The molecule of the year, *Science* 258:1861, 1992.
4. Culotta E, Koshland DE: NO news is good news, *Science* 258:1862, 1992.
5. Chowienczyk P, Ritter J: Arginine: NO more than a simple amino acid? *Lancet* 350(Sept 27):901, 1997.
6. Service RF: Folding proteins caught in the act, *Science* 273(5271):29, 1996.
7. Service RF: Amino acid alchemy transmutes sheets to coils, *Science* 277(5323):179, 1997.
8. Guyton AC, Hall JE: *Textbook of medical physiology,* ed 9, Philadelphia, 1996, Saunders.
9. Shils ME, Olson JA, Shike M: *Modern nutrition in health and disease,* ed 8, vol 1, Philadelphia, 1994, Lea & Febiger.
10. Young VR, Pellett PL: Plant proteins in relation to human protein and amino acid nutrition, *Am J Clin Nutr* (suppl 5S):1203S, 1994.
11. Liu K: Storage proteins and hard-to-cook phenomenon in legume seeds, *Food Tech* 51(5):58, 1997.
12. Phillips RD: Nutritional quality of cereal and legume storage proteins, *Food Tech* 51(5):62, 1997.
13. Manary MJ et al: Protein metabolism in children with edematous malnutrition and acute lower respiratory infection, *Am J Clin Nutr* 65:1005, 1997.
14. Manary MJ et al: Whole-body protein kinetics in children with kwashiorkor and infection: a comparison of egg white and milk as dietary sources of protein, *Am J Clin Nutr* 66:643, 1997.
15. Food and Nutrition Board, National Academy of Sciences—National Research Council: *Recommended dietary allowances,* ed 10, Washington, DC, 1989, National Academy Press.
16. Messina VK, Burke KI: Position of the American Dietetic Association: vegetarian diets, *J Am Diet Assoc* 47(11):1317, 1997.

■ FURTHER READING

Messina VK, Burke KI: Position of The American Dietetic Association: vegetarian diets, *J Am Diet Assoc* 97(11):1317, 1997.

This statement provides a sound basis for well-planned vegetarian diets, which clarifies the different types and eating patterns involved, as well as health advantages.

Radetsky P: Kim's coils, *Discover* 16(6):112, 1995.

This interesting article from a well-known popular science magazine relates experiences of a young biochemist, Peter Kim, working in the field of protein biology, whose discoveries illuminate the fundamental nature of proteins and their structures, especially how viruses like flu and HIV manage to work their way into our cells. The secret, he discovered, lies in the shapes protein take when they fold and coil. Excellent illustrations of the gene-regulated process provide clear views of this protein capacity to shape and reshape itself through coils and pleated sheets. It's worth a search through the library stacks!

Issues & Answers

Vegetarian food patterns: harmful or healthy?

At least 7 million Americans have become vegetarians, replacing meats as a main entree item with legumes, grains, and vegetables. Their meals follow a variety of patterns.

I. "True vegetarians"

Some groups call themselves "true" vegetarians because they allow no animal products in their diets. But their highly restrictive "dietary laws" have caused serious malnutrition problems. These problems are found among the following persons:

Zen macrobiotics, who eat only brown rice and drink herbal tea to achieve a perfect balance of yin and yang in order to fend off disease.

Vegans, who rely on fruits, vegetables, nuts, and seeds and use no source of animal protein, fortified foods, or nutritional supplements.

Fruitarians, who eat only fresh and dried fruits, nuts, honey, and sometimes olive oil.

II. Alternate animal-product vegetarians

Other vegetarian diets, however, as well as a strict vegan diet—if well planned—can be very nutritious. These alternate forms of "animal-product" vegetarianism include:

Lactovegetarians, who allow milk, cheese, yogurt, and other milk products as the only animal protein in their diets.

Ovovegetarians, who use eggs as their only source of animal protein.

Ovolactovegetarians, who include milk, cheese, and other dairy products, as well as eggs.

Pollovegetarians, who allow only poultry in a plant-based diet.

Pescovegetarians, who allow only fish in a plant-based diet.

"Red meat abstainers," who eat any animal product except red meat, may also consider themselves to be vegetarians.

The reasons people give for becoming vegetarian are as varied as these diets. Often they may result from personal beliefs or convictions, living situations, or health problems:

Religion. Religious communities, such as the Seventh-Day Adventists, use vegetarianism as a means of self-discipline, as well as to promote good health. Other vegetarians may or may not be religious but feel it is "sinful" to kill a living animal for food.

Ecology. Approximately half of the world's grain output is used to feed livestock. Some vegetarians feel it could be better used to feed people so that less land would be used to meet the world's protein needs. Some also feel that using less land would result in a reduction in the use of pesticides now used to ensure large crops.

Economics. Beans, grains, and vegetables are cheaper than meat. Some vegetarians are on limited incomes, concerned with saving money for their personal or family needs. Others are also concerned about finding a way to meet food shortages in poor nations throughout the world.

Health. Another common reason for selecting vegetarianism is to achieve good health. By avoiding animal products, vegetarians manage to reduce their intake of cholesterol and saturated fats, thus perhaps gaining some protection against heart disease.

Does a vegetarian diet offer other important nutrients besides protein?

Yes. Vegetarians can meet the recommended dietary allowance (RDA) for most major nutrients without taking supplements. However, a few key nutrients create problems if the vegetarian is not careful:

- **Vitamin B_{12}.** This vitamin is found only in animal products. People who follow veganism or the macrobiotic diets are at the greatest risk for a deficiency. Vegans may be at special risk because they take in a large amount of folacin, another B vitamin that can mask signs of B_{12} deficiency. A deficiency can be avoided, however, by including fortified foods or taking a B_{12} supplement along with sufficient complete protein from complementary amino acids to ensure synthesis of the intrinsic factor (a mucoprotein) necessary for B_{12} absorption.

- **Vitamin A.** Vegetarians tend to get more provitamin A, carotene, than they need. This usually isn't a problem, unless they are also taking supplements that include vitamin A. One study shows that 85% of vegetarians take supplements. These may include as much as 10 times the RDA for vitamin A! As a fat-soluble vitamin, vitamin A

Continued

can build up in body tissues and reach toxic levels. The result could be anorexia, irritability, dry skin, and hair loss.

- **Iron.** Grains and legumes have iron but much of it is poorly absorbed from the gut. Absorption can be enhanced, however, by including a good source of vitamin C in the same meal.

Can vegetarian women get enough protein for a successful pregnancy?

Yes, though including animal products—as in ovolac-tovegetarianism—may become essential to meet extra nutritional needs. Supplements are recommended also for such hard-to-get nutrients as iron.

Is the vegetarian diet safe for children?

Children manage to grow and develop fairly well on a vegetarian diet that includes the nonmeat animal proteins milk, cheese, and eggs. They tend to be a little shorter than average but this may be the result of other genetic or environmental factors. Vegetarian children also tend to be mildly anemic, probably because of the poor availability of iron from grains and legumes. Again, including a source of vitamin C with meals may be helpful. The vegan diet, unless it is carefully planned and monitored, and all levels of macrobiotic diets are too poor in required nutrients to sustain childhood growth needs.

Can you lose weight on a vegetarian diet?

Yes, definitely. Eliminating meats automatically removes a major source of fat in the diet. Since fats provide more than twice the number of kcalories per gram than carbohydrates or protein, the vegetarian diet is usually much lower in kcalories than the "meat-and-potatoes" diet. In fact, some vegetarians—especially pregnant women, children, and athletes—have to be careful to get *enough* kcalories.

The well-planned vegetarian diet can be nutritious. If used wisely, especially in its ovolacto form, it can offer many advantages in terms of health, economy, and ecology.

References

Franklin TL, Kolasa KM et al: Adherence to very low fat diet by a group of cardiac rehabilitation patients in the rural southeastern United States, *Arch Fam Med* 4:551, 1995

Jacob RA, Burri BJ: Oxidative damage and defense, *Am J Clin Nutr* 63(suppl):985S, 1996.

Key TH et al: Dietary habits and mortality in 11,000 vegetarian and health conscious people: results of a 17-year follow-up, *Br Med J* 13:775, 1996.

Messina VK, Burke KI: Position of The American Dietetics Association: vegetarian diets, *J Am Diet Assoc* 97(11):1317, 1997.

Pagenkemper J: The impact of vegetarian diets on renal disease, *Top Clin Nutr* 10:22, 1995.

Roberts WC: Preventing and arresting coronary atherosclerosis, *Am Heart J* 130:580, 1995.

Chapter

6

Energy Balance and Weight Management

In Chapter 2, we reviewed the overall digestion-absorption-metabolism continuum in our bodies for handling the three energy nutrients. In this chapter we consider the relationship between body energy balance and body weight, problems of overweight and underweight, and their effects on health.

We will find, however, that this balance is not a simple matter. We are not all alike, and our energy needs vary in different circumstances and different body types. Each of us is unique, and our varying body weights may reflect this fact. This individual view of weight patterns is difficult for many modern societies to accept, and the social norm of thinness creates undue pressure for many whose natural weight cannot conform.

Here we will seek an improved goal of weight management based on sound nutrition, physical and emotional health, and physical fitness. This approach is important for all persons, but especially for those with health risks related to excess body weight.

THE HUMAN ENERGY SYSTEM

ENERGY CYCLE AND TRANSFORMATION

Forms of human energy

It is clear that in our physical world **energy**, like matter, is neither created nor destroyed. When we speak of energy "production," what we really mean is that it is being *transformed*. Energy is being changed in form and cycled throughout a system. In the human body the various metabolic processes convert stored chemical energy in our food to other forms of energy for the body's work. In our bodies, energy is available in four basic forms for life processes: *chemical, electrical, mechanical,* and *thermal.* Our ultimate source of power is the sun with its vast reservoir of nuclear reactions (Figure 6.1). Then through the process of photosynthesis, as shown in the chapter on carbohydrates (see Figure 3.1), using water and carbon dioxide as raw materials, plants transform the sun's energy into food storage forms of chemical energy. In the body these stored food fuels are converted to the basic energy unit glucose, which together with fatty acids is metabolized to release its energy to be transformed and cycled through body systems. Water and carbon dioxide, the initial materials used by the plants, are retrieved as end products of this process of oxidation in the body. And so the cycle goes on and on.

Transformation of energy

Through the many processes of metabolism, after stored chemical energy in food is taken into the body, it is converted further to chemical energy in other metabolic products to do the body's work. This chemical energy is then changed still further to other forms of energy as this work is performed. For example, chemical energy is changed to electrical energy in brain and nerve activity. It is changed to mechanical energy in muscle contraction. It is changed to thermal energy in the regulation of body temperature. It is changed to still other types of chemical energy in the synthesis of new compounds. In all these work activities of the body, heat is given off to the surrounding atmosphere and larger biosphere.

In human *metabolism*, as in any energy system, energy is always present as either *free energy* or *potential energy*. Free energy is the energy involved at any given moment in the performance of a task. It is unbound and in motion. Poten-

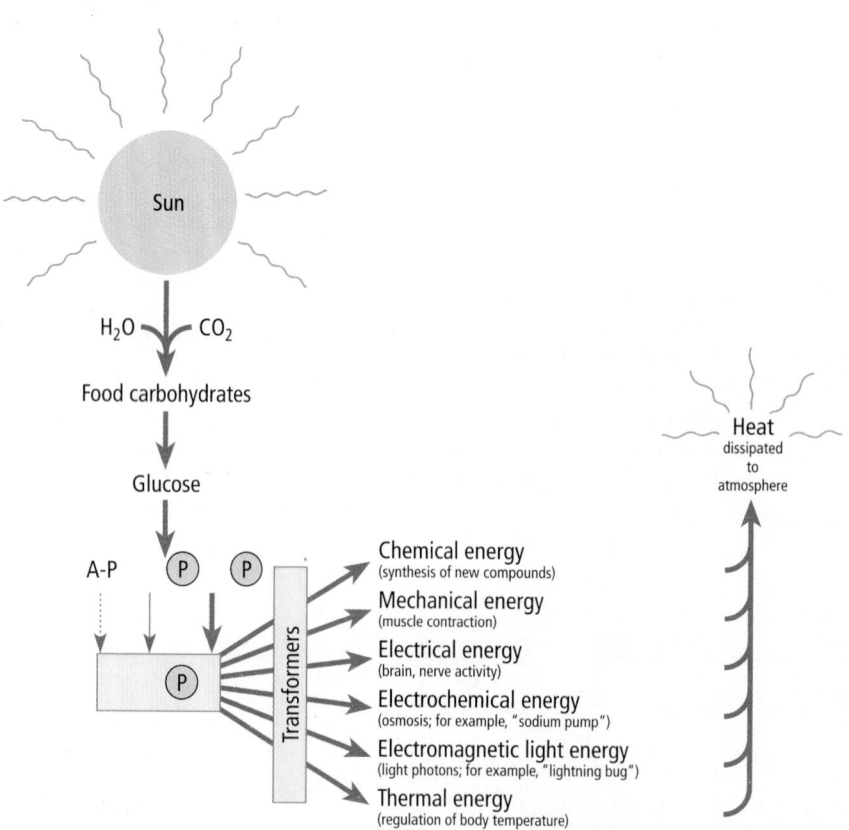

Figure 6.1   Transformation of energy from its primary source (the sun) to various forms for biologic work by means of metabolic processes ("transformers").

tial energy is the energy that is stored or bound in the various chemical compounds, available for conversion to free energy as needed for work. For example, energy stored in sugar is potential energy. When we eat it and it is metabolized, free energy is released and body work results. As work is done, energy in the form of heat is released.

Energy balance: input and output

Whether the energy system is electrical, mechanical, thermal, or chemical, in the course of the many reactions that comprise its internal operation the body's free energy supply is decreased by this essential body work and the reservoir of potential energy is secondarily diminished. Therefore the system must be constantly refueled from some outside source. In the human energy system this basic input of fuel is our food.

The energy demands of the body require a constant supply of available energy. These energy needs support the body's total basic metabolic needs, as well as the additional physical activity requirements. In the human energy system this physical energy output is evident in our activities. But energy output to an even larger degree is also going on internally at all times to meet our basal or resting energy needs.

ENERGY CONTROL IN HUMAN METABOLISM

In the human body the energy produced in its many chemical reactions, if "exploded" all at once, would be destructive. There must be some mechanism therefore by which energy is controlled in the human system, so that it may support life and not destroy it. Several basic means of control, chemical bonding and controlled reaction rates, accomplish this task.

Chemical bonding

The main mechanism controlling energy in the human system is **chemical bonding**. The chemical bonds that hold elements of compounds together consist of energy. As long as the compound remains constant, energy is being exerted to maintain it. When the compound is taken into the body and broken into its parts, this energy is released and available for body work. Three basic types of chemical bonds transfer energy in the body:

- *Covalent bonds.* These are regular bonds, based on relative **valence** of constituent elements, that link the elements of a chemical compound together—for example, such as those that hold carbon atoms together in the core of an organic compound.
- *Hydrogen bonds.* Weaker than covalent bonds, these bonds are nonetheless significant because they can be formed in large numbers. Also, the very fact that they are less strong and can be broken easily makes them important because they

can be transferred or passed readily from one substance to another to help form still another substance.

- *High-energy phosphate bonds.* A main example of these high-energy phosphate bonds at work is the compound **adenosine triphosphate (ATP)**, which is the unique compound the human body uses to store energy for its cell work. Like storage batteries for electrical energy, these bonds become the controlling force for ongoing energy needs.

Controlled reaction rates

The many chemical reactions that make up the body's energy system must also have controls. Some of the reactions that break down proteins if left to themselves—for example, as in sterile decomposition—would span several years. Such reactions must be accelerated, or getting the needed energy from eating a meal would take years. At the same time, they must be regulated so that too fast a reaction will not produce a burst of energy in a single "explosion." Control agents regulating these cell activities are the enzymes, coenzymes, and hormones.

---

adenosine triphosphate (ATP) The high-energy compound formed in the cell and called the "energy currency" of the cell because of the binding of energy in its high-energy phosphate bonds for release for cell work as these bonds are split. A compound of adenosine (a nucleotide containing adenine and ribose) that has three phosphoric acid groups. ATP is a high-energy phosphate compound important in energy exchange for cellular activity. The splitting off of the terminal phosphate bond (PO_4) of ATP to produce adenosine diphosphate (ADP) releases bound energy and transfers it to free energy available for body work. The reforming of ATP in cell oxidation again stores energy in high-energy phosphate bonds for use as needed. They may be charged and discharged according to conditions in the cell.

chemical bonding Process of linking the radicals, chemical elements, or groups of a chemical compound.

energy The capacity of a system for doing work; available power. Energy is manifest in various forms—motion, position, light, heat, and sound. Energy is interchangeable among these various forms and is constantly being transformed and transferred among them.

valence Power of an element or a radical to combine with or to replace other elements or radicals. Atoms of various elements combine in definite proportions. The valence number of an element is the number of atoms of hydrogen with which one atom of the element can combine.

1. *Enzymes.* Many specific **enzymes** in every cell control specific cell reactions. All enzymes are protein compounds. They are produced in the cells under control of specific genes. One specific gene controls the making of one specific enzyme, and there are thousands of enzymes in each cell. Each enzyme works on its own particular substance, which is called its **substrate**. The enzyme and its substrate lock together to produce a new reaction product, and the original enzyme remains unchanged, ready to do its specific work over and over again (Figure 6.2).

2. *Coenzymes.* Many reactions require a partner to assist the enzyme in completing the reaction. These coenzyme factors in many instances involve several of the vitamins, especially the B-complex vitamins and some of the minerals. It may be helpful to think of the coenzyme as another substrate, since in receiving the material transferred, the coenzyme is changed or reduced.

3. *Hormones.* In energy metabolism **hormones** act as messengers to trigger or control enzyme action. For example, the rate of oxidative reactions in the tissues—the body's metabolic rate—is controlled by the *thyroid-stimulating hormone (TSH)* from the anterior pituitary gland. Another familiar example is the controlling action of insulin from the pancreas islet cells on the rate of glucose utilization in the tissues. Steroid hormones also have the capacity to regulate the cell's ability to synthesize enzymes.

Types of metabolic reactions

The two types of reaction constantly going on in energy metabolism are anabolism and catabolism. Each requires energy. The processes of *anabolism* synthesize new and more complex substances. The processes of *catabolism* break down more complex substances to simpler ones. These processes release free energy, but the work also uses up some free energy. Therefore there is a constant energy deficit, which must be supplied by food.

Sources of stored energy

When food is not available, as in periods of fasting or starvation, the body must draw on its own stores for energy:

1. *Glycogen.* Only a 12- to 48-hour reserve of glycogen exists in liver and muscle and is quickly depleted.

2. *Muscle mass.* Storage of energy as protein exists in limited amounts in muscle mass, but in greater volume than glycogen stores.

3. *Adipose fat tissue.* Although fat storage may be larger, the supply varies from person to person and from circumstance to circumstance.

MEASUREMENT OF ENERGY BALANCE

Kilocalorie

Because the body performs work only as energy is released by chemical reactions, and because all work takes the form of heat production, energy may be measured in terms of heat equivalents. Such a heat measure is the **calorie**. To avoid using large numbers, the professional nutritionist and biochemist use the term **kilocalorie** (1000 calories), abbreviated kcalorie or kcal. This is the amount of heat required to raise 1 kg of water 1° C.

Joule (J)

The international (SI) unit of energy measurement is the **joule**. It expresses the amount expended when 1 kg of a substance is moved 1 meter by a force of 1 newton. It was named for James Prescott Joule (1818-1889), an English physicist who discovered the first law of thermodynamics and invented an electromagnetic engine. The conversion factor for changing kilocalories (kcalories or kcal) to kilo-

Figure 6.2   Lock-and-key concept of the action of enzyme, coenzyme, and substrate to produce a new reaction product.

joules (kJ) is 4.184—1 kcal equals 4.184 kJ. Because the conversion product of energy values of diets in kilojoules renders large numbers, a simpler term is the megajoule (MJ)—1 MJ equals 239 kcal.

FOOD ENERGY MEASURE

The energy in various foods is generally measured in two basic ways: calorimetry and computing the approximate composition.

Calorimetry

The caloric values of various foods expressed in food value tables have usually been determined by direct **calorimetry**.[1] In this process a metal container called a *bomb calorimeter* is used. The name comes from its long tubular shape. A weighed amount of food is placed inside, and the instrument is immersed in water. The food is then ignited by an electric spark in the presence of oxygen and burned. The increase in the temperature of the surrounding water indicates the number of kcalories given off by the oxidation of the food. Remember when you use food value tables, however, that these values represent averages of a number of samples of the given food tested. The value of a particular serving of that food varies around that figure.

Approximate composition

An alternate method of measuring food energy is by computing the approximate nutrient composition of a given food using values in food value tables or databases. These values are based on the average kcalorie value of each of the three energy-yielding macronutrients. These values are known as their respective **fuel factors**: 1 g of carbohydrate yields 4 kcal, 1 g of fat yields 9 kcal, and 1 g of protein yields 4 kcal. In comparison, 1 g of beverage alcohol yields 7 kcal.

TOTAL ENERGY REQUIREMENTS

The total energy expended by an individual supports three essential energy uses: (1) basal metabolic needs (basal energy expenditures [BEE] or resting energy expenditures [REE]), (2) food intake effect, and (3) physical activities.

---

calorie A unit of heat energy. The calorie used in the study of metabolism is the large calorie, or kilocalorie, defined as the amount of heat required to raise the temperature of 1 kg of water 1° Celsius (centigrade).

calorimetry Measurement of amounts of heat absorbed or given out. *Direct method:* measurement of amount of heat produced by a subject enclosed in a small chamber. *Indirect method:* measurement of amount of heat produced by a subject by the quantity of nitrogen and carbon dioxide eliminated.

enzyme Various complex proteins produced by living cells that act independently of these cells. Enzymes are capable of producing certain chemical changes in other substances without themselves being changed in the process. Their action is therefore that of a catalyst. Digestive enzymes of the gastrointestinal secretions act on food substances to break them down into simpler compounds and greatly accelerate the speed of these chemical reactions. An enzyme is usually named according to the substance (substrate) on which it acts, with the common suffix *-ase*; for example, sucrase is the specific enzyme for sucrose and breaks it down to glucose and fructose.

fuel factor The kilocalorie value (energy potential) of food nutrients; that is, the number of kilocalories that 1 g of the nutrient yields when oxidized. The kilocalorie fuel factor for carbohydrate is 4; for protein, 4; and for fat, 9. The basic figures are used in computing diets and energy values of foods. (For example, 10 g of fat yields 90 kcal.)

hormones Various internally secreted substances from the endocrine organs, which are conveyed by the blood to another organ or tissue on which they act to stimulate increased functional activity or secretion. This tissue or substance is called its target organ or substance.

joule The internal (SI) unit of energy and heat, defined as the work done by the force of 1 newton acting over the distance of 1 meter. A newton (named for Sir Isaac Newton, 1643-1727, English mathematician, physicist, and astronomer) is the international unit of force, defined as the amount of force that, when applied in a vacuum to a body having a mass of 1 kg, accelerates it at the rate of 1 meter per second. These are examples of the exactness with which terms and values used by the world's scientific community must be defined, as illustrated in the *Système International d'Unités (SI)*.

kilocalorie The general term calorie refers to a unit of heat measure and is used alone to designate the *small calorie*. The calorie used in nutritional science and the study of metabolism is the *large calorie,* 1000 calories, or kilocalorie, to be more accurate and avoid use of very large numbers in calculations.

substrate The specific organic substance on which a particular enzyme acts to produce new metabolic products.

Basal metabolic rate (BMR)

The sum of all internal chemical activities that maintain the body at rest comprise its basal metabolism. The **basal metabolic rate (BMR)**, frequently referred to as **resting metabolic rate (RMR)**, is a measure of the energy required by these activities of resting tissue. Certain small but vitally active tissues—brain, liver, gastrointestinal tract, heart, and kidneys—together make up less than 5% of the total body weight, yet they contribute about 60% of the total basal metabolic processes. This resting metabolic rate is the largest component of energy expenditure in humans, constituting about 60% to 70% of the daily energy expenditure of individuals, and is influenced by the state of fitness and the pretesting environment.[2]

Measuring BMR

Direct and indirect methods of measuring BMR are used:
1. *Direct calorimetry*. In direct methods, a chamber large enough for a person to enter is used, and the body's heat production at rest is measured. This instrument is large and costly and is therefore limited to research studies.[2]
2. *Indirect calorimetry*. In this indirect method, a smaller portable instrument, sometimes called a *metabolator*, can be brought to the side of the bed or chair on a cart. The person breathes into the instrument through a mouthpiece, and the exchanges of gases in respiration, the *respiratory quotient* (CO_2/O_2), is measured while the subject is at rest. The metabolic rate is calculated with a high degree of accuracy from the rate of oxygen utilization because more than 95% of the energy expended by the body is derived from metabolic reactions with oxygen.[1,2] Energy (BMR) measured in this manner is equivalent to the heat released by the body.
3. *Indirect laboratory tests*. Since the thyroid hormone regulates BMR, thyroid function tests are used in clinical practice to serve as indirect measures of BMR. These tests include measures of serum protein-bound iodine (PBI), and serum thyroxin levels, both triiodothyronine (T_3) and thyroxin (T_4), as well as the radioactive iodine uptake test. The free thyroxin index (FTI) is an overall measure based on the product of T_3 and T_4. These two compounds are produced in the final two stages of thyroid hormone synthesis. This product ($T_3 \times T_4$) reflects the relative functioning of the thyroid gland and the amount of hormone activity influencing the BMR.

Factors influencing BMR

The four main factors influencing BMR are lean body mass, growth, fever and disease, and cold climate.

1. *Lean body mass*. Lean body mass is the major factor influencing BMR because of its greater level of metabolic activity than that of less active tissues such as fat and bones. Differences, for example, in metabolic requirements for women are primarily related to their generally lower amount of lean muscle mass in comparison with men.
2. *Growth*. Growth during childhood and pregnancy, as well as milk production during lactation, requires anabolic work under the influence of growth hormone.
3. *Fever and disease*. Fever increases BMR about 7% for each 0.83° C (1° F) rise. In addition, diseases involving increased cell activity—such as cancer, certain anemias, cardiac failure, hypertension, and respiratory problems such as emphysema—usually increase BMR. Conversely, the abnormal states of starvation and malnutrition lower BMR because the lean body mass is diminished.
4. *Cold climate*. BMR rises in response to lower temperatures as a compensatory mechanism to maintain body temperature.

Food intake effect

Food ingestion stimulates metabolism and requires energy to meet the multiple activities of digestion, absorption, and transport of nutrients. This overall metabolic stimulation is called the **thermic effect of food (TEF)**. About 10% to 15% of the body's total energy needs are used in activities related to metabolizing food.

Physical activity needs

Exercise involved in work and recreation or in physical training and competition accounts for wide individual variations in energy requirements (see Chapter 14). The effects of various activities on energy metabolism have been measured by the oxygen consumption method of indirect calorimetry. Some of these representative kcalorie expenditures in various types of work and recreation are given in Table 6.1. The feelings of fatigue after periods of study are not caused by vast cerebral activity but by the various amounts of muscle tension or moving about involved. Heightened emotional states alone do not increase the metabolic activity, but they may bring additional energy needs because they involve increased muscle tension, restlessness, and agitated movements.

In summary, the basic components of energy expenditure required during weight maintenance are (1) *resting metabolic rate (RMR)*, the energy demands of the basal metabolic activity—about 70% of the total; (2) the *thermic effect of food (TEF)*—about 10% of the total; and (3)

Table			
6.1 Energy expenditure/hour during various activities*			

Light activities (120-150 kcal/hr)	Light to moderate activities (150-300 kcal/hr)	Moderate activities (300-400 kcal/hr)	Heavy activities (420-600 kcal/hr)
Personal care	**Domestic work**	**Yard work**	**Yard work**
Dressing	Ironing	Digging	Chopping wood
Shaving	Making beds	Mowing lawn (not	Digging holes
Washing	Sweeping floors	motorized)	Shoveling snow
	Washing clothes	Pulling weeds	
Sitting			**Walking**
Peeling potatoes	**Yard work**	**Walking**	5 mph
Playing cards	Light gardening	3½ to 4 mph on level	Up stairs
Playing piano	Mowing lawn (power mower)	surface	Up hills
Rocking		Up and down small hills	Climbing
Sewing	**Light work**		
Typing	Auto repair	**Recreation**	**Recreation**
Writing	Painting	Badminton	Bicycling 11 to 12 mph
	Shoe repair	Ballet exercises	or up and down hills
Standing or slowly	Store clerk	Calisthenics	Cross-country skiing
moving around	Washing car	Canoeing 4 mph	Jogging 5 mph
		Dancing (waltz, square)	Swimming
Billiards	**Walking**	Golf (no cart)	Tennis (singles)
	2 to 3 mph on level surface	Ping-Pong	Waterskiing
	or down stairs	Tennis (doubles)	
		Volleyball	
	Recreation		
	Archery		
	Bicycling 5½ mph on level surface		
	Bowling		
	Canoeing 2½ to 3 mph		

*Energy expenditure depends on the physical fitness (that is, amount of lean body mass) of the individual and continuing of exercise. Note that some of these activities can be used as aerobic activities to promote cardiovascular fitness.

the variable requirements of *physical activity*. To these factors another factor called *adaptive thermogenesis* is sometimes added. This is defined as the change in resting metabolic rate associated with adaptation to environmental stress, such as changes in dietary intake, area temperature, and emotional state.

Obesity, in the traditional sense, represents an energy imbalance resulting from an excess of energy input (fuel from food) over energy output (energy requirement or expenditure). However, investigators are increasingly recognizing a genetic-based low resting metabolic rate characteristic of an inherited obesity disorder—perhaps better termed *essential obesity*—which is approached and understood much like essential hypertension, for example.[3] The opposite body weight disorder, extreme weight loss as seen in anorexia nervosa, results from a deficit of energy input to meet the body's energy requirement (see *Issues & Answers*, p. 108).

Where do you stand in your own energy balance? Try estimating your own energy requirement using the two useful calculations indicated here: (1) total energy output per day and (2) body mass index (see *Practical Application*

box, p. 92). Compare your estimate with your general energy needs as indicated in the RDA standards, or Table 6.2, and your Body Mass Index (see *To Probe Further* box, p. 104).

---

basal metabolic rate (BMR)   Amount of energy required to maintain the resting body's internal activities after an overnight fast. See also resting metabolic rate (RMR).

resting metabolic rate (RMR)   Amount of energy required to maintain the resting body's internal activities when in a normal environment temperature. Because of small differences in measuring techniques, RMR may be slightly different from the same person's **basal metabolic rate (BMR)**. In practice, however, RMR and BMR measurments may be used interchangeably.

thermic effect of food   Body heat produced by food; amount of energy required to digest and absorb food and transport nutrients to the cells. This basic preparatory work accounts for about 10% of the day's total energy (kcalories) requirement.

Two useful calculations: total energy output per day and body mass index (BMI)

A. Calculate your own total energy output per day (in kcal)

Your total energy output (in kcal) per day is the sum of your body's three uses of energy:

1. Resting metabolic rate
2. Thermic effect of food
3. Physical activity

1. Resting metabolic rate (RMR)

Use general formula:

Women: 0.9 kcal/kg/hr
Men: 1 kcal/kg/hr

Convert weight (lb) to kg: 1 kg = 2.2 lb

Multiply by formula:

RMR (kcal) = 1 (or 0.9) × kg weight × 24 (hours in day)

2. Thermic effect of food intake (TEF)

The thermic effect of food is the energy the body uses in the process of digestion and absorption. It averages 10% of the energy in the food.

Record your food intake for 1 day (24 hours) and calculate approximate energy value (kcal), using either the Table of Food Values in Appendix K or a simple computer program.

Find energy cost of thermic effect of food (TEF):

TEF (kcal) = 10% of total kcal in food consumed

3. Physical activity

Estimate your general average level of physical activity.

The energy used by physical activity can be approximated as a percentage of your RMR and varies with the degree of physical activity. Use this list to select your activity level:

Average Activity Level	Energy Cost: % of RMR
Sedentary	20%
Very light	30%
Moderate	40%
Heavy	50%

Find the energy cost of your activity level:

Physical activity energy cost (kcal) = RMR × your activity %

For example, if you are sedentary (mostly sitting): RMR × 20%

4. Calculate your total energy output

Total energy output (kcal) = **RMR + TEF + physical activity**

Example 1

A woman who weighs 130 lb (59 kg), who eats an average of 1800 kcalories per day, and who has started and maintains a regular physical exercise program.

RMR = 0.9 × 59 × 24 = 1274 kcal
TEF = 1800 × 10% = 180 kcal
Activity = RMR × 40% = 510 kcal
Total energy output = 1964 kcal

Result: This woman will lose weight. Her energy output is around 150 kcalories per day greater than her food intake. Since 1 lb of body weight equals approximately 3500 kcalories, she will lose about 1 lb every 20 to 30 days with the above eating and exercise routine.

Example 2

A man who weighs 180 lb (82 kg), who eats an average of 2700 kcalories per day, and who has a sedentary lifestyle.

RMR = 1 × 82 × 24 = 1968 kcal
TEF = 2700 × 10% = 270 kcal
Activity = RMR × 20% = 394 kcal
Total energy output = 2632 kcal

Result: This man will tend to gain weight slowly over time. What would your clinical advice be to him?

B. Calculate your own body mass index (BMI)

Body mass index (BMI) is usually calculated in metric terms, as follows:

$$BMI = weight\ (kg) \div height\ (meters)^2$$

BMI may also be calculated using weight in pounds and height in inches, using a mathematical calculation factor, as follows:

BMI =

Step 1 *Multiply* weight (lb) × 705
Step 2 *Divide* result of Step 1 by height (inches)
Step 3 *Divide* result of Step 2 by height (inches)

Most adults have a BMI in the 20s. Health risks associated with obesity begin with a BMI above 25.

Example:

Weight	= 160 lb
Height	= 62 inches
160 × 705	= 112,800
112,800 ÷ 62	= 819
1819 ÷ 62	= 29
BMI	= 29

BODY COMPOSITION: FATNESS AND LEANNESS

BODY WEIGHT VERSUS BODY FAT

Sometimes the common terms *obesity* and *overweight* are used without the necessary attention to *body composition*. It is helpful to consider first the distinct meanings and concepts embodied in each of these terms.

Obesity

As it is used in the traditional medical model, the word **obesity** is a clinical term for excess body weight, defining it in the sense of a disease. It is generally applied to a person who is 20% to 30% or more above a so-called standard weight, usually displayed in weight-height tables. These Metropolitan tables were constructed a number of years ago from information obtained from life insurance holders, largely white middle-aged males, hardly representative of our current diverse and aging United States population. Thus they tell us little about particular individuals. The problem lies in defining the word *standard*. This term is usually defined in reference to average weight according to height and frame. But even this is not much help because an average person does not really exist. Every person is individual, a unique and complex human being, and *normal* values in healthy persons vary over a relatively wide range. Age plays a large role in this variance.

Overweight versus overfat

We often use the term *overweight* as a synonym for obesity. But the two terms are not interchangeable, and the distinction is important. For example, a football player in peak condition can be markedly "overweight" according to standard weight-height charts. That is, he can weigh considerably more than the "average" man of the same height, but much of his greater weight is not fat at all. In clinical usage, the term *overweight* refers to persons with body weight in excess of the weight-height standard but below the 20% excess designated as obesity. In relation to health, however, the term *overfat* would be a more correct designation because it refers to the percentage of excess body fat in the overall total body composition. As a result of this understanding, experts in the field of nutrition have defined *obesity* in relation to severe obesity and its implications for health as "an excess of body *fat* frequently resulting in a significant impairment of health."[4]

Body composition

What is critical, then, in determining a reasonable body weight is **body composition**. In relation to our concern about body weight and health, we need to know what the body composition is, how much of the body weight comes from fat, and how much is from lean body mass. It is much more precise to talk in terms of *fatness* and *leanness* than overweight. When speaking of weight, we need to ask for whom, under what circumstances, and by what measures. We need to consider individual body composition and use some practical means of determining it as a guideline for planning individual care. On the basis of metabolic activity—hence energy (kcalories) demand—and comparative size, the four-compartment model of body composition is divided into lean body mass, body fat, body water, and mineral mass—mainly bone. In this basic model, based on laboratory studies with adults, approximately 50% of the body weight is contributed by water, 25% by fat, 20% by lean body mass, and 5% by mineral mass.[5]

1. *Lean body mass (LBM).* This major body component of active fat-free cell mass largely determines the basal metabolic rate and energy and nutrient need. It changes through the life cycle and in adulthood accounts for some 30% to 65% of the total body weight. In any person it accounts for almost all of the energy requirement. When persons lose weight from changes in their diet, the loss reflects changes not only in body fat but also in LBM. Physical activity and exercise are essential for developing and maintaining the relative LBM size.

2. *Body fat.* Gross body fat varies widely with individual degrees of fatness or leanness. These differences reflect the number and size of fat cells, the **adipocytes**, that make up the adipose tissue. In an adult man, for example, fat accounts for a range of 14% to 28% of total body weight. In a woman, it is somewhat larger, about 15% to 29% of body weight. These amounts vary with age, climate, exercise, and fitness. About half the body fat is in the subcutaneous fat layers as insulation, thus providing a useful measure—the triceps skinfold—for estimating body fat in relation to LBM.

3. *Body water.* The body water content varies with relative leanness or fatness and with age, hydration, and health status. Generally it makes up

---

adipocyte A fat cell. All cell names end in the suffix *-cyte,* with the type of cell indicated by the root word to which it is added.

body composition The relative sizes of the four basic body compartments that make up the total body: lean body mass (muscle mass), fat, water, and bone.

obesity Fatness; an excessive accumulation of fat in the body.

Table

6.2   Good body weights-for-height for adults, expressed in pounds (for height, in feet-inches) and kilograms (for height, in centimeters) and related to BMI*

Height (ft-in)†	19-34 years Average weight (lb)	19-34 years Range (lb)	35 years + Average weight (lb)	35 years + Range (lb)	Centimeters	19-34 years Average weight (kg)	19-34 years Range (kg)	35 years + Average weight (kg)	35 years + Range (kg)
5'0"	112	97-128	123	108-138	152	51	44-58	55	49-62
5'1"	116	101-132	127	111-143	155	53	46-60	58	50-65
5'2"	120	104-137	131	115-148	157	54	47-62	59	52-67
5'3"	124	107-141	135	119-152	160	56	49-64	61	54-69
5'4"	128	111-146	140	122-157	163	58	51-66	64	56-72
5'5"	132	114-150	144	126-162	165	60	52-68	65	57-74
5'6"	136	118-155	148	130-167	168	62	54-71	68	59-76
5'7"	140	121-160	153	134-172	170	64	55-72	69	61-78
5'8"	144	125-164	158	138-178	173	66	57-75	72	63-81
5'9"	149	129-169	162	142-183	175	67	58-77	74	64-83
5'10"	153	132-174	167	146-188	178	70	60-79	76	67-86
5'11"	157	136-179	172	151-194	180	71	62-81	78	68-88
6'0"	162	140-184	177	155-199	183	74	64-84	80	70-90
6'1"	166	144-189	182	159-205	185	75	65-86	82	72-92
6'2"	171	148-195	187	164-210	188	78	67-88	85	74-95
6'3"	176	152-200	192	168-216	191	80	69-91	88	77-99
6'4"	180	156-205	197	173-222	193	82	71-93	89	78-101
6'5"	185	160-211	202	177-228	196	85	73-96	92	81-104
6'6"	190	164-216	208	182-234	198	86	75-98	94	82-106
					BMI (kg/m²)	22	19-25	24	21-27

Data adapted from US Department of Agriculture, US Department of Health and Human Services: *Nutrition and your health: dietary guidelines* for *Americans,* ed 3, Washington, DC, 1990, US Government Printing Office; and from Bray GA: Pathophysiology of obesity, *Am J Clin Nutr* 55:448S, 1992.
*Without clothes
†Without shoes.

about 50% to 65% of body weight. Lean persons have a somewhat larger proportion of body water than do fat persons because lean muscle tissue contains more water than does any other body tissue except blood.

4. *Bone.* The remaining mineral mass, largely in the skeletal structure, accounts for only about 4% to 6% of the total body weight. The major mineral component is calcium, as you would expect, which makes up about 75% of the body mineral mass in bone and other body cells and fluids.

In free-living populations, however, individuals vary widely around these body composition proportions. A number of factors influence these variances[5]:

*   *Gender.* Women have more fat tissue, and men have more muscle mass.
*   *Age.* Younger adults have more lean body mass and less fat than do older adults.
*   *Physical exercise.* Persons physically fit from daily work and other physical activities have less fat

and more relative lean body mass than do those leading sedentary lives.

*   *Race.* Black women have more mineral mass than do white women.
*   *Climate.* Those in cold climates have somewhat more subcutaneous fat than those in hot tropical areas to protect body temperature.
*   *Weight extremes.* Obese persons have excess fat in relation to lean body mass.

Measuring body composition

Various indirect methods of measuring body composition have been developed. These include such classic means as water displacement (weighing under water) and measuring radioactive body emissions. Newer methods include ultrasonics, light absorption and reflection, electrical conductivity and resistance, radioactive absorption, and other research techniques.[6] In clinical practice related estimates are made from various measurements of body circumferences and skinfold thicknesses.

STANDARD WEIGHT-FOR-HEIGHT MEASUREMENTS

Two basic approaches have been used to evaluate body weight. These are (1) standard weight-height tables and (2) National Research Council tables and body mass index (BMI).

Weight-height tables

Most of the standard United States tables, as indicated, are based on the Metropolitan Life Insurance Company's so-called ideal weight-for-height charts, derived from life expectancy data gathered by the company since the 1930s. (These tables are printed inside the back book cover for reference.) But there are problems with this information base for today's diverse total population. Also, investigators have found that health risks are as great—if not greater—in the thin, low-weight range as for the obese group. Within each age group, extremely thin—as well as extremely fat—persons have higher mortality rates. The message seems to be that persons should strive to be neither excessively overweight nor excessively underweight and that the multitude of health problems attributed to moderate amounts of overweight are unfounded.[7]

National Research Council tables and body mass index

Other, more recent height-weight tables have been developed that are more realistic for practitioners. They are based on the National Research Council data on weight and health and the dietary guidelines.[8,9] These guides, shown in Table 6-2, relate height and adult age ranges to good ranges of body weight, as well as to body mass index (BMI).[10] The BMI can be calculated as follows:

$$BMI = weight (kg) \div height (meters)^2$$

The metric conversion factors involved are: (1) 1 kg equals 2.2 lb, and (2) 1 meter (m) equals 39.37 in. The desired health maintenance BMI range for adults is 20 to 25 kg/m². Health risks associated with obesity begin at about 30 kg/m². Values above 40 kg/m² indicate severe obesity.

INDIVIDUAL VARIATION

"Ideal" weight versus good individual body weight

The basic problem with "ideal" weight, as we have seen, is that it really doesn't exist. A person's ideal body weight depends on many different factors, including age, body shape, metabolic rate, genetic makeup, gender and physical activity, among many others. Persons need varying amounts of weight and can carry different amounts of weight in good health. It is the position of The American Dietetic Association that successful weight management for adults requires a lifelong commitment to healthful lifestyle behaviors emphasizing eating practices and daily physical activity that are sustainable and enjoyable.[11]

Necessity of body fat

Some body fat is necessary to survival. This has been demonstrated in times of human starvation. Such victims die of fat loss, not protein depletion. For mere survival, men require 3% body fat and women require 12%. However, we need to do more than just stay alive. For the human race to continue, we need to be able to work and reproduce. The additional body fat carried by women has evolved to enable them to bear children. Especially for reproductive capacity, women require about 20% body fat. Menstruation—**menarche**—begins when the female body reaches a certain size or, more precisely, when the young girl's body fat reaches this critical proportion of body weight, somewhere near 20%. Approximately this amount is needed for ovulation and thus for eventual pregnancy. Most women gain body fat during pregnancy. This fat storage is important for lactation because the production of breast milk requires energy. Usually the lactation process then brings a gradual loss of these body fat stores. Dieting during pregnancy in an attempt to avoid storing this needed body fat is extremely dangerous and leads to a low-birth-weight baby at risk for developmental difficulties.

HEALTH, OBESITY, AND SOCIAL IMAGES

OBESITY AND HEALTH

Many common beliefs about the relation of obesity and health conflict with data available from scientific studies.

Common beliefs

Common folk beliefs hold that being fat is "bad for you." This view is reinforced by traditional medical opinion of many years that obesity is an illness and contributes to a wide number of health problems, including hyperlipidemia, carbohydrate intolerance, surgical risk, anesthesia risk, pulmonary and renal problems, pregnancy complications, diabetes, and hypertension. Generally, this broad "medicalization" of obesity views all fatness as an unhealthy condition that must be *controlled*—prevented or treated indefinitely, with drugs if necessary.[11]

Conflicting data

Often in such broad statements the distinction is not made between moderate overweight states and massive or morbid variances. Both the extremes of fatness and thinness pose medical problems. The major issue relates to

---

menarche   The beginning of first menstruation with the onset of puberty.

the effect of degrees of general overweight in the population and requires closer study. Clear health risks exist in *extreme* obesity, but unless a person is at least 30% *overfat*, the relationship of "overweight" to disease or mortality is questionable. This significant obesity is at least 20% above the ideal body weight in standard tables.[6] This weight correlates approximately with a body mass index (BMI) of 27 (see pp. 94, 95).

Specific health implications

However, there are important health implications of obesity. An earlier National Institutes of Health (NIH) consensus development conference of experts identified adverse effects of obesity on health in three main areas:

1. *Hypertension, hypercholesterolemia, and diabetes.* In the three health problems of essential hypertension, elevated serum cholesterol levels, and non-insulin-dependent diabetes mellitus (NIDDM) the evidence indicates a strong association with obesity, varying directly with the extent of the obesity and being reversible with weight reduction.[12] There is a genetic factor in each of these chronic conditions. Thus early intervention follows in developing health habits in diet and exercise to maintain optimal weight, especially in high-risk families.
2. *Coronary heart disease.* Although the evidence was not as strong, the NIH panel agreed that sufficient long-term data from the classic Framingham study shows association of degree of obesity with coronary heart disease (CHD), independent of other risk factors. In any event, the primary conditions of hypertension, elevated blood cholesterol, and NIDDM are strong risk factors for CHD, thus linking obesity indirectly to CHD.
3. *Cancer.* Evidence indicates associations between some types of cancer with dietary fat and obesity.[13] These data show that obese men, regardless of smoking habits, had a higher mortality from cancer of the colon, rectum, and prostate. Obese women had a higher mortality from cancer of the breast (postmenopausal), uterus (including cervix and endometrium), and ovaries, as well as the gallbladder and biliary passages.

Currently, physicians indicate that being substantially overweight, having a BMI of about 30 or so, correlates with serious health problems such as coronary heart disease, hypertension, and diabetes, as well as a variety of musculoskeletal problems.[12] Even smaller amounts of weight loss of 10% to 15% of body weight have been shown to improve these conditions.[13]

Emerging attitude change in obesity and its treatment

A major shift, one that focuses on a philosophy of *trust* rather than *control*, is emerging among health professionals with a deeper understanding of attitudes about obesity or fatness and its treatment, especially with children.[14,15] Also, increasingly, wise professionals are seeing the "other side of obesity" and asking questions such as: "What is the health status of obese persons who are not in treatment programs?" and "If obesity is such a serious health hazard, why are Americans living longer at the same time they are getting fatter?"[16]

SOCIAL IMAGES: FEAR OF FATNESS AND EATING DISORDERS

The thinness model

A model of thinness, especially directed toward women, pervades American society. Fueled by capital investment in New York City's Madison Avenue advertising, successful use of an exaggerated image of thinness has been the drive for marketing many products. The "ideal" woman has been remade in the eyes of America. The gaunt, almost cadaverous models adorning the covers of many glamour magazines seem to mock most women's attempts to feel good about themselves and their bodies. In many instances, these social pressures have created a fear of fatness that leads to a persistent pursuit of the abnormally thin ideal marketed constantly in the media. These fears of fatness can develop early, as observed especially among fourth-grade 9-year-old girls. By senior high school, a number of middle-class adolescent girls have already developed a fear of fatness and begun to develop disordered eating, including restraint and binge eating.

Evolutionary conflict and social pressure

This extreme degree of thinness now popular in America, however, goes against evolutionary body wisdom. It took the human species thousands of centuries to evolve the greater fat-carrying capacity of women for reproductive purposes. The largely futile and often dangerous attempts to lower body weight drastically have damaged the self-image of many women and men alike. Strong prejudice exists against obese persons, regardless of their age, gender, race, or socioeconomic status. But some people, try as they might, simply cannot and do not lose weight, or they live "yo-yo" lives with a perpetual cycling of ups and downs of weight—an even greater threat to their physical and emotional health.[3] They do not and cannot conform to the social norms, no matter how hard they try, and are somehow blamed for their condition. Many people see fat people as (1) *gluttonous*—they eat more than they should; (2) *lazy*—if they wanted to, they could lose weight; (3) *neurotic*—they have an oral fixation caused by arrested development during childhood; or (4) *unhappy*—they eat because they are depressed. Many studies of comparative behavior have shown no evidence for any of these stereotyped beliefs about overweight persons. Rather, there is now considerable evidence that human obesity can have a significant genetic component, in youth as well as at middle age, as indicated in the recent discoveries of the new obesity genes, especially the *obese* gene that produces *leptin*.[17,18] In tests with genetically obese mice, leptin causes reduced food intake, loss of body weight, and decreased body weight. The human leptin has demonstrated the same function.

Eating disorders

Numerous reports indicate that about 80% of young women and 30% of young men in America are dieters.[19,20] These young people, as well as adolescents, and even younger children, are at risk of developing eating disorders. A recent study identified community groups most important to reach for prevention of eating disorders: junior high school students, coaches, and parents.[20] These eating disorders have been described by the American Psychiatric Association, edition IV: anorexia nervosa, bulimia nervosa, eating disorder not otherwise specified, and binge eating disorder.[21] The American Dietetic Association, in its current position paper on eating disorders, includes an excellent full page box giving a descriptive summary of each condition.[22] Nutrition education and nutrition intervention should be integrated into the team treatment of patients with eating disorders during the assessment and treatment phases of outpatient and/or inpatient therapy.

1. *Anorexia nervosa,* a form of self-induced starvation, has reached alarming proportions among adolescent girls. They become terrified of gaining weight and refuse to eat, even though they may be hungry. They often perceive themselves to be "fat," "gross," and "ugly," even if they are severely underweight or emaciated. This condition can become life-threatening, inducing malnutrition and requiring hospitalization (see *Issues & Answers,* p. 108). A small percentage of these young victims eventually die from this disorder.
2. *Bulimia nervosa,* a gorging-purging syndrome, also creates both emotional and physical problems. It is increasingly common among young women. Some estimate that as many as 20% of college women engage in bulimic behavior. In a sense, a bulimic person is a "failed anorectic" one. Unable to go without eating, these persons engage in the practice of gorging themselves with large amounts of food and subsequently purging themselves, usually by induced vomiting.
3. *Eating disorder not otherwise specified,* as indicated, covers similar disorders that do not meet the criteria for any specific one. For example, the person's eating behavior is like that of anorexia nervosa except that despite substantial weight loss the current weight is in the normal range and she still has regular menses. It is like bulimia nervosa except that binges occur less frequently, body weight remains normal as a result of constant self-induced vomiting and spitting out chewed food without swallowing it, and there are frequent episodes of binge eating without the purging or induced vomiting of bulimia nervosa.
4. *Binge eating disorder,* characterized by recurrent episodes of binge eating, differs from bulimia nervosa in that the recurrent episodes of binge eating are not followed by compensatory behaviors such as purging by self-induced vomiting or laxative use. The person eats rapidly and alone from embarrassment and deep distress about the problem, quickly consuming large amounts of food until feeling uncomfortably full, and afterward has a deep sense of guilt. There is marked distress and self-disgust about the binge eating.

THE PROBLEM OF WEIGHT MANAGEMENT

How does a person go about managing excess weight, or more correctly, excess fat? Simple, you say—just reverse the process by which it was gained. Everybody knows that on the energy balance sheet, when energy taken in does not equal energy expended, the difference is reflected in weight either stored or lost, and 3500 kcalories is the equivalent of 0.45 kg (1 lb) of body fat. That is part of the answer, but altogether it is not quite that simple.

INDIVIDUAL VARIANCES

Energy balance factors

Keeping a weight balance score in such arithmetic terms is not that easy. First, it's difficult to know *precisely* how many kcalories are in the food you are eating. Second, it's even more difficult to know how many kcalories you are

---

anorexia nervosa Extreme psychophysiologic aversion to food, resulting in life-threatening weight loss. A psychiatric eating disorder caused by a morbid fear of fatness, in which the person's distorted body image is reflected as fat when the body is actually malnourished and extremely thin from self-starvation.

bulimia nervosa A psychiatric eating disorder related to the person's fear of fatness, in which cycles of gorging on large quantities of food are followed by self-induced vomiting and use of diuretics and laxatives to maintain a "normal" body weight.

burning up. This depends on your basal metabolic activity, the resting metabolic rate and thermic effect of food, body size, amount of lean body mass, age, gender, and physical activity, among other things.

Metabolic efficiency

Some persons have proclaimed for years, "It's not fair! She can eat twice as much as I can and never gains an ounce." The medical rejoiner has been, until recently, "She gets more exercise than you do." That may be true in some cases, but not all. Some people do metabolize food more easily than others, while in others a low metabolic rate—especially a low thermic effect of food (see pp. 90, 91)—contributes to their overweight state.

EXTREME APPROACHES

For such "lazy," "weak-willed," and "morally inferior" creatures, as some deride them, overweight persons endure rather incredible experiences in their constant struggle to lose weight, including some of the following.

Fad diets

A constant array of various "diet books" floods the American market. They usually sell briefly and then fade away, largely because their "quick fix" does not work. Moreover, nutritional science finds itself caught in the "diet wars" because there are no magic, simple answers to a far more complex problem. Most of the fad diets fail on three counts: (1) they are based on scientific inaccuracies and misinformation; hence they are often nutritionally inadequate; (2) they do not address the basic behavioral problem involved and the lifelong food and exercise habit change, actually a new lifestyle, required to maintain a healthy weight for a given individual once it is achieved; and (3) they do not recognize that some persons' natural healthy weight may exceed these rigid extremes. For some persons the degree of kilocaloric restriction required places impossible demands, and they find themselves caught in the **chronic dieting syndrome** with its harmful physical and psychologic effects. To conform to society's thinness values, they are often consigned to a lifetime battle against biologic mechanisms that operate within their bodies to return them to their natural weight, or metabolic set-point—a high price for false hope.[6] In some instances, they often become caught up in various schemes and scams in our burgeoning United States diet industry, where it is estimated that in a year some $51 billion will be spent on a wide range of weight loss diets, products, and services.[6,12]

Fasting

This drastic approach takes many forms, from literal fasting to use of very-low-calorie diets of special formulas. Effects may be those of semi-starvation: acidosis, postural hypotension, increase in urinary loss of important electrolytes, increase in serum uric acid, constipation, and a decrease in basal metabolic rate (BMR). In past use of such extreme practices, there has been sufficient loss of heart muscle to cause death. And, at best, more recent programs have failed in the critical period after initial weight loss to help persons maintain the new weight when refeeding began.

Special clothing and body wraps

Special "sauna suits" are claimed to help weight loss in specific spots of the body or to help clear up so-called "cellulite" tissue. To the scientific community "spot reduction" is a fabrication, as is "cellulite," which is a word coined some years ago in Europe by a "beauty operator" and has no factual basis. This mummylike wrapping is endured by some persons in an attempt to reduce body size. What small weight loss may result is usually caused by temporary water loss. The only way to lose weight is to metabolize more kcalories than are consumed.

Drugs

The amphetamines, commonly called "speed," and over-the-counter drugs such as *phenylpropanolamine (PPD)* (Dexatrim), a stimulant similar to amphetamine, were once popular in the treatment of obesity. They are no longer used because their abuse was a danger to health. However, the disordered metabolism of severe obesity, with its high risk in chronic disease, has renewed medical interest in drug research for its treatment. Two newer drugs that increase the activity of the neurotransmitter serotonin have been used in combination, *fenfluramine* (Pondimin)-*phentermine* (Fastin), commonly called "fen-phen." However, on September 15, 1997, fenfluramine and a similar drug *dexfenfluramine* (Redux), were recalled from the global market by the United States Food and Drug Administration (FDA) because of continuing reports from physicians that their use was contributing to heart valve defects and primary pulmonary hypertension (PPH) in some users.[23-27] Currently, these drugs are under further study and development. Nutrition and food behavior counseling and daily walking exercise remain the core of healthy weight management.

Surgery

Surgical intervention is usually reserved for medical treatment of severely obese persons after more traditional methods have failed. They include earlier procedures such as intestinal bypass, which resulted in serious side effects and is no longer used. Current procedures focus on gastric bypass, including several forms of gastroplasty (Figure 6.3), as well as jejunoileal bypass, but these surgeries are not without problems and require skilled team management, including nutritional care.[28,29]

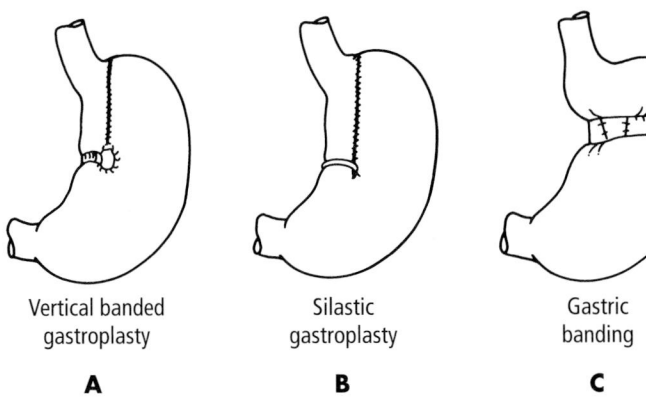

Vertical banded gastroplasty	Silastic gastroplasty	Gastric banding
A	**B**	**C**

Figure 6.3 Simple gastric-restriction procedures for treatment of obesity in order of frequency in current practice. **A**, Vertical banded gastroplasty—50%. **B**, Silastic ring gastroplasty—5%. **C**, Gastric banding—4%. More complex procedures that bypass part of the digestive tract are reserved for treating severe, massive obesity. (Adapted from Grace DM: Gastric restriction procedures for treating severe obesity, *Am J Clin Nutr* 55:556S, 1992 and Mason EE et al: Perioperative risks and safety of surgery for severe obesity, *Am J Clin Nutr* 55:573S, 1992.)

A more limited type of cosmetic surgery, developed in the 1980s and still in current vogue, is a form of local fat removal, lipectomy, commonly called *liposuction*. It is used to remove fat deposits under the skin in places of cosmetic or figure concern such as the hip and thigh areas. A thin tube is inserted through a small incision in the skin, and a desired amount of the fat deposit is suctioned away. However, this procedure is quite painful and carries risks of infection, large disfiguring skin depressions, or blood clots that lead to dangerous circulatory problems and possible kidney failure. Any surgical procedure carries risk and may cause other problems as side effects.

TYPES AND CAUSES OF OBESITY

Theories about the cause of obesity have varied in recent years. The prior simplistic terms "exogenous" (external cause) and "endogenous" (internal cause) are too vague to be useful and have been discarded. Rapidly developing research, however, is providing better knowledge of the types and causes of various obesities, which is gradually dispelling some of the longstanding social myths and prejudices about obesity. We are beginning to understand that there are different forms of obesity, which vary in extent, body distribution, and underlying genetic-metabolic factors. This knowledge provides a more realistic individual approach to care. Four basic factors may be identified: genetic-metabolic, psychologic, social, and physiologic.

Genetic-metabolic factors

There is increasing evidence that familial tendencies probably influence a person's chances of becoming fat more than any other basic factor. A genetic base may regulate differences in body fat, including gender variances. Numerous studies have confirmed that gene-controlled low resting metabolic rate (RMR) is a contributor to obesity, not a result, and that adaptive thermic effect of food (TEF) has genetic influences.[6] The semistarvation of rigorous dieting reduces the RMR even further as an adaptive response to the dietary restriction. Further validation studies on the metabolic set-point for adipocyte or total body fat that predisposes an individual for a particular natural weight level are continuing. In any event, this genetic-metabolic variability should not lead such persons into inadequate diets, but instead guide them into developing wise dietary and exercise habits. Of course, overweight is not *strictly* a genetic condition, but in some persons this factor may well relate to food habits learned over time, as other factors discussed here indicate.

Psychologic factors

The public perceives fat persons as having less control over their appetites and as being more responsive to external cues than to internal ones. That is, some believe obese persons eat (1) when it's mealtime by the clock or when they're surrounded by tasty foods, instead of when they're really hungry, (2) when they're unhappy, or (3) because as children they associated food with maternal love. It is true that reactive eating from stress or anxiety contributes to obesity. However, these factors cannot be applied to *all* fat persons as a group. They have no more tendency to these actions and feelings than anyone else. But there is no question about the role that psychology must play in any wise weight management program. Our cultural ideal thin body type and social discrimination against obese persons have created psychologic problems in many individuals that need to be addressed. Psychosocial support—in the form of counselor, support group, friends, or family—is critical for a successful weight management program.

---

chronic dieting syndrome A compulsive eating disorder, commonly referred to as **compulsive overeating**. It includes binge eating episodes, but without the purging behavior of persons with bulimia nervosa. This is an emotional, reactive eating pattern occurring in response to stress or anxiety and used to soothe painful feelings.

Social factors

The class values placed on the obese state by different social groups also influence its frequency. As a person moves upward in social class, there is a tendency to be more highly motivated to maintain a moderate or normal body weight. In lower socioeconomic status groups obesity is more common and considered normal. In higher-level groups greater social value is usually placed on the nonobese state. The length of exposure to these values and their pressure on individuals in any social class determines reaction to them. Other social and environmental factors associated with obesity include cultural and family food patterns, job environments and recreational eating that encourage use of kcalorie-dense foods, the social role of eating, the sedentary patterns of recreation and employment, and television viewing time, with its inactivity and constant snacking.

Physiologic factors

Normal physiology during the growth years contributes to accumulation of fat tissue deposits. There are critical periods during growth for the development of obesity, such as early childhood and early stages of puberty. Early and middle adulthood are other potential periods because of reduced physical activity with no adjustment of caloric intake. For women other times may be during pregnancy and after menopause, resulting from hormonal changes. For men a critical period is early to middle adulthood, generally resulting from decreasing activity with no change in food habits formed during adolescence, when the body has high energy needs. Both men and women tend to gain weight after age 50 years because of the lower resting metabolic rate (RMR), decreased physical exercise, and failure to adjust food habits accordingly.

A significant physiologic factor in obesity is fat cell increase. Normally, the full genetic complement of fat cells is reached by puberty and then remains constant. After puberty, these fat cells may increase in mass within limits, rarely exceeding about 1.5 μg, but not usually in number. However, if overeating continues after the fat cells have reached their maximal capacity, cell proliferation is triggered again. Once this increased cell number has occurred, it is not reversed. In extreme obesity, for example, the number of fat cells may increase from a norm of about 30 billion to approximately 120 billion, each one of which is also increased in size. The only means of weight reduction then is to diminish individual cell size. Once the body has added fat cells to accommodate extra fuel storage, these cells remain and store varying amounts of fat. A similar harmful pattern of increased fat storage occurs in individuals whose natural metabolic set-point for body weight is higher than cultural ideals of thinness when they respond to unrealistic weight goals and constant diets. Hunger and frustration are inevitable, and rebound overeating follows in a repeated cycling of weight loss and regain in the chronic dieting syndrome.

Increased fat cell formation also affects body fat distribution. A form of localized fat cell increase occurs in women over the lower body areas of thighs and hips, called *gynecoid*—or lower body—obesity. This form of obesity is benign and unrelated to the metabolic complications of obesity. However, a second type of central abdominal fat deposit—called *android* because it is the usual pattern of adult male fat distribution—is a typical pattern that also occurs in women and is associated with metabolic complications, such as non-insulin-dependent diabetes mellitus (NIDDM) in males and females.

THE HEALTH MODEL: A POSITIVE PERSONAL APPROACH

GENERAL COMPONENTS

Healthful adult weight management is based on combined wisdom from nutritional and behavioral research. A well-balanced, individually tailored food plan, together with a gradually increased exercise program and supportive behavioral change measures, can be effective and personally rewarding. In health care practice the general approach to weight management is based on underlying sound nutrition and energy balance and the client's personal situational needs. It focuses on two main aspects: (1) motivation and support and (2) a personalized program.

Motivation and support

The degree of personal motivation is a prime factor. Through initial interviews, the nutrition counselor—usually a specially trained registered dietitian (RD)—seeks to determine individual needs, attitudes toward food and weight, and the meaning food has for the client. Recognition is given to emotional factors involved, and support is provided by the nutritionist—together with the nurse and the physician—to meet the client's particular needs.

Personal program

To be successful, a weight management program must meet personal needs and goals. Such a program has some form of the following parts:

1. *Food behaviors.* Note the quantity of food served and eaten. Use moderate to small portions, attractively served. Take time to eat *slowly* and savor the food taste and texture. Reduce hidden factors added in food preparation, mainly fat. Increase fiber content. Choose a variety of foods from a basic food guide, which serves as a focus for sound realistic nutrition education. Empha-

size whole primary foods and a minimum of processed foods. Plan a fairly even food distribution throughout the day.

2. *Exercise behaviors.* Plan for regular daily exercise. Start with walking, building to a brisk aerobic pace, for about a half hour a day. Aerobic exercise benefits a person in a weight-management program because it (1) lowers the body-weight set-point, (2) suppresses appetite, (3) reduces body fat, (4) increases basal metabolic rate, (5) increases energy expenditure, and (6) retains and builds lean body mass (LBM). Then gradually increase the time of the exercise period to 45 to 60 minutes, and add other activities that can have aerobic value, such as swimming, or develop a set of body exercises, including stretching, body and muscle development, aerobic periods, and a cool-down period. High heart rate intensity exercise, especially, has been shown to decreases body fat.[30] Set occasional goals and keep a record of progress. Use variety in your program and enjoy it.

3. *Stress reduction exercises.* Practice progressive muscle relaxation and stress-reduction exercises. Learn an appropriate pattern as a guide, using imagery as a mental focusing device, or use tapes of environmental recordings if they are helpful. Select a suitable time and stay with it for daily practice. Start with a brief 10-minute period and increase as desired. In our stress-filled modern environment many persons really do not know how to relax.

4. *Personal interest area.* Develop some creative interest area for intellectual stimulation, personal enjoyment, and fulfillment. Explore various community groups or resources to support such activities.

5. *Follow-up program.* A follow-up schedule of appointments with the nutrition counselor is then outlined, and its values are discussed with the client. On subsequent visits, progress can be reviewed, problems discussed, and solutions explored. Continuing support can be provided. Practical suggestions for dealing with such things as realistic goals, food and exercise behaviors, meals at home and away from home, and any other special situations can be discussed. This follow-up support helps the client anticipate needs, reinforce new learnings, avoid pitfalls, sustain motivation, and deal positively with periods of frustration.

BEHAVIORAL ASPECTS

Behavioral change in respect to food and exercise is an important component of long-term weight management. It requires family, individual, or group support. Experienced and sensitive practitioners in health care settings recognize increasingly the need to provide ongoing training and support for the obese client, both individually and in peer support groups, to modify undesirable food behaviors and lack of physical activity that may have contributed to the obesity, if long range success is to be achieved. Food behavior particularly is rooted in many human experiences and associations and environmental situations. These experiences often produce addictive forms of eating response. Behavior-oriented therapies are designed to help the person change food, eating, and exercise patterns that contribute to the excessive fat and weight. These strategies help to increase insight, awareness, and understanding of present behaviors; to motivate toward positive change; and to recondition behaviors into new ones to meet personal goals. When the person changes associations with the undesirable habit patterns, he or she can then plan a means of constructive action. Supportive behavioral change activities are directed toward (1) self-management of eating behavior—the when, what, why, where, how, and how much, and (2) promotion of physical activity and increased energy output, providing a better total energy balance, as well as an added means of reducing stress.

PRINCIPLES OF A SOUND FOOD PLAN

On the basis of careful interviewing, body composition measures, and evaluation of available laboratory data, the nutritionist makes a comprehensive assessment of nutritional and health status, food and physical activity habits and behaviors, and living situation. Details for such full assessment are described in Chapter 15. Then, on the basis of this individual assessment, personal needs and goals can be established with the client. An appropriate food plan is developed together to meet normal nutritional needs and any necessary therapeutic modification for health problems that are present. Such a personal plan has several basic parts.

Energy balance

The energy intake level is adjusted to meet individual weight management needs. A moderate personal eating pattern is outlined. This gradual process is best for long-term success and health. On the average, for women, a sound plan for energy needs is based on about 1200 to 1500 kcal/day. For larger women and for men, a plan of about 1500 to 1800 kcal/day would meet gradual weight adjustment energy needs. It may be helpful to some persons to determine what their basal and activity needs are as a basis for understanding their overall energy expenditure factors (Table 6.3). The full newly expanded food exchanges are given in Appendix L.

Table 6.3	General approximations for daily adult basal and activity needs	
Basal energy needs (avg. 1 kcal/kg/hr)	**Male (70 kg) kcal** $70 \times 24 = 1680$	**Female (58 kg) kcal** $58 \times 24 = 1392$
Activity energy needs		
Very sendentary + 20% basal	$1680 + 336 = 2016$	$1392 + 278 = 1670$
Sedentary + 30% basal	$1680 + 504 = 2184$	$1392 + 418 = 1810$
Moderately active + 40% basal	$1680 + 672 = 2352$	$1392 + 557 = 1949$
Very active + 50% basal	$1680 + 840 = 2520$	$1392 + 696 = 2088$

Nutrient balance

Basic energy nutrients are outlined to achieve the following nutrient balance:

1. *Carbohydrate.* About 50% to 55% of total kcalories, with emphasis on complex forms, such as starches with fiber, and moderation of sugars.
2. *Protein.* Approximately 20% of total kcalories, with emphasis on lean food choices and small portions to curtail fat.
3. *Fat.* About 25% to 30% of total kcalories, with emphasis on plant fats, scant use, and alternate seasonings.

In general, this nutrient balance approximates the recommendations of the United States Dietary Guidelines for Healthy Americans. Review these guidelines in Chapter 1. They are helpful as a good basic nutrition education tool.

Distribution balance

Spread food fairly evenly through the day to meet energy needs. Consider any daily "problem times" and plan simple snacks to meet such needs.

Food guide

Use some type of general food reference lists from which the client can make a variety of food choices to fulfill the basic personal food plan. The food exchange system provides such a guide (see *To Probe Further* box, p. 104). This system draws on a broad database to provide a good general reference guide for comparative food values and portions, variety in food choices, and basic meal planning.[31] Food items can easily be combined into desired dishes. To lower fat in food preparation, use alternate seasonings, such as herbs and spices, onion and garlic, lemon juice, vinegar, wine, fat-free broth, mustard, and other condiments.

PERSONAL NEEDS

Individual adaptations

Throughout the planning, remember to focus on the individual client and personal needs. If the plan is unrealistic, whatever its form or basis, it will not be followed. Some persons find it helpful to keep a daily journal, which can include notes of food intake, environmental food cues, feelings, physical symptoms, and any stress factors related to food behavior. It may also include notes about other activities such as physical exercise or stress-reduction practice. A periodic review of such notes may help in making general observations, determining problem areas, monitoring progress, and gaining insights for setting personal goals to achieve desired health and fitness behavior changes. Essential parts of all programs are nutrition counseling and education—especially in reducing total fat, but also assessing quantity in all foods, protein and carbohydrates as well, and ongoing support for behavioral change, and increased physical activity.

Currently in the United States, there is a healthy growing awareness among health professionals, their clients, and the public in general that the modern phenomenon of constant restrictive "dieting" and the United States diet industry is counterproductive and harmful in the long run to many persons, especially to growing children and adolescents, as well as overweight women whose natural body weight levels do not conform to society's thinness model. As a result, health professionals are developing alternative approaches, based on a health and fitness model, for persons who benefit from a more supportive gradual plan with emphasis on exercise and gradual diet changes focused first on fat, but remembering that excess carbohydrate and protein add more kcalories also. The American Dietetics Association defines healthy weight management as the adoption of "healthful and sustainable eating and exercise behaviors indicated for reduced disease risk and improved feelings of energy and well-being."[11] Thus, at the very least, all healthy weight management will include the following goals:

1. Gradual development of a healthful eating style with increased use of whole grains, fruits, and vegetables.
2. A nonrestrictive approach to eating based on internal regulation of food—hunger and satiety.

3. Gradual increase to at least 30 minutes of enjoyable physical activity each day.

Such health and fitness models provide needed help with positive behavioral changes through ongoing supportive counseling and peer group support.

EARLY HEALTHY WEIGHT MANAGEMENT APPROACH

In the last analysis, it seems that the most constructive activity lies in early healthful weight *management* that centers on trust, which builds self-esteem and responsibility as children experience normal growth as a basis for prevention of obesity as they grow older, whereas most current prevention models focus on weight *control*, which builds self-doubt and dependency.[14,15] Thus the wise goal is to achieve and maintain an inherently appropriate body weight and maintain it through a healthy balance between energy intake in wise food choices and energy output in enjoyable physical exercise, recognizing all the while that fatness is a normal condition for *some* people. Early nutrition education, positive food and fitness behavior, and habit formation in the family—with support and guidance for young parents and children before an obese condition develops—will help prevent many problems in later adulthood.

THE PROBLEM OF UNDERWEIGHT

We have discussed at length the major problem of excess weight. But conversely, what about the state of less-than-adequate weight? Excluding the self-imposed eating disorders, what dangers lie in being generally underweight? What are some of its causes and approaches to treatment?

DEFINITION

Extremes in underweight, just as in overweight, bring or accompany serious health problems.[32] Although general underweight is a less common problem in the American population than is overweight, it does occur in a small percentage—estimated at somewhat less than 10%—among persons who have trouble gaining and maintaining weight. Some seem to lack control over how much they eat at a meal and reach a full feeling with less food than do persons of normal weight. The underweight condition may be associated with poverty, poor living conditions, or long-term disease. A person with more than 10% below the average weight for height and age is considered underweight; 20% or more is cause for concern. Serious problems may result in these persons, especially young children who may suffer long-term growth retardation or failure to thrive. Resistance to infection is lowered, general health is poor, malnutrition develops, and strength is reduced.

GENERAL CAUSES

In general, underweight is associated with conditions that cause basic malnutrition, such as the following:

- *Wasting disease.* Long-term hypermetabolic disease such as cancer, or short- or long-term infection and fever, place metabolic demands on the body that drain the body's resources.
- *Poor food intake.* Diminished food intake results from physiologic causes suggested before or from other situations, such as (1) psychologic factors that cause a person to refuse to eat, (2) loss of appetite or imbalance in the brain's hunger-satiety centers, or (3) personal poverty and limited food supply.
- *Malabsorption.* Poor nutrient absorption results from (1) prolonged diarrhea, (2) gastrointestinal disease, or (3) abuse of laxatives.
- *Hormonal imbalance.* Hyperthyroidism or other abnormalities may increase the needs of the body.
- *Energy imbalance.* Greatly increased physical activity without a corresponding increase in food brings an energy balance deficit.
- *Poor living situation.* An unhealthy home environment or no home at all results in irregular and inadequate meals, or in some persons, an indifferent or defeated attitude toward food.

NUTRITIONAL CARE

Underweight persons require special nutritional care to rebuild their body tissues and nutrient stores and regain their health. Any food plan needs to be adapted for each person's unique situation, whether it involves personal or economic needs, living situation, or underlying disease. The dietary goal, according to each person's tolerance, is to increase energy and nutrient intake in a diet that is (1) high-calorie, at least 50% above standard needs, (2) high-protein, to rebuild tissue, (3) high-carbohydrate, to provide a primary energy source in easily digested form, (4) moderate-fat, to add kcalories but not exceed toleration limits, and (5) a good source of all the vitamins and minerals, including individual supplements where deficiencies require them. Good food of wide variety, well-prepared and seasoned, and attractively presented helps revive lagging appetites and increases the desire to eat. Frequent small nourishing meals and snacks spread through the day, including favorite foods, stimulate interest in eating and increase optimal use of foods and their nutrients. To achieve the desired increase in kcalories, use (1) food seasonings, such as margarine or butter, sauces, and dressings, and (2) a food supplement such as Ensure (Ross) to add kcalories and key nutrients.

A basic aim is to help build the best food habits possible, within any limitations that may exist, so that the improved nutritional status and weight can be main-

To Probe Further

Food guide: the exchange system of dietary management

The exchange system of dietary management, developed by two professional organizations, the American Dietetic Association and the American Diabetes Association, is based on the concept of nutritional equivalency. Thus its basic food lists are simple groupings of common foods according to their generally equivalent nutritional values. This system may be used for any situation requiring a balance of the energy nutrient foods—carbohydrates, fats, and proteins.

The foods are divided into basic groups (with subgroups), called the "exchange lists." Each food item within a group or subgroup contains about the same food value as other food items in that group, allowing for exchange within groups, thus providing for variety in food choices as well as food value control. Hence the term *food exchanges* is sometimes used to refer to food choices or servings. The total number of "exchanges" per day depends on individual nutritional needs, based on normal nutritional standards. There is some variation in the composition of foods within each exchange group. The full listings of foods in each exchange group is given in Appendix H. Food listings may be used as reference, along with current nutrient values on food product labels, for controlling a particular nutrient such as grams of fat consumed each day

---

tained once it is regained. This rehabilitation process requires much creative counseling with each individual and family, with attention to the underlying socioeconomic or disease conditions. Practical personal guides and ongoing support are needed to counteract root causes of the malnutrition. In some extreme cases, tube feeding or total parenteral nutrition (TPN) may be necessary (see Chapter 17).

TO SUM UP

Energy is that force or power that enables the body to maintain it life-sustaining metabolic work, as well as all its physical work and activity. The energy provided by food is measured in *kilocalories* or *joules*. Body energy cycles among various basic forms such as chemical, electric, mechanical, and thermal. *Metabolism* is the body's way of changing the chemical energy of food into these cycling forms of body energy according to body needs. When food is not available, the body draws on its own stores to meet energy needs: glycogen from carbohydrate stores, fatty acids from fat tissue, and amino acids from lean body mass.

Total energy needs are based on basal (maintenance) and nonbasal (exercise) requirements. The basal metabolic rate (BMR)—or the currently used term resting metabolic rate (RMR), the amount of energy required to maintain the body at rest after a 12-hour fast—and the added thermic effect of food (TEF) comprise the body's metabolic energy needs, with variable needs for work and other physical activities. The four main compartments of body composition are lean body mass, body fat, body water, and mineral mass. Body composition is measured by a number of methods developed for research, population surveys, and clinical practice.

Body weight has traditionally been used as an indicator of obesity, which raises the risk of health problems. But it is the *composition* of the weight, lean versus fat tissue, that is the most important aspect. Weight-management programs have traditionally been designed for obese persons. However, a growing modern obsession with thinness has created new weight-management problems—the development of the *chronic dieting syndrome*, which leads to ever increasing cycles of dieting and regaining and decreasing self-esteem, as well as fostering eating disorders that result in semi-starvation.

In general, the health and fitness model of weight management is based on personal motivation and support for the individual. Aspects of such a program include changing food attitudes and behaviors, increasing physical activity, learning and practicing relaxation techniques, and developing personal interests. Behavioral strategies, with counselor and group support, help the individual examine the effect of life situations on eating habits and change those situations that encourage overeating. According to individual needs, sound weight management is based on an adjusted energy level, mainly in decreasing fat and increasing exercise, that allows for (1) gradual small to moderate rates of loss, or in some instances a more healthful holding pattern that recognizes individual natural weight levels, (2) sound nutrition, and (3) support for food and exercise behavior changes. The ideal plan begins with prevention, stressing positive food habits and physical fitness from early childhood to help prevent major problems later in life.

The opposite problem of underweight also brings food problems. It results from physiologic, psychosocial, economic, or disease causes. A nutrient- and energy-rich diet supplied through multiple small meals is needed, with ongoing counseling to help with the underlying causes and rehabilitation process.

■■ QUESTIONS FOR REVIEW

1. What does the term *fuel factor* mean? What is this comparative factor for each of the energy-yielding nutrients?

2. Define *resting metabolic rate.* What factors influence this rate? Which body tissues contribute most of the body's basal metabolic needs and what approximate percentage of the total energy expenditure do these internal basal metabolic activities require?

3. What factors influence nonbasal energy needs?

4. Calculate your own energy balance for 1 day based on your energy input (food) and your energy output (RMR + TEF + physical activity). (See *Practical Application* box, p. 92)

5. Describe the major eating disorders associated with America's growing obsession with thinness. What social factors contribute to this obsession? Compare these to the factors that contribute to the growing tendency of overweight.

6. Discuss the safety of five popular means of trying to lose weight.

7. Describe four basic types of causes for obesity.

8. Describe five components of the "health model" for weight management. How does it differ from the traditional medical model?

9. What are the basic principles of a sound food-exercise plan for weight management programs?

10. List some ways of increasing energy intake for an underweight person.

■■ REFERENCES

1. Guyton AC, Hall JE: *Textbook of medical physiology,* ed 9, Philadelphia, 1996, Saunders.

2. Schutz Y, Jéquier E: Energy needs: assessment and requirements. In Shils ME, Olson JA, Shike M, eds: *Modern nutrition in health and disease,* ed 8, vol 1, Philadelphia, 1994, Lea & Febiger.

3. Gibbs WW: Gaining on fat, *Sci Am* 275(2):88, 1996.

4. Behme MT: Symposium on diet, nutrition, and health, *Nutr Today* 32(1):23, 1997.

5. Forbes GB: Body composition: influence of nutrition, disease, growth, and aging. In Shils ME, Olson JA, Shuke M, eds: *Modern nutrition in health and disease,* ed 8, vol 1, Philadelphia, 1994, Lea & Febiger.

6. Phinney SD, Halsted CH: Obesity, anorexia nervosa, and bulimia. In Feldman M, Scharschmidt BF, Sleisenger MH, eds: *Gastrointestinal and liver disease,* ed 6, vol 1, Philadelphia, 1998, Saunders.

7. Schwartz MW, Seeley RJ: The new biology of body weight regulation, *J Am Diet Assoc* 97(1):54, 1997.

8. US Department of Agriculture, US Department of Health and Human Services: Nutrition and your health: dietary guidelines for Americans, *Home and Garden Bulletin No 232,* ed 4, Washington, DC, 1995, US Government Printing Office.

9. Bray GA: Pathophysiology of obesity, *Am J Clin Nutr* 55:488S, 1992.

10. Cummings SM, Goodrick GK, Foreyt JP: Position of the American Dietetic Association: weight management, *J Am Diet Assoc* 97(1):71, 1997.

11. Kassirer JP, Angell M: Losing weight—an ill-fated New Year's resolution, *N Engl J Med* 338(1):52, 1998.

12. Colditz GA et al: Weight gain as a risk factor in clinical diabetes mellitus in women, *Ann Intern Med* 122:481, 1995.

13. Hynder EL: Primary prevention of cancer: planning and policy considerations, *J Natl Cancer Inst* 83(7):475, 1991.

14. Satter EM: Internal regulation and the evolution of normal growth as the basis for prevention of obesity in children, *J Am Diet Assoc* 96(9):860, 1996.

15. Evers C: Empower children to develop healthful eating habits, *J Am Diet Assoc* 97(10S):S116, 1997.

16. Duran N: The other side of obesity, *Nutr Today* 31(2):80, 1996.

17. Behme MT: Leptin: product of the *obese* gene, *Nutr Today* 31(4):138, 1996.

18. Roberts SB, Greenberg AS: The new obesity genes, *Nutr Rev* 54(2):41, 1996.

19. Peters PK et al: Questionable dieting behaviors are used by young adults regardless of sex and student status, *J Am Diet Assoc* 96(7):709, 1996.

20. Whisenant SL, Smith BA: Eating disorders: current nutrition therapy and perceived needs in dietetics education and research, *J Am Diet Assoc* 95(10):1109, 1995.

21. American Psychiatric Association: *Diagnostic criteria for eating disorders,* ed 4 revised (DSM IV-R), Washington, DC, 1994, The Association.

22. Reiff DW, Reiff KL: Position of the American Dietetic Association: nutrition intervention in the treatment of anorexia nervosa, bulimia nervosa, and binge eating, *J Am Diet Assoc* 94(8):902, 1994.

23. Ault A: Anti-obesity drugs recalled from the global market, *Lancet* 350(Sept 20):867, 1997.

24. Connolly HM et al: Valvular heart disease associated with fenfluramine-phentermine, *N Engl J Med* 337(9):581, 1997.

25. Saltzman E, Siegel RD: Update: cardiopulmonary risks of appetite suppressant drugs, *Nutr Today* 32(5):210, 1997.

26. Bray G: Drug treatment of obesity: don't throw the baby out with the bath water, *Am J Clin Nutr* 67(1):1, 1998.

27. Halstead CH: Controversies: should drugs be used in the treatment of obesity? *Am J Clin Nutr* 67(1):1, 1998.

28. Atkinson RL: Obesity surgery as a model for understanding the regulation of food intake and body weight, *Am J Clin Nutr* 66:184, 1997.

29. Näslund E et al: Reduced food intake after jejunoileal bypass: a possible association with prolonged gastric emptying and changed gut hormone patterns, *Am J Clin Nutr* 66:26, 1997.

30. Bryner RW et al: The effects of exercise intensity on body composition in women, *J Am Coll Nutr* 16(1):68, 1997.

31. Wheeler ML, Franz M et al: Macronutrient and energy database for the 1995 Exchange Lists for Meal Planning: a rationale for clinical practice decisions, *J Am Diet Assoc* 96(11):1167, 1996.

32. Klein S, Jeejeebhoy KN: The malnourished patient: nutritional assessment and management. In Feldman M, Scharschmidt BF, Slesenger MH, eds: *Gastrointestinal and liver disease,* ed 6, vol 1, Philadelphia, 1998, Saunders.

■■■ FURTHER READING

American Dietetic Association: *The healthy weight: a practical food guide,* Chicago, 1995, The Association.

Cummings SM, Goodrick K, Foreyt JP: Position of The American Dietetic Association, *J Am Diet Assoc* 97(1):71, 1997.

The practical food guide, available from ADA, explains why popular diets often fail and provides a plan for a healthy weight. The excellent ADA position paper on weight management provides background and guidance for healthy weight management based on good eating practices and daily physical activity that one can live with and enjoy.

Cameron KE, Dwyer JT et al: Prescription appetite suppressants in weight management, *Nutr Today* 32(5):202, 1997.

Saltzman E, Siegel RD: Update: cardiopulmonary risks of appetite suppressant drugs: new concerns and unanswered questions, *Nutr Today* 32(5):210, 1997.

These two timely articles in a single issue discuss the background history and current status and use of appetite-suppressant drugs in weight management.

Berg FM: *Afraid to eat: children and teens in weight crisis,* Hettinger, ND, 1997, Healthy Weight Publishing Network.

Duran N: The other side of obesity, *Nutr Today* 31(2):80, 1996.

Parham ES: Is there a new weight paradigm? *Nutr Today* 31(4):155, 1996.

Satter EM: Internal regulation and the evolution of normal growth as the basis for prevention of obesity in children, *J Am Diet Assoc* 96(9):860, 1996.

These authors, nutritionists and family therapists, indicate the growing awareness of a new paradigm of healthy body weight that puts us in the midst of a major shift in our understanding and attitudes about fatness and the treatment of obesity. This new awareness is especially focused on the emerging change in the way we see and treat childhood obesity. This is important reading in these growing areas.

Case study

The obese patient with hypertension

Rosanna Giovanni is a 45-year-old woman, mother of three children, first seen in the clinic 6 months ago for a routine checkup. At that time she weighed 90 kg (200 lb) and had a blood pressure reading of 152/88 mm Hg. She is 155 cm (5 ft 2 in) tall. At the initial visit she had no serious complaints other than a bad cold. Her physician warned her that her blood pressure was somewhat elevated and scheduled a return visit for another reading the following week. After two more readings of 160/95 and 155/89 mm Hg consecutively, Mrs. Giovanni was told that she had hypertension. No medication was prescribed. However, she was referred to the nutritionist to begin weight management and sodium control.

During the assessment interview the clinic nutritionist discovered that Mrs. Giovanni ate two meals at home and one at work. Breakfast usually consisted of scraps of food left on plates by her school-age children. Lunch was a hot meal with dessert purchased in the cafeteria of the hospital where she worked part-time as an admissions clerk. Dinner was almost always an Italian-style meal, often including pasta with rich sauces and cheese or filled with meat, plus a variety of vegetables and salads. Desserts, usually made from scratch, were served with every dinner.

Mrs. Giovanni was very interested in gradually losing some weight to avoid taking antihypertensive medication if possible. However, she was apprehensive about the possibility of having to give up her favorite foods to do so. The nutritionist reassured her. With Mrs. Giovanni, the nutritionist helped with a food preparation plan to reduce fat and salt by using a number of alternative seasonings in the family recipes. Then she arranged for Mrs. Giovanni to join one of the clinic's peer support groups where she could experience some stress reduction exercises and new ways of looking at food.

Three months later Mrs. Giovanni had lost 8 kg (18 lb). She reported feeling much better and said her family was very supportive of her efforts. As a result of new cooking methods, her overweight husband had finally started to lose weight as well. She continued to lose an average of 0.7 kg (1.4 lb) per week for another month, but suddenly she gained 2.5 kg (5 lb) in a 2-week period. At a nutrition interview conducted shortly after that time, she revealed that her husband had recently been hospitalized with a stroke. Apparently he also had hypertension but had refused to see a physician for many years.

The effects of the stroke were very mild; however, Mrs. Giovanni continued to worry about her husband's health. She began to eat desserts with lunch again and kept nuts, candies, and other snack foods at home for "nibbling." The nutritionist provided personal support in the office and suggested adding exercise to the routine as a good form of healthy weight and stress management. Mrs. Giovanni resisted the idea at first, saying that she could not fit it into her current schedule of caring for three children and her husband and working part-time at the hospital. However, after bringing the subject up in her weight management group meeting, she gained positive feedback and practical ideas for fitting some aerobic activities into her busy schedule.

During the next 3 months, Mrs. Giovanni resumed her previous weight loss pattern and has begun to feel better. The exercise routine has also helped her to look better and to feel better about herself. She informed the nutritionist that, aside from her appearance, she is most proud of the effect of her healthy diet program on her family. Her children have reduced their junk food intake, and her husband has even begun exercising with her almost every day.

Questions for analysis

1. How do you think Mrs. Giovanni's lifestyle, meal pattern, food habits, and food preparation methods influenced her weight status?

2. What is hypertension? What roles does weight management play in controlling it? Why did Mrs. Giovanni's physician recommend nondrug methods of control through diet?

3. In developing a meal plan with Mrs. Giovanni, what advice would you offer to help her retain the cultural flavor of her meals while reducing her kcalorie intake?

4. What are some ways that Mrs. Giovanni may strengthen her behavioral changes toward food and exercise? What other behavioral approaches may be useful?

5. What is aerobic exercise? Why is it effective for a weight management program?

6. What practical suggestions would you offer to Mrs. Giovanni for helping her incorporate exercise time into her busy routine? Why?

Issues Answers

Eating disorders: the high price of our drive for thinness

"Bean lean, slender as the night, narrow as an arrow, pencil thin, get the point?" So reads the clever advertising copy of a well-known New York fashion house, one of many such Madison Avenue reflections of our American culture's obsession with thinness, especially for women. Many of these women are paying a heavy price in physical and psychologic illness from eating disorders.

America's developing thinness drive

This obsessive cultural drive for thinness is, in fact, a comparatively recent social phenomenon in the American experience. At the beginning of the 1900s, the skinny woman would have been seen as awkward, unsightly, perhaps piteously at risk for disease, and certainly not a standard of beauty. Even in the 1950s, Marilyn Monroe had an hourglass figure that would be considered overweight by today's standards. Then in the 1960s, the fashion world discovered a model named "Twiggy" from her small, straight-as-a-stick, little-girl figure. The thinner form became the ideal, and fashions were developed based on her thin type of body shape. But Twiggy was *naturally* thin, and many naturally moderate-weight women could only reach that ideal by becoming *unnaturally* thin through constant dieting. Thus the trend to be acceptable by reshaping the body through weight loss and restrained eating became entrenched, fueled by a growing diet industry, the profits of which made its purveyors willing partners. This trend strengthened through the 1970s and 1980s. Now in the 1990s, the model form is somewhat more "athletic" in appearance but still thin, so women must add workouts to dieting to meet society's ideals. The notion is perpetuated that personal worth and self-esteem derive from how we look rather than who we are.

General nature and extent of thinness pressure and disordered eating

The drive for thinness is now appearing even in very young girls early in their initial grade school social experiences. Nine-year-olds in the fourth grade, for example, are already saying that they want to be thinner, and are beginning to restrict normal eating of foods they label as "bad." By high school years, the pressure to be thin intensifies. Adolescents learn early, even before puberty and its rapid growth effects, that thinness in women and athletic leanness and muscle development in men are major cultural criteria for determining attractiveness and social acceptability. Unfortunately, however, many soon learn that it is difficult to meet these standards because genetic inheritance plays a major role in determining body size and shape. They also find themselves in a double bind with the inactivity and snacking that accompany watching television. Dieting may appear an attractive tool to offset these effects and reshape their bodies, including practices such as fasting, low-energy deficit diets, heavy workouts, and purging behavior such as induced vomiting and use of laxatives, diuretics, and diet pills. An increasing number of boys, especially those in wrestling and bodybuilding activity, and girls practice such on-and-off cycles of dieting and purging to accomplish this body reshaping. Students are waving red flags for eating problems, such as preoccupation with food and body weight, inappropriate body image, and reluctance to eat.

Researchers studying eating disorders tell us that the percentage of persons with eating problems is increasing, and that this is a true increase and not just a factor of increased reporting. Most scientific evidence indicates that both biologic and psychosocial factors are involved, especially impaired family communication patterns. Eating moderately to maintain a natural weight level is perfectly healthy and promotes wellness of mind and body. For some individuals, however, who are sensitive to family and social pressures about acceptably thin body weight and labels of "good" and "bad" food, dieting begins to serve other purposes of achieving acceptance and a sense of self-worth. This pattern of chronic restrictive dieting has been strongly related to the development of eating disorders, in which feelings about self and body image are projected to food. Eating, then, becomes fueled by emotional rather than actual physiologic needs.

American Psychiatric Association criteria for eating disorders

Four forms of such eating disorders are now recognized and described by the American Psychiatric Association (AHA) in its guidelines for medical therapy teams— Diagnostic criteria for eating disorders, *Diagnostic and Statistical Manual*, edition 4, Washington, D.C., 1994, APH. These four forms, revised DSM IV-R, are anorexia nervosa, bulimia nervosa, eating disorder not otherwise specified, and binge eating disorder. Each has distinctive characteristics, based on APA's diagnostic criteria and symptoms.

Anorexia nervosa

The eating disorder anorexia nervosa—"appetite loss from nervous disease"—is actually misnamed. It is starvation with excessive weight loss, self-imposed at great physical and psychologic cost, leading to body weight less than 85% of that expected. Through their distorted body image, those with anorexia nervosa have intense fear of gaining weight or becoming fat. They do not see themselves as underweight and emaciated but as always fat, and they continue to restrict their eating in ritualistic ways. Anorexia nervosa affects about 1% of young women, but its dangerous path can lead to sudden death from severe hypoglycemia and cardiac arrest. Significant deficits of bone mass occur as a frequent and often early complication of anorexia nervosa in adolescence, so that osteoporosis and bone fractures have become a "new morbidity" for dieting adolescent girls.

Diagnostic criteria. DSM IV-R describes the following states as being diagnostic for anorexia nervosa:

1. Refusal to eat sufficient food to maintain body weight over a minimal normal weight for age and height, for example, weight loss leading to maintenance of body weight 15% below that expected; or failure to make expected weight gain during a period of growth, leading to body weight 15% below that expected.
2. Intense fear of gaining weight or becoming fat, even though underweight.
3. Disturbance in the way in which one's body weight, size, or shape is experienced: for example, the person claims to "feel fat" even when emaciated and believes that one area of the body is "too fat" even when obviously underweight.
4. In females, absence of at least three consecutive menstrual cycles when otherwise expected to occur.

Bulimia nervosa

Bulimia, literally "ox-hunger," is descriptive of the massive amounts of food sometimes consumed and has been called the binge-and-purge syndrome. Because the person is eating, although in a disorderly manner, a fairly normal weight level is usually maintained and the underlying problem is a guilt-ridden secret. Control is lost when eating, and extremely large amounts of food are consumed. Then in response the individual attempts to purge the body from the effects of the large amount of food by self-induced vomiting, fasting, excessive exercise, or using laxatives, diuretics, or diet pills. The emotional and physical cost of maintaining such disordered behavior is great.

Diagnostic criteria. The DSM IV-R describes specific behavioral criteria for bulimia nervosa and the psychologic and physical effects:

1. Recurrent episodes of binge eating—rapid consumption of a large amount of food in a single, relatively short period of time.
2. A feeling of loss of control over eating behavior during the binges.
3. Regular self-induced vomiting; use of laxatives or diuretics; strict dieting or fasting; or vigorous exercise to prevent weight gain. In the nonpurging type, the person uses other compensatory behaviors, such as fasting and excessive exercise.
4. Minimum average of 2 binge eating episodes a week for at least 3 months.
5. Persistent overconcern with body shape and weight.

Eating disorder not otherwise specified

Diagnostic criteria. This newly developed third eating disorder category, as its name indicates, lists eating behaviors that do not meet descriptions for other eating disorders.

1. It is like anorexia nervosa except that regular menses continue and despite substantial weight loss the current weight is within normal range.
2. It is like bulimia nervosa except that binges occur less than twice a week and the pattern lasts less than 3 months.
3. The person usually maintains a normal weight by self-induced vomiting after eating even small amounts of food, such as two cookies.
4. The person repeatedly chews and spits out large amounts of food but does not swallow.

Binge eating disorder

This eating disorder, commonly referred to as compulsive overeating, includes binge eating episodes without the purging behavior of bulimia nervosa. This type of eating usually occurs in response to stress or anxiety as an emotional eating pattern to soothe or relieve painful feelings. The binges may be triggered in part by physiologic factors. Dietary restriction and failure to achieve satiety precede binges and probably help drive them in a cyclic pattern.

Diagnostic criteria. The DSM IV-R describes specific criteria for binge eating disorder:

1. Eating within any 2-hour period large amounts of food until feeling uncomfortably full.
2. Eating large amounts of food when not feeling hungry and eating alone as a result of feeling embarrassed by the amount.
3. Feelings of self-disgust, depression, or guilt after each bingeing episode, which occur at least 2 days a week.

Continued

4. Marked distress about the binge eating, but no compensatory behaviors such as purging, fasting, or excessive exercise.

Whatever form it takes, the chronic dieting syndrome fueled by our cultural drive for thinness contributes to these compulsive eating disorders. Persons who attempt to reach these unrealistic, and for them unnatural, weight goals are "forever dieting" and inevitably experience hunger and frustration. Rebound eating in some form usually occurs, followed by more attempts to lose weight, creating the characteristic weight cycling with its physiologic effects compounding the psychologic problem. With each successive weight loss, the resting metabolic rate (RMR) drops more quickly; thus the weight comes off with greater difficulty. Evidence now suggests that lean body mass lost with such dieting cycles may not be recovered with each regain in weight, thus altering body composition. Even if the final weight achieved is in a so-called normal range, the increased percentage of body fat can cause abnormalities, creating the "metabolically obese" individual of normal weight.

Treatment approaches

Eating disorders take a high toll in both physical and psychologic health of many adolescent girls and young women and require individualized care. First, the best chance for success in improving their condition lies with team care by a sensitive, experienced group of health professionals, including a physician, clinical psychologist, clinical nutritionist, and nurse. Outpatient services may provide needed care for less serious cases of bulimia nervosa, but often for life-threatening anorexia nervosa more intense inpatient care is essential. Second, with an individualized approach, especially for bulimia nervosa, a "stepped-care" program at five levels of intervention may provide appropriate options. At least five levels may be used: (1) some form of self-help with written material; (2) nutrition and diet education and counseling, either individual or group; (3) antidepressant drug therapy in combination with counseling and support; (4) individual outpatient psychologic treatment, including cognitive behavior therapy; and (5) a period of day patient or inpatient care, with follow-up outpatient care.

These are serious health matters. How long are we willing to pay this heavy price for distorted societal images of personal worth based on how we look instead of who we are? Change in any area is difficult, but it rests on a foundation of awareness and knowledge of the problem; then changes in attitude can come. Only then will we see a weakening of America's drive for thinness and its feeding of serious eating disorders. Certainly, we need to seek more ethical practices in our own work, as well reforms in the diet industry. More realistic individualized approaches to help persons with weight and health will follow and will help to reduce the risks for serious eating disorders.

References

American Psychiatric Association: *Diagnostic and statistical manual,* ed 4, Washington, DC, 1994, The Association.

Bruce B, Wilfley D: Binge eating among the overweight population: a serious and prevalent problem, *J Am Diet Assoc* 96(1):58, 1996.

Eiger MR, Christie BW, Sucher KP: An outcome measure of patients with eating disorders, *J Am Diet Assoc* 96(1):62, 1996.

Foreyt JP et al: Future directions in obesity disorders, *Addict Behav* 21:767, 1996.

Moukaddem M et al: Increase in diet-induced thermogenesis at the start of refeeding in severely malnourished anorexia nervosa patients, *Am J Clin Nutr* 66(2):133, 1997.

Neumark-Sztainer D, French SA, Feffery RW: Dieting for weight loss: associations with nutrient intake among women, *J Am Diet Assoc* 96(11):1172, 1996.

Orphanidou CI et al: Changes in body composition and fat distribution after short-term weight gain in patients with anorexia nervosa, *Am J Clin Nutr* 65(6):1034, 1997.

Rees JM: Eating disorders in adolescents: a model for broadening our perspective, *J Am Diet Assoc* 96(1):22, 1996.

Chapter

7

Vitamins

Here we begin a two-chapter sequence on the non-energy-yielding micronutrients, the vitamins and minerals. First, we look at the vitamins.

Probably no other group of nutritional elements has so captured the interest of scientists, health professionals, and the general public as has the vitamin group. Attitudes toward vitamins have varied widely, running the gamut from wise functional use to wild flagrant abuse.

In this chapter we will review both fat- and water-soluble vitamins. We will focus on why we need them and how we may obtain them.

The Study of Vitamins

General Nature and Classification

During the five decades of vitamin discovery in the first half of the 1900s, the remarkable nature of these vital agents became more and more apparent. Three key characteristics were evident: (1) they were not metabolized to yield energy as were the energy nutrients carbohydrate, fat, and sometimes protein; (2) they were vital to life; and (3) often not a single substance but a group of related substances turned out to have the particular metabolic activity. The name *vitamin* developed during initial research years when one of the early scientists working with a nitrogen-containing chemical substance called an **amine** thought that this was the common nature of these vital agents. So he named his discovery *vitamine* (vital amine). Later the final "e" was dropped when other similarly vital substances turned out to be a variety of organic compounds. The name vitamin has been retained to designate compounds of this class of essential substances. At first, letter names were given to individual vitamins discovered. But as the number of them increased rapidly, this practice created confusion. Thus in recent years more specific scientific names based on structure or function developed. However, for fat-soluble vitamins, although their chemical structures are now well known, their letter names have been retained for clarity because in each case a number of closely related compounds with similar properties are also well known.[1]

Definition of a Vitamin

As the vitamins were discovered one by one and the list of them grew, two basic characteristics clearly emerged to define a compound as a vitamin:

1. It must be a vital organic dietary substance that is not an energy-producing carbohydrate, fat, or protein, and is usually necessary in only very small quantities to perform a particular metabolic function or to prevent an associated deficiency disease.
2. It cannot be manufactured by the body and therefore must be supplied in food.

Classification

Vitamins are usually grouped and distinguished according to their solubility in either fat or water:

Fat-soluble

The fat-soluble vitamins are A, D, E, and K. They are closely associated with lipids in their fate in the body. They can be stored, and their functions are generally related to structural activities.

Water-soluble

The water-soluble vitamins are C and the B-complex family. These have fewer problems in absorption and transport. They cannot be stored except in the general "tissue saturation" sense. The B vitamins function mainly as coenzyme factors in cell metabolism. Vitamin C is a vital structural agent.

Current Concepts and Key Questions

To clarify current concepts concerning each known vitamin, consider these key questions as the basis for your study:

Nature. What is the vitamin's general structural nature?

Absorption and transport. How does the body handle this particular vitamin?

Function. What does this vitamin do? This is, perhaps, the most significant question.

Requirement and sources. How much of this vitamin do we need and where can we obtain it?

Here, then, we will briefly review each of the vitamins in turn—four fat-soluble (A, D, E, K) and nine water-soluble (C and B vitamins). In each case we will identify the specific chemical name, a more common usage now in the case of water-soluble vitamins, and review answers to the key questions above. In some cases, a group of similar substances have the vitamin activity, not just a single substance bearing the specific name.

Fat-Soluble Vitamins

Vitamin A

Chemical and physical nature

Vitamin A is a generic term for a group of compounds having similar biologic activity. These compounds include **retinol, retinal,** and retinoic acid. The term *retinoids* refers to both the natural forms of retinol and its synthetic copies. Chemically, retinol is a primary alcohol of high molecular weight ($C_{20}H_{29}OH$). Because it has a specific function in the retina of the eye and is an alcohol, vitamin A has been given the specific chemical name *retinol*. It is soluble in fat and in ordinary fat solvents. Because it is insoluble in water, it is fairly stable in cooking.

Forms

There are two basic dietary forms of vitamin A:

1. *Preformed vitamin A: retinol.* This is the natural form of vitamin A, found only in animal food sources and usually associated with fats. Vitamin A compounds are deposited primarily in the liver but also in small amounts in the kidneys, lungs, and fat tissue. In this form, its dietary sources are mainly the fat portion of dairy products, egg yolk, and storage organs such as liver.

2. *Provitamin A: beta-carotene.* This is the original substance, the "provitamin A," behind the animal sources of vitamin A itself, in plants that animals have eaten and converted to the vitamin. This original plant source is beta-carotene ($C_{40}H_{56}$), which is found in plant pigments. It is called carotene because one of its main sources is the yellow pigment of carrots and other vegetables and fruits. Beta-carotene is significant in human nutrition and is the common precursor of vitamin A.[1,2] It supplies about two thirds of the vitamin A necessary in human nutrition. These yellow and red carotenoid pigments, which occur in abundance in many vegetable foods and can be changed to vitamin A in the liver, continue to be the main sources of vitamin A for most of the world's population.[3]

ABSORPTION AND STORAGE

Substances that aid absorption

Vitamin A enters the body as the preformed vitamin A from animal sources and the precursor carotene from plant sources. Several substances aid in the absorption of vitamin A and carotene by the body:

1. **Bile salts.** With fat and other fat-related compounds, bile transports vitamin A in micelles, minute fat globules formed in the small intestine after initial digestion and then carried into the intestinal wall for further preparation. Clinical conditions affecting the biliary system, such as obstruction of the bile ducts, infectious hepatitis, and liver cirrhosis, hinder vitamin A absorption.
2. **Pancreatic lipase.** This fat-splitting enzyme is necessary for initial hydrolysis in the upper small intestine of fat emulsions or oil solutions of the vitamin. Water-based preparations of retinol are available for use in conditions where secretion or absorption of pancreatic lipase is curtailed, such as in cystic fibrosis or pancreatitis.[1]
3. **Dietary fat.** Some fat in the food mix, simultaneously absorbed, stimulates bile release for effective absorption of vitamin A.

Carotene conversion

In the intestinal wall during absorption some of the carotene is converted to vitamin A. The remainder is absorbed and transported as such, dissolved in the fat part of lipoproteins.

Transport and storage

The route of absorption of both vitamin A and carotene parallels that of fat. In the intestinal mucosa all the retinol, from both natural preformed animal sources and from plant carotene conversion, is incorporated into the chylomicrons.[1] In this form it enters the bloodstream via the lymphatic system and is carried to the liver for storage and distribution to the cells. The liver, by far the most efficient storage organ for vitamin A, contains about 90% of the body's total quantity. This amount is sufficient to supply the body's needs for about 6 to 12 months, and some persons have been known to store as much as a 4-year supply. These stores are reduced, however, during infectious disease, especially in childhood infections such as measles. For example, among malnourished nonimmunized children in many parts of the world, measles has become a leading killer disease and is now designated by the WHO Expanded Program on Immunization as a target for both vitamin A supplementation and immunization. Age is also a factor in absorption. For example, in the newborn, especially the premature infant, absorption is poor. With advancing age, elderly persons may experience increasing difficulties with absorption. In addition, chronic use of mineral oil as a laxative hinders vitamin A absorption.

FUNCTIONS OF VITAMIN A

Vitamin A's role in visual adaption to light and dark has been well established. It also has a number of more generalized functions that influence vision, the health of body coverings and linings (epithelial tissue), the process of growth, antioxidant capacity, and reproductive functions.

Vision

The eye's ability to adapt to changes in light depends on a light-sensitive pigment, rhodopsin—commonly known as visual purple—in the rods of the retina (Figure 7.1). Rhodopsin is composed of the vitamin A substance, retinal, and the protein, opsin (Figure 7.2). When the body is deficient in vitamin A, the normal rhodopsin cannot be

---

amine An organic compound containing nitrogen. There are many different amine organic compounds.

retinal Organic compound that is the aldehyde form of retinol, derived by the enzymatic splitting of absorbed carotene. It performs vitamin A activity. In the retina of the eye, retinal combines with opsins to form visual pigments. In the rods it combines with scotopsin to form rhodopsin (visual purple). In the cones it combines with photopsin to form the three pigments responsible for color vision.

retinol Chemical name for vitamin A derived from its function relating to the retina of the eye and light-dark adaptation. Daily RDA standards are stated in retinol equivalents (RE) to account for sources of the preformed vitamin A and its precursor provitamin A, beta-carotene.

Figure 7.1   Structure of the eye. (From Seeley RR, Stephens TD, Tate PP: *Anatomy and physiology,* ed 2, New York, 1992, McGraw-Hill.)

Figure 7.2   The vision cycle: light-dark adaptation role of vitamin A.

Without vitamin A, the epithelial cells become dry and flat. They gradually harden to form keratin, a process called **keratinization**. Keratin is a protein that forms dry, scalelike tissue, normal in the case of nails and hair but abnormal in the case of skin and mucosal membranes. When the body is deficient in vitamin A, many such abnormal epithelial tissue changes may occur:

1. *Eye.* The cornea dries and hardens, a condition called xerophthalmia (Figure 7.3). In extreme deficiency the process may progress to blindness. This progressive blindness resulting from vitamin A deficiency is a serious public health problem; it affects the health and sight of a staggering number of persons in many parts of the world. The tear ducts dry, robbing the eye of its cleansing and lubricating means, and infection follows easily.
2. *Respiratory tract.* Ciliated epithelium in the nasal passages dries and the cilia are lost, thus removing a barrier to entry of infection. The salivary glands dry, and the mouth becomes dry and cracked, open to invading organisms.
3. *Gastrointestinal tract.* Mucosal membrane secretions decrease so that tissues dry and slough off, affecting digestion and absorption.
4. *Genitourinary tract.* As epithelial tissue breaks down, problems such as urinary tract infections, calculi, and vaginal infections increase.

made and the rods and cones of the retina become increasingly sensitive to light changes, causing **night blindness**. This condition can usually be cured in about 30 minutes by an injection of vitamin A (retinol), which is readily converted into retinal and then into rhodopsin.

Epithelial tissue

Vitamin A is necessary to build and maintain healthy epithelial tissue, which provides our primary barrier to infections. The epithelium includes not only the outer skin but also the inner mucous membranes. This function of vitamin A is the basis for current study of retinoids and carotene in relation to cancers of epithelial origin (see *Issues & Answers,* p. 145).

Figure 7.3 Xerophthalmia. (From McLaren DS: *A colour atlas and text of diet-related disorders,* ed 2, 1992, Mosby–Year Book Europe Limited.)

Figure 7.4 Follicular hyperkeratosis caused by vitamin A deficiency. (From McLaren DS: *A colour atlas and text of diet-related disorders,* ed 2, 1992, Mosby–Year Book Europe Limited.)

5. *Skin.* As skin becomes dry and scaly, small pustules or hardened, pigmented, papular eruptions appear around hair follicles, a condition called *follicular hyperkeratosis* (Figure 7.4).
6. *Tooth formation.* Specific epithelial cells surrounding tooth buds in fetal gum tissue that normally become specialized cup-shaped organs called *ameloblasts* may not develop properly. These little organs form the enamel of the developing tooth.

Growth

Vitamin A is essential for the growth of bones and soft tissues. This effect is probably caused by the vitamin's influence on protein synthesis, mitosis (cell division), or stability of cell membranes. Growth and maintenance of

bone require constant remodeling of the bone tissue according to growth and repair needs. To accomplish this constant reshaping and balance task, continuous growth of new bone and removal of old bone must occur. Vitamin A participates in the important job of tunneling out old bone to make way for new bone; the tunnels are filled in to accommodate growth needs, all the while maintaining the precise pattern set in the initial embryonic cartilage model.

Antioxidant capacity

The provitamin A, beta-carotene, has been shown to have **antioxidant** capacity, raising interest in its ability to protect persons as they grow older from cell damage caused by free radicals.[4] The free radicals are parts of compounds that are by-products of normal metabolism in cells, or they may be created by environmental exposure to sunlight, tobacco smoke, car exhaust fumes, ozone, or x-rays. In any case, free radicals damage the DNA, cell membranes, and cell compounds, or kill the cell outright. These accumulative effects advance the aging process of cell deterioration. Antioxidant substances help to neutralize free radicals in the cell, protecting those persons susceptible to such oxidative stress by grabbing an electron from another molecule. Chemists have likened this action to a "bucket brigade" that takes the dangerous chemical property and passes it from one molecule to the next, thus hindering its harmful action.

Reproduction

The retinoids, except for retinoic acid, are necessary to support normal sexual maturation during adolescence and function of the adult reproductive system. Vitamin A deficiency causes glandular degeneration and sterility.

VITAMIN A REQUIREMENT

Influencing factors

A number of variables modify vitamin A needs. Although the vitamin is generally ample in most diets, many factors may alter need in a given individual: (1) amount stored in the liver, (2) form in which it is taken

---

antioxidant A substance that inhibits oxidation of polyunsaturated fatty acids and formation of free radicals in the cells.

keratinization The process of creating the protein keratin, which is the principal constituent of skin, hair, nails, horny tissues, and the organizing matrix of the enamel of the teeth. It is a very insoluble protein.

night blindness Inability to see well at night in diminished light, resulting from lack of required vitamin A.

(carotene or vitamin A), (3) illness, and (4) gastrointestinal or hepatic defects. Vitamin A deficiency may occur as a result of (1) inadequate dietary intake, (2) poor absorption resulting from lack of bile or defective absorbing surface, and (3) inadequate conversion of carotene because of liver or intestinal disease.

Units of measure

To cover such variables, the RDA standard recommends a margin of safety above minimal needs. Traditionally, vitamin A has been measured in international units (IU). Currently, the RDA uses the measure of **retinol equivalents (RE)**. These RDA standards, continuing in use until the new Recommended Dietary Intake (RDI) standards are completed, are printed inside this book's covers for quick reference, with footnotes giving the weight equivalents for retinol and beta-carotene. The RE provides a more accurate measure because it accounts for individual absorption and conversion variances. All other countries and international agencies have also adopted the retinol equivalent (RE) measure.

Hypervitaminosis A

Because the liver can store large amounts of vitamin A, and many persons take additional megadose supplements, it is clearly possible to consume a potentially toxic quantity. Hypervitaminosis A is manifested by joint pain, thickening of long bones, loss of hair, and jaundice. Excess vitamin A may also cause liver injury with resulting portal hypertension and ascites.

FOOD SOURCES OF VITAMIN A

There are few animal sources of natural preformed vitamin A: liver, kidney, cream, butter, and egg yolk. Our main dietary sources are the yellow and green vegetable and fruit sources of carotene. In addition, commercial

Table 7.1	Food sources of vitamin A (RDA for adults: women 800 µg RE; men, 1000 µg RE)				
	Quantity	Vitamin A (µg RE)		Quantity	Vitamin A (µg RE)
Bread, cereal, rice, pasta			Avocado	1 med	189
This food group is not an important source of vitamin A.			Banana	1 med	69
			Cantaloupe	1/4 med	1386
Vegetables			Grapefruit (pink)	1/2 med	162
Asparagus	1/2 cup	196	Orange juice	1/2 cup	75
Beet greens	1/2 cup	1110	Papaya	1 cup (cubes)	735
Bok choy cabbage	1/2 cup	790	Peach	1 med	399
Broccoli (fresh)	1 med stalk	1350	Prunes (dried)	4 prunes	207
Broccoli (frozen)	1/2 cup (chopped)	721	Tangerine	1 med	108
Brussels sprouts	1/2 cup (4 sprouts)	121	Watermelon	1 wedge (4 × 8 in)	753
Carrots (raw)	1/2 cup (1 med)	2379	**Meat, poultry, fish, dry beans, eggs, nuts**		
Collard greens	1/2 cup	2223	Clams (canned)	3 oz	144
Corn	1 sm cob	93	Egg, whole	1 large	78
Dandelion greens	1/2 cup	1843	Liver, beef	3.5 oz	10,831
Green beans	1/2 cup	102	Liver, chicken	3.5 oz	4912
Green peas	1/2 cup	144	Salmon, pink (raw)	3 oz	30
Kale	1/2 cup	1369	**Milk, dairy products**		
Lima beans	1/2 cup	60	Cheddar cheese	1 oz	90
Mustard greens	1/2 cup	1218	Milk, lowfat 2% (fortified)	8 fl oz	150
Pumpkin (canned)	1/2 cup	2352	Milk, skim (fortified)	8 fl oz	150
Romaine lettuce	1/2 cup (chopped)	157	Milk, whole (unfortified)	8 fl oz	101
Spinach	1/2 cup	2187	Ricotta cheese, whole milk	1/2 cup	182
Summer squash	1/2 cup	123	Swiss cheese	1 oz	72
Sweet potato (baked, in skin)	1 med	2769	Yogurt, whole	8 fl oz	84
Tomato (cooked)	1/2 cup	325	**Fats, oils, sugar**		
Winter squash	1/2 cup	1021	Butter	1 tbsp	138
Fruits			Margarine	1 tbsp	141
Apricot (dried)	4 halves	490			
Apricot (fresh)	3 med	867			

products such as margarine are fortified with vitamin A. The vitamin A values of selected foods are given in Table 7.1.

VITAMIN D

CHEMICAL AND PHYSICAL NATURE

Early investigators wrongly classed this substance as a vitamin. But it is now clear that it is really a prohormone of a sterol type and in its active form is viewed as a hormone. The precursor base in human skin is the lipid cholesterol material **7-dehydrocholesterol**. Thus all forms of these compounds with vitamin D activity are soluble in fat but not in water. They are heat stable and are not easily oxidized.

FORMS

Two compounds with vitamin D activity are involved in nutrition: *ergocalciferol (vitamin D_2)* and *cholecalciferol (vitamin D_3)*. Vitamin D_2 is formed by irradiating ergosterol (provitamin D_2), which is found in ergot (a fungus growth on rye and other cereal grains) and yeast. The much more significant product in human nutrition is D_3, **cholecalciferol**, which is formed by irradiating 7-dehydrocholesterol (provitamin D_3) in the skin. D_3 occurs also in fish liver oils.

ABSORPTION, TRANSPORT, AND STORAGE

Absorption

The absorption of dietary vitamin D_3 occurs in the small intestine with the aid of bile. It mixes with the intestinal bile-fat complex and is absorbed in these fat packets. Malabsorption diseases such as celiac syndrome, colitis, and Crohn's disease hinder vitamin D absorption.

Active hormone synthesis

The synthesis of the active hormonal form of *1,25-dihydroxycholecalciferol {1,25(OH)$_2$D$_3$}* is accomplished by the combined action of skin, liver, and kidneys, an overall process now called the vitamin D endocrine system.[1-3]

1. *Skin.* In the skin, 7-dehydrocholesterol, the precursor cholesterol compound, is irradiated by the sun's ultraviolet rays to produce vitamin D_3. The amount of D_3 produced by this irradiation in the skin depends on a number of variables, including length and intensity of sunlight exposure and color of the skin (see *To Probe Further* box, p. 142). For example, heavily pigmented skin can prevent up to 95% of ultraviolet radiation from reaching the deeper layer of the skin for adequate synthesis of the steroid hormone. Also, persons who lack exposure to sunlight—house-bound, or nursing home elderly persons or those living in crowded city areas with high air pollution rates—would fail to receive adequate skin irradiation.[4,5]

2. *Liver.* After synthesis in the skin, vitamin D_3 is transported by its special globulin protein carrier to the liver. Here a special liver enzyme converts D_3 to **25-hydroxycholecalciferol [25(OH)D$_3$]**, the intermediate product. This intermediate product is then transported by the same serum protein carrier to the kidney for final activation.

3. *Kidneys.* In the kidney a special renal enzyme, 1-alpha-hydroxylase, forms the physiologically active vitamin D hormone, *1-alpha,25-dihydroxycholecalciferol {1α,25(OH)$_2$ D$_3$}*. In general usage, the chemical name of the active vitamin D hormone is **calcitriol**.

FUNCTIONS OF VITAMIN D HORMONE

Vitamin D in the body is predominantly associated with calcium and phosphorus metabolism. It influences the absorption of these minerals and their deposit in bone tissue.

Calcium and phosphorus absorption and bone mineralization

In balance with the parathyroid hormone, the vitamin D endocrine system based in the kidneys stimulates the active transport of calcium and phosphorus in the small

---

calcitriol Activated hormone form of vitamin D [1,25(OH)$_2$D$_3$]—1,25-dihydroxycholecalciferol.

cholecalciferol Chemical name for vitamin D in its inactive dietary form (D$_3$). When the inactive cholecalciferol is consumed or its counterpart cholesterol compound is developed in the skin, its first stage of activation occurs in the liver and then is completed in the kidney to the active vitamin D hormone form *calcitriol,* 1,25-dihydroxycholecalciferol, or shorter form 1,25(OH)$_2$D$_3$.

7-dehydrocholesterol A precursor cholesterol compound in the skin that is irradiated by sunlight to produce an initial stage in the process of forming activated vitamin D hormone.

retinol equivalent (RE) Unit of measure for dietary sources of vitamin A, both preformed vitamin, retinol, and the precursor provitamin, beta-carotene. 1 RE = 1 μg retinol or 6 μg beta-carotene.

25-hydroxycholecalciferol [25,(OH)D$_3$] Initial product formed in the liver in the process of developing the active vitamin D hormone.

intestine and promotes normal bone mineralization. First, vitamin D stimulates calcium and phosphorus absorption in the intestine and their deposit in bone tissue. Second, balanced with this action, parathyroid hormone stimulates calcium withdrawal from the bone and excretion of phosphorus in the urine to help maintain the normal calcium-phosphorus balance in the blood. A third hormone participates in this triad of regulatory agents in calcium metabolism. This is calcitonin, a polypeptide secreted by connective tissue cells in the thyroid gland.

Role in bone disease

When the body does not have enough vitamin D, it cannot build normal bones. In children this vitamin D deficiency disease is called *rickets*. In the growing child the condition is characterized by malformation of skeletal tissue (Fig 7.5). In adults the disease is called *osteomalacia*. It occurs mostly in women of childbearing age who get little exposure to sunlight, have poor diets, or have frequent pregnancies, each followed by periods of lactation. The wide use of vitamin D-fortified foods, especially milk, has nearly eliminated common vitamin D deficiency rickets in developed countries, but it does occur, most frequently in infants 6 to 18 months of age. Cases in the United States have occurred among breast-fed infants who were not receiving the recommended vitamin D supplements.[5] In other parts of the world, rickets remains a public health problem. It occurs more often in northern countries with limited winter sunlight or in dark-skinned persons whose skin pigmentation inhibits passage of the sun's ultraviolet rays.

In addition, because of the active regulatory role of vitamin D as a balancing hormone, it has been used to treat the bone disease secondary to kidney failure, renal **osteodystrophy**, which is characterized by defective bone formation. Vitamin D also contributes to the treatment of **osteoporosis**, a bone loss disease common in older women that leads to fractures. Increasing awareness of this postmenopausal bone-thinning disease has led to interesting generational mother-daughter studies to reduce risks in later years.[6]

Basic cell processes

Beyond this role in bone and mineral metabolism, evidence is growing that the vitamin D hormone system is involved in widespread basic cell processes with targets in a number of organ tissues, such as brain, kidney, liver, skin, and reproductive tissue; hormone-secreting glands; and certain cells of the immune system. Investigators suggest that these expanded metabolic activities probably relate to an active hormonal role in controlling basic cell functions such as cell reproduction and spread, as well as cell differentiation. This ongoing work may lead to possible use of the vitamin D analogs in treatment of some types of leukemias and the persistent skin disorder psoriasis.

Figure 7.5   Bowlegs in rickets.   (From McLaren DS: A *colour atlas and text of diet-related disorders,* ed 2, 1992, Mosby–Year Book Europe Limited.)

VITAMIN D TOXICITY

Toxic amounts of vitamin D build up in the body easily because vitamin D is stored in adipose tissue and is released slowly. Toxic intakes of vitamin D may result from self-administered large doses of the vitamin supplement or from unknowing intake of large amounts in fortified foods such as milk. In the United States milk has been fortified with vitamin D since the 1930s, which has had the result of largely eradicating common rickets. The United States federal regulations specify that each quart of milk contain 10 μg (400 IU). However, experience has shown that vitamin D has to be used cautiously and carefully. Adults taking continued megadoses of 1500 μg (60,000 IU) have shown signs of severe intoxication.

Cases of intoxication do sometimes occur, usually from excessively fortified food. For example, a previous 1992 United States outbreak of vitamin D intoxication was traced to a single local dairy's sporadic addition of excessive vitamin D to milk during the fortification process.[7] Symptoms included failure to thrive and calcium deposits in soft tissue of the kidney nephrons in a 15-month-old child and progressive weakness, bone pain, and hypercalcemia in adults. A follow-up investigation of fortified milk and infant formula from supermarkets in five Eastern states showed similar irregularities in fortification from their labeled content of vitamin D addition.[7] General infant feeding poses special problems. Excess intake is possible in infant feeding practices where fortified milk, fortified cereal, plus variable vitamin supplements are used. The infant needs only 10 μg (400 IU) daily, whereas the amount in all of these items can easily total 100 μg (4000 IU).

Fortunately, however, excess vitamin D in dairy products is not a far-reaching problem. A larger problem relates to lactose intolerance. Greater skin pigmentation may interfere with natural synthesis of 7-dehydrocholesterol in populations that are also least likely to consume dairy products as a result of this intolerance.

VITAMIN D REQUIREMENT

Influencing factors

Difficulties exist in setting requirements for vitamin D. Variables arise from numerous sources: a limited number of food sources available, lack of knowledge of precise body needs, and differing degrees of skin synthesis by irradiation. Needs vary between winter and summer in northern climates. Also, a person's way of living and working determines the degree of sunlight exposure and thus influences individual need. Persons living and working indoors need more than someone who works outside all day. Elderly people or invalids who do not go out-of-doors may need supplementary vitamin D. Growth demands in childhood and in pregnancy and lactation necessitate increased intake.

RDA standard

The RDA standard is 10 μg of cholecalciferol (400 IU) daily for children and for women during pregnancy and lactation. The daily allowance for persons from 6 months to 24 years of age is the same—10 μg (400 IU)—and for all adults 25 years of age and older it is 5 μg (200 IU). Questions are raised about the adequacy of this allowance for older adults above age 65, especially elderly homebound persons for whom there is as yet no consensus of need. However, these needs are currently under study for the new projected Recommended Dietary Intakes to replace the Recommended Dietary Allowances (see Chapter 1).

FOOD SOURCES OF VITAMIN D

Few natural food sources of vitamin D exist. The two basic substances with vitamin D activity, D_2 and D_3, occur only in yeast and fish liver oils. The main food sources are those to which crystalline vitamin D has been added. Milk, because it is commonly used, has proved to be the most practical carrier. However, such food must be fortified accurately and consistently and the products monitored regularly by public health officials to avoid toxic excesses. It is now a widespread commercial practice to standardize the added vitamin content of milk at 10 μg (400 IU)/qt. Milk is also a good carrier for the vitamin because it contains calcium and phosphorus as well. Margarines are also fortified with 37.5 μg (1500 IU)/lb to serve as butter substitutes. A summary of food sources of vitamin D is given in Table 7.2.

VITAMIN E

CHEMICAL AND PHYSICAL NATURE

Vitamin E was discovered in connection with studies concerning the reproductive responses of rats and was identified as an alcohol. Because of this rat reproductive function and its chemical nature as an alcohol, it was named **tocopherol** from the Greek word *tokos,* meaning "childbirth." Since then, tocopherol has come to be commonly known as the antisterility vitamin, but this effect has been demonstrated only in rats and not in humans, despite all advertising claims for its contribution to sexual powers.

FORMS

Vitamin E is the generic name for a group of compounds with similar physiologic activity. It is the collective term for 8 or so fat-soluble 6-hydroxychroman compounds that show the biologic activity of alpha-tocopherol, the most significant of the group in human nutrition.[1,8] It is a pale yellow oil, stable to acids and heat and insoluble in water. It oxidizes very slowly, which gives it an important role as an antioxidant, to "neutralize" free cell radicals, and a protective role in preventing oxidation of the unsaturated fats. This oxidative capacity gives it widespread clinical application.[9]

---

osteodystrophy Defective bone formation.

osteoporosis Abnormal thinning of bone, producing a porous, fragile, latticelike bone tissue of enlarged spaces, prone to fracture of deformity.

tocopherol Chemical name for vitamin E. It was so named by early investigators because their initial work with rats indicated a productive function, which did not turn out to be the case with humans. In humans it functions as a strong antioxidant to preserve structural membranes, such as cell walls.

Table 7.2	Food sources of vitamin D (RDA for adults: 5 μg)		
		Quantity	**Vitamin D (μg)**

	Quantity	Vitamin D (μg)
Bread, cereal, rice, pasta		
Corn flakes	1 cup (1 oz)/28 g	1.00
Granola	$1/4$ cup (1 oz)/28g	1.23
Raisin bran	$1/2$ cup (1 oz)/28g	1.23
Vegetables		
This food group is not an important source of vitamin D.		
Fruits		
This food group is not an important source of vitamin D.		
Meat, poultry, fish, dry beans, nuts		
This food group is not an important source of vitamin D.		
Eggs		
Egg, whole	1 large/50 g	0.68
Egg yolk	Yolk of 1 large egg/17 g	0.68
Milk, dairy products		
Cheddar cheese	1 oz/28 g	0.08
Cream cheese	1 oz/28 g	0.05
Evaporated milk (vitamin D fortified)	$1/2$ cup (4 fl oz)/126 g	2.50
Milk, whole or nonfat (vitamin D fortified)	1 qt/960 g	10.00
Milk, whole or nonfat (vitamin D fortified)	1 cup (8 fl oz)/240 g	2.50
Fats, oils, sugar		
Margarine	1 tbsp	1.50

ABSORPTION, TRANSPORT, AND STORAGE

Vitamin E is absorbed with the aid of bile. With other lipids in the chylomicrons, it is transported out of the intestinal wall into body circulation in the blood plasma lipoproteins. Accumulated intake is stored in the liver and mainly in fat tissue. In adipose tissue, vitamin E is held mainly in bulk liquid droplets, and mobilization of alpha-tocopherol from these droplets is slow.

FUNCTIONS OF VITAMIN E

Antioxidant

Vitamin E acts as nature's most potent fat-soluble antioxidant. The polyunsaturated fatty acids in the structural lipid membranes of cells are particularly vulnerable to oxidative breakdown by free radicals in the cell, especially in the aging immune system.[8,10] The tocopherols can interrupt this oxidation process, protecting the cell membrane fatty acids from the oxidative damage.

Selenium relationship

Even with adequate vitamin E intake, some damaging cell peroxides may be formed, so a second line of defense is needed to destroy them before they can damage the cell membrane. The agent providing this added defense is a selenium-containing enzyme. Thus the trace element selenium spares vitamin E by reducing the vitamin's requirement. Similarly, in this partnership role, vitamin E helps reduce the selenium requirements.

VITAMIN E DEFICIENCY

When adequate vitamin E is not available, the cells are more vulnerable to oxidative attack and damage. For example, if vitamin E is deficient, the lipid membranes of red blood cells are exposed to oxidation of their structural polyunsaturated fatty acids. The membranes are broken, the contents lost, and the cells destroyed. The continued loss of red blood cells leads to anemia. This vitamin E deficiency disease is thus called **hemolytic anemia**. Premature infants are especially vulnerable because they missed the last month or two of fetal life, when vitamin E stores are normally built up.

In older children and adults, vitamin E deficiency presents a different set of symptoms, sometimes called *neurologic syndrome of vitamin E deficiency*.[11] These symptoms are associated with functions of the nervous system. The main nerves involved are (1) spinal cord fibers that affect physical activity such as walking, and (2) the retina of the eye, which affects vision. This group of neurologic problems has been recognized since medical advances have enabled children, such as those with cystic fibrosis and pancreatic insufficiency, to live longer with chronic defective absorption of fats and fat-soluble vitamins. The loss of the pancreatic fat-digesting enzyme lipase and its associated emulsifying agent bile leads to a chronic fatty diarrhea and inability to absorb fat and fat-soluble nutrients such as vitamin E. This vitamin E deficiency disrupts the making of **myelin**, the protective fat covering for the long axons of nerve cells that help pass messages along to muscles they serve. In children and adults this neurologic disorder, the lack of vitamin E, causes pigment degeneration of the retina's rods and cones. These light-sensitive cell membranes are rich in polyunsaturated fatty acids, and vitamin E is critical for preventing oxidation damage. There are also increasing population studies that link vitamin E to protection against cardiovascular disease. The ongoing research suggests that vitamin E inhibits the lipoprotein oxidation that initiates the atherosclerosis process[12] (see Chapter 20).

VITAMIN E REQUIREMENT
RDA standard

The requirements for vitamin E vary with the amount of polyunsaturated fatty acids in the diet. The RDA standard for adults in alpha-tocopherol equivalents (α-TE) is 10 mg for men and 8 mg for women. Needs during childhood growth years range from 3 to 10 mg. These stated allowances are based on an estimate of a diet composed of 80% α-TE and 20% other tocopherols with varying potencies.

Special clinical needs

Since vitamin E protects cellular and subcellular membranes and hence tissue health, it is an important nutrient in the diets of pregnant and lactating women, and especially for newborn infants. Two medical problems found in infants, particularly premature ones, have responded positively to vitamin E therapy: (1) retrolental fibroplasia, a condition causing severely limited vision or complete blindness from the effect of excess oxygen therapy following birth; and (2) hemolytic anemia, a condition in which fragile erythrocyte membranes break down because of high cell peroxide levels and the induced deficiency of vitamin E. Also, older persons may require more vitamin E in relation to heart disease. For example, it has been proved effective for those suffering circulatory disturbances such as pain in the legs (intermittent claudication) after walking has begun. This therapy helps reduce the arterial blockage causing the pain.

Vitamin E is the only one of the fat-soluble vitamins for which no toxic effect in humans is known. Its use as a supplement has shown no harmful effects. Regular vitamin E replacement therapy is needed for the chronic pancreatic insufficiency and malabsorption conditions described. Current interest in ongoing research concerning vitamin E and its antioxidant role in decreasing free radical damage to cells has led researchers and clinicians to recommend use of moderate supplements of 200 to 300 mg α-TE/day for many middle-aged and older adults.[12] The RDA level is an arbitrary practical allowance, for example, for male adults of 10 mg α-TEs. Compared with other fat-soluble vitamins, vitamin E is relatively nontoxic by mouth and most adults appear to tolerate oral doses of 100 to 800 mg/day with no gross signs or evidence of toxicity.[13]

FOOD SOURCES OF VITAMIN E

The richest dietary sources of vitamin E are the vegetable oils. Together, soybean oil at 29% and palm oil at 21% comprise 50% of the world's consumption (USDA, 1995).[8,9] Curiously enough, these are also the richest sources of polyunsaturated fatty acids, which

vitamin E protects from oxidation. Other food sources include nuts, certain vegetables and fruits, and only small amounts in cereals, dairy products, and meats. A summary of main food sources of vitamin E is given in Table 7.3.

VITAMIN K
CHEMICAL AND PHYSICAL NATURE

The studies of Henrik Dam, a biochemist at the University of Copenhagen, working with a hemorrhagic disease in chicks that were fed a fat-free diet led to the discovery of vitamin K. He found that the absent factor responsible was a fat-soluble blood-clotting vitamin. Because of its blood clotting function, he called it *koagulationsvitamin*, or vitamin K, from this Swedish word for its physiologic action. Later he succeeded in isolating and identifying the compound from alfalfa, for which he received the Nobel Prize in physiology and medicine. This major form of the vitamin found in plants has been named **phylloquinone** (K_1) for its chemical structure. This is our dietary form of vitamin K; its name is generally used as the vitamin's basic chemical name.[14] **Menaquinone** (K_2) is synthesized by intestinal bacterial flora and contributes about half our daily supply. **Menadione** (K_3) is the parent compound in the body; water-soluble derivatives are reformed in the liver to biologically active menaquinones.

Forms

As with most of the vitamins, several forms of vitamin K comprise a group of substances with similar biologic activity in blood-clotting. There are two main forms of vitamin K:

1. K_1, which is the major form found in plants, phytomenadione.

---

hemolytic anemia An anemia (reduced number of red blood cells) caused by breakdown of red blood cells and loss of their hemoglobin.

menadione The parent compound of vitamin K in the body; also called *vitamin K_3*.

menaquinone Form of vitamin K synthesized by intestinal bacteria; also called *vitamin K_2*.

myelin High lipid-to-protein substance forming a fatty sheath to insulate and protect neuron axons and facilitate their neuromuscular impulses.

phylloquinone A fat-soluble vitamin of the K group (K_1) $C_3H_{46}O_2$, found in green plants or prepared synthetically.

Table 7.3	Food sources of vitamin E as alpha-tocopherol (RDA for adults: women, 8 mg; men, 10 mg)	
	Quantity	Vitamin E (mg α-TE)
Bread, cereal, rice, pasta		
This food group is not an important source of vitamin E.		
Vegetables		
Asparagus (raw)	4 spears/58 g	1.15
Avocado (raw)	1 med/173 g	2.32
Brussels sprouts (boiled)	1/2 cup (4 sprouts)/78 g	0.66
Cabbage, green (raw)	1/2 cup shredded/35 g	0.58
Carrot (raw)	1 med/72 g	0.32
Lettuce, iceberg (raw)	1/4 head/135 g	0.54
Spinach (raw)	1/2 cup chopped/28 g	0.53
Sweet potato (raw)	1 med/130 g	5.93
Fruits		
Apple (raw, with skin)	1 med/138 g	0.81
Apricot (canned)	4 halves/90 g	0.80
Banana (raw)	1 med/114 g	0.31
Mango (raw)	1 med/207 g	2.32
Pear (raw)	1 med/166 g	0.83
Meat, poultry, fish, dry beans, eggs		
This food group is not an important source of vitamin E.		
Nuts		
Almonds (dried)	1 oz (24 nuts)/28 g	6.72
Hazelnuts (dried)	1 oz/28 g	6.70
Peanut butter	1 tbsp/16 g	3.00
Peanuts (dried)	1 oz/28 g	2.56
Walnuts (dried)	1 oz (14 halves)/28 g	0.73
Milk, daily products		
This food group is not an important source of vitamin E.		
Fats, oils, sugar		
Corn oil	1 tbsp/14 g	1.90
Cottonseed oil	1 tbsp/14 g	4.80
Olive oil	1 tbsp/14 g	1.60
Palm oil	1 tbsp/14 g	2.60
Peanut oil	1 tbsp/14 g	1.60
Safflower oil	1 tbsp/14 g	4.60
Soybean oil	1 tbsp/14 g	1.50

2. K_2, which is synthesized by intestinal bacteria, so vitamin K is not required directly in the diet, the menaquinones.

A water-soluble analog, which does not require bile for absorption, goes directly into the portal blood system.

ABSORPTION, TRANSPORT, AND STORAGE

K_1 and K_2 require bile salts and pancreatic secretions for absorption as with other fat-related products.[1,14] They are packaged in the intestinal chylomicrons and travel via the abdominal lacteals into the lymphatic system and then into the portal blood for transport to the liver. In the liver, vitamin K is stored in small amounts, although its concentration there declines rapidly. It is excreted in considerable quantity after administration of therapeutic doses.

FUNCTIONAL ROLES OF VITAMIN K

Blood clotting

A major function of vitamin K is to catalyze the synthesis of blood-clotting factors by the liver. Vitamin K is essential for maintaining normal levels of four blood-clotting factors: (1) factor II, **prothrombin**; (2) factor VII, serum prothrombin conversion accelerator (SPCA); (3) factor IX, plasma thromboplastin component (PTC); and (4) factor X, Stuart-Prower factor.[15] Each of these specific clotting factors is a protein synthesized by the liver in an inactive precursor form dependent on vitamin K for activation. Vitamin K acts as an essential cofactor with a carboxylase enzyme to produce the active form of these precursors, mainly prothrombin, by adding a carboxyl (COOH) radical to the amino acid glutamic acid (Glu). This process converts specific glutamic acid residues in vitamin K–dependent proteins to gamma-carboxyglutamic acid (Gla). The activated clotting factors can then combine with calcium (factor IV), an element essential in the clotting process. In the absence of functioning liver tissue, vitamin K cannot act. When liver damage has caused decreased blood levels of prothrombin, and this problem in turn has led to hemorrhage, vitamin K is ineffective as a therapeutic agent.

Skeletal metabolism

Numerous vitamin K–dependent proteins have been found in bone, including osteocalcin and matrix Gla protein. There is evidence linking vitamin K status to bone mineral density and the risk of hip fracture.[16-18]

Neonatology

The sterile intestinal tract of the newborn can supply no vitamin K during the first few days of life until normal bacterial flora develop. During this immediate postnatal period, therefore, hemorrhagic disease of the newborn can occur. To prevent this result, a prophylactic dose of vitamin K is usually given to the infant soon after birth.

Malabsorption disease

Any defect in fat absorption will cause a failure in vitamin K absorption, resulting in prolonged blood clotting time. For example, patients with bile duct obstruction are usually given vitamin K before surgery. Also, after a cholecystectomy, which hinders normal bile release, vitamin K, which requires bile and fat for normal absorption, is not readily absorbed.

Drug therapy

Several drug-nutrient interactions involve vitamin K. An anticlotting drug such as bishydroxycoumarin (Dicumarol) or warfarin acts as an **antimetabolite**, preventing the liver from making substances needed to form blood clots and thus inhibiting the action of vitamin K. When a drug of this nature is used for treating conditions such as blood clots in the lung or blood vessels, vitamin K may be used as a balancing "antidote" to the drug in the management of blood clotting time.[19,20] Also, in extended use of antibiotics, the intestinal bacterial flora is diminished, thus reducing one of the body's main sources of vitamin K.

VITAMIN K REQUIREMENT

In past years, it has been difficult to determine a specific dietary level for vitamin K for several reasons: (1) part of the body's apparent need is supplied by bacterial synthesis, (2) our body reserves are small and turn over rapidly, and (3) instruments for measuring such small amounts were just developing. Also, we lacked reliable food source information. Now, however, with increasing knowledge and advances in laboratory equipment for measuring small amounts, a more specific RDA has recently been established. Thus based on an approximate need in adults of 1 μg/kg body weight per day, the current RDA for men is stated as 80 μg/day, and for women, it is 65 μg/day. The average daily intake of vitamin K by surveyed individuals in the United States seems to be more than adequate.[21] Therefore, no additional amount is stated for pregnancy and lactation or for older adults. However, older adults who have chronic diseases, are on drug therapy, or are consuming poor diets may need more. Newborns require a vitamin K injection shortly after birth. The RDA standard during the first 6 months of life is 5 μg/day, and during the second 6 months of the first year, it is 10 μg/day. Persons who are taking antibiotics, who are being fed by tube or total parenteral nutrition (TPN) by vein for long periods, or who have biliary obstruction or chronic malabsorption disease require monitoring and therapeutic supplementation as indicated.

A deficiency of vitamin K is unlikely except in the clinical conditions indicated. An adequate amount is usually ensured because intestinal bacteria synthesize an added supply and the amount needed is apparently quite small. Toxicity from vitamin K, even with large amounts taken over extended periods, has not been observed.

Table
7.4 Food sources of vitamin K (RDA for adults: women, 65 μg; men, 80 μg)

	Quantity	Vitamin K (μg)
Bread, cereal, rice, pasta		
Oats (dry)	100 g	63
Wheat bran	100 g	83
Whole wheat flour	100 g	30
Vegetables		
Broccoli (raw)	100 g	132
Cabbage (raw)	100 g	149
Cauliflower (raw)	100 g	191
Lentils (dry)	100 g	223
Lettuce, iceberg (raw)	100 g	112
Spinach (raw)	100 g	266
Turnip greens (raw)	100 g	650
Fruits		
This food group is not an important source of vitamin K.		
Meat, poultry, fish, dry beans, eggs, nuts		
Beef liver	100 g	104
Chicken liver	100 g	80
Pork liver	100 g	88
Milk, dairy products		
This food group is not an important source of vitamin K.		
Fats, oils, sugar		
Corn oil	100 g	60
Soybean oil	100 g	540

FOOD SOURCES OF VITAMIN K

Dietary vitamin K, phylloquinone, is present to some degree in most vegetables. It is found especially in green vegetables and liver. A recent American survey of food habits found that for both men and women, the top four contributors of vitamin K_1 were dark-green vegetables—spinach, collards, lettuce, and broccoli.[21] A summary of main food sources is given in Table 7.4.

A summary of the fat-soluble vitamins is given in Table 7.5.

antimetabolite A substance bearing a close structural resemblance to one required for normal physiologic functioning and exerting its effect by interfering with the utilization of the essential metabolite.

prothrombin Blood-clotting factor (number II) synthesized in the liver from glutamic acid and CO_2, catalyzed by vitamin K.

Table 7.5	Summary of fat-soluble vitamins			
Vitamin	Physiologic functions	Results of deficiency	Requirement	Food sources
Vitamin A Provitamin: beta-carotene Vitamin: retinol	Production of rhodopsin and other light-receptor pigments Formation and maintenance of epithelial tissue Growth Reproduction Toxic in large amounts	Poor dark adaptation, night blindness, xerosis, xerophthalmia Keratinization of epithelium Growth failure Reproductive failure	Adult male: 1000 μg or RE (5000 IU) Adult female : 800 μg or RE (4000 IU) Pregnancy: 1000 μg or RE (5000 IU) Lactation 1200 μg or RE (6000 IU) Children: 400 μg or RE (2000 IU) to 800 or RE (4000 IU)	Liver, cream, butter, whole milk, egg yolk Green and yellow vegetables, yellow fruits Fortified margarine
Vitamin D Provitamins: ergosterol (plants); 7-dehydrocholesterol (skin) Vitamins: D$_2$ (ergocholecalciferol) and D$_3$ (cholecalciferol)	Calcitriol a major hormone regulator of bone mineral (calcium and phosphorus) metabolism Calcium and phosphorus absorption Toxic in large amounts	Faulty bone growth; rickets, osteomalacia	Adult: 5-10 μg cholecalciferol (200-400 IU) Pregnancy and lactation: 10-12.5 μg (400-500 IU) depending on age Children: 10 μg (400 IU)	Fortified milk Fortified margarine Fish oils Sunlight on skin
Vitamin E Tocopherols	Antioxidant Hemopoiesis Related to action of selenium	Anemia in premature infants	Adult: 8-10 mg α-TE Pregnancy and lactation: 10-11 mg α-TE Children: 3-10 mg α-TE	Vegetable oils
Vitamin K K$_1$ (phylloquinone) K$_2$ (menaquinone) Analog: K$_3$ (menadione)	Activates blood-clotting factors (for example, prothrombin) by alpha-carboxylating glutamic acid residues Toxicity can be induced by water-soluble analogs	Hemorrhagic disease of the newborn Defective blood clotting Deficiency symptoms are produced by coumarin anticoagulants and by antibiotic therapy	Adult: 70-140 μg Children: 15-100 μg Infants: 12-20 μg	Cheese, egg yolk, liver Green leafy vegetables Synthesized by intestinal bacteria

WATER-SOLUBLE VITAMINS

VITAMIN C

CHEMICAL AND PHYSICAL NATURE

The recognition of vitamin C is associated with the history of an unrelenting search for the cause of the ancient hemorrhagic disease **scurvy**. Early observations, mostly among British sailors and explorers, led to the American discovery of an acid in lemon juice that prevented or cured scurvy. The specific chemical name of vitamin C is ascorbic acid, given to this substance because of its anti-

scorbutic, or antiscurvy, properties. The structure of vitamin C is similar to that of glucose, its metabolic precursor in most animals, but humans lack a specific enzyme needed to change glucose to ascorbic acid. Thus, human scurvy can be called a disease of distant genetic origin, an inherited metabolic defect.

Vitamin C is an unstable, easily oxidized acid. It can be destroyed by oxygen, alkalis, and high temperatures. Thus, cook vitamin C foods in as little water as possible for brief periods and keep covered. Do not cut vegetables into small pieces until time of use, to curtail cut surface exposure to the air. Keep juices tightly closed.

ABSORPTION, TRANSPORT, AND STORAGE

Vitamin C is easily absorbed from the small intestine. But this absorption is hindered by a lack of hydrochloric acid or by bleeding from the gastrointestinal tract. Vitamin C is not stored in single tissue deposits as is vitamin A. Rather it is more generally distributed throughout the body tissues, maintaining a tissue saturation level. Any excess is excreted in the urine. The tissue levels relate to intake, and the size of the total body pool adjusts to maintain balances. The total amount in adults varies from about 4 g to as little as 0.3 g. Tissue levels diminish slowly, so with no intake, deficiency symptoms would not appear for approximately 3 months. This explains why generally healthy people in more isolated living situations can survive the winter without eating many fresh fruits and vegetables. Sufficient vitamin C for early infancy needs is present in breast milk if the mother has a good lactation diet. Cow's milk, however, contains very little vitamin C; remember that these animals have the enzymes to make their own vitamin C from glucose. Because of this, human infant formulas made from cow's milk are supplemented with ascorbic acid.

FUNCTIONS OF VITAMIN C

General antioxidant capacity

In general, along with vitamins A and E, vitamin C is an antioxidant. This means that vitamin C also takes up free oxygen in the cells resulting from cell metabolism. This action prevents oxygen from feeding hungry oxygen-free radicals that also result from normal metabolism in cells but damage or destroy cells if they are not defused.

Intercellular cement substance

We require vitamin C to build and maintain body tissues in general, including bone matrix, cartilage, dentin, collagen, and connective tissue. When vitamin C is absent, the important ground substance does not develop into collagen; the collagen fibers formed in most body tissues remain defective and weak.[3,22] When the vitamin is given, formation of cartilaginous tissue follows quickly. **Collagen** is a protein substance that exists in many body tissues, such as the white fibers of connective tissue. Blood vessel tissue particularly is weakened without the cementing substance from vitamin C's metabolic action that helps provide firm capillary walls. Thus vitamin C deficiency is characterized by fragile capillaries, easily ruptured by blood pressure or trauma, resulting in diffuse tissue bleeding. Deficiency signs include easy bruising, pinpoint hemorrhages of the skin, bone and joint hemorrhages, easy bone fracture, poor wound healing, and soft bleeding gums, a condition called gingivitis. Cigarette smoking and alcohol have adverse effects on serum carotenoids.[23,24]

General body metabolism

The concentration of vitamin C is greater in the more metabolically active tissue such as the adrenal glands, brain, kidney, liver, pancreas, thymus, and spleen than in less active tissues. More vitamin C is also present in a child's actively multiplying tissue than in adult tissue. Vitamin C helps in the formation of hemoglobin and the development of red blood cells in two ways: (1) it aids in the absorption of iron, and (2) it influences the removal of iron from ferritin, the protein-iron-phosphorus complex in which iron is stored, so that more iron is made available to tissues producing the hemoglobin.

Vitamin C also participates in other tissues in numerous processes that have clinical implications. For example, in addition to its role in collagen formation, vitamin C is needed for the synthesis of carnitine, an amino acid that transports long-chain fatty acids into cell mitochondria where they are used to produce energy (see *Practical Application* box, Chapter 5, p. 74). Also, vitamin C is necessary for synthesis of many peptide hormones, the hormone norepinephrine, and many receptors for the neurotransmitter acetylcholine.

Clinical problems and normal growth

Some basic clinical problems, as well as normal growth, require additional vitamin C:

1. *Wound healing.* The significant role of vitamin C in cementing the ground substance of supportive tissue makes it an important agent in wound healing. This creates added demands for vitamin C in traumatic injury or surgery, especially where extensive tissue regeneration is involved.

2. *Fevers and infections.* Infectious processes deplete tissue stores of vitamin C. Optimal tissue stores help maintain resistance to infection. Just how large an amount may be required to maintain this protection is not known. Fevers also deplete tissue stores of vitamin C as they accompany the infectious processes and produce a catabolic effect.

---

collagen The protein substance of the white fibers (collagenous fibers) of skin, tendon, bone, cartilage, and all other connective tissue; it is converted into gelatin by boiling.

scurvy A hemorrhagic disease caused by lack of vitamin C. Diffuse tissue bleeding occurs, limbs and joints are painful and swollen, bones thicken because of subperiosteal hemorrhage, ecchymoses (large, irregular, discolored skin areas resulting from tissue hemorrhages) form, bones fracture easily, wounds do not heal well, gums are swollen and bleeding, and teeth loosen.

3. *Growth periods.* Additional vitamin C is required during the growth periods of infancy and childhood. It is also needed during pregnancy to supply demands for rapid fetal growth and development of maternal tissues.

4. *Stress and body defense.* Body stress from injury, fracture, general illness, or shock calls on vitamin C tissue saturation. A large amount of vitamin C is present in the adrenal glands, which play a primary role in the stress response pattern.

VITAMIN C REQUIREMENT

Difficulties in establishing requirements for vitamin C involve questions about individual tissue needs and whether minimum or optimum intakes are desired. From numerous studies, estimates of a desired body pool size of vitamin C in healthy adults average 1500 mg, which an intake of about 45 mg/day will maintain. The RDA standard for adults is 60 mg/day for an optimal margin to cover variances in tissue demand. Cigarette smokers require about twice as much—100 mg/day.[23,24] Additional amounts are added for pregnancy and lactation needs. Gradual increases during childhood support growth needs.

Although pharmacologic doses of 1 g or more daily have been reported to reduce frequency and severity of symptoms of the common cold and other respiratory problems, controlled trials have not supported this claim. Thus such amounts are not recommended for the entire population. Nonetheless, many persons do habitually ingest this dose daily without developing any toxic effects. On the other hand, others have experienced adverse effects such as gastrointestinal problems. Because the risk is unknown, routine use of such large doses is not recommended.

FOOD SOURCES OF VITAMIN C

Vitamin C can be oxidized easily. Thus the handling, preparation, cooking, and processing of any food source of the vitamin should be considered in evaluating that food's contribution of the vitamin to the diet. Well known sources include citrus fruit and tomatoes. Less regarded but good additional sources include white potatoes, sweet potatoes, cabbage, broccoli, and other green and yellow vegetables and fruits. A summary of food sources of vitamin C is given in Table 7.6.

A summary of vitamin C and its role in the body is given in Table 7.7.

Some guidelines for vitamin supplementation are provided (see *Practical Application* box, p. 128).

Table 7.6	Food sources of vitamin C (RDA for adults: 60 mg)				
	Quantity	**Vitamin C (mg)**		**Quantity**	**Vitamin C (mg)**
Bread, cereal, rice, pasta			**Fruits—cont'd**		
This food group is not an important source of vitamin C.			Orange, navel	1 med	80
			Papaya (raw)	1 med	188
Vegetables			Pineapple (raw)	1/2 cup	12
Asparagus (boiled)	1/2 cup (6 spears)	18	Raspberries (raw)	1/2 cup	15
Avocado (raw)	1 med	14	Strawberries (raw)	1/2 cup	44
Broccoli (raw)	1/2 cup	41	Tangerine (raw)	1 med	26
Brussels sprouts (boiled)	1/2 cup (4 sprouts)	48	**Meat, poultry, fish, dry beans, eggs, nuts**		
Cauliflower (raw)	1/2 cup, pieces	38	Beef liver (fried)	3.6 oz	23
Green pepper (raw)	1/2 cup, chopped	64	Ham, lean	3.5 oz	27
Kale (boiled)	1/2 cup	27	(canned; vitamin C added)		
Potato (baked, with skin)	1 med	26	Lentils (boiled)	1 cup	3
Sweet potato (baked)	1 med	28	Soybeans (boiled)	1 cup	3
Tomato (raw)	1 med	22	**Milk, dairy products**		
Fruits			Milk, skim	8 fl oz	2
Cantaloupe (raw)	1/2 cup, pieces	34	Milk, whole	8 fl oz	4
Grapefruit, white	1/2 med	39	**Fats, oils, sugar**		
Kiwi (raw)	1 med	75	This food group is not an important source of vitamin C.		
Lemon	1 med	31			
Lemon juice (fresh)	8 fl oz	112			
Orange juice (fresh)	8 fl oz	124			

Table 7.7 Summary of vitamin C (ascorbic acid)			
Physiologic functions	**Clinical applications**	**Requirement**	**Food sources**
Antioxidation	Scurvy (deficiency)	60 mg	Fresh fruits, especially citrus
Collagen biosynthesis	Wound healing, tissue formation		Vegetables, such as tomatoes, cabbage, potatoes, chili peppers, and broccoli
General metabolism	Fevers and infections		
Makes iron available for hemoglobin synthesis	Stress reactions		
Influences conversion of folic acid to folinic acid	Growth		
Oxidation-reduction of the amino acids, phenylalanine and tyrosin			

B VITAMINS

DEFICIENCY DISEASE AND VITAMIN DISCOVERIES

The story of the B vitamins is a compelling one. It is a story of persons dying of a puzzling, age-old disease for which there was no cure. It was eventually learned that common, everyday food held the answer. The paralyzing disease was **beriberi**, which had plagued the Orient for centuries and caused persons in many places to search for its solution (Figure 7.6). Early observations and studies provided important clues, but application of the "vitamine" connection to this human sickness was needed. This was finally achieved when an American chemist, R.R. Williams, and his associates with the Philippine Bureau of Science used extracts of rice polishings and cured the epidemic infantile *beriberi*, a paralysis named by the repeated native words, "I can't, I can't," describing its crippling effects. The food factor was named water-soluble B because it was thought to be a single vitamin. Now we know it consists of a large group of individual B vitamins, all water soluble but each having unique metabolic functions in human health. The original letter-naming scheme has long since become meaningless and we are now accustomed to calling the B vitamins by their familiar specific chemical names.

VITAL COENZYME ROLE

The B vitamins, originally believed to be important only in preventing the deficiency diseases that led to their discovery, have now been identified in relation to many important metabolic functions. As vital control agents, they serve in many specific reactions as **coenzyme** partners with key cell enzymes in energy metabolism and tissue building.

    Here we will review briefly the eight basic vitamins in this group of water-soluble compounds. First we will look at the three classic deficiency disease factors—thiamin, riboflavin, and niacin. Then we will explore more

Figure 7.6   Beriberi is a thiamin deficiency characterized by extreme weakness, paralysis, anemia, and wasting away (for example, decreased metabolic function in the liver). (From McLaren DS: *A colour atlas and text of diet-related disorders*, ed 2, 1992, Mosby–Year Book Europe Limited.)

recently discovered coenzyme factors—pyridoxine, pantothenic acid, and biotin. Finally, we will examine the important blood-forming factors—folic acid and cobalamin.

---

beriberi   A disease of the peripheral nerves caused by a deficiency of thiamin (vitamin B_1). It is characterized by pain (neuritis) and paralysis of the extremities, cardiovascular changes, and edema. Beriberi is common in the Orient, where diets consist largely of milled rice with little protein.

coenzyme factors   A major metabolic role of the micronutrients, vitamins and minerals, as essential partners with cell enzymes in a variety of reactions in both energy and protein metabolism.

Nutrient or drug?

In 1954 researchers found out that large doses, 10 to 1000 times the RDA, of specific nutrients helped alleviate symptoms in certain genetic disorders. Later the public got the idea that this would be helpful for healthy people, too. So they began using nutrients as drugs.

A similarity does exist. Both nutrients and drugs are used by the body in specific amounts to control or improve a physiologic condition or illness, to prevent a disease, or to relieve symptoms. But the similarity ends there for many people. They know that too much of any drug can be harmful, but they fail to apply this wise logic to nutrients, too. As a result, some persons have had to learn the hard way.

Some bad results

Toxic effects of vitamin megadoses

Physicians may prescribe large doses of water-soluble vitamins, believing them safe because they are not stored in the body. However, they have recently discovered the potential toxicity of at least one such vitamin—pyridoxine (B_6). Gynecologists had been prescribing this vitamin at levels that were 1000 to 2700 times its RDA to help patients relieve the discomfort of edema during their menstrual cycle. The patients eventually developed unstable gaits, with such numbness in the hands that they were unable to walk or carry out their usual duties at work. To make matters worse, the prescription did nothing to relieve their discomfort.

"Artificially induced" deficiency symptoms

These occur when blood levels of one nutrient rise above normal, resulting in an increased need for other nutrients with which it interacts. Deficiencies also occur when large doses are suddenly removed, creating a "rebound effect." This effect has been seen in infants born to mothers who took megadoses of vitamin C during pregnancy, yet the infants developed scurvy after birth when their high nutrient supply was cut off.

Wise warnings

The megavitamin lesson is not easily taught. Megadose salespersons frequently have more time, money, and better "selling" techniques with which they can misinform the public. Nonetheless, for your client's welfare, you will still want to warn them:

Vitamins, like drugs, can be harmful in large amounts

The only time megadoses are helpful is when the body already has a severe deficiency or is unable to absorb or metabolize the nutrient efficiently.

All nutrients work in harmony to promote good health

Adding large amounts of only one makes the body believe that it isn't getting enough of the others and increases the risk of developing deficiency symptoms.

Supplements should not be taken without first analyzing nutrient levels currently in the diet

This helps avoid problems of excess, which may increase with a cumulative effect over time.

Food remains the best source of nutrients

Most food items provide a wide variety of nutrients in every bite, as opposed to the dozen or so found in a vitamin bottle. By itself a vitamin can actually do very little. Its action is catalytic and so it requires a substrate to work on. These necessary substrates are the energy nutrients—carbohydrate, protein, fat—and their metabolites. With careful selection of a variety of foods and wise storage, meal-planning, and preparation, most people can still secure an ample amount of essential nutrients. Food provides these necessities and a great deal of pleasure as well.

A last word on balance

Remember that as more is known about the *pharmacologic* effects of some vitamins, special use of them in larger prescribed *therapeutic* doses will occur. For example, niacin is already being used as a drug in medical care of cardiovascular disease to effectively lower elevated blood cholesterol levels. Some physicians have suggested increased use of vitamin E to decrease free radical cell damage, as well as more vitamin B_6 to counter the large loss induced by the drug theophylline, which is used to treat respiratory problems such as asthma. Such therapeutic use is not to be equated with nutritional needs or effects. As with any drug, pharmacologic use follows regular testing and approval procedures for designated medical therapy.

References

Berman MK et al: Vitamin B_6 in premenstrual syndrome, *J Am Diet Assoc* 90(6):859, 1990.

Thomas PR: Food for thought about dietary supplements, *Nutr Today* 31(2):46, 1996.

Slesinski MJ et al: Trends in use of vitamin and mineral supplements in the United States: the 1987 and 1992 National Health Surveys, *J Am Diet Assoc* 95(8):921, 1995.

Ubbink JB et al: Relationship between vitamin B_6 status and elevated pyridoxal kinase levels induced by theophylline therapy in humans, *J Nutr* 120:1359, 1990.

THIAMIN

The search of many persons for the cause of beriberi led eventually to a successful conclusion with the identification of thiamin as the control agent involved. Its basic nature and metabolic function were then clarified in the early 1930s.

CHEMICAL AND PHYSICAL NATURE

Thiamin is a water-soluble, fairly stable vitamin. However, it is destroyed by alkalis. Its name comes from its chemical ringlike structure. One of its major parts is a thiazole ring: *thi*(o + vit)*amin.*

ABSORPTION AND STORAGE

Thiamin is absorbed more readily in the acid medium of the first section of the small intestine, the duodenum. In the lower duodenum the acidity of the food mass is buffered by the alkaline intestinal secretions. Thiamin is not stored in large quantities in the tissues; thus a continuous supply of thiamin is necessary.[25] The tissue content is highly relevant to increased metabolic demand, as in fever, increased muscular activity, pregnancy, and lactation. The tissue stores also depend on the adequacy of the diet and on its general composition. For example, carbohydrate increases the need for thiamin, whereas fat and protein spare thiamin. Any unused thiamin is constantly excreted in the urine.

FUNCTION OF THIAMIN

Basic coenzyme role

The main function of thiamin as a metabolic control agent relates to energy metabolism. When actively combined with phosphorus as the coenzyme **thiamin pyrophosphate (TPP)**, thiamin serves as a coenzyme in key reactions that produce energy from glucose or that convert glucose to fat for tissue energy storage. About 80% of the body's total thiamin is in its vital energy coenzyme TPP.[25] Thus the symptoms of beriberi—muscle weakness, gastrointestinal disturbances, and neuritis—can be traced to problems related to these basic energy functions of thiamin.

Clinical problems

Inadequate thiamin to provide the key energizing coenzyme factor in the cells produces broad clinical effects:

1. *Gastrointestinal system.* Various symptoms such as anorexia, indigestion, constipation, gastric atony, and deficient hydrochloric acid secretion may result from thiamin deficiency. When the cells of the smooth muscles and the secretory glands do not receive sufficient energy from glucose, they cannot do their work in digestion to provide still more glucose. A vicious cycle ensues as the deficiency continues.

2. *Nervous system.* The central nervous system depends on glucose to do its work. Without sufficient thiamin to help provide this constant fuel, neuronal activity is impaired, alertness and reflex responses are diminished, and general apathy and fatigue result. If the deficiency continues, lipogenesis is hindered and damage or degeneration of myelin sheaths—lipid tissue covering the nerve fibers—follows. This causes increasing nerve irritation, pain, and prickly or deadening sensations. Paralysis results if the process continues unchecked, as in the classic thiamin deficiency disease beriberi.

3. *Cardiovascular system.* With continuing thiamin deficiency, the heart muscle weakens and cardiac failure results. Also, smooth muscle of the vascular system may become involved, causing dilation of the peripheral blood vessels. As a result of cardiac failure, edema appears in the lower legs.

4. *Musculoskeletal system.* A chronic painful musculoskeletal condition called primary fibromyalgia results from inadequate amounts of TPP in muscle tissue. The widespread muscle pain responds to TPP therapy, as indicated by measuring the activity of a key related enzyme, transketolase, in red blood cells, a common test for individual thiamin status.[25]

THIAMIN REQUIREMENT

RDA standard

The thiamin requirement in human nutrition is stated in terms of carbohydrate and energy needs, as expressed in kcaloric intake. On this basis, the current RDAs for adults are 0.5 mg/1000 kcalories daily, with a minimum of 1 mg/day, even for those consuming less than 2000 kcalories daily. An increase of 0.4 mg/day is needed for pregnancy, and an added 0.5 mg/day is needed for lactation. The allowance for children and teenagers is the same as for adults. For infants the need is 0.4 mg/1000 kcalories, the same as that recommended by the American Academy of Pediatrics. Since excess thiamin is easily cleared by the kidneys, there is no evidence of toxicity from oral doses.

Special needs

Several important conditions influence thiamin requirements:

1. *Alcoholism.* Thiamin is most important in nutritional therapy for persons with alcoholism.[25]

---

thiamin pyrophosphate (TPP) Activating coenzyme form of thiamin that plays a key role in carbohydrate metabolism.

Table

7.8   Food sources of thiamin (RDA for adults: women, 1.0 mg; men, 1.4 mg)

	Quantity	Thiamin (mg)		Quantity	Thiamin (mg)
Bread, cereal, rice, pasta			**Meat, poultry, fish, dry beans, eggs, nuts**		
Bran flakes	1 cup	0.46	Beef liver (fried)	3.5 oz	0.21
Bread, whole wheat	1 slice	0.10	Black-eyed peas (boiled)	1 cup	0.35
Corn muffin	1 muffin	0.10	Cashews (roasted)	1 oz	0.12
Egg noodles, enriched	1 cup	0.20	Chicken, light and dark		
Pasta, enriched	1 cup	0.23	(roasted, without skin)	3.5 oz	0.07
Rice, enriched	1 cup	0.23	Chicken liver (simmered)	3.5 oz	0.18
Wheat flakes	1 cup	0.40	Ham (canned)	3.5 oz	0.88
			Kidney beans (boiled)	1 cup	0.28
Vegetables			Lentils (boiled)	1 cup	0.34
Asparagus (boiled)	1/2 cup (6 spears)	0.09	Lima beans (boiled)	1 cup	0.30
Avocado (raw)	1 med	0.19	Navy beans (boiled)	1 cup	0.37
Brussels sprouts (boiled)	1/2 cup (4 sprouts)	0.08	Peanuts (roasted)	1 oz	0.12
Corn, yellow (boiled)	1/2 cup	0.18	Pecans (dried)	1 oz	0.24
Green peas (boiled)	1/2 cup	0.21	Pinto beans (boiled)	1 cup	0.32
Potato (baked, with skin)	1 med	0.22	Sirloin steak (broiled)	3.5 oz	0.13
			Soybeans (boiled)	1 cup	0.27
Fruits			Top round (broiled)	3.5 oz	0.12
Figs (dried)	10 figs	0.13	Tuna (baked)	3 oz	0.24
Orange juice (fresh)	8 fl oz	0.22			
Orange, navel (raw)	1 med	0.13	**Milk, dairy products**		
Raisins, seedless	2/3 cup	0.16	Milk, skim	8 fl oz	0.09
			Milk, whole	8 fl oz	0.09
			Fats, oils, sugar		
			This food group is not an important source of thiamin.		

Both a primary (lack of adequate diet) and a conditioned (effect of alcohol itself) malnutrition may develop and bring serious neurologic disorders.

2. *Other disease.* Fevers and infections increase cellular energy requirements. Persons with chronic illness, especially older adults, require particular attention to prevent deficiencies.

3. *Normal growth and development.* About a 50% increase in thiamin requirement accompanies pregnancy and lactation, demanded by the rapid fetal growth, the increased metabolic rate during pregnancy, and the production of milk. Continuing growth during infancy, childhood, and adolescence requires attention to thiamin needs. At any point in the life cycle, the larger the body and its tissue volume is, the greater are cellular energy requirements and thus thiamin needs.

Food sources of thiamin

Although thiamin is widespread in almost all plant and animal tissues commonly used as food, the content is usually small. Deficiency of thiamin is a distinct possibility when kcalories are markedly curtailed, as in alcoholism or anorexia, and when persons are following some highly inadequate special diet. Good food sources include lean pork, beef, and liver, but major sources are seeds of plants—whole and enriched grains, and legumes.[1] Thiamin is extremely water soluble and thus is readily lost in cooking water. Table 7.8 provides some comparative food sources of thiamin.

Riboflavin

Discovery

As early as 1897 a London chemist first observed in milk whey a water-soluble pigment with peculiar yellow-green fluorescence. But it was not until 1932 that riboflavin was actually discovered by researchers in Germany.[26] The vitamin was given the chemical group name flavins from the Latin word for yellow. Later, because the vitamin was found also to contain a sugar named ribose, the name riboflavin was officially adopted.

CHEMICAL AND PHYSICAL NATURE

Riboflavin is a yellow-green fluorescent pigment that forms yellowish brown, needlelike crystals. It is water-soluble and relatively stable to heat but easily destroyed by light and irradiation.

ABSORPTION AND STORAGE

Absorption of riboflavin occurs readily in the upper section of the small intestine, assisted by combination with phosphorus in the intestinal mucosa. Long-term laxative use of some bulk fiber supplements such as psyllium gum, especially when taken with milk or near meals, can hinder riboflavin absorption and contribute to its deficiency in body metabolism. Storage is limited, although small amounts are found in liver and kidney. Day-to-day tissue turnover needs must be supplied in the diet.

FUNCTIONS OF RIBOFLAVIN

Basic coenzyme role

The cell enzymes of which riboflavin is an important part are called flavoproteins. Riboflavin enzymes, flavin mononucleotide (FMN) and flavin adenine dinucleotide (FAD), operate at vital reaction points in the process of energy metabolism and in deamination. This is the key reaction that removes the nitrogen-containing amino group from certain amino acids. Thus riboflavin acts as a control agent in both energy production and tissue building. In its important coenzyme role in FMN and FAD, riboflavin acts as an antioxidant.[27]

Clinical problems

Problems associated with riboflavin deficiency include the following two conditions.
1. *Ariboflavinosis.* A deficiency of riboflavin, or **ariboflavinosis**, brings a combination of symptoms, which centers on tissue inflammation and breakdown and poor wound healing. Even minor injuries easily become aggravated and do not heal easily. The lips become swollen, cracking easily, and characteristic cracks develop at the corners of the mouth, a condition called cheilosis. Cracks and irritation develop at nasal angles. The tongue becomes swollen and reddened, a condition called **glossitis** (Figure 7.7). Extra blood vessels develop in the cornea, creating corneal vascularization, and the eyes burn, itch, and tear. A scaly, greasy skin condition, seborrheic dermatitis, may develop, especially in skin folds. Since nutritional deficiencies are usually multiple rather than single, riboflavin deficiencies seldom occur alone. They are especially likely to occur in conjunction with deficiencies of other B vitamins.

Figure 7.7 Glossitis. (From McLaren DS: *A colour atlas and text of diet-related disorders,* ed 2, 1992, Mosby–Year Book Europe Limited.)

2. *Deficiency in newborns.* Because riboflavin is light sensitive, newborn infants with elevated blood levels of bilirubin treated with phototherapy have shown signs of riboflavin deficiencies even when supplements were provided.

RIBOFLAVIN REQUIREMENT

Influencing factors

The body's riboflavin requirement is related to total energy needs, level of exercise, body size, metabolic rate, and rate of growth—all of which are related to protein intake.

RDA standard

For practical purposes the general RDA standard for riboflavin is based on 0.6 mg/1000 kcalories for all ages.

Risk groups

Persons in certain risk groups or clinical situations may require increased riboflavin. These include persons living in poverty or following bizarre food habits. It also applies to those with gastrointestinal disease or chronic illness where poor appetite and malabsorption exist. In addition, people who have poor wound healing and those persons in growth periods such as in childhood, pregnancy, and lactation are at risk.

---

ariboflavinosis Group of clinical manifestations of riboflavin deficiency.

glossitis Swollen, reddened tongue; riboflavin deficiency symptom.

FOOD SOURCES OF RIBOFLAVIN

The most important source of riboflavin is milk. There are several flavins in milk. The most abundant one, initially named lactoflavin, has been renamed specifically riboflavin, to distinguish it from the others.[27] Each quart of milk contains 2 mg of riboflavin, which is more than the daily requirement. Other good sources are organ meats such as liver, kidney, and heart; whole or enriched grains; and vegetables. Because riboflavin is destroyed by light, milk is now sold in cardboard or opaque plastic containers. It is stable to heat and not easily destroyed in proper cooking. Table 7.9 gives some food sources of riboflavin.

NIACIN

The age-old disease related to niacin (nicotinic acid) is *pellagra* (Figure 7.8). It is characterized by a typical dermatitis and often has fatal effects on the nervous system.[28] Pellagra was first observed in 18th century Europe, where it was endemic in populations subsisting largely on corn. Later the American physician Goldberger, who made his now classic observations while studying the problem in America's Southern states, found further clues among children in an orphanage. He noticed that although the majority of the children had pellagra to some degree, a few of them did not. He discovered that the few who were free of pellagra were sneaking into the pantries at night and eating the orphanage's limited supply of milk and meat. His investigation established the relation of the disease to a certain food factor. But it was not until 1937 that University of Wisconsin scientist Elvehjem definitely associated niacin with pellagra by using it to cure a related disease—black tongue in dogs. Correlation between human pellagra and niacin deficiency was then rapidly secured.[28,29]

CHEMICAL AND PHYSICAL NATURE

Further study of niacin and pellagra made clear a close connection of niacin to the essential amino acid tryptophan.

Table 7.9	Food sources of riboflavin (RDA for adults: women, 1.2 mg; men, 1.6 mg)				
	Quantity	Riboflavin (mg)		Quantity	Riboflavin (mg)
Bread, cereal, rice, pasta			**Meat, poultry, fish, dry beans, eggs, nuts—cont'd**		
Bran flakes	1 cup	0.40	Chicken liver (simmered)	3.5 oz	1.76
Bread, whole wheat	1 slice	0.05	Clams (baked)	3 oz (9 small)	0.36
English muffin, plain	1 muffin	0.18	Egg, fresh	1 large	0.18
Noodles, enriched	1 cup	0.18	Ground beef, regular (broiled)	3.5 oz	0.19
Spaghetti, enriched	1 cup	0.11	Ham loin, lean (broiled)	3.5 oz	0.31
Wheat flakes	1 cup	0.42	Kidney beans (boiled)	1 cup	0.10
			Lentils (boiled)	1 cup	0.18
Vegetables			Lima beans (boiled)	1 cup	0.10
Asparagus (boiled)	1/2 cup (6 spears)	0.11	Mackerel (baked)	3 oz	0.35
Avocado (raw)	1 med	0.21	Rainbow trout (baked)	3 oz	0.19
Mushrooms (boiled)	1/2 cup pieces	0.23	Sirloin steak (broiled)	3.5 oz	0.30
Spinach (boiled)	1/2 cup	0.21	Soybeans (boiled)	1 cup	0.49
Sweet potato (baked)	1 med	0.15	Top round (broiled)	3.5 oz	0.27
Fruits			**Milk, dairy products**		
Blueberries (raw)	1 cup	0.07	Brie cheese	1 oz	0.15
Figs (dried)	10 figs	0.17	Buttermilk	8 fl oz	0.38
Pear (raw)	1 med	0.07	Cheddar cheese	1 oz	0.11
Prunes (dried)	10 prunes	0.14	Cottage cheese, creamed	1 cup	0.34
Raspberries (raw)	1 cup	0.11	Cottage cheese, 2% fat	1 cup	0.42
			Milk, skim	8 fl oz	0.34
Meat, poultry, fish, dry beans, eggs, nuts			Milk, whole	8 fl oz	0.39
Almonds (oil roasted)	1 oz	0.28	Ricotta cheese, whole milk	1 cup	0.48
Beef liver (fried)	3.5 oz	4.14	Yogurt, whole	8 fl oz	0.32
Chicken, dark (roasted, without skin)	3.5 oz	0.23	**Fats, oils, sugar**		
Chicken, light (roasted, without skin	3.5 oz	0.12	This food group is not an important source of riboflavin.		

1. *Precursor role of tryptophan.* Curious observations were made by early investigators that raised puzzling questions. Why was pellagra rare in some population groups whose diets were actually low in niacin, whereas the disease was common in other groups whose diets were higher in niacin? And why did milk, which is low in niacin, cure or prevent pellagra? Furthermore, why was pellagra so common in groups subsisting on diets high in corn? In 1945, scientists at the University of Wisconsin finally made the key discovery—tryptophan can be used by the body to make niacin; it is a **precursor** of niacin. Milk prevents pellagra because it is high in tryptophan. Almost exclusive use of corn contributes to pellagra because it is low in tryptophan. And some populations with diets low in niacin may never have pellagra because they happen also to be consuming adequate amounts of tryptophan.

2. *Niacin equivalent.* This tryptophan-niacin relation led to the development of the unit of measure called **niacin equivalent (NE)**. In persons with average physiologic needs, approximately 60 mg of tryptophan produces 1 mg of niacin, the amount designated as a niacin equivalent. Dietary requirements are now given in terms of total milligrams of niacin equivalents.

Figure 7.8 Pellegra. (From McLaren DS: *A colour atlas and text of diet-related disorders,* ed 2, 1992, Mosby–Year Book Europe Limited.)

FORMS

Two forms of niacin exist. Niacin (nicotinic acid) is easily converted to its amide form, nicotinamide, which is water soluble, stable to acid and heat, and forms a white powder when crystallized.

FUNCTIONS OF NIACIN

Basic coenzyme role

Niacin has two coenzyme forms, NAD (nicotinamide-adenine dinucleotide), which is catabolic, and NADP (nicotinamide-adenine dinucleotide phosphate), which is anabolic. In these forms, niacin is a partner with riboflavin in the cellular coenzyme systems that convert proteins, and the small amount of glycerol from fats, to glucose and then oxidize glucose to release energy.

Drug therapy

High doses of nicotinic acid act as vasodilators and cause skin flushing, gastrointestinal distress, and itching. Such a dosage has been effective in lowering serum cholesterol.

Clinical problems

Generally niacin deficiency appears as weakness, anorexia, indigestion, and various skin eruptions. More specific symptoms involve the skin and nervous system. Skin areas exposed to sunlight develop a dark, scaly dermatitis. If deficiency continues, the central nervous system becomes involved, and confusion, apathy, disorientation, and neuritis occur.

NIACIN REQUIREMENT

Influencing factors

Factors such as age and growth periods, pregnancy and lactation, illness, tissue trauma, body size, and physical activity affect the niacin requirement.

RDA standard

The current RDAs for adults of all ages are 6.6 mg/1000 kcalories and not less than 13 niacin equivalents at intakes of less than 2000 kcalories. These recommendations allow for the contribution of tryptophan, in terms of niacin equivalents, from the dietary protein sources.

niacin equivalent (NE) A measure of the total dietary sources of niacin equivalent to 1 mg of niacin. Thus an NE is 1 mg of niacin or 60 mg of tryptophan.

precursor Something that precedes; in biology, a substance from which another substance is derived.

<table>
<tr><td colspan="3">**T a b l e**</td></tr>
<tr><td colspan="3">**7.10**   Food sources of niacin (RDA for adults: women, 13 mg NE; men, 18 mg NE)</td></tr>
</table>

	Quantity	Niacin (mg)
Bread, cereal, rice, pasta		
Bread, whole wheat	1 slice	1.0
Corn meal, yellow, enriched	1 cup	4.8
Cream of wheat (regular, cooked)	$^3/_4$ cup	1.1
Oatmeal (cooked)	$^3/_4$ cup ($^1/_3$ cup dry)	0.2
Rice, white, enriched (cooked)	$^1/_2$ cup	1.1
Wheat flour, all-purpose, enriched	1 cup	4.8
Vegetables		
Asparagus (boiled)	$^1/_2$ cup (6 spears)	0.9
Avocado (raw)	1 med	3.3
Broccoli (raw)	$^1/_2$ cup chopped	0.3
Carrot (raw)	1 med	0.7
Corn, yellow (boiled)	$^1/_2$ cup	1.3
Mushrooms (raw)	$^1/_2$ cup pieces	1.4
Peas, green (boiled)	$^1/_2$ cup	1.8
Potato (baked, with skin)	1 med	3.3
Tomato (boiled)	$^1/_2$ cup	0.9
Tomato juice	6 fl oz	1.2
Fruits		
Banana (raw)	1 med	0.8
Figs (dried)	10 figs	1.3
Mango (raw)	1 med	1.2
Raspberries (raw)	1 cup	1.1
Meat, poultry, fish, dry beans, eggs, nuts		
Beef liver (fried)	3.5 oz	14.4
Chicken liver (simmered)	3.5 oz	4.6
Ground beef, regular (broiled)	3.5 oz	6.8
Ham, cured, regular	3.5 oz	4.8
Peanut butter	1 tbsp	2.2
Peanuts (dry roasted)	1 oz	3.8
Salmon (baked)	3 oz	5.7
Sirloin steak (lean, broiled)	3.5 oz	4.3
Swordfish (baked)	3 oz	10.0
Top round, lean (broiled)	3.5 oz	6.0
Milk, dairy products		
Milk, skim	8 fl oz	0.2
Milk, whole	8 fl oz	0.2
Fats, oils, sugar		
This food group is not an important source of niacin.		

FOOD SOURCES OF NIACIN

Meat is a major source of niacin. Good sources include peanuts, dried beans and peas. Enrichment makes good sources of all grains. Otherwise corn and rice are poor food sources of niacin because they are low in tryptophan. Table 7.10 gives some comparative food sources of niacin.

PYRIDOXINE

CHEMICAL AND PHYSICAL NATURE

The chemical structure of pyridoxine, a pyridine ring, accounts for its specific name. It is water soluble and heat stable, but sensitive to light and alkalis.

FORMS

Vitamin B_6 is a generic term for a group of vitamins with a similar function. Three forms occur in nature—pyridoxine, pyridoxal, and pyridoxamine. In the body all three forms are equally active as precursors of the potent pyridoxine coenzyme pyridoxal phosphate (B_6-PO_4)—PLP.

ABSORPTION AND STORAGE

Pyridoxine is easily absorbed in the upper portion of the small intestine. It is "stored" in the tissue saturation sense and found throughout the body, evidence of its many essential metabolic activities.

FUNCTIONS OF PYRIDOXINE

Coenzyme in protein metabolism

In its active phosphate form (PLP), pyridoxine is a coenzyme in many types of amino acid reactions:

1. *Neurotransmitters.* Converts glutamic acid to gamma-aminobutyric acid (GABA), a substance found in the gray matter of the brain, and converts the essential amino acid tryptophan to serotonin, a potent regulatory substance in brain activity.
2. *New amino acids.* Transfers nitrogen from amino acids to form new ones and releases carbon residues for energy.
3. *Sulfur transfer.* Moves sulfur from an essential sulfur-containing amino acid (methionine) to form other sulfur compounds.
4. *Niacin.* Controls formation of niacin from tryptophan.
5. *Hemoglobin.* Incorporates amino acids into heme, the essential nonprotein core of hemoglobin.
6. *Amino acid transport.* Actively transports amino acids from the intestine into circulation and across cell walls into the cells.

Coenzyme in carbohydrate and fat metabolism

PLP provides metabolites for energy-producing fuel. It also converts the essential fatty acid, linoleic acid, to another fatty acid, arachidonic acid.

Clinical problems

It is evident from this sample list of metabolic activities that pyridoxine holds a key to a number of clinical problems.

1. *Anemia.* A hypochromic type of anemia relates to the role of pyridoxine in heme formation. It can occur even in the presence of a high serum iron level. Such deficiency of pyridoxine has been demonstrated by a special test and the anemia cured by supplying the deficient vitamin.
2. *Central nervous system problems.* Through its role in the formation of the two regulatory compounds in brain activity, serotonin and GABA, pyridoxine controls related neurologic conditions. In infants deprived of the vitamin, as was the case when a batch of hospital formula was mistakenly autoclaved at high temperature, there is increased irritability progressing to convulsions. Immediate supplementation with the vitamin restores function.
3. *Physiologic demands in pregnancy.* Pyridoxine deficiencies during pregnancy have been demonstrated by special tests and subsequently alleviated by supplementation. Fetal growth creates greater maternal metabolic needs and increases pyridoxine requirement.
4. *Oral contraceptive use.* Women taking estrogen-progesterone oral contraceptives require additional pyridoxine. An abnormal state of tryptophan metabolism contributes to the increased need.
5. *Drug therapy.* The drug isoniazid (isonicotinic acid hydrazide, or INH), used as a chemotherapeutic agent for tuberculosis, is an antagonist to pyridoxine. Also, it inhibits the conversion of glutamic acid, the only amino acid the brain metabolizes, and causes a side effect of neuritis. Treatment with large doses of pyridoxine, 50 to 100 mg/day, prevents this effect.

PYRIDOXINE REQUIREMENT

RDA standard

A deficiency of pyridoxine is unlikely because the amounts present in the general diet are large relative to the requirement. Since pyridoxine is involved in amino acids metabolism, the need varies with dietary protein intake. The RDA standard is 2 mg/day for men and 1.6 mg/day for women, with additions for pregnancy and lac-

tation. Amounts for infants and children are shown in the RDA tables inside the book covers.

Toxic effects

Acute toxicity of pyridoxine is rare.[30] However, when pyridoxine is taken in larger amounts, up to 5 g/day, for long periods of time, as in therapy for premenstrual syndrome (PMS), it causes lack of muscular coordination and in some cases severe nerve damage. Symptoms disappear when the large supplement is discontinued.

FOOD SOURCES OF PYRIDOXINE

Pyridoxine is widespread in foods, but many sources provide only very small amounts. Good sources include grains, seeds, liver and kidney, and other meats. Table 7.11 gives some comparative food sources of pyridoxine.

PANTOTHENIC ACID

DISCOVERY

Pantothenic acid was isolated and synthesized between 1938 and 1940.[31] Because it occurs in all forms of living things and is an acid, it was named **pantothenic acid**. True to its name, it is widespread in nature and in body functions. Intestinal bacteria synthesize considerable amounts. This source, together with its widespread natural occurrence, makes deficiencies unlikely.

Chemical and physical nature

Pantothenic acid is a white crystalline compound. It is readily absorbed in the intestine, and combines with phosphorus to form the active acetyl coenzyme A. It is in this key controlling compound of coenzyme A that pantothenic acid has such widespread metabolic presence and use throughout the body. There is no known toxicity or a natural deficiency.

FUNCTIONS OF PANTOTHENIC ACID

In its one basic role as an essential constituent of the body's key activating agent acetyl-coenzyme A (Co-A), pantothenic acid is vital to metabolic reactions involving carbohydrate, fat, and protein metabolism.[31]

pantothenic acid A B vitamin found widely distributed in nature and occurring throughout the body tissues. Pantothenic acid is an essential constituent of coenzyme A, which has extensive metabolic responsibility as an activating agent of a number of compounds in many tissues.

Table 7.11	Food sources of pyridoxine (vitamin B_6) (RDA for adults: women, 1.6 mg; men, 2.0 mg)	
	Quantity	Pyridoxine (mg)
Bread, cereal, rice, pasta		
Wheat germ (toasted)	1/4 cup (1 oz)	0.28
Vegetables		
Avocado (raw)	1 med	0.48
Asparagus (boiled)	1 med	0.13
Broccoli (boiled)	1/2 cup	0.15
Carrot (raw)	1 med	0.11
Potato (baked, with skin)	1 med	0.70
Fruits		
Apple (raw, with skin)	1 med	0.07
Banana (raw)	1 med	0.66
Figs (dried)	10 figs	0.42
Grape juice (bottled)	8 fl oz	0.16
Meat, poultry, fish, dry beans, eggs, nuts		
Beef liver (fried)	3.5 oz	0.27
Cashews (roasted)	1 oz	0.07
Chicken light meat (roasted, without skin)	3.5 oz	0.60
Chicken liver (simmered)	3.5 oz	0.68
Ground beef, regular (broiled)	3.5 oz	0.27
Ham (canned)	3.5 oz	0.48
Kidney beans (boiled)	1 cup	0.21
Lentils (boiled)	1 cup	0.35
Lima beans (boiled)	1 cup	0.30
Navy beans (boiled)	1 cup	0.30
Peanut butter (chunk style)	1 tbsp	0.14
Peanut butter (creamy)	1 tbsp	0.06
Peanuts (roasted)	1 oz	0.07
Pinto beans (boiled)	1 cup	0.27
Sirloin steak (broiled)	3.5 oz	0.45
Soybeans (boiled)	3 oz	0.40
Swordfish (baked)	3 oz	0.32
Top round (broiled)	3.5 oz	0.61
Walnuts (dried)	1 oz	0.18
Milk, dairy products		
Milk, skim	8 fl oz	0.10
Milk, whole	8 fl oz	0.10
Fats, oils, sugar		
This food group is not an important source of pyridoxine.		

PANTOTHENIC ACID REQUIREMENT

Since deficiency is unknown, a requirement for pantothenic acid has not been stated. The RDA's estimated safe and adequate range for adults is 4 to 7 mg. The daily intake in an average American diet ranges from about 5 to 10 mg. Thus a deficiency is unlikely with the widespread occurrence of the vitamin in food sources.

FOOD SOURCES OF PANTOTHENIC ACID

Sources of pantothenic acid are equally as widespread as its occurrence in body tissue. Rich sources include metabolically active tissue such as liver and kidney. Egg yolk and milk contribute more. Table 7.12 shows some food sources of pantothenic acid.

BIOTIN

GENERAL NATURE OF BIOTIN

The minute traces of biotin in the body perform multiple metabolic tasks. Its potency is great, and natural deficiency is unknown. But some cases of induced deficiency have occurred in patients on long-term total parenteral nutrition (TPN), and several inborn errors of biotin metabolism have been defined according to the specific enzyme that is lacking.[32] There is no known toxicity. It is an essential sulfur-containing vitamin.

FUNCTIONS OF BIOTIN

Biotin functions as a partner with acetyl-coenzyme A in reactions that transfer carbon dioxide from one compound and fix it onto another. Examples of this combination of cofactors at work include (1) initial steps in synthesis of some fatty acids, (2) conversion reactions involved in synthesis of some amino acids, and (3) carbon dioxide fixation in forming purines.

BIOTIN REQUIREMENTS

Since the amount needed for metabolism is so small, the human requirement for biotin has not yet been established in specific terms. The RDA adult estimate is 30 to 100 μg/day, but human requirements for biotin at various ages remain uncertain.[33] Obvious biotin deficiency has never been reported during a normal pregnancy.[34] Intestinal bacteria synthesis contributes to the body's supply of biotin, but the amount is uncertain.

FOOD SOURCES OF BIOTIN

Biotin is widely distributed in natural foods, but its bioavailability is highly variable in different foods. For example, the biotin of corn and soy meals is completely

Table

7.12 Food sources of pantothenic acid (RDA for adults: 4-7 mg)

	Quantity	Pantothenic acid (mg)		Quantity	Pantothenic acid (mg)
Bread, cereal, rice, pasta			**Meat, poultry, fish, dry beans, eggs, nuts—cont'd**		
All-bran	1/3 cup (1 oz)	0.49	Chicken, dark meat (roasted without skin)	3.5 oz	1.21
Bagel	1 bagel	0.20			
Bread, whole wheat	1 slice	0.18	Chicken, light meat (roasted without skin)	3.5 oz	0.97
English muffin, plain	1 muffin	0.29			
Oatmeal, regular (quick)	3/4 cup (1 oz)	0.35	Chicken liver (simmered)	3.5 oz	5.41
Shredded wheat	1 oz	0.24	Egg, fresh	1 large	0.85
Soybean flour (defatted)	1/2 cup	1.00	Egg yolk, fresh	Yolk of 1 large egg	0.76
Wheat germ (toasted)	1/4 cup (1 oz)	0.39	Garbanzo beans (boiled)	1/2 cup	0.24
Vegetables			Ground beef, regular (broiled)	3.5 oz	0.38
Avocado (raw)	1 med	1.68	Ham, cured, regular	3.5 oz	0.50
Broccoli (raw)	1/2 cup, chopped	0.24	Lentils (boiled)	1/2 cup	0.83
Corn, yellow (boiled)	1/2 cup	0.72	Lima beans (boiled)	1/2 cup	0.36
Potato (baked, with skin)	1 med	1.12	Peanut butter (chunk style)	2 tbsp	0.31
Squash, winter, all varieties, (baked)	1/2 cup	0.36	Peanuts (roasted)	1 oz	0.39
			Pinto beans (boiled)	1/2 cup	0.26
Sweet potato (boiled)	1/2 cup, mashed	0.87	Salmon (smoked)	3 oz	0.74
Tomato (boiled)	1/2 cup	0.35	Sirloin steak (broiled)	3.5 oz	0.35
			Top round (broiled)	3.5 oz	0.48
Fruits			Turkey, light meat (roasted without skin)	3.5 oz	0.63
Apricots (raw)	3 med	0.25			
Banana (raw)	1 med	0.30			
Figs (dried)	10 figs	0.81	**Milk, dairy products**		
Orange juice (fresh)	8 fl oz	0.47	American cheese, processed	1 oz	0.14
Orange, navel (raw)	1 med	0.35	Blue cheese	1 oz	0.49
Papaya (raw)	1 med	0.86	Cheddar cheese	1 oz	0.12
Pomegranate (raw)	1 med	0.92	Milk, skim	8 fl oz	0.81
			Milk, whole	8 fl oz	0.76
Meat, poultry, fish, dry beans, eggs, nuts			Yogurt, whole	8 fl oz	0.88
Almonds (dried)	1 oz (24 nuts)	0.13			
Beef liver (fried)	3.5 oz	5.92	**Fats, oils, sugar**		
Black beans (boiled)	1/2 cup	0.24	This food group is not an important source of pantothenic acid.		
Black-eyed peas (boiled)	1/2 cup	0.35			
Cashews (roasted)	1 oz (16 med nuts)	0.34			

available, whereas that of wheat is almost unavailable. Excellent food sources include egg yolk, liver, kidney, and other animal tissues, as well as tomatoes and yeast. Fruit and meat are poor sources. The biotin in general United States diets ranges from about 30 to 45 μg/day.

FOLATE

DISCOVERY

Folate is the generic name for a group of substances that have similar nutritional properties and chemical structures. One of these substances was first extracted from dark green, leafy vegetables such as spinach and thus initially given the name folic acid, or folacin, from the Latin word *folium*, meaning

"leaf."[35] The reduced form of folic acid is folinic acid. Folic acid was then identified and isolated in laboratory studies of anemias and growth factors in animals. In 1945 folic acid was obtained from liver and finally synthesized. The term *folate* refers to 1, the salt form of folic acid, and both terms are often used interchangeably for the vitamin.

CHEMICAL AND PHYSICAL NATURE

Folic acid forms yellow crystals and is a conjugated substance made up of three acids: (1) pteroic acid, (2) para-aminobenzoic acid (PABA), and (3) glutamic acid (an amino acid). The chemical name for folic acid, from its structure, is pteroylglutamate (PGA).

PABA is sometimes touted in nutrition supplement claims as a separate essential factor in human nutrition, but it is not. Its only role in human nutrition is that of a component of the vitamin, folic acid. Animal and human cells are capable neither of synthesizing PABA nor of attaching it to the rest of the vitamin molecule. Only plants and certain bacteria can do this. Thus dietary folic acid, preformed by plants, is the essential substance in human nutrition, and the major source of this folic acid is green leafy vegetables.

FUNCTIONS OF FOLATE

Basic coenzyme role

Folates function as necessary coenzyme agents in the important task of attaching single carbons to many metabolic compounds. Several key compounds are examples:

1. *Purines*. Nitrogen-containing compounds essential to all living cells, involved in cell division and in the transmission of inherited traits.
2. *Thymine*. Essential compound forming a key part of deoxyribonucleic acid (DNA), the important material in the cell nucleus that controls and transmits genetic characteristics.
3. *Hemoglobin*. Heme, the iron-containing nonprotein portion of hemoglobin.

Clinical problems

Some clinical problems associated with folate follow:

1. *Anemia*. A nutritional **megaloblastic anemia** may occur in simple folate deficiency. Since tissue growth requires additional folate, this folate deficiency anemia is a special risk in pregnant women, growing infants, and young children, as well as adolescent "dieting" girls, especially those who also smoke.[36]
2. *Sprue*. Folate is an effective agent in the treatment of **sprue**, a gastrointestinal disease characterized by intestinal lesions, malabsorption defects, diarrhea, macrocytic anemia, and general malnutrition. The vitamin corrects both the blood-forming and the gastrointestinal defects of the disease.
3. *Chemotherapy*. The drug amethopterin (Methotrexate), used in cancer chemotherapy, acts as a folate antagonist to reduce the tumor growth. The effect of this action is to prevent synthesis of DNA and purines.
4. *Growth and stress*. Increased folate is needed during periods of rapid growth, especially during fetal development.

Heart disease and folate

Current reports of 5-year investigations among participants in the Physicians' Health Study have found that elevated blood levels of homocysteine were associated with increased risk of myocardial infarction or death resulting from cardiac disease.[37] Although many factors

may contribute to heart disease, in these large long-term studies there was a significant association with plasma levels of folate, as well as vitamin B_{12} and vitamin B_6, which in turn resulted from low intakes of these vitamins, especially folate. These results have led researchers to suggest that folic acid intake among the general population may be too low.[37-39]

FOLATE REQUIREMENT

Average American and Canadian diets contribute about 0.3 μg/kg body weight of folate and provide approximately 90% of the adult population with sufficient absorbable folate to meet daily needs and maintain adequate storage. On this basis, the current RDA for folate is 200 μg for men and 180 μg for women. Based on a 50% food folate absorption, the RDA for folate is 400 μg/day for women during pregnancy to meet increased needs for fetal and maternal tissue growth. Increases are also indicated for lactation. In addition, the United States Public Health Service recently expanded its folate fortification to grain food products, indicating that all women of childbearing age should regularly have a dietary folate intake of at least 400 μg/day to protect against the risk of having a pregnancy with spina bifida or other neural tube defect.[40] The varying needs of infants, children, and adolescents are indicated in the summary RDA tables inside the book cover.

This current RDA for folate is about 50% lower than the amounts previously recommended. This reduction has raised some concern that this allowance may not provide adequate safety allowance for specific population groups at risk, such as pregnant women, adolescents, and older adults, especially those with the added burdens of low socioeconomic status.[41,42]

FOOD SOURCES OF FOLATE

Folate is widely distributed in foods. Good sources include green leafy vegetables, liver, legumes and a few fruits such as orange, orange juice, and cantaloupe. Table 7.13 gives a summary of food sources of folate. However, household preparation plus food processing and storage may destroy as much as 50% of the folate. Since there is potential for toxicity from the increased intake of folate, excessive supplemental use is not recommended.

COBALAMIN

DISCOVERY

The discovery of cobalamin (vitamin B_{12}) was associated with the search for the specific agent responsible for control of **pernicious anemia**.[35,43,44] At first the disease was thought to be related to a deficiency of folate. However,

Table 7.13 Food sources of folate (RDA for adults: women, 180 μg; men, 200 μg)	Quantity	Folate (μg)
Bread, cereal, rice, pasta		
Bread, whole wheat	1 slice	14
Wheat germ (toasted)	$^1/_4$ cup (1 oz)	100
Vegetables		
Asparagus (boiled)	$^1/_2$ cup (6 spears)	88
Avocado (raw)	1 med	113
Peas, green (boiled)	1 cup	51
Spinach (boiled)	1 cup	262
Fruits		
Banana (raw)	1 med	22
Figs (dried)	10 figs	14
Orange (raw)	1 med	47
Strawberries (raw)	1 cup	26
Meat, poultry, fish, dry beans, eggs, nuts		
Beef liver (fried)	3.5 oz	220
Black beans (boiled)	1 cup	256
Black-eyed peas (boiled)	1 cup	358
Chicken liver (simmered)	3.5 oz	770
Chick-peas (boiled)	1 cup	282
Egg, whole	1 large	32
Green beans (boiled)	1 cup	42
Kidney beans (boiled)	1 cup	229
Lima beans, baby (boiled)	1 cup	273
Navy beans (boiled)	1 cup	255
Peanut butter	1 tbsp	13
Peanuts (dry roasted)	1 oz	41
Pinto beans (boiled)	1 cup	794
Milk, dairy products		
Milk, whole	8 fl oz	12
Yogurt, whole	8 fl oz	17
Fats, oils, sugar		
This food group is not an important source of folate.		

although folate helped the initial red blood cell regeneration, it was not permanently effective and did not control the nerve problems associated with the disease. When folate was found to be lacking in full effectiveness, the search continued for the remaining piece of the disease puzzle.

In 1948 two groups of workers, one in America and one in England, crystallized a red compound from liver, which they then numbered B$_{12}$. In the same year it was clearly shown that this new vitamin could control both the blood-forming defect and the neurologic involvement in pernicious anemia. Soon afterward, the working groups of scientists were able to produce the vitamin through a process of bacterial fermentation. This process remains the main source of commercial supply today. The scientists named their vitamin discovery cobalamin because of its unique structure with a single brilliant red atom of the trace element cobalt at its center.

CHEMICAL AND PHYSICAL NATURE

Cobalamin is a complex red crystalline compound of high molecular weight, with a single cobalt atom at its core. It occurs as a protein complex in foods, so its food sources are mainly of animal origin. The ultimate source, however, may be designated as the synthesizing bacteria in the intestinal tract of herbivorous animals. Some synthesis is done by human intestinal bacteria.

ABSORPTION, TRANSPORT, AND STORAGE

Absorption

Intestinal absorption takes place in the ileum. Cobalamin is first split from its protein complex by the gastric hydrochloric acid and then bound to a specific glycoprotein called intrinsic factor, secreted by the gastric mucosal cells. This cobalamin-intrinsic factor complex then moves into the intestine, where it is absorbed by special receptors in the ileal mucosa.

Storage

Cobalamin is stored in active body tissues. Organs holding the greatest amounts are the liver, kidney, heart, muscle, pancreas, testes, brain, blood, spleen, and bone marrow. These amounts are minute, but the body holds them tenaciously and the stores are only slowly depleted. For example, a typical postgastrectomy anemia does not become apparent until 3 to 5 years after removal of the organ and subsequent loss of its secretions.

FUNCTIONS OF COBALAMIN

Basic coenzyme role

As an essential coenzyme factor, cobalamin is closely related to amino acid metabolism and the formation of the heme portion of hemoglobin. Its requirement increases as protein intake increases.

---

megaloblastic anemia Anemia resulting from faulty production of abnormally large immature red blood cells, caused by a deficiency of vitamin B$_{12}$ and folate.

pernicious anemia A chronic macrocytic anemia occurring most commonly after age 40. It is caused by absence of the intrinsic factor normally present in the gastric juices and necessary for the absorption of cobalamin (B$_{12}$) and is controlled by intramuscular injections of vitamin B$_{12}$.

sprue Alternate term for adult celiac disease, a malabsorption syndrome.

Clinical problems

Special needs for cobalamin occur in several problems related to blood-forming:

1. *Pernicious anemia.* In the absence of the intrinsic factor–specific component of gastric secretion required for cobalamin absorption, pernicious anemia develops. The vitamin is then not available for its key role in heme formation, and adequate hemoglobin cannot be synthesized.

   Conversely, however, folate is not the primary agent for treating pernicious anemia. As indicated, although folate results in blood cell regeneration in persons with pernicious anemia, its effect is not permanent, nor does it control the degenerative neurologic problems. This is the critical distinction between cobalamin and folate in the diagnosis and treatment of this anemia. Therefore, the American Medical Association and the United States Food and Drug Administration have recommended that no more than 0.4 mg of folate be included in multivitamin preparations, as this amount would suffice for common needs and not mask the development of pernicious anemia or prevent its diagnosis.

   A person with defective cobalamin absorption, and hence pernicious anemia, can be given from 15 to 30 μg/day of cobalamin in intramuscular injections during a relapse and can be maintained afterward by an injection of about 30 μg every 30 days. This treatment controls both the blood-forming disorder and the degenerative effects on the nervous system.

2. *Megaloblastic anemia.* Since cobalamin shares close metabolic relations with folate, a megaloblastic anemia develops when either of the vitamins is deficient. Cobalamin indirectly affects blood formation by providing an activated form of folate.

3. *Sprue.* Like folate, cobalamin is effective in the treatment of the intestinal syndrome of **sprue**. However, it is most effective when used in conjunction with folate because its role is indirect activation of folic acid.

COBALAMIN REQUIREMENT

The amount of dietary cobalamin needed for normal human metabolism is very small. Reported minimum needs have been from 0.6 to 1.2 μg/day, with a range upward to approximately 2.8 μg to allow for individual variances. The ordinary diet easily provides this much and more. For example, 1 cup of milk, one egg, and 4 oz meat provide 2.4 mg. The RDA standard recommends an intake of 3 μg/day for adults. This amount allows a safety margin to cover variances in individual need, absorption, and body stores.

Table 7.14	Food sources of vitamin B_{12} (RDA for adults: 2 μg)	
	Quantity	**Vitamin B_{12} (mg)**
Bread, cereal, rice, pasta		
This food group is not an important source of vitamin B_{12}.		
Vegetables		
This food group is not an important source of vitamin B_{12}.		
Fruits		
This food group is not an important source of vitamin B_{12}.		
Meat, poultry, fish, dry beans, eggs, nuts		
Beef liver (fried)	3.5 oz	111.80
Chicken liver (simmered)	3.5 oz	19.39
Chicken, white meat (roasted)	3.5 oz	0.34
Clams (steamed)	3 oz (9 small)	84.05
Egg, fresh	1 large	0.77
Ground beef, regular (broiled)	3.5 oz	2.93
Ham, cured, regular	3.5 oz	0.80
Mackerel (baked)	3 oz	16.18
Oysters (steamed)	3 oz (12 med)	32.63
Salmon (baked)	3 oz	4.93
Sirloin steak (lean, broiled)	3.5 oz	2.86
Swordfish (baked)	3 oz	1.72
Top round, lean (broiled)	3.5 oz	2.48
Milk, dairy products		
Cheddar cheese	3.5 oz	0.83
Milk, skim	8 fl oz	0.83
Milk, whole	8 fl oz	0.87
Swiss cheese	3.5 oz	1.86
Yogurt, whole	8 fl oz	0.84
Fats, oils, sugar		
This food group is not an important source of vitamin B_{12}.		

FOOD SOURCES OF COBALAMIN

Cobalamin is supplied by animal foods. The richest sources are liver and kidney, lean meat, milk, egg, and cheese. Natural dietary deficiency is rare. It has only been observed in some groups of strict vegetarians, who displayed symptoms of nervous disorders, sore mouth and tongue, neuritis, and amenorrhea. Table 7.14 gives food sources of cobalamin.

A summary of the water-soluble B vitamins is given in Table 7.15.

PHYTOCHEMICALS

DEFINITIONS AND DEVELOPMENT

The term "phytochemical" comes from the Greek word *phyton* meaning "plant," and it pertains to the chemical nature of the compound. It describes a wide vari-

Table

7.15 Summary of B-complex vitamins

Vitamin	Coenzyme: physiologic	Clinical applications	Requirement	Food sources
Thiamin	Carbohydrate metabolism Thiamin pyrophosphate (TPP): oxidative decarboxylation	Beriberi (deficiency) Neuropathy Wernicke-Korsakoff syndrome (alcoholism) Depressed muscular and secretory symptoms	0.5 mg/1000 kcal	Pork, beef, liver, whole or enriched grains, legumes
Riboflavin	General metabolism Flavin adenine dinucleotide (FAD) Flavin mononucleotide (FMN)	Cheilosis, glossitis, seborrheic dermatitis	0.6 mg/1000 kcal	Milk, liver, enriched cereals
Niacin (nicotinic acid, nicotinamide)	General metabolism Nicotinamide adenine dinucleotide (NAD) Nicotinamide adenine dinucleotide phosphate (NADP)	Pellagra (deficiency) Weakness, anorexia Scaly dermatitis Neuritis	6.6 NE/1000 kcal	Meat, peanuts, enriched grains (protein foods containing tryptophan)
Vitamin B_6 (pyridoxine, pyridoxal, pyridoxamine)	General metabolism Pyridoxal phosphate (PLP): transamination and decarboxylation	Reduced serum levels associated with pregnancy and use of oral contraceptives Antagonized by isoniazid, penicillamine, and other drugs	2 mg (men) 1.6 mg (women)	Wheat, corn, meat, liver
Pantothenic acid	General metabolism CoA (coenzyme A): acetylation	Many roles through acyltransfer reactions (for example, lipogenesis, amino acid activation, and formation of cholesterol, steroid hormones, heme)	4 to 7 mg	Liver, egg, milk
Biotin	General metabolism N-Carboxybiotinyl lysine: CO_2 transfer reactions	Deficiency induced by avidin (a protein in raw egg white) and by antibiotics Synthesis of some fatty acids and amino acids	30 to 100 μg	Egg yolk, liver Synthesized by intestinal microorganisms
Folate (folic acid, folacin)	General metabolism Single carbon transfer reactions (for example, purine nucleotide, thymine, heme synthesis)	Megaloblastic anemia	200 μg (men) 180 μg (women)	Liver, green leafy vegetables
Cobalamin	General metabolism Methylcobalamin: methylation reactions (for example, synthesis of amino acids, heme)	Pernicious anemia induced by lack of intrinsic factor Megaloblastic anemia Methylmalonic aciduria Homocystinuria Peripheral-neuropathy (strict vegetarian diet)	2 μg	Liver, meat, milk, egg, cheese

ety of chemical compounds produced by plants that act either as antioxidants or hormones in the originating plants or in persons eating the plants.[45,46] Expanding scientific evidence supports the role of phytochemicals, as well as functional foods modified to provide specific health benefits, in the prevention and treatment of disease.[47] The term "carotinoids" describes a group of pigments in fruits and vegetables, including alpha- and beta-carotene, so-named from the Latin word *carota* meaning "carrot" from the vegetable's deep yellow color. In its current usage, carotinoids include a number of pigments found in plants but not synthesized in animals.[48]

MAJOR DIETARY CAROTINOIDS

Some major carotinoids in the American diet and their food sources include the following examples:

1. Alpha-carotene: carrots
2. Beta-carotene: broccoli, cantaloupe, carrots, spinach
3. Beta-cryptoxanthin: oranges and orange juice, peaches, tangerines
4. Lutein: broccoli, corn, green beans, green peas, spinach and other greens
5. Lycopene: tomatoes and tomato products

TO SUM UP

A vitamin is an organic, noncalorigenic food substance that is required in small amounts for certain metabolic functions and cannot be manufactured by the body. Vitamins may be fat or water soluble, and their solubility affects their absorption and mode of transport to target tissues.

The fat-soluble vitamins are A, D, E, and K. Their metabolic tasks are mainly structural in nature, and their

To Probe Further

Sunlight—or the Milky Way?

Sunlight and milk, that is, *fortified* milk, are the primary sources of vitamin D. But can we rely on them to supply our needs?

Sunlight, we have long held, is the least constant of the two because of the number of factors that can affect its absorption and ability to transform cholesterol into provitamin D_3, a precursor to vitamin D. However, we are now learning, after United States milk fortification regulations have been in place since the early 1930s, that we can't always count on milk either.

Season of the year

Ultraviolet exposure varies by season, depending on the type of activity (especially indoor versus outdoor) of the individual and the type of clothing worn. Studies of older persons with hip fractures show high correlation with very little exposure to sunshine.

Body composition

It has also been shown that gross obesity, which reduces the person's mobility and often confines them indoors, decreases exposure to ultraviolet light, even to the point of increasing the risk of a vitamin D deficiency.

Let us consider milk as an alternate source. We have looked to milk as the most reliable source of vitamin D, especially for persons at risk for deficiency problems (for example, postmenopausal women, especially those who spend much of their time indoors, and infants). However, as we have known, the milk must be *fortified* with vitamin D, 10 μg (400 IU)/quart by United States regulations, to provide necessary amounts with a reasonable intake.

However, we now find that we can't always rely on the fortification process either. Recent news of an outbreak of vitamin D toxicity from drinking milk traced to a single dairy raises questions about how reliable milk really is as a consistent source of vitamin D. Not so reliable, subsequent investigations proved through sampling milk and infant formulas in five adjacent states. Labels on these random products showed the required amount of fortification, but in fact actual analysis indicated a wide range of added vitamin D from toxic levels to *none*.

It seems that the answer to our initial question is "both." We need to benefit from both sunlight and milk, but in controlled amounts. Just as we have learned that too little or too much sunlight can do harm, we are now learning the same thing about milk fortification. Vigilant monitoring and enforcement of regulations is necessary if fortification of milk and other foods is to remain a reliable source of vitamin D.

References

Holick MF et al: The vitamin D content of fortified milk and infant formula, *N Engl J Med* 326(18):1178, April 30, 1992.

Jacobus CH et al: Hypervitaminosis D associated with drinking milk, *N Engl J Med* 326(18):1173, April 30, 1992.

fate in the body is associated with lipids. The possibility of toxicity is enhanced for fat-soluble vitamins because the body can store them. Such toxicity is no longer rare because of the current popularity of vitamin A supplements.

The remaining vitamins are water soluble: ascorbic acid (C) and the B-complex vitamins. These vitamins share three characteristics: (1) synthesis by plants and thus dietary supply by plant foods or animal foods (except vitamin B_{12}); (2) no stable "storage" form and therefore must be provided regularly in the diet (except vitamin B_{12}); and (3) function as a coenzyme factor in cell metabolism (except vitamin C). Toxicity levels are usually not associated with water-soluble vitamins because excess is easily excreted in the urine. However, two vitamins have shown toxic effects when taken in megadoses (i.e., in gram amounts): pyridoxine (B_6), which can result in severe nerve damage, and ascorbic acid (C), which has been associated with gastrointestinal disturbances, renal calculi, and lowered resistance to infection. All water-soluble vitamins, especially vitamin C and folate, are easily oxidized, and care must be taken in food storage and preparation practices to preserve them. A number of recently discovered phytochemicals in foods have important functions in the body.

■ QUESTIONS FOR REVIEW

1. List and describe three health problems caused by a vitamin A deficiency. Give three possible causes of a deficiency.

2. How do the absorption and storage of a vitamin affect its potential deficiency or toxicity? Give several examples to illustrate.

3. Describe the function of vitamin D hormone, calcitriol. Who is at risk for developing a deficiency? Why?

4. List three conditions that increase the risk for vitamin K deficiency. How do these deficiencies develop?

5. What three characteristics are shared by most water-soluble vitamins? Identify an exception to each and explain the reason.

6. Define the term *coenzyme factor* as applied to the role of vitamins, especially water-soluble vitamins. Give several examples to illustrate.

7. Which water-soluble vitamins are potentially toxic? Why? What signs of toxicity have been observed for each?

8. Which B vitamins play significant roles in blood formation? Describe their roles and interactions.

9. Define the term phytochemical and give examples with food sources of each.

■ REFERENCES

1. Marsh MN, Riley SA: Digestion and absorption of nutrients and vitamins. In Feldman M, Scharschmidt BF, Sleisenger MH, eds: *Gastrointestinal and liver disease,* ed 6, vol 2, Philadelphia, 1998, Saunders.

2. Olson JA: Vitamin A, retinoids, and carotenoids. In Shils ME, Olson JA, Shike M, eds: *Modern nutrition in health and disease,* ed 8, vol 1, Philadelphia, 1994, Lea & Febiger.

3. Guyton AC, Hall JE: *Textbook of medical physiology,* ed 9, Philadelphia, 1996, Saunders.

4. Kinyamu HK et al: Serum vitamin D metabolites and calcium absorption in normal young and elderly free-living women and in women living in nursing homes, *Am J Clin Nutr* 65:790, 1997.

5. Holick MF: Vitamin D. In Shils ME, Olson JA, Shike M, eds: *Modern nutrition in health and disease,* ed 8, vol 1, Philadelphia, 1994, Lea & Febiger.

6. Couturier M, Imbach A: Calcium and vitamin A intake in women and their daughters: distribution by food groups and meals, *J Can Diet Assoc* 58(2):77, 1997.

7. Jacobus CH et al: Hypervitaminosis D from drinking milk, *N Engl J Med* 326(18):1173, 1992.

8. Farrell PM, Roberts RJ: Vitamin E. In Shils ME, Olson JA, Shike M, eds: *Modern nutrition in health and disease,* ed 8, vol 1, Philadelphia, 1994, Lea & Febiger.

9. Entenmiller RR: Vitamin E content of fats and oils—nutritional implications, *Food Technology* 51(5):78, 1997.

10. Meydani SN: Vitamin E enhancement of T cell-mediated function in healthy elderly: mechanisms of action, *Nutr Rev* 53(4):S52, 1995.

11. Howard IJ: The neurologic syndrome of vitamin E deficiency: laboratory and electrophysiologic assessment, *Nutr Rev* 48(4):169, 1990.

12. Tangney CC: Vitamin E and cardiovascular disease, *Nutr Today* 32(1):13, 1997.

13. Food and Nutrition Board, National Research Council: *Recommended dietary allowances,* ed 10, 1989, National Academy Press.

14. Olson RE: Vitamin K. In Shils ME, Olson JA, Shike M, eds: *Modern nutrition in health and disease,* ed 8, vol 1, Philadelphia, 1994, Lea & Febiger.

15. Shearer MJ: Vitamin K, *Lancet* 345:229, 1995.

16. Sokoll LJ et al: Changes in osteocalcin, plasma phylloquinone, and urinary γ-carboxyglutamic acid in response to altered intakes of dietary phylloquinone in human subjects, *Am J Clin Nutr* 65:779, 1997.

17. Rucker RB: Editorial—improved functional endpoints for use in vitamin K assessment: important implications for bone disease, *Am J Clin Nutr* 65:883, 1997.

18. Binkley NC, Suttie JW: Vitamin K nutrition and osteoporosis, *J Nutr* 125:1812, 1995.

19. Weibert RT et al: Correction of excessive anticoagulation with low-dose oral vitamin K, *Ann Intern Med* 126(12):959, 1997.

20. Lipkin R: How vitamin K helps prevent hemorrhaging, *Sci News* 148(13):199, 1995.

21. Booth SL et al: Food sources and dietary intakes of vitamin K_1 (phylloquinone) in the American diet: data from the FDA Total Diet Study, *J Am Diet Assoc* 96(2):149, 1996.

22. Jacob RA: Vitamin C. In Shils ME, Olson JA, Shike M, eds: *Modern nutrition in health and disease,* Philadelphia, 1994, Lea & Febiger.

23. Lykkesfeldt J et al: Ascorbic acid and dehydroascorbic acid as biomarkers of oxidative stress caused by smoking, *Am J Clin Nutr* 65:959, 1997.

24. Albanes D et al: Effects of supplemental β-carotene, cigarette smoking, and alcohol consumption on serum carotenoids in the Alpha-Tocopherol, Beta-Carotene Cancer Prevention Study, *Am J Clin Nutr* 66:366, 1997.

25. Tanphaichitr V: Thiamin. In Shils ME, Olson JA, Shike M, eds: *Modern nutrition in health and disease,* ed 8, Philadelphia, 1994, Lea & Febiger.

26. McCormick DB: Riboflavin. In Shils ME, Olson JA, Shike M, eds: *Modern nutrition in health and disease,* ed 8, vol 1, Philadelphia, 1994, Lea & Febiger.

27. Rivlin RS, Dutta P: Vitamin B_2 (riboflavin): relevance to malaria and antioxidant activity, *Nutr Today* 30(2):62, 1995.

28. Swendseid ME, Jacob RA: Niacin. In Shils ME, Olson JA, Shike M: eds: *Modern nutrition in health and disease,* ed 8, vol 1, Philadelphia, 1994, Lea & Febiger.

29. Klevay LM: And so spake Goldberger in 1916: pellagra is not infectious! *J Am Coll Nutr* 16(3):290, 1997.

30. Leklem JE: Vitamin B_6. In Shils ME, Olson JA, Shike M, eds: *Modern nutrition in health and disease,* ed 8, vol 1, Philadelphia, 1994, Lea & Febiger.

31. Plesofsky-Vif N: Pantothenic acid and coenzyme A. In Shils ME, Olson JA, Shils M, eds: *Modern nutrition in health and disease,* ed 8, vol 1, Philadelphia, 1994, Lea & Febiger.

32. Dakshinamurti K: Biotin. In Shils ME, Olson JA, Shike M, eds: *Modern nutrition in health and disease,* ed 8, vol 1, Philadelphia, 1994, Lea & Febiger.

33. Mock NI et al: Increased urinary excretion of 3-hydroxy-sovaleric acid and decreased urinary excretion of biotin status in experimental biotin deficiency, *Am J Clin Nutr* 65:951, 1997.

34. Mock DM, Stadler DD: Conflicting indicators of biotin status from a cross-sectional study of normal pregnancy, *J Am Coll Nutr* 16(3):252, 1997.

35. Herbert V, Das KC: Folic acid and vitamin B_{12}. In Shils ME, Olson JA, Shike M, eds: *Modern nutrition in health and disease,* ed 8, vol 1, Philadelphia, 1994, Lea & Febiger.

36. Green TJ et al: Oral contraceptives did not affect biochemical folate indexes and homocysteine concentrations in adolescent females, *J Am Diet Assoc* 98(1):49, 1998.

37. Herzlich BC: Editorial: Plasma homocyst(e)ine, folate, vitamin B_6 and coronary artery disease risk, *J Am Coll Nutr* 15(2):109, 1996.

38. Chasan-Taber L et al: A prospective study of folate and vitamin B_6 and risk of myocardial infarction in US physicians, *J Am Coll Nutr* 15(2):136, 1996.

39. Boushey CJ et al: A quantitative assessment of plasma homocysteine as a risk factor for vascular disease: probable benefits of increasing folic acid intakes, *JAMA* 274:1049, 1995.

40. Staff report—Nutrition science and policy: folic acid fortification, *Nutr Rev* 54(3):94, 1996.

41. Koehler KM et al: Folate nutrition and older adults: challenges and opportunities, *J Am Diet Assoc* 97(2):167, 1997.

42. Koehler KM et al: Vitamin supplementation and other variables affecting serum homocysteine and methyl-malonic acid concentrations in elderly men and women, *J Am Coll Nutr* 15(4):364, 1996.

43. Herbert V: Vitamin B_{12}. In Zeigler EE, Filer LJ Jr, eds: *Present knowledge in nutrition,* ed 7, Washington, D.C., 1996, ILSI Press.

44. Toh B-H, van Driel IR, Gleeson PA: Pernicious anemia, *N Engl J Med* 337(20):1441, 1997.

45. Gopsalan C: Dietetics and nutrition: impact of scientific advances and development, *J Am Diet Assoc* 97(7):737, 1997.

46. Rock CL et al: Update on the biological characteristics of the antioxidant micronutrients: vitamin C, vitamin E, and the carotenoids, *J Am Diet Assoc* 96(7):693, 1996.

47. Bloch A, Thomson CA: Position of the American Dietetics Association: phytochemicals and functional foods, *J Am Diet Assoc* 95(4):493, 1995.

48. Wu C: How antioxidants defend cells, *Sci News* 151(7):111, 1997.

■ FURTHER READING

Abbey M: The importance of vitamin E in reducing cardiovascular risk, *Nutr Rev* 53(9):S28, 1995.

Gaziano JM: Antioxidants in cardiovascular disease: randomized trials, *Nutr Rev* 54(6):175, 1996.

These articles provide helpful background concerning possible antioxidant roles of vitamins A (beta-carotene), C, and E in reducing risk of cardiovascular disease.

Campbell MK et al: Assessing fruit and vegetable consumption in a 5-A-Day study targeting rural blacks: the issue of portion size, *J Am Diet Assoc* 96(10):1040, 1996.

Havas S et al: 5-A-Day for Better Health: a new research initiative, *J Am Diet Assoc* 94(1):32, 1994.

These articles describe the recent research program conducted by the National Cancer Institute, National Institutes of Health (NHI), in a public-private partnership between NIH and the Produce for Better Health Foundation (PBH). Havas' group reports on community-research projects in nine of the state programs involved, which were designed to encourage Americans to eat 5 or more servings of fruits and vegetables every day, one of the nation's health promotion and disease prevention objectives.

Booth SL et al: Food sources and dietary intakes of vitamin K_1 (phylloquinone) in the American diet: data from the FDA Total Diet Study, *J Am Diet Assoc* 96(2):149, 1996.

Suttie JW: Vitamin K and human nutrition, *J Am Diet Assoc* 92(5):585, 1992.

Suttie, a leader in vitamin K research, provides information about the role of vitamin K in bone growth, as well as the status of food analysis to produce needed food value tables. Booth and her colleagues follow with important information concerning main food sources of vitamin K_1 in the American diet to help meet these needs.

Thomas PR: Food for thought about dietary supplements, *Nutr Today* 31(2):46, 1996.

This excellent first-person article provides healthy skepticism and stimulates critical thought with eight cogent points to consider concerning the use of dietary supplements. (Also see *Issues & Answers.*)

Issues Answers

Guidelines for vitamin supplementation

"Charlatan!" cry the conservative health workers at anyone who suggests a need for vitamin supplements.

"Fuddy-duddy!" reply the self-proclaimed "nutrition experts" who prescribe megadoses of everything from A through Zinc to cure anything that ails you.

Who's right? Probably someone who suggests something between these two extremist views. The RDAs are based on the average needs of a healthy population, not on specific individual needs, which can vary widely. But extremists may take these concepts too far. Extreme "traditionalists" try to apply these standards rigidly to every individual. "Pill-pushers" recommend megadoses of everything "to cover all the bases" and increase their profits.

Biochemical individuality is a real concept. It cannot be overlooked when assessing an individual's nutritional needs. Since it is influenced by health status, personal habits, age, and other factors, the assessment process should consider at least the following conditions.

Pregnancy and lactation

The RDA takes into account increased nutrient requirements for these situations. But individual food preferences and food availability may make meeting these increased nutrient needs by diet alone difficult. Supplements then become a more reasonable way of ensuring an adequate intake to meet the increased nutrient demands.

Oral contraceptive use

The use of oral contraceptives lowers serum levels of several B vitamins, including vitamin B_6 (pyridoxine) and niacin, as well as vitamin C. If nutrient intake levels are marginal, some supplements may be necessary. Of course, it is more important to encourage the client to improve her diet or assist her in obtaining nutritious foods.

Aging

The aging process may increase the need for some nutrients because of decreased food intake and impaired nutrient metabolism. Marginal or so-called subclinical deficiencies of ascorbic acid, thiamin, riboflavin, and pyridoxine are seen in the elderly, even among individuals using supplements. This suggests that current RDA standards may be too low to meet their particular needs.

Studies of the nutrient needs of an aging United States population are currently in progress and will be reflected in the new Recommended Dietary Intakes (RDIs) replacing the longstanding RDAs (see Chapter 1).

Restricted diets

Persons who are eternally "dieting" may find it difficult to meet many of the nutrient standards if they take in less than 1200 kcal/day. Strict diets are not recommended; however, carefully assess and counsel with anyone on a weight-reduction regimen.

Exercise

Persons involved in physical exercise programs have been shown to require increased riboflavin to maintain normal tissue levels. Most people who exercise consume adequate amounts of food to compensate for this possible deficit. But the combination of restricting kcalories and exercising accentuates this need even more and may indicate the need for a B-complex supplement, especially in women who do not tolerate milk (the major source of riboflavin) well.

Smoking

This unhealthful, addictive habit reduces ascorbic acid levels by as much as 30%. If dietary intake is marginal, a small supplement (for example, 100 mg/day) may help compensate for the reduction. Of course, stopping the harmful habit helps even more.

Alcohol

Chronic or abusive use of alcohol impedes absorption and utilization of the B-complex vitamins, especially thiamin, and it even destroys folate. Supplements of multivitamins rich in B-complex vitamins, as well as ascorbic acid, help. However, a change in alcohol consumption must accompany nutritional therapy to prevent recurrence of deficiency signs.

Caffeine

Taken in large quantities, caffeine flushes water-soluble vitamins from the body faster than usual. Small supplements of B-complex and ascorbic acid may help. Reduced caffeine intake helps even more.

Continued

Disease

In a state of disease, malnutrition, debilitation, or hypermetabolic demand, each patient must of course be carefully assessed to determine just what degree of overall nutrient supplementation and diet modification may be indicated for clinical purposes. These needs are particularly evident in long-term illness.

Once all these conditions are carefully evaluated, a wise nutrition program can be developed. In many situations, supplementation can be avoided by a change in personal habits. Best of all, people in general are better served by changing personal habits. They are able to maintain good health while avoiding artificially induced deficiencies and expensive health food store bills.

References

Bogden JD: Studies on micronutrient supplements and immunity in older people, *Nutr Rev* 53(4):S59, 1995.

Porter DV: Dietary supplements: recent chronology and legislation, *Nutr Rev* 53(2):31, 1995.

Slesinski MJ et al: Trends in use of vitamin and mineral supplements in the United States: the 1987 and 1992 National Health Interview Surveys, *J Am Diet Assoc* 95(8):921, 1995.

Thomas PR: Food for thought about dietary supplements, *Nutr Today* 31(2):46, 1996.

Chapter

8

Minerals

In this chapter we look at the remaining micronutrients, the minerals. They may seem simple in comparison to the complex organic vitamin compounds, but they fulfill a variety of metabolic functions.

Elements for which the requirement is greater than 100 mg/day are called major minerals, not because they are more important, but because there are more of them in the body. Those needed in much smaller amounts are called trace elements, of which a few that are needed in only minute amounts are called ultratrace elements.

Here we will review each of these groups of minerals. As with the vitamins, we will focus on why we need them and how we may obtain them.

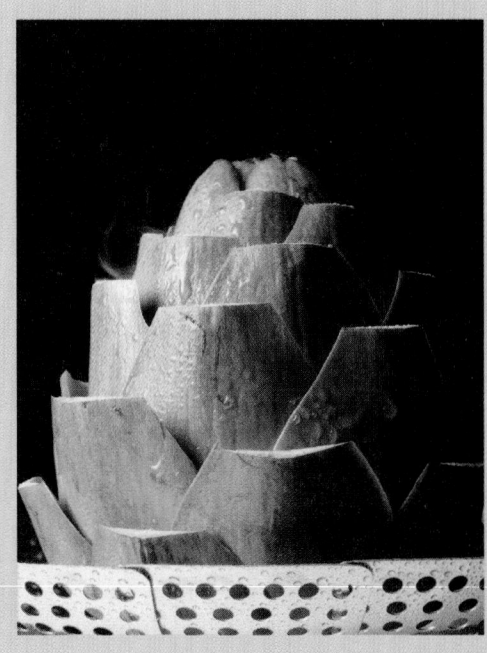

MINERALS IN HUMAN NUTRITION

OUR CYCLE OF MINERALS

On Earth, we live within a vast slow-motion cycle of minerals essential to our existence as humans. Over eons of time, shifting oceans and mountains have deposited an array of elements that move from rock to soil, to plants, to animals and humans.[1,2] Until recent times our access to some of these elements in sufficient measure for health has depended on luck—where we happened to live. But over time, with more knowledge of how they can be processed, transported, and used in agriculture, better distribution has developed.

METABOLIC ROLES

Variety of functions

Minerals are inorganic elements widely distributed in nature. They have vital roles in human metabolism that are as varied as are the minerals themselves. These substances, which appear so inert in comparison with the complex organic vitamin compounds, fulfill an impressive variety of metabolic functions: building, activating, regulating, transmitting, and controlling. For example, ionized sodium and potassium exercise all-important control over shifts in body water. Dynamic calcium and phosphorus provide structure for the body's framework. Oxygen-hungry iron gives a core to heme in hemoglobin. Brilliant red cobalt is the atom at the core of cobalamin (vitamin B_{12}). Iodine is the necessary constituent of the thyroid hormones, which in turn control the rate of body metabolism. Far from being static and inert, minerals are active participants, helping to control many of the metabolic processes in the body.

Variety in amount needed

Minerals also differ from vitamins in another way. Vitamins, as you saw in the previous chapter, are all required in very small amounts to do their metabolic jobs. Minerals, however, are required in varying amounts, from the relatively large amounts of the major minerals to the exceedingly small amounts of the trace elements. For example, the major mineral calcium forms a relatively large amount of body weight—about 2%. Most of this is in skeletal tissue. Thus an adult weighing 150 lb has about 3 lb of calcium in the body. On the other hand, the trace element iron is present in small amounts. This same adult has only about 3 g (about $1/10$ oz.) of iron in his body, mostly in the hemoglobin of red blood cells.

CLASSIFICATION

In your study you will find these important mineral elements grouped in three main sections, one major and two trace. These commonly used divisions are based on (1) how much of the mineral is required by the body and (2)

Table 8.1 Major minerals and trace elements in human nutrition		
	Trace elements	
Major minerals (required intake over 100 mg/day)	**Essential (required intake under 100 mg/day)**	**Essentiality unclear**
Calcium (Ca)	Iron (Fe)	Silicon (Si)
Phosphorus (P)	Iodine (I)	Vanadium (V)
Magnesium (Mg)	Zinc (Zn)	Nickel (Ni)
Sodium (Na)	Copper (Cu)	Tin (Sn)
Potassium (K)	Manganese (Mn)	Cadmium (Cd)
Chloride (Cl)	Chromium (Cr)	Arsenic (As)
Sulfur (S)	Cobalt (Co)	Aluminum (Al)
	Selenium (Se)	Boron (B)
	Molybdenum (Mo)	
	Fluoride (F)	

how much we know at this point about its essentiality, (in cases of some of the trace elements).

Major minerals

Seven minerals present in the body in large amounts are called the major minerals. These include calcium, magnesium, sodium, potassium, phosphorus, sulfur, and chloride.

Trace elements

The remaining minerals are present in smaller amounts and are called trace elements. The essential nature of 10 of these has been determined. For the remaining eight, their precise functioning is as yet not entirely clear.

In Table 8.1 you will find a listing of the minerals in each group. We briefly review each, looking at (1) balance controls maintaining the body's needed amount, (2) physiologic function, (3) associated clinical problems, (4) the body's requirement, and (5) food sources.

MAJOR MINERALS
CALCIUM

Of all the minerals in the body, calcium by far occurs in the largest amount. The total amount of body calcium is in constant balance with food sources from the outside as well as with tissue calcium within the body among its various parts. A number of dynamic balance mechanisms are constantly at work to maintain these levels within normal ranges. The balance concept, therefore, can be applied at three basic levels: (1) the intake-absorption-output balance, (2) the bone-blood balance, and (3) the calcium-phosphorus blood serum balance.

INTAKE-ABSORPTION-OUTPUT BALANCE

Calcium intake

The average adult American diet contains about 700 to 1200 mg of calcium. Most of this comes from dairy products and some from green leafy vegetables and grains. However, the absorption of minerals in general is less efficient than that of the vitamins and macronutrients. Not all of the food intake of minerals is necessarily available. The term **bioavailability** refers to the degree to which the body uses a particular nutrient, such as calcium in this case, which depends on many factors that influence its absorption-excretion balance or its balance in body tissues. For example, skeletal growth during childhood, especially the tremendous growth spurt during puberty, makes tremendous calcium demands.[3,4] This skeletal bone growth demand for calcium is particularly evident in adolescents, especially in boys.[5,6] This is one of the basic facts that makes the setting of precise requirements for minerals difficult. Stated requirements for many of these elements are given as estimated ranges of need rather than as precise figures.

Absorption of calcium

Only about 10% to 30% of the calcium in an average diet is absorbed. Most food calcium occurs in complexes with other dietary components. These complexes must be broken down and the calcium released in a soluble form before it can be absorbed. Absorption takes place in the small intestine, chiefly in the first section, the duodenum, where the gastric acidity is still effective rather than being buffered as the food mass moves along.

Factors increasing calcium absorption

The following factors increase calcium absorption:

1. *Vitamin D hormone.* An optimum amount of this control agent is necessary for calcium absorption. This agent controls the synthesis of a calcium-binding protein carrier in the duodenum that transports the mineral into the mucosal cells and blood circulation.[7]
2. *Body need.* During periods of greater body demand, such as growth or depletion states, more calcium is absorbed. Physiologic states in the life cycle—growth, pregnancy and lactation, and old age—have a strong influence on the amount of absorption needed to meet body requirements. In elderly persons in general, and in postmenopausal women in particular, the ability to absorb calcium is reduced.[8,9]
3. *Dietary protein and carbohydrate.* A greater percentage of calcium is absorbed when the diet is high in protein. However, this larger amount absorbed results in increased renal excretion, with a negative calcium balance following. Thus, in essence, high-protein diets only induce increased calcium requirements to maintain cal-

cium balance. Lactose enhances calcium absorption through the action of the lactobacilli, which produce lactic acid and lower intestinal pH. However, this effect is not always consistent.[10]

4. *Acidity.* Lower pH (increased acidity) favors solubility of calcium and consequently its absorption.

Factors decreasing calcium absorption

The following factors decrease calcium absorption:

1. *Vitamin D deficiency.* Vitamin D hormone, along with parathyroid hormone, is essential for calcium absorption.
2. *Dietary fat.* Excess dietary fat or poor absorption of fats results in an excess of fat in the intestine. This fat combines with calcium to form insoluble soaps. These insoluble soaps are excreted, with consequent loss of the incorporated calcium.
3. *Fiber and other binding agents.* An excess of dietary fiber binds calcium and hinders its absorption. Other binding agents include oxalic acid, which combines with calcium to produce calcium oxalate, and phytic acid, which forms calcium phytate. Oxalic acid is a constituent of green leafy vegetables, but the amount of oxalates in them varies, making some of them better sources of calcium than others. Phytic acid is found in the outer hull of many cereal grains, especially wheat.
4. *Alkalinity.* Calcium is insoluble in an alkaline medium and consequently is poorly absorbed.

Calcium output

The overall body calcium balance is maintained first, therefore, at the point of absorption. A large unabsorbed amount—some 70% to 90%, varying according to body need—remains to be eliminated in the feces. A small amount of calcium may be excreted in the urine, about 200 mg/day, to maintain normal levels in the body fluids.

BONE-BLOOD BALANCE

Calcium in the bones

In a healthy state the body maintains a constant turnover of the calcium in the bone tissue, which is the major site of calcium storage. Calcium in the bones and teeth is about 99% of that in the entire body. However, this is not a static storage. Bone tissue is constantly being built and reshaped according to various body needs and stresses (Figure 8.1). As much as 700 mg calcium enters

---

bioavailability Amount of a nutrient ingested in food that is absorbed and thus available to the body for metabolic use.

and leaves the bones each day. And all the while the body maintains a dynamic equilibrium. But in certain conditions or disease, withdrawals may exceed deposits and a state of calcium imbalance occurs. For example, conditions such as immobility from a body cast or diseases such as osteoporosis would cause excess bone calcium withdrawals.

Calcium in the blood

The remaining small amount of calcium not in bone tissue—about 1%—circulates in the blood and other body fluids. Despite its small amount, however, this serum calcium plays a vital role in controlling body functions. Calcium in the blood occurs in two main forms:

1. *Bound calcium.* About half the calcium in the blood is bound in the plasma proteins, hence it is not free or diffusible, that is, able to move about or to enter into other activities.
2. *Free ionized calcium.* Free particles of calcium, carrying electrical charges and hence in an active ionized form, move freely about and diffuse through membranes to control a number of body functions. These functions include blood clotting, transmission of nerve impulses, muscle contraction and relaxation, membrane perme-

ability, and enzyme activation. This is a good illustration of a small amount of a nutrient doing a great deal of metabolic work because it is in an activated form.

CALCIUM-PHOSPHORUS SERUM BALANCE

A final level of calcium balance is that which calcium maintains with phosphorus in the blood serum. Amounts of these two minerals in the blood are normally maintained in a definite relationship because of their relative solubility. This relationship is called the *calcium-phosphorus serum balance.* This serum balance is the solubility product of calcium × phosphorus, expressed in milligrams per deciliter of each mineral. Normal serum levels are 10 mg/dl of calcium in children and adults, and 4 mg/dl of phosphorus in adults and 5 mg/dl in children. Thus the normal serum calcium-phosphorus solubility products are $10 \times 4 = 40$ for adults and $10 \times 5 = 50$ for children. Any situation that causes an increase in the serum phosphorus level would cause a resulting decrease in the serum calcium level to hold the calcium-phosphorus solubility product constant. In such a case, the decreased serum calcium may bring on signs of tetany from lack of neuromuscular controls. To help maintain

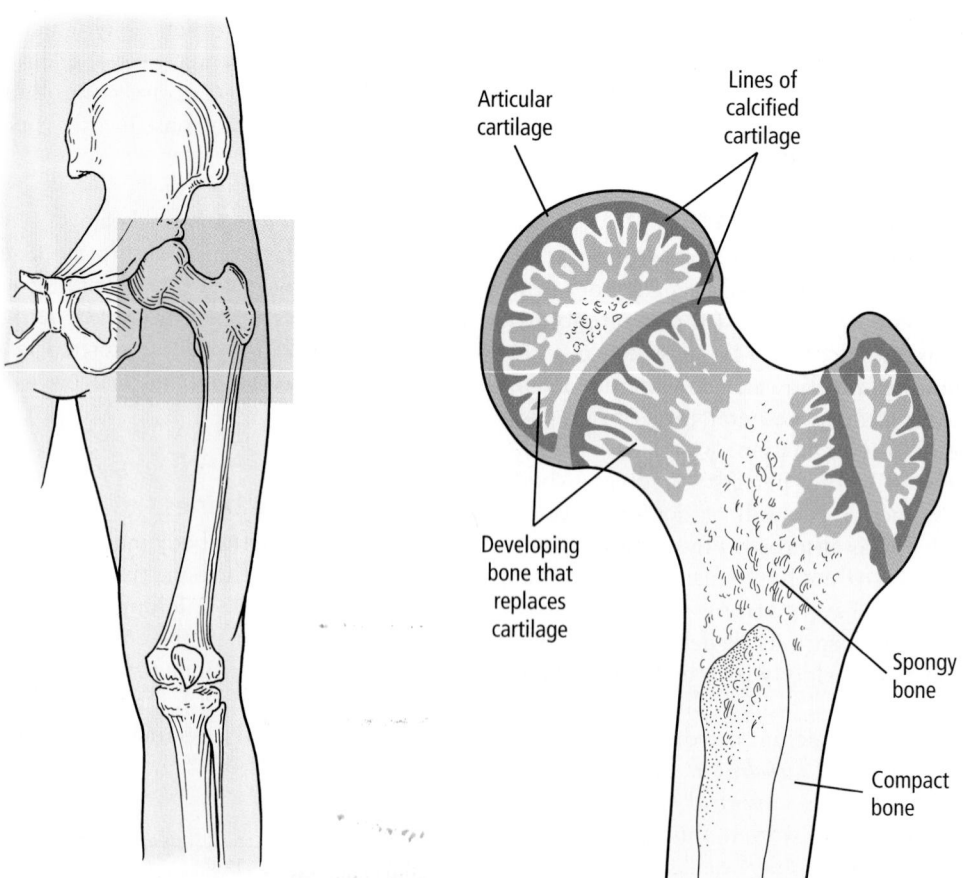

Figure 8.1   Bone and cartilage development.

the normal calcium-phosphorus serum balance, the ideal dietary calcium-phosphorus balance is 1 to 1.5 for children and women during pregnancy and lactation. Other adults require a 1 to 1 dietary balance, meaning equal amounts of dietary calcium and phosphorus, for ideal absorption and utilization.

Control agents for calcium balance

Two main control agents work together to maintain these vital levels of calcium balance in the body: parathyroid hormone and vitamin D hormone *(calcitriol)*. The cooperative action of these two factors is a good example of the **synergistic** behavior of metabolic controls. Consider the interdependent relationship of these agents:

1. *Parathyroid hormone.* The parathyroid glands, lying adjacent to the thyroid glands, are particularly sensitive to changes in the circulating blood level of free ionized calcium. When this level drops, the parathyroid gland releases its hormone, which then acts in three ways to restore the normal blood calcium level: (1) it stimulates intestinal mucosa to absorb more calcium, (2) it withdraws more calcium rapidly from the bone **compartment**, and (3) it causes kidneys to excrete more phosphate. These combined activities then restore calcium and phosphorus to their correct balance in the blood.

2. *Vitamin D hormone.* In general, along with parathyroid hormone, vitamin D hormone controls absorption of calcium. It also, with the help of parathyroid hormone, affects the deposit of calcium and phosphorus in bone tissue. Thus these two agents balance each other, with vitamin D hormone acting more to control calcium absorption and bone deposit and parathyroid acting more to control calcium withdrawal from bone and kidney excretion of its partner serum phosphorus.

A third hormonal agent, **calcitonin**, is also involved in calcium balance. Produced by special C cells in the thyroid gland, it prevents abnormal rises in serum calcium by modulating release of bone calcium. Thus its action counterbalances that of parathyroid hormone to help regulate serum calcium at normal levels in balance with bone calcium.

The overall balance relationship of the various factors involved in calcium metabolism is illustrated in Figure 8.2.

PHYSIOLOGIC FUNCTIONS OF CALCIUM

Bone formation

The physiologic function of 99% of the body calcium is to build and maintain skeletal tissue. This is done by special types of cells that are in constant balance between depositing and withdrawing bone calcium.

Tooth formation

Special tooth-forming organs in the gums deposit calcium to form teeth. The mineral exchange continues as in bone. This exchange in dental tissue occurs mainly in the dentin and cementum. Very little deposit occurs in the enamel once the tooth is formed.

General metabolic functions

The remaining 1% of the body's calcium performs a number of vital physiologic functions.

1. *Blood clotting.* In the blood clotting process, serum calcium ions are required for cross-linking of fibrin, giving stability to the fibrin threads.

2. *Nerve transmission.* Normal transmission of nerve impulses along axons requires calcium. A current of calcium ions triggers the flow of signals from one nerve cell to another and on to the waiting target muscles.

3. *Muscle contraction and relaxation.* Ionized serum calcium helps initiate contraction of muscle fibers and control following the contraction. This catalyzing action of calcium ions on the muscle protein filaments allows the sliding contraction between them to occur (see Chapter 14). This action of calcium is particularly vital in the constant contraction-relaxation cycle of the heart muscle.

4. *Cell membrane permeability.* Ionized calcium controls the passage of fluids and solutes through cell membranes by affecting membrane permeability. It influences the integrity of the intercellular cement substance.

5. *Enzyme activation.* Calcium ions are important activators of specific cell enzymes, especially ones that release energy for muscle contraction. They play a similar role with other enzymes, including lipase, which digests fat, and with some members of the protein-splitting enzyme system.

---

calcitonin A polypeptide hormone secreted by the thyroid gland in response to hypercalcemia, which acts to lower both calcium and phosphate in the blood.

compartment The collective quantity of material of a given type in the body. The four body compartments are *lean body mass* (muscle), *bone, fat,* and *water.*

synergism The joint action of separate agents in which the total effect of their combined action is greater than the sum of their separate actions. (Adjective: synergistic.)

Figure 8.2   Calcium metabolism. Note the relative distribution of calcium in the body.

CLINICAL PROBLEMS

A number of clinical problems may develop from imbalances that interfere with the various physiologic and metabolic functions of calcium.

Tetany

A decrease in ionized serum calcium causes tetany, a state marked by severe, intermittent spastic contractions of the muscle and by muscular pain.

Rickets

A deficiency of vitamin D hormone causes rickets. When there is inadequate exposure to sunlight or deficient dietary intake of vitamin D, proper bone formation cannot take place.

Osteoporosis

The usual form of **osteoporosis**, which is characterized by bone mineral loss, occurs mainly in older persons, especially in postmenopausal women. In women affected, the most rapid rate of loss occurs in the first 5 years after menopause. There is a negative calcium balance of about 40 to 120 mg/day, indicating loss from both the outer bone layer—*cortex*—and the small developing needlelike projections of bone—*trabecula*—into the central marrow forming the calcium anchoring network of bone matrix. Afterward the rate of bone loss is

about 1% a year. In some patients it is not corrected by increased dietary calcium alone but is often improved by exercise and sometimes coupled cautiously with vitamin D supplements under medical/nutrition supervision.[10] Outpatient clinic programs usually center on individual assessment and nutrition care plans, with focus on sufficient protein, energy calories, and vitamin D, with a regular individual exercise program.[11-13] Current medical approaches to stimulate new bone growth involve hormonal therapy with both vitamin D hormone and estrogen.[14] An idiopathic osteoporosis occurring in young adults does not respond to calcium therapy.

Resorptive hypercalciuria and renal calculi

These two conditions can tilt the usually fine-tuned calcium deposition-mobilization balance maintained by the controlling hormones. When this normal balance is disturbed, resorption of calcium from bone and subsequent increased urinary calcium excretion occurs. A main factor leading to such a condition is prolonged immobilization. Such an imbalance may occur, for example, from a full body cast after orthopedic surgery or a spinal cord injury, or with a body brace following a back injury. In such cases, normal muscle tension on bones that is necessary for calcium balance is lessened, and the risk of renal stones from increased urinary calcium is increased.

Table 8.2 Food sources of calcium (RDAs for adults: 800 mg)

	Quantity	Calcium (mg)		Quantity	Calcium (mg)
Bread, cereal, rice, pasta			**Fruits—cont'd**		
Bran muffin, homemade	1 muffin	54	Raspberries (raw)	$^1/_2$ cup	14
Bread, whole wheat	1 slice	18	Strawberries (raw)	$^1/_2$ cup	11
Corn muffin, from mix	1 muffin	96	Tangerine (raw)	1 med	12
Cream of wheat (cooked)	$^3/_4$ cup	38	**Meat, poultry, fish, dry beans, eggs, nuts**		
Pasta, enriched (cooked)	1 cup	16	Almonds (roasted)	1 oz	148
Rice, enriched	1 cup	21	Beef liver (fried)	3.5 oz	11
Wheat flakes	1 cup	43	Cashews (roasted)	1 oz	13
Vegetables			Chicken, dark (roasted, without skin)	3.5 oz	179
Artichoke (boiled)	1 med	47	Chicken, light (roasted, without skin)	3.5 oz	216
Asparagus (boiled)	$^1/_2$ cup (6 spears)	22	Egg, whole	1 large	90
Avocado (raw)	1 med	19	Ham (canned)	3.5 oz	6
Broccoli (raw)	$^1/_2$ cup	21	Kidney beans (boiled)	1 cup	50
Brussels sprouts (boiled)	$^1/_2$ cup (4 sprouts)	28	Lentils (boiled)	1 cup	37
Carrots (raw)	1 med	19	Lima beans (boiled)	1 cup	32
Collards (boiled)	1 cup	148	Peanuts (roasted)	1 oz	15
Corn, yellow (boiled)	$^1/_2$ cup	2	Soybeans (boiled)	1 cup	175
Kale (chopped)	$^1/_2$ cup	47	**Milk, dairy products**		
Peas, green (boiled)	$^1/_2$ cup	19	Milk, skim	8 fl oz	302
Potato (baked, with skin)	1 med	115	Milk, whole	8 fl oz	290
Tomato (raw)	1 med	8	Yogurt, whole	8 fl oz	355
Fruits			**Fats, oils**		
Apricots (raw)	3 med	15	This food group is not an important source of calcium.		
Banana (raw)	1 med	7	**Sugar**		
Cantaloupe (raw)	$^1/_2$ cup	8	Brown sugar	1 cup	123
Figs (dried)	10 figs	269	Molasses, barbados	1 tbsp	49
Orange juice (fresh)	8 fl oz	27			
Orange, navel (raw)	1 med	56			
Papaya (raw)	1 med	72			

CALCIUM REQUIREMENT

Recognizing that peak bone mass is attained by about age 25, the RDA standard has been raised for young adults. An intake of 1200 mg/day for both sexes from ages 11 to 24 has been recommended to cover the important accelerated growth years of adolescence and early adulthood. A conservative estimate of a 40% absorption rate is assumed. The previous allowance for older adults is continued at 800 mg/day. An allowance of 1200 mg/day is made for pregnancy and lactation, irrespective of age. The standard for formula-fed infants is 400 mg/day for the first 6 months and 600 mg/day for the remainder of the first year. For children ages 1 to 10, the standard is 800 mg/day.

In comparison, the new report on standards for calcium and related nutrients has just been submitted from the related subcommittee to the larger comprehensive Scientific Evaluation of Dietary Reference Intakes (DRI) Committee.[15] American nutritional scientists and national health policy organizations, working with Health Canada, have just submitted their report of these new reference values in this first full report of the working DRI committees. This report is the first of a series of reports that will now serve as the new reference values for the intake of nutrients by healthy Americans and Canadians.

FOOD SOURCES OF CALCIUM

Dairy products provide the bulk of dietary calcium. One quart of milk contains about 1 g of calcium. Cheese is also a major source. Other sources, including eggs, green leafy vegetables, broccoli, legumes, nuts, and whole grains, contribute smaller amounts. Table 8.2 provides some comparative food sources of calcium.

---

osteoporosis Abnormal thinning of bone, producing a porous, fragile, latticelike bone tissue of enlarged spaces that is prone to fracture or deformity.

PHOSPHORUS

Phosphorus makes up about 1% of total body weight. It is closely associated with calcium in human nutrition and has been called its metabolic twin. However, it has some unique characteristics and functions of its own.

ABSORPTION-EXCRETION BALANCE

Absorption

The same factors that control calcium absorption also regulate phosphorus. Free phosphate is absorbed in the jejunum of the small intestine in relation to calcium and is also regulated by active vitamin D hormone, although the hormonal effect is greater on calcium absorption than on phosphorus.[16] Equal amounts of calcium and phosphorus should exist in the diet for an optimal ratio. Since phosphate occurs in food as a phosphate compound, mainly with calcium, the first step for its absorption is its splitting off as the free mineral. Factors similar to those that influence calcium absorption also affect phosphorus absorption. For example, an excess of calcium or other binding material, such as aluminum or iron, inhibits phosphorus absorption.

Excretion

The kidneys provide the main excretion route for regulation of the serum phosphorus level. Usually, 85% to 95% of plasma phosphate is filtered at the renal glomeruli and largely reabsorbed at the tubules, along with calcium, under the influence of vitamin D hormone. But when increased phosphate excretion is needed to maintain the normal serum calcium-phosphate balance, parathyroid hormone acts to override the effect of vitamin D hormone. The amount of phosphorus excreted in the urine of a person ingesting an average diet is 0.6 to 1.8 g/day.

BONE-BLOOD-CELL BALANCE

Bone

From 80% to 90% of the body's phosphorus is in the skeleton, including the teeth, compounded with calcium. This bone compartment of phosphorus is in constant interchange with the rest of the body's phosphorus, which is circulating in the blood and other body fluids.

Blood

The serum phosphorus level normally ranges from 3 to 4.5 mg/dl in adults and somewhat higher, 4 to 7 mg/dl, in children. The higher range during the growth years is a significant clue to its role in cell metabolism.

Cells

In its active phosphate form phosphorus plays a major role in the structure and function of all living cells.

Here it works with proteins, lipids, and carbohydrates to produce energy, build and repair tissues, and act as a buffer.

Hormonal controls

Because calcium and phosphorus work closely together, phosphorus balance is under the direct control of the same two hormones controlling calcium—vitamin D hormone and parathyroid hormone. A deficiency or depletion of phosphate occurs from dietary lack, diminished absorption from the intestine, or excessive wasting through the kidney.

PHYSIOLOGIC FUNCTIONS OF PHOSPHORUS

The plasma concentration of phosphorus ranges from 2.5 to 4 mg/dl, with higher mean values in young adults than in the elderly and no difference between genders until menopause, when serum values increase in women.[17] This body phosphorus serves many diverse roles, both inside and outside of cells, and enters practically every cell metabolic pathway.

Bone and tooth formation

About 80% to 90% of the body phosphorus helps make bones and teeth. As a component of calcium phosphate, it is constantly being deposited and reabsorbed in the process of bone formation.

General metabolic activities

Far out of proportion to the relatively small remaining amount, the rest of the phosphorus is intimately involved in overall human metabolism in every living cell. It has several vital roles.

1. *Absorption of glucose and glycerol.* Phosphorus combines with glucose and glycerol to assist in their intestinal absorption. It also promotes renal tubular reabsorption of glucose to return this sugar to the blood.
2. *Transport of fatty acids.* Phospholipids provide a form of fat transport.
3. *Energy metabolism.* Phosphorus-containing compounds, for example, adenosine triphosphate (ATP), are key cell substances in energy metabolism.
4. *Buffer system.* The phosphate buffer system of phosphoric acid and phosphate helps control acid-base balance in the blood.

Physiologic changes

Situations involving physiologic and clinical changes in serum phosphorus level include the following:

1. *Recovery from diabetic acidosis.* Active carbohydrate absorption and metabolism use much phosphorus, depositing it with glycogen and causing temporary hypophosphatemia.

2. *Growth.* Growing children usually have higher serum phosphate levels, resulting from high levels of growth hormone.
3. *Hypophosphatemia.* Low serum phosphorus levels occur in intestinal diseases such as sprue and celiac disease, which hinder absorption; in bone disease such as rickets or osteomalacia, which upset the calcium-phosphorus serum balance; and in primary hyperparathyroidism, in which the excess secretion of parathyroid hormone causes excess renal tubular excretion of phosphorus. Symptoms of hypophosphatemia include muscle weakness because the cells are deprived of phosphorus essential for energy metabolism.
4. *Hyperphosphatemia.* Both renal insufficiency or hypoparathyroidism cause excess accumulation of serum phosphate. As a result, the calcium side of the serum calcium-phosphorus balance is low, causing tetany.

PHOSPHORUS REQUIREMENT

Dietary ratio

During growth, pregnancy, and lactation the balance of dietary phosphorus to calcium should ideally be 1:1. In ordinary adult life the intake of phosphorus is about one and a half times that of calcium. In general, since these two minerals are found in the same food sources, if calcium needs are met, adequate phosphorus will be ensured.

RDA standard

The current RDA standard for phosphorus is 800 mg for children 1 to 10 years of age, 1200 mg for ages 11 to 24 years, and 800 mg for all adults beyond the age of 24. For formula-fed infants from birth to 6 months of age the standard is 300 mg/day, and for infants ages 6 to 12 months, 500 mg/day. Compare these RDA standards with the new Dietary Reference Intakes (RDIs) developed with Health Canada, to serve the needs of Americans and Canadians.[15]

FOOD SOURCES OF PHOSPHORUS

Milk and milk products are the most significant sources of phosphorus, as they are for calcium. However, because phosphorus plays such a large role in cell metabolism, it is also found in lean meats. Table 8.3 provides a list of food sources of phosphorus.

SODIUM

As the major cation of the extracellular body fluid, sodium is one of the most plentiful minerals in the body. About 120 mg (4 oz) is in the body of an adult, with one

third in the skeleton as inorganic bound material. The remaining two thirds is free ionized sodium.

ABSORPTION-EXCRETION BALANCE

Absorption

Sodium intake is readily absorbed from the intestine. Normally only about 5% remains for elimination in the feces. Larger amounts are lost in abnormal states such as diarrhea.

Excretion

The major route of excretion is through the kidney, under the powerful hormonal control of **aldosterone**, the sodium-conserving hormone from the adrenal glands.

PHYSIOLOGIC FUNCTIONS OF SODIUM

Water balance

Ionized sodium is the major guardian of body water outside of cells. Variations in its body fluid concentrations largely determine the distribution of water by *osmosis* from one body area to another.

Acid-base balance

In association with chloride and bicarbonate ions, ionized sodium helps regulate acid-base balance.

Cell permeability

The sodium pump in all cell membranes helps exchange sodium and potassium and other cellular materials. A major substance carried into cells by this active transport system is glucose.

Muscle action

Sodium ions play a large part in transmitting electrochemical impulses along nerve and muscle membranes and help maintain normal muscle action. Potassium and sodium ions balance the response of nerves to stimulation, the travel of nerve impulses to muscles, and the resulting contraction of the muscle fibers.

Hypertension

Several large studies, including a worldwide epidemiologic study (the international INTERSALT Study) with a sample size of 10,079 subjects, ages 20 to 59 years from 32 countries, have clearly related an increas-

---

aldosterone Potent hormone of the cortex of the adrenal glands, which acts on the distal renal tubule to cause reabsorption of sodium in an ion exchange with potassium. The aldosterone mechanism is essentially a sodium-conserving mechanism but indirectly also conserves water, since water absorption follows the sodium reabsorption.

Table

8.3   Food sources of phosphorus (RDAs for adults: 800 mg)

	Quantity	Phosphorus (mg)		Quantity	Phosphorus (mg)
Bread, cereal, rice, pasta			**Meat, poultry, fish, dry beans, eggs, nuts—cont'd**		
Bran flakes	3/4 cup	158	Chicken, dark (roasted, without skin)	3.5 oz	179
Bran muffin, homemade	1 muffin	111	Chicken, light (roasted, without skin)	3.5 oz	216
Bread, whole wheat	1 slice	65	Chick-peas (boiled)	1 cup	275
Cream of wheat (cooked)	3/4 cup	31	Clams, canned	3 oz	287
English muffin, plain	1 muffin	64	Cod (baked)	3 oz	117
Oatmeal (cooked)	3/4 cup	133	Crab, Alaska king (steamed)	3 oz	238
Pasta, enriched (cooked)	1 cup	70	Egg, whole	1 large	90
Rice, enriched (cooked)	1 cup	57	Ground beef, regular (broiled)	3.5 oz	170
Wheat flakes	1 cup	98	Halibut (baked)	3 oz	242
			Ham, canned (lean)	3.5 oz	224
Vegetables			Lentils (boiled)	1 cup	356
Artichoke (boiled)	1 med	72	Lobster (steamed)	3 oz	157
Avocado (raw)	1 med	73	Oysters (steamed)	3 oz (12 med)	236
Brussels sprouts (boiled)	1/2 cup (4 sprouts)	44	Peanut butter, creamy	1 tbsp	60
Carrots (raw)	1 med	32	Peanuts (roasted)	1 oz	100
Corn, yellow (boiled)	1/2 cup	84	Pinto beans (boiled)	1 cup	273
Peas, green (boiled)	1/2 cup	94	Sirloin steak, lean (broiled)	3.5 oz	244
Potato (baked, with skin)	1 med	115	Sole (baked)	3.5 oz	344
Spinach (boiled)	1/2 cup	50	Soybeans (boiled)	1 cup	421
Sweet potato (baked)	1 med	62	Trout, rainbow (baked)	3 oz	272
			Tuna, light, canned in water	3 oz	158
Fruits			Walnuts, dried	1 oz	132
Figs (dried)	10 figs	128			
Kiwi fruit (raw)	1 med	31	**Milk, dairy products**		
Orange juice (fresh)	8 fl oz	42	Cheddar cheese	1 cup	145
Orange, navel (raw)	1 med	27	Cottage cheese, creamed	1 cup	277
Raisins, seedless	2/3 cup	97	Milk, skim	8 fl oz	247
			Milk, whole	8 fl oz	227
Meat, poultry, fish, dry beans, eggs, nuts			Swiss cheese	1 oz	171
Almonds (roasted)	1 oz (22 nuts)	156	Yogurt, whole	8 fl oz	215
Bacon (fried)	3 med	64			
Beef liver (fried)	3.5 oz	461	**Fats, oils, sugar**		
Beef top round, lean (broiled)	3.5 oz	246	This food group is not an important source of phosphorus.		
Black-eyed peas (boiled)	1 cup	266			

ing dietary salt (NaCl) intake, mainly in the increasing use of processed foods, to the increasing incidence of hypertension.[18] Other studies include (1) the Dietary Approaches to Stop Hypertension (DASH), based on functional foods containing phytochemicals in a diet rich in vegetables, fruits, and low-fat dairy products, and containing an average sodium intake of 3 g/day[19]; (2) the Trials of Hypertension Prevention (TOHP), held in a large number of American study sites, and including positive responses in weight management and sodium reduction[20]; and (3) a smaller study in a London medical school with untreated hypertensive elderly adults, which demonstrated a blood pressure reduction with only modest reductions of salt.[21]

SODIUM REQUIREMENT

RDA standard

The body can function on a rather wide range of dietary sodium by mechanisms designed to conserve or excrete the mineral. Thus there is no specific stated requirement. However, the RDAs do include a table of estimated minimum requirements of the three minerals—sodium, chloride, and potassium—that are major electrolytes in body fluid balance. This RDA standard estimates a minimum sodium requirement for healthy persons over age 18 to be about 500 mg/day to cover wide variations in individual patterns of physical activity and climate, which influence relative losses in perspiration. Thus a safe

Table

8.4 Food sources of sodium (estimated safe and adequate daily intakes for adults: 1100-3300 mg)

	Quantity	Sodium (mg)		Quantity	Sodium (mg)
Bread, cereal, rice, pasta			**Meat, poultry, fish, dry beans, eggs, nuts—cont'd**		
Bran flakes	¾ cup	264	Halibut (baked)	3 oz	59
Bran muffin, homemade	1 muffin	168	Ham, canned (lean)	3.5 oz	1255
Bread, whole wheat	1 slice	159	Lentils (boiled)	1 cup	4
Corn flakes	1 cup	310	Lobster (steamed)	3 oz	323
Wheat flakes	1 cup	270	Mackerel (baked)	3 oz	71
			Oysters (steamed)	3 oz (12 med)	190
Vegetables			Peanut butter, creamy (unsalted)	1 tbsp	3
Artichoke (boiled)	1 med	79			
Broccoli (boiled)	½ cup	12	Peanut butter, creamy (with salt)	1 tbsp	131
Brussels sprouts (boiled)	½ cup	17			
Carrot (raw)	1 med	25	Shrimp (steamed)	3 oz (15 large)	190
Potato (baked, with skin)	1 med	16	Sirloin steak, lean (broiled)	3.5 oz	66
Spinach (boiled)	½ cup	63	Soybeans (boiled)	1 cup	1
Tomato (raw)	1 med	10	Tuna, light, canned in water (with salt)	3 oz	303
Fruits					
This food group is not an important source of sodium.			**Milk, dairy products**		
			Cheddar cheese	1 oz	176
Meat, poultry, fish, dry beans, eggs, nuts			Cottage cheese, creamed	1 cup	850
Almonds (roasted, unsalted)	1 oz (22 nuts)	3	Milk, skim	8 fl oz	126
Bacon (broiled/fried)	3 med pieces	303	Milk, whole	8 fl oz	119
Beef liver (fried)	3.5 oz	106	Swiss cheese	1 oz	74
Beef top round, lean (broiled)	3.5 oz	61	Yogurt, whole	8 fl oz	105
Black-eyed peas (boiled)	1 cup	6			
Chicken, dark (roasted, without skin)	3.5 oz	93	**Fats, oils, sugar**		
			Butter (salted)	1 tbsp	123
Chicken, light (roasted, without skin)	3.5 oz	77	Butter (unsalted)	1 tbsp	2
			Margarine, stick, corn oil (salted)	1 tbsp	132
Clams (steamed)	3 oz (9 small)	95			
Crab, blue (steamed)	3 oz	237	Margarine, stick, corn oil (unsalted)	1 tbsp	3
Egg, whole	1 large	69			
Ground beef, regular (broiled)	3.5 oz	83	Molasses, black	1 tbsp	19
			Sugar, brown	1 cup	44

and adequate sodium intake for adults has been set at approximately 1100 to 3300 mg/day.

General dietary intake

Sodium in the average American diet, mainly in processed foods, usually far exceeds the RDA estimate of adequate intake, even excluding the added amount in table salt. There is about 4 g sodium in the average 10 g of table salt consumed daily. A wiser adult intake of about 2 g sodium would equal about 5 g (1 teaspoon) of salt.

FOOD SOURCES OF SODIUM

The main dietary source of sodium is common salt used in cooking, seasoning, and processing of foods. Natural food sources include milk, meat, eggs, and certain vegetables such as carrots, beets, leafy greens, and celery.

Some comparative food sources of sodium are provided in Table 8.4.

POTASSIUM

Potassium is about twice as plentiful as sodium in the body. An adult body contains about 270 mg (9 oz, 4000 mEq). By far the greater portion is found inside the cells, since potassium is the major guardian of the body water inside cells. However, the relatively small amount in fluid outside cells has a significant effect on muscle activity, especially heart muscle.

ABSORPTION-EXCRETION BALANCE

Absorption

Dietary potassium is easily absorbed in the small intestine. Potassium also circulates in the gastrointestinal secretions and is reabsorbed in the digestive process. However, diseases such as prolonged diarrhea cause dangerous losses.

Excretion

Urinary excretion is the principle route of potassium loss. There is excess loss with some diuretic drugs. Since maintenance of serum potassium within the narrow normal range is vital to heart muscle action and electrolyte balance, the kidneys guard potassium carefully. However, they cannot guard potassium as effectively as sodium. In the renal aldosterone mechanism for sodium conservation, potassium is lost in exchange for sodium. The normal obligatory loss is about 160 mg/day.

PHYSIOLOGIC FUNCTIONS OF POTASSIUM

Water and acid-base balance

As the major guardian of cell water, potassium inside the cells balances with sodium outside the cells to maintain normal osmotic pressures and water balance to protect cellular fluid. Potassium also works with sodium and hydrogen to maintain acid-base balance.

Muscle activity

Potassium plays a significant role in the activity of skeletal and cardiac muscle. Together with sodium and calcium, potassium regulates neuromuscular stimulation, transmission of electrochemical impulses, and contraction of muscle fibers. This effect is particularly notable in the action of the heart muscle. Even small variations in serum potassium concentration are reflected in electrocardiographic (ECG) changes. Variations in serum levels or low serum potassium may cause muscle irritability and paralysis. The heart may even develop a gallop rhythm and finally cardiac arrest.

Carbohydrate metabolism

When blood glucose is converted to glycogen for storage, 0.36 mmol of potassium is stored for each 1 g glycogen. When a patient in diabetic acidosis is treated by insulin and glucose, rapid glycogen production draws potassium from the serum. Serious hypokalemia can result unless adequate potassium replacement accompanies treatment.

Protein synthesis

Potassium is required for the storage of nitrogen in muscle protein and general cell protein. When tissue is broken down, potassium is lost together with the nitrogen. Amino acid replacement includes potassium to ensure nitrogen retention.

POTASSIUM REQUIREMENT

As with sodium, no specific dietary requirement is given for potassium. However, based on balance studies of the amount needed to replace losses and maintain normal body stores and plasma levels, the RDA standard estimates a minimum safe daily intake for adults of approximately 1600 to 2000 mg. In light of considerable evidence that dietary potassium has a beneficial effect on hypertension, in its report *Diet and health: implications for reducing chronic disease risk*, the National Research Council has recommended an increase in potassium by eating more fruits and vegetables. The RDA has stated a safe and adequate range of daily potassium intake for adults of 1875 to 5625 mg. The usual diet contains from 2000 to 4000 mg/day, which is ample for common needs.

FOOD SOURCES OF POTASSIUM

Potassium is widely distributed in natural foods, since it is an essential constituent of all living cells. Legumes, whole grains, fruits such as oranges and bananas, leafy green vegetables, broccoli, potatoes, meats, and milk products supply considerable amounts. People who eat large amounts of fruits and vegetables have a high potassium intake of about 8 to 11 g/day, well above the minimum safe level of 2 g/day. Table 8.5 gives some comparative food sources of potassium.

OTHER MAJOR MINERALS

Three additional minerals are assigned to the major minerals group because of the extent of their occurrence in the body. These are magnesium, chloride, and sulfur.

MAGNESIUM

Magnesium has widespread metabolic functions and is present in all body cells. An adult body contains about 25 g of magnesium or a little less than an ounce. About 70% of this small but vital amount is combined with calcium and phosphorus in the bone.[22] The remaining 30% is distributed in various tissues and body fluids, where it has widespread metabolic use in all cells as a control agent. It acts as an enzyme activator for energy production and building tissue protein. It also aids in normal muscle action. The RDA standard is 350 mg/day for men and 300 mg for women. The new American recommended Dietary Reference Intakes (DRI) for magnesium, developed jointly with Health Canada, have just been issued among the National Academy of Sciences first new values report of the working DRI nutrient-energy committees.[15]

Magnesium is relatively widespread in nature and thus in unprocessed foods. For example, large concentrations of magnesium occur in unmilled grains, but more

Table 8.5 Food sources of potassium (estimated safe and adequate daily intake for adults: 1875-5625 mg)

	Quantity	Potassium (mg)		Quantity	Potassium (mg)
Bread, cereal, rice, pasta			**Meat, poultry, fish, dry beans, eggs, nuts**		
Bran flakes	3/4 cup	184	Black-eyed peas (boiled)	1 cup	476
Bran muffin, homemade	1 muffin	99	Chicken, dark (roasted, without skin)	3.5 oz	240
Bread, whole wheat	1 slice	44	Chicken, light (roasted, without skin)	3.5 oz	247
Oatmeal (cooked)	3/4 cup	99	Clams (steamed)	3 oz (9 small)	534
Pasta, enriched (cooked)	1 cup	85	Crab, blue (steamed)	3 oz	275
Rice, white, enriched	1 cup	57	Egg, whole	1 large	65
Wheat flakes	1 cup	110	Ground beef, regular (broiled)	3.5 oz	292
Wheat germ, toasted	1/4 cup (1 oz)	268	Halibut (baked)	3 oz	490
Vegetables			Ham, canned (lean)	3.5 oz	364
Artichoke (boiled)	1 med	316	Lentils (boiled)	1 cup	731
Asparagus (boiled)	1/2 cup (6 spears)	279	Lima beans (boiled)	1 cup	955
Avocado (raw)	1 med	1097	Lobster (steamed)	3 oz	299
Broccoli (raw)	1/2 cup, chopped	143	Mackerel (baked)	3 oz	341
Brussels sprouts (boiled)	1/2 cup (4 sprouts)	247	Oysters (steamed)	3 oz (12 med)	389
Carrot (raw)	1 med	233	Peanut butter, creamy	1 tbsp	110
Corn, yellow (boiled)	1/2 cup	204	Peanuts (dry roasted)	1 oz	184
Mushrooms (boiled)	1/2 cup, pieces	277	Pinto beans (boiled)	1 cup	800
Potato (baked, with skin)	1 med	844	Salmon (baked)	3 oz	319
Spinach (boiled)	1/2 cup	419	Sirloin steak, lean (broiled)	3.5 oz	403
Sweet potato (baked)	1 med	397	Soybeans (boiled)	1 cup	886
Tomato (raw)	1 med	254	Trout, rainbow (baked)	3 oz	539
Fruits			Tuna, light, canned in water (with salt)	3 oz	267
Apple (raw, with skin)	1 med	159	**Milk, dairy products**		
Banana	1 med	451	Cottage cheese, creamed	1 cup	177
Cantaloupe	1 cup, pieces	494	Milk, skim	8 fl oz	406
Dates (dried)	10 dates	541	Milk, whole	8 fl oz	368
Figs (dried)	10 figs	1332	Yogurt, whole	8 fl oz	351
Orange juice (fresh)	8 fl oz	486	**Fats, oils**		
Orange, navel	1 med	250	This food group is not an important source of potassium.		
Prunes (dried)	10 prunes	626	**Sugar**		
Prune juice (canned)	8 fl oz	706	Molasses, black	1 tbsp	585
Raisins, seedless	2/3 cup	751	Sugar, brown	1 cup	499
Meat, poultry, fish, dry beans, eggs, nuts					
Almonds (dry roasted)	1 oz (22 nuts)	219			
Beef liver (fried)	3.5 oz	364			
Beef top round, lean (broiled)	3.5 oz	442			

than 80% is lost by removal of the germ and outer layers of the grain. Its main food sources include nuts, soybeans, cocoa, seafood, whole grains, dried beans and peas, and green vegetables. Most fruits, except bananas, are relatively poor sources, as are milk, meat, and fish. Thus, on the whole, diets rich in vegetables and unrefined grains are much higher in magnesium than are diets made up mostly of refined foods, meat, and dairy products. Table 8.6 gives some comparative food sources of magnesium.

CHLORINE (CHLORIDE)

Chlorine appears in the body as the chloride ion (Cl^-). Chlorine accounts for about 3% of the body's total mineral content, mainly as a part of the fluid outside of cells, where it helps control water and acid-base balances. Spinal fluid has the highest concentration. A relatively large amount of ionized chloride is found in the gastrointestinal secretions, especially as a component of gastric hydrochloric acid (HCl).

Table 8.6	Food sources of magnesium (RDAs for adult women, 300 mg; for adult men, 350 mg)				
	Quantity	**Magnesium (mg)**		**Quantity**	**Magnesium (mg)**
Bread, cereal, rice, pasta			**Meat, poultry, fish, dry beans, eggs, nuts—cont'd**		
Bran flakes	3/4 cup	68	Chick-peas (boiled)	1 cup	78
Bran muffin, homemade	1 muffin	35	Cod (baked)	3 oz	36
Bread, whole wheat	1 slice	23	Crab, blue (steamed)	3 oz	28
Oatmeal (cooked)	3/4 cup	42	Egg, whole	1 large	6
Pasta, enriched (cooked)	1 cup	28	Ground beef, regular (broiled)	3.5 oz	20
Wheat flakes	1 cup	31	Halibut (baked)	3 oz	91
Vegetables			Ham, canned (lean)	3.5 oz	17
Artichoke (boiled)	1 med	47	Lentils (boiled)	1 cup	71
Avocado (raw)	1 med	70	Lobster (steamed)	3 oz	30
Corn, yellow (boiled)	1/2 med	26	Mackeral (baked)	3 oz	83
Okra (boiled)	1/2 cup	46	Oysters (steamed)	3 oz (12 med)	92
Peas, green (boiled)	1/2 cup	31	Peanut butter, creamy	1 tbsp	28
Potato (baked, with skin)	1 med	55	Peanuts (roasted)	1 oz	49
Spinach (boiled)	1/2 cup	79	Pinto beans (boiled)	1 cup	95
Sweet potato (baked)	1 med	23	Sirloin steak, lean (broiled)	3.5 oz	32
Fruits			Soybeans (boiled)	1 cup	95
Figs (dried)	10 figs	111	Trout, rainbow (baked)	3 oz	33
Kiwi (raw)	1 med	23	Tuna, light, canned in water	3 oz	25
Orange juice (fresh)	8 fl oz	27	Walnuts, dried	1 oz	57
Raisins, seedless	2/3 cup	33	**Milk, dairy products**		
Meat, poultry, fish, dry beans, eggs, nuts			Cheddar cheese	1 oz	8
Almonds (roasted)	1 oz (22 nuts)	86	Cottage cheese, creamed	1 cup	11
Beef liver (fried)	3.5 oz	23	Milk, skim	8 fl oz	28
Beef top round, lean (broiled)	3.5 oz	31	Milk, whole	8 fl oz	33
Black-eyed peas (boiled)	1 cup	91	Swiss cheese	1 oz	10
Chicken, dark (roasted, without skin)	3.5 oz	23	Yogurt, whole	8 fl oz	26
Chicken, light (roasted without skin)	3.5 oz	27	**Fats, oils, sugar**		
			This food group is not an important source of magnesium.		

SULFUR

Sulfur is present in all body cells, usually as a constituent of cell protein. Elemental sulfur occurs in sulfate compounds with sodium, potassium, and magnesium. Organic forms occur mainly with other protein compounds: (1) sulfur-containing amino acids, such as methionine and cystine; (2) glycoproteins in cartilage, tendons, and bone matrix; (3) detoxification products formed in part by bacterial activity in the intestine; (4) other organic compounds such as heparin, insulin, coenzyme A, lipoic acid, thiamin, and biotin; and (5) keratin in hair and nails.

The major minerals are summarized in Table 8.7.

TRACE ELEMENTS: THE CONCEPT OF ESSENTIALITY

By the simplest definition, an essential element is one required for existence; conversely, its absence brings death. For major elements that occur in relatively large amounts in the body, as we have seen, such determinations can be made easily because the quantity present is sufficiently available for study. However, for things that occur in very small amounts, this determination of essentiality is not easy to make. For example, of the 54 known chemical elements in the major part of the periodic table, 27 have been determined to be essential to

Table
8.7 Summary of major minerals (required intake over 100 mg/day)

Mineral	Metabolism	Physiologic functions	Clinical applications	Requirements	Food sources
Calcium (Ca)	Absorption according to body need; requires Ca-binding protein and regulated by vitamin D, parathyroid hormone, and calcitonin; absorption favored by protein, lactose, acidity. Excretion chiefly in feces: 70%-90% of amount ingested. Deposition-mobilization is bone tissue constant, regulated by vitamin D and parathyroid hormone	Constituent of bones and teeth. Participates in blood clotting, nerve transmission, muscle action, cell membrane permeability, enzyme activation	Tetany (decrease in serum Ca). Rickets, osteomalacia. Osteoporosis. Resorptive hypercalcinuria, renal calculi. Hyperthyroidism and hypothyroidism	Adults: 800 mg. Pregnancy and lactation: 1200 mg. Infants: 400-600 mg. Children: 800-1200 mg	Milk, cheese. Green, leafy vegetables. Whole grains. Egg yolk. Legumes, nuts
Phosphorus (P)	Absorption with Ca aided by vitamin D and parathyroid hormone as for calcium; hindered by binding agents. Excretion chiefly by kidney according to serum level, regulated by parathyroid hormone. Deposition-mobilization in bone compartment constant	Constituent of bones and teeth, ATP, phosphorylated intermediary metabolites. Participants in absorption of glucose and glycerol, transport of fatty acids, energy metabolism, and buffer system	Growth. Recovery from diabetic acidosis. Hypophosphatemia: bone disease, malabsorption syndromes, primary hyperparathyroidism. Hyperphosphatemia: renal insufficiency, hypothyroidism, tetany	Adults: 800 mg. Pregnancy and lactation: 1200 mg. Infants: 300-500 mg. Children: 800-1200 mg	Milk, cheese. Meat, egg yolk. Whole grains. Legumes, nuts
Magnesium (Mg)	Absorption according to intake load; hindered by excess fat, phosphate, calcium, protein. Excretion (regulated by kidney)	Constituent of bones and teeth. Coenzyme in general metabolism, smooth muscle action, neuromuscular irritability. Cation in intracellular fluid	Low serum level following gastrointestinal losses. Tremor, spasm in deficiency induced by malnutrition, alcoholism	Adults: 280-350 mg. Pregnancy and lactation: 290-355 mg. Infants: 40-60 mg. Children: 80-170 mg	Milk, cheese. Meat, seafood. Whole grains. Legumes, nuts
Sodium (Na)	Readily absorbed. Excretion chiefly by kidney, controlled by aldosterone	Major cation in extracellular fluid, water balance, acid-base balance. Cell membrane permeability, absorption of glucose. Normal muscle irritability	Losses in gastrointestinal disorders, diarrhea. Fluid-electrolyte and acid-base balance problems. Muscle action	Adults: 500 mg. Infants: 120-200 mg. Children: 225-500 mg	Salt (NaCl). Sodium compounds in baking and processing. Milk, cheese. Meat, eggs. Carrots, beets, spinach, celery

Continued

Table 8.7	Summary of major minerals (required intake over 100 mg/day)—cont'd				
Mineral	**Metabolism**	**Physiologic functions**	**Clinical applications**	**Requirements**	**Food sources**
Potassium (K)	Readily absorbed Secreted and resorbed in gastrointestinal circulation Excretion chiefly by kidney, regulated by aldosterone	Major cation in intracellular fluid, water balance, acid-base balance Normal muscle irritability Glycogen formation Protein synthesis	Losses in gastrointestinal disorders, diarrhea Fluid-electrolyte, acid-base balance problems Muscle action, especially heart action Losses in tissue catabolism Treatment of diabetic acidosis: rapid glycogen production reduces serum potassium level Losses with diuretic therapy	Adults: 2000 mg Infants: 500-700 mg Children: 1000-2000 mg	Fruits Vegetables Legumes, nuts Whole grains Meat
Chloride (Cl)	Readily absorbed Excretion controlled by kidney	Major anion in extracellular fluid, water balance, acid-base balance, chloride-bicarbonate shift Gastric hydrochloride—digestion	Losses in gastrointestinal disorders, vomiting, diarrhea, tube drainage Hypochloremic alkalosis	Adults: 750 mg Infants: 180-300 mg Children: 350-750 mg	Salt (NaCl)
Sulfur (S)	Elemental form absorbed as such; split from amino acid sources (methionine and cystine) in digestion and absorbed into portal circulation Excreted by kidney in relation to protein intake and tissue catabolism	Essential constituent of protein structure Enzyme activity and energy metabolism through free sulfhydryl group (—SH) Detoxification reactions	Cystine renal calculi Cystinuria	Diet adequate in protein contains adequate sulfur	Meat, eggs Milk, cheese Legumes, nuts

human life and function. By far, most living matter as we know it is made up of five fundamental elements: hydrogen (H), carbon (C), nitrogen (N), oxygen (O), and sulfur (S). We know these elements well because their concentrations are relatively large, hence more easily studied, and their requirements for human function can be stated in multiples of grams per gram of body weight. This is a recognizable quantity with which we can be comfortable. We have means for analysis of such quantities and can easily see that these are essential elements. Also, the major minerals you have just reviewed here occur in respectable amounts in the body, so their essentiality has been more easily studied and determined.

A much larger number of elements—microelements or trace elements—occur in biologic matter in such small amounts that measurement and analysis are exceedingly difficult. In many cases we know little about them and understand even less. It is much harder to determine the essentiality of these trace elements because we apparently require so little of them. In general, trace elements have been defined as those having a required intake of less than 100 mg/day. Yet some of them exist in fairly large amounts in our diet and our environment.

Essential function

Despite difficulties in determining the essentiality of these very small amounts of trace elements in our bodies, Mertz, a leading researcher and authority in trace element metabolism, has left us much knowledge about these important minerals.[23,24] He taught us early and lasting lessons that essentiality can be determined on the basis of function and effect of deficiency, and that safe, recommended dietary intakes must be safe from toxicity but adequate to meet nutrition requirements. This is no small task.[23,24]

1. *Basic functions of trace elements.* An element is essential when a deficiency causes an impairment of function and supplementation with that substance, but not with others, prevents or cures this impairment. Studies in this field have identified the two basic functions of trace elements in terms of *catalytic* and *structural* components of larger molecules.
2. *Deficiency and requirement.* Because these small amounts of trace elements are not easily measured, specific needs have been stated only for the following: (1) iron (Fe) because it has a long history, (2) zinc (Zn) because it occurs in higher concentration than some of the others, (3) iodine (I) because it has only one specific known function, and (4) selenium (Se) because of its recently recognized partnership with vitamin E as an antioxidant agent. Thus far the RDA standard only estimates requirements for the others in terms of a general range of need.

On the basis of current knowledge, these small trace elements may be classed in two groups: those that are definitely essential and those that are probably essential.

Definitely essential elements

Ten trace elements have been assigned essential roles in human nutrition based on defined function and need determined from research. This group includes: iron (Fe), iodine (I), zinc (Zn), copper (Cu), manganese (Mn), chromium (Cr), cobalt (Co), selenium (Se), molybdenum (Mo), and fluoride (Fl).

Probably essential elements

All the remaining eight trace elements are probably essential, but a more complete understanding requires the development of better means of analysis and tests for function. These elements include: silicon (Si), vanadium (V), nickel (Ni), tin (Sn), cadmium (Cd), arsenic (As), aluminum (Al), and boron (B).

We look first at iron and iodine because of their long history and clearly defined specific function. Then we will briefly review the remainder. These essential elements are summarized in Table 8.8.

IRON

Of all the micronutrients, iron has the longest and best described history, and its essential mechanisms for body regulation to avoid both iron overload and iron deficiency have been well described.[25]

FORMS OF IRON IN THE BODY

The human body contains only about 45 mg iron/kg body weight. This iron is distributed in four forms that point to its basic metabolic function:

Transport iron

A trace of iron, 0.05 to 0.18 mg/dl, is in plasma and bound to its transport carrier protein *transferrin*.

Hemoglobin

Most of the body's iron, about 70%, occurs in red blood cells as a vital constituent of the heme portion of **hemoglobin**. Another 5% is a part of the muscle oxygen-carrying hemoglobin *myoglobin*.

Storage iron

About 20% of the body iron is stored as the protein-iron compound **ferritin**, mainly in the liver, spleen, and bone marrow. Excess iron is stored in the body as **hemosiderin**, interchanging with ferritin as needed.

Cellular tissue iron

The remaining 5% of body iron is distributed throughout all cells as a major component of oxidative enzyme systems for the production of energy.

---

ferritin Protein-iron compound in which iron is stored in tissues; the storage form of iron in the body.

hemoglobin Oxygen-carrying pigment in red blood cells; a conjugated protein containing four heme groups combined with iron and four long polypeptide chains forming the protein globin, named for its ball-like form; made by the developing red blood cells in bone marrow, hemoglobin carries oxygen in the blood to body cells.

hemosiderin Insoluble iron oxide–protein compound in which iron is stored in the liver if the amount of iron in the blood exceeds the storage capacity of ferritin, for example, during rapid destruction of red blood cells (malaria, hemolytic anemia).

Table

8.8   Summary of trace elements (required intake less than 100 mg/day)

Element	Metabolism	Physiologic functions	Clinical applications	Requirements	Food sources
Iron (Fe)	Absorption controls bioavailability; favored by body need, acidity, and reduction agents such as vitamins; hindered by binding agents, reduced gastric HCl, infection, gastrointestinal losses Transported as transferrin, stored as ferritin or hemosiderin Excreted in sloughed cells, bleeding	Hemoglobin synthesis, oxygen transport Cell oxidation, heme enzymes	Anemia (hydrochromic, microcytic) Excess: hemosiderosis, hemochromatosis Growth and pregnancy needs	Adults: men—10 mg, women—15 mg Pregnancy and lactation: 30 and 15 mg, respectively Infants: 6-10 mg Children: 10-12 mg	Liver, meats, eggs Whole grains Enriched breads and cereals Dark green vegetables Legumes, nuts (iron cookware)
Iodine (I)	Absorbed as iodides, taken up by thyroid gland under control of thryoid-stimulating hormone (TSH) Excretion by kidney	Synthesis of thyroxin, which regulates cell metabolism, basal metabolic rate (EMR)	Endemic colloid goiter, cretinism Hypothyroidism and hyperthyroidism	Adults: 150 μg Infants: 40-50 μg Children: 70-150 μg	Iodized salt Seafood
Zinc (Zn)	Absorbed with zinc-binding ligand (ZBL) from pancreas Transported in blood by albumin; stored in many sites Excretion largely intestinal	Essential coenzyme constituent: carbonic anhydrase, carboxypeptidase, lactic dehydrogenase	Growth: hypogonadism Sensory impairment: taste and smell Wound healing Malabsorption disease	Adults: 12-15 mg Infants: 5 mg Children: 10-15 mg	Widely distributed Seafood, oysters Liver, meat Milk, cheese, eggs Whole grains
Copper (Cu)	Absorbed with copper-binding protein metallothionein Transported in blood by histidine and albumin Stored in many tissues	Associated with iron in enzyme systems, hemoglobin synthesis Metalloprotein enzyme constituent	Hypocupremia: nephrosis and malabsorption Wilson's disease, excess copper storage	Adults: 1.5-3 mg Infants: 0.4-0.7 mg Children: 0.7-2.5 mg	Widely distributed Liver, meat Seafood Whole grains Legumes, nuts (Copper cookware)
Manganese (Mn)	Absorbed poorly Excretion mainly by intestine	Enzyme component in general metabolism	Low serum levels in diabetes, protein-energy malnutrition Inhalation toxicity	Adults: 2-5 mg Infants: 0.3-1.0 μg Children: 1-5 μg	Cereals, whole grains Legumes, soybeans Leafy vegetables
Chromium (Cr)	Absorbed in association with zinc Excretion mainly by kidney	Associated with glucose metabolism; improves faulty glucose uptake by tissues; glucose tolerance factor	Potentiates action of insulin in persons with diabetes Lowers serum cholesterol, LDL-cholesterol* Increases HDL*	Adults: 50-200 μg Infants: 10-60 μg Children: 2-200 μg	Cereals Whole grains Brewer's yeast Animal protein

*LDL, Low-density lipoprotein; HDL, high-density lipoprotein.

Table					

8.8 Summary of trace elements (required intake less than 100 mg/day)—cont'd

Element	Metabolism	Physiologic functions	Clinical applications	Requirements	Food sources
Cobalt (Co)	Absorbed as component of food source, vitamin B_{12} Elemental form shares transport with iron Stored in liver	Constituent of vitamin B_{12}, functions with vitamin	Deficiency associated only with deficiency of vitamin B_{12}	Unknown, evidently minute	Vitamin B_{12} source
Selenium (Se)	Absorption depends on solubility of compound form Excreted mainly by kidney	Constituent of enzyme glutathione peroxidase Synergistic antioxidant with vitamin E Structural component of teeth	Marginal deficiency when soil content is low Deficiency secondary to parenteral nutrition (TPN), malnutrition Toxicity observed in livestock	Adults: 55-70 μg Infants: 10-15 μg Children: 20-50 μg	Varies with soil content Seafood Legumes Whole grains Low-fat meats and dairy products Vegetables
Molybdenum (Mo)	Readily absorbed Excreted rapidly by kidney Small amount excreted in bile	Constituent of oxidase enzymes, xanthine oxidase	Deficiency unknown in humans	Adults: 75-250 μg Infants: 15-30 μg Children: 25-250 μg	Legumes Whole grains Milk Organ meats Leafy vegetables
Fluoride (F)	Absorption in small intestine; little known of bioavailability Excreted by kidney—80%	Accumulates in bones and teeth, increasing hardness	Dental caries inhibited Osteoporosis: may help control Excess: dental fluorosis	Adults: 1.5-4 mg Infants: 0.1-0.5 mg Children: 0.5-2.5 mg	Fish Fish products Tea Foods cooked in fluoridated water Drinking water

LDL, Low-density lipoprotein; *HDL,* high-density lipoprotein.

ABSORPTION-TRANSPORT-STORAGE-EXCRETION BALANCE

In the body, iron follows a unique system of interrelated absorption-transport-storage-excretion. Optimal levels of body iron are not maintained by urinary excretion as is the case with most plasma constituents. Rather, the mechanisms of iron control lie in the absorption-transport-storage complex.

Absorption

The main control of the body's iron balance is at the point of intestinal absorption. Dietary iron enters the body in two forms: **heme** and **nonheme** (Table 8.9). By far the larger portion is nonheme—all plant sources plus 60% of animal sources. But it is absorbed at a much slower rate than the smaller heme portion because nonheme iron is tightly bound in its food sources to organic molecules in the form of ferric iron (Fe^{+++}). In the acidic

medium of the stomach, it must be disassociated and reduced to the more soluble ferrous iron (Fe^{++}). This is a source of nutritional concern because of nonheme's greater quantity in the diet.

heme iron Dietary iron from animal sources, from the heme portion of hemoglobin in red blood cells. Heme iron is more easily absorbed and transported in the body than nonheme iron from plant sources, but it supplies the smaller portion of the body's total dietary iron intake.

nonheme iron The larger portion of dietary iron, including all the plant food sources and 60% of the animal food sources, which lacks the more easily absorbed and bioavailable heme iron in the remaining 40% of the animal food sources that contain hemoglobin residues or iron containing heme.

Table 8.9	Characteristics of heme and nonheme portions of dietary iron	
	Dietary iron	
	Heme (smallest portion)	Nonheme (largest portion)
Food sources	None in plant sources; 40% of iron in animal sources	All plant sources of iron; 60% of iron in animal sources
Absorption rate	Rapid; transported and absorbed intact	Slow; tightly bound in organic molecules

Control of iron distribution and transfer in the absorbing cell involves several receiving substances. Iron is never allowed to travel about the body unescorted. First, the iron, all now in ferric form, is bound by an initial intracellular molecule (ICM). This ICM leaves a portion of the iron to serve needs of the absorbing cell's mitochondria, then delivers specific proportions to its regular receptors and carriers: (1) apoferritin (*apo-*, meaning derived or separated from something), the cell's special protein receptor with which iron combines to form the immediate holding compound, epithelial ferritin, and (2) apotransferrin, the blood's special protein receptor with which iron combines to form its circulating carrier compound, serum transferrin.

The amount of ferritin already present in the intestinal mucosa determines the amount of ingested iron that is absorbed or rejected. When all available apoferritin has been bound to iron to form ferritin, any additional iron that arrives at the binding site is rejected, returned to the lumen of the intestine, and passed on for excretion in the feces. In all, only 10% to 30% of the ingested iron is absorbed, mostly in the duodenum. The remaining 70% to 90% is eliminated.

The following factors favor absorption:

1. *Body need.* In deficiency states or in periods of extra demand, as in growth or pregnancy, mucosal ferritin is lower and more iron is absorbed. When tissue reserves are ample or saturated, iron is rejected and excreted.
2. *Acidity and reduction agents.* Vitamin C (ascorbic acid) aids iron absorption by its reducing action and effect on acidity. Other metabolic reducing agents have similar effects, as does the gastric hydrochloric acid, which provides the optimal acid medium for preparing iron for use.
3. *Calcium.* An adequate amount of calcium helps bind and remove agents such as phosphate and phytate, which would combine with iron and prevent its absorption.

The following factors hinder absorption:

1. *Binding agents.* Materials such as phosphate, phytate, and oxalate bind iron and remove it from the body. Tea and coffee have also been shown to inhibit nonheme iron absorption.
2. *Reduced gastric acid secretion.* Surgical removal of stomach tissue (gastrectomy) reduces the number of cells that secrete hydrochloric acid, thus reducing the necessary acid medium for iron reduction.
3. *Infection.* Severe infection hinders iron absorption.
4. *Gastrointestinal disease.* Malabsorption or any disturbance that causes diarrhea or *steatorrhea* (fatty diarrhea) hinders iron absorption.

Thus the bioavailability of iron essentially depends on its absorption, which in turn depends on a number of influencing factors in the body. This is a unique and precarious arrangement.

Transport

As we have seen in the mucosal cells of the duodenum and proximal jejunum, iron is oxidized and bound with the plasma transferrin for transport to body cells. Normally, only about 20% to 35% of the iron-binding capacity of transferrin is filled. The remaining capacity forms an unsaturated plasma reserve for handling variances in iron intake.

Storage

Bound to plasma transferrin, iron is delivered to its storage sites in bone marrow and to some extent in the liver. Here it is transferred to apoferritin again to form ferritin for storage and use as needed in synthesizing hemoglobin for red blood cells. This binding with apoferritin provides a stable, exchangeable storage form for the body needs. A second, less soluble storage compound, hemosiderin, provides reserve storage in the liver. From these storage compounds, iron is mobilized for hemoglobin synthesis as needed. In the average adult, 20 to 25 mg/day of iron are used in hemoglobin synthesis. However, the body avidly conserves the iron in hemoglobin, recycling the iron when red blood cells are destroyed after their average life span of about 120 days. These interrelationships of body iron absorption-transport-storage mechanisms are diagrammed in Figure 8.3.

Excretion

Because the main regulatory mechanism controlling iron levels in the body occurs at the point of absorption, only minute amounts are lost by renal excretion. Essentially none is in the urine, as opposed to other circulating minerals, which are often excreted in the urine. Rather, the small amounts of iron excreted normally come from the

Figure 8.3 Summary of iron metabolism, showing its absorption, transport, main use in hemoglobin formation, and its storage forms (ferritin and hemosiderin).

sloughing off of skin tissue, gastrointestinal cells, and normal gastrointestinal and menstrual blood loss. Unusual blood loss such as that from heavy menstrual flow, childbirth, surgery, acute and chronic hemorrhage, gastrointestinal disease, or parasitic infestation may bring severe iron loss.

PHYSIOLOGIC FUNCTIONS OF IRON

Oxygen transport

Iron is "pocketed" within the heme molecule, which is the fundamental nonprotein part of hemoglobin in the red blood cells. As such, iron functions as a major transporter of vital oxygen to the cells for respiration and metabolism. Iron is also a constituent of the similar compound myoglobin in muscle tissue.

Cellular oxidation

Although in smaller amounts, iron also functions in the cells as a vital component of enzyme systems for oxidation of glucose to produce energy.

Growth needs

During growth, positive iron balance is imperative. At birth, the infant has a small 4- to 6-month supply of iron stored in the liver from fetal development. Breast-fed infants obtain some iron in breast milk. However, since cow's milk does not supply iron, iron is added to commercial formulas. Supplementary iron-rich and fortified foods are added to the diet at about 4 to 6 months of age. In this way the classic milk anemia of young children is prevented. Iron is also needed for continued growth and to build up reserves for the physiologic stress of adolescence, especially the onset of menses in girls. The woman's need for iron is increased greatly during pregnancy to maintain the increased number of red blood cells in an expanded circulating blood volume and to supply the iron needed for storage in the developing fetal liver. Normal blood loss during delivery reduces iron stores further.

CLINICAL PROBLEMS

Because of the unique physiologic controls of the body's iron content, clinical abnormalities may result from either a deficiency or an excess of iron.

Iron deficiency

Surprisingly, iron deficiency occurs in both developed and underdeveloped countries for two main reasons: (1) the modest dietary supply is not readily absorbed, and (2) the body holds to its iron, and it is excreted not through the urine but rather through a number of avenues of potential loss. Iron deficiency then results in a hypochromic microcytic anemia. This deficiency may result from several causes[26]:

1. *Nutritional anemia* is an inadequate dietary supply of iron and other nutrients needed for hemoglobin and red blood cell production. Hemoglobin's role in providing oxygen to the cells is important in understanding the symptoms of anemia.
2. *Hemorrhagic anemia* occurs when there is excessive blood iron loss.
3. *Postgastrectomy anemia* occurs because of the lack of gastric hydrochloric acid necessary to liberate iron for absorption.
4. *Malabsorption anemia* occurs in the presence of iron-binding agents that prevent absorption of iron or mucosal lesions that affect the absorbing surface.

5. *Chronic disease anemia* is caused by abnormalities in the recycling of iron from hemoglobin of old blood cells that frequently accompany infections, inflammatory disorders, or connective tissue diseases such as arthritis. Anemia of chronic disease also occurs in renal disease.

The world problem of iron-deficiency anemia

Nutritional anemias, of which iron-deficiency is the greatest, constitute the second most prevalent nutritional deficiency in the world, second only to protein-energy malnutrition. More than 2 billion persons around the world are anemic or iron deficient, with women and children most likely to be affected.[27] Iron-deficiency anemia respects neither social class nor geographic situation; general iron balance in many places is often precarious. Vulnerable life cycle periods include infancy and early childhood, adolescence, the reproductive years of women from menses to menopause, pregnancy, and older adulthood.[28-31]

IRON REQUIREMENT

Iron stores vary widely, from about 300 mg in women to 1000 mg in men. Iron losses in healthy men average about 1 mg/day; in women the loss is about 1.5 mg/day. The addition for women is based on usual menstrual losses averaged over the month. Considering the iron balance studies, usual United States surveys of intake from the general food supply, and the need to maintain adequate iron reserves, the current RDAs are set at 15 mg/day for women and 10 mg/day for men. Studies have shown a relation between excess iron and heart disease, especially in men. Also, acute iron deficiency has occurred in obese persons on a very low-kcalorie diet.[32,33] In general, the needs of postmenopausal women are about the same as the standard for men. During pregnancy, the total allowance increases to 30 mg/day, but no addition is necessary during lactation because the menses is usually absent during this period. The growth needs of children are indicated in the RDA table inside the book covers.

IRON TOXICITY

Iron toxicity has not been observed in the general population from dietary sources, except for ingestion of food cooked in iron vessels and in stainless steel cookware.[34] However, there are some 2000 cases of iron poisoning every year in the United States, second only to aspirin poisoning, that occur among small children who pick up and eat the bright-colored adult-dose iron tablets carelessly left within their reach. At all times, caution concerning iron supplements is vital. The only other cause of iron overload is the genetic disease hemochromatosis, which afflicts about 1.5 million persons in the United

States. Researchers have just recently identified the gene that causes this disease.[35] Although iron is absolutely necessary, caution should be used because it can be toxic as well.

FOOD SOURCES OF IRON

The typical Western diet provides an average of 6 mg of heme and nonheme iron per 1000 kcalories of energy intake.[25] Heme iron is an important dietary source of iron because it is more effectively absorbed than nonheme iron. From 5% to 35% of heme iron is absorbed from a single meal; nonheme absorption from a single meal ranges from 2% to 20%. Thus although heme iron makes

up about 10% of the total dietary iron, it may provide up to one third of the total absorbed iron.[25] Nonheme iron, which makes up about 90% of the remaining dietary iron, accounts for 60% of the iron from animal sources and 100% of the iron found in plant sources.

Iron is widespread among foods in the United States food supply, especially in meats (particularly in organ meats such as liver), eggs, vegetables, and cereals (fortified cereal products). Fortification of grain products such as flour, breads, and cereals has at times been controversial among some nutritionists and policy makers. Nonetheless, it has helped to reduce our incidence of childhood iron-deficiency anemia. Table 8.10 gives some comparative food sources of iron.

Table
8.10 Food sources of iron (RDAs for adult women, 15 mg; for adult men, 10 mg)

	Quantity	Iron (mg)		Quantity	Iron (mg)
Bread, cereal, rice, pasta			**Meat, poultry, fish, dry beans, eggs, nuts—cont'd**		
Bran flakes	3/4 cup	4.50	Chick-peas (boiled)	1 cup	4.74
Bran muffin, homemade	1 muffin	1.26	Clams (steamed)	3 oz (9 small)	23.76
Bread, whole wheat	1 slice	0.86	Crab, blue (steamed)	3 oz	0.77
Cream of wheat, regular (cooked)	3/4 cup	7.70	Egg, whole	1 large	1.04
Oatmeal (cooked)	3/4 cup	1.19	Ground beef, regular (broiled)	3.5 oz	2.44
Pasta, enriched (cooked)	1 cup	2.40	Halibut (baked)	3 oz	0.91
Rice, white, enriched (cooked)	1 cup	1.80	Ham, canned (lean)	3.5 oz	0.94
Wheat flakes	1 cup	4.45	Lentils (boiled)	1 cup	6.59
			Lima beans (boiled)	1 cup	4.50
Vegetables			Mackerel (baked)	3 oz	1.33
Artichoke (boiled)	1 med	1.62	Oysters (steamed)	3 oz (12 med)	11.39
Avocado (raw)	1 med	2.04	Pinto beans (boiled)	1 cup	4.47
Broccoli (boiled)	1/2 cup	0.89	Shrimp (steamed)	3 oz (15 large)	2.62
Brussels sprouts (boiled)	1/2 cup	0.94	Sirloin steak, lean (broiled)	3.5 oz	3.36
Peas, green (boiled)	1/2 cup	1.24	Sole (baked)	3.5 oz	1.40
Potato (baked, with skin)	1 med	2.75	Soybeans (boiled)	1 cup	8.84
Spinach (boiled)	1/2 cup	3.21	Trout, rainbow (baked)	3 oz	2.07
			Tuna, light, canned in water	3 oz	2.07
Fruits					
Dates (dried)	10 dates	0.96	**Milk, dairy products**		
Figs (dried)	10 figs	4.18	Cheddar cheese	1 oz	0.19
Prune juice (canned)	8 fl oz	3.03	Cottage cheese, creamed	1 cup	0.29
Prunes (dried)	10 prunes	2.08	Milk, skim	8 fl oz	0.10
Raisins, seedless	2/3 cup	2.08	Milk, whole	8 fl oz	0.12
			Yogurt, whole	8 fl oz	0.11
Meat, poultry, fish, dry beans, eggs, nuts					
Almonds (roasted)	1 oz (22 nuts)	1.08	**Fats, oils, sugar**		
Beef liver (fried)	3.5 oz	6.28	This food group is not an important source of iron.		
Beef top round, lean (broiled)	3.5 oz	2.88			
Black-eyed peas (boiled)	1 cup	4.29	**Sugar**		
Cashews (roasted)	1 oz	1.70	Molasses, black	1 tbsp	3.20
Chicken, dark (roasted, without skin)	3.5 oz	1.33	Sugar, brown	1 cup	4.90
Chicken, light (roasted, without skin)	3.5 oz	1.06			

IODINE

Iodine shares with iron a longer history of study than that of other trace minerals. Its function and requirement are clearly defined. The basic function of iodine is to participate in the synthesis of the hormone *thyroxine* by the thyroid gland.

The body of the average adult contains a small amount of the trace element iodine, from 20 to 50 mg. Approximately 50% of this is in the muscles, 20% in the thyroid glands, 10% in the skin, and 6% in the skeleton. The remaining 14% is scattered in other endocrine tissue, in the central nervous system, and in plasma transport. By far, the greatest iodine tissue concentration is in the thyroid glands, where its one function is to participate in the synthesis of the thyroid hormone thyroxine.[36]

ABSORPTION-EXCRETION BALANCE

Absorption

Dietary iodine is absorbed in the small intestine in the form of iodides. These are loosely bound with proteins and carried by the blood to the thyroid gland. About one third of this iodide is selectively absorbed by the thyroid cells and removed from circulation.

Excretion

The remaining two thirds of the iodide is usually excreted in the urine within 2 to 3 days after ingestion.

Hormonal control

A pituitary hormone, thyroid-stimulating hormone (THS), stimulates the uptake of iodine by the thyroid cells in direct feedback response to the plasma levels of the hormone. This normal physiologic feedback mechanism maintains a healthy circular balance between supply and demand. This is a characteristic pattern for governing all the hormones from the several endocrine glands that are controlled by the pituitary master gland.

PHYSIOLOGIC FUNCTION OF IODINE

Thyroid hormone synthesis

The only known function of iodine in human metabolism is its participation in the synthesis of the thyroid hormone thyroxine. The hormone thyroxine in turn stimulates cell oxidation and regulates basal metabolic rate (BMR), apparently by increasing oxygen uptake and reaction rates of enzyme systems handling glucose. In this role iodine indirectly exerts a tremendous influence on the body's total metabolism.

Plasma thyroxine

The free thyroxine, with its associated iodine, is secreted into the bloodstream and bound to plasma protein for transport to body cells as needed. After being used to stimulate oxidation in the cell, the hormone is degraded in the liver and the iodine is excreted in bile as inorganic iodine.

CLINICAL NEEDS

Abnormal thyroid function

Both hyperthyroidism and hypothyroidism affect the rate of iodine uptake and use and subsequently influence the body's overall metabolic rate.

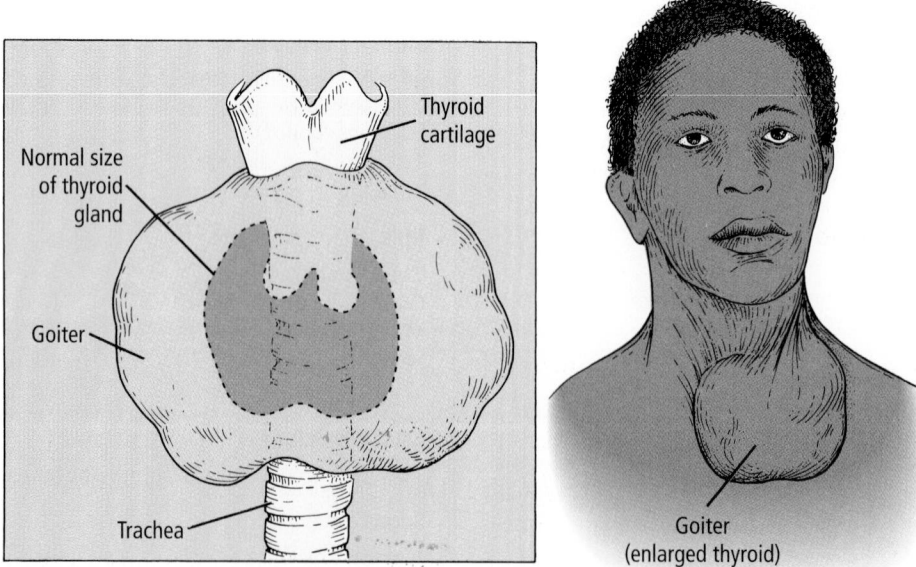

Figure 8.4   Goiter. The extreme enlargement shown here is a result of extended duration of iodine deficiency.

Goiter

Endemic colloid **goiter**, characterized by great enlargement of the thyroid gland, occurs in persons living where water and soil and thus locally grown foods contain little iodine. Some 800 million people live in iodine-deficient areas in underdeveloped countries of the world where endemic goiter is a large health problem. In such situations the iodine-starved thyroid gland cannot produce a normal quantity of thyroxine. As a result, the blood level of the thyroid hormone is too low to shut off TSH secretion by the pituitary gland. The pituitary gland continues putting out TSH, and these large quantities of TSH continue to stimulate the thyroid gland, calling on it to produce the thyroxine that it cannot supply. In this iodine-deficient state, the only response that the thyroid makes is to increase the amount of thyroglobulin (colloid), which then accumulates in the thyroid follicles. Such a gland becomes increasingly engorged and may attain a tremendous size, weighing 500 to 700 g (1 to 1½ lb) or more (Figure 8.4). Some areas of the world have severe iodine deficiency, with related disease and mortality rates. For example, in a western desert area of China, a place of severe iodine deficiency, replacement through iodination of the irrigation water has successfully reduced the high infant mortality rates.[37] Also, in the west Africa goiter belt, iodized rapeseed oil has eradicated severe endemic goiter.[38]

Iodine overload

An excessive incidental dietary intake of iodine may occur occasionally through methods used in dairy farming. These dairy farm sources include iodized salt licks for the animals and the use of iodophors, iodine-containing chemicals used to sanitize udders, milking machines, and milk tanks. Other iodine-containing compounds are the iodates used as dough conditioners in breads, erythrosin used as food colorings, and derivatives of iodine supplements added to animal feeds. Various case reports of iodine toxicity and population studies have indicated that levels of iodine through foods, dietary supplements, or topical medications may exceed by many times the recommended dietary allowances.

IODINE REQUIREMENT

Tests for urinary iodide excretion are used to indicate iodine intake and status, as well as the risk for goiter and a wide spectrum of other iodine deficiency disorders. These disorders can range from severe **cretinism** with mental retardation to barely visible enlargement of the thyroid gland. Balance studies indicate that an adult needs a minimum of 50 to 75 µg/day of iodine to maintain desirable tissue levels as measured by urinary excretion rates. Based on these findings, the current RDA standard sets an allowance for all adults of 150 µg/day to provide an extra margin of safety. An added 25 µg/day is recommended during pregnancy to cover fetal requirements. The extra need during lactation is 50 µg/day to meet infant growth needs. The demand is increased during periods of accelerated adolescent growth. Thus the allowance for older children ages 11 years and above is set at 150 µg/day, the same as that for adult maintenance.

FOOD SOURCES OF IODINE

Seafood provides a considerable amount of iodine. The quantity in natural sources varies widely depending on the iodine content of the soil and the iodine compounds used in food processing. The commercial iodizing of table salt (1 mg to every 10 g of salt) provides a main dietary source. Some iodine deficiencies have been observed in persons who avoid salt.

OTHER ESSENTIAL TRACE ELEMENTS

ZINC

Zinc has come to nutritional prominence as an essential trace element with wide clinical significance. Its wide tissue distribution reflects its broad metabolic activity as a component of key cell enzymes. An adult's total zinc content ranges from about 2.3 mmol (1.5 g) in women to 3.8 mmol (2.5 g) in men.[39] It is present in minute quantities in all body organs, tissues, fluids, and secretions. Although it is vital throughout life, it is especially important through growth periods such as pregnancy and lactation, infancy and childhood, and adolescence.[40-42] It has vital maturation functions at each stage.

Clinical problems

Because of its widespread metabolic use, a number of clinical problems caused by zinc deficiency (see *Practical Application* box, p. 172) can occur:

1. *Hypogonadism.* Diminished function of the gonads and dwarfism can result from pronounced human zinc deficiency during critical growth periods.

---

cretinism A congenital disease resulting from absence or deficiency of normal thyroid secretion, characterized by physical deformity, dwarfism, mental retardation, and often goiters.

goiter Enlargement of the thyroid gland caused by lack of sufficient available iodine to produce the thyroid hormone thyroxine.

Zinc barriers

Are people eating more zinc but absorbing it less? Current trends toward a "heart-healthy" diet may be the reason why. Some Americans may be at risk for developing a zinc deficiency, not because they are avoiding zinc-rich foods, but because they are choosing foods and supplements that reduce its availability for absorption. For example:

- Animal foods, rich in readily available zinc, are consumed less by an increasingly cholesterol-conscious public.
- Dietary fiber, being promoted by some persons as a cardiovascular panacea, may hinder absorption and create a negative zinc balance.
- Phytates and oxalates, components of fiber-rich foods, may also hinder absorption and present other zinc antagonists.
- Food processing may make zinc less available.
- Vitamin-mineral supplements may contain iron/zinc ratios greater than 3:1 and provide enough iron to inhibit zinc absorption.

Other factors that reduce zinc availability include such unusual cravings as pica, the eating of non-food material such as clay, practiced primarily by children and pregnant women. Also, such clinical conditions as cystic fibrosis, alcohol cirrhosis, celiac disease, and diarrhea limit zinc absorption.

The risk for deficiency is greatest among pregnant and breast-feeding women. Low levels of zinc can reduce the amount of protein available to carry iron and vitamin A to the target tissues and reduce the mother's appetite and taste for foods. As a result, the fetus is at even greater risk for inadequate growth and development.

All these conditions, plus milling processes that remove excessive amounts of zinc from grains, have resulted in an average per capita intake of 12.5 mg/day. This is less than the 15 mg/day recommended for most persons and far less than the 20 and 25 mg/day recommended for pregnancy and lactation, respectively.

To put more zinc in individual diets:

- Include some form of animal food—meat, milk, and eggs—in the diet every day to ensure a minimal intake of zinc.
- Avoid extensive use of alcohol.
- Avoid "crash" diets.

Signs of zinc deficiency are still fairly rare in the United States, so there is no need for persons to overprotect themselves with massive doses. These large doses may compete with other elements such as iron and create still other deficiency problems. Excess zinc can lead to nausea, abdominal pain, and anemia. As with all other nutrients, too much of a good thing can sometimes be as bad as too little—or even worse.

References

King JC, Keen L: Zinc. In Shils ME, Olson JA, Shike M, eds: *Modern nutrition in health and disease,* ed 8, vol 1, Philadelphia, 1994, Lea & Febiger.

Marsh MN, Riley SA: Digestion and absorption of nutrients and vitamins. In Feldman M, Scharschmidt BF, Sleisenger MH, eds: *Gastrointestinal and liver disease,* ed 6, vol 2, Philadelphia, 1998, Saunders

2. *Taste and smell defects.* Hypogeusia (diminished taste) and hyposmia (diminished smell) in a number of clinical situations are improved with zinc supplementation.
3. *Wound healing.* The healing of wounds, or any other tissue injury from physiologic stress, inflammation, or hormonal changes, is retarded in zinc-deficient persons. This defect seems to be common in most hospitals, and patients benefit from zinc supplementation. Frequently, hospital diets, especially when combined with poor consumption by ill persons, provide limited amounts of dietary zinc.
4. *Growth and development and life cycle needs.* Special needs during growth periods include pregnancy and lactation, infants and children, rapid adolescent growth, and sexual function. Also, older persons with poor appetites who subsist on marginal diets or who have unhealed wounds or debilitating illness are particularly vulnerable to zinc deficiency. As a result of such deficiency, they often suffer from reduced immune function.

5. *Malabsorption disease.* Zinc deficiency can occur with malabsorption diseases such as Crohn's disease. The ulcerative lesions in the mucosal surface hinder the absorption of zinc, and zinc intake is low as a result of anorexia or selection of foods low in zinc.

Zinc requirement and food sources

As with the trace element iron, an optimal intake of zinc in the United States population cannot be assumed. The current adult RDAs are set at 15 mg for men and 12 mg for women (the requirement for women is lower because of their lower weight). The RDA table (see inside book cover) gives remaining allowances based on age and sex. The best sources of dietary zinc are seafood (especially oysters), meat, and eggs. Additional less rich sources are legumes and whole grains. Since animal food sources supply the major portion of dietary zinc, pure vegetarians (especially women) may be at risk for development of marginal zinc deficiency. Table 8.11 gives some comparative food sources of zinc. Although zinc deficiency should be avoided, excess zinc interferes with the absorption of copper, the next trace element we will discuss.

COPPER

This trace element has frequently been called the "iron twin." The two elements are metabolized in much the same way and share functions as cell enzyme components. Both are related to energy production and hemoglobin synthesis. Copper is widely distributed in natural foods, so a general dietary deficiency is rare.[43] It has only been observed during unsupplemented total parenteral nutrition (TPN) feeding, high levels of zinc intake, or general malnutrition. The RDAs estimate a safe and adequate range of dietary copper intake for adults at 1.5 to 3 mg/day, which regular United States diets supply. Copper is widely distributed in natural foods. Its richest sources are organ meats (especially liver), seafoods (especially oysters), nuts, and seeds, and in smaller amounts in whole grains and legumes.

MANGANESE

The total adult body content of manganese is about 20 mg, occurring mainly in the liver, bones, pancreas, and pituitary. Although it is considered a dietary essential, it is toxic at high levels.[44] It functions like other trace elements as an essential part of cell enzymes that catalyze a number of important metabolic reactions. Manganese deficiency, evidenced by low serum levels, has been reported in diabetes and pancreatic insufficiency, as well as in protein-energy malnutrition states such as kwashiorkor. Toxicity occurs as an industrial disease syndrome, inhalation toxicity, in miners and other workers who have prolonged exposure to manganese dust. In such

cases, excess manganese accumulates in the liver and central nervous system, producing severe neuromuscular symptoms that resemble those of Parkinson's disease. The RDA estimates a safe and adequate dietary intake of manganese at 2 to 5 mg/day, which regular United States diets easily supply. The best food sources of manganese are plant foods—cereal grains, legumes, seeds, nuts, leafy vegetables, tea, and coffee. Animal foods are relatively poor sources.

CHROMIUM

The precise amount of chromium present in body tissues is not well defined because of difficulties in analysis. Although large geographic variations occur, the total body content is small, less than 6 mg. The highest concentrations have been found in skin, adrenal glands, brain, muscle, and fat. Serum levels are usually less than 10 mg/ml. Chromium functions as an essential component of the organic complex **glucose tolerance factor (GTF)**, which facilitates the action of insulin.[45] The amount of chromium needed by the body is controversial.[46] Thus the RDA standard estimates a wide safe and adequate intake of chromium for adults at a range of 50 to 200 μg/day. Studies indicate that a chromium intake of less than 20 μg/day is generally inadequate.[46] Brewer's yeast is a rich source. Good food sources include liver, cheddar cheese, and wheat germ. Most grain products, especially whole grains, provide additional sources.

COBALT

Cobalt occurs in only minute trac...

Table	
8.11	Food sources of zinc (RDAs for adults: women, 12 mg; men, 15 mg)

	Quantity	Zinc (mg)		Quantity	Zinc (mg)
Bread, cereal, rice, pasta			**Meat, poultry, fish, dry beans, eggs, nuts**		
Bran muffin, homemade	1 muffin	1.08	Almonds (roasted)	1 oz (22 nuts)	1.39
Bread, whole wheat	1 slice	0.42	Beef liver (fried)	3.5 oz	6.07
Cream of wheat (cooked)	¾ cup	0.24	Cashews (roasted)	1 oz	1.59
English muffin, plain	1 muffin	0.41	Chicken, dark (roasted, without skin)	3.5 oz	2.80
Oatmeal (cooked)	¾ cup	0.86	Chicken, light (roasted without skin)	3.5 oz	1.23
Pasta, enriched (cooked)	1 cup	0.70	Chick-peas (boiled)	1 cup	2.51
Wheat flakes	1 cup	0.63	Clams, canned	3 oz	2.32
Vegetables			Crab, Alaska king (steamed)	3 oz	6.48
Artichoke (boiled)	1 med	0.43	Egg, whole	1 large	0.72
Asparagus (boiled)	½ cup (6 spears)	0.43	Ham, canned (lean)	3.5 oz	1.93
Avocado (raw)	1 med	0.73	Kidney beans (boiled)	1 cup	1.89
Broccoli (raw)	½ cup	0.18	Lentils (boiled)	1 cup	2.50
Brussels sprouts (boiled)	½ cup (4 sprouts)	0.25	Lima beans (boiled)	1 cup	1.79
Carrots (raw)	1 med	0.14	Lobster (steamed)	3 oz	2.48
Collards (boiled)	½ cup	0.23	Oysters (steamed)	3 oz (12 med)	154.62
Kale (boiled chopped)	½ cup	0.15	Peanuts (roasted)	1 oz	0.93
Peas, green (boiled)	½ cup	0.95	Soybeans (boiled)	1 cup	1.98
Potato (baked, with skin)	1 med	0.65	**Milk, dairy products**		
Tomato (raw)	1 med	0.13	Milk, skim	8 fl oz	0.98
Fruits			Milk, whole	8 fl oz	0.93
Apricots (raw)	3 med	0.28	Yogurt, whole	8 fl oz	1.34
Banana (raw)	1 med	0.19	**Fats, oils, sugar**		
Cantaloupe (raw)	½ cup	0.25	This food group is not an important source of iron.		
Figs (dried)	10 figs	0.94			
Orange juice (fresh)	8 fl oz	0.13			
Orange, navel (raw)	1 med	0.08			

...NIUM

...m is deposited in all body tissues except fat. High-
...entrations occur in the liver, kidney, heart, and
...rum levels are about 0.22 μg/dl. Selenium func-
...integral component of an antioxidant enzyme
...cells and lipid membranes against oxidative
...is role, selenium balances with tocopherol
...h sparing the other. This protective func-
...d, since the enzyme is found in most
...dies have found that selenium com-
...east milk are more biologically avail-
...tion than those in formulas.[47] Sele-
...ructural component, incorporated
...of the teeth. The RDA standard
...uate adult intake of selenium at
...ood sources vary with the sele-
...good sources include seafood,
...t meats, and dairy products,
...g in vegetables.

MOLYBDENUM

Molybdenum functions as an enzyme cofactor in numerous metabolic activities to catalyze the hydroxylation of various substrates.[48] The precise occurrence of molybdenum in human tissues and its clear coenzyme roles are under continuing investigation. The body tissue amount of molybdenum is exceedingly small, 0.1 to 1 μg/g of wet tissue. The largest amounts are deposited in the liver, kidney, adrenal glands, and bone, with lesser but significant quantities in the lungs, spleen, and muscle. The RDA standard estimates a safe and adequate allowance for adults and older children of 75 to 250 μg/day. The ranges for other age groups are derived on the basis of weight. The amounts of molybdenum in foods vary considerably, depending on the environment in which the food is grown. In general, however, the richest sources include legumes, whole grains, milk, leafy vegetables, and organ meats. The poorer sources include fruits, stem and root vegetables, and muscle meats.

FLUORIDE

The trace element fluoride accumulates in all body tissues showing calcification, mostly in bones and teeth. In human nutrition, fluoride functions mainly to inhibit *dental caries*. The principal cause of caries is acid dissolution of tooth enamel. This acid is produced by microorganisms feeding on fermentable carbohydrates adhering to the teeth after a meal or snack. Fluoride therapy enhances the ability of the tooth structure to withstand the erosive effect of the bacterial acid. Establishment of a fluoride requirement is difficult because it appears to be retained in the bones regardless of the intake level. The RDA adult standard estimates a need in the range of 1.5 to 4 mg/day. Fish, fish products, and tea contain the highest concentration of fluoride. Cooking in fluoridated water raises the level in many foods. The public health measure of fluoridation of public water supply to 1 ppm provides adequate amounts, and has largely been responsible for the remarkable decline in dental caries.

PROBABLY ESSENTIAL TRACE ELEMENTS

The remaining trace elements that have been found in human tissue have less well-defined metabolic functions. However, they have been found to be essential in animal nutrition and are probably essential in human nutrition in a similar manner, both as cofactors for cell enzymes in key metabolic reactions and as structural components in special tissues, for example, the role of boron with calcium in bone-building.[48,49] These eight trace elements are silicon (Si), vanadium (V), nickel (Ni), tin (Sn), cadmium (Cd), arsenic (As), aluminum (Al), and boron (B). Apparently, most of these trace elements are needed in such minute amounts that primary dietary deficiency is highly unlikely. However, with increased use of long-term total parenteral nutrition (TPN) therapy, induced deficiencies may be of increasing clinical concern.

WATER-ELECTROLYTE BALANCE

A number of the major minerals described above have basic functions as electrolytes in controlling the body's vital water balance. This collective function is fundamental to health and often a vital part of patient care. In brief summary here, we will look at the three basic interdependent factors that control this balance: (1) the water itself (the solvent base for solutions), (2) the various particles (solutes) in solution in the water, and (3) the separating membranes that control the flow.

WATER BALANCE

Body water distribution

If you are a woman, your body is about 50% to 55% water. If you are a man, your body is about 55% to 60% water. The higher water content in most men is a result of their greater muscle mass. Striated muscle contains more water than any body tissue other than blood. The remaining 40% of a man's weight is about 18% protein and related substances, 15% fat, and 7% minerals. A woman's remaining body composition is about the same except for a somewhat smaller muscle mass and a larger fat deposit.

Water functions

Body water performs three essential functions: (1) helps give structure and form to the body through the turgor it provides for tissues, (2) creates the water-based environment necessary for the vast array of chemical actions and reactions that comprise the body's metabolism and sustain life, and (3) provides the means for maintaining a stable body temperature.

Water compartments

Consider the water in your body in two compartments, as shown in Figure 8.5: (1) the total water outside of cells— the extracellular fluid compartment (ECF), and (2) the total water inside of cells—the intracellular fluid compartment (ICF).

1. *Extracellular fluid (ECF).* Water outside of cells makes up about 20% of the total body weight. It consists of four parts: (1) blood plasma, which accounts for about 25% of the ECF and 5% of body weight; (2) **interstitial fluid**, the water surrounding the cells; (3) secretory fluid, the water circulating in transit; and (4) dense tissue fluid, water in dense connective tissue, cartilage, bone.
2. *Intracellular fluid (ICF).* Water inside cells makes up about 40% to 45% of the total body weight. Since the body cells handle our vast metabolic activity, it is no surprise that the total water inside cells is about twice the amount outside.

OVERALL WATER BALANCE: INTAKE AND OUTPUT

The average adult metabolizes from 2.5 to 3 L of water per day in a constant turnover balanced between intake and output. This water enters and leaves the body by var-

---

interstitial fluid The fluid situated between parts or in the interspaces of a tissue.

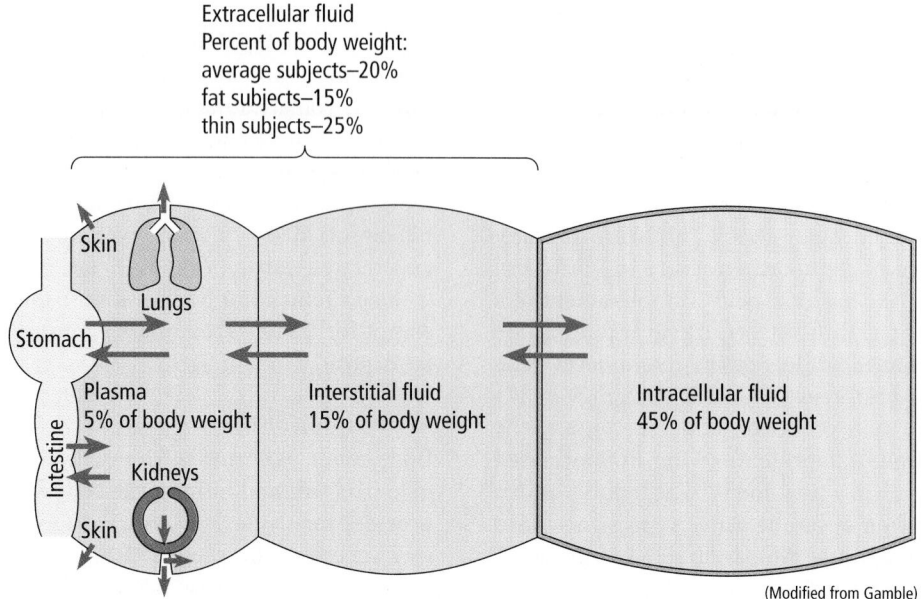

Figure 8.5　Body fluid compartments. Note the relative total quantities of water in the intracellular compartment and in the extracellular compartment. (Modified from Gamble JL: Chemical anatomy, physiology, and pathology of extracellular fluid, Cambridge, MA, 1964, Harvard University Press.)

ious routes, controlled by basic mechanisms such as thirst and hormonal activity.

Water enters the body in three main forms: (1) preformed water as water and in other beverages that are consumed, (2) preformed water in foods that are eaten, and (3) metabolic water, a product of cell oxidation.

Water leaves the body through the kidneys, skin, lungs, and fecal elimination through the large intestine.

These routes of intake and output must be in constant balance. This balance is summarized in Table 8.12. Abnormal conditions, such as diarrhea or dysentery, produce much greater losses, causing serious clinical problems if prolonged. Extensive loss of body fluids can be especially dangerous in infants and children. Their bodies contain a greater percentage of the total body water, and much more of the water is outside of cells and easily available for loss.

FORCES CONTROLLING WATER DISTRIBUTION

Forces that influence and control the distribution of body water revolve around two factors: (1) the **solutes**, particles in solution in body water, and (2) the separating membranes between water compartments.

Solutes

A variety of particles with varying concentrations occur in the body. Two main types, electrolytes and plasma protein, control water balance.

Electrolytes. Several minerals provide major electrolytes for the body. In this role, these small inorganic elements

Table 8.12	Approximate daily adult intake and output of water			
			Output (loss)	
	Intake (replacement) ml/day		**Obligatory (insensible) ml/day**	**Additional (according to need) ml/day**
Preformed		Lungs	350	
Liquids	1200-1500	Skin		
In foods	700-1000	Diffusion	350	
Metabolism	200-300	Sweat	100	± 250
(oxidation		Kidneys	900	± 500
of food)				
		Feces	150	
TOTAL	2100-2800	TOTAL	1850	750
	(approx. 2600 ml/day)		(approx. 2600 ml/day)	

are called **electrolytes** because they are free in solution and carry an electrical charge. These free, charged forms are called ions, that is, atoms, elements, or groups of atoms that, in solution, carry either a positive or negative electrical charge. An ion carrying a positive charge is called a cation; examples are sodium (Na^+)—major cation of water outside cells, potassium (K^+)—major cation of water inside cells, calcium (Ca^{++}), and magnesium (Mg^{++}). Conversely, an ion carrying a negative charge is called an anion; examples are chloride (Cl^-), carbonate (HCO_3^-), phosphate (HPO_4^{--}), and sulfate (SO_4^{--}). Because of their small size, these ions or electrolytes can diffuse freely across body membranes. Thus they produce a major force controlling movement of water within the body.

Plasma proteins. Organic substances of large molecular size, mainly albumin and globulin of the plasma proteins, influence the shift of water in and out of capillaries in balance with their surrounding water. In this function, these plasma proteins are called colloids (from the Greek word *kolla*, glue) and form colloidal solutions. Because of their large size, these particles or molecules do not pass readily through separating capillary membranes. Therefore they normally remain in the blood vessels where they exert **colloidal osmotic pressure (COP)** to maintain the vascular blood volume.

Organic compounds of small molecular size. Other organic compounds of small size, such as glucose, urea, and amino acids, diffuse freely but do not influence shifts of water unless they occur in abnormally large concentrations. For example, the large amount of glucose in the urine of a patient with uncontrolled diabetes mellitus causes an abnormal osmotic diuresis or excess water output.

Water and solutes move across the body's separating membranes by the basic physiologic mechanisms that operate fluid balances according to body need. These mechanisms include osmosis, diffusion, filtration, active transport, and pinocytosis.

INFLUENCE OF ELECTROLYTES ON WATER BALANCE

Measurement of electrolytes
The concentration of electrolytes in a given solution determines the chemical activity of that solution. It is the number of particles in a solution that is the important factor in determining chemical combining power. Thus electrolytes are measured according to the total number of particles in solution, each one of which contributes chemical combining power according to its valence, rather than the total weight. The unit of measure commonly used is an equivalent. Since small amounts are usually in question, most physiologic measurements are expressed in terms of *milliequivalents (mEq)*. The term refers to the number of ions—cations and anions—in solution, as determined by their concentration in a given volume. This measure is expressed as the number of milliequivalents per liter *(mEq/L)*.

Electrolyte balance
Electrolytes are distributed in the body water compartments in a definite pattern, which has physiologic significance. This distribution pattern maintains stable electrochemical neutrality in body fluid solutions.

According to biochemical and electrochemical laws, a stable solution must have equal numbers of positive and negative particles. It must be electrically neutral. When shifts and losses occur, compensating shifts and gains follow to maintain this dynamic balance, essential electroneutrality.

Electrolyte control of body hydration
As stated earlier, ionized sodium is the chief cation of ECF, and ionized potassium is the chief cation of ICF. These two electrolytes control the amount of water retained in any given compartment. The usual bases for these shifts in water from one compartment to the other are ECF changes in concentration of these electrolytes. The terms *hypertonic* and *hypotonic* dehydration refer to the electrolyte concentration of the water outside the cell, which in turn causes a shift of water into or out of the cell to maintain balance.

INFLUENCE OF PLASMA PROTEIN ON WATER BALANCE

Capillary fluid shift mechanism
Water is constantly circulated throughout the body by the blood vessels. However, it must get out of the vessels to service the tissues and then be drawn back into circulation to maintain the normal transporting flow. Two main opposing pressures—colloidal osmotic pressure (COP) from plasma protein (mainly albumin) and hydrostatic pressure (blood pressure) of the capillary blood flow—provide balanced control of water and solute movement across capillary membranes. The body maintains this constant flow of water and the materials it is carrying to and from the cell by means of a shifting balance of these two pressures. It is a filtration process oper-

colloidal osmotic pressure (COP) Pressure produced by the protein molecules in the plasma and in the cell. Because proteins are large molecules, they do not pass through the separating membranes of the capillary cells. Thus they remain in their respective compartments, exerting a constant osmotic pull that protects vital plasma and cell fluid volumes in these compartments.

electrolytes A chemical element or compound, which in solution dissociates as ions carrying a positive or negative charge (for example, H^+, Na^+, K^+, Ca^{++}, Mg^{++}, and Cl^-, HCO_3^-, $HPO_4^=$, $SO_4^=$). Electrolytes constitute a major force controlling fluid balances within the body through their concentrations and shifts from one place to another to restore and maintain balance—*homeostasis*.

solutes Particles of a substance in solution; a solution consists of a substance and a dissolving medium (solvent), usually a liquid.

To Probe Further

Losing by a hair

Many Americans, at one time or another, have spent a great deal of money getting their hair analyzed. For a few strands of hair and a sizable fee they have been told they can find out if their potassium levels are low, their lead levels are high, or their sodium levels are just right. Or can they?

Hair is dead tissue. It starts out as living cells, full of vitamins and minerals found in the rest of the body. The dead cells are "glued" together with a sulfur-rich protein called *keratin,* and they continue to "grow" as a single strand of hair. Vitamins disappear when the cells die and are not found in hair, but the minerals linger on. Yet even with the detection of minerals there are problems:

- Some minerals are lost when hair cells die. The keratin is so rich in sulfur that it masks the presence of some minerals and attracts others in levels that exceed those found in the body.
- Hair can be "contaminated" by shampoos, hard or soft water, dyes, or even air pollution, thereby skewing laboratory calculations.
- Science doesn't know what the relationship is between hair levels and blood levels for certain nutrients.
- Some persons don't even know how to wash hair samples before testing, so large amounts of contaminants get "analyzed" too.
- There are no standard laboratory values for minerals found in hair. Laboratories can simply state that levels are higher, lower, or the same as those seen previously.

But hair analysis is not totally worthless. Coroners use it all the time to find out if a person has died from arsenic, lead, or other poisons. Public health workers use it to compare mineral levels in populations in different parts of the country if they suspect that soil depletion, water contamination, or other environmental changes have affected nutrient levels in local food supplies. Also, it can help researchers and individual practitioners monitor changing nutrient levels over a period of time.

The usefulness of hair analysis in general practice, however, is overshadowed by strong condemnation from the American Medical Association and health professionals. This negative response comes not only because of its shortcomings, but also because mail-order hair analysis companies use it to diagnose conditions (that often don't exist) and "suggest" (being careful to avoid the term *prescribe*) treatments with a variety of supplements, which frequently are sold by the same companies doing the analysis, in amounts that are often potentially dangerous.

So, unless you're due for a haircut, have some money you don't need, and feel the need to purchase and use unnecessary supplements, hair analysis is probably not the most productive thing you could choose to do.

References

Barrett S, Herbert V: Fads, frauds, and quackery. In Shils ME, Olson, JA, Shike M, eds: *Nutrition in health and disease,* ed 8, vol 1, Philadelphia, 1994, Lea & Febiger.

---

ating according to the differences in osmotic pressure on either side of the capillary membrane.

When blood first enters the capillary system, the greater blood pressure forces water and small solutes (glucose, for example) out into the tissues to bathe and nourish the cells. The plasma protein particles, however, are too large to go through the pores of capillary membranes. Hence the protein remains in the vessel and exerts the now greater colloidal osmotic pressure that draws the returning fluid and its materials back into circulation from the cells. This process is called the **capillary fluid shift mechanism.** It provides one of the most important and widespread homeostatic mechanisms in the body to maintain water balance, without which cells would die.

Cell fluid control

Much as plasma protein provides colloidal osmotic pressure to maintain the volume of extracellular fluid, cell protein helps to provide the osmotic pressure that maintains the volume of fluid inside the cell. Also, ionized potassium within the cell guards cell water in balance with ionized sodium guarding water outside the cell. This balance supports the flow of water, nutrients, and metabolites in and out of cells to sustain life.

INFLUENCE OF HORMONES ON WATER BALANCE

Antidiuretic hormone mechanism

The antidiuretic hormone (ADH), also called *vasopressin*, is secreted by the posterior lobe of the pituitary gland. It causes reabsorption of water by the kidney according to body need. Thus it is a water-conserving mechanism. In any stress situation with threatened or real loss of body water, this hormone is triggered to hold on to precious body water.

Aldosterone mechanism

Aldosterone is primarily a sodium-conserving hormone, related in its operation to the renin-angiotensin system, but in doing this job it also exerts a secondary control over water loss. This mechanism's full name is the **renin-angiotensin-aldosterone mechanism** because renin, an enzyme from the kidney, and angiotensin, the active product of its substrate (angiotensinogen) from the liver, are the intermediate substances used to trigger the adrenal glands to produce the aldosterone hormone. Both aldosterone and ADH are activated by stress situations such as injury or surgery.

TO SUM UP

Minerals are inorganic substances that are widely distributed in nature. They build body tissues; activate, regulate, and control metabolic processes; and transmit neurologic messages.

Minerals are classified as (1) major minerals, required in relatively large quantities, which make up 60% to 80% of all the inorganic material in the body, and (2) trace elements, required in quantities as small as a microgram (μg), which make up less than 1% of the body's inorganic material. Seven major minerals and ten trace

minerals are known to be essential in human nutrition, with another eight trace elements probably essential, and still others constantly being examined for possible essentiality.

Overall water balance in the body is controlled by fluid intake and output. The distribution of body fluids is mainly controlled by two types of solutes: (1) electrolytes, which are charged mineral elements and other particles derived from inorganic compounds, and (2) plasma protein, which is mainly albumin, consisting of particles too large to pass through capillary membranes but capable of influencing the flow of fluid from one compartment to another. These solute particles influence the distribution of fluid passing across cell or capillary membranes, separating body fluid into its two compartments.

QUESTIONS FOR REVIEW

1. List the 7 major minerals, describing physiologic function and problems created by dietary deficiency or excess.
2. List the 10 trace elements with proven essentiality for humans. Which have established RDA standards? Which have "safe and adequate intake" limits established. Why is it difficult to establish RDAs for everyone?
3. What accounts for the edema of starvation?
4. Why does potassium depletion occur in prolonged diarrhea?

REFERENCES

1. Eaton SB, Nelson DA: Calcium in evolutionary perspective, *Am J Clin Nutr* 54 (suppl):281s, 1991.
2. Kirshner RP: The earth's elements, *Sci Am* 271(4):59, 1994.
3. Prentice A: Calcium requirements of children, *Nutr Rev* 53(2):37, 1995.
4. Abrams SA et al: Calcium and magnesium balance in 9-14-yr-old children, *Am J Clin Nutr* 66:1172, 1997.
5. Jackman LA et al: Calcium retention in relation to calcium intake and postmenarchal age in adolescent females, *Am J Clin Nutr* 66:327, 1997.
6. Martin AD et al: Bone mineral and calcium accretion during puberty, *Am J Clin Nutr* 66:611, 1997.
7. Fullmer CS: Intestinal calcium absorption: calcium entry, *J Nutr* 122:644, 1992.
8. Wood RJ et al: Mineral requirements of elderly people, *Am J Clin Nutr* 62(3):493, 1995.
9. Porter DV: Washington update: NIH Consensus Development Conference state optimal calcium intake, *Nutr Today* 29(5):1994.
10. Marriot BM: Editorial—vitamin D supplement: a word of caution, *Ann Intern Med* 127(3):231, 1997.
11. Packard PT, Heaney RP: Medical nutrition therapy for patients with osteoporosis, *J Am Diet Assoc* 97(4):414, 1997.

capillary fluid shift mechanism Process that controls the movement of water and small molecules in solution (electrolytes, nutrients) between the blood in the capillary and the surrounding interstitial area. Filtration of water and solutes out of the capillary at the arteriole end and reabsorption at the venule end are accomplished by shifts in balance between the intracapillary hydrostatic blood pressure and the colloidal osmotic pressure exerted by the plasma proteins.

renin-angiotensin-aldosterone mechanism Three-stage system of sodium conservation, hence control of water loss, in response to diminished filtration pressure in the kidney nephrons: (1) pressure loss causes kidney to secrete the enzyme renin, which combines with and activates angiotensinogen from the liver; (2) active angiotensin stimulates of the adjacent adrenal gland to release the hormone aldosterone; (3) the hormone causes reabsorption of sodium from the kidney nephrons and water follows.

12. Holick M: Vitamin D and bone health, *J Nutr* 126:1159S, 1996.

13. Bromer F: Calcium and osteoporosis, *Am J Clin Nutr* 69(6):831, 1994.

14. Tepper BJ, Nayga RM: Awareness of the link between bone disease and calcium intake is associated with higher dietary calcium intake in women aged 50 years and older: results of the 1991 CSFII-DHKS, *J Am Diet Assoc* 98(2):196, 1998.

15. Food and Nutrition Board, Institute of Medicine: Dietary Reference Intakes (DRIs) for calcium, phosphorous, magnesium, vitamin D, and fluoride, *Nutr Today* 32(5):182, 1997.

16. Allen LH, Wood RJ: Calcium and phosphorous. In Shils ME, Olson JA, Shike M, eds: *Modern nutrition in health and disease,* ed 8, vol 1, Philadelphia, 1994, Lea & Febiger.

17. Anderson JJB, Barrett CJH: Dietary phosphorous: the benefits and the problems, *Nutr Today* 29(2):29, 1994.

18. Stamler J: The INTERSALT Study: background, methods, findings, and implications, *Am J Clin Nutr* 65(suppl):626S, 1997.

19. Blackburn GL: Functional foods in the prevention and treatment of disease: significance of the Dietary Approaches to Stop Hypertension Study, *Am J Clin Nutr* 66:1067, 1997.

20. Whelton PK et al: Efficacy of nonpharmacologic interventions in adults with high-normal blood pressure: results from phase 1 of the Trials of Hypertension Prevention, *Am J Clin Nutr* 65(suppl):652S, 1997.

21. Cappuccio FP et al: Double-blind randomized trial of modest salt restriction in older people, *Lancet* 350(Sept 20):850, 1997.

22. Dreosti IE: Magnesium status and health, *Nutr Rev* 53(9):S23, 1995.

23. Mertz W: The essential trace elements, *Science* 213:1332, 1981.

24. Mertz W: Risk assessment of essential trace elements: new approaches to setting recommended dietary allowances and safety limits, *Nutr Rev* 53(7):1995.

25. Beard JL, et al: Iron metabolism: a comprehensive review, *Nutr Rev* 54(10):295, 1996.

26. Fleming D: Plasma transferrin receptor helps to predict iron deficiency in the anemia of chronic disease, *Nutr Rev* 53(6):167, 1995.

27. Gallowat R, McGuire J: Daily versus weekly: How many iron pills do pregnant women need? *Nutr Rev* 54(10):318, 1996.

28. Preziosi P et al: Effect of iron supplementation on the iron status of pregnant women: consequences for newborns, *Am J Clin Nutr* 66:1178, 1997.

29. Ziegler EE, Fomon SJ: Strategies for the prevention of iron deficiency: iron in infant formulas and baby foods, *Nutr Rev* 54(11):348, 1996.

30. Sargent JD et al: Iron deficiency in Massachusetts communities: socioeconomic and demographic risk factors among children, *Am J Pub Health* 86(4):544, 1996.

31. Connor JR, Beard JL: Dietary iron supplements in the elderly: to use or not to use? *Nutr Today* 32(3):102, 1997.

32. Beguin Y et al: Acute functional iron deficiency in obese subjects during a very-low-energy all-protein diet, *Am J Clin Nutr* 66:75, 1997.

33. Beard J et al: Changes in iron status during weight loss with very-low-energy diets, *Am J Clin Nutr* 66:104, 1997.

34. Park J, Brittin HC: Increased iron content of food due to stainless steel cookware, *J Am Diet Assoc* 97(6):659, 1997.

35. Facelmann K: Rusty organs: researchers identify the gene for iron overload disease, *Sci News* 151(3):46, 1997.

36. Clugston GA, Helzel BS: Iodine. In Shils ME, Olson JA, Shike M, eds: *Modern nutrition in health and disease,* ed 8, vol 1, Philadelphia, 1994, Lea & Febiger.

37. Delong GR et al: Effect on infant mortality of iodination of irrigation water in a severely iodine-deficient area of China, *Lancet* 350(13):771, 1997.

38. Ingenbleek Y et al: Iodized rapeseed oil for eradication of severe endemic goitre, *Lancet* 350(22):1542, 1997.

39. King JC, Keen CL: Zinc. In Shils ME, Olson JA, Shike M, eds: *Modern nutrition in health and disease,* ed 8, vol 1, Philadelphia, 1994, Lea & Febiger.

40. Fung EB et al: Zinc absorption in women during pregnancy and lactation: a longitudinal study, *Am J Clin Nutr* 66:80, 1997.

41. Nishi Y: Zinc and growth, *Am J Clin Nutr* 15(4):340, 1996.

42. Prasad AS: Zinc deficiency in women, infants, and children, *J Am Coll Nutr* 15(2):113, 1996.

43. Percival SS: Neutropenia caused by copper deficiency, *Nutr Rev* 53(3):59, 1995.

44. Greger JL, Malecki EA: Manganese: How do we know our limits? *Nutr Today* 32(3):116, 1997.

45. Anderson RA: Nutrition factors influencing the glucose/insulin system: chromium, *J Am Coll Nutr* 16(5):404, 1997.

46. Nielsen FH: Controversial chromium: Does the superstar mineral of the Mountebanks receive appropriate attention from clinicians and nutritionists? *Nutr Today* 31(6):226, 1996.

47. Alaejos MS, Romero CD: Selenium in human lactation, *Nutr Rev* 53(6):159, 1995.

48. Nielsen FH: Ultratrace minerals. In Shils ME, Olson, JA, Shike M, eds: *Modern nutrition in health and disease,* ed 8, vol 1, Philadelphia, 1994, Lea & Febiger.

49. Naghii MR et al: The boron content of selected foods and the estimation of its daily intake among free-living subjects, *Am J Coll Nutr* 15(6):614, 1996.

■ FURTHER READING

Aggett PJ, Comerford JG: Zinc and human health, *Nutr Rev* 53(9):S17, 1995.

Ziegler EE, Foman SJ: Strategies for the prevention of iron deficiency: iron in infant formulas and baby foods, *Nutr Rev* 54(11):348, 1996.

These authors, experienced in research and clinical practice, provide valuable background for relating basic knowledge of zinc and iron to their fundamental roles in cellular metabolism and ways of meeting these needs.

Nishi Y: Anemia and zinc deficiency in the athlete, *J Am Coll Nutr* 15(4):323, 1996.

Nishiyama S et al: Zinc status relates to hematologic deficits in women endurance runners, *J Am Coll Nutr* 15(4):359, 1996.

These authors apply knowledge of zinc metabolism to the endurance demands of athletes in long-distance running. The usual low consumption of essential trace elements results in reduced peak athletic performance.

Fackelmann K: Hypertension's lead connection, *Sci News* 149(24):382, 1996.

Lanphear BP et al: Lead-contaminated house dust and urban children's blood lead levels, *Am J Pub Health* 86(10):1416, 1996.

Mushak P, Crocetti A: Lead and nutrition: biologic interactions of lead with nutrients, *Nutr Today* 31(1):12, 1996.

Stanek K et al: Lead consumption of 18- to 36-month-old children as determined from duplicate diet collections: nutrient intakes, blood lead levels, and effects on growth, *J Am Diet Assoc* 98(2):155, 1998.

These four articles by experienced clinicians in pediatrics, toxicology, nutritional epidemiology, and public health provide valuable information concerning the results of excessive intake of the dangerous element lead on the metabolism of nutrients, especially on the development of young children, who are particularly vulnerable to its toxic impact.

Issues & Answers

Guidelines for trace element supplementation

Currently in the marketplace, trace elements have become popular in both sales and discussions of supplementation. Are there any reasonable guidelines for supplementation based on reliable and current research?

Ten trace elements have generally been identified as essential for optimal health, although this designation for some of them still awaits a full scientific consensus. These elements are chromium, cobalt, copper, fluoride, iodine, iron, manganese, molybdenum, selenium, and zinc. Public health workers are concerned about toxic levels of several elements, especially arsenic, manganese, vanadium, and nickel. Nutritionists must also be concerned about toxicity, in terms of dietary and supplemental contributions leading to excess intake, as well as deficiency, in terms of deciding whether to eliminate factors interfering with bioavailability and/or to evaluate the possible need for supplements.

The following list may serve as a basic guide for examining the need for supplementation of the United States diet with trace minerals.

Iron is provided by organ meats, dried fruits, whole grains, fortified breakfast cereals, legumes, and dark green leafy vegetables. Men require 10 mg/day; women require 15 mg. The RDA for pregnant women is doubled to 30 mg/day, but since this increased pregnancy requirement cannot be met by the iron content of usual United States diets, or by the iron stores of many women, **daily iron supplements are recommended**. Other high-risk groups may need to supplement their diets: adolescent girls, low-income adolescent boys, athletes, and elderly blacks. Before recommending a supplement to these individuals, however, you will want to evaluate their intake of iron antagonists such as fiber and caffeine.

Iodine is provided by foods grown in iodine-rich soil, seafood, and iodized salt. Daily adult requirements are 150 μg/day, although the average intake is several times that amount because of the widespread use of iodine-containing compounds in the dairy and baking industries. Since greater levels can result in thyrotoxicosis, **supplementation is not recommended**.

Zinc is supplied by oysters, whole grains, legumes, nuts, and meats. The recommended intake is 15 mg/day for men and 12 mg/day for women. Pregnancy only increases the need 3 mg/day, and early and late lactation increases the needs to 7 mg/day and 4 mg/day, respectively, to avoid deficiency signs of slow growth, impaired taste and smell, poor wound healing, and skin problems. Others at risk include alcoholics and individuals on long-term low-calorie diets. It takes 3 to 24 weeks for symptoms to appear, but supplementation relieves deficiency symptoms in a matter of days. To avoid an overdose, characterized by gastrointestinal upset, nausea, and bleeding, eating habits should be checked for zinc antagonists, for example, an excessive intake of fiber or iron.

Copper is widely available in liver, oysters, shellfish, nuts, whole grains, and legumes. The average diet was previously believed to provide 2 to 5 mg/day, easily meeting the minimum RDA standard of 2 to 3 mg/day. Intake levels are now believed to range from less than 1 mg to no more than 2 mg/day, based on new analysis methods, thus placing a larger segment of the population at risk for developing a mild deficiency. Before recommending supplements, however, examine factors that reduce copper bioavailability, such as a low protein intake or high levels of zinc, cadmium, fiber, or ascorbic acid.

Chromium is provided by brewer's yeast, animal products, and whole grains. Daily requirements have been estimated between 50 to 200 μg. Deficiency signs include resistance to insulin and other signs of diabetes. Supplementation not only reduces insulin resistance, but also increases HDL-cholesterol, thereby offering some protection against coronary heart disease. Although reliable diagnostic tests have not been developed yet, it is estimated that current intakes fall below recommended levels. However, because it has only shown effectiveness in small, controlled studies, supplementation recommendations have not been made yet for any population groups.

Selenium is provided by fish, whole wheat, and plants grown in selenium-rich soil. RDAs of 70 and 55 μg/day are stated for men and women, respectively, but the average diet provides this much and more. Selenium is believed to offer protection against breast cancer. One group of researchers believes that "optimal cancer protection" is provided at levels of 150 to 300 μg/day, although the connection between blood levels in cancer patients and cancer-free individuals has not been established. In addition to cancer, selenium is believed to protect against heart disease, arthritis, heavy metal poisoning, sexual dysfunction, and aging. As there is no current evidence of selenium deficiency in the general population, **supplementation is not recommended.**

Manganese is provided by whole grain, green vegetables, and dried beans. Safe intakes are estimated in the range of 2.5 to 5 mg/day. Deficiency signs in humans have not been reported, but signs of toxicity have. Toxicity is associated mainly with industrial exposure. However, the possibility of an excess suggests that **supplementation is not recommended.**

Silicon requirements for humans are not known, nor are reliable food sources. Deficiency has been associated with poor bone growth in chicks and statistically correlated with cardiovascular disease in humans. However, the need for supplementation has not been established.

Nickel is provided by legumes, cocoa, wheat, shellfish, milk, meats, and a variety of vegetables and fresh fruits. Requirements are estimated at about 75 μg/day, although United States intakes have been estimated between 300 to 600 μg/day. In light of this excessive intake, plus the existence of at least one sign of toxicity (a nickel-sensitivity dermatitis), **supplementation is not recommended.**

Vanadium requirements and reliable food sources are both unknown. However, it is estimated that the average American diet provides 1 to 2 mg/day. Some individuals are apparently sensitive to this amount, exhibiting severe depression. They improve when given megadoses of vitamin C, which blocks vanadium activity. The need for supplementation is not indicated because of its potential for toxicity in this sensitive population group.

References

Gable CB: Hemochromatosis and dietary iron supplements: implications from US mortality, morbidity, and health survey data, *J Am Diet Assoc* 92(2):208, 1992.

Marsh MN, Riley SA: Digestion and absorption of nutrients and vitamins. In Feldman M, Scharschmidt BF, Sleisenger MH, eds: *Gastrointestinal and liver disease,* ed 6, vol 2, Philadelphia, 1998, Saunders.

Nielsen FH: Ultratrace minerals. In Shils ME, Olson JA, Shike M, eds: *Modern nutrition in health and disease,* ed 8, vol 1, Philadelphia, 1994, Lea & Febiger.

Pennington JAT: A review of iodine toxicity reports, *J Am Diet Assoc* 90(11):1571, 1990.

Community Nutrition: The Life Cycle

Part 2

The Food Environment and Food Habits

This chapter begins the second part of your study of nutrition with a two-chapter sequence on food habits and family nutrition counseling. Here we seek to apply the nutritional science principles you have learned to personal and family needs.

The science of human nutrition only comes alive in terms of personal need. Human compassion and concern are as necessary as practical guides and skills to apply knowledge in a useful and helpful manner.

Here we begin with a look at our changing food environment and the web of influences that determine personal food choices and habits.

THE ECOLOGY OF HUMAN NUTRITION

THE FOOD ENVIRONMENT AND MALNUTRITION

Out of necessity our food habits are inevitably linked to our environment. As a result, our rapidly changing human environment, with its problems of imbalance, such as pollution, and malnutrition, often threatens health. The word **ecology** comes from a Greek word, *oikos*, meaning "house." Just as many factors and forces within a family interact to influence its members, so even greater forces in our physical environment and social system can interact to produce disease.

The public health significance of malnutrition, local and worldwide, continues to grow.[1] Globally, maldistribution of income leaves a fifth of the world's population, a billion people, living in absolute poverty.[2] It is estimated that each day 35,000 persons (14 million per year) die of hunger, malnutrition, and its preventable burden of disease.[3] Protein-energy malnutrition continues to rank first among the world's nutritional deficiency diseases. Observation and experience have brought deepened awareness of two important interrelated facts: (1) having adequate food alone is not the complete answer, although it fulfills a fundamental need for all persons, and (2) a national high standard of living does not necessarily eliminate the problem of malnutrition. Even in the midst of plenty in America, malnutrition exists.[4] Many malnourished people live in high-risk conditions of poverty, which influences the health of everyone involved. Among young pregnant women, malnutrition brings rising infant mortality rates. It occurs among vulnerable groups such as elderly and hospitalized persons. It is found among persons suffering from alcoholism and drug addition. Malnutrition is associated with poverty and homelessness. In other cases, it is partner to a distorted obsession with thinness. Human misery and human waste of life from malnutrition, more prevalent in some regions of our country and regions of the world than in others, occurs nonetheless in both world hemispheres. The extent of this human suffering is impossible to quantify.

At its fundamental biologic level, malnutrition results from an inadequate supply of nutrients to the cells. However, this lack of essential nutrients at the cell level is by no means a simple problem. It is caused by a complex web of factors: physical, psychologic, personal, social, cultural, economic, political, and educational. Each of these factors is more or less important at a given time and place for a given individual. If these factors are only temporarily adverse, the malnutrition may be short term, alleviated rapidly, and cause no longstanding results or harm to life. But if malnutrition continues unrelieved, it becomes chronic. Irreparable harm to life follows, and eventually death ensues. For the **epidemiol-**ogist a triad of variables influences disease: (1) agent, (2) host, and (3) environment. These three factors describe malnutrition.

Agent

The fundamental agent in malnutrition is lack of food. Because of this lack, certain food nutrients that are essential to maintaining cell activity are missing. As indicated, many factors may interact to cause or modify this lack of food: inadequate quantity and quality of food, insufficient amounts for children during critical growth periods, loss of supply through famine, poverty, maldistribution, war, or unwise choices made from foods available.

Host

The host is the person—infant, child, or adult—who suffers from malnutrition. Various personal characteristics may influence the disease: presence of other diseases, increased need for food during times of growth; pregnancy or heavy labor; congenital defects or prematurity; and personal factors such as emotional problems and poverty.

Environment

Many environmental factors influence malnutrition. These include sanitation, social problems, culture, economic and political structure, and agriculture.

The classic interactive and tangled web of some of these factors leading to malnutrition, as experienced by pioneer British pediatrician Cecily Williams in her early work in Africa with kwashiorkor, is shown in Figure 9.1. This debilitating web of malnutrition factors, in one combination or another, is still being experienced in numerous places around the world everyday.

ECONOMIC AND POLITICAL ENVIRONMENT

Food availability and use

In any society, at both governmental and personal levels, food availability and use involve both money and politics. It is plainly evident that money is a basic necessity for getting an adequate food supply. Sometimes, however, the role of politics and government structure and policies is not always as evident. Nonetheless, both are always intertwined in securing human nutrition.

Government food and agriculture programs

In any country, food and agricultural programs at any level of government influence food availability and distribution. A number of factors may be involved, such as land management practices and erosion, water distribution, water pollution from long-term use of questionable pesticides, food production and distribution policies, and food assistance programs for persons in need.

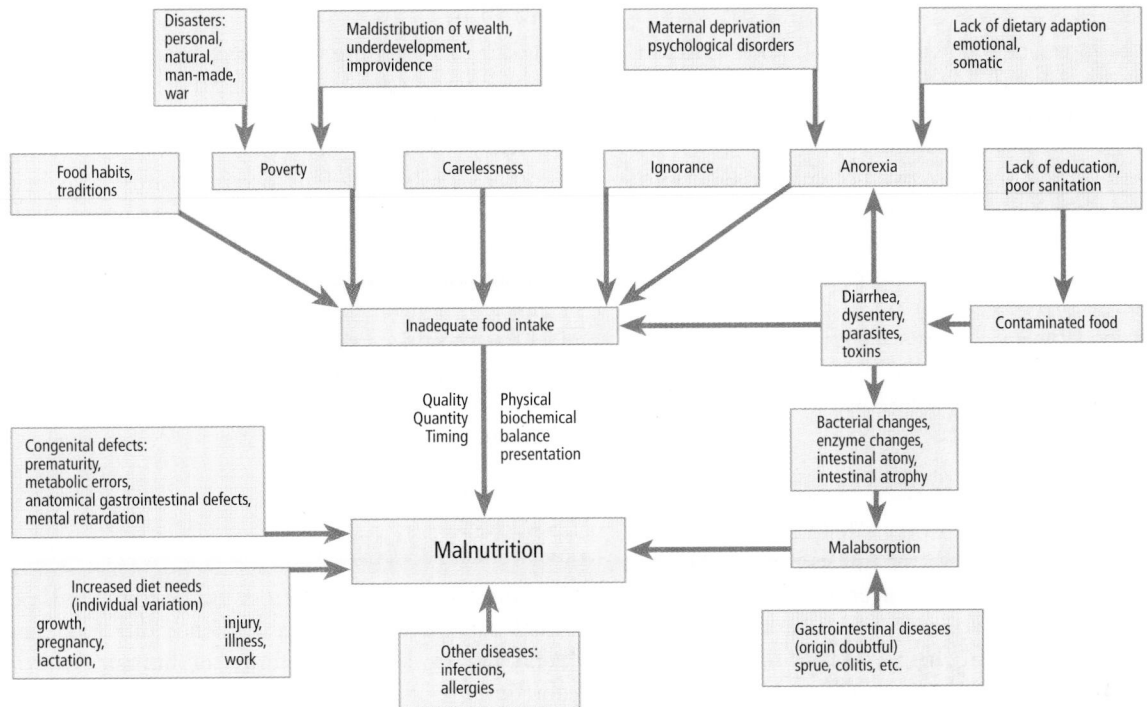

Figure 9.1   The multiple etiology of malnutrition. (Modified from Williams CD: Malnutrition, *Lancet* 2:342, 1962.)

THE PROBLEM OF POVERTY

We are all made increasingly aware through the daily news that malnutrition, even famine and death, exists in many countries that are hard-pressed by social conditions such as war, inequity, and desperate poverty. But even here, in the United States, one of the wealthiest world nations, many studies document widespread hunger and malnutrition among the poor, especially among minority groups, with increasing numbers of infants and young children involved.[5,6] For example, black infants in the United States still have twice the chance of dying in their first year as white infants do, one of five United States children under age 18 lives in poverty, and black and Hispanic children are nearly three times more likely to live in poverty as white children.[6]

Tremendous problems exist among the poor and at times they seem almost insurmountable. Often a culture of poverty develops and is reinforced and perpetuated by society's values and attitudes, which wall off such persons more completely than do physical barriers. As a result of extreme pressures caused by living conditions, poverty-stricken persons become victims of negative attitudes and characteristics, feeling isolated, powerless, and insecure, feelings that influence their use of community health services.

Isolation

Strong feelings of alienation from mainstream society are common among the poor. In many communities, few if any channels of communications are open between the lowest income groups and the rest of society. In most instances a poor person responds to such feelings of alienation by further withdrawal. Each person feels isolated and alone and concludes that no one is concerned. Hazards to health are inherent in poor housing and poor nutrition and are often compounded by distance from the sources of health care.

Powerlessness

It is ironic that often those persons most exposed to risks and emergencies have the fewest coping resources. Extreme frustration is inevitable and persons become overwhelmed. Why try, they conclude, if they have no control over the situation? Why plan, if there is no future different from today? In such a day-to-day struggle to exist, poor persons often see little value in long-range preventive health measures.

---

ecology   Relations between organisms and their environments

epidemiology   The study of factors determining the frequency, distribution, and strength of diseases in population groups.

Insecurity

Subjected to forces outside their control, poor individuals and families have little or no security. Insecurity and anxiety often incapacitate them. In such a setting, where hunger may be a constant companion, food—which has for poor people the same deep psychologic and emotional meaning that it has for all people—assumes even greater meaning than it has for persons who rarely know hunger. The United States Department of Agriculture (USDA) defines food security as "access by all people at all times to enough food for an active, healthy life."[9] Minimally, this means ready availability of nutritionally adequate and safe foods in socially accepted ways.[9,10]

ROLE OF THE HEALTH WORKER

How can concerned health workers help individuals and families conditioned by years of poverty or crushed by new poverty? In the face of such overpowering feelings of isolation, helplessness, and insecurity, what attitudes are necessary to be of real help? What methods and approaches are most likely to reach our clients and patients and supply their needs? Some basic principles can help.

Self-awareness

First, we must explore our own feelings about the poor. We must be aware of our own distorted vision, our own class values and attitudes. If we are to be agents of constructive change, true helping vehicles, we must first have some understanding of the person's situation and its broad social setting. We must also understand ourselves better and confront our own cultural conditioning and biases.

Rapport

Genuine warmth, interest, friendliness, and kindness grow from within. Rapport is that feeling of relationship between persons that is born of mutual respect, regard, and trust. This sense of relationship gives both helper and helped a deep feeling of working together. Its most basic ingredient is a concern for people and persons, a positive orientation toward human beings in general and concern for individuals in particular. It is born of a deep knowledge of what it means to be human.

Acceptance

This term is another way of stating the principle that one must begin where the client or patient is. Each person's own concerns should be the primary consideration. Often we work with other team specialists to cut through the maze of factors involved in a given situation before the client or patient is ready to accept or even to consider the health practice or diet counsel that is needed or desired. Much time may have to be spent, for example, in coming to understand the meaning of food to this person, before practical dietary matters can begin to be explored.

Listening

The art of listening—positive, active, creative listening—is vital. Clients must tell their story in their own way, with no interruption by distracting statements or questions and no deflecting of the conversation to another's problems. This listening must also be observant. Sequence of statements, subjects introduced, areas of intense feeling, and areas ignored give clues to needs. Throughout we must proceed with sensitivity and create a relaxed, nonthreatening atmosphere, in which persons feel free to talk—*and we must listen*. The reason that some frustrated persons finally take their problems to the streets may well be that no one listens to them unless they do.

DEVELOPMENT OF FOOD HABITS

In addition to these factors of poverty and politics, other aspects of our lives influence our food patterns. Food habits, like other forms of human behavior, do not develop in a vacuum. They result from many personal, cultural, social, and psychologic influences. For each of us these factors are interwoven to develop a unique individual.

CULTURAL INFLUENCES

Strength of personal culture

Often the most significant thing about a society's *culture* is what it takes for granted in daily life. Culture involves not only the more obvious and historical aspects of a person's communal life, that is, language, religion, politics, technology, and so on, but also all the little habits of everyday living, such as preparing and serving food and caring for children, feeding them, and lulling them to sleep. These many facets of a person's culture are learned gradually as a child grows up in a society. Through a slow process of conscious and unconscious learning, we take on our culture's values, attitudes, habits, and practices through the influence of our parents, teachers, and others. Whatever is invented, transmitted, and perpetuated, socially acquired knowledge and habits, we learn as part of our culture. These elements become internalized and entrenched.

Food in a culture

Food habits are among the oldest and most deeply rooted aspects of many cultures and exert deep influence on the behavior of the people. The cultural and subcultural background determines what shall be eaten as well as when and how it shall be eaten. There is, of course, considerable variation. But rational and irrational, beneficial and injurious customs are found in every part of the world. Nevertheless, food habits are primarily based on food availability, economics, and personal food meanings and beliefs. Included among these influential factors are the geography of the land, the agriculture practiced by the people, their economic and marketing practices, their view about healthy or safe food, and their history and traditions. Within every culture certain foods are deeply infused with symbolic meaning. These symbolic foods are related to major life experiences from birth through death, to religion, to politics, and to general social organization. From early times, ceremonies and religious rites have surrounded certain events and seasons. Food gathering, preparing, and serving have followed specific customs and commemorated special events of religious and national significance and heritage. Many of these customs remain today (see *Issues & Answers,* p.207).

SOCIAL INFLUENCES

Social organization

The study of human group behavior reveals numerous activities, processes, and structures by which social life goes on. Human behavior can be understood in terms of social phenomena and problems, such as social change, urbanism, rural life, the family, the community, race relations, delinquency, drugs, and crime. These social problems carry nutritional implications. Two aspects of social organization concern health professionals: class structure and value systems.

1. *Class structure.* The structure of a society is largely formed by groupings according to such factors as economic status, education, residence, occupation, or family. Within a given society many of these groups exist, and their values and habits vary widely. Subgroups develop on the basis of region, religion, age, sex, social class, health concerns, occupation, or political affiliation. Within these subgroups there may be still smaller groupings with distinct attitudes, values and habits. A person may be a member of several subcultural groups, each of which influences values, attitudes, and habits. Our democratic philosophy, as well as the humanitarian ideals on which the health professions have been nurtured, combine to make the reality of class differences difficult for us to accept.

2. *Value systems.* A society's value systems develop as a result of its history and heritage. Traditionally, four basic premises have influenced American value systems and have affected attitudes toward health care and food habits:
   - *Equality.* A high value on equality leads health workers to establish quality health care standards for all people, although in reality this does not always occur.
   - *Sociality.* The high respect accorded to a social nature builds peer group pressures and status-seeking within social groups. Foods may be

accepted because they are high-status foods or rejected because they are low-prestige foods. Even the use of dietary supplements has been associated with the desire for prestige, along with health concerns.
   - *Success.* The esteem in which success is held often leads persons to measure life in terms of competitive superlatives. They want to set the best table, provide the most abundant supply of food for the family, or to have the biggest eater and the fattest baby of any in the neighborhood.
   - *Change.* The value placed on change leads families and individuals to seek constant variety in their diets, to be geared for action, to be a mobile society, and to seek quick-cooking, conveniently prepared foods. In response to such marketing demands, food technologists continually produce an array of new food products.

Food and social factors

Food habits in any setting are highly socialized. These habits perform significant social functions, some of which may not always be evident. First, within social relationships, food is a symbol of social acceptance, warmth, and friendliness. People tend to accept food more readily from those persons they view as friends or allies. They accept advice about food from persons they consider to be authorities or with whom they can feel warm relationships.

Second, within family relationships, the primary social unit, strong food patterns develop. Food habits that are most closely associated with family sentiments are the most tenacious throughout life. Long into adulthood, certain foods trigger a flood of childhood memories and are valued for reasons totally apart from any nutritional value. Strong religious factors associated with food tend to have their origin and reinforcement within the family meal circle. Also, family income, community sources of food, and market conditions influence food habits and ultimately food choices. Persons eat foods that are readily available to them and that they have the money to buy.

PSYCHOLOGIC INFLUENCES

Social psychology

Social psychology is concerned with (1) social interaction in terms of its effect on individual behavior, and (2) the social influences of individual perception, motivation, and action. How does a particular individual perceive a given situation? What basic needs motivate action and response? What social factors surround a particular action? Issues of particular concern include the effect of culture on personality, the socialization of the child, differences in individuals in groups, group dynamics, group attitudes and opinions, and leadership. The methods of social psychology have made important contributions to nutrition, medicine, nursing, and allied health care, especially to problems of human behavior under stress.

Food and psychologic factors

Individual behavior patterns, especially those related to eating, result from many interrelated psychosocial influences. Factors that are particularly pertinent to the shaping of food habits are motivation and perception.

1. *Motivation.* People are not the same the world over. Those of differing cultures are not motivated by the same needs and goals. Even primary biologic drives such as hunger and sex are modified in their interpretation, expression, and fulfillment by many cultural, social, and personal influences. The kinds of food sought, prized, or accepted by one individual at one time and place may be rejected by another living in different circumstances. For persons existing in a state of basic hunger or semistarvation, food is the whole perception and motivation. Such a person thinks, talks, and dreams about food. Under less severe circumstances, however, the concern for food may be on a relatively abstract level and may involve symbolism that is associated with other needs. For example, Maslow's classic hierarchy of human needs illustrates these human strivings.[9] He described five levels of need that operate in turn, each building on the previous ones:

   - *Basic physiologic needs.* Hunger, thirst.
   - *Safety needs.* Physical comfort, security, protection.
   - *"Belongingness" needs.* Love, giving and receiving affection.
   - *Recognition needs.* Self-esteem, status, sense of self-worth, strength, self-confidence, capability, adequacy.
   - *Self-actualization needs.* Self-fulfillment, creative growth.

   Of course, these levels of need overlap and vary with time and circumstance. But we can use them to help us understand the needs of our clients and plan care accordingly.

2. *Perception.* To make sense out of an otherwise chaotic assortment of impressions, we perceive our environment in different ways. These perceptions enable us to live in an environment that feels relatively stable. However, perception also limits understanding. Every phenomenon that the outer world offers is filtered through our own social and personal lenses. In every experience of our lives, we perceive a blend of three facets: (1) the *external* reality, (2) the *message* of the stimulus that is conveyed by the nervous system to the integrative centers of the brain where thinking and evaluation go on, and (3) the *interpretation* that we put on every part of our personal experience. A host of subjective ele-

ments—hunger, thirst, hate, fear, love, self-interest, values, temperament—influence our response to the outer world's phenomena.

On the basis, then, of personal motivation and perception, personal learning takes place. In the final analysis, each person must learn in his or her own way according to need. It is this personal human dimension that makes a health professional's work profound. Persons learn because they have an urgent need to know. They learn because their curiosity is aroused. They learn because they want to make meaning out of their lives. They learn by exploring, making mistakes and correcting them, testing, verifying. All of these things individuals must do for themselves. This is true of everyone's learning. It is true of the learning we desire for our clients. It is true of our own learning.

Health concerns: misinformation and food safety

Food misinformation

Unscientific statements about food and nutrition often mislead the public and contribute to poor food habits. Persons have often surrounded their cultural eating habits with myths of various sorts. Some scientifically unsubstantiated beliefs about certain foods may be harmless, but others may have more serious implications for health and well-being. Claims about foods or supplements that are not based on scientific evidence, such as heavy use of vitamin supplements for general health maintenance, often mislead the public and contribute to poor food habits.[10] False information may come from folklore, or it may be built on half-truths, innuendoes, and outright deception, as in cases of fraud.

In contrast, nutritional science is a growing body of knowledge built on vigorously examined scientific evidence. Concern for food safety and wholesomeness clearly existed long before the scientific method was known. Nonetheless, in this rapidly changing world, it is only on the sound basis of scientific knowledge that we may make wise food choices and recognize misinformation as such.

Types of food faddist claims

Food faddists make exaggerated claims for certain types of food. These claims fall into four basic groups: (1) certain foods will cure specific conditions, (2) certain foods are harmful and should be avoided, (3) special food combinations are very effective as reducing diets or have special therapeutic effects, and (4) other "natural" foods can meet body needs and prevent disease. A basic error can be found when we examine these claims carefully. Notice that each one focuses on foods as such, not on the chemical components—the nutrients—that are the actual physiologic agents of life and health. It is true, of course, that certain individuals may be allergic to specific foods and obviously should avoid them. It is also true that certain foods have particularly high concentrations of certain nutrients and are therefore good sources of such nutrients. But it is the nutrients, not the specific foods, that have specific functions in the body. And furthermore, each of these nutrients may be found in a number of different foods. Persons require specific nutrients, never specific foods.

Why should the health worker be concerned about food faddism and its effects on food habits? What harm may food faddism do? Essentially, food fads involve three basic dangers that concern all members of the health care team.

- *Dangers to health.* Responsibility for one's health is fundamental. However, self-diagnosis and self-treatment can be dangerous, especially where health problems are concerned. When such action is based on questionable sources, the dangers are multiplied. By following such a course, a person with a real illness may fail to seek appropriate medical care. Many anxious patients who have cancer, diabetes, or arthritis have been misled by fraudulent claims of cures and postponed effective therapy. Superstitions that are perpetuated counteract scientific progress and sound health teaching.

- *Money spent needlessly.* Some of these foods and supplements used by faddists are harmless, but most are expensive. As much as $2.5 billion per year has been spent by consumers on nutrient supplements. Such money may be wasted. When dollars are scarce, the family may neglect to buy foods that fill its basic needs, opting instead to purchase a "guaranteed cure" (see *Case Study,* p. 205).

- *Distrust of the food market.* Our food environment is rapidly changing. We need intelligent concern and rational problem solving to meet nutritional requirements. A wise course is to select a variety of primary foods "closer to the source"—having minimal processing—adding a few carefully selected processed items for specific uses. Blanket erroneous teaching concerning food and health breeds public suspicion and distrust of the common food market and of food technology and agriculture in general. Each food product must be evaluated on its own merits in terms of individual needs. These needs include nutrient contribution, aesthetic values, safety, and cost.

Groups vulnerable to food fads

Food fads appeal especially to certain groups of people with particular needs and concerns. Among these are older adults, adolescents, obese persons, athletes, and those whose living depends on their physical appearance.

- *Older persons.* Fear of changes that come as youth and potency wane leads many middle-aged persons to grasp at exaggerated claims that some product will restore their youthful vigor. Elderly persons in pain and discomfort, perhaps living alone with chronic illness, may respond to the hope that the special supplement holds a sure cure.[10] Desperately ill and lonely individuals are easy prey for exaggerated health claims.

- *Young persons.* Figure-conscious adolescent girls and muscle-minded rapidly growing boys frequently respond to advertisements for crash programs to attain the perfect body. Young people, particularly those who are lonely or have exaggerated ideas of glamour, hope to achieve peer-group acceptance by these means.

- *Obese persons.* One of the most disturbing and frustrating health problems in America is obesity. Obese persons, faced with a bewildering barrage of propaganda advocating diets, pills, and devices, are likely to respond to the fad of the moment to solve everything (see Chapter 6).

- *Athletes and coaches.* Athletes and their coaches are prime targets for those who push supplements. Always looking for the added something to give them the competitive edge, athletes can be lured by nutrition myths and hoaxes (see Chapter 14).

- *Entertainers.* Persons in the public eye, such as entertainers, may look for certain foods, drugs, or dietary combinations that will help them retain the physical appearance and strength on which their careers depend; they may easily believe false claims about these foods.

These various groups are vulnerable for obvious reasons. No segment of the population, however, seems to be completely free from food faddism's appeal. Particularly in metropolitan areas, "health food," with its attendant supplements, is a large industry, bigger in the United States than in any other country.

The answer

How do we respond to food habits associated with food faddism, misinformation, or even deception? What can health professionals do? What should they do? Several things merit consideration:

1. *Assess your own attitudes and habits.* We cannot counsel or teach others until we have first examined our own position. Instruction based on personal conviction, practice, and enthusiasm will achieve far more than teaching that says, in effect, "Do as I say, not as I do."

2. *Use reliable sources.* Two types of background knowledge are vital: (1) knowledge of the product and the persons behind it, and (2) knowledge of human nutritional physiology and the scientific method of problem-solving.

3. *Recognize human needs.* Observe these needs in yourselves and in others to understand how psychologic

and cultural factors affect food habits. Consider the emotional needs that are symbolically fulfilled by foods, the eating of foods, and by the rituals surrounding the process. Respect personal needs. Welcome the positive power that food and eating rituals possess for filling these needs. Even when there is reason to believe that the client is using food as a crutch for emotional adjustment, the value of such an adjustment must be considered. A wise teacher of mine once put it well: "We must avoid 'breaking crutches' without providing alternative support."

4. *Be alert to community opportunities*. Grasp any opportunity that arises to present sound health information to groups or individuals, formally or informally. Learn of available community resources and use them. Develop communication skills. Avoid monotony. Use a well-disciplined imagination. Without these things, the message will not convince.

5. *Think scientifically*. We can teach young children to use the problem-solving approach to everyday situations. Children are naturally curious. With their eternal *"Why?"* they often seek evidence to support statements made to them. We need to teach them and ourselves the value of asking three significant questions: "What do you mean?" "How do you know?" and "What is your evidence?"

6. *Know responsible authorities*. The Food and Drug Administration (FDA) has the legal responsibility of controlling the quality and safety of food and drug products marketed in the United States. But it needs the vigilance of consumers to help fulfill so large a task. Other governmental, professional, and private organizations also provide resources for consumer education. The American Dietetic Association has provided guidance for a United States national policy on enrichment and fortification of the food supply that protects against nutrient insufficiencies and toxicities.[11]

INFLUENCE OF FOOD SAFETY CONCERNS ON FOOD HABITS

America's food supply has radically changed over the past years. These changes, which have swept the food-marketing system, are rooted in widespread social change and scientific advance. The agricultural and food processing industries have developed a wide variety of chemicals to increase and preserve our food supply and to create new products. In the process, however, critics have increasingly voiced concerns about how these changes may affect food safety, food habits, and the overall environment.[12] Concerns have centered on pesticides and food additives.

Plant pesticides and animal drugs

For the most part, over the past few decades, American agriculture has developed into a modern mechanized business structure. As a whole, it has brought large crop yields to feed a growing population. To accomplish this task, a growing chemical industry has supplied an increasing number of plant pesticides and herbicides to produce large crops, as well as animal antibiotics and growth hormones to develop livestock for market. Bovine somatotropin (bST)—growth hormone—has been approved by the FDA for commercial use by dairy farmers to increase milk production, and similarly porcine somatotropin (bBT) is used with pigs to produce far less body fat and leaner cuts of pork. Large American agricultural corporations, as well as individual farmers, use a number of chemicals to advance food production. They use them for a variety of reasons—to control a wide number of destructive insects, kill weeds, control plant diseases, stop fruit from dropping prematurely, cause leaves to fall and thus facilitate harvesting, make seeds sprout, keep seeds from rotting before they sprout, increase yield, and improve marketing quality.

Over time, however, problems from the frequent use of pesticides have developed in four main areas: (1) pesticide residues on food, (2) leaching of the chemicals into ground water and surrounding wells, (3) increased exposure of farm workers to the strong chemicals, and (4) increased amount of chemicals required as insect tolerance for pesticides develops. The task of assessing health risks for the thousands of pesticides in use or being developed is difficult. The current FDA routine screening assays detect only part of all United States pesticides.

An increasing number of concerned farmers, with help from soil scientists, are developing alternative systems of sustainable agriculture that do not rely on heavy pesticide use. Instead, they combine conservative practices and modern technology, including the biotechnology of **agrogenetics**, which grows safe, quality produce from resistant strains of genetically modified foods, thus reducing the need for toxic pesticides and herbicides.[13,14] A variety of new plants are being developed that protect resources, preserve the environment, reduce the need for toxic pesticides and herbicides, and are still profitable. Other local farmers have introduced the concept of regional eating that reconnects people to a locally produced food supply.[15]

Food processing additives

In addition, over the past few decades, chemicals intentionally added to foods during processing have become an integral part of our food supply. Our present variety of food market items would be impossible without them. For example, additives enrich food with added nutrients, produce uniform qualities of food products, standardize functional factors such as thickening and stabilization, preserve foods, and improve flavor and texture. Table 9.1 lists some examples of these additives. A number of micronutrients and antioxidants are being added to pro-

Table 9.1 Some examples of intentional food additives		
Function	**Chemical compounds**	**Common food uses**
Acids, alkalis, buffers	Sodium bicarbonate	Baking powder
	Tartaric acid	Fruit sherbets
		Cheese spreads
Antibiotics	Chlortetracycline	Dip for dressed poultry
Anticaking agents	Aluminum calcium silicate	Table salt
Antimycotics	Calcium propionate	Bread
	Socium propionate	Bread
	Sorbic acid	Cheese
Antioxidants	Butylated hydroxyanisole (BHA)	Fats
	Butylated hydroxytoluene (BHT)	Fats
Bleaching agents	Benzoyl perioxide	Wheat flour
	Chlorine dioxide	
	Oxides of nitrogen	
Color preservative	Sodium benzoate	Green peas
		Maraschino cherries
Coloring agents	Annotto	Butter, margarine
	Carotene	
Emulsifiers	Lecithin	Bakery goods
	Monoglycerides, diglycerides	Dairy products
	Propylene glycol alginate	Confections
Flavoring agents	Amyl acetate	Soft drinks
	Benzaldehyde	Bakery goods
	Methyl salicylate	Candy, ice cream
	Essential oils, natural extracts	Canned meats
	Monosodium glutamate	
Nonnutritive sweeteners	Saccharin	Diet packed canned fruit
	Aspartame	Low-kcalorie soft drinks
Nutrient supplements	Potassium iodide	Iodized salt
	Vitamin C	Fruit juices
	Vitamin D	Milk
	Vitamin A	Margarine
	B vitamins, iron	Bread and cereal
Sequestrants	Sodium citrate	Dairy products
	Calcium pyrophosphoric acid	
Stabilizers and thickeners	Pectin	Jellies
	Vegetable gums (carob bean, carrageenan, guar)	Dairy desserts and chocolate milk
	Gelatin	Confections
	Agar-agar	Low-kcalorie salad dressings
Yeast foods and dough conditioners	Ammonium chloride	Bread, rolls
	Calcium sulfate	
	Calcium phosphate	

cessed foods, not for increasing the nutrient content but for their technical effects.

Food additives have served many useful purposes, but problems also have developed. Initial control of food safety began in 1938 with the establishment of the Federal Food, Drug, and Cosmetic Act. Such control continued in 1960 with amendments regulating the use of food additives. These amendments created what has become known as the *GRAS list*—Generally Recognized As Safe additives. Rigid testing to determine their true safety, however, was lacking. Any additive developed after 1960

required this rigid testing before approval. The now famous Delany Clause, named for the congressman who proposed it, was attached in the final hours of congressional debate on the legislation. This clause banned food additives found to cause cancer "in man or animal." Today, however, advanced testing procedures and new knowledge of natural food constituents and metabolic processes make the zero-risk Delany clause seem outdated and inconsequential in terms of its intent over three decades ago. The 1977 congressional directive to FDA to test the thousands of GRAS items is ongoing.

Research has always been a large part of the FDA's work. Along with the USDA's Agricultural Research Service, FDA scientists continually evaluate foods and food components through their own research (Figure 9.2). In the past, FDA views and policies have varied with administrators and sometimes left much to be desired. Nevertheless, broader views more in tune with today's needs seem to prevail now. Today people want to know more than just that a given food will not kill them. They want to know whether it has any positive nutritional value. Thus for a more health-conscious public and a changed marketplace, the FDA has recently developed expanded nutrition guidelines for food labels on a variety of food products.

FDA FOOD LABELING REGULATIONS

Prior nutrition label information

In the mid 1970s, the FDA began describing general nutrition information on food labels, and some producers added limited information on their own in response to increasing market demand. Nutrients and food constituents that consumer groups wanted listed on labels included the macronutrients (carbohydrates, fat, and pro-

Figure 9.2   Research in food chemistry. A chemist in the US Department of Agriculture's Agricultural Research Service makes an adjustment on a molecular still used in a project to aid in manufacturing dry milk. (Courtesy USDA.)

tein) and their total energy value (kcalories), key micronutrients (vitamins and minerals), sodium, cholesterol, and saturated fat.

Current FDA food label regulations

In November of 1990 a new law, the Nutrition Labeling and Education Act of 1990 (NLEA), was enacted by Congress and signed by the President. The NLEA requires mandatory labeling of most processed foods under the jurisdiction of the FDA and forms the core of the FDA's reform effort. It also includes voluntary labeling of fresh fruits, vegetables, and seafood. The USDA is responsible for standards and consumer information concerning other meat and poultry, as well as dairy products. Over a 3-year process, involving consumers and producers, as well as health professionals, the new food labels emerged. Basic features of the revised labeling regulations now include guidelines to define the following items: kcalories and nutrients, descriptive terms, serving sizes and number of servings per container, health claims, and a standardized label format based on results of consumer research (see *To Probe Further* box, p. 201).

Major food label changes

Consumers began seeing the new nutrition label (Figure 9.3) on food products in the summer of 1994. The most visible changes now in practice are how food is advertised and marketed. For example, manufacturers no longer can claim that a product does not contain an ingredient that has never been contained in that product. This means that products that never contained cholesterol cannot make the claim "no cholesterol." Descriptors—such as "light," and "low fat," or "reduced kcalories"—now have legal definitions that are universal to all products.

The current Nutrition Facts label (Figure 9.3), now familiar on food products in all food markets and grocery stores, uses the term Daily Reference Value (DRV) rather than the former outdated values.[16] DVRs are now listed for carbohydrates, proteins, total fat, saturated fat, fiber, cholesterol, sodium, and potassium. DVRs for energy sources (fats, carbohydrates, protein) are based on percentages of 2000 and 2500 kcalorie diets, and DVRs for other food components represent the uppermost limit that is considered desirable. Table 9.2 shows a comparison of the nutrition information on the former (old) food labels and the current ones. FDA guidelines for the new nutrient labeling regulations are defined in the *To Probe Further* box, p. 201. In August 1996, the FDA completed and published final regulations for the nutrition labeling of raw fruits, vegetables, and fish.[17] Recently, in 1994, the trilateral North American Free Trade Agreement (NAFTA) was enacted, committing Canada, the United States, and Mexico to work toward harmonized consumer labeling standards.[18]

GOVERNMENT FOOD SAFETY CONTROL AGENCIES

General agency controls

Several government agencies help control the safety and quality of our food supply. Concerned sections of the United States Department of Health and Human Services (DHHS) are the FDA and the Public Health Service (PHS). The USDA controls pesticide use in farming; related work is assigned to the Agricultural Research Service and the Consumer Marketing Service. The Federal Trade Commission and the National Bureau of Standards also protect the consumer. Of these various agencies, however, the one specifically controlling food safety is the FDA.

Food and Drug Administration

The Food and Drug Administration (FDA) is a law enforcement agency charged by Congress to ensure, among other things, that our food supply is safe, pure, and wholesome. The agency enforces federal food safety regulations through various activities including, (1) food sanitation and quality control, (2) control of chemical contaminants and pesticides, (3) control of food additives, (4) regulation of movement of food across state lines, (5)

nutrition and nutrition labeling of foods, (6) safety of public food service, and (7) safety of meat and milk. The most common means of enforcement is use of recalls and seizures of contaminated food.

The FDA's division of consumer education conducts an active program of protection through public education and general information. Special attention is given to nutrition misinformation. Materials are prepared and distributed to individuals, students, and community groups. Consumer specialists work through all FDA district offices.

FOODBORNE DISEASE

Costs

Another large factor affecting food safety and food choice is foodborne disease. Many disease-bearing organisms inhabit our environment and can contaminate our food and water. Lapses in their control still occur, resulting in high incidences of illness, death, and economic costs. For example, estimates of foodborne disease in the United States are approximately 12.6 million cases per year, costing about $8.4 billion. Microbiologic diseases, bacterial and viral, represent 84% of these costs, compared with 88% in Canada. The most economically significant United States diseases are salmonellosis and staphylococcal poisoning, costing annually about $4 billion and $1.5 billion, respectively. Other costly types include listeriosis, trichinosis, *Clostridium perfringens* enteritis, and botulism. Approximately 9000 Americans die each year of foodborne disease, and an estimated 80 million become ill.[19]

Food sanitation

Strict sanitation measures and rigid personal hygiene are essential. Throughout all preparation, the food and everything that touches it must be scrupulously clean. Cooking procedures and temperature standards must be followed, all serving equipment must be kept clean, leftover food must be stored and reused appropriately or discarded, and garbage must be contained and disposed of in a sanitary manner. We know all these measures, but some persons do not always practice them. These rules are especially important for food handlers working in any phase of public food service operations, food processing and packaging plants, public markets, or delicatessen shops or counters. Also, persons with any infectious disease or hand injury, however small, should not work with food.

Bacterial food infections

Bacterial food infections result from eating food contaminated by large colonies of bacteria. Specific bacteria cause specific diseases. Four examples are *Escherichia coli 0157:H7*, salmonellosis, shigellosis, and listeriosis.

1. *Escherichia coli 0157:H7. Escherichia coli 0157:H7* microorganisms inhabit the intestines of animals

---

Nutrition Facts

Serving Size: 1/2 cup (114 g)
Servings Per Container: 4

Amount per Serving

kcalories 260
kcalories from fat 120

	% Daily Value*
Total Fat 13 g	20%
Saturated Fat 5 g	25%
Cholesterol 30 mg	10%
Sodium 660 mg	28%
Total Carbohydrates 31 g	11%
Sugars 5 g	
Dietary Fiber 0 g	0%
Protein 5 g	

Vitamin A 4% • Vitamin C 1% •
Calcium 15% • Iron 4%

*Percents (%) of a Daily Value are based on a 2,000 kcalorie diet. Your Daily Values may vary higher or lower depending on your kcalorie needs

Nutrient	2,000 kcalories	2,500 kcalories
Total Fat	65 g	80 g
Saturated Fat	20 g	25 g
Cholesterol	300 mg	300 mg
Sodium	2,400 mg	2,400 mg
Total Carbohydrate	300 g	375 g
Fiber	25 g	30 g

1 g Fat = 9 kcalories
1 g Carbohydrate = 4 kcalories
1 g Protein = 4 kcalories

Figure 9.3   Example of a current food label.

Table

9.2 Selected examples of bacterial foodborne disease

Foodborne disease	Causative organisms (genus and species)	Food source	Symptoms and course
Bacterial food infections			
Salmonellosis	Salmonella *S. typhi* *S. paratyphi*	Milk, custards, egg dishes, salad dressings, sandwich fillings, polluted shellfish	Mild to severe diarrhea, cramps, vomiting; appears 12-24 hours or more after eating; lasts 1-7 days
Shigellosis	Shigella *S. dysenteriae*	Milk and milk products, seafood, salads	Mild diarrhea to fatal dysentery (especially in young children); appears 7-36 hours after eating; lasts 3-14 days
Listeriosis	Listeria *L. monocytogenes*	Soft cheese, poultry, seafood, raw milk, meat products (paté)	Severe diarrhea, fever, headache, pneumonia, meningitis, endocarditis; symptoms begin after 3-21 days
Bacterial food poisoning (Enterotoxins)			
Staphylococal	Staphylococcus *S. aureus*	Custards, cream fillings, processed meats, ham, cheese, ice cream, potato salad, sauces, casseroles	Severe abdominal pain, cramps, vomiting, diarrhea, perspiration, headache, fever, prostration; appears suddenly 1-6 hours after eating; symptoms subside generally within 24 hours
Clostridial Perfringens enteritis Botulism	Clostridium *C. perfringens* *C. botulinum*	Cooked meats, meat dishes held at warm or room temperature Improperly home-canned foods; smoked and salted fish, ham, sausage, shellfish	Mild diarrhea, vomiting; appears 8-24 hours after eating; lasts a day or less Symptoms range from mild discomfort to death within 24 hours; initial nausea, vomiting, weakness, dizziness, progressing to motor and sometimes fatal breathing paralysis

and humans. Most types of *E. coli* intestinal bacteria are benign; some do nutritionally important tasks such as bacterial fermentation of resistant starch (see Chapter 3). However, some strains, such as *E. coli* serotype O157:H7, produce toxins that cause serious disease. Over the past decade, *E. coli O157:H17* has emerged as a major cause of individual cases and large outbreaks of diarrhea, both bloody and non-bloody.[20]

Physicians at the United States Centers for Disease Control and Prevention (CDC) in Atlanta who tracked this virulent microorganism indicate that from a clinical and public health standpoint it is by far the most important *E. coli* serotype in North America. In the United States alone, it is estimated to cause more than 20,000 infections and as many as 250 deaths each year. Major outbreaks have resulted from eating beef, mainly undercooked ground beef. The largest North American outbreak affected over 700 persons, 4 of whom died, in four western states and was traced to undercooked hamburgers from a fast-food restaurant chain.[21] As a result of this outbreak, the public has recognized the need for adequate cooking of ground beef patties to ensure safety against *E. coli*.[21,22]

2. *Salmonellosis*. Salmonellosis is caused by the bacteria *Salmonella*, named for the American veterinarian-pathologist Daniel Salmon (1850-1914), who first isolated and identified species commonly causing human foodborne infections, *S. typhi* and *S. paratyphi*. These organisms grow readily in common foods such as milk, custards, egg dishes, salad dressings, and sandwich fillings. Seafood, especially shellfish such as oysters and clams, from polluted waters may also be a source of infection. A large number of recently reported United States cases have been traced to shelled (or cracked) eggs. Salmonellosis continues to be one of the main causes of foodborne disease world wide. Unsanitary handling of foods and utensils can spread the bacteria. Resulting cases of gastroenteritis may vary in intensity from mild diarrhea to severe attacks. Practices of immunization, pasteurization, and sanitary regulations involving community water and food supplies as well as food handlers help to control such outbreaks. Incubation and multiplication of the bacteria take time after the food is eaten, so symptoms of food infection develop slowly, usually 12 to 24 hours after ingestion.

3. *Shigellosis*. Shigellosis is caused by the bacteria *Shigella*, named for the Japanese physician Kiyoshi

Shiga (1870-1957), who first discovered a main species of the organism—*S. dysenteriae*—during a **dysentery** epidemic in Japan in 1898. Shigellosis is usually confined to the large intestine and may vary from a mild transient disturbance in adults to fatal dysentery in young children. The bacteria grow easily in foods, especially in milk, a common carrier to infants and children. Reported outbreaks have been traced to uncooked tofu salad and to shredded lettuce and cabbage packaged for restaurants and the retail market.[23] The boiling of water or the pasteurization of milk kills the organisms, but the food or milk can easily be reinfected by unsanitary handling by a carrier. The disease is spread in much the same way as salmonellosis is transmitted, by unsanitary handling of food.

4. *Listeriosis.* Listeriosis is caused by the bacteria *Listeria*, named for the English surgeon Baron Joseph Lister (1827-1912), who first applied knowledge of bacterial infection to principles of antiseptic surgery in a benchmark 1867 publication, which led to "clean" operations and the development of modern surgery. Only within the past few decades, however, has knowledge of the role of *Listeria* in directly causing foodborne disease in humans, both occasional illness and disease epidemics, increased and the major species causing human illness—*L. monocytogenes*—been identified.[24,25] Before 1981 *Listeria* was thought to be only an animal disease organism transmitted to humans only by direct contact with infected animals. Now we know that these organisms occur widely in the environment. In high-risk individuals such as elderly persons, pregnant women, infants, or persons with suppressed immune systems, the organisms can produce a rare but often fatal illness, with severe symptoms such as diarrhea, flulike fever and headache, pneumonia, **sepsis**, **meningitis**, and **endocarditis**. Foodborne disease has been traced to a variety of foods, including raw milk, raw eggs, seafood, chicken, turkey, meat, and meat products.

Bacterial food poisonings

Food poisoning is caused by the ingestion of bacterial toxins that have been produced in foods by the growth of specific kinds of bacteria before the food is eaten. The powerful toxin is ingested directly, and symptoms therefore develop rapidly, usually within 1 to 6 hours after the food is eaten. Two types of bacterial food poisoning are most commonly responsible, staphylococcal and clostridial.

1. *Staphylococcal food poisoning.* Named for the shape of the main causative organism *Staphylococcus aureus*, staphylococcal food poisoning is by far the most common form of bacterial poisoning observed in the United States. Powerful preformed toxins contaminate the food, producing rapid illness within 1 to 6 hours after ingestion. Symptoms come on suddenly—severe cramping and abdominal pain with vomiting and diarrhea, usually accompanied by sweating, headache, and fever. In some cases there may be shock and prostration. Recovery is fairly rapid, however, depending on the amount of toxin ingested. The source of contamination is usually an infection on the hand of a worker preparing the food, often minor or unnoticed. Foods that are particularly effective culture beds include custard- and cream-filled bakery goods, chicken and ham salads, processed meats, cheese, sauces, and combination dishes. The toxin makes no change in the normal odor, taste, or appearance of the food, so the person eating it is not warned.

2. *Clostridial food poisoning.* Named for the shape of the bacterium *Clostridium*, mainly *C. perfringens* and *C. botulinum*, clostridial food poisoning is caused by powerful toxins in contaminated foods. The *C. perfringens* spores are in soil, water, dust, and refuse, that is, virtually everywhere. The organism multiplies in cooked meat and meat dishes and develops its toxin in foods held for extended periods at warming or room temperatures. Thus, many reported outbreaks occur from food eaten in school cafeterias, college dining rooms, and restaurants. In each case, cooked meat was improperly handled in preparation and refrigeration. Control rests mainly on careful preparation and adequate cooking of meats, prompt service, and immediate refrigeration at sufficiently low temperatures. *C. botulinum* causes far more serious, often fatal food poisoning from eating food containing its powerful toxin. Depending on the dose of toxin taken and the individual response, the illness may vary from mild discomfort to death within 24 hours. Mortality rates are high. Vomiting, weakness,

---

dysentery A general term given to a number of disorders marked by inflammation of the intestines, especially of the colon, and attended by abdominal pain and frequent stools containing blood and mucus. The causative agent may be chemical irritants, bacteria, protozoa, or parasites.

endocarditis Inflammation of the *endocardium,* the serous membrane that lines the cavities of the heart.

meningitis Inflammation of the *meninges,* the three membranes that envelop the brain and spinal cord, caused by a bacterial or viral infection and characterized by high fever, severe headache, and stiff neck or back muscles.

sepsis Presence in the blood or other tissues of pathogenic microorganisms or their toxins; conditions associated with such pathogens.

and dizziness are initial complaints. Progressively, the toxin irritates motor nerve cells and blocks transmission of neural impulses at the nerve terminals, causing gradual paralysis. Sudden respiratory paralysis with airway obstruction is the major cause of death, especially in infants and young children.[27]

C. botulinum spores are widespread in soil throughout the world and may be carried on harvested food to the canning process. Like all clostridia, this species is anaerobic (develops in the absence of air) or nearly so. The relatively air-free can and the canning temperatures (above 27° C [80° F]) provide good conditions for toxin production. The development of high standards in the commercial canning industry has eliminated this source of botulism, but cases still result each year, mainly from eating carelessly home-canned foods. Boiling for 10 minutes destroys the toxin (not the spore), so all home-canned food, no matter how well preserved, should be boiled at least 10 minutes before eating. In the United States, Alaska and Washington have the highest incidence. Alaska has the greater number of botulism cases because of the native habits of eating uncooked or partially cooked meat that has been fermented, dried, or frozen.

Table 9.2 summarizes these bacterial sources of food contamination.

Viruses

Illnesses caused by viral contamination are few compared with those caused by bacterial contamination. Illnesses caused by viruses include upper respiratory infections, such as colds and influenza, and infections from hepatitis A virus (see Chapter 18). Explosive epidemics of infectious hepatitis have occurred in schools, towns, and other communities after fecal contamination of water, milk, or food. Contaminated shellfish from polluted waters have caused several outbreaks. Again, stringent control of community water and food supplies, as well as personal hygiene and sanitary practices of food handlers, are essential for prevention of disease.

CHANGES IN PERSONAL FOOD HABITS

BASIC DETERMINANTS OF FOOD CHOICE

We have discussed the broad areas of environment, culture, and psychosocial development, as well as modern food safety concerns, in terms of their influence on food habits. Clearly, some of the basic determinants of food choice focus on a variety of interacting physical, social, and physiologic factors, as summarized in Table 9.3. It is difficult to change some of our own eating patterns for health needs or personal desires. It is even more difficult to help our health care clients modify some of their habits, even when we understand their cultural patterns. We need to understand just how complex the factors are that influence the food choices persons make when they eat what they do (see *Practical Application* box, p. 203).

IMMIGRATION AND ETHNIC DIVERSITY

The story of immigration to the United States and our growing ethnic diversity is hardly a new one. It is one of the fundamental themes of this country's development. We have discussed the importance of these ethnic, cultural, and religious identities. In the United States we have many cultures and subcultures that have remained distinct or have become assimilated in varying degrees. Every group has contributed parts of its food habits to the general culture. In turn, American food patterns have infused into these new cultures, so that lines of difference are less distinct.

Americans of many different ethnic backgrounds have enriched our overall cultural patterns. We find varied and intermingling foods and food patterns blending with those of our own particular background (see *Issues & Answers*, p. 207). However, sometimes this happy intermingling of different cuisine has a cost. It does not always occur without difficulty and cultural dislocation.

Table
9.3   Factors determining food choices

Physical factors	Social factors	Physiologic factors
Food supply available	Advertising	Allergy
Food technology	Culture	Disability
Geography, agriculture, distribution	Education, nutrition, and general	Health-disease status
Personal economics, income	Political and economic policies	Personal food acceptance
Sanitation, housing	Religion and social customs	Needs, energy, or nutrients
Season, climate	Social class role	Therapeutic diets
Storage and cooking facilities	Social problems, poverty, or alcoholism	

To Probe Further

Food and Drug Administration guidelines for nutrition labeling regulations

Implementation of the 1990 Nutrition Labeling and Education Act (NLEA) has changed the way consumers look at food labels. This law, NLEA, was developed by the Food and Drug Administration (FDA) through a painstaking public process with consumers, food industry, and health professionals. It now empowers the FDA to enforce these regulations for the food industry and the public to help consumers make wise food choices.

The FDA label guidelines cover five main areas: nutrients and energy (as kcalories), serving sizes, definitions for terms used, label format, and health claims.

Nutrients and kcalories

The NLEA requires a food product to provide nutrient and energy information for the following:
- Protein (in terms of amino acid quality)
- Energy (as kcalories)
- Fat-soluble vitamins A, D, E, and K
- Water-soluble vitamins C, thiamin, riboflavin, niacin, pyridoxine (B_6), folate, and cobalamin (B_{12})
- Calcium, phosphorus, magnesium, iron, zinc, iodine, and selenium

On the revised label, new reference nutrient values have replaced the outdated and confusing term "U.S. RDAs." Instead, the terms now used are Reference Daily Intake (RDI) and Daily Reference Value (DRV). The RDIs are derived from the current 1989 RDAs and are population-based averages for all the age and sex groups of the current RDAs (excluding pregnant and lactating women, for whom the stated current RDAs apply). The DRV of a given nutrient in a food product is its content in that product expressed as a percentage of the RDI for that nutrient.

Serving sizes

Under the revised label rules, a standardized reference serving size is set for a large number of food categories in quantities customarily eaten. These portions are expressed in common household measures. The USDA has standardized serving sizes for meat and poultry products.

Descriptors

To improve communication between producers and consumers, everyone must work from the same FDA-supplied "dictionary." In this "dictionary" nine core terms have been defined: free, low, light or lite, less, high, source of, more, fresh, and reduced. The following are examples:
- *Fat free*—less than 0.5 g of fat per serving.
- *Low cholesterol*—20 mg of cholesterol or less per serving and per 100 g; 2 g saturated fat or less per serving. Any label claim about cholesterol is prohibited for all foods that contain more than 2 g of saturated fat per serving.
- *Light or lite*—at least a one-third reduction in kcalories (40 kcalories with minimum fat reduction of 3 g; if fat contributes 50% or more of kcalories, fat content must be reduced by 50% compared with the reference food).
- *Less sodium*—at least a 25% reduction or more than 140 mg per serving.
- *High*—20% or more of the RDI or DRV per serving.
- *Reduced saturated fat*—saturated fat content reduced by 50% or more, with a minimum reduction of more than 1 g per serving.

Nutrition label format

The standardized nutrition labeling format provided by the FDA is mandatory for all food producers and marketing agents. This format resulted from consumer research for developing sound nutrition information the consumers want and readily understand. It continues to serve as an important vehicle for nutrition education, as the law (NLEA) mandated.

The FDA guidelines indicate that any label health claim must be supported by substantial scientific evidence and has found that only four proposals meet this test and can be used: (1) sodium and hypertension, (2) calcium and osteoporosis, (3) lipids and cancer, and (4) lipids and cardiovascular disease.

References

FDA staff: The new food label: your guide to better nutrition, *Nutr Today* 25(1):37, 1992.

Legislative News: Terms on food labels: ADA comments on proposals from FDA and USDA, *J Am Diet Assoc* 2(3):543, 1992.

Pennington JAT, Wilkening VL: Final regulations for the nutrition labeling of raw fruits, vegetables, and fish, *J Am Diet Assoc* 97(11):1299, 1997.

Salton E et al: The new food label as a tool for healthy eating, *Nutr Today* 29(3):18, 1994.

Ethnic groups within the United States encounter a new world. Their lifestyles often undergo dramatic alterations, and the cultural integrity of the group can be severely shaken. Every group adapts in a unique way specific to its original culture and to the historic circumstances in which it undergoes the change.

CHANGING AMERICAN FOOD PATTERNS

Some traditional American food patterns are also changing. The stereotype of the all-American family with parents and two children eating three meals a day with a ban on snacking is no longer the common pattern. In the past two decades we have experienced far-reaching changes in our way of living and, subsequently, in our food patterns.

Households

The number of households is gradually increasing, and the alternate pattern of nontraditional households that are not families—that is, groups of unrelated persons or persons living alone—continues. By the year 2000 the average household size is expected to decline from 2.69 to 2.48, with husband-wife households decreasing from 58% to 53% of all households.[27,28] The number of children under age 5 will decline through this decade. The number of adults over age 65 will increase, and the greatest increase will be among those "oldest old" persons over age 85 years, who will have increased by 30%. The racial and ethnic population pattern will also have changed by the year 2000. Whites, not including Hispanics, will decline from 76% to 72% of the American population. Hispanics, the fastest growing population group, will increase from 8% to 11%. Blacks will increase from 12.4% to 13%. Other racial groups, including Native Americans, Alaskan natives, Asians, and Pacific Islanders, will increase from 3.5% to 4%.[28,29] These continuing trends indicate significant changes in the American social picture, part of a dynamic and rapidly changing society.

WORKING COUPLES

The number of women in the work force continues to increase rapidly. The increasing number of working couples is a trend that is not likely to reverse. By the year 2000, women of all racial and ethnic groups will be the major source of new entrants into the labor market, comprising 47% of the total work force, compared with 45% in 1988.[28,30] Between 1988 and 2000 white men will make up only 25% of the net growth of the labor force. There is a correlation between the education of women and their presence in the labor force; about 51% of college undergraduates are women. In general, women account for 30% of the enrollment in law schools, 25% in medical schools, 30% in business schools, and 12% in technical graduate schools. This phenomenon of working couples is not restricted to one social, economic, or eth-

nic group. It is a widespread societal change, bringing with it changes in the functioning of the family. Working parents rely on food items and cooking methods that save time and labor.

FAMILY MEALS

Family meals are less common. Many persons rarely eat breakfast and lunch in the family setting, but family dinners occur about 75% of the time. Often both parents work or the single parent works, and many late afternoon sports or other activities among the children curtail the time available for meal preparation and having the whole family sit down to eat at the same time.

HEALTH CONSCIOUSNESS

The interest of Americans in physical fitness continues. This has taken primarily two forms. First, there is more general nutrition awareness. Consumers have an increased interest in the nutrition content of their food, an expressed concern about a wholesome and safe food supply, and a strong support of the new nutrition labeling regulations. Interest in health claims on food products has increased, but there is some uncertainty about how to evaluate them. Second, there is more attention to weight watching, although not always through a healthy approach that includes regular meals with less fat combined with moderate regular physical exercise. More than half of the American population at any given time is on a weight-reducing diet. Consumers are interested in "light" foods perceived to be lower in kcalories.

ECONOMY

More and more Americans are economizing on food. Many supermarket shoppers are changing their diets primarily to save money. Consumers are stocking up on bargains and cutting back on expensive convenience foods. They are buying items in larger packages and in bulk and doing much less store hopping for bargains, staying with the store they consider to have the lowest overall prices. Brand loyalty has declined, and the purchase of generic products has increased. Consumers look more carefully at labels to gain information about comparative products.

GOURMET COOKING

The use of gourmet foods and specialty ethnic dishes has risen, and food specialty shops have sprung up in every shopping center. Gourmet cooking has become a popular hobby, and entertaining guests at home over a gourmet meal often displays the chef's skills in the elegance and quality of the food. This phenomenon parallels the general trend toward meals that are easy to fix, take little time, and fulfill the consumers' nutrition needs. Super-

Cultural sensitivity in nutritional care in a multicultural society: "Walk a mile in my shoes"

This familiar line from a popular American song of years past is a concise statement of deep truth: "You can never really know me and my life, my needs and inner thoughts, my joys and sorrows, my feelings and desires, my health or illness—until you walk a mile, many miles, in my shoes." It speaks volumes about the cultural sensitivity American health workers of all kinds need in order to do their work in an increasingly multicultural society.

Too often, pressures of time and circumstance mean that a health professional's individual culture may conflict with professional community nutrition health services or clinical medical nutrition therapy for persons of another culture. To apply the principles of cultural sensitivity embodied in the lines of the song quoted above, we need to understand and incorporate cultural awareness in all our nutrition work. This opportunity comes first in nutrition assessment, always the necessary basis for the nutritional care that is developed together with the client or family.

Nutrition assessment

Cultural knowledge is a needed foundation for sound nutritional care. We need to gather basic information about the client's culture, foods most frequently used, and how the culture influences food environment and behavior. Aspects of the family and community food environment that must be understood to provide relevant individual medical nutrition therapy and family guidance include the following:

- Types of food available
- Which foods are accepted and/or preferred
- Safety of food supply and related health problems
- Energy and nutrient quality of major foods chosen

Aspects of family and community food behaviors that must also be understood include the following:

- Most commonly used foods, who selects them, how and where they are obtained
- Food preparation, how divided among family/community
- Food eaten, how much, when, with whom, where
- Food storage, facilities and methods, food safety, garbage disposal

Skills needed for culturally sensitive care

Discovering special cultural knowledge is no small task. It may begin with regular library research, but it must broaden with techniques such as observation, participant observation, and informal interviewing.

Observation

Observe the neighborhood and homes in which clients live as well as where they shop for foods and the types of food available. If possible, a home visit may be planned, where facilities for food storage, food preparation, and eating may be informally discussed.

Participant observation

Learn more about the client group by participating in their activities. For example, read the same newspaper, listen to the same radio sta- tions, go to the same community meetings, and shop in the same food markets that clients use.

Informal interviewing

Learn more about the client group by interviewing individuals from or closely associated with the client group. Ask relevant questions about food and health behaviors or other health care professionals who serve the cultural group, any community leaders among the group, and any other members of the group.

Recognizing the rapidly changing United States environment for health care, public health leaders, through a national survey, have recently identified future training needs for all nutrition practitioners by the year 2005. In both categories surveyed—health education changes needed and the most important routine knowledge areas and skills required— one repeated specific statement stood out among the top responses: "Greater cultural sensitivity and skills to develop culturally relevant programs and services; bilingual practitioners."

References

Cassidy CM: Walk a mile in my shoes: culturally sensitive food-habit research, *Am J Clin Nutr* 59(suppl 1S): 190S, 1994.

Pobocik RS, Shovic AC: Development of a nutrition exchange booklet for Guam using culturally accepted foods, *J Am Diet Assoc* 96(3):285, 1996.

Shovic AC: Development of a Samoan nutrition exchange list using culturally accepted foods, *J Am Diet Assoc* 94(5):541, 1994.

Terry RD: Needed: a new appreciation of culture and food behavior, *J Am Diet Assoc* 94(5):501, 1994.

markets are establishing special gourmet deli shops and specialty fast-foods, take-out picnic baskets, and other creative items.

FAST-FOODS

Today approximately one third of all food that Americans eat is eaten away from home, much of it from fast-food restaurants. About 46 million people eat at a fast-food restaurant each day, about 1 out of every 12 meals.[30] Several factors have contributed to this phenomenal increase in the use of fast-food, including a greater number of working women, dual-career families, more diverse schedules of family members, an aging population, and an increasing number of one- and two-person households. Fast-foods meet the needs of many people because they are quick, reasonably priced, and readily available. Also, currently these restaurants are responding to the health concerns of their customers by changing some of their practices, such as the continued trend toward the use of vegetable oils instead of animal fats for frying, an increase in the number of low-fat menu items, and more fruits and vegetables available at salad bars. Food industry analysts even paint a future of increasing home delivery services, high-quality vending machine foods, and ready-to-eat packages for microwave-equipped homes.[30]

TO SUM UP

We all grow up and live our lives in a social context. We each inherit at least one cultural background and live in our particular society's social structure, complete with food habits and attitudes about eating. It is from a social perspective that we can best examine changes in food habits. We need to understand the effects on health that are associated with major social and economic shifts. We also need to understand current social forces to best help persons make new dietary changes that will benefit their health. We must meet concerns about food misinformation and food safety.

The United States has a long history of immigration. Every new group has adjusted to life in the new country in its own way. They have contributed a unique ethnic diversity to American life and food patterns.

Traditional American food patterns are changing in a number of ways. We increasingly rely on food technology in our fast, complex life. More women are employed, households are getting smaller, more and more persons are living alone, and our meal patterns are different. We search for less fancy, lower-cost food items, and also creative gourmet cooking for special occasions. In general we are more nutrition and health conscious. Fast-food outlets have increased and become a large factor in our changing food patterns.

QUESTIONS FOR REVIEW

1. Describe some ways in which environmental factors interact to produce malnutrition and give examples.
2. What is the meaning of culture? How does it affect our food patterns?
3. What are some social and psychologic factors that influence our food habits? Give examples of personal meanings related to food.
4. Why does the public tend to accept nutrition misinformation so easily? What groups are more susceptible? Select one such group and give some effective approaches you might use in reaching them with sound nutrition information.
5. How do food misinformation and concerns about food safety affect food habits?
6. What is the basis of concern about food additives and pesticide residues?
7. In what ways does ethnic diversity enrich American food patterns? Give several examples.
8. Name several trends in America's changing food patterns and discuss their implications for nutrition and health.

REFERENCES

1. Jelliffe DB, Jelliffe EFP: Causation of kwashiorkor: toward a multi-factorial consensus, *Pediatrics* 90:110, 1992.
2. Godal T: Fighting the parasites of poverty: public research, private industry, and tropical diseases, *Science* 264(5167):1864, 1994.
3. Beckman D et al: Position of the American Dietetic Association: world hunger, *J Am Diet Assoc* 95(10):1160, 1995.
4. Vozenilek GP: Dietetics in the fight against domestic hunger, *J Am Diet Assoc* 98(3):266, 1998.
5. Singh GK, Yu SM: Infant mortality in the United States: trends, differentials, and projections, 1950 through 2010, *Am J Public Health* 85(7):957, 1995.
6. Bird ST, Bauman KE: The relationship between structural and health services variables and state-level infant mortality in the United States, *Am J Public Health* 85(1):26, 1995.
7. Staff report: Public policy news: ADA action on food security and proposed federal regulations, *J Am Diet Assoc* 97(9):952, 1997.
8. Kendall A, Kennedy E: Position of the American Dietetic Association: Domestic food and nutrition security, *J Am Diet Assoc* 98(3):337, 1998.
9. Maslow AH: *Motivation and personality*, New York, 1954, Harper & Row.
10. Thomas PR: Food for thought about dietary supplements, *Nutr Today* 31(2):46, 1996.
11. Stephenson MG, Guthrie HA: Positions of the American Dietetic Association: enrichment and fortification of foods and dietary supplements, *J Am Diet Assoc* 94(6):661, 1994.

12. Hillars VN et al: Roles of food and nutrition educators in food safety discussions, *J Nutr Ed* 26(5):246, 1994.

13. FDA Backgrounder Statement: Biotechnology of food, *Nutr Today* 29(4):19, 1994.

14. Schmidt K: Genetic engineering yields first pest-resistant seeds, *Science* 265(5190):1472, 1994.

15. Hahn NI: Growing a healthy food system, *J Am Diet Assoc* 97(9):950, 1997.

16. Legislative Highlights: Final food labeling regulations, *J Am Diet Assoc* 93(2):146, 1993.

17. Pennington JAT, Wilkening VL: Final regulations for the nutrition labeling of raw fruits, vegetables, and fish, *J Am Diet Assoc* 97(11):1299, 1997.

18. Staff report, nutrition science and policy: Food labeling: a Canadian and international perspective, *Nutr Rev* 53(4):103, 1995.

19. Conkling W: Uninvited guests, *Am Health* 13(8):50, 1994.

20. Boyce TG et al: *Escherichia coli 0157:H7* and the hemolytic-uremic syndrome, *N Engl J Med* 333(6):364, 1995.

21. Buchanan RL, Doyle MP: Foodborne disease significance of *Escherichia coli 0157:H7* and other enterohemorrhagic *E. coli*, *Food Technology* 51(10):69, 1997.

22. Juneja VK et al: Thermal destruction of *Escherichia coli 0157:H7* in hamburger, *J Food Protection* 60(10);1163, 1997.

23. Mohle-Boetani JC et al: Community-wide shigellosis: control of an outbreak and risk factors in child day-care centers, *Am J Public Health* 85(6):812, 1995.

24. Armstrong D: Listeria monocytogenes. In Mandel GL, Bennett JE, eds: *Principles and practice of infectious diseases*, ed 4, New York, 1995, Churchill Livingstone.

25. Hedberg K et al: Listeriosis in Minnesota, January 1986 through May 1988, *Am J Public Health* 85(9):1293, 1995.

26. Schreiner MJ et al: Infant botulism: a review of 12 years' experience at Children's Hospital of Philadelphia, *Pediatrics* 87(2):159, 1991.

27. Bureau of the Census: *Projects of households and families:1886 to 2000*, Washington, DC, 1986, US Department of Commerce.

28. US Department of Health and Human Services, Public Health Services: *Healthy people 2000: national health promotion and disease prevention objectives*, Pub No 91-50212, Washington, DC, 1990, US Government Printing Office.

29. Spencer G: *Projections of the population of the United States by age, sex, and race: 1985 to 2080, current population reports, population estimates and projections*, Series P-25, No 1018, Washington, DC, 1989, US Department of Commerce, Bureau of the Census.

30. Price K et al: Fast foods: the current state of affairs, *Diet Curr* 18(4):1, 1991.

■ FURTHER READING

Cieslak PR et al: Hamburger-associated *Escherichia coli* O157:H7 infection in Las Vegas: a hidden epidemic, *Am J Public Health* 87(2):176, 1997.

Tilden J Jr et al: A new route of transmission for *Escherichia coli*: infection from dry fermented salami, *Am J Public Health* 86(8):1142, 1996.

Angulo FJ et al: A community waterborne outbreak of Salmonellosis and the effectiveness of a boil water order, *Am J Public Health* 87(4):580, 1997.

These three reports of community disease outbreaks describe the intense investigations of infection sources, two with meat—hamburgers and salami—and one with a community water source. Rapid public response in the meat cases helped investigators stop further spread quickly. But in the case of the contaminated water supply, even after immediate and continuous warnings via local radio to boil all drinking water, a number of persons became seriously ill, their foolish and dangerous excuses for not complying being "I forgot" and "I didn't believe it."

Ingham S, Thies ML: Position of the American Dietetic Association: food and water safety, *J Am Diet Assoc* 97(2):184, 1997.

This professional statement outlines the responsibility of all collaborating health workers to maintain a safe food and water supply, and describes ways in which all persons involved can work together to ensure this safety level at all times. A current list of food safety education resources for professionals is provided.

Case study

Faddism and economic problems: a young family trying to cope

Helen Brown, age 20, and her husband Charles, age 21, live in a small flat in the low-rent district of the city with their three children—a boy of 3, a girl of 18 months, and their new baby of 6 weeks. Helen has gained weight, so that she now weighs 93 kg (205 lb). She feels old and unattractive. She has always been rather dependent on her mother and lately on her husband, but now she seems less and less able to cope.

Charles works in a gas station during the day and sometimes gets extra mechanic work at night, but he barely makes enough to meet expenses. Many bills are unpaid, friction between Charles and Helen has increased, and Charles is increasingly away from home.

About the time that Helen came home from the county hospital with the new baby, Helen's mother, Mrs. Miller, age 50, came to live with the Brown fam-

Continued

Case study

Faddism and economic problems:
a young family trying to cope—cont'd

ily. She had been living alone, but her arthritis had begun to cripple her, so she could no longer work or care for herself.

A district public health nurse in the county, Miss Jordan, visited Helen and her new baby for a 6-week checkup. When Miss Jordan arrived at the apartment, she found Helen distraught and in tears. Charles, she said, had gone off to work that morning angrily saying that he might not return until she grew up and learned how to manage things better. Helen was wearing an old housecoat, and her hair was uncombed. She had a formula bottle in her hand, seemingly not knowing quite what to do with it. The apartment was crowded and cluttered. Dishes filled the small kitchen sink, and every available space seemed taken up with used utensils. The two older children were thin and fretful, hitting at each other over a toy both wanted and pulling at their mother's housecoat for her attention.

Although it was midmorning, the children had had no breakfast. The baby was crying in the crib in the corner of the room, waiting for the bottle that Helen was trying to fix to feed her. Helen's mother was lying on the sofa with her crutches close by.

Miss Jordan offered to feed the baby. After the feeding Miss Jordan weighed the baby and found that she was not gaining weight as she should. Helen said that none of the formula seemed to agree with the baby and she was constantly spitting it up.

At this point, Mrs. Bryant, who lived in the flat above, knocked on the door. She brought a bottle of food supplement to Helen, for which Helen, after searching and finally finding her purse, gave her a $10 bill. While Helen was searching for her purse, Mrs. Bryant enthusiastically told Miss Jordan about her special health food products.

"This is a special high-protein food supplement. It isn't sold through stores but only through special agents like me who know its real worth. You know, all this processed food you buy in markets is worthless. There's no food value left in it. It's no wonder everybody's half sick. It's all caused by bad diet. But this supplement will make the difference. It's a natural food substance, organically grown. It's the very thing Helen needs to get her strength back and help her lose weight. As for the children," she continued, "it's just what they need, too, to put some meat on their bones."

Then Mrs. Bryant turned to Helen's mother and patted her arm. "You poor dear. As soon as you start using this, too, a double dose daily for awhile, your arthritis will be cured."

As she was leaving, Mrs. Bryant said to Miss Jordan, "You look a little peaked yourself. You could use some, too. Here let me leave this leaflet with you that tells all about it."

After Mrs. Bryant left, Helen explained that Charles' anger that morning resulted from her buying the expensive special food supplement when their family budget was so tight.

After talking with Helen and her mother, Miss Jordan made definite arrangements to return the following week. As she drove away from the apartment building, she was thinking about her observations and the problems she had encountered in the Brown family. Already she had decided that when she returned to the district public health office, she would consult with the nutritionist and leave the supplement pamphlet with her to investigate. She also decided to speak with the psychiatric nursing consultant and a social worker in the social services department.

Questions to Guide Your Inquiry

1. Imagine you are the nutritionist or the nurse. What important questions come to your mind from your observations?

2. What problems do you identify? What are Helen's needs? What are her husband's needs?

3. What solutions do you propose? How would you involve other health department persons in you plan of action?

4. Consider each of the children. What growth and development needs—physical, psychosocial, and nutritional—does each child have? What food and feeding practices are related? (See Chapter 12.)

5. What actions do you propose to meet each child's needs?

6. What are Mrs. Miller's needs? Do you think nutrition is related to arthritis?

7. Why is this family vulnerable to the "health food" sales pressures of the neighbor, Mrs. Bryant?

8. What food myths or misinformation did you find? What dangers are involved in such food fads or misinformation? Why does food faddism exist? What can health workers do about food fads?

9. What additional information would you need to work with this family toward some positive goals? What possible sources or means would you use to obtain this information?

Issues Answers

The spice of ethnic diversity in American food patterns

In the area of good food, the increasing ethnic diversity in the United States population is cause for celebration! Our taste buds celebrate the spice such ethnic diversity brings to American food patterns. Older American traditions from a variety of cultures mingle with more recent arrivals to provide a smorgasbord of ethnic experiences. Each reflects the culture in which it developed, based on both religious laws and regional influences.

Religious Dietary Laws

Jewish

Observance of Jewish food laws differs among the three basic groups within Judaism: (1) Orthodox—strict observance, (2) conservative—less strict, and (3) reform—less ceremonial emphasis and minimum general use. The basic body of dietary laws is called the Rules of Kashruth. Foods selected and prepared according to these rules are called kosher, from the Hebrew word meaning "fit, proper." Originally these laws had special ritual significance. Present Jewish dietary laws apply this significance to laws governing the slaughter, preparation, and serving of the meat, to the combining of meat and milk, to fish, and to eggs. Various food restrictions exist.

1. *Meat.* No pork is used. Forequarters of other meats are allowed, as well as all commonly used forms of poultry. All forms of meat used are rigidly cleansed of all blood.
2. *Meat and milk.* No combining of meat and milk is allowed. Orthodox homes maintain two sets of dishes, one for serving meat and the other for meals using dairy products.
3. *Fish.* Only fish with fins and scales are allowed. These may be eaten with either meat or dairy meals. No shellfish or eels may be used.
4. *Eggs.* No egg with a blood spot may be eaten. Eggs may be used with either meat or dairy meals.

Many of the traditional Jewish foods relate to festivals of the Jewish calendar that commemorate significant events in Jewish history. Often special Sabbath foods are used. A few representative foods include:

- **Bagels**— Doughnut-shaped, hard yeast rolls.
- **Blintzes** —Thin filled and rolled pancakes.
- **Borscht (borsch)**—Soup of meat stock, mixed with beaten egg or sour cream, beets, cabbage, or spinach. Served hot or cold.
- **Challah**—Sabbath loaf of white bread, shaped as a twist or coil, used at the beginning of the meal after the kiddush, the blessing over wine.
- **Gefullte (gefilte fish)**—From a German word meaning "stuffed fish," usually the first course of Sabbath evening meal, made of fish fillet, chopped and seasoned and stuffed back into the skin or rolled into balls.
- **Kasha**—Buckwheat groats (hulled kernels), used as a cooked cereal or as a potato substitute with gravy.
- **Knishes**—Pastry filled with ground meat or cheese.
- **Lox**—Smoked, salted salmon.
- **Matzo**—Flat unleavened bread.
- **Strudel**—Thin pastry filled with fruit and nuts, rolled and baked.

Moslem

Moslem dietary laws are based on restrictions or prohibitions on some foods and promotion of others, derived from Islamic teachings in the Koran. The laws are binding and must be followed at all times, even during pregnancy, hospitalization, or travel. The general rule is that "all foods are permitted" unless specifically conditioned or prohibited.

1. *Milk products.* Permitted at all times.
2. *Fruits and vegetables.* Except if fermented or poisonous.
3. *Breads and cereals.* Unless contaminated or harmful.
4. *Meats.* Seafood, including fish, shellfish, eels, and sea animals, and land animals except swine; pork is strictly prohibited.
5. *Alcohol.* Strictly prohibited.

Any food combinations are used as long as no prohibited items are included. Milk and meat may be eaten together, in contrast to Jewish kosher laws. The Koran mentions certain foods as being of special value: figs, olives, dates, honey, milk, and buttermilk. Prohibited foods in the Moslem dietary laws may be eaten when no other sources of food are available.

Continued

Among the Moslem people, a 30-day period of daylight fasting is required during Ramadan, the ninth month of the Islamic lunar calendar, thus rotating through all seasons. The fourth pillar of Islam commanded by the Koran is fasting. Ramadan was chosen for the sacred fast because it is the month in which Mohammed received the first of the revelations that were subsequently compiled to form the Koran and also the month in which his followers first drove their enemies from Mecca in AD 624. During the month of Ramadan, Moslems throughout the world observe daily fasting, taking no food or drink from dawn to sunset. Nights, however, are often spent in special feasts. First, an appetizer is taken, such as dates or a fruit drink, followed by the family's "evening breakfast," the *iftar*. At the end of Ramadan a traditional feast lasting up to 3 days climaxes the observance. Special dishes mark this occasion. There are delicacies such as thin pancakes dipped in powdered sugar, savory buns, and dried fruits.

Spanish (Hispanic) and Native American influences
Mexican
Food habits of early Spanish settlers and Indian nations form the basis of present food patterns of persons of Mexican (Hispanic) heritage who now live in the United States, chiefly in the Southwest. Three foods are basic to this pattern: dried beans, chili peppers, and corn. Variations and additions may be found in different places or among those of different income levels. Relatively small amounts of meat and occasional eggs are used. Fruit, such as oranges, apples, and bananas, or papayas and mangos are used, depending on availability. For centuries corn has been the basic grain used as bread in the form of tortillas, which are flat cakes baked on a hot griddle. Some wheat is used in making tortillas; rice and oat are added cereals. Coffee is a main beverage. Major seasonings are chili peppers, onions, and garlic; the basic fat is lard.

Puerto Rican
The Puerto Rican people share a common heritage with the Mexicans, so much of their food pattern is similar. They add tropical fruits and vegetables, many of which are available in their neighborhood markets in the United States. A main type of food is *viandas*, starchy vegetables and fruits such as plantain and green bananas. Two other staples of the diet are rice and beans. Milk, meat, yellow and green vegetables, and other fruits are used in limited quantities, but dried codfish is a staple food. Coffee is a main beverage. Lard is the main cooking fat.

Native American
The Native American population, Indian and Alaskan Natives, is composed mainly of more than 500 federally recognized diverse groups living on reservations, in small rural communities, or in metropolitan areas. Despite their individual diversity, the various groups share a spiritual attachment to the land and a determination to retain their culture. Food has great religious and social significance, and is an integral part not only of celebrations and ceremonies but also of everyday hospitality, which includes a serious obligation for serving food. Foods may be prepared and used in different ways from region to region and vary according to what can be grown locally, harvested or hunted on the land or fished from its rivers, or is available in food markets. Among the Native American groups of the southwest United States, the food pattern of the Navajo people, whose reservations extend over a 25,000–square mile area in the junction of three states—New Mexico, Arizona, and Utah, may serve as an example.

Historically, the Navajos learned farming from the early Pueblo people, establishing corn and other crops as staples. Later they learned herding from the Spaniards, making sheep and goats available for food and wool. Some families also raised chickens, pigs, and cattle. Currently, Navajo food habits combine traditional dietary staples with modern food products available from supermarkets and fast-food restaurants. Meat is eaten daily—fresh mutton, beef, pork, chicken, or smoked or processed meat. Other staples include bread—tortillas or fry bread, blue cornbread, and cornmeal mush; beverages—coffee, soft drinks, and fruit-flavored drinks; eggs; vegetables—corn, potatoes, green beans, tomatoes; and some fresh or canned fruit. Frying is a common method of food preparation; lard and shortening are main cooking fats. There is an increased use of modern snack foods high in fat, sugar, calories, and sodium, especially among children and teenagers.

Southern United States influences
African Americans
The black populations, especially in the Southern states, have contributed a rich heritage of American food patterns, particularly to Southern cooking as a whole. Like their moving original music of spirituals, blues, gospel, and jazz, Southern black food patterns were born of hard times, and developed through a creative ability to turn any basic staples at hand into memorable food. Although regional differences occur as with any basic food pattern, surveys indicate representative use of foods from basic food groups:
1. *Breads/cereals.* Traditional breads include hot breads such as biscuits, spoonbread (a souffle-like dish of cornmeal mush with beaten eggs), cornmeal muffins, and skillet cornbread. Commonly used cereals are cooked cereals such as cornmeal mush, hominy grits (ground corn), and oatmeal. In general, more cooked cereal is used than ready-to-eat dry cereals.
2. *Eggs/dairy products.* Eggs are used and some cheese, but little milk, probably as a result of the greater prevalence of lactose intolerance among blacks than among whites.

3. *Vegetables.* A frequent type of vegetable is leafy greens: turnip greens, collards, mustard greens, and spinach, usually cooked with bacon or salt pork. Cabbage is used boiled or chopped raw with a salad dressing (cole slaw). Other vegetables used include okra (coated with cornmeal and fried), sweet potatoes (baked whole or sliced and candied with added sugar), green beans, tomatoes, potatoes, corn, butterbeans (lima), and dried beans such as black-eyed peas or red beans cooked with smoked ham hocks and served over rice. The black-eyed peas over rice is a dish called Hopping John, traditionally served on New Year's Day for good luck in the new year.
4. *Fruits.* Commonly used fruits include apples, peaches, berries, oranges, bananas, and juices.
5. *Meat.* Pork is a common meat, including fresh cuts and ribs, sausage, and smoked ham. Some beef is used, mainly ground for meat loaf or hamburgers. Poultry is used frequently, mainly fried chicken, and baked holiday turkey. Organ meats such as liver, heart, intestines (chitterlings), or poultry giblets (gizzard and heart) are used. When it is available, fish used includes catfish, some flounder, and shellfish such as crab and shrimp. Frying is a common method of cooking; fats used are lard, shortening, or vegetable oils.
6. *Desserts.* Favorites include pies—pecan, sweet potato, pumpkin, and deep-dish peach or berry cobblers; cakes such as coconut and chocolate; and bread pudding to use leftover bread.
7. *Beverages.* Coffee, apple cider, fruit juices, lemonade, iced tea, carbonated soft drinks, and buttermilk, a better-tolerated form of milk.

French Americans

The Cajun people of the southwestern costal waterways in southern Louisiana have contributed a unique cuisine and food pattern to America's rich and varied fare. It provides a model for learning about rapidly expanding forms of American ethnic food. The Cajuns are descendants of the early French colonists of Acadia, a peninsula on the eastern coast of Canada now known as Nova Scotia. In the pre-Revolutionary wars between France and Britain, both countries contended for the area of Acadia. However, after Britain finally gained control of all of Canada, fear of an Acadian revolt led to a forcible deportation of French colonists in 1755. After a long and difficult journey down the Atlantic coast, then westward along the Gulf of Mexico, a group of the impoverished Acadians finally settled along the bayou country of what is now Louisiana. To support themselves, they developed their unique food pattern from seafood at hand and what they could grow and harvest. Over time they blended their own French culinary background with the Creole cookery they found in their new homeland around New Orleans, which had descended from classical French cuisine combined with other European, American Indian, and African dishes.

Thus the unique Cajun food pattern of the southern United States represents an ethnic blending of cultures using basic foods available in the area. Cajun foods are strong-flavored and spicy, with the abundant seafood as a base, usually cooked as stew and served over rice. The well-known hot chili sauce, made of crushed and fermented red chili peppers blended with spices and vinegar and sold world wide under the trade name Tabasco sauce, is still made by generations of a Cajun family on Avery Island on the coastal waterway of southern Louisiana. The most popular shellfish native to the region is the crawfish, now grown commercially in the fertile rice paddies of the bayou area. Other seafood used includes catfish, red snapper, shrimp, blue crab, and oysters. Cajun dishes usually start with a *roux* made from heated oil and flour mixed with liquid to form a sauce base, to which vegetables, then meat or seafood, and seasonings are added to form a stew. Vegetables used include onions, bell peppers, parsley, shallots, and tomatoes; seasonings are cayenne (red) pepper, hot pepper sauce (Tabasco), crushed black pepper, white pepper, bay leaves, thyme, and *filé* powder. *Filé* powder is made from ground sassafras leaves and serves both to season and to thicken the dish being made. Some typical Cajun dishes include seafood or chicken gumbo, jambalaya (dish of Creole origin, combining rice, chicken, ham, pork, sausage, broth, vegetables, and seasonings), red beans and rice, blackened catfish or red snapper (blackened with pepper and seasonings and seared in a hot pan), barbecued shrimp, breaded catfish with Creole sauce, and boiled crawfish. Breads and starches include French bread, hush puppies (fried cornbread-mixture balls), cornbread muffins, cushcush (cornmeal mush cooked with milk), grits (hominy, ground corn), rice, and yams. Vegetables include okra, squash, onions, bell peppers, and tomatoes. Desserts include ambrosia (fresh fruits such as oranges and bananas with grated coconut), sweet potato pie, pecan pie, berry pie, bread pudding, or pecan pralines.

Eastern-Oriental food patterns

Chinese

Chinese cooks believe that refrigeration diminishes natural flavors. Therefore they select the freshest foods possible, hold them the shortest time possible, then cook them quickly at a high temperature in a *wok* with only small amounts of fat and liquid. This basic round-bottom pan allows control of heat in a quick stir-frying method that preserves natural flavor, color, and texture. Vegetables cooked just before serving are still crisp and flavorful when served. Meat is used in small amounts in combined dishes rather than as a single main entree. Little milk is used but eggs and soybean products such as tofu add protein. Foods that have been dried, salted, pickled, spiced, candied, or canned may be added as garnishes or relishes to mask some flavors or textures or to enhance other. Fruits are usually eaten fresh. Rice is the staple

Continued

grain used at most meals. The traditional beverage is unsweetened green tea. Seasonings include soy sauce, ginger, almonds, and sesame seed. Peanut oil is a main cooking fat.

Japanese

In some ways, Japanese food patters are similar to those of the Chinese. Rice is a basic grain at meals, soy sauce is used for seasoning, and tea is the main beverage. The Japanese diet contains more seafood, especially raw fish items, which may be used in dishes such as *sashimi* and *sushi*. Many varieties of fish and shellfish are used. Vegetables are usually steamed; some are pickled. Fresh fruit is eaten in season, a tray of fruit being a regular course at main meals.

Southeast Asian

Since 1971, in the wake of the war in Vietnam, more than 340,000 Southeast Asians have come to the United States as refugees. The largest group are Vietnamese; others have come from the adjacent war-torn countries of Laos and Cambodia. They have settled mainly in California, with other groups in Florida, Texas, Illinois, and Pennsylvania. Their basic food patterns are similar. They are making an impact on American diet and agriculture, and Asian grocery stores stock many traditional Indo-Chinese food items. Rice, both long-grain and glutinous, forms the basis of the Indonesian food pattern, and it is eaten at most meals. The Vietnamese usually eat rice plain in a separate rice bowl and not mixed with other foods, whereas other Southeast Asians may eat rice in mixed dishes. Soups are also commonly used at meals. Many fresh fruits and vegetables are used along with fresh herbs and other seasonings such as chives, spring onions, chili peppers, ginger root, coriander, turmeric, and fish sauce. Many kinds of fish and shellfish are used, as well as chicken, duck, pork, and beef. Stir-frying in a wok-type pan with a small amount of lard or peanut oil is a common method of cooking. A variety of vegetables and seasonings are used, with small amounts of seafood or meat added. Since coming to the United States, the Indonesians have made some diet changes that reflect American influence. These include use of more eggs, beef and pork, but less seafood, more candy and other sweet snacks, bread, fast-foods, soft drinks, butter and margarine, and coffee.

Mediterranean influences

Italian food patterns

The sharing of food is an important part of Italian life. Meals are associated with warmth and fellowship, and special occasions are shared with families and friends. Bread and pasta are basic foods. Milk, seldom used alone, is typically mixed with coffee in equal portions. Cheese is a favorite food, with many popular varieties. Meats, poultry, and fish are used in many ways, and the varied Italian sausages and cold cuts are famous. Vegetables are used alone, in mixed main dishes or soups, in sauces, and in salads. Seasonings include herbs and spices, garlic, wine, olive oil, tomato puree, and salt pork. Main dishes are prepared by initially browning vegetables and seasonings in olive oil; adding meat or fish for browning as well; covering with such liquids as wine, broth, or tomato sauce; and simmering slowly on low heat for several hours. Fresh fruit is often the dessert or a snack.

Greek

Everyday meals are simple, but Greek holiday meals are occasions for serving many delicacies. Bread is always the center of every meal, with other foods considered accompaniments. Milk is seldom used as a beverage, but rather as the cultured form of yogurt. Cheese is a favorite food, especially *feta*, a white cheese made from the sheep's milk and preserved in brine. Lamb is a favorite meat, but others, especially fish, are used also. Eggs are sometimes a main dish, never a breakfast food. Many vegetables are used, often as a main entree, cooked with broth, tomato sauce, onions, olive oil, and parsley. A typical salad of thinly sliced raw vegetables and feta cheese, dressed with olive oil and vinegar, is often served with meals. Rice is a main grain in many dishes. Fruit is an everyday dessert, but rich pastries, such as *baklava* are served on special occasions.

References

Broussard-Marin L, Hynak-Hankinson MT: Ethnic food, the use of Cajun cuisine as a model, *J Am Diet Assoc* 89(8):1117, 1989.

Chau P et al: Dietary habits, health beliefs, and food practices of elderly Chinese women, *J Am Diet Assoc* 90(4):579, 1990.

For your information: a look at Japanese Dietary Guidelines, *J Am Diet Assoc* 90(11):1527, 1990.

Monsen ER: Respecting diversity helps America eat right, *J Am Diet Assoc* 92(3):282, 1992.

Nobmann ED et al: The diet of Alaska Native adults, *Am J Clin Nutr* 55:1024, 1992.

Nomani MZA et al: Effects of Ramadan fasting on plasma uric acid and body weight in healthy men, J Am Diet Assoc 90(10):1435, 1990.

Stowers SL: Development of a culturally appropriate food guide for pregnant Caribbean immigrants in the United States, *J Am Diet Assoc* 92(3):331, 1992.

Chapter

10

Family Nutrition Counseling: Food Needs and Costs

This chapter continues the two-chapter opening sequence on food habits and family nutrition counseling that introduces Part 2 of your study on Community Nutrition and the Life Cycle.

In the previous chapter we considered the food environment and influences that shape food habits. Here we continue with family counseling and education approaches to meeting health problems, frequently in the face of economic hardships.

Often in our clinics and communities we must interpret complex information in a variety of settings to meet numerous family health and nutrition needs. Here, then, we seek approaches and resources to help meet these needs.

FAMILY NUTRITION COUNSELING

Community health workers frequently need to apply the principles of health teaching in family nutrition counseling. Health and nutrition are inseparable, and the term *counseling* is appropriate.[1] If we work with the family on the basis of counseling principles, various members are led to explore their own situation, to express their needs, and to find ways of meeting those needs that are best suited to their particular life situation. It has long been evident that societies shape their own patterns of disease; sociodemographic factors largely determine health at all ages.[2-4] Our job is to help persons and families explore their options and make decisions in the light of knowledge and personal support.

PERSON-CENTERED GOALS

Realistic family diet counseling must be person-centered. It involves close attention to personal and family needs, nutrition and health problems, and food choices and costs. In our work we have three main goals: (1) to obtain basic information about the client and the living situation that relates to nutrition and health needs, (2) to provide basic health teaching to help meet these needs, and (3) to support the client and family in all personal efforts to meet needs through encouragement, reinforcement, general caring and concern, and practical resources. A basic skill that all health workers must learn, therefore, is the skill of talking with clients in a helpful manner.

INTERVIEWING

Skills in interviewing are essential in health care. Interviewing does not necessarily mean only the more formal or structured history-taking activity; frequently it means a purposeful planned conversation either in the hospital, clinic, or home. It may be a simple telephone call to the home to determine ongoing needs or progress. General principles of interviewing should guide these activities, including the purpose or focus, means used to achieve the purpose, and measuring results.

Focus and purpose

As indicated, the focus of all health care is the individual client and personal health needs. It may be a small intermediate goal relating to some aspect of the overall care, or it may be a long-term goal. Our ultimate purpose is to provide whatever help the individual or family may need to determine personal health needs and goals and to work with the person or family in finding ways of meeting these needs and goals.

Means used to achieve purpose

Health workers use various means of accomplishing these purposes—building a helping relationship, creating a comfortable climate, and developing positive attitudes.

1. *Relationship.* Counseling is a dynamic person-centered process built on a helping relationship. This is reflected in the common use of the word *services* for all health care–related activities. The most important means of helping a person is establishing a relationship of mutual trust and respect. The most significant tool we ever have for helping others is ourselves. Our role is that of a helping vehicle. Within this kind of relationship, true healing can take place.

2. *Climate.* The kind of climate we create involves both the physical setting and the psychologic feelings involved. The physical setting should be as comfortable as possible in relation to space, ventilation, heating, lighting, and sitting or lying down. Other important factors include providing sufficient time for the interview in a quiet setting free from interruptions and with sufficient privacy to assure confidentiality. If it is in an office setting, the desk should be to the side, not between the therapist and client.

3. *Attitudes.* The word *attitude* refers to that aspect of personality that accounts for a consistent behavior toward persons, situations, or objects. Our attitudes are learned. Hence they develop from life experiences and influences. Because they are learned, they can be examined. We can become more aware of them. We can try to strengthen those attitudes that are desirable and constructive, and at the same time seek to change or modify those attitudes that are less desirable and more destructive. If a health worker is to be able to help meet clients' needs, certain attitudes are necessary components of behavior:
   - *Warmth.* A genuine concern for the client or patient is displayed by interest, friendliness, and kindness; we convey warmth by being thoughtful.
   - *Acceptance.* We must meet clients as they are and where they are. To accept the client does not necessarily mean approval of behavior. It does mean a realization that clients or patients usually regard their behavior as purposeful and meaningful. It may be a means of handling stress. An attitude of acceptance conveys that a person's thoughts, ideas, and actions are important and worth attention simply because a human being has the right to be treated as having worth and dignity.
   - *Objectivity.* To be objective is to be free of bias. It is having a nonjudgmental attitude. Of course, complete objectivity is impossible, but reasonable objectivity is certainly a goal that can be attained. We must be aware of our own feelings and biases, and we should attempt to control them. The evaluation of a situation must be based on what is actually happening, that is, the facts as we perceive them, not on mere opinions, assumptions, or inferences.

- *Compassion.* An attitude of compassion enables us to feel with and for another person or oneself. It means accepting the impact of an emotion, holding it long enough to absorb its meaning, and entering into a kind of fellowship of feeling with the person who is moved by the emotion. There is nothing easy in developing the attitude of compassion; it requires emotional maturity.

Measuring results

Continuous and terminal evaluation of our interviews is an ongoing part of our activity. Evaluation is measuring how behavioral changes in the client and in ourselves are related to the needs and goals that have been identified. In summary, therefore, health workers will always be dealing with the following sequence of questions in interviewing:

1. *Need.* What is wrong? What is the health problem or need of the client or patient?
2. *Goal.* What does the client want to do about it? What is the client's immediate goal? What is the long-range goal?
3. *Information.* What information do I need to know to help the client? What does the client need to know to help take care of personal needs? What knowledge and skills are necessary to solve the health problem?
4. *Action.* What has to be done to help meet the need? What plan of action is best for solving the health problem and meeting the client's personal needs?
5. *Result.* What happened? What was the result of the action planned and carried out? Did it solve the problem or meet the need? If not, why not? What change in plan is indicated?

IMPORTANT ACTIONS OF THE INTERVIEW

Five important actions of an interview can be identified: observing, listening, responding, terminating, and recording. Each of these requires study, practice, and development of skills.

Observing

Ordinarily we do not deliberately and minutely look at all the persons we meet. However, in the care of persons with health needs the helping role requires such behavior. Our purpose is to gather information that will guide us in understanding clients and their environment. Valid observation is a skill that is developed through concentration, study, and practice. Areas of such needed observation include the following:

1. *Physiologic functioning and features.* Refer to Table 1-1 in the first chapter and review the clinical signs of nutritional status. Such features as these may be used as a basis for making detailed observations of physical features. Learning to take an organized look at the person may help develop greater accuracy and objectivity. We tend to see what we have the mindset, sensitivity, or awareness to see. Therefore, we need to develop certain sensitivities to detect pertinent details that can provide important clues to real needs.

2. *Behavior patterns.* Observe closely not only the physical features but also the immediate behavior of the client or patient in the health care situation. Attempt to look at the behavior in terms of its meaning to the person in relation to self-concept and the illness. From these observations, certain assumptions or educated guesses can be made. But realize all the while that these are only assumptions and hence need to be validated and clarified with the client to determine whether they are indeed factual. This action helps us to understand our own feelings and rule out our own biases, prejudices, or distortions of the situation.

3. *Environment.* Observing the client's immediate environment in an organized manner is also helpful. This may be the home and community environment on a visit, or it may be the immediate environment in a clinic or hospital setting.

Listening

Hearing and listening are not the same thing. Hearing is purely a physiologic function, only the first phase of the listening process. The function of the listening is to hear, to identify the sound, to understand its meaning, and to learn by it.

Although the senses have amazing powers of perception, they are limited. The nervous system must constantly select and discriminate among the millions of bits of information it confronts. Listening is also limited. A large part of communication time is spent in listening, but the average person without special training has only about 25% listening efficiency. In other words, one hears only a small percent of the total surrounding communication.

The task of the health worker is to learn the art of creative listening. First of all, we must learn to be comfortable as a listener. Usually our lives are so filled with activity and noise that to sit and listen quietly is often difficult. Actually, most of us have had little experience during our own development of being listened to, so listening to others must be learned. We practice listening by staying close by, assuming a comfortable position, and giving our full attention to the person who is speaking. We show genuine interest by indicating agreement or understanding with a nod of the head or making such sounds as "Uh-huh," "I see," or "And then?" at the appropriate moments in the conversation. We must learn to remain silent when the other person's comment jogs some personal memory or parallel experience of our own. We learn to listen not only for the words the patient uses but also for the repetition of key words, the rise and fall of the tone of voice, hesitant or aggressive expression of words and ideas, and the softness or harshness of tone. We listen to the overall content of what is being said, to the main ideas being expressed, and to the topics chosen for discussion. We listen for the feelings, needs, and goals that are being stated. We learn to listen to the silences and to be comfortable with them, giving the person time to frame thoughts and express them.

Responding

The responses we give to the client or patient may be verbal or nonverbal. Nonverbal responses include signs and actions, such as gestures and movements, silences, facial expressions, nods of the head, and touch. Verbal responses make use of language—words and meanings (Table 10.1). But we must remember that we give our own meanings to the words we use. A word is only a symbol, not the thing itself. Thus we must give attention to our choice of words—we must "begin where the person is." And all the while we must provide a supportive environment for responses (see *Practical Application* box). Also, we must watch the level and pace of our speaking. Questions should be clear, concise, free from bias, and always nonthreatening. Sometimes a verbal response may be a simple restatement of what the client has said. This enables the person to hear the statement again, think about it, and thus reinforce, expand, or correct it. At other times the response may be a reflection of what the expressed feelings seem to be. This enables the client to respond, to verify or to deny that this was indeed the feeling. We must never act on our assumptions about the client's feelings without verifying them first.

Terminating the interview

The close of the interview should meet several needs. It may be used to summarize the main points covered or to reinforce learning. If contact with the client is to continue, it can include plans for the follow-up visits or activities. It should always leave the person with the sense that the health worker's concern has been sincere and that the door is always open for further communication, should the person so desire.

Recording

Some means of recording the important points of the interview should be arranged. This should be as unobtrusive as possible, with little note-taking, if any, during the interview itself and completion of the record immediately afterward. If some recording device is used, the client's permission must always be obtained. Give full assurance that identity will be erased and that the recording will only be used for a specific purpose, such as to help the health worker improve interviewing skills or to learn the health needs of a particular group of people, as in gathering research data.

Various members of the health care team contribute information about the client or patient and the health problem in a system of written reports. This is the patient's chart, a legal document, which, in case of litigation, could be used in court. There is an obligation to the client or patient to respect confidentiality and to determine what and how much information is shared and with whom. At the same time health care workers have a responsibility for relaying to other health team members pertinent information to aid in the total planning of care.

What aspects of the interview should be recorded? Data from two basic areas of communication are needed: (1) a description of the client or patient's general phys-

Table 10.1 Verbal responses used by the helping professions

Purpose of response	Type of response	Description
Clarification	Content	Counselor summarizes content of conversation up to that point
	Affective	Counselor paraphrases or defines concern that client has implied but not actually stated
Leading	Closed question	Question that can be answered with "yes" or "no" or with very few words
	Open question	Question that cannot be answered briefly; often triggers discussion or a flow of information
	Advice	Provision of an alternative type of behavior by counselor for client; may be an activity or thought
	Teaching	Information presented by counselor with intention of helping client acquire knowledge and skills to perform appropriate nutrition-related behaviors
Self-revealing	Self-involving	Response made to client's statements that reflects the personal feelings of counselor
	Self-disclosing	Response made to client's statements that reflects factual information about counselor
	Aside	Statement counselor makes to self

ical and emotional status and concerns, followed in some instances by judgment of the immediate and ongoing care needs, and (2) description of whatever care and teaching was given and results observed. In addition, we may sometimes include follow-up plans made with the patient and the family or notes concerning needs that were passed on to other health care team members or to other agencies. Similar information is often communicated through oral team reports and various case conferences.

---

practical application

Creating a supportive nutrition counseling environment

Over 50 years ago a sensitive physician named Dr. Henderson expressed truths about the client interview in a healing environment; his thoughts are as applicable today as they were then. Perhaps they are even more true in today's far more complex world. He reminds us anew that we must truly listen to our clients and patients every day if we are to help them.

Listening

"Now hear this," he seems to be imploring us still. "We must listen," he is saying, "for what the client wants to tell us, for what he does not want to tell us, and for what he cannot tell us. He does not want to tell things that are shameful or painful. And he cannot tell us his implicit assumptions that even he does not know." It sounds like the creative listening that a more modern philosopher and counselor, Carl Rogers, used to call it. This is no passive activity; it is an active counseling skill. Only by using it can we really hear and respond wisely.

Also, nutrition counselors may inadvertently close communication channels by failing to ask questions or otherwise verbally discouraging the client from expressing real concerns and expectations or by using body language that is distracting, inappropriate, or misinterpreted by the client because of cultural differences.

Questions and reflections

Questions or statements that reflect what the client says or feels and that encourage further expression are usually open-ended, making a simple yes-or-no response inadequate, or they are affective, reflecting feelings that the client may have implied but not expressed directly. Closed questions and self-directed statements do little to encourage the person to "open up" (see Table 10-1).

Body language

Body language can be distracting or intimidating, or it can make the client feel at home. The key is to understand the client's concept of the following communication factors:

- *Personal space.* Americans like a lot of room. Try sitting next to the only passenger on a city bus and note the amount of anxiety created! In other cultures, such as the Middle East, closeness, even to the point of pushing and shoving, is considered acceptable behavior. Thus we must understand that our distance from our clients may affect their sense of comfort.
- *Eye contact.* Americans show respect by looking at each other straight in the eye. Asians, for example, do the same by looking downward. Attempts to interchange these behaviors can be interpreted as being rude.
- *Speech inflection.* The tone of voice and its loudness and inflection may be interpreted as threatening or comforting depending on the region or country of origin of the listener.

You cannot always be aware of your clients' attitudes toward body language ahead of time. However, you can take note of any signs of uneasiness and at least invite them to discuss anything about the interview that may be causing concern.

Yes, Dr. Henderson, we still hear you. We can—and must—listen.

References

Henderson L: Physician and patient as a social system, *N Engl J Med* 212: 819, 1935.

Heppner PP et al: Carl Rogers: reflections on his life, *J Counsel Dev* 63:14, 1984.

Jerome NW: Culture-specific strategies for capturing local dietary intake patterns, *Am J Clin Nutr* 65(suppl): 1166S, 1997.

NUTRITION HISTORY AND ANALYSIS

Personal life situation and food patterns

Working closely with the nutritionist on the health care team, learn the family's situation and values and identify health and nutrition needs through a general nutrition history and analysis. Several methods for such interviewing may be used, either separately or in combination, depending on the circumstances and the need.

1. *24-hour recall.* Ask the person to recall all food and drink consumed during the previous day, noting the nature and amount of each item.[5] This method has disadvantages with some persons whose memory may be limited, such as elderly people or young children, and it does not reveal long-term food habits. Simple food models in pictorial form can be used successfully to help quantify the reported food intake.[6]

2. *Food records.* Persons are asked to record their food intake for a brief period of time, usually about 3 days. Each person is taught how to describe the food items used singly or in combination and how to measure amounts consumed. Often a 3-day record is used following an initial diet history as a periodic monitoring tool.

3. *Food frequency.* Use a structured questionnaire that lists common food items or food groups to obtain information about quantity and frequency of use.[7] This tool may be helpful in relation to a particular disease risk or incidence by helping to determine use of specific groups of foods over an extended period of time.

4. *Diet history.* At the initial individual or family contact, a nutrition interview provides needed information for planning continuing care. Professional nutritionists and dietitians use a comprehensive form of this approach in a variety of clinical and community settings, usually evaluating their findings by detailed computer analysis. Other health care team members working with the dietitian may contribute helpful nutrition information through use of a simplified version, such as the activity-associated general day's food pattern given in Figure 10.1. Most people eat in relation to activity or work throughout the day, where they are, what they are doing, and whom they are with at the time. Using such an activity-associated guide through the day gives both interviewer and client a structure and provides a series of memory jogs to flesh out the information in greater detail to permit constructive counseling. With respect to each item, questions are asked in terms of general habits—nature of food items, form, frequency, preparation,

---

Name _____   Date _____

Height _____ Weight (lb) _____ (kg) _____ Age _____

Referral   Ideal weight _____
Diagnosis
Diet order
Members of household
Occupation
Recreation, physical activity

Present food intake	Place	Hour	Frequency, form, and amount checklist
Morning			Milk
			Cheese
			Meat
			Fish
			Poultry
Noon			Eggs
			Cream
			Butter, margarine
			Other fats
Evening			Vegetables, green
			Vegetables, other
			Fruits (citrus)
			Legumes
			Potato
			Bread–kind
			Sugar
			Desserts
Summary			Beverages
			Alcohol
			Vitamins
			Candy

Figure 10.1   Nutrition history: activity-associated general day's food pattern. Also record general activity pattern throughout the day.

portion, seasoning—not in terms of a specific day's intake. All through such an interview important clues to food attitudes and values can be communicated. Note these for later thought and exploration. An added practical method that may be helpful is a brief informal household food inventory, for example, a short checklist of high-fat foods, in conjunction with assessment of how often each item is eaten.[8] If your manner is interested and accepting, the information should be valid and straightforward. Conversely, if you are judgmental and authoritarian, persons will probably tell you only what they think you want to hear.

Changing American eating behavior

A basic reason for using an activity-associated general day's food intake as the structure for a diet history is that America's eating behavior is changing from traditional patterns. Surveys indicate that current eating behavior has become much more fragmented into frequent light feedings—called "grazing" by many observers—than the traditional family meals. Actually, studies of American eating patterns over the past 20 years have consistently found that the smallest and fastest shrinking population segment (only about 15%) is composed of those who still cook three regular meals a day, and the largest and most rapidly growing group is composed of those who eat easily portable items that don't take much time to cook or consume.

Plan of care

On the basis of the diet history and review of any health problems requiring diet modification, a realistic personal food plan can be developed with the individual and family. Then any related follow-up care as needed can be developed. This may take the form of return visits to the clinic, home visits, consultation and referral with other members of the health care team, or use of community resources. Follow-up work requires patience and a steady focus on the goal, knowing that there are options of reaching it. Imagination and good humor are invaluable. Take one step at a time; guide the client and family in applied nutrition principles, give support as needed, help with adjustments of the plan, provide reinforcement of prior learning, and continue to add new learning opportunities as the family's needs develop.

THE TEACHING-LEARNING PROCESS

LEARNING AND CHANGED BEHAVIOR

There is far more to teaching and learning than merely dispensing information, but the myth still prevails in much of health education that if enough information is provided, harmful health practices will be changed. This is not always the case. There is a vast difference between a person who has learned and a person who has only been informed. Learning must ultimately be measured in terms of changed behavior. As with counseling, valid education focuses not on the practitioner or teacher or the content but on the learner. The health teacher's major task is to create situations in which clients and their families can learn, succeed, and develop self-direction, self-motivation, and self-care. These learning goals are especially important in dealing with adult patients and clients[9] (see *To Probe Further* box, p. 224).

ASPECTS OF HUMAN PERSONALITY INVOLVED IN LEARNING

The teaching-learning experience involves three fundamental aspects of the human personality—thinking, feeling, and the will to act.

Thinking

We grasp information through our personal thinking process. We take in information selectively, then process and shape it according to our needs. The total thought process provides the background knowledge that is the basis for reasoning and analysis. The learner senses the contribution of this thinking to the learning process as "I know how to do it."

Feeling

In each of us specific feelings and responses are associated with given items of knowledge and situations. These emotions reflect desires and needs that are aroused. Emotions provide impetus, creating the tensions that spur us to act. The learner senses the contribution of emotion to the learning process as "I want to do it."

Will to act

The will to act arises from the conviction that the knowledge discovered can fulfill the felt need and relieve the symptoms of tension. The will focuses the decision to act on the knowledge received so that attitude, value, thought, or pattern of behavior can be changed. The learner senses the contribution of the will to the learning process as "I will do it."

PRINCIPLES OF LEARNING

Learning follows three basic laws: (1) learning is *personal*, occurring in relation to perceived personal needs; (2) learning is *developmental*, building on prior knowledge and experience; and (3) learning means change, resulting in some form of *changed behavior*.

Individuality

Learning can only be individual. We must all learn for ourselves, according to our own needs, in our own way and time, and for our own purpose. The teacher must discover who the learner is by asking questions that clarify the learner's relationship to the problem. New approaches to realistic nutrition education can help teachers vary teaching-learning strategies to meet the differing needs of learners and learning situations.

Need fulfillment

An important initial force in learning is personal **motivation**. Persons learn only what they believe will be useful to them, and they retain only what they think they need. The more immediately persons can put new learning to use, the more readily they grasp it. The more it satisfies their immediate goals, the more effective the learning will be.

Contact

Learning starts from a point of contact between prior experience and knowledge, an overlap of the new with the familiar. Find out what the individual already knows and to what past experiences the present situation can be related. Start the process of learning at this point. Search for the areas of association that are present, then relate your teaching to that point of contact.

Active participation

Since learning is an active process through which behavior can change, learners must become personally involved. They must participate actively. Indeed, effective teaching strategies require active participation of learners to bring about desired changes in attitudes and behaviors.[10] One means of securing participation is through planned feedback. Feedback may take several forms:

1. Ask questions that require more than a "yes" or "no" answer and that reveal a degree of understanding and motivation, such as those in Table 10-1.
2. Use guided return demonstrations, which are brief periods in which procedures are practiced and skills discussed. Such guided practice develops ability, self-confidence, and security. It enables the learner to clarify the principles involved as a basis for decision-making about particular situations and actions.
3. Have the learner try out the new learning in personal experiences outside the teacher-directed situation. Alternate such trials with return visits to review these experiences. Answer, or help the person to answer, any questions raised and provide continued support and reinforcement.

Appraisal

At appropriate intervals take stock of the changes that your clients have made in outlook, attitude, and actions toward their specific goals in health and nutrition care and education. Careful, sympathetic questioning may reveal any blocks to learning. In addition to speeding the learning process, such concern will show you whether you are communicating clearly, making contact, or choosing the best method. It may help you to recall principles that you may have glossed over. In the final analysis, the measure of success in teaching lies not in the number of facts transferred, but in the change for the better that has been initiated in your client.

In all, the nutrition educator who builds on clients' needs and goals, imparts a strong knowledge and interest in the subject, shows respect and concern for each individual in the program, and projects self-confidence has the greatest chance for success. In the long run, clients following a personal goal-setting approach in their nutrition counseling and education will have more opportunity to develop self-care responsibility and personal choice than those following a purely diet-prescription approach. (See *Issues & Answers*, p. 227.) Initially the personal goal-setting approach may take longer, but it achieves far greater long-term results.

In its position paper on nutrition education for the public the American Dietetic Association has summed up its key education philosophy in four brief statements concerning food choices to maintain good nutrition: (1) the focus should be on total diet rather than on individual foods, (2) there are no good or bad foods, (3) the keys to a good diet are balance, variety, and moderation, and (4) a positive approach to foods should be emphasized.[11]

FAMILY ECONOMIC NEEDS: FOOD ASSISTANCE PROGRAMS

In your counseling you will discover economic stress among many clients and their families. Some may need financial help. In such situations you will need to discuss available food assistance programs and make appropriate referrals, through your team nutritionist and social worker or directly to community agencies and programs involved.

COMMODITY DISTRIBUTION PROGRAM

In the post-Depression years, legislation was initiated to stabilize agricultural prices. This legislation provided for the federal government to purchase market surpluses of perishable goods. Later the resulting accumulation of food stocks led to the creation of distribution programs as a means of disposing of the stored products (Figure 10.2). Such surplus has been defined as either physical (exceeding requirements) or economic (prices below desired levels). Foods coming under these regulations include meat and poultry, fruits and vegetables, eggs, dried beans, and peas. Most of these items purchased under this program have been donated by the Food and Nutrition Service of the United States

Department of Agriculture (USDA) to schools through the National School Lunch and School Breakfast Programs. Foods accumulated through other aspects of the legislation are price-supported basic and nonperishable items. These foods have been donated to child-feeding programs, summer camps, Indian reservations, trust territories, nutrition programs for the elderly, charities, disaster-feeding programs, and the Commodities Supplemental Food Program (Figure 10.3).

Figure 10.2   Warehouse for food surplus goods used in Commodity Distribution Program. (US Department of Agriculture.)

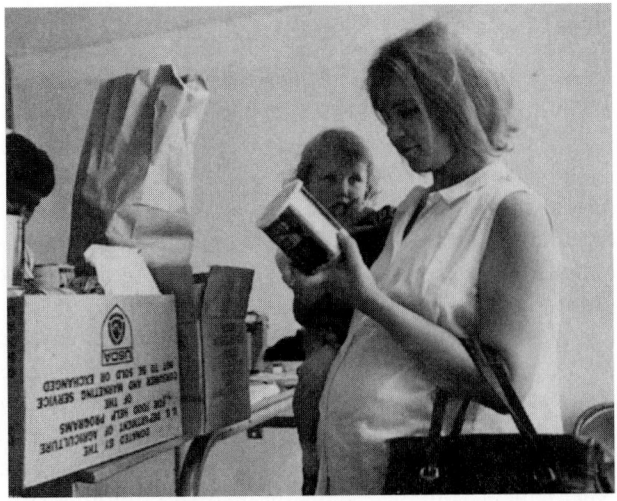

Figure 10.3   Pregnant mother and her child participating in Commodities Supplemental Food Program. (US Department of Agriculture.)

FOOD STAMP PROGRAM

Also growing out of the post-Depression years, the Food Stamp Program was founded to help low-income families purchase needed food. The program became part of permanent legislation by the Food Stamp Act of 1964, which made the program available to all counties wishing to participate. The program has developed from a $13 million program in 1961 to a nearly $12 billion program in 1985. Although it has suffered Federal Administration budget cuts through the past two decades, it remains the largest United States food assistance program. The eligible income is adjusted annually; for example, eligible net monthly income for a four-person household was $1,263 in fiscal year 1996.[12] Under this program participants are issued coupons or food stamps. The coupons are distributed to participating households, defined by the program as a group of people living in the same house who buy, store, and eat food together. These coupons are supposed to be sufficient to cover the household's food needs for 1 month. These households must have a net monthly income below the program's eligibility limit in order to qualify. This limit is quite low, and usually families who qualify simply aren't making enough money to buy food. Eligibility is based on gross, not actual net, income. For example, the Poverty Index Ratio (PIR) used, as is that with the United States Department of Health and Human Services (DHHS) for its National Health and Nutrition Examination Survey (NHANES), is calculated on gross family income.[13] This PIR compares household income to three times the cost of the lowest USDA Thrifty Food plan. Households with a PIR of less than 1 are below the official poverty line. The need to measure food insecurity accurately among low-income families was officially recognized in 1993, and a validated food insecurity or food insufficiency questionnaire followed as part of the United States Census Bureau's April 1995 Current Population Survey.[14]

CHILD NUTRITION PROGRAMS

After the Surplus Commodities Program was started, the government faced a glut of accumulated food items and needed a means of disposing of them. During World War II the military discovered a distressing rate of nutrition-related disorders that prevented a number of its draftees from serving in the army. Out of these two situations the National School Lunch Program of 1946 was born. From this initial program came all of today's child nutrition programs.

motivation   Forces that affect individual goal-directed behavior toward satisfying needs or achieving personal goals.

National school lunch and breakfast programs

These programs provide financial assistance to schools to enable them to provide nutritious lunches and breakfasts to their students. The program allows poor children to eat free meals or meals at reduced prices, and other students pay somewhat less than the full cost of the meal. Commodity foods, as described previously, are available to participating schools, and the programs usually entail minimal costs to the school district. All public and private nonprofit schools are eligible to participate in the program if their average tuition per student does not exceed $1500. Children's residential institutions, preschools, and the Head Start programs run as part of a school system are also eligible. Lunches served must fulfill approximately one third of the child's Recommended Dietary Allowance (RDA) for nutrients.

Child care food program

This program provides USDA food commodities, cash equivalents, and meal reimbursements for most or all of the meal and administration costs of feeding children up to 12 years of age who are enrolled in organized child care programs. These settings include day care centers, recreation centers, settlement houses, and some Head Start programs. The children's eligibility for free and reduced-price meals is the same as for the school lunch and breakfast programs.

WOMEN, INFANTS, AND CHILDREN PROGRAM

The Special Supplemental Food Program for Women, Infants, and Children (commonly called *WIC*) provides nutritious foods to low-income women who are pregnant or breast-feeding and to their infants and children under the age of 5 years. The food is either distributed free or purchased by free vouchers (Figure 10.4). It is designed to supplement the diet with rich sources of iron, protein, and certain vitamins. The vouchers are good for such foods as milk, eggs, cheese, juice, fortified cereals, and infant formulas. The program includes funding to cover clinic visits for medical checkups and for nutrition education and counseling by public health nutritionists. It is administered by the USDA through state health departments and Native American tribes, bands, or groups, run locally by public health facilities or organizations.

WIC participants must be pregnant or postpartum mothers (up to 6 months), lactating mothers (up to 12 months), or women having children under the age of 5 years. They must be at nutritional risk and must have an income under the reduced-price guidelines for the school lunch program. Factors indicating nutritional risk include evidence of an inadequate diet, poor growth patterns, a lack of nutrition understanding, or a medical history of nutrition-related problems, such as low–birth

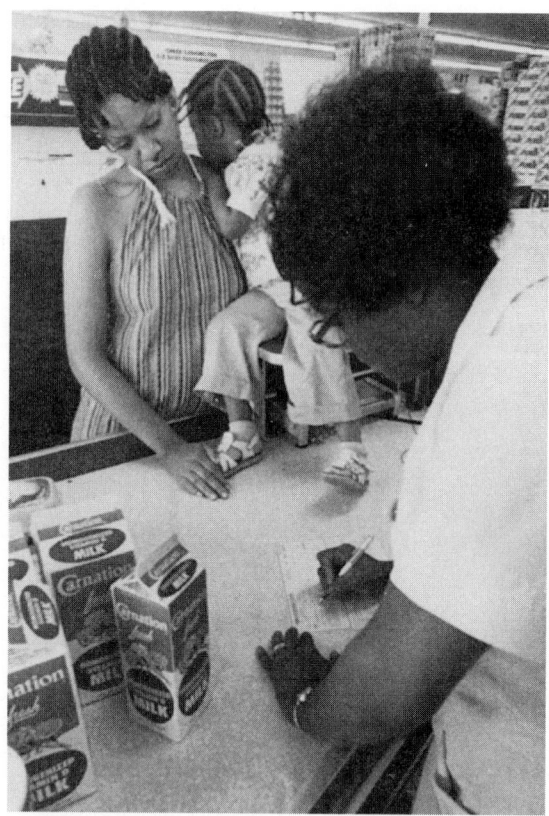

Figure 10.4   Mother in WIC program using program vouchers at a supermarket to buy groceries. (US Department of Agriculture.)

weight or premature infants, pregnancy-induced hypertension (toxemia), spontaneous abortions (miscarriages), and anemia. The prevalence of anemia among infants and children in low-income families has steadily declined over the past decade. The decline is largely a result of the positive impact of public health programs such as WIC, which includes both food support and continuing nutrition education. A specially developed "Simple-Easy" education plan provides the WIC client with personalized action plans they need to achieve needed behavior change.[15] Also, WIC prenatal supplementation has helped reduce the incidence of lowbirth weight and raise the mean birth weight.

Since its legislation by the United States Congress in 1972, the WIC program has served the needs of millions of women and children who have received benefits at over 1000 clinics across the United States.[16] Unlike the food stamp or school lunch programs, however, WIC is not an "entitlement" program. This means that eligibility does not automatically entitle one to benefits. There is an absolute ceiling each year on funding and therefore on participation.

NUTRITION PROGRAM FOR ELDERLY PERSONS

Congress has provided two types of food programs to benefit the growing numbers of elderly citizens in the United States. Regardless of their income level, all persons over 60 years of age are eligible to receive meals from the Congregate Meals Program or the Home-Delivered Meals Program. Elderly persons often face many social, physical, and economic difficulties and do not eat adequately to fulfill their nutritional needs. Many of them suffer from isolation and social deprivation. The main difference in these two programs is their setting and social aspect. The Congregate Meals Program provides ambulatory elderly persons with a hot nourishing noon meal at a community center where they can share food once a day, 5 days a week, with a group of their peers at no charge. Free transportation is often provided. Social events and nutrition information accompany the meals. The nutrition education component often includes, for example, one of a special series of brief 10-statement self-check reviews of true-false questions, each designed to correct misconceptions about the relationship between diet and one of the common chronic diseases among the elderly.[17] In comparison, the Home-Delivered Meals Program, sometimes called Meals-on-Wheels, provides homebound elderly persons who have difficulty preparing their own meals with at least one nutritious meal delivered to them in their home Monday through Friday.[18] A special concern in this program centers on the very frail elderly persons being served who are most needy. Both programs may accept voluntary contributions for meals from those who are able to do so.

All of the food assistance programs reviewed here provide a base of food security for many low-income families. However, studies indicate that family food shortages in general have increased during the past decade among low-income families who are barely subsisting, as well as among participants in these government assistance programs who also experience food shortages, especially during the last week of each monthly cycle of stamps, coupons, or vouchers.[19] United States populations most at risk for these food shortages include the elderly, single parent families, and children.

FOOD BUYING GUIDES

General family nutrition counseling may also involve guidance in planning for control of family food costs.

UNITED STATES DEPARTMENT OF AGRICULTURE FOOD PLANS

The USDA periodically issues low-cost food plans to serve as guides for food assistance programs. These plans are called liberal, moderate, low, and thrifty or very low-cost food plans, but in comparison to modern consumer food costs in general they are all low-cost plans. These very low-cost food plans are developed by nutritionists, economists, and computer experts at USDA on the basis of a predetermined level of spending appropriate to the prevailing policy identifying the poverty threshold. The lowest of all these low-cost plans is used to determine allotments of food stamp coupons to poor households.

FAMILY FOOD COSTS

A number of factors influence the way a family divides its food dollar. Some of these factors as listed here can help your client's family work out their household food plan.

1. Family income
2. Number, sex, ages, and general activities of family members
3. Any family food produced or preserved at home
4. Likes and dislikes of family members and special family dishes
5. Special dietary needs of any family member
6. Time, transportation, and energy for food shopping and preparation
7. Skill and experience in food management: planning, buying, cooking
8. Storing and cooking facilities in the home
9. Amount and kind of entertaining, if any
10. Meals eaten away from home
11. Value family places on food and eating

GOOD SHOPPING AND FOOD HANDLING PRACTICES

Today's American family spends more time shopping for food than cooking it. Food marketing is big business, and buying food for a family may seem to be a more complex affair than the preparation of food at home. A large American supermarket may stock some 8000 or more different food items, and more are being added daily. A single food item may be marketed in a dozen different ways at as many different prices. Frequently client families ask for more help with food buying than with any other aspect of fulfilling their diet needs, in terms of both cost and nutrition.[20,21] The following four food handling practices will help to control costs.

Plan ahead

Use market guides in newspapers, plan general menus, keep a kitchen supply checklist, and make out a market list ahead of time according to location of items in a regularly visited market. Such planning helps avoid impulse buying and extra trips.

Buy wisely

Know the market, market items, packaging, grades, brands, portion yields, measures, and food value in a market unit. Watch for sale items and buy in quantity if it results in savings and the food can be adequately stored or used. Be cautious in selecting convenience foods. The added timesaving may not be worth the added cost.

Store food safely

The kitchen waste that results from food spoilage and misuse can be controlled. Conserve food by storing items according to their nature and use, using dry storage, covered containers, and refrigeration as needed. Keep opened and partly used food packages at the front of the shelf for early use. Avoid plate waste by preparing only the amount needed by the family and use leftovers intelligently and creatively.

Cook food well

Retain maximum food value in cooking processes and prepare food with imagination and good sense. Give zest and appeal to dishes by using a variety of seasonings and combinations.

In all family nutrition counseling, however, we must remember that as much as the family may have learned about nutrition this is not always a primary factor. Family members usually eat because they are hungry or because the food looks and tastes good, not necessarily because it is nutritious.

THE BEST FOOD BUYS

Vegetables and fruits

In addition to minerals, these foods supply vitamins A and C, two nutrients found in surveys to be most often lacking in the average American diet. Give your clients the following guidelines:

1. Buy fresh items in season to avoid costs of out-of-season foods transported in from warmer, distant places.
2. Select fresh produce that is firm, crisp, and heavy for size. Medium-size items are usually better buys than large items, most of which may need to be discarded in preparation.
3. Distinguish between types of fresh produce defects. Small surface defects do not affect quality or food value and may cost less. Many or deep defects cause more waste, as does decay that is even slightly evident.
4. Compare costs of fresh produce sold by weight or count. The resulting price per item can be computed by each method of sale to make the best choice.
5. Avoid fancy grades in canned vegetables and fruits. Grading is based on shape, size, and perfection of pieces. Lower grades contain small, broken, or imperfect pieces, but they are equal in taste and food value and thus are good buys.
6. Buy vegetable and fruits in large cans, if family size warrants it.
7. Select low-cost dried foods. Dehydrated foods vary in

price. Dried beans, peas, and lentils are excellent food buys. But specialty dried foods, such as potatoes or dried fruits, are usually more expensive than fresh ones.
8. Compare cost of frozen, canned, and fresh vegetable and fruit items. Frozen items are usually more expensive. However, specials and family-sized packages can be compared weight for weight with canned or fresh items in season.
9. Cook vegetables with care. Excess cooking water and time destroy or eliminate vitamins and minerals and rob the vegetable of color, texture, and taste. Such unappetizing food often goes uneaten and causes costly waste.

Breads and Cereals

Most bread and cereal products are well liked, inexpensive, and fit easily into meal plans. This group of foods, along with potatoes and other vegetables, provides complex carbohydrates, which nutritionists advise should be the staple food of most persons' diets. Whole-grain foods are good sources of dietary fiber and are high in important vitamins and minerals. They are also important sources of amino acids and, in combination with other grains and legumes, form complete proteins. Many foods in this group can be excellent bargains:

1. Whole-grain or enriched products are much more nutritious than refined grains and products and are usually no more expensive.
2. Enriched specialty breads, such as French or Italian, cost up to three times more than whole-grain bread with similar or better nutritive value.
3. Precooked rice is much more expensive than unprocessed and often lacks many of the nutrients lost in processing.
4. Many cereals have nutrients added. Cereals that advertise 100% of the RDA for vitamins and minerals are usually more expensive. If the diet is adequate, such levels of supplementation are unnecessary.
5. Ready-to-eat cereals, instant hot cereals, and those packaged for individual servings are usually much more expensive. Buy grains in bulk if adequate storage can be provided.
6. Baked goods made at home, from scratch or even from some mixes, are usually much cheaper than bakery goods.
7. A large loaf of bread may not weigh more than a small loaf. Compare prices of equal weights of bread to find the better buy.
8. Try unusual forms of grains. For example, bulgur, buckwheat groats (hulled kernels), barley, and millet are excellent grains and can be used in many meals. Bulgur, which is cooked like rice, has a toastlike color, is rich in wheat flavor, and is equal in food value to whole wheat.

PROTEIN FOODS

Plant proteins

Dried beans and peas, grains, nuts, and seeds are inexpensive sources of proteins. Legumes and grains contribute needed amino acids to provide food sources of protein. These foods store well, are versatile in preparation, low in fat, and free of cholesterol, which is purely an animal product. They are also good sources of vitamins and minerals, including iron, zinc, and the B vitamins. For example, tofu, a curd made from soybean milk, has been the low-cost protein backbone of the East Asian diet for more than 2000 years.

Eggs

Eggs provide high-quality complete protein and are sold according to grade and size, neither of which is related to food value. Egg grades are based on qualities such as firmness of egg white, appearance, and delicacy of flavor, not on food value or quality. Shell color varies with species and has no effect on quality.

Milk and cheese

Dairy products are good sources of high-quality complete protein. However, whole milk products carry saturated fat, so distinguish among them those that are lower in fat as well as lower in price:

1. Fluid nonfat milk, buttermilk, and canned evaporated milk cost less than whole, fluid milk. Low-fat milks may be 1% or 2% butterfat; whole milk is 4%. To produce these lower fat milks, part of the butterfat is removed and dry milk solids are added. For example, whole milk contains 170 kcal/cup, 2% milk contains 135 kcal/cup, and nonfat milk contains 80 kcal/cup.
2. Nonfat dried milk is the best bargain of all forms of milk. Reconstituted with water, it provides a fluid nonfat milk at less than half the cost of the fresh form. It can also be used in many ways in cooking to add valuable nutrition, as well as the base for making yogurt.
3. If family size warrants it, buy milk in bulk containers.
4. If cheese is used often, buy it in bulk. It costs less per unit of weight and keeps better. Cheese standards set by the FDA are based on percentage of fat and moisture. The most commonly used, cheddar cheese (American, Daisy, Longhorn), is 50% fat and 30% moisture. Spread cheeses and imported cheeses are much more expensive.
5. Cottage cheese is an unripened, soft curd (80% moisture) and hence a rapidly perishable item. Buy it only as used to avoid waste from spoilage.

Poultry

Buy poultry by the whole bird. Usually the larger, more mature birds cost less than the young broilers and fryers, and they can be made equally tender with longer, moist cooking methods, such as braising, stewing, or pressure cooking.

Organ meats

Liver, kidney, and heart carry many nutrients, especially iron, although liver is high in cholesterol. However, in some areas they may actually be more expensive than some other boneless cuts of meat. A good cookbook will have appetizing ways of cooking them for family acceptance.

Fish

This is sometimes a fairly expensive food in many areas, depending on the season and the kind. Shellfish is more costly. Less expensive packed styles of canned fish may be available. For example, tuna is packed according to sizes of pieces, with fancy or solid pack (large pieces) being most expensive.

Red meats

Since meat is commonly one of the most costly food items, learn how it is graded, cut, processed, and marketed. Excellent learning material is available through the local county home advisor, USDA Extension Service. Avoid cuts with large amounts of gristle, bone, and fat. The lower grades provide good quality and less fat, and they cost less.

ADDITIONAL RESOURCES

Farmers' markets

In community farmers' markets local produce is made available directly to consumers. This outlet has the advantage of fresh produce at prices lower than those found in the supermarket. It also offers opportunities for socializing experiences between growers and consumers and gives a sense of community cohesion.

Consumer cooperatives

Consumer cooperatives focus on the economics of food marketing as well as on the issues of nutrition and ecology. The newer food cooperatives usually deal in bulk sales of whole or minimally processed foods. Belonging to a food cooperative increases personal responsibility and individual choice, and brings food issues into the hands of the consumer. Many of these food cooperatives stress the purchase of locally grown foods, thus strengthening local farmers while providing very fresh foods for consumers.

Home gardens

With a little effort any extra yard space may be turned into a home garden. Many persons are now turning to their backyards, interspacing vegetable plants among flowers and shrubbery in front yards, using allotted com-

To Probe Further

Effect of adult learning concepts on the nutrition interview

The adult client's openness to new knowledge and openness to a change of behavior is influenced by attitudes, educational background, physical characteristics, and economic situations. Teaching adults is quite different from teaching preadults.

We often say that a child is not a miniature adult, and we treat them accordingly. But we sometimes forget that an adult is not just a larger child, and we may be condescending—even insulting—without being aware of it. This is equally true in the nutrition interview and in a more formal educational setting.

The successful counselor considers these seven most prevalent *attitudes* affecting the counseling session with an adult client or patient:

- *Clients want to be treated as adults*. Clients do not appreciate being reprimanded or "talked down to."
- *Every client is an individual*. No matter how many clients you see with a particular health problem, each client wants to be treated as though his or her condition presents unique needs.
- *Most adult clients prefer objectivity and a business-like approach*. Although warmth and empathy are appropriate, do not forget the fact that the counseling session is a "role-playing" situation. Some degree of formality, such as the use of titles and surnames (not first-name familiarity), creates a structured environment to which most working adults are accustomed. If the client prefers a more relaxed atmosphere, he or she should be the one to steer the session in that direction.
- *Clients often resist change*. Change is threatening, especially when it involves something as personal as eating habits. An explanation of the need for change accomplishes more than *insisting* on change.
- *Some clients lack confidence*. Lack of education, fear of failure, distrust of the medical community, and other factors may reduce the client's confidence in his or her ability to follow diet plans. Patience, answering questions appropriately, and setting realistic goals may help promote a sense of confidence, as well as initiate therapy.
- *Some clients are overconfident*. Some clients expect too much from their diet plan or themselves. This is sometimes a mask for a fear of failure. Again, setting realistic goals may help the client become a bit more realistic and avoid disappointment.
- *Clients need positive reinforcement and feedback*. Some clients need help to overcome fear and anxiety and guidance to promote adherence to a food plan.

To accommodate *educational factors*, the counselor should consider the following:

- *Educational levels vary*. A lack of education may strip a client of the courage to ask questions or verbalize feelings and concerns. The counselor should make the client more comfortable by avoiding jargon and responding to every question on the level on which it is asked.
- *Isolated facts are difficult to remember*. The counselor must be familiar with the client's values and experiences to relate individual nutrition concepts, thus making them more meaningful.
- *Many adults have been exposed to years of incorrect or out-of-date information*. This may be difficult to overcome because of the effective teaching skills of persons dispensing misinformation. However, a professionally conducted session in which the correct information is presented in a nonintimidating way may be helpful in convincing the client that your message is more reliable than those provided by, for example, a television commercial.

Additional considerations include physical and economic factors such as the following:

- *Physical factors*. Physical factors affecting the counseling session, such as limited or no vision, limited hearing ability, illiteracy, or language barrier, may require more time, patience, or specially designed audiovisuals to facilitate learning. Involving a friend or family member in the session to interpret or learn may help reinforce the food behavior changes at home.
- *Economic factors*. Economic factors influence the outcome of counseling if the client believes that the new food choices are expensive. Explaining wise buying practices and the benefits of dietary changes versus the cost of continued health care, always in a supportive, nonintimidating way, may help the client overcome this anxiety. If cost is a barrier, the counselor may refer the client to a social worker or any social service organization that could provide assistance.

Above all, counselors and teachers of adult clients must treat them as the adults they are. Wise practitioners develop approaches and methods that help their adult learners enhance their own creative thinking and problem-solving skills. At the beginning of every counseling or teaching session they strive to establish the empathy and good rapport that is essential for effective communication. Only in this way is sufficient information obtained about the clients concerns and expectations and learning needs to develop an effective plan for solving nutrition-related problems. Nutrition counseling that influ-ences health behavior changes starts where the client is, then matches stages of interventions to help moti-vate and prepare each individual in steps toward per-sonal health goals.

References

Kicklighter JR: Characteristics of older adult learners: a guide for dietetics practitioners, *J Am Diet Assoc* 91(11):1418, 1991.

Sigman-Grant M: Stages of change: a framework for nutrition interventions, *Nutr Today* 31(4):162, 1996.

munity spaces, window boxes, planter boxes on porches, and even indoor potted plots to grow at least a portion of their own produce.

TO SUM UP

A major role of health care professionals is to translate the large amount of nutrition information available so that it can meet the needs of clients and families. They must present it in such a way that it is easily understood, is retained and applied by the learner, and can be evaluated to improve its effectiveness and ability to meet continu-ing care needs. Valid health and nutrition education must focus on the needs of the learner. Goals for planning counseling and educational activities and the methods for meeting these goals must be based on identifiable client and family needs.

Families and individuals under economic stress need counseling concerning financial assistance. Various United States food assistance programs operate to help families in need. Referrals to appropriate agencies may be made. The nutrition counselor may also need to assist the family in planning the most economic and nutritious meals possible within their limited circumstances. The family may need help in learning good shopping and food handling practices—planning ahead, buying wisely, storing safely, and cooking appropriately to preserve nutritional values and make food appetizing.

QUESTIONS FOR REVIEW

1. Identify and describe the skills necessary for an effec-tive nutrition counseling session.
2. Identify the basic principles of learning and describe how they may be used in planning nutrition educa-tion for one of your clients and his or her family.
3. What government food assistance programs are available to help low-income families? What other local food resources are available in your commu-nity?
4. List and discuss the "best food buys" described in this chapter. How many of the recommended prac-tices do you follow in selecting, storing, and prepar-ing foods?

REFERENCES

1. Helm KK, Klawitter B: *Nutrition therapy,* Lake Dallas, TX, 1995, Helm Seminars.
2. Link BG, Phelan JC: Understanding sociodemographic differences in health—the role of fundamental social causes, *Am J Public Health* 86(4):471, 1996.
3. Miller CA: A contract on America's children, *Am J Public Health* 86(4):473, 1996.
4. Jefferys M: Social inequalities in health—do they dimin-ish with age? *Am J Public Health* 86(4):474, 1996.
5. Smith GJ et al: Survey of the diet of Pima Indians using quantitative food frequency assessment and 24-hour recall, *J Am Diet Assoc* 96(8):778, 1996.
6. Posner BM et al: Validation of two-dimensional models for estimation of portion size in nutrition research, *J Am Diet Assoc* 92(6):738, 1992.
7. Zulkifli SN: The food frequency method for dietary assess-ment, *J Am Diet Assoc* 82(6):681, 1992.
8. Patterson RE et al: Using a brief household inventory as an environmental indicator of individual dietary practices, *Am J Public Health* 87(2):272, 1997.
9. Kicklighter JR: Characteristics of older adult learners: a guide for dietetics practitioners, *J Am Diet Assoc* 91(11):1418, 1991.
10. Johnson CC et al: Behavioral counseling and contracting as methods for promoting cardiovascular health in fami-lies, *J Am Diet Assoc* 92(4):479, 1992.
11. Shafer L, Gillespie A, Wilkins JL, Borra ST: Position of the American Dietetic Association: nutrition education for the public, *J Am Diet Assoc* 96(11):1183, 1996.
12. Legislative Highlights: Welfare reform law specifies changes and budget cuts for Food Stamps and child nutri-tion programs, *J Am Diet Assoc* 96(10):999, 1996.
13. Wotecki CE et al: Selection of the nutrition status indica-tors for field surveys: the HANES III design, *J Nutr* 120:1440, 1990.

14. Kendall A et al: Relationship of hunger and food insecurity to food availability and consumption, *J Am Diet Assoc* 96(10)1019, 1996.

15. Erickson K: Effective education: make it simple—make it easy, *J Nutr Ed* 23:40A, 1991.

16. Owen AL, Owen GM: Twenty years of WIC: a review of some effects of the program, *J Am Diet Assoc* 97(7):777, 1997.

17. Magnus MH: Self-check, group-check: congregate meal site nutrition education, *J Nutr Ed* 22:310D, 1990.

18. Coulston AM et al: Meals-on-Wheels applicants are a population at risk for poor nutritional status, *J Am Diet Assoc* 96(6):570, 1996.

19. Taren DL et al: Weekly food servings and participation in social programs among low-income families, *Am J Public Health* 80(11):1376, 1990.

20. Burro ST, Wellman NS: "Checking out" the supermarket shopper, *J Am Diet Assoc* 91(12):1511, 1991.

21. Carson CA et al: Putting nutrition on the grocery shelf, *J Am Diet Assoc* 92(2):159, 1992.

■ FURTHER READING

Coulston AM et al: Meals-on-Wheels applicants are a population at risk for poor nutritional status, *J Am Diet Assoc* 96(6):570, 1996.

Shovic A, Geoghegan P: Assessment of meal portion, food temperature, and select nutrient content of the Hawaii Meals-on-Wheels program, *J Am Diet Assoc* 97(5):530, 1997.

These two articles describe current services of the Meals-on-Wheels program for homebound elderly persons, who are often frail and malnourished.

Kendall A et al: Relationship of hunger and food insecurity to food availability and consumption, *J Am Diet Assoc* 96(10):1019, 1996.

Lee JD et al: Implementing the community-university model: dietetics students collaborate with Volunteers of America, *J Am Diet Assoc* 97(3):297, 1997.

These two articles describe the severe problems of hunger in a rural community and the hands-on experience of nutrition students with congregate meal sites for older adults.

Issues Answers

A person-centered model applied to diabetes education

A recently developed **paradigm** for nutrition education called *holistic education* can well apply to teaching good self-care practices to clients with chronic disorders such as diabetes.

This approach draws from good management and good medicine: (1) it varies its style to meet the situation, and (2) it focuses on the whole person—mind-body-spirit, well-being, and wellness. Holistic education regards clients or patients as active partners in the mutual goal of good health care. And further, it teaches persons to use their "boxes and their bubbles"—an excellent thinking model. Our "box" is our rational left side of the brain. Our "bubbles" emerge from our intuitive right side of the brain. We need both. We need to combine rational processes and intuitive ones to build creative thinking skills. Activity that just provides information or shows techniques does not help clients build creative thinking skills for themselves.

Investigations of national patient education programs indicate that many of them provide information and skills training without incorporating learning theories in the design of the program. They also lack a systematic way of assessing and influencing learner attitudes.

Learning theories are usually based on the psychosocial needs of the persons involved as well as their educational needs. In this instance, the person with diabetes has the major responsibility for the day-to-day management of the disease in order to maintain health and avoid complications. Thus diabetes education serves as a model for all good nutrition education and counseling in health care. With approximately 75% of all treated persons with diabetes failing to follow their prescribed diets, we should examine what we are doing in designing instruction for the person with diabetes. Ask yourself these questions.

Is the teaching process effective?

Does the teaching process take into account the following:
- How do people learn?
- What is worth learning?
- Who really is responsible for a person's health?
- What responsibilities for learning lie within the learner versus the instructor?

Is the learning process effective?

Does the learning process consider the following:
- How significant is the condition to the person at that point in his or her life?
- Does the person have a sense of psychologic safety, that is, does the person feel accepted well enough to discuss diabetes control problems openly and honestly?
- How will the instructor know if the person's attitude has changed toward receiving or using new information?

These questions are important reminders to consider factors that influence learning behavior when planning any health care and education program. Although this may seem to be immediately beyond the realm of nutrition, it is extremely important in any aspect of the care plan and learning process precisely because self-care control of any chronic disease lies primarily in the hands of the person with the disease. This is especially true in diabetes care. No matter how much information is provided, it is ultimately up to the individual to decide what foods are selected, how much is eaten, and when it is consumed.

Diabetes educators, for example, often fail to consider major aspects of the person's own individual and unique personal life that may influence these decisions, such as family finances, work situation, or social activities. They may also fail to recognize the effect of these activities on the individual's sense of personal responsibility for his or her own health. This may also influence the type of instruction provided or even the decision to provide instruction at that time at all.

The educator must be able to assess the person's sense of responsibility and capacity for continuing self-care daily and use this information to develop or revise instruction and counseling that leads to positive behaviors. Dietitians and other health care workers may benefit from the systematic methods of assessment that have already been developed in the field of clinical psychology. Therapists have identified five levels of responsibility and client characteristics, with possible intervention methods for each level, as shown in Table 10.2.

---

paradigm   A pattern or model serving as an example; a standard or ideal practice or behavior based on a fundamental value or theme.

Table

10.2   Levels of personal responsibility and relevant intervention methods for diabetes

Level of personal responsibility	Client characteristics	Intervention method
1. Being diabetic is a disaster	Feels hopeless, helpless, defeated; self-care may be impossible	Educate family member or other caregivers
2. Being diabetic is a burden	Blames problem on others; expects others to feel sorry for him or her; feels angry, threatened	Provide emotional support; help client accept anger in order to move on
3. Being diabetic is a problem	Blames self as often as others; personal growth is possible	Reinforce attitudes that reflect sense of responsibility; examine irresponsibility; examine irresponsible attitude in nonjudgmental way
4. Being diabetic is a challenge	Rarely blames others for problem; recognizes responsibility, but does not act on it; good self-care expected	Point out discrepancies between stated need and actual behavior
5. Being diabetic is an opportunity	Takes total responsibility for the problem; acts positively on decisions; optimal self-care is expected	Provide tools required for good self-care

Such a system for assessing client attitudes has specific benefits. These benefits can guide client education in good self-care involving food habits not only in diabetes but also in other chronic conditions in families, such as hypertension and cardiovascular disease. Benefits of such a system include the following:

1. It recognizes, and reinforces in the instructor, that the client is ultimately responsible for his or her health.
2. It gives the instructor an objective, measurable way of assessing client attitudes that can be compared and evaluated for progress.
3. It serves as a basis for selecting appropriate teaching methods or counseling techniques, which can then be changed to match the client's current level of responsibility.

References

American Medical Association: Council on scientific education for health, *JAMA* 263:1816, 1990.

Johnson CC et al: Behavioral counseling and contracting as methods for promoting cardiovascular health in families, *J Am Diet Assoc* 92(4):479, 1992.

Leontos C et al: National Diabetes Education Program: opportunities and challenges, *J Am Diet Assoc* 98(1):73, 1998.

McNutt K: Why some consumers don't believe some nutrition claims, *Nutr Today* 32(6):252, 1997.

Rinke WJ: Holistic education: a new paradigm for nutrition education, *J Nutr Ed* 18(4):151, 1986.

Nutrition During Pregnancy and Lactation

In this chapter we begin a three-chapter sequence on nutrition in health care throughout the life cycle. In each chapter, we will relate principles of nutrition to the remarkable process of human growth and development.

As we focus first on the beginning of new life, we examine the prenatal nutritional demands of the pregnant mother and her developing child. Mother and child possess great powers of adaptation to meet these demands.

Here we explore these tremendous physiologic changes during pregnancy and some possible complications. You will see how vital a role nutritional support plays in a successful course and outcome.

MATERNAL NUTRITION AND THE OUTCOME OF PREGNANCY

EARLY MEDICAL PRACTICE

For centuries, in all cultures, a great body of folklore has surrounded pregnancy. Various traditional practices and diets have been followed, many of which have had little basis in fact, and much clinical advice has been based only on supposition. For example, early obstetricians even held the notion that semistarvation of the mother was really a blessing in disguise because it produced a small baby of light weight who would be easier to deliver. To this end they used diets restricted in kcalories, protein, water, and salt. Despite the lack of any scientific evidence to support such ideas, two assumptions, now known to be false, governed practice: (1) the parasite theory: whatever the fetus needs it draws from the stores of the mother despite the maternal diet, and (2) the maternal instinct theory: whatever the fetus needs, the mother instinctively craves and consumes.

HEALTHY PREGNANCY

It is clear now that until recently much of the counsel given to pregnant women over the past few decades has been based more on tradition than on scientific fact. Increasing evidence indicates that positive nutritional support of pregnancy, rather than past negative restrictions born of limited knowledge and false assumptions, promotes a positive successful outcome with increased health and vigor of mothers and infants alike. This struggle over the past few decades, particularly to define the "healthy pregnancy," has not been easy. Now a healthy pregnancy is described in broader terms of mother and infant and family. We are beginning to understand more about what this really means, especially as we see around us the current fetal damages from malnutrition and drug abuse. We know that we must assess and support more fully the quality of life of each mother and her family if we are to approach the healthy pregnancy we desire for all mothers.

DIRECTIONS FOR CURRENT PRACTICE

Clinical observations and developing science in both nutrition and medicine have provided directions for healthier pregnancies. They have long refuted previous false ideas and laid a sound base for our current practice. A benchmark report of the National Research Council (NRC) first reflected this applied scientific base and led the way. This report, *Maternal Nutrition and the Course of Human Pregnancy*, was a clear turning point and provided undeniable direction for a new positive approach to the management of pregnancy.[1] Indeed, continuing research has reinforced this positive direction. On the basis of the significant NRC findings, guidelines for nutritional care of pregnant women were then issued by the American College of Obstetrics and Gynecology and the American Dietetic Association.[2-4] These reports have continued to provide guidelines for physicians, nutritionists, dietitians, and nurses in their prenatal care. We are reminded by these guides that a child is nutritionally 9 months old at birth, even older when we consider the significance of the mother's preconception status. Ancient Chinese wisdom has embodied this truth in their counting of age at birth as 1 year.

FACTORS DETERMINING NUTRITIONAL NEEDS

It is now evident from increased knowledge and the wide experience of many clinicians that maternal nutrition is critically important to both the mother and the child. It lays the fundamental foundation for the successful outcome of pregnancy—a healthy and happy mother and child. Several vital considerations emerge as factors that determine the nutritional requirements of the mother during her pregnancy.

Age, gravida, and parity

Age plays a major role in pregnancy; the teenage mother adds her own immaturity and growth needs to those imposed by pregnancy. At the other end of the reproductive cycle, hazards increase with age. Also, the number of pregnancies (**gravida**) and the number of viable offspring (**parity**), as well as the time intervals between them, greatly influence the mother's nutrient reserves, her increased nutritional needs, and the outcome of the pregnancy.

Preconception nutrition

The mother brings to each pregnancy all of her previous life experiences, including her diet and food habits. Her general health and fitness and her state of nutrition at the time of conception are products of her lifelong dietary habits and her genetic heritage.

Complex physiologic interactions of gestation

Three distinct biologic entities are involved during **gestation**: the mother, the **fetus**, and the **placenta**, which nourishes fetal growth.[5] Together they form a unique biologic whole. Constant metabolic interactions go on among them. Their functions, while unique, are at the same time interdependent. It is this unique biologic **synergism** that nourishes and sustains the pregnancy.

BASIC CONCEPTS INVOLVED

As a result of our increased knowledge of pregnancy and nutrition, we can provide better nutritional guidance. Three basic concepts form a fundamental framework for assessing maternal nutrition needs and for planning supportive prenatal care for both parents.

Perinatal concept

The prefix *peri-* comes from the Greek root meaning "around, about, or surrounding." Thus the word *perinatal* refers more broadly to the scope of factors that surround a birth than merely the 9 months of the physical gestation. Certainly, as nutrition knowledge and understanding have increased, health professionals realize that all of a woman's life experiences surrounding her pregnancy need to be considered. Her nutritional status and food patterns, which have developed over a number of years, and the degree to which she has established and maintained nutritional reserves are all important factors. Cultural and social influences have shaped beliefs and values of both parents about pregnancy. All of these influences come to bear on any pregnancy.

Synergism concept

The word **synergism** is a term used to describe biologic systems in which the cooperative action of two or more factors produces a total effect greater than and different from the mere sum of the parts. In short, a new whole is created by the unified, joint effort of blending the parts in which each part makes more powerful the action of the others. Of the many biologic and physiologic examples of synergism, pregnancy is a prime case in point. Maternal organism, fetus, and placenta combine to produce a new whole, a system not existing before and producing a total effect greater than and different from the sum of the parts, all for the sole purpose of sustaining and nurturing the pregnancy and its offspring. Physiologic measures change. Blood volume increases, cardiac output increases, ventilation rate and tidal volume of breathing increase, and basal metabolic rate increases. The physiologic norms of the nonpregnant women do not apply.

Thus the normal physiologic adjustments of pregnancy cannot be viewed as pathologic with application of treatment procedures for that same type of response in the nonpregnant state. For example, a normal physiologic generalized edema of pregnancy is a protective response. It reflects the normal increase in total body water necessary to support the increased metabolic work of pregnancy and is associated with enhanced reproductive performance.

Life continuum concept

In a real sense, throughout her life a woman is providing for the ongoing continuum of life through food that she eats. Each child obviously becomes a part of this continuing process during the pregnancy when the mother's diet directly sustains growth. But in the broader sense both parents carry over their nutritional heritage, practices, and beliefs in the teaching of their growing children, who in the next generation pass on this heritage both genetically and culturally.

POSITIVE NUTRITIONAL DEMANDS OF PREGNANCY

BASIC NUTRIENT ALLOWANCES AND INDIVIDUAL VARIATION

The period of gestation is an exceedingly rapid growth period. During this brief 9 months, the human life grows from a single fertilized egg cell (ovum) to a fully developed infant weighing about 3 kg (7 lb). On the basis of this intense physiologic growth and development of the fetus, what nutrients must the mother supply? What must her diet provide to meet the nutritional demands of the fetus and of her own changing body during this critical period of human growth?

Throughout the pregnancy there is an increased need for all the basic nutrients, as indicated by the current Recommended Dietary Allowances (RDAs) outlined by the National Research Council (NRC) (Table 11.1).[4] But it is important to remember that these are guidelines, and individual variances in need must be examined for each pregnancy. Individual variations such as body size, activity, and multiple pregnancy would need to be considered. Also, quantitative need for nourishment of pregnant adolescents must be noted. The need for individual counseling and for correct use of the Recommended Dietary Allowances (RDAs) as guidelines is clearly stated by the NRC: "They are not called 'requirements,' because they are not intended to represent merely literal (minimal) requirements of average individuals, but to cover

---

fetus   The unborn offspring in the postembryonic period, after major structures have been outlined; in humans the growing offspring from 7 to 8 weeks after fertilization until birth.

gestation   The period of embryonic and fetal development from fertilization to birth; pregnancy.

gravida   A pregnant woman.

parity   The condition of a woman with respect to having borne viable offspring.

placenta   Special organ developed in early pregnancy that provides nutrients to the fetus and removes metabolic waste.

synergism   The joint action of separate agents in which the total effect of their combined action is greater than the sum of their separate actions.

Table

11.1 RDAs of some selected nutrients for pregnancy and lactation (National Research Council, 1989 Revision)

Nutrients	Nonpregnant girl		Nonpregnant woman	During pregnancy	Lactation	
	11-14 yr 46 kg 101 lb	15-18 yr 55 kg 120 lb	25 yr 63 kg 138 lb	All ages	(600 ml/day) First 6 months	(750 ml/day) Second 6 months
Kcalories	2200	2200	2200	No change in the first trimester; add 300 kcal/day for second and third trimesters	2840	2710
Protein (g)	46	44	50	Add 10 g/day	Add 15 g/day	Add 12 g/day
Calcium (mg)	1200	1200	800	1200 mg throughout		
Iron (mg)	15	15	15	30 mg throughout	15	15
Vitamin A μg RE)	800	800	800	800 μg RE throughout	1300	1200
Thiamin (mg)	1.1	1.1	1.1	1.5 mg throughout	1.6 mg throughout	
Riboflavin (mg)	1.3	1.3	1.3	1.6 mg throughout	1.8	1.7
Niacin (mg NE)	15	15	15	17 mg NE throughout	20 mg NE throughout	
Ascorbic acid (mg)	50	60	60	70 mg throughout	95	90
Vitamin D (μg)	10	10	5	10 μg throughout	10 μg throughout	

substantially the individual variations in the requirements of healthy people."[4] In considering the needs of the healthy pregnant woman, we will review here the nutrient elements in terms of general amounts of increased intake indicated, why this increase is recommended, and how it may be obtained in basic foods.

ENERGY NEEDS

Kcalories must be sufficient to (1) supply the increased energy and nutrient demands created by the increased metabolic workload, including some maternal fat storage and fetal fat storage to ensure an optimal newborn size for survival, and (2) spare protein for tissue-building. A minimum of about 36 kcal/kg is required for efficient use of protein during pregnancy. The current RDA standard recommends an additional amount of energy, 300 kcalories during the second and third trimesters of rapid growth, making a total of about 2200 to 2500 kcalories, about a 10% to 15% increase over the mother's general prepregnant need. This amount may be insufficient for active, large, or nutritionally deficient women, who may need as much as 2500 to 3000 kcalories. Remember that a minimum of 1800 kcalories is required just to avoid negative nitrogen balance, to say nothing of the added pregnancy and activity needs. This primary positive emphasis on sufficient kcalories is critical to ensure nutrient and energy needs to support the pregnancy. Appropriate weight gain during the pregnancy indicates whether sufficient kcalories are being provided.

PROTEIN NEEDS

The total amount of protein recommended (RDA) for the pregnant woman is about 60 g/day, an increase of about 10 to 15 g/day. Protein, with its essential nitrogen, is the nutrient basic to tissue growth. Nitrogen balance studies give some indication of the large amounts of nitrogen used by the mother and child during pregnancy and emphasize the importance of maternal reserves to meet initial needs even before the pregnancy is confirmed. More protein is necessary to meet tissue demands posed by (1) rapid growth of the fetus, (2) enlargement of the uterus, mammary glands, and placenta, (3) increase in maternal circulating blood volume and subsequent demand for increased plasma proteins to maintain colloidal osmotic pressure and circulation of tissue fluids to nourish cells, and (4) formation of **amniotic fluid** and storage reserves for labor, delivery, and lactation.

Milk, egg, cheese, and meat are complete protein foods of high biologic value. Protein-rich foods also contribute other nutrients such as calcium, iron, and B vitamins. Additional protein may be obtained from legumes and whole grains, with lesser amounts in other plant sources.

MINERAL NEEDS

All of the major and trace minerals play roles in maternal health. Two that have special functions in relation to pregnancy—calcium and iron—deserve particular attention.

Calcium

The pregnant woman requires (RDA) 1200 mg of calcium daily, an increase of 400 mg/day for women age 25 or older, to match the general recommendation for all adolescents and young women ages 19 to 25. Calcium is the essential element for the construction and maintenance of bones and teeth. It is also an important factor in the blood-clotting mechanism and is used in normal muscle action and other essential metabolic activities. The rapid fetal mineralization of skeletal tissue during the final period of rapid growth demands more calcium.

Dairy products are a primary source of calcium. Some increase in milk or equivalent in milk foods (cheese, or nonfat milk powder used in cooking) is recommended. Additional calcium is obtained in whole or fortified cereal grains and in green leafy vegetables.

Iron

The pregnant woman needs 30 mg/day of iron, a 50% increase over her general RDA needs. Some pregnant women may need supplementary iron in addition to increased dietary sources to meet the additional requirement of pregnancy. The iron cost of pregnancy is high. With increased demands for iron, often insufficient maternal stores, and inadequate provision through the usual diet, a daily supplement of 30 to 60 mg of iron may be prescribed. If the woman is anemic at conception, a larger therapeutic amount of 120 to 200 mg of iron is recommended.

To obtain the needed amount of iron, check the percentage of elemental iron in the iron preparation being used. For example, the commonly used compound ferrous sulfate is a hydrated salt ($FeSO_4\ 7H_2O$), which contains 20% iron. It is usually dispensed in tablets containing 195, 300, or 325 mg of the ferrous sulfate compound. Each tablet, then, would contain 39, 60, or 65 mg of iron, respectively. Thus to supply a regular daily supplement of 60 mg of iron, one 300-mg tablet of ferrous sulfate is required, and for a therapeutic dose of 120 mg iron, two 300-mg tablets are required.

However, there are problems with routine iron supplementation for all pregnant women, such as unpleasant gastrointestinal side effects and less motivation to maintain a good diet. Also, there may be imbalances with other trace elements, such as zinc, which competes with iron for absorption. Actually, excess iron intake when not needed may potentially mask inadequate pregnancy-induced hemodilution, a normal pregnancy adaptation that puts less strain on the maternal heart, minimizes hemoglobin loss with blood loss at delivery, and increases nutrient flow to the fetus. Thus some prenatal clinics follow protocols that prescribe regular prenatal vitamins with iron at the first clinic visit. Then individual additional iron supplementation is used only if hemoglobin falls to 10.5 g/dl or less at any time during the pregnancy.

During pregnancy, the maternal circulating blood volume normally increases from 40% to 50%, and may increase more with multiple births. An individual mother's iron supplement need must be assessed accordingly. Maternal iron is also needed to supply iron stores for the developing fetal liver. Adequate maternal iron stores also help fortify the mother against serum iron losses at delivery.

It is no surprise, then, that our major food source of iron is liver. Its use can be encouraged by suggesting appetizing ways of preparing it. Other food sources include meat, legumes, dried fruit, green vegetables, eggs, and enriched bread and cereals (see list of iron-containing foods in Chapter 8, p. 169).

VITAMIN NEEDS

Increased amounts of vitamins A, B-complex, C, and D are needed during pregnancy. If these needs are met, sufficient amounts of vitamins E and K are also available.

Vitamin A

The daily amount of vitamin A recommended (RDA) for pregnancy is 800 μg of retinol equivalents (RE), a continuance of the woman's regular need. For most women in the United States, no extra amount is needed. However, malnourished, underweight women, as well as those with multiple pregnancies, need more. Vitamin A is an essential factor in cell development, maintenance of strong epithelial tissue, tooth formation, and normal bone growth. Liver, egg yolk, butter and fortified margarine, dark-green and yellow vegetables, and fruits are good food sources.

B vitamins

There is a special need for the various B vitamins during pregnancy. These are usually supplied by a well-balanced diet that is increased in quantity and quality to supply needed energy and nutrients. The B vitamins are important as coenzyme factors in a number of metabolic activities related to energy production, tissue protein synthesis, and function of muscle and nerve tissue; therefore they play key roles in the increased metabolic work of pregnancy.

There is a special increased metabolic need for the B vitamin folate during pregnancy. Folate deficiency usually occurs in conjunction with general malnutrition, making the pregnant woman in low-socioeconomic conditions especially vulnerable. A specific megaloblastic anemia caused by maternal folate deficiency sometimes

---

amnionic fluid The watery fluid within the membrane enveloping the fetus, in which the fetus is suspended occurs and warrants supplementation of the diet with folic acid. This added amount is particularly needed where such demands are greater, as in a multiple pregnancy. The RDA standard recommends a supplement of 400 μg/day of folate, more than twice the regular adult need of 180 μg/day, to prevent such deficiencies.

Also, special knowledge and use of folic acid has recently been recommended by the United States Department of Health and Human Services, Public Health Services for all women of childbearing age to protect against the risk of the serious defects of spina bifida and anencephaly.[6] These congenital defects in the formation of the spine develop in early embryonic life, when the neural tube, which forms the spinal cord, does not close completely, leaving part of one or more vertebrae of the spinal cord exposed at birth (see Chapter 25). Each year in the United States approximately 2500 infants are born with spina bifida and anencephaly, and an estimated 1500 affected fetuses are aborted.[7]

Vitamin C

Special emphasis must be given to the pregnant woman's need for ascorbic acid. Vitamin C is essential to the formation of intercellular cement substance in developing connective tissues and vascular systems. It also increases the absorption of iron that is needed for the increasing quantities of hemoglobin. The RDA standard recommends 70 mg/day for the pregnant women, an increase of 10 mg/day over the regular adult need of 60 mg/day. Additional food sources such as citrus fruit and other vegetables and fruits should be included in the mother's diet.

Vitamin D

Adults who lead active lives involving adequate exposure to sunlight probably need little additional vitamin D. However, during pregnancy the increased need for calcium and phosphorus presented by the developing fetal skeletal tissue requires additional vitamin D to promote the absorption and utilization of these minerals. The recommended (RDA) amount for pregnancy is 10 μg cholecalciferol (400 IU/day). Food sources include fortified milk, liver, egg yolk, and fortified margarine.

DIETARY PATTERNS: GENERAL AND ALTERNATIVE

General daily food pattern

A variety of familiar foods usually supplies the mother's need for added nutrients and makes eating a pleasure. The increased quantities of essential nutrients needed during pregnancy may be met in many ways by planning around a daily food pattern and using key types of suggested core foods. A general daily food pattern that meets basic nutrient needs is suggested in Table 11.2. Compare the increases in each food group suggested for the preg-

nant or lactating adolescent or woman during the reproductive cycle with the basic amounts for the nonpregnant woman. Comparison indicates the need for increased amounts of basic foods during pregnancy to meet increased key nutrient needs. It may be used as a guide, with additional foods added according to individual energy needs and personal desires. This pattern represents the "orthodox middle-class American diet." It has been labeled the "biomedically recommended prenatal diet," which is generally used worldwide by most health professionals in industrialized, affluent countries.

Alternative food patterns

With the increasing ethnic diversity in our American culture, it is especially important to use the mother's personal cultural food patterns in dietary counseling. We are ethnocentric if we rigidly adhere to the orthodox pattern previously discussed as the pattern for all pregnant women. It is but one alternative diet pattern among many others from different cultures, belief systems, and lifestyles. We need to remind ourselves that an extreme, unquestioning pursuit of "science versus magic" may lead us to label any alternative practice as unscientific and unreasonable, thus closing our minds to some possibly fruitful avenues of scientific exploration. We must always remember that specific nutrients, not specific foods, are required for a successful pregnancy and that these nutrients are found in a wide variety of food choices. If we are wise we will encourage our clients to use foods that serve their nutritional needs, whatever those foods might be. A number of resources have been developed to serve as guides for a variety of alternative food patterns, ethnic and vegetarian.

In essence, then, two important principles govern the diet: (1) that the pregnant woman eat a sufficient quantity of food and (2) that she eat regularly, avoiding any habit of fasting or skipping meals, especially breakfast.

GENERAL DIETARY PROBLEMS

FUNCTIONAL GASTROINTESTINAL PROBLEMS

Nausea and vomiting

Symptoms of nausea and vomiting are usually mild and short-term, the so-called morning sickness of early pregnancy because it occurs more often on arising than later in the day. At least 50% of all pregnant women, most of them in their first pregnancy, experience this condition, beginning during the fifth or sixth week of the pregnancy and usually ending about the fourteenth to sixteenth week. A number of factors may contribute to the situation. Some are physiologic, based on hormonal changes that occur early in pregnancy, or from low blood sugar that is relieved by carbohydrate foods but symptoms return within 2 to 3 hours after a meal. Others may be psychologic, based on situational tensions or anxieties about the pregnancy itself. Still others may be dietary problems, based on poor food habits. Simple treatment generally improves food toleration. Frequent small low-fat meals and snacks, fairly dry and consisting chiefly of easily digested energy-yielding foods such as carbohydrates (mainly starches), are usually more readily tolerated. Also, it may help to avoid cooking odors as much as possible. Liquids are best taken between meals instead of with meals.

Hyperemesis

In a small number of pregnant women, about 3.5 per 1000 pregnancies, a severe form of persistent nausea and vomiting occurs that does not respond to usual treatment. This condition, hyperemesis, begins early in the pregnancy and may last throughout. It may develop into the more serious pernicious form of **hyperemesis gravidarum**.[8] This persistent condition causes severe alterations in fluids and electrolytes, weight loss, and nutritional deficits, sometimes requiring alternative feeding by enteral or parenteral methods to sustain the pregnancy (see Chapter 18, p. 348). If the condition is unchecked, the mother is usually hospitalized and receives peripheral parenteral nutrition, followed by careful oral refeeding or tube feeding. In any case, continued personal support and reassurance are important.

Constipation

The complaint of constipation is seldom more than minor, but it contributes to discomfort and concern. Placental hormones relax the gastrointestinal muscles, and the pressure of the enlarging uterus on the lower portion of the intestine may make elimination somewhat difficult. Increased fluid intake; use of naturally laxative foods containing dietary fiber, such as whole grains, fruits and vegetables; dried fruits (especially prunes and figs); and other fruits and juices generally induce regularity. Laxatives should be avoided. Appropriate daily exercise is essential for overall health during pregnancy.

Hemorrhoids

A fairly common complaint during the latter part of pregnancy is that of hemorrhoids. These are enlarged veins in the anus, often protruding through the anal sphincter. This vein enlargement is usually caused by the increased weight of the fetus and its downward pressure. The hemorrhoids may cause considerable discomfort, burning, and itching. Occasionally, they may rupture and bleed under pressure of a bowel movement, causing the mother still more anxiety. The problem is usually controlled by the dietary suggestions given for constipation. Also, sufficient rest during the latter part of the day may help relieve some of the downward pressure of the uterus on the lower intestine.

Heartburn or gastric pressure

The related complaints of heartburn or a full feeling are sometimes voiced by pregnant women. These discomforts occur especially after meals and are usually caused by the pressure of the enlarging uterus crowding the stomach. Gastric reflux of some of the food mass, now a liquid chyme mixed with stomach acid, may occur in the lower esophagus, causing an irritation and burning sensation. Obviously, this common complaint has nothing to do with heart action, but is so called because of the close proximity of the lower esophagus to the heart. The full feeling comes from general gastric pressure, lack of normal space in the area, a large meal, or gas formation. These complaints are usually remedied by dividing the day's food into a series of small meals, avoiding eating large meals at any time, and not lying down after a meal. Comfort is also improved by wearing loose-fitting clothing.

Effects of iron supplements

During pregnancy an iron supplement in the form of ferrous sulfate may be given to counteract the physiologic dilution anemia of pregnancy because of the increased circulating blood volume. The effects of added iron medication include gray or black stools and sometimes nausea, constipation, or diarrhea. To help avoid food-related effects, the iron supplement should be taken an hour before a meal or 2 hours after with liquid such as water or orange juice but not with milk or tea. The iron effect in the body is increased with vitamin C and decreased with milk, other dairy foods, eggs, whole-grain bread and cereal, and tea.

WEIGHT GAIN DURING PREGNANCY

General amount of weight gain

Healthy women produce healthy babies over a wide range of total weight gain. It is the individual assessment of need and the quality of the weight gain that is of paramount importance. Optimal weight gain from a quality diet throughout pregnancy makes an important contribution to a successful course and outcome. It should not be a problem or a source of contention. An average weight gain during normal pregnancy is about 11 to 16 kg (25 to 35 lb).[9] Around this average many individual variations occur. There is no specific rigid norm or restriction to which all women should be held regardless of individual needs. Such a course is obviously unwise and unscientific. Current recommendations are therefore usually stated in terms of ranges to accommodate variances in needs. An initial base for evaluation,

---

hyperemesis gravidarum Severe vomiting during pregnancy, which is potentially fatal.

Table

11.2 Daily food guide for women

Food group	One serving equals		Recommended minimum servings		
			Nonpregnant		Pregnant/ lactating
			11-24 yr	25+ yr	
Protein foods Provide protein, iron, zinc, and B vitamins for growth of muscles, bone, blood, and nerves; vegetable protein provides fiber to prevent constipation	*Animal protein:* 1 oz cooked chicken or turkey 1 oz cooked lean beef, lamb, or pork 1 oz or 1/4 cup fish or other seafood 1 egg 2 fish sticks or hot dogs 2 slices luncheon meat	*Vegetable protein:* 1/2 cup cooked dry beans, lentils, or split peas 3 oz tofu 1 oz or 1/4 cup peanuts, pumpkin seeds, or sunflower seeds 1 1/2 oz or 1/3 cup other nuts 2 tbsp peanut butter	5 A half serving of vegetable protein daily	5	7 One serving of vegetable protein daily
Milk products Provide protein and calcium to build strong bones, teeth, and healthy nerves and muscles and to promote normal blood clotting	8 oz milk 8 oz yogurt 1 cup milk shake 1/2 cup cream soup (made with milk) 1 1/2 oz or 1/3 cup grated cheese (like cheddar, Monterey, mozzarella, or Swiss)	1 1/2-2 slices presliced American cheese 4 tbsp Parmesan cheese 2 cups cottage cheese 1 cup pudding 1 cup custard or flan 1 1/2 cups ice milk, ice cream, or frozen yogurt	3	2	3
Breads, cereals, grains Provide carbohydrates and B vitamins for energy and healthy nerves; also provide iron for healthy blood; whole grains provide fiber to prevent constipation	1 slice bread 1 dinner roll 1/2 bun or bagel 1/2 English muffin or pita 1 small tortilla 3/4 cup dry cereal 1/2 cup granola 1/2 cup cooked cereal	1/2 cup rice 1/2 cup noodles or spaghetti 1/4 cup wheat germ 1 4-inch pancake or waffle 1 small muffin 8 medium crackers 4 graham cracker squares 3 cups popcorn	7 Four servings of whole grain products daily	6	7
Vitamin C–rich fruits and vegetables Provide vitamin C to prevent infection and to promote healing and iron absorption; also provide fiber to prevent constipation	6 oz orange, grapefruit, or fruit juice enriched with vitamin C 6 oz tomato juice or vegetable juice cocktail 1 orange, kiwi, or mango 1/2 grapefruit or cantaloupe 1/2 cup papaya 2 tangerines	1/2 cup strawberries 1/2 cup cooked or 1 cup raw cabbage 1/2 cup broccoli, brussels sprouts, or cauliflower 1/2 cup snow peas, sweet peppers, or tomato puree 2 tomatoes	1	1	1

NOTE: The Daily Food Guide for Women may not provide all the kcalories you require. The best way to increase your intake is to include more than the minimum servings recommended.

Modified from California Department of Health Services, Maternal and Child Health: *Nutrition during pregnancy and postpartum period: a manual for health care professionals,* Sacramento, 1990, CDHS.

Table

11.2   Daily food guide for women—cont'd

Food group	One serving equals		Recommended minimum servings		
			Nonpregnant		Pregnant/ lactating
			11-24 yr	25+ yr	
Vitamin A-rich fruits and vegetables					
Provide beta-carotene and vitamin A to prevent infection and to promote wound healing and night vision; also provide fiber to prevent constipation	6 oz apricot nectar or vegetable juice cocktail 3 raw or 1/4 cup dried apricots 1/4 cantaloupe or mango 1 small or 1/2 cup sliced carrots 2 tomatoes	1/2 cup cooked or 1 cup raw spinach 1/2 cup cooked greens (beet, chard, collards, dandelion, kale, mustard) 1/2 cup pumpkin, sweet potato, winter squash, or yams	1	1	1
Other fruits and vegetables					
Provide carbohydrates for energy and fiber to prevent constipation	6 oz fruit juice (if not listed above) 1 medium or 1/2 cup sliced fruit (apple, banana, peach, pear) 1/2 cup berries (other than strawberries) 1/2 cup cherries or grapes 1/2 cup pineapple 1/2 cup watermelon	1/2 cup dried fruit 1/2 cup sliced vegetable (asparagus, beets, green beans, celery, corn, eggplant, mushrooms, onion, peas, potato, summer squash, zucchini) 1/2 artichoke 1 cup lettuce	3	3	3
Unsaturated fats					
Provide vitamin E to protect tissue	1/8 medium avocado 1 tsp margarine 1 tsp mayonnaise 1 tsp vegetable oil	2 tsp salad dressing (mayonnaise-based) 1 tbsp salad dressing (oil-based)	3	3	3

however, may be the average weight of the products of pregnancy as shown in Table 11.3. In addition to the components of growth and development usually attributed to a pregnancy, an important part is maternal stores. This laying down of extra adipose fat tissue is necessary for maternal energy reserves to sustain rapid fetal growth during the latter half of pregnancy and for labor and delivery and maintaining lactation after birth. About 2 to 3.5 kg (4 to 8 lb) of adipose tissue are commonly deposited for these needs. An important report of the National Academy of Sciences, *Nutrition During Pregnancy*, recommends setting weight gain goals together with the pregnant woman according to her prepregnant nutritional status and weight-for-height[9]:

1. Normal weight women: 11.5 to 16 kg (25 to 35 lb)
2. Underweight women: 13 to 18 kg (28 to 40 lb)
3. Overweight women: 7 to 11.5 kg (15 to 25 lb)

The recommendation for adolescent mothers is that they should strive for the upper end of the range, 16 kg (35 lb). The recommendation for a woman carrying twins to avoid complications is a target weight gain of 16 to 20.5 kg (35 to 45 lb).[9] Compared with single birth infants twin birth infants are five times more likely to be born premature (less than 37-week gestation), nine and a half times more likely to be very low birth weight (less than 1500 g), and eight and a half times more likely to be low birth weight (less than 2500 g).[10]

Quality of weight gain

The important consideration, as indicated, lies in the nutritional quality of the gain. Specifically, the foods consumed should be nutrient dense. They should be nutritious foods to meet the nutrient requirements, not foods contributing only empty kcalories. Also, there has been failure in some cases to distinguish between weight

Table 11.3 Approximate weight of products of normal pregnancy	
Products	**Weight**
Fetus	3400 g (7.5 lb)
Placenta	450 g (1 lb)
Amniotic fluid	900 g (2 lb)
Uterus (weight increase)	1100 g (2.5 lb)
Breast tissue (weight increase)	1400 g (3 lb)
Blood volume (weight increase)	1800 g (4 lb) (1500 ml)
Maternal stores	1800-3600 g (4-8 lb)
TOTAL	10,850-12,650 g (10.8-12.7 kg; 24-28 lb)

gained as a result of edema and that as a result of deposition of fat—maternal stores for energy to sustain rapid fetal growth during the latter part of pregnancy and energy for lactation to follow. Analysis of the total tissue gained in an average pregnancy shows that the largest component, 62%, is water. Fat accounts for 31% and protein for 7%. Water is also the most variable component of the tissue gained, accounting for a range of 8 kg (18 lb) to as much as 11 kg (24 lb). Of the 8 kg of water usually gained, about 5.5 kg (12 lb) is associated with fetal tissue and other tissues gained in pregnancy. The remaining 2.5 kg (6 lb) accumulates in the maternal interstitial tissues.[10] Gravity causes the maternal tissue fluids to pool more in the lower extremities, leading to general swelling of the ankles, which is seen routinely in pregnant women. This fluid retention is a normal adaptive phenomenon designed to support the pregnancy and exert a positive effect on fetal growth. The connective tissue becomes more **hygroscopic** as a result of the estrogen-induced changes in the ground substance. The connective tissue thus becomes softer and more easily distended to facilitate delivery through the cervix and the vaginal canal. Also, the increased tissue fluid during pregnancy provides a means for handling the increased metabolic work and circulation of numerous metabolites necessary for fetal growth.

Clearly, severe kcaloric restriction is harmful to the developing fetus and the mother. It is inevitably accompanied by restriction of the vitally needed nutrients essential to the growth process. Thus *weight reduction should never be undertaken during pregnancy*. To the contrary, sufficient weight gain should be encouraged with the use of a nourishing diet as outlined.

Rate of weight gain

On the whole, about 1 to 2.3 kg (2 to 5 lb) is an average weight gain during the first trimester. Thereafter, an average weight gain of about 0.5 kg (1 lb) per week during the remainder of the pregnancy is usual, although some women may need to gain more. There is no scientific justification for routinely limiting weight gain to lesser amounts. Moreover, an individual woman who needs to gain more should not have unrealistic grid patterns imposed on her. It is only unusual patterns of gain, such as a sudden sharp increase in weight after the twentieth week of pregnancy, which may signal abnormal water retention, that should be monitored closely, especially if it occurs in conjunction with blood pressure elevation and proteinuria.

Weight gain and sodium intake

Sometimes in relation to weight gain, questions are raised about the use of salt during pregnancy. A moderate amount of dietary sodium is needed for two essential reasons: (1) it is the major mineral required for controlling the extracellular fluid compartment and (2) this vital body water is increased during pregnancy to support its successful outcome. Current practice usually follows a regular diet with moderate sodium intake, 2 to 3 g/day, with light use of salt to taste. Limiting sodium beyond this general use is contrary to physiologic need in pregnancy and is unfounded. The National Research Council and professional obstetric guidelines have labeled routine salt-free diets and diuretics as potentially dangerous.[1-4] Maintaining the needed increase in circulating blood volume during pregnancy requires adequate amounts of sodium and protein.

HIGH-RISK MOTHERS AND INFANTS

IDENTIFY RISK FACTORS INVOLVED

To avoid the consequences of poor nutrition during pregnancy, a first procedure is to identify mothers at risk (see *Practical Application* box, p. 240). In a joint report, the American College of Obstetrics and Gynecology and the American Dietetic Association have issued a set of risk factors as shown in Table 11.4 that identify women with special nutritional needs during pregnancy.[3] These nutrition-related factors are based on clinical evidence of inadequate nutrition. However, rather than waiting for clinical symptoms of poor nutrition to appear, a better approach would be to identify poor food patterns that will bring on nutritional problems and prevent these problems from developing. On this basis, three types of dietary patterns predict failure to support optimal maternal and fetal nutrition: (1) insufficient food intake, (2) poor food selection, and (3) poor food distribution throughout the day. These patterns, added to the list of risk factors in Table 11.4, are much more sensitive for nutritional risk.

Table 11.4 Nutritional risk factors in pregnancy	
Risk factors present at the onset of pregancy	**Risk factors occuring during pregnancy**
Age	Low hemoglobin or
15 years or younger	hematocrit
35 years or older	Hemoglobin less than
Frequent pregancies; three or	12 g
more during a 2-year period	Hematocrit less than
Poor obstetric history or poor	35 mg/dl
fetal performance	Inadequate weight gain
Poverty	Any weight loss
Bizarre or faddist food habits	Weight gain of less than
Abuse of nicotine, alcohol, or	1 kg (2 lb) per month
drugs	after the first
Therapeutic diet required for	trimester
a chronic disorder	Excessive weight gain:
Inadequte weight: less than	greater than 1 kg (2 lb)
85% of standard weight	per week after the first
Excessive weight: more than	trimester
120% of standard weight	

PLAN PERSONAL CARE

Once early assessment identifies risk factors, practitioners can then give more careful attention to these women. By working closely with each mother and her personal food pattern and living situation, a food plan can be developed with her to ensure an optimal intake of energy and nutrients to support her pregnancy and its successful outcome.

RECOGNIZE SPECIAL COUNSELING NEEDS

Several special needs require sensitive counseling. These areas of need include the age and parity of the mother; any use of harmful agents such as alcohol, cigarettes, drugs, or pica; and socioeconomic problems.

Age and parity

Pregnancies at either age extreme of the reproductive cycle pose special problems. The adolescent pregnancy carries many social and nutrition-related risks. Imposed on a still immature teenage body are the additional demands of the pregnancy. The obstetric history of a woman is expressed in terms of number and order of pregnancies, or her **gravida** status. **Nulligravidas** (no prior pregnancy) 15 years old and younger are especially at risk, since their own growth is incomplete, so sufficient weight gain and the quality of their diet are particularly important.[10,11] Sensitive counseling provides both information and emotional support. It should involve family or other persons significant to the young mother.

On the other hand, the older **primigravida** (first pregnancy), over 35 years of age, also requires special attention. She may be more at risk for hypertension, either preexisting or pregnancy-induced, and may need more attention to rate of weight gain and amount of sodium used, as well as any drug therapy prescribed.[12] In addition, several pregnancies within a limited number of years leave a mother drained of nutritional resources and entering each successive pregnancy at a higher risk. Counseling may well include discussions of acceptable means of contraception and nutrition information and support.

Social habits: alcohol, cigarettes, drugs, and pica

These four personal habits cause fetal damage and are contraindicated during pregnancy. Even moderate prenatal alcohol exposure is associated with low birth weight and has effects on children's psychomotor development.[13] Extensive or habitual alcohol use leads to the well-described and documented fetal alcohol syndrome (FAS), which is currently a leading cause of mental retardation. Cigarette smoking during pregnancy is also contraindicated.[14] Harmful substances in tobacco cause fetal damage and special problems of placental abnormalities, including prematurity and low birth weight (see *Practical Application* box, p. 240), largely as a result of impaired oxygen transport. Counseling with mothers who smoke should stress the importance of quitting.

Drug use, both recreational and medicinal, also poses numerous problems. Self-medication with over-the-counter drugs carries potential adverse effects. The use of street drugs is especially hazardous, exposing the developing fetus to the risks of addiction and possibly AIDS from the mother's use of contaminated needles in her drug injections. Dangers come not only from the drug itself or contaminated needles but also from the impurities such street drugs contain. In addition, drug abuse from megadosing with basic nutrients such as vitamin A during pregnancy may also cause fetal damage.[15] Especially dangerous are drugs made from vitamin A compounds, retinoids such as Accutane or etretinate, prescribed for severe acne, which have caused spontaneous abortion of malformed infants by women who conceived during such acne treatment. Thus the use of these drugs without contraception is definitely contraindicated.

---

hygroscopic   Taking up and retaining moisture readily.

nulligravida   A woman who has never been pregnant.

primigravida   A woman pregnant for the first time.

Who will have the low birth weight baby?

The number of babies weighing less than 2500 g (5 lb) at birth is on the rise. It is a leading cause of infant mortality in the United States. It also contributes to poor cognitive abilities and learning problems in the school-age children who survive.

Perinatal nutritionists are well aware of the dietary factors that may influence this increase, especially poor weight gain during pregnancy. The prevalence of that turn-of-the-century adage to "grow the baby to fit the pelvis" continues to influence some physicians, nurses, and expectant mothers to limit prenatal weight gain to 9 kg (20 lb) or less to avoid obstetric problems, especially at delivery. This practice is harmful and is refuted by recent evidence that a gain of 11 to 15 kg (25 to 35 lb) is correlated with birth weights of greater than 2500 g (5 lb).

The obsession with weight control during pregnancy can lead to harmful restrictions of vital energy and nutrients. Weight reduction should *never* be attempted during pregnancy. Such regimens are extremely dangerous to the fetus. Even the common practice of skipping breakfast, especially late in pregnancy, may potentially impair intellectual development by inducing a ketotic, pseudostarvation state very quickly. Increased ketoacidosis from fat breakdown can cause neurologic damage to the fetus.

Nondietary factors influencing the incidence of lowbirth weight (LBW) or premature babies have been identified in numerous studies:

- Rise in number of older primigravidas (that is, over 35 years of age)
- Rise in number of teenage pregnancies
- Low socioeconomic status, low educational level
- History of obstetric problems, such as prior LBW birth or reproductive loss
- Poor nutritional status, including low prepregnant weight for height, low-energy intake during pregnancy, low hemoglobin level and hematocrit, inadequate early weight gain
- Clinical problems such as pregnancy-induced hypertension (PIH)
- Behavioral/environmental risk factors, smoking, alcohol and drug abuse.
- Single marital status (often an indicator of low economic status)
- Technologic advances in neonatal care, which keep premature infants alive longer
- Race: nonwhites have higher rates of LBW infants than whites do, which is more a function of poverty, limited education, or young age than race as such

To reduce the risk of LBW infants in populations being served by your facility, you may want to do the following:

- Explain the rationale for gaining around 11 to 15 kg (25 to 30 lb).
- Discourage the use of cigarettes, alcohol, and drugs.
- Monitor excessive weight gain and sodium intake in older primigravidas, who are often at risk for prenatal essential hypertension and obesity.
- Explore eating habits of adolescents in the local community, working with the girl and her significant others to incorporate nutrient-dense foods into her meal and snack selections.
- Keep abreast of federal, state, and local supplemental food programs (for example, WIC) available to low-income women to ensure an adequate intake of nutrients and kcalories.
- Encourage regular eating patterns throughout pregnancy.

References

Hack M et al: Effect of very low birth weight and subnormal head size on cognitive abilities at school, *N Engl J Med* 325(4):231, 1991.

Haughton B et al: Public health nutrition practices to prevent low birth weight in eight southeastern states, *J Am Diet Assoc* 92(2):187, 1992.

Porter DV: WIC nutrition risk criteria: a scientific assessment, *Nutr Today* 31(5):216, 1996.

Caffeine

Although milder in its effect (depending on extent of use) than agents discussed above, caffeine is still a widely used drug that can cross the placenta and enter fetal circulation. Its use at pharmacologic levels has been associated with low birth weight.[16] A pharmacologic dose of caffeine—250 mg—is contained in 2 cups of coffee, 3.5 cups of tea, or five 12-oz colas, so such use is not recommended. Most responsible health agencies have recommended that pregnant women avoid caffeine-containing beverages and that products containing caffeine be plainly labeled to inform consumers.

Pica

Pica is the craving and consuming of unusual nonfood substances such as laundry starch, clay, dirt, or ice. This practice during pregnancy is more widespread than health care workers have believed. The eating of clay or dirt may indicate an iron deficiency anemia.[17,18] Where these unusual practices exist they must be understood as deep-rooted cultural patterns that require a respectful approach by health workers who seek to negotiate appropriate behavior changes.[17]

Socioeconomic problems

Special counseling is required for women and young girls living in low-income situations or extreme poverty. Numerous studies and clinical observations indicate that lack of prenatal care, often associated with racial prejudices and fears as well as poverty, places the expectant mother in grave difficulty. Special counseling, sensitive to personal needs, is needed to help plan resources for care and financial assistance. Resources include programs such as WIC and the Commodity Distribution Program, both of which are described in the previous chapter.

COMPLICATIONS OF PREGNANCY

ANEMIA

Anemia is common during pregnancy. It is often associated with a normal maternal blood volume increase of about 50% and a disproportionate increase in red cell mass of about 20%. About 10% of all women in large prenatal clinics in the United States have hemoglobin concentrations of less than 10 g/dl and a hematocrit reading below 32%. Anemia is far more prevalent among the poor, many of whom live on diets barely adequate for subsistence. However, anemia is by no means restricted to lower economic groups.

Iron-deficiency anemia

A deficiency of iron is by far the most common cause of anemia in pregnancy. The total cost of a single normal pregnancy in iron stores is large—about 500 to 800 mg. Of this amount nearly 300 mg is used by the fetus. The remainder is used in the expanded maternal blood volume and its increased red blood cells and hemoglobin mass. This iron requirement exceeds the available reserves in the average woman. Thus in addition to including iron-rich foods in the diet, a daily supplement of 30 to 60 mg is usually recommended. Treatment of highly deficient states requires daily therapeutic doses of 120 to 200 mg, which is usually continued for 3 to 6

months after the anemia has been corrected in order to replenish the depleted stores.

Folate-deficiency anemia

A less common megaloblastic anemia of pregnancy results from folate deficiency. During pregnancy, the fetus is sensitive to folate inhibitors and therefore has increased metabolic requirements for folate. To prevent this anemia, the RDA standard recommends 400 μg of folate daily. Women with poor diets will need supplementation to reach this intake goal.

Hemorrhagic anemia

Anemia caused by blood loss is more likely to occur during labor and delivery rather than during pregnancy. Blood loss may occur earlier, as a result of abortion or ruptured tubular pregnancy. Most patients undergoing these physiologic problems receive blood by transfusion, and iron therapy may be indicated for adequate replacement hemoglobin formation.

PREGNANCY-INDUCED HYPERTENSION

Relation to nutrition

A number of clinicians have presented clinical and laboratory evidence that pregnancy-induced hypertension, or PIH (formerly labeled toxemia), is a disease principally affecting young mothers with their first pregnancy. It is especially related to diets poor in protein, kcalories, calcium, and salt. Such malnutrition affects the liver and its metabolic activities. Whatever its underlying causes and multiorgan effects, nutritional support of the pregnancy is, as always, a primary concern. Certainly, as many practitioners have observed, PIH is classically associated with poverty, inadequate diet, and little or no prenatal care. Much of the PIH problem, which seems to develop early from the time of implantation of the fertilized ovum into the uterine lining, may be reduced by good prenatal care from the beginning of the pregnancy, which inherently includes attention to sound nutrition. It is this sound nutritional status, which a woman brings to her pregnancy and maintains throughout, that provides her with optimal resources for adapting to the physiologic stress of gestation. Her fitness during pregnancy is a direct function of her past state of nutrition and her optimal nutrition throughout pregnancy.

Clinical symptoms

PIH is defined according to its manifestations, which generally occur in the third trimester toward term. These symptoms are hypertension, abnormal and excessive edema, albuminuria, and in severe cases, convulsions or coma, a state called **eclampsia**.

---

eclampsia Advanced pregnancy-induced hypertension (PIH), manifested by convulsions.

Treatment

Specific treatment varies according to the individual patient's symptoms and needs. Optimal nutrition is a fundamental aspect of therapy in any case. Emphasis is given to a regular diet with adequate dietary protein and calcium. Correction of plasma protein deficits stimulates the capillary fluid shift mechanism and increases circulation of tissue fluids, with subsequent correction of the **hypovolemia**. In addition, adequate salt and sources of vitamins and minerals are needed for correction and maintenance of metabolic balance.

MATERNAL DISEASE CONDITIONS

Preexisting clinical conditions in the mother further complicate pregnancy. In each case, management of these conditions is based on general principles of care related to both pregnancy and the particular disease involved. Examples of three such maternal conditions are reviewed here. They are hypertension, diabetes mellitus, and phenylketonuria.

Hypertension

Preexisting hypertension in the pregnant woman can cause considerable maternal and fetal consequences. Many of these problems can be prevented by initial screening and continued monitoring by the prenatal nurse, with referral to the clinical nutritionist for a plan of care. The hypertensive disease process begins long before signs and symptoms appear, and later symptoms are inconsistent. Risk factors for hypertension before and during pregnancy are given in Table 11.5. Nutritional therapy centers on (1) prevention of weight extremes, underweight or obesity; (2) correction of any dietary deficiencies and maintenance of optimal nutritional status during pregnancy; and (3) management of any related preexisting disease such as diabetes mellitus or hyperlipidemia. Sodium intake may be moderate but should not be unduly restricted because of its relation to fluid and electrolyte balances during pregnancy and its controversial therapy in hypertension in general. Initial and continuing client education and a close relationship with the nurse-nutritionist care team contribute to successful management of the hypertension and prevent problems that may occur.

Diabetes mellitus

The management of preexisting diabetes in pregnancy presents special problems. Today, however, improved expectations for the diabetic mother's pregnancy constitute one of the success stories of modern medicine. Contributing factors to this improved outlook include advances in technology for monitoring fetal development, increased knowledge of nutrition and diabetes, and management refinements in tight blood glucose control through self-monitoring.[19,20] Routine screening is necessary to detect gestational diabetes, and team

Table 11.5	Risk factors in pregnancy-induced hypertension	
Before pregancy	**During pregnancy**
Nulligravida	Primigravida
Diabetes	Large fetus
Preexisting condition (hypertension, renal or vascular disease)	Glomerulonephritis
Family history of hypertension or vascular disease	Fetal hydrops
Diagnoses of pregnancy-induced hypertension in a previous pregnancy	Hydramnios
Dietary deficiencies	Multiple gestation
Age extremes 20 years or younger 35 years or older	Hydatidiform mole

management is required for preexisting insulin-dependent diabetes mellitus (IDDM).[21,22] During pregnancy, glycosuria is not uncommon because of the increased circulating blood volume and its load of metabolites. Gestational diabetes occurs in 2% to 13% of the pregnant population. But only 20% to 30% of these women showing this pregnancy-induced abnormal glucose tolerance subsequently develop diabetes. Nonetheless, follow-up is important because of the higher risk these women carry for fetal damage during this gestational period. Refer to Chapter 21 for a detailed discussion of diabetes care.

Maternal phenylketonuria

Successful detection and management of phenylketonuria (PKU) babies through United States newborn screening programs in all states has ensured their normal growth and development to adulthood. PKU is a genetic metabolic disease caused by a missing enzyme for the metabolism of the essential amino acid phenylalanine. It is controlled by a special low-phenylalanine diet initiated at birth. Now a new generation of young women with PKU since birth are beginning to have children of their own. However, maternal PKU presents potential fetal hazards. Experience has shown how crucial it is for the mother to follow a strict low-phenylalanine diet before conception, whenever possible, to minimize risks of fetal damage in the early cell differentiation weeks of pregnancy.

NUTRITION DURING LACTATION

CURRENT BREAST-FEEDING TRENDS

An increasing number of mothers in America and other developed countries are choosing breast-feeding for their infants (see *To Probe Further* box, p. 245). Sev-

Figure 11.1 Nurse discussing postpartum and infant care with new mother. (David York, Medichrome.)

Table 11.6 Nutritional components of human milk (per 100 ml)				
Milk component	**Colostrum**	**Transitional**	**Mature**	**Cow's milk**
Kilocalories	57.0	63.0	65.0	65.0
Vitamins, fat-soluble:				
A (μg)	151.0	88.0	75.0	41.0
D (IU)	—	—	5.0	2.5
E (mg)	1.5	0.9	0.25	0.07
K (μg)	—	—	1.5	6.0
Vitamins, water-soluble:				
Thiamin (μg)	1.9	5.9	14.0	43.0
Riboflavin (μg)	30.0	37.0	40.0	145.0
Niacin (μg)	75.0	175.0	160.0	82.0
Pantothenic acid (μg)	183.0	288.0	246.0	340.0
Biotin (μg)	0.06	0.35	0.6	2.8
Vitamin B_{12} (μg)	0.05	0.04	0.1	1.1
Vitamin C (mg)	5.9	7.1	5.0	1.1

eral factors have contributed to this choice: (1) more mothers are informed about the benefits of breast-feeding (Figure 11.1), (2) practitioners recognize the ability of human milk to meet infant needs (Table 11.6), (3) maternity wards and alternative birth centers are being modified to facilitate successful lactation, and (4) community support is more available, even in work places. Exclusive breast-feeding by well-nourished mothers can be adequate for periods ranging from 2 to 15 months.[23] Solid foods are usually added to the baby's diet at about 6 months of age.

NUTRITIONAL NEEDS

The physiologic needs of lactation are greater than those of pregnancy, and they demand adequate nutritional support (see Tables 11.1 and 11.2). The basic nutritional needs for lactation include the following additions to the mother's prepregnant needs.

hypovolemia Abnormally decreased volume of circulating blood in the body.

Protein

The RDA standard for protein needs during lactation is 65 g/day during the first 6 months and 62 g/day during the second 6 months. This is an increase of about 15 to 20 g/day from the regular needs of the adolescent girl (44 to 46 g/day) and the adult woman (46 to 50 g/day).

Energy

The recommended kcaloric increase is 500 kcalories more than the usual adult allowance. This makes a daily total of about 2500 to 2700 kcalories. This additional energy need for the overall total lactation process is based on three factors:

1. *Milk content.* An average daily milk production for lactating women is 850 ml (30 oz). Human milk has a kcalorie range of 20 to 70 kcal/oz or an average of 24 kcal/oz. Thus 30 oz of milk has a value of about 700 kcalories.
2. *Milk production.* The metabolic work involved in producing this amount of milk requires from 400 to 450 kcalories. During pregnancy the breast is developed for this purpose, stimulated by hormones from the placenta, forming special milk-producing cells called lobules (Figure 11.2). After birth the mother's production of the hormone prolactin con-

tinues this milk-production process, which the suckling infant stimulates. Thus milk production depends on the demand of the infant. The suckling infant stimulates the brain's release of the hormone oxytocin from the pituitary gland to initiate the let-down reflex for the release of the milk from storage cells to travel down to the nipple. This reflex is easily inhibited by the mother's fatigue, tension, or lack of confidence, a particular source of anxiety in the new mother. She may be reassured that a comfortable and satisfying feeding routine is usually established in 2 to 3 weeks (Figure 11.3).

3. *Maternal adipose tissue storage.* The additional energy need for lactation is drawn from maternal adipose tissue stores deposited during pregnancy in normal preparation for lactation to follow in the maternal cycle. Depending on the adequacy of these stores, additional energy input may be needed in the lactating woman's daily diet.

MINERALS

The RDA standard for calcium during lactation is 1200 mg/day, the same as for the nonpregnant adolescent girl and the young adult woman, but a 400-g increase from the regular adult need of 800 mg. The calcium needs of the breast-feeding mother are not greater than those during pregnancy. The increased amount of calcium that was required during gestation for the mineralization of the fetal skeleton is now diverted into the mother's milk production. Iron, because it is not a principal mineral component of milk, need not be increased for the production of milk.

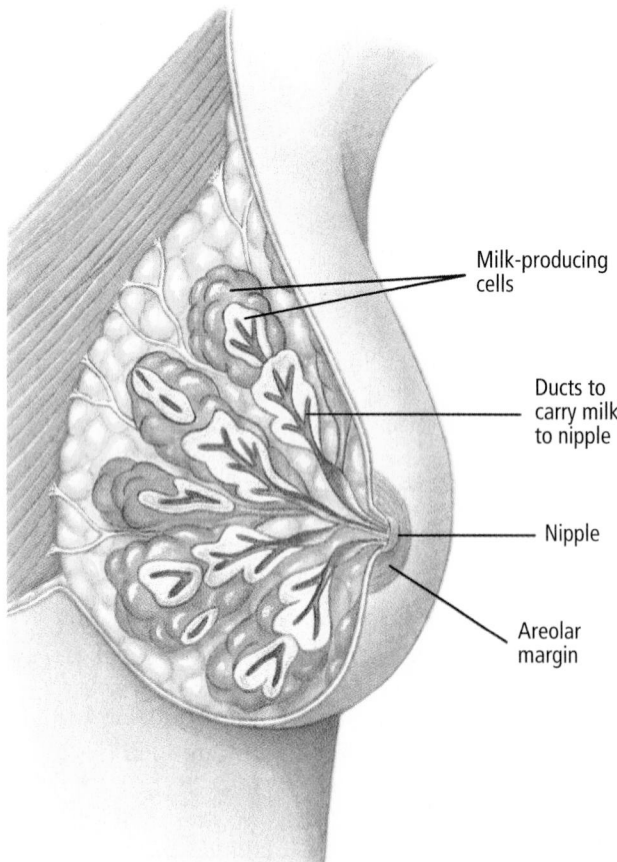

Figure 11.2   Anatomy of the breast. (From Wardlaw G, Insel P: *Perspectives in nutrition,* ed 2, New York, 1993, McGraw-Hill.)

Milk-producing cells

Ducts to carry milk to nipple

Nipple

Areolar margin

Figure 11.3   Breast-feeding the newborn infant. Note that the nurse, in assisting the mother, avoids touching the infant's outer cheek so as not to counteract his natural rooting reflex at the touch of the breast.

To Probe Further

Breast-feeding: the dynamic nature of human milk

There is no question that human milk is the ideal first food for human infants. Its dynamic nature changes to match growth needs. The mother's choice to breast-feed her infant depends on a number of factors, however, especially for new mothers, who often need information and counseling from early pregnancy.

Even premature infants can thrive on human milk. Mothers and physicians have sometimes been reluctant to consider breast-feeding for babies born prematurely or delivered by cesarean section, fearing that there may be some negative effect on the quantity or quality of human milk. This uncertainty about the nutritional quality of mother's milk has also led them to encourage adding formula and/or solid foods to the diet to make sure the baby is well-fed. These practices are usually unnecessary. They often contribute to allergies, obesity, and digestive problems because of the extra stress placed on an immature gut.

Breast milk for the preterm infant

Levels of nutrients in mother's milk shift according to the gestational age of the infant at birth. The preterm infant is often denied its mother's milk by some hospital workers because they think of it as mature milk having too little protein and too much lactose to meet the child's needs. An analysis of the nutritional quality of preterm milk, however, reveals energy and fat concentrations that are 20% to 30% higher, protein levels 15% to 20% higher, and lactose levels 10% lower than those found in mature milk. Premature milk can meet the preterm infant's needs.

Breast milk during weaning

Nutrient levels continue to change with time to match changing growth patterns and developing digestive abilities. Mother's milk does provide sufficient kcalories and nutrients to keep babies well-fed without supplemental formula or food. Even when the infant is being weaned, the nature of human milk ensures adequate nutrients, just in case the new, solid-food diet can't meet the child's needs. Human milk collected during gradual weaning has been found to have higher concentrations of protein, sodium, and iron. Lactose levels are lower, possibly so that higher amounts of kcalories can be supplied by fats, a more concentrated source.

Breast milk and the cesarean-section infant

The quality of human milk is not influenced by the way the baby comes into the world. Many women fear that a baby born by cesarean section cannot be nursed because they think that this method of delivery delays or prevents the production of mature milk. Milk production is stimulated by the release of the placenta, which occurs whether the delivery is vaginal or not. Studies confirm that there is no significant difference in the length of time it takes for mature milk to come in after vaginal or cesarean deliveries.

Thus premature or cesarean deliveries should not discourage women from breast-feeding. Mothers should not underestimate the nutritive quality of their milk simply because it does not appear as rich and thick as cow's milk. After all, cow's milk is made for young calves who are up and running around after birth and have a much shorter, faster growth period. But for the human infant, in both nutritional and immunologic terms, breast milk remains the best milk.

Mothers' fact and fancy about breast-feeding

In early counseling, mothers express a variety of concerns about breast-feeding. These are a few such statements:

"My breasts aren't big enough." When it comes to breast-feeding, all women are created equal. The only parts of the breast that participate in milk production are the glandular and nervous tissue, as well as the nipple; these are basically the same in healthy women. The only difference between a 32A and a 42DD is the amount of fat the breast contains.

"Breast-feeding causes cancer." Actually, in recent years, investigators have been looking to breast-feeding as a possible means of preventing breast cancer. At this point, however, no studies exist that convincingly show that breast-feeding either helps or hinders a woman from developing this disease.

"Breast-feeding will ruin my figure." Breast-feeding might actually help a woman regain her figure more quickly. Because the caloric demand of breast-

Continued

feeding exceeds that of the nonpregnant woman by about 500 kcalories, a slightly faster rate of weight loss may be expected. Furthermore, oxytocin, the hormone manufactured to stimulate milk production, also stimulates uterine contractions, helping reduce the uterus to its prepregnant size more rapidly.

"Breast-feeding is painful." It can be if the baby is nursed infrequently or the mother's hygienic practices leave much to be desired. However, if milk is not allowed to collect in the breast to the point of engorgement, if the nipples are kept clean and dry, and if proper latch-on techniques are used while nursing, the chances for having a painful experience will be relatively small.

"Breast milk isn't nutritious." The thin, bluish appearance of breast milk has some women convinced that it is no more nourishing than water. Let them look at Table 13-6; they'll be pleasantly surprised at how well breast milk meets the nutritional needs of the infant.

"I can't go to work or school if I breast-feed." Breast milk can be stored for 24 hours in the refrigerator or several months in the freezer. Many working mothers take advantage of this by expressing their milk and storing it for use by a baby-sitter. In fact, women often express milk on their breaks at school or work. (Some employers even provide breast pumps at the workplace.) Not only does this relieve the pressure of buildup, but it also allows the milk to be stored for later use at home.

Other women would like to breast-feed, but are worried about special "what if" situations, such as:

"What if I need a cesarean section?" The method of delivery does not affect the quality or quantity of milk produced. The baby can be held in such a way (the football hold) that he or she does not rest on the mother's abdominal stitches.

"What if the baby is premature?" Mother's milk changes to meet the infant's needs at all stages of development.

"What if the baby has a birth defect such as Down syndrome?" This baby can be nursed; however, it does require time, patience, and the use of slightly different nursing techniques. The mother should be told about the special nursing needs of this infant to avoid disappointment or a feeling of failure in case breast-feeding becomes impractical for her particular living situation.

"What if I have twins?" Believe it or not, it has been done. It takes time, patience, and good coordination, but it can be done. Triplets, however, are another matter altogether. Women have successfully nursed triplets, but often they did very little else until the babies were weaned. This mother will need emotional support whether she attempts to nurse or, finding the amount of time and patience required overwhelming, is forced to bottle-feed.

Some women may purposefully choose to breast-feed to avoid pregnancy. But this is by no means a dependable contraception method. The more well-nourished women of the world tend to be more fertile and have been surprised to find themselves pregnant and breast-feeding at the same time. Women who breast-feed must understand that the lack of a menstrual period during lactation does not mean they cannot become pregnant. Contraceptives, preferably barrier types, may be required if another pregnancy is not desired at that time.

Advantages and barriers to breast-feeding

These factors need to be reviewed with each individual mother in her particular situation. Only on this basis can she make the informed decision best for the baby and for her.

There are many nutritional, physiologic, psychologic, and practical advantages to breast-feeding:

1. *Human milk changes* to meet changing nutrient and energy needs of both the newborn and the maturing infant during the first months of life. It is always there in the correct form to meet the growing infant's needs.
2. Infants experience *fewer infections*, since the mother transfers certain antibodies or immune properties in human milk to her nursing infant. Also, there is no exposure of the infant to infectious organisms in the environment that can contaminate preparation and equipment for bottle-feeding, especially in poorer living situations.
3. *Fewer allergies and intolerances* occur, especially in allergy-prone infants, since cow's milk contains a number of potentially allergy-causing proteins that human milk does not have.
4. *Ease of digestion* is greater with breast milk, since human milk forms a softer curd in the gastrointestinal tract that is easier for the infant to digest.
5. The *convenience and economy* of breast milk is greater, since the mother is free from the time and expense involved in buying and preparing formula, and her breast milk is always ready and sterile.
6. Breast-feeding provides *psychologic bonding*, since the mother and infant relate to one another during feeding, regular times of rest and enjoyment, cuddling and fulfillment.

Despite the advantages of breast-feeding, some women do have to deal with perceived barriers associated with misinformation, personal feelings of modesty, family pressures, or outside employment.

1. *Misinformation*, a major barrier, creates negative impressions and ideas. Women in today's world often lack positive role models in extended families or experienced friends with whom they can discuss their feelings and obtain much practical guidance. Experienced breast-feeding mothers can fill this need, especially for young first-time mothers.

2. *Personal modesty and anxiety*, or a fear of appearing immodest in breast exposure, may hinder some young mothers from breast-feeding. Sensitive counseling, especially with a positive role model as described, can help to allay some of these personal fears. Most of women's breast-feeding is in the privacy of the home, rather than around others, so early support during initial experiences would be helpful.

3. *Family pressures*, especially from the husband, not to breast-feed have strong influence on the young first-time mother, even though she may want to do so. Initial counseling and education about breast-feeding should include both parents whenever possible. Reasons for negative attitudes can be explored and misinformation clarified with sound education.

4. *Outside employment*, with a limited maternity leave and job loss if the mother does not return to work at that time, can complicate the mother's deci-sion, even though she may want to breast-feed her baby. However, if the mother does have the will, there are ways to do both. After breast-feeding is well established during her maternity leave, she can regularly express milk by hand or with a breast pump into sterile disposal nursing bags to use with disposal holder, cap, and nipple ensemble. Rapid chilling and strict sanitation are required, but it can be planned, given the commitment. Some companies provide child care facilities for their employees, recognizing this modern need as good business. The mother can plan occasional formula feeds to fill in with the sustained breast-feeding.

All of these approaches to breast-feeding have real rewards for the infant. In addition, they can strengthen the mother's confidence in her own maternal capabilities. The importance even of these intangible benefits should not be underestimated.

References

American Academy of Pediatrics Work Group on Breast-feeding: Policy statement on breast-feeding, *Pediatrics* 100(Dec):1035, 1997.

Armotrading DC et al: Impact of WIC utilization rate on breast-feeding among international students at a large university, *J Am Diet Assoc* 92(3):352, 1992.

Ghaemi-Ahmadi S: Attitudes toward breast-feeding among Iranian, Afghan, and Southeast Asian immigrant women in the United States: implications for health and nutrition education, *J Am Diet Assoc* 92(3):354, 1992.

Krebs NF, Murtaugh MA: Position of the American Dietetic Association: promotion of breast feeding, *J Am Diet Assoc* 97(6):662, 1997.

In addition, for the breast-feeding infant, the American Academy of Pediatrics recommends a fluoride supplement of 0.25 mg/day because lactating mothers produce milk that is low in fluoride (about 16 μg/L).

VITAMINS

The RDA standard for vitamin C during lactation is 95 mg/day during the first 6 months and 90 mg/day for the second 6 months. This is a considerable increase from the regular 50 to 60 mg/day for adolescent girls and 60 mg/day for adult women. Increases over the mother's prenatal intake are also recommended for vitamin A, since it is a constituent of milk, and for the B-complex vitamins, since they are involved as coenzyme factors in energy metabolism. The quantities of vitamins needed therefore invariably increase as the kcalorie intake increases.

FLUIDS

Ample fluid intake is needed, 8 to 10 glasses/day, before and during lactation. Also, the critical factor necessary for successful milk production is the increased energy intake. The basis for this increased caloric need is described in the previous discussion. Additional beverages such as juices and milk contribute both fluid and kcalories.

REST AND RELAXATION

In addition to the increased diet, the nursing mother requires rest, moderate exercise, and relaxation. Both parents may benefit from counseling focused on reducing the stresses of their new family situation, as well as meeting their own personal needs.

TO SUM UP

Pregnancy involves synergistic interactions among three distinct biologic entities: the fetus, the placenta, and the mother. Maternal needs reflect the increasing nutritional needs of the fetus and the placenta, as well as the need to meet maternal needs and to prepare for lactation. An optimal weight gain of about 11 kg (25 lb), or more as needed, is recommended during pregnancy to accommodate the rapid growth taking place. Even more significant than the actual weight gain is the quality of the diet.

Common problems occurring during pregnancy include nausea and vomiting, heartburn, or constipation. In most cases they are easily relieved without medication by simple, often temporary, changes in the diet. Serious problems with pregnancy may be associated with preexisting chronic maternal conditions, for example, diabetes mellitus, or conditions arising as a result of physical or metabolic demands of pregnancy, for example, iron-deficiency anemia and PIH. Unusual or erratic eating habits, age, parity, prepartum weight status, and low income are among the many related factors that also place the mother at risk for complications.

In its current position paper, the American Dietetic Association strongly encourages public health and clinical efforts that promote breast-feeding to optimize the indisputable nutritional, immunologic, psychologic, and economic benefits.[24] The ultimate goal of prenatal care is a healthy infant and a mother physically capable of breast-feeding her child, should she choose to do so. Human milk provides essential nutrients in quantities required for optimal infant growth and development. It also supplies immunologic factors that offer protection against infection. Lactation requires an increase in kcalories beyond the needs of pregnancy. Adequate fluid intake is guided by the mother's natural thirst.

QUESTIONS FOR REVIEW

1. List and discuss five factors that influence the nutritional needs of the woman during pregnancy. Which factors would place a woman in a high-risk category? Why?

2. List six nutrients that are required in larger amounts during pregnancy. Describe their special role during this period. Identify four food sources of each.

3. Identify two common problems associated with pregnancy and describe the dietary management of each.

4. List and describe the screening indicators and risk factors for hypertension and diabetes mellitus during pregnancy.

5. List and discuss five major nutritional factors of lactation.

REFERENCES

1. Food and Nutrition Board, Committee on Maternal Nutrition, National Research Council—National Academy of Sciences: *Maternal nutrition and the course of human pregnancy,* Washington, DC, 1970, National Academy Press.

2. American College of Obstetricians and Gynecologists, Committee on Nutrition: *Nutrition in maternal health care,* Chicago, 1974, The College.

3. American College of Obstetricians and Gynecologists and American Dietetic Association, Task Force on Nutrition: *Assessment of maternal nutrition,* Chicago, 1978, The College and Association.

4. Food and Nutrition Board, National Academy of Sciences—National Research Council: *Recommended dietary allowances,* ed 10, Washington, DC, 1989, National Academy Press.

5. Garnica AD, Chan W-Y: The role of the placenta in fetal nutrition and growth, *J Am Coll Nutr* 15(3):206, 1996.

6. US Department of Health and Human Services, Public Health Service, Center for Disease Control: Knowledge and use of folic acid by women of childbearing age-United States, 1995, *Morbidity and Mortality Weekly Report* 44(38):716, 1995.

7. Worthington-Roberts, B: The role of maternal nutrition in the prevention of birth defects, *JADA* 97(10, suppl 2):S184, 1997.

8. Erick M: Hyperolfaction and hyperemesis gravidarum: what is the relationship? *Nutr Rev* 53(10):289, 1995.

9. Food and Nutrition Board, Institute of Medicine, National Academy of Sciences: *Nutrition during pregnancy,* Washington, DC, 1990, National Academy Press.

10. Luke B, Leurgans S: Maternal weight gains in ideal twins outcomes, *J Am Diet Assoc* 96(2):178, 1996.

11. Johnson CS et al: Pregnancy weight gain in adolescents and young adults, *J Am Coll Nutr* 10(3):185, 1991.

12. Walker JJ: Hypertensive drugs in pregnancy, *Clin Perinatol* 18(4):845, 1991.

13. Larroque B et al: Moderate prenatal alcohol exposure and psychomotor development at preschool age, *Am J Public Health* 85(12):1654, 1995.

14. Hellerstadt WL et al: The effects of cigarette smoking and gestational weight change on birth outcome in obese and normal weight women, *Am J Public Health* 87(4):591, 1997.

15. Watson RR: Vitamin A and teratogenesis: recommendations for pregnancy, *J Am Diet Assoc* 88(3):364, 1988.

16. Hinds TS et al: The effect of caffeine on pregnancy outcome variables, *Nutr Rev* 54(7):203, 1996.

17. Kolasa KM, Weismiller DG: Nutrition during pregnancy, *Am Fam Physician* 56(1):205, 1997.

18. Rainville AJ: Pica practices of pregnant women are associated with lower maternal hemoglobin level at delivery, *J Am Diet Assoc* 98(3):293, 1998.

19. Pasui K, McFarland KF: Management of diabetes in pregnancy, *Am Fam Physician* 55(8):2731, 1997.

20. Jovanovic-Peterson L, Peterson CM: Vitamin and mineral deficiencies that may predispose to glucose intolerance of pregnancy, *J Am Coll Nutr* 15(1):14, 1996.

21. Naylor CD et al: Selective screening for gestational diabetes mellitus, *N Engl J Med* 337(22):1591, 1997.

22. Green MF: Screening for gestational diabetes mellitus, *N Engl J Med* 337(22):1625, 1997.

23. American Academy of Pediatrics Work Group on Breast-feeding: Policy statement on breast-feeding, *Pediatrics* 100(Dec):1035, 1997.

24. Krebs NF, Murtaugh: Position of the American Dietetic Association: promotion of breast feeding, *J Am Diet Assoc* 97(6):662, 1997.

■ FURTHER READING

Jack BW, Culpepper L: Preconception care, risk reduction and health promotion in preparation for pregnancy, *JAMA* 264(9):1147, 1990.

These physicians discuss the priority of the 1990s, as identified in the Institute of Medicine's *Preventing Low Birth Weight*, through preconception nutrition assessment, improving risk status, and preparing families for childbearing.

Krebs NF, Murtaugh MA: Position of the American Dietetic Association: promotion of breast feeding, *J Am Diet Assoc* 97(6):662, 1997.

This current position paper of the ADA clearly outlines the numerous values of breast-feeding and the roles and responsibilities of all health care professionals to provide encouragement and support through active lactation management.

Carruth BR, Skinner JD: Practitioners beware: regional differences in beliefs about nutrition during pregnancy, *J Am Diet Assoc* 91(4):435, 1991.

Rainville AJ: Pica practices of pregnant women are associated with lower maternal hemoglobin level at delivery, *J Am Diet Assoc* 98(3):293, 1998.

These articles provide information about various food beliefs and practices that need to be investigated during the prenatal period.

Haughton B et al: Public health nutrition practices to prevent low birth weight in eight southeastern states, *J Am Diet Assoc* 92(2):187, 1992.

Kolasa KM, Weismiller DG: Nutrition during pregnancy, *Am Fam Physician* 56(1):205, 1997.

The first of these two articles discusses the problem of low birth weight, a leading cause of infant mortality in the United States, and the second one provides an excellent summary resource for all health practitioners in the vital role of nutrition during pregnancy.

Case study

A baby for the Delgados

Felicia Delgado is a 19-year-old married primigravida who tested positive for urinary human chorionic gonadotropin (HCG) 2 weeks ago. Mrs. Delgado is 151 cm (5 ft, 5 in) tall with an average pregravid weight of 57 kg (125 lb). Her current gestational age is 6 weeks. Her history for chronic disorders and other serious health problems is negative.

During her initial nutrition interview, Mrs. Delgado indicated that the pregnancy was unplanned. She seemed especially worried about the effects of her irregular diet on the baby. As college students, she and her 21-year-old husband had erratic meals, dominated by junk food. Mrs. Delgado's 24-hour diet history revealed an inadequate intake of dark green or yellow vegetables and milk products, as well as meat or eggs and citrus fruits. The couple realized that these types of foods were an important part of a nutritious diet but were felt inexperienced as cooks and they lack the time and money to prepare healthful meals every day.

At the end of the initial counseling session, the nutritionist told the couple about a series of prenatal group discussions conducted by members of the clinic's perinatal health team, including sessions on pregnancy, labor and delivery, and the care and feeding of the infant. These are attended primarily by a mixture of experienced parents and young, first-time parents-to-be and are offered as a means of introducing practical aspects of pregnancy and parenting.

The Delgados attended every prenatal group meeting and kept all consequent diet-counseling sessions. Their food choices improved in time, and Mrs. Delgado's

weight gain progressed normally, to a total of 12 kg (28 lb) by the time of delivery. The Delgados had a healthy 4 kg (8 lb, 2 oz) baby girl.

Questions for analysis

1. What health professional ideally should be included on the health care team caring for Mrs. Delgado? Describe the significance of each role to the outcome of her pregnancy. What roles do Mr. and Mrs. Delgado have?
2. What nutritional deficiencies would you expect in Mrs. Delgado's diet? What practical problems would you expect her to encounter in attempting to improve her diet?
3. Write a 1-day meal plan for Mrs. Delgado, taking into account her lifestyle and schedule, as well as the amounts of nutrients considered adequate for pregnancy.
4. Write a lesson plan for a group session on nutrition during pregnancy. Include a general description, behavioral objectives, content outline, teaching methods and materials, and evaluation tool(s) you would use.
5. Would you encourage Mrs. Delgado to breast-feed? If so, why? What factors would you expect might discourage her from trying? How would you discuss these factors?
6. Write a lesson plan for an infant feeding session, addressing breast- and-bottle-feeding methods. Include the components listed in questions 3 and 4.

Issues Answers

Drug use and the outcome of pregnancy

Since the tragic discovery a number of years ago of the teratogenic effects of thalidomide, the interest in the effects of drugs used during pregnancy has risen dramatically among health workers and the general public. The tragic consequences of inappropriate drug use make it of quintessential importance that the nutritionist or nurse, while obtaining a dietary history, also gather a complete history of drug use, both licit and illicit, to warn the mother of the potential dangers involved and have her discuss in detail any prescribed drugs with her physician. Listed here are descriptions of the effects of a variety of common drugs on the pregnant woman, the fetus, and the outcome of pregnancy.

Alcohol

No safe level of alcohol consumption has yet been found for pregnant women, despite a recent claim that pregnant women can safely have up to two drinks a day. Even moderate social drinking has been associated with subclinical signs of fetal alcohol syndrome (FAS). This disorder is characterized by growth retardation, malformed facial features, joint and limb abnormalities, cardiac defects, mental retardation, and, in serious cases, death. FAS signs have been seen in tests with rats as early as the human equivalent of the third week of gestation, when most women are unaware of their pregnancies. Thus moderate-to-heavy drinking among sexually active women of childbearing age may carry potential danger.

The nutritional problems of FAS are similar to those seen in chronic alcoholism. A zinc deficiency has specifically been associated with congenital defects and impaired immune function among children born to alcohol abusers. Alcohol has also induced signs of secondary hyperparathyroidism in pregnant animals, thus potentially affecting serum calcium levels.

Psychotropic drugs

A number of drugs have routinely been prescribed for female patients to treat a variety of neuroses and psychoses. If taken during pregnancy, they exhibit teratogenic effects.

Lithium has recently been associated with an increased risk for Epstein's anomaly (a rare cardiovascular abnormality), goiter, and diabetes insipidus, as well as neonatal toxic disturbances such as cyanosis, hypothermia, and bradycardia. A diminished suck reflex will impede attempts to nourish the infant exposed to lithium in utero.

Diazepam (Valium) is associated with an abnormal fetal heart rate. The neonate risks delivery by cesarean section, with oral-facial malformations, a depressed Apgar score, and a reluctance to feed. Rats exposed to diazepam in utero have exhibited abnormal motor skills and arousal processes.

Tricyclic antidepressants (for example, Imipramine) have led to morphologic and behavioral abnormalities in rats.

Anticonvulsants

Phenytoin (Dilantin, Hydantoin) is prescribed to control seizures caused by epilepsy and other conditions. Even though this drug has caused malformations in the offspring of rats, physicians are reluctant to discontinue it for their patients with epilepsy during pregnancy. Because only 7% of children born to mothers using the drug develop malformations, and significantly more develop malformations and developmental disabilities when the mother's epilepsy goes untreated, this may be one case in which prenatal drug use is more beneficial than not using it.

Caffeine

It is wise to avoid this very commonly used stimulant, at least during pregnancy. Pregnant women who are heavy coffee drinkers are considered at risk for miscarriages, premature deliveries, and small-for-gestational age infants. Therefore intake of caffeinated foods, beverages (coffee, tea, cocoa, cola), and medications should be avoided.

Marijuana

Evaluation of the effects of street drugs (marijuana, LSD, heroin, methadone) on nutritional status is difficult because of multiple drug use, uncertain purity, unknown dosage and timing, and inadequate nutritional status of many drug users. A 1982 report on a study of marijuana use in 35 pregnancies revealed a higher incidence of meconium staining (which could relate to fetal damage), poor prenatal weight gain, very short (less than 3 hours) or prolonged labor, operative delivery (cesarean, forceps), and other perinatal problems among marijuana users. Although the researchers admitted flaws in their study (for example, the use of subjects who chose to participate or not), the outcome indicates a need to investigate these potentially fatal effects further.

Nicotine

Cigarette smoking has been well documented for its association with low–birth weight infants, impairment of mental and physical growth, and increased potential mortality. The dietary implications of prenatal smoking are presented in at least one study showing that although the smokers may eat more than nonsmokers, they still deliver smaller babies. In addition, nicotine's ability to increase heart rate, blood pressure, and fat breakdown compromises the health and nutritional status of mother and infant alike.

Thus with the exception of those used to treat individuals with seizure disorders or natural replacement therapy (for example, insulin for persons with type I diabetes), drugs should be avoided at all costs during pregnancy to ensure the health of the mother and a safe and healthy outcome of the pregnancy. The nutrition counselor is well-advised to keep up with the most recent findings regarding medications (prescribed, over-the-counter, and street drugs) to evaluate the nutritional status of the mother using them and warn her of the potential harm they may pose for her and her baby.

References

Frank DA et al: Cocaine and marijuana use during pregnancy by women intending and not intending to breast-feed, *J Am Diet Assoc* 92(2):215, 1992.

Hellerstedt WL et al: The effects of cigarette smoking and gestational weight change on birth outcomes in obese and normal-weight women, *Am J Public Health* 87(4):591, 1997.

Hinds TS et al: The effect of caffeine on pregnancy outcome variables, *Nutr Rev* 54(7):203, 1996.

Larroque B et al: Moderate prenatal alcohol exposure and psychomotor development at preschool age, *Am J Public Health* 85(12):1654, 1995.

Nutrition for Growth and Development

In this second chapter in our life cycle series, we look at growing infants, children, and adolescents. We consider their physical growth and their inseparable psychosocial development at each progressive stage.

This unified growth and development nurtures the integrated nature of the child into that of the adult. The whole process produces the whole person.

Within this dual framework, we consider food and feeding as a vital part of the whole development of the child. In each age group, we relate nutritional needs and the food that supplies them to the normal physical maturation and psychosocial development achieved at each stage.

HUMAN GROWTH AND DEVELOPMENT

INDIVIDUAL NEEDS OF CHILDREN

Growth may be defined as an increase in size. Biologic growth of an organism occurs through cell multiplication. Development is the associated process in which growing tissues and organs take on increased complexity of function. Both of these processes are part of one whole, forming a unified inseparable concept of growth and development. Through these changes a small dependent newborn is transformed into a fully functioning independent adult. However, each child is a unique individual with individual needs. This is a paramount principle in working with children. Thus we must always seek to discover these individual human needs if we are to help each child reach his or her greatest growth and development potential.[1,2]

NORMAL LIFE CYCLE GROWTH PATTERN

The normal human life cycle follows four general stages of overall growth and development: infancy, childhood, adolescence, and adulthood.

Infancy

Growth velocity is rapid during the first year of life, with the rate tapering off in the latter half of the year. At the age of 6 months an infant has probably doubled the birth weight and at 1 year he or she may have tripled it.

Childhood

During the latent period of childhood between infancy and adolescence, the growth rate slows and becomes erratic. At some periods there are plateaus. At other times small spurts of growth occur. The overall **growth deceleration** affects appetite accordingly. At times children will have little or no appetite, and at other times they will eat voraciously. Parents who know that this is a normal pattern should relax and avoid making eating a battleground with their children.

Adolescence

With the beginning of puberty the second **growth acceleration** period occurs. Because of the hormonal influences involved, enormous physical changes develop. These changes include the development of long bones, sex characteristics, and fat and muscle mass.

Adulthood

In the final stage of a normal life cycle, growth levels off on the adult plateau. Then it gradually declines during old age—the period of senescence.

MEASURING CHILDHOOD PHYSICAL GROWTH

Growth charts

Children grow at widely varying individual rates. In clinical practice a child's pattern of growth is compared with **percentile** growth curves derived from measurement of numbers of children throughout the growth years. Contemporary **growth chart grids** have been developed by the National Center for Health Statistics (NCHS) and reflect a broad base for growth patterns in children today. These charts are based on data from large numbers of a nationally representative sample of children. Two age intervals are used: birth to 36 months and 2 to 18 years, with separate curves for boys and for girls (see Appendix I, *Physical Growth NCHS Percentiles*).

Anthropometry

Practitioners use **anthropometry** to monitor a child's growth, with the growth charts and other clinical standards as reference. A number of methods and measures may be employed:

1. *Weight and height*. These are common general measures of physical growth. They provide a basic measure but give only a crude index of growth without showing finer details of individual variations. They are used mainly to look for patterns of growth over time, as the individual child's pattern is plotted on the related age group chart. The recumbent length of infants and small children is measured initially, then standing height as they grow older.

2. *Body circumferences and skinfolds*. The head circumference is a valuable measure in infants, but it is seldom taken routinely after 3 years of age. Measures of

---

anthropometry   The science of measuring the size, weight, and proportions of the human body.

growth acceleration   Period of increased speed of growth at different points of childhood development.

growth chart grids   Grids comparing stature (length), weight, and age of children by percentile; used for nutritional assessment to determine how their growth is progressing. The most commonly used grids are those of the National Center for Health Statistics (NCHS), published by the Fels Research Institute.

growth deceleration   Period of decreased speed of growth at different points of childhood development.

growth velocity   Rapidity of motion or movement; rate of childhood growth over normal periods of development, as compared with a population standard.

percentile   One of 100 equal parts of measured series of values; rate or proportion per hundred.

abdomen, chest, and leg at its maximal girth of the calf are usually included at periodic intervals. Other measures for monitoring muscle mass growth and **body composition** include the midarm circumference and the triceps skinfold at the same point. Using these two measures, the midarm muscle circumference can be calculated easily (see Chapter 15, p. 319). Skinfold measures, including a number of body sites, are done with special calipers and require skill and practice for accuracy. Longitudinal growth studies in research centers employ many measures of development in addition to these basic monitoring ones used in general practice.

Clinical signs

Various clinical signs of optimal growth may be observed as measures of a child's nutritional status. These include such factors as general vitality; a sense of well-being; good posture; healthy gums, teeth, skin, hair, and eyes; muscle development; and nervous control. Refer to Table 1.1 (Chapter 1) for a review of these general signs and observations.

Laboratory tests

In addition, other measures of growth can be obtained by various laboratory tests. These may include studies of blood and urine to determine levels of hemoglobin, vitamins, and similar substances (see Appendix K, *Normal Constituents of Blood and Urine in Adults*). X-ray films of the hand and wrist may be used to measure degree of bone development.

Nutritional analysis

A nutritional analysis of general eating habits (see Chapter 10) provides helpful information for assessing growth needs. A diet history form (see Figure 10.1) and food value tables (see Appendix A) may be used. In clinical practice, however, diet evaluations are usually done by computer. The nutritionist uses information from a variety of methods for a basic food intake analysis to use in diet counseling with the parents.

MENTAL AND PSYCHOSOCIAL DEVELOPMENT

Mental growth

Measures of mental growth usually involve abilities in speech and other forms of communications, as well as the ability to handle abstract and symbolic material in thinking. Young children think in very literal terms. Then, as they develop in mental capacity, they can handle more than single ideas and form constructive concepts.

Emotional growth

Emotional growth is measured in the capacity for love and affection, as well as the ability to handle frustration and its anxieties. It also involves the child's ability to control aggressive impulses and to channel hostility from destructive to constructive activities.

Social and cultural growth

Social development of a child is measured in terms of the ability to relate to others and to participate in group living and cultural activities. These social and cultural behaviors are first learned through relationships with parents and family, all of which have much influence on food habits and feeding patterns. As the child's horizon broadens, relationships are developed with those outside the family, with friends, and with others in the community, at school, church, or other social gatherings. For this reason a child's play during the early years is a highly purposeful activity.

NUTRITIONAL REQUIREMENTS FOR GROWTH

ENERGY NEEDS

During childhood the demand for kcalories is relatively great. However, there is much variation in need with age and condition. For example, the total daily kcaloric intake of a 5-year-old child is spent in the following way: (1) about 50% supplies basal metabolic requirements (BMR), (2) 5% is involved in the thermic effect of food (TEF) that is eaten, that is, in the work of digestion, absorption, and general stimulation of metabolism, (3) various physical activities require about 25%, (4) 12% is needed for tissue growth, and (5) about 8% is represented in fecal loss. Of these kcalories, carbohydrate is the primary energy source, and it is also important to spare protein for its essential growth needs rather than having it spent for energy. Fat kcalories are important as backup energy sources, but particularly as sources of essential fatty acids such as linoleic acid needed for growth. However, an excess of fat, especially from animal sources, should be avoided.

PROTEIN NEEDS

Protein provides the essential building materials for tissue growth—amino acids. As a child grows, the requirements per unit of body weight gradually decrease. For example, during the first 6 months of life an infant requires 2.2 g/kg. This amount gradually decreases until adulthood, when protein needs are only about 0.8 g/kg. Usually the healthy, active, growing child will consume the necessary amount of kcalories and protein in the variety of foods provided.

WATER REQUIREMENTS

The infant's relative need for water is greater than that of the adult. The infant's body content of water is from

70% to 75% of the total body weight, whereas in the adult water constitutes only about 60% to 65% of the total body weight. Also, a large amount of the infant's total body water is *outside* the cell and more easily lost. The child's water need is related to the kcaloric intake and the urine concentration. Generally an infant drinks daily an amount of water equivalent to 10% to 15% of body weight, whereas the adult's daily amount equals 2% to 4% of the body weight. A summary of approximate daily fluid needs during the growth years is given in Table 12.1.

MINERAL AND VITAMIN NEEDS

In your previous study of minerals and vitamins, you learned of their essential roles in tissue growth and maintenance and in overall energy metabolism. Positive childhood growth and development depend on an adequate amount of these essential substances. For example, rapidly growing young bones require calcium and phosphorus. An x-ray film of a newborn's body would reveal a skeleton appearing as a collection of disconnected, separate bones requiring mineralization. Calcium is also needed for the developing teeth, muscle contraction, nerve irritability, blood coagulation, and heart muscle action. Another mineral of concern is iron, essential for hemoglobin formation. The infant's fetal store is diminished in 4 to 6 months. Thus solid food additions at that time help supply needed iron. Such initial foods as enriched cereal and egg and later meat accomplish this. The use of iron-fortified formulas and foods, especially by high-risk children enrolled in the WIC program, has greatly reduced the incidence of iron-deficiency anemia among children.

Excess amounts of two vitamins, A and D, are of concern in feeding children. Excess intake of these vitamins may occur over prolonged periods because of misunderstanding, ignorance, or carelessness. Parents must be carefully instructed to use only the amount directed and no more. These excesses bring clear toxic symptoms:

1. *Vitamin A.* Symptoms of toxicity from excess vitamin A include lack of appetite, slow growth, drying and cracking of the skin, enlargement of the liver and spleen, swelling and pain of long bones, and bone fragility.
2. *Vitamin D.* Symptoms of toxicity from excess vitamin D include nausea, diarrhea, weight loss, excess urination especially at night, and eventual calcification of soft tissues, including those of renal tubules, blood vessels, bronchi, stomach, and heart.

A summary of the Recommended Dietary Allowances (RDAs) for overall nutritional needs for growth, as indicated by the National Research Council, is given in Table 12.2.

STAGES OF GROWTH AND DEVELOPMENT: AGE GROUP NEEDS

THE STAGES OF HUMAN LIFE

Throughout the human life cycle food and feeding not only serve to meet nutritional requirements for physical growth, but they also relate intimately to personal psychosocial development. The nutritional age-group needs of children cannot be understood apart from the child's overall maturation as a unique person. Over the past years, Erik Erikson's theory of human development has come to play a significant role in our view of the human life cycle.[3] A leading American psychoanalyst, Erikson has contributed much insight to our understanding of human personality and growth throughout critical periods of our development.

Psychosocial development

Erikson has identified eight stages in human growth and a basic psychosocial developmental problem for the crisis the person struggles with at each stage. The developmental problem at each stage has a positive ego value and a conflicting negative counterpart:

1. *Infancy*—Trust versus distrust
2. *Toddler*—Autonomy versus shame and doubt
3. *Preschooler*—Initiative versus guilt
4. *School-age child*—Industry versus inferiority
5. *Adolescent*—Identity versus role confusion
6. *Young adult*—Intimacy versus isolation
7. *Adult*—Generativity versus stagnation
8. *Older adult*—Ego integrity versus despair

Table 12.1 Approximate daily fluid needs during growth years	
Age	**ml/kg**
0-3 months	120
3-6 months	115
6-12 months	100
1-4 years	100
4-7 years	95
7-11 years	90
11-19 years	50
>19 years	30

body composition   The relative sizes of the four basic body compartments that make up the total body: lean body mass (muscle mass), fat, water, and bone.

Table

12.2   RDA for growth (National Research Council, 1989 version)

Age	Weight		Height		Energy	Protein	Fat-soluble vitamins			
(yr)	(kg)	(lb)	(cm)	(in)	(kcal)	(g)	Vit. A (μg RE)	Vit. D (μg)	Vit. E (mg α-TE)	Vit. K (μg)
Infants										
0-0.5	6	13	60	24	650	13	375	7.5	3	5
0.5-1	9	20	71	28	850	14	375	10	4	10
Children										
1-3	13	29	90	35	1300	16	400	10	6	15
4-6	20	44	112	44	1800	24	500	10	7	20
7-10	28	62	132	52	2000	28	700	10	7	30
Males										
11-14	45	99	157	62	2500	45	1000	10	10	45
15-18	66	145	176	69	3000	59	1000	10	10	65
Females										
11-14	46	101	157	62	2200	46	800	10	8	45
15-18	55	120	163	64	2200	44	800	10	8	55

Given favorable circumstances, a growing child develops positive ego strength at each life stage and therefore builds increasing inner resources and strengths to meet the next life crisis. The struggle at any age, however, is not forever won at that point. A residue of the negative remains, and in periods of stress, such as an illness, regression in some degree usually occurs. But as the child gains mastery at each stage of development, assisted by significant positive relationships of support, integration of self-controls takes place. Various related developmental tasks surround each of these stages. These are learnings that, when accomplished, contribute to successful resolution of the core problem.

Physical growth

The developmental tasks of childhood food choices and feeding practices are intimately related. Food habits do not develop in a vacuum. They flow as an integral part of physical and psychosocial development. In this section we relate these two influences to the general age group's developmental characteristics.

At each of the age group stages of childhood we discuss, food and feeding practices are integrated and associated with the normal physical and psychosocial maturation. Various neuromuscular motor skills enable the child to accomplish related physical activities. Psychosocial development influences food attitudes, behavior, patterns, and habits.

INFANT (BIRTH TO 1 YEAR)

Physical characteristics of a full-term infant

The full-term infant is born after successful growth and development during a normal gestation period of about 40 weeks (280 days), weighing approximately 3.2 kg (7 lb). During the first year of life, the infant grows rapidly, from this average birth weight to a 1-year-old child ready

to walk and weighing about 9 kg (20 lb). Thus energy requirements during this first year of tremendous growth are high.

Full-term infants have the ability to digest and absorb protein, a moderate amount of fat, and simple carbohydrates. They have some difficulty with starch, since amylase, the starch-splitting enzyme, is not being produced at first. However, as starch is introduced, this enzyme begins to function. The renal system functions well, but more water relative to size is needed than in an adult to manage urinary excretion. Their first baby teeth do not erupt until about the fourth month, so initial food must be liquid or semiliquid. They have limited nutritional stores from gestation, especially in iron. Thus they need supplements of vitamins and minerals, first in concentrated drops and later in semisolid food additions to their first food—breast milk or a substitute infant formula. The newborn's **rooting reflex** and somewhat recessed lower jaw are natural adaptations for feeding at the breast.

Psychosocial development

The core psychosocial developmental task during infancy is the establishment of trust versus distrust. Much of the infant's early psychosocial development is **tactile** in nature, from touching and holding, especially in feeding. Feeding is the infant's main means of establishing human relationships. The close mother-infant bonding in the feeding process fills the basic need to build trust. The need for sucking and the development of the oral organs, lips and mouth, as sensory organs represent adaptations to ensure an adequate early food intake for survival. As a result, food becomes the infant's general means of exploring the environment and is one of the early means of communication. The infant has additional "nonnutritive" sucking need that is satisfied especially with the extra effort required in sucking while breast-feeding, or in using a nipple such as the "Nuk" variety. As muscular

Water-soluble vitamins						Minerals							
Vit. C (mg)	Thiamin (mg)	Riboflavin (mg)	Niacin (mg NE)	Vit. B$_6$ (mg)	Folate (μg)	Vit. B$_{12}$ (μg)	Calcium (mg)	Phosphorus (mg)	Magnesium (mg)	Iron (mg)	Zinc (mg)	Iodine (μg)	Selenium (μg)
30	0.3	0.4	5	0.3	25	0.3	400	300	40	6	5	40	10
35	0.4	0.5	6	0.6	35	0.5	600	500	60	10	5	50	15
40	0.7	0.8	9	1.0	50	0.7	800	800	80	10	10	70	20
45	0.9	1.1	12	1.1	75	1.0	800	800	120	10	10	90	20
45	1.0	1.2	13	1.4	100	1.4	800	800	170	10	10	120	30
50	1.3	1.5	17	1.7	150	2.0	1200	1200	270	12	15	150	40
60	1.5	1.8	20	2.0	200	2.0	1200	1200	400	12	15	150	50
50	1.1	1.3	15	1.4	150	2.0	1200	1200	280	15	12	150	45
60	1.1	1.3	15	1.5	180	2.0	1200	1200	300	15	12	150	50

coordination involving the tongue and the swallowing reflex develops, infants gradually learn to eat a variety of semisolid foods, beginning at about 6 months of age. As physical and motor maturation develop, they begin to show a desire for self-feeding. When these stages of development occur, the exploration of new powers should be encouraged. If their needs for food and love are fulfilled in this early relationship with the mother, father, or other feeding adult, as well as in broadening relationships with other family members, trust is developed. They evidence this trust by an increasing capacity to wait a bit for feedings until they are prepared.

Breast-feeding

The ideal food for the human infant is human milk. It has specific characteristics that match the infant's nutritional requirements during the first year of life. The process of breast-feeding today, as in the past, is successfully initiated and maintained by most women who try. However, sometimes there are problems, as well as a high degree of variability among nursing mothers as to frequency of feedings and intake and growth indexes. Thus in providing support for mothers who want to breast-feed their babies, experienced nutritionists and nurses, many of whom are certified professional lactation counselors, advise flexibility rather than a rigid approach.

The mother's breasts, or mammary glands, are highly specialized secretory organs, as indicated in the previous chapter, illustrated in Figure 11.1. They are composed of glandular tissue, fat, and connective tissue. The secreting glandular tissue has 15 to 20 lobes, each containing many smaller units called lobules. In the lobules secretory cells called alveoli or acini form milk from the nutrient material supplied to them by a rich capillary system in the connective tissue. During pregnancy the breasts are prepared for lactation. The alveoli enlarge and multiply and toward the end of the prenatal period secrete a thin, yellowish fluid called **colostrum**, which contains important antibodies and proteins. As the infant grows, the breast milk develops, adapting in composition to meet growth needs.

Breast milk is produced under the stimulating influence of the hormone prolactin from the anterior pituitary gland. After the milk is formed in the mammary lobules by the clusters of secretory cells (alveoli or ancini), it is carried through converging branches of the **lactiferous ducts** to reservoir spaces called **ampullae** under the **areola**, the pigmented area of skin surrounding the nipple. Two other pituitary hormones, principally oxytocin and, to a lesser extent, vasopressin, stimulate the ejection of the milk from the alveoli to the ducts, releasing it to the baby.

ampullae A general term for a flasklike wider portions of a tubular structure; spaces under the nipple of the breast for storing milk.

areola A defined space; a circular area of different coler surrounding a central point, such as the darkened pigmented ring surrounding the nipple of the breast.

colostrum Thin yellow fluid first secreted by the mammary gland a few days before and after childbirth, preceding the mature breast milk. It contains up to 20% protein including a large amount of lactalbumin, more minerals and less lactose and fat than does milk, and immunoglobulins representing the antibodies found in maternal blood.

lactiferous ducts Branching channels in the mammary gland that carry breast milk to holding spaces near the nipple ready for the infant's feeding.

rooting reflex A reflex in a newborn which stimulation of the side of the cheek or the upper or lower lip causes the infant to turn its mouth and face to the stimulus.

tactile Pertaining to the touch.

This is commonly called the let-down reflex. It causes a tingling sensation in the breast and the flow of milk. The initial sucking of the baby stimulates this reflex. The newborn rooting reflex, oral needs for sucking, and the basic hunger drive usually induce and maintain normal relaxed breast-feeding for the healthy mother.

The mother should follow the baby's lead with an on-demand schedule. The baby's continuing rhythm of need establishes feedings, usually about every 3 to 4 hours. The mother can feed the baby for about 5 to 10 minutes on each breast, burping the baby gently between each period of sucking to expel swallowed air and noting when the baby is satisfied and removing him from the breast. The nipple should air dry to prevent irritation and soreness. Interval use of a pacifier provides more sucking if needed.

The mother's diet and rest are important factors in establishing lactation and breast feeding. Table 11.2, p. 236 indicates a balanced diet to support ample milk production, including food choices from various food groups for meals and snacks. Natural thirst guides adequate fluid intake. Adequate rest and relaxation for the mother are essential. She should be guided not to allow an undue concern about the usually slow rate of weight loss after childbirth to lead her to curtail her diet and thus compromise her milk supply. This energy supply is especially important in the early weeks of establishing the regular milk production. Afterward, a gradual weight loss occurs naturally, but the mother should not unrealistically expect a rapid return to her prepregnant weight. Breast-feeding is simple and enjoyable for the healthy, relaxed mother and infant. A nutritionally adequate diet ensures ample milk production. Infant supplements of vitamins K and D are usually given, but supplements of iron and fluoride are controversial.

However, for the premature and low–birth weight baby, feeding through the first year of life poses more problems. These special needs are discussed in *Issues & Answers* (p. 270).

Bottle-feeding

Formula feeding by bottle may be preferred by some mothers. If the mother does not choose breast-feeding or stops early, bottle feeding of an appropriate formula is an acceptable alternative. A variety of commercial formulas that approximate human milk composition are available, as well as special formulas for allergies, lactose intolerance, diarrhea, and other infant problems. Several types of constituent protein are used, as shown in Table 12.3, including cow's milk base, soy protein, **casein hydrolysate, elemental** amino acids, or meat base. Some of the cow's milk–based formulas are whey-adjusted to more nearly approximate the protein ratio in human milk. Standards for levels of nutrients required in infant formulas are based on recommendations from the American Academy of Pediatrics. Minimum levels are established for 29 nutrients, and maximum levels for 9 nutrients.

When formula is given, the baby should be cradled by the arm, as in breast-feeding, keeping the baby's head upright as much as possible to avoid milk running into the ear canals, resulting in a possible ear infection. The close human touch and warmth are important. When the infant is obviously satisfied, extra milk should not be forced, regardless of the amount remaining in the bottle. Any remaining formula should be thrown away and not refrigerated for reuse. Infants usually take the amount of formula they need. Today most infants are fed on a so-called demand schedule, which works out to about every 3 to 4 hours. A healthy infant will soon establish an individual pattern according to growth requirements.

Cow's milk

Regular unmodified cow's milk is not suitable for infants for three reasons: (1) it causes gastrointestinal bleeding, (2) its **renal solute load** is too heavy for the infant's renal system to handle, leaving too small a margin of safety for maintaining water balance during illness, diarrhea, or hot weather, and (3) it affects iron status, not only because of the gastrointestinal bleeding and blood loss but also because it is low in iron and its high calcium and phosphorus levels inhibit iron absorption.[4] In addition, infants should not use reduced fat milks, such as nonfat or 2% fat, for two reasons: (1) insufficient energy is provided to support requirements, causing body fat to be used to make up the deficit, and (2) linoleic acid in the fat portion of milk is the essential fatty acid needed for growth and development of body tissues.[4] A specific form of eczema has been observed in infants deficient in linoleic acid, and a low-fat diet in infancy may harm physical and intellectual development. To meet the special needs of infants, the American Academy of Pediatrics recommends breast milk or formulas up to 1 year of age, with a gradual addition of appropriate foods beginning at 6 months. There is no need for special formulas for older infants and they are an added expense.[5]

Beikost: solid food additions

No nutritional need exists for introducing solid foods to infants earlier than 4 to 6 months of age, although studies of adolescent mothers of low-socioeconomic status report such additions as early as 2 months.[5,6] Earlier use may contribute to allergies. Nutritional and medical authorities agree that for the first 6 months of life the optimal single food for the infant is human milk or alternative feeding of appropriate formula. Until that time the infant does not need any additional food and is not able to adequately handle them. On the contrary, there are advantages to delaying the introduction of solid foods until this time. Six-month-old infants have reached the stage of development in which they can communicate desire and interest in food and thus participate in the feeding process. Self-feeding efforts begin first with a

Table 12.3	A comparison of types of formulas manufactured for full-term infants			
Type of formula used		**Protein content**	**Fat content**	**Carbohydrate content**
Milk-based routine	Source:	Nonfat cow's milk	Vegetable oils	Lactose
	g/100 kcal:	2.2-2.3	5.4-5.5	10.5-10.8
	% Kcal:	9	48-50	41-43
Whey-adjusted routine	Source:	Nonfat cow's milk plus demineralized whey	Vegetable and oleo oils	Lactose
	g/100 kcal:	2.2	5.4	10.8
	% Kcal:	9	48	43
Soy isolate (cow's milk sensitivity)	Source:	soy isolate	Vegetable oils	Corn syrup solids and/or sucrose
	g/100 kcal:	2.7-3.2	5.1-5.6	9.9-10.2
	% Kcal:	12-13	45-51	39-40
Casein hydrolysate (protein sensitivity, galactosemia)	Source:	Casein hydrolysate	Corn oil or corn oil and MCT*	Tapioca starch and glucose, sucrose, or corn syrup solids
	g/100 kcal:	2.8-3.3	3.9-4.0	13.1-13.6
	% Kcal:	11-13	35	52-54
Meat-based (cow's milk, sensitivity, galactosemia)	Source:	Beef hearts	Sesame oil and beef heart fat	Tapioca starch and sucrose
	g/100 kcal:	4.0	4.8	9
	% Kcal:	16	47	37

*Medium-chain triglycerides.

whole hand **palmar grasp**, and then a more refined **pincer grasp** is developed by the end of the first year. There is also less tendency at this time to overfeed the infant. As solid food is gradually added, the amount of milk consumed is reduced accordingly.

No one sequence of food additions must be followed. A general guide is given in Table 12.4. Individual responses and needs may be a basis for choices, as food becomes a source of enjoyment and a new means of bonding warm family relationships. Single foods are given first, one at a time in small amounts, so that adverse reactions can be identified. The traditional initial transition food is fortified infant cereal, specifically infant rice cereal as it has the least potential for allergic reaction, mixed with a little milk or formula, then fruits, vegetables, egg, potato, and finally meat. Small amounts are given at first, usually offered before the milk feeding. Over time the child will learn to eat and enjoy a wide variety of foods, which is the basic goal. Many commercial baby foods are available, prepared today without the formerly used ingredients of sugar, salt, or monosodium glutamate. Some mothers prefer preparing their own baby food. This can easily be done by cooking and straining vegetables and fruits in a clean environment, freezing a batch at a time in ice cube trays, then storing the cubes in plastic bags in the freezer. Then a single cube can be reheated conveniently for use at a feeding.

Two basic principles should guide the feeding process: (1) necessary nutrients are needed, not any specific food; and (2) food is a main basis of early learning. Food not only serves for physical sustenance but also supplies other personal development and cultural needs. Good food habits begin early in life and continue as a child grows older. By the time infants are

casein hydrolysate formula Infant formula composed of hydrolyzed casein, major milk protein, produced by partially breaking down the casein into smaller peptide fragments, making a product that is more easily digested.

elemental formula A nutrition support formula composed of single elemental nutrient components that require no further digestive breakdown and are thus readily absorbed. Infant formula produced with elemental, ready-to-be-absorbed components free of amino acids and carbohydrate as simple sugars.

palmar grasp Early grasp of the young infant, clasping an object in the palm and wrapping the whole hand around it.

pincer grasp Later digital grasp of the older infant, usually picking up smaller objects with a precise grip between thumb and forefinger.

renal solute load Collective number and concentration of solute particles in a solution carried by the blood to the kidney nephrons for excretion in the urine. The particles are usually nitrogenous products from protein metabolism and the electrolyte Na.

Table 12.4	Guideline for adding solid foods to infant's diet during the first year*	
When to start	**Foods added**	**Feeding**
Fifth to sixth month	Cereal and strained cooked fruit	10 AM and 6 PM
	Egg yolk (at first, hard boiled and sieved; soft boiled or poached later)	
	Strained, cooked vegetable and strained meat	2 PM
	Zwieback or hard toast	At any feeding
Seventh to ninth month	Meat: beef, lamb, or liver (broiled or baked and finely chopped)	10 AM and 6 PM
	Potato: baked or boiled and mashed or sieved	

Suggested meal plan for age 8 months to 1 year or older

7 AM	Milk	240 ml (8 oz)
	Cereal	2-3 tbsp
	Strained fruit	2-3 tbsp
	Zwieback or dry toast	
12 NOON	Milk	240 ml (8 oz)
	Vegetables	2-3 tbsp
	Chopped meat or one whole egg	
	Puddings or cooked fruit	2-3 tbsp
3 PM	Milk	120 ml (4 oz)
	Toast, zwieback, or crackers	
6 PM	Milk	240 ml (8 oz)
	Whole egg or chopped meat	
	Potato: baked or mashed	2 tbsp
	Pudding or cooked fruit	2-3 tbsp
	Zwieback or toast	

*Semisolid foods should be given immediately before milk feeding. One or two teaspoons should be given first. If food is accepted and tolerated well, the amount should be increased to 1 to 2 tablespoons per feeding.

NOTE: Banana or cottage cheese may be used as substitution for any meal.

approximately 8 or 9 months old, they should be able eat family foods—chopped, cooked foods, simply seasoned—without needing special infant foods. Throughout the first year of life the infant's needs for physical growth and psychosocial development will be met by breast milk or formula, a variety of solid food additions, and a loving, trusting relationship between parents and child (Figure 12.1).

TODDLER (1 TO 3 YEARS)

Physical characteristics and growth

After the rapid growth of the first year the growth rate of children slows. But although the rate of gain is less, the pattern of growth produces significant changes in body form. The legs become longer, and the child begins losing baby fat. There is less body water and more water inside the cells. The young child begins to look and feel less like a baby and more like a child. Energy demands are fewer because of the slackened growth rate. However, important muscle development is taking place. In fact, muscle mass development accounts for about one half the total gain during this period. As the child begins to walk and stand erect, more muscle is needed to strengthen the body. There is special need, for example, for big muscles

in the back, the buttocks, and the thighs. The overall rate of skeletal growth slows, but there is more deposit of mineral rather than lengthening of the bones. The increased mineralization strengthens the bones to support the increasing weight. The child has 6 to 8 teeth at the beginning of the toddler period. By 3 years of age the remainder of the deciduous teeth have erupted.

Psychosocial development

The psychosocial development of toddlers is pronounced. The core developmental problem they struggle with is the conflict of autonomy versus shame. Each child has a profound increasing sense of self, of being a distinct and individual person apart from the parents, not just an extension of them. As physical mobility increases, the sense of **autonomy** and independence increases. A growing curiosity leads to much exploration of the environment, and increasingly the mouth is used as a means of exploring. Touch is important, providing the means of learning what objects are like. Often the constant use of "no" is not a perverse negativism as much as it reflects a significant struggle with newly emerging ego needs in conflict with the parents' control efforts. The child wants to do more and more, but the attention span is fairly short and interest shifts to other things.

Figure 12.1 **A,** Six-month-old boy taking a variety of solid food additions and developing wide tastes. Here feeding has become a bond of relationship between parent and child and is serving as a source not only of physical growth but also of psychosocial development. **B,** Optimum physical development and security are evident, the result of sound nutrition and loving care.

Food and feeding

Physical growth and psychosocial development during the toddler period influence nutrient needs (Table 12.2) and food patterns (see the *Practical Application* box, p.262).

1. *Energy*. The need for kcalories is not high because of the relatively decreased growth rate after the first year of life. The energy need now increases very slowly in small spurts. At about 1 year of age children need approximately 850 to 1000 kcalories, and only 1300 to 1500 kcalories by age 3. From age 1 to 2 some children do not eat as much as they did in the second half of infancy. Parents will avoid conflict with their toddler about eating if they remember this normal decreased need for kcalories, resulting from the slowed growth rate, and the child's necessary struggle for autonomy and selfhood, which often involves refusal of food. The child varies in appetite, so food intake may be irregular between "appetite eating" and "nonappetite eating". Encouragement and support are needed from caretakers but never the battleground trap that some parents fall into. Some wise parents have prepared a special plate of small snacks, often small finger-food pieces of raw vegetables and fruits kept in the refrigerator or a few crackers on a special low surface, both on a special colorful plate, so the child may have a measure of positive control when hungry. They will eat when they are hungry and have encouraging positive feed-

back. Positive early learning and experiences help develop food acceptance patterns.[7]

2. *Protein*. In relation to energy (kcalorie) needs, protein needs are relatively increased. The toddler requires a total of about 16 g/day. Muscle and other body tissues grow rapidly. At least half of this protein should be of animal origin because animal protein has high biologic value. This does not mean that meat itself is necessary. Families following a balanced ovolactovegetarian diet have shown that children grow just as well and attain similar heights as do their nonvegetarian counterparts.[8]

3. *Minerals*. Calcium and phosphorus are needed for bone mineralization. The bones are strengthening to keep pace with the muscle development and increasing activity. Iron is needed to maintain adequate hemoglobin levels in an increasing blood volume as the body size increases.

4. *Food choices*. About 2 to 3 cups of milk daily are sufficient for the young child's needs. Sometimes excess milk intake, a habit carried over from infancy, may exclude many solid foods from the diet. As a result,

---

autonomy The state of functioning independently, without extraneous influence.

Toddler feeding made simple

Parents waste a lot of time coaxing, arguing, begging, and even threatening their 2- to 5-year-olds to eat more than 1½ green peas at dinner. You can help them save time by developing child-feeding strategies based on the developmental needs of their toddlers.

The first step is to remind them that their children are not growing as fast as they did during the first year of life. Consequently, they need less food. Also, a child's energy needs are sporadic. Parents should watch toddlers' activity levels. Food should be provided to help their bodies keep up with the myriad of activities they have planned each day.

Next, offer a few suggestions that make child-feeding easier:

- Serve small portions, not much more than a baby-food jar could hold. Let them ask for seconds if they're still hungry.
- Guide them in serving themselves small amounts. This takes a while because, like adults, children's eyes tend to be bigger than their stomachs. Constant, gentle reminders will eventually help them learn when to stop.
- Keep quick-fix, nutritious foods around for off-hour meals. The term *snack* isn't appropriate for the amount of food some youngsters put away between meals. To keep from turning into a permanent short-order chef, the parent should consider

keeping food such as fruit, cheese, and peanut butter to serve between meals and to provide essential nutrients.

- Don't put away the main meal before serving dessert. Amazing but true: some children will ask for main meal foods *after* finishing dessert, if they're still hungry.
- Avoid overseasoning. If it's too spicy, no amount of screaming and cajoling will make them eat it.
- Don't force foods that the child dislikes. Individual food dislikes usually don't last very long. If the child shuns one food, offer a similar one—*if* it's available at that meal; for example, a fruit if the child shuns vegetables. If not, ignore it and don't worry about malnutrition. At this rate, there's little chance of deficiency signs cropping up soon.
- Enroll the child in nursery school. Because food is not always available in the classroom, toddler students learn to eat at regular times. They also tend to try foods that are abhorred at home, probably because of peer pressure or a desire to impress a new authority figure—the teacher.
- Be patient. While adults are discussing world events over broccoli, toddlers are learning how to pick it up with their forks.

Remember that beginning at about age 4 years young children are able to perceive relationships of food to positive concepts of health and nutrition. They are ready to learn more about food in these positive relations, so cash in on these rapidly developing capacities and explorations. Also, remember that the child's social and emotional environment surrounds food and positive attitudes and behaviors relate to improved dietary quality.

Yes, toddlers might take longer; they might not eat. But with flexibility, time, patience, and a sense of humor, most parents find they can get enough nutrients into their children to keep them healthy and happy throughout the preschool years.

References

Birch LL: Children's food acceptance patterns, *Nutr Today* 31(6):234, 1996.

Kennedy E, Powell R: Changing eating patterns of American children: a view from 1996, *J Am Coll Nutr* 16(6):524, 1997.

Satter EM: Internal regulation and the evolution of normal growth as the basis for prevention of obesity in children, *J Am Diet Assoc* 96(9):860, 1996.

Singleton JC et al: Role of food and nutrition in the health perceptions of young children, *J Am Diet Assoc* 92(1):67, 1992.

Stanek K et al: Diet quality and the eating environment of preschool children, *J Am Diet Assoc* 90(11):1582, 1990.

the child may lack iron and develop a so-called milk anemia. On the other hand, a child may dislike milk as a beverage and replacement can be made in soups, puddings, or custards, or dry milk can be used in cooked cereals, mashed potatoes, meatloaf, and the

like. Offering the child an increasing variety of foods will help to develop good food habits, for such food habits are learned and there is little opportunity for learning if a child is not exposed to a wide variety of foods. An emphasis on refined sweets is best avoided, reserving them for special occasions, not for habitual use or for bribes to get a child to eat.

Summary principles

Two important principles, which parents should know and understand, can guide wise feeding practices during this period:

1. The child needs fewer kcalories but relatively more protein and minerals for physical growth. Therefore a variety of foods should be offered in smaller amounts to provide key nutrients. Young children of mothers working outside the home meet these nutritional needs for growth just as well. Studies of United States children have shown that maternal employment status has no detrimental effects on young children's diets.

2. The child is struggling for selfhood in normal psychosocial development. This struggle often takes the form of refusal of food and a desire to do things for self before being fully able to do them completely. If parents are patient, offer a variety of foods in small amounts, and encourage some degree of food choice and self-feeding in the child's own ceremonial manner, eating can be a happy, positive means of development. It can help satisfy the child's growing need for independence and ritual. Parents need to maintain a calm, relaxed attitude of sympathetic interest, to understand the child's struggle and give help where needed. But they must be careful to avoid both overprotection and excessive rigidity.

PRESCHOOLER (3 TO 6 YEARS)

Physical characteristics and growth

As shown in normal childhood growth charts (see Appendix I, *Physical Growth NCHS Percentiles*), each child tends to settle into a regular genetic **growth channel** as physical growth continues in spurts. On occasion the child bounds with energy. Play is hard play—running, jumping, and testing new physical resources. At other times the child will sit for increasing periods of time engrossed in passive types of activities. Mental capacities are developing, and there is more thinking and exploring of the environment. Energy needs, about 1800 kcal/day, as well as specific nutrients, as shown in Table 12-2, need emphasis. Protein requirements continue to increase as the child grows older. Preschool children need about 24 g/day of good, quality protein such as is found in milk, egg, meat, and cheese. They continue to need calcium and iron for storage. Since vitamins A and C may be lacking in the diets of preschool growing children, a variety of fruits and vegetables should be provided.

Psychosocial development

Each age group builds on the previous one. The core psychosocial developmental problem preschool children struggle with is essentially that of initiative versus guilt. They are beginning to develop the superego—the conscience. As powers of active movement increase, they have increasing imagination and curiosity. This very capacity often leads them into troubled feelings about their changing attitudes, especially toward parents. This is a period of increasing imitation and of sex identification. The little boy imitates his father or other male role models. The little girl imitates the mother or other female role models. In their play much of this becomes evident in the use of grown-up clothes and role-playing in domestic or job situations. Wise parents will avoid sex stereotyping responses, especially during this formative period. Self-feeding skills increase and eating assumes greater social aspects. The family mealtime is an important means of socialization and sex identification, as the children imitate their parents and others at the table.

Food and feeding

The preschool child is beginning to form definite responses to various types of foods:

1. *Vegetables and fruits.* Fruits are usually well liked. However, of all the food groups, vegetables usually are the least well liked by children, yet these foods contain many vitamins and minerals needed for growth. Where there is space or opportunity, involving the young child in planting and growing vegetables in a small garden is an excellent early learning experience. Trips to the market can also help the child see a variety of shapes and colors in vegetables and discover new ones, as each in turn can be prepared at home in a variety of tasteful ways. Children usually dislike strong vegetables such as cabbage and onions. They have a keen sense of taste, so flavor and texture are important. They like pieces of crisp raw vegetables or fruits to eat as finger foods. Tough strings cause problems, and tough parts are hard to manage and therefore should be removed. For example, it is easy to break a crisp piece of celery and remove the strings before giving it to the child. Children also react to consistency of vegetables, disliking them overcooked.

2. *Milk, cheese, egg, and meat.* It is helpful if children can set their own goals in quantities of food. Portions need to be relatively small. Often children can pour their own milk from a small pitcher into a small glass and subsequently drink more. The quantity of milk needed usually declines during these years. The child will drink 2 or 3, rarely 4, cups of milk during the day. Smaller children like their milk more room

---

growth channel The progressive regular growth pattern of children, guided along individual genetically controlled channels, influenced by nutritional and health status.

temperature, not icy cold. Also, they prefer it in small glasses that hold about 4 to 6 oz rather than in large, adult-sized glasses. Cheese is a favorite finger food or snack. Egg is usually well liked if cooked with sufficient body to pick up with the fingers, such as scrambled or boiled. Meat should be tender, easy to chew or cut; hence ground meat is popular, but must be well cooked to make it safe.

3. *Grains.* The wide variety in which grains can be eaten adds to their appeal to children, who enjoy various breads, cereals, and crackers.

4. *Temperature.* Since children prefer their foods lukewarm, not hot, some foods may remain on their plates and become dry and gummy such that the child refuses to eat it. Thus very small portions should be served at first.

5. *Single foods.* Children usually prefer single foods to combination dishes such as casseroles or stews. This is a period of language learning for children. They like to learn names of foods, and be able recognize and name them from their shape, color, texture, taste. So these identifiable characteristics need to be retained as much as possible.

6. *Finger foods.* Children like to eat food they can pick up with their fingers. Frequently when appetites lag, fruits can be substituted for vegetables. Often a variety of raw fruits and vegetables cut into finger-sized pieces and offered to children for their own selection provides a resource of needed nutrition.

7. *Food jags.* Because of developing social and emotional needs, preschool children frequently follow "food jags," eating only a particular food. This may last for several days. But it is usually short-lived and is of no major consequence.

The preschool period is one of increasing growth for the young child. Lifetime food habits are forming. Food continues to play an important part in the developing personality, and group eating becomes significant as a means of socialization. The social and emotional environment and companionship at mealtimes, with family or other caretakers, greatly influence the young child's food intake and quality of the diet.[9] The child learns food patterns at the family table or in group situations away from home. For example, if the family is vegetarian, they will need to give special attention to the child's energy and protein needs for growth. The child may be involved in a child care or preschool situation in which group eating occurs. Food habits of preschoolers are greatly affected by peer modeling, and food preferences grow according to what the group is eating. In such situations the child learns a widening variety of family food habits and forms new social relationships and food patterns. Study shows that young children also include a relationship to health in their perceptions of food and are more ready to understand and learn more about food, nutrition, and health than we have previously thought.

THE SCHOOL-AGE CHILD (6 TO 12 YEARS)

Physical characteristics and growth

The school-age period has been called the latent time of growth. The rate of growth slows, and body changes occur gradually. However, resources are being laid down for the rapid adolescent growth ahead. Sometimes this has been called the lull before the storm. By now the body type has been established, and growth rates vary widely. Girls usually outdistance boys in the latter part of this period.

Psychosocial development

The core psychosocial developmental problem children struggle with during these early school years is the tension between industry versus inferiority. They have widening horizons, new school experiences, and challenging learning opportunities. They develop increased mental powers and ability to work out problems and face competitive activities. They develop abilities to cooperate in group activities and begin to experience a sense of adequacy and accomplishment, and sometimes the frustration of not winning. The child begins moving from a dependence on parental standards to those of peers, first steps in preparing for coming maturity and self-growth. Pressures are generated for self-control of a growing body. These pressures produce changes in previously learned habits, and negative attitudes sometimes expressed are evidence of these struggles for growing independence. There is a temporary disorganization of previous learning and personality, a sort of loosening up of the pattern for the inevitable changes ahead in adolescence. It is a diffuse period of gangs, cliques, hero worship, pensive daydreaming, emotional stresses, and learning to get along with other children.

Food and feeding

The slowed rate of growth during this period results in a gradual decline in the food requirement per unit of body weight. This decline continues up to the latter part of the period just before approaching adolescence. Likes and dislikes are a product of earlier years. Family food attitudes are imitated, but increasing outside activities often compete with family mealtimes, and family conflicts arise. Research has firmly established the close relation of sound nutrition and childhood learning. Breakfast is particularly important for a school-age child. It breaks the fast of the sleep hours and prepares the child for problem-solving and memory spans in the learning hours at school. The School Breakfast and Lunch Programs provide nourishing school meals that many children would not otherwise have (see Chapter 10). Numerous school programs help to maintain sound nutrition through such efforts as implementing the United States dietary guidelines into child nutrition programs, new lower-fat desserts in school lunch programs, and reducing food waste by having recess before lunch.[8,10,11] In school a child can observe many food attitudes and taste new foods that he or she may not normally

Table 12.5	Favorite food choices of American children (listed in order of preference)					
Breakfast	**Lunch or dinner**	**Vegetables**	**Fruits**	**Beverages**	**Desserts**	**Sandwiches**
Cereal	Steak or roast beef	Corn	Apple	Cola or soda	Ice cream	Peanut butter and jelly
Pancakes and waffles	Pizza	Carrots	Orange	Milk	Cake	Meat or cold cuts
Eggs	Spaghetti	Beans	Peach	Fruit punch	Pie	Ham
French toast	Chicken	Tomatoes	Grapes	Root beer	Pudding	Tuna fish
Toast	Hamburger	Peas	Banana	Juices (other than orange)	Gelatin dessert	Cheese
Sweet rolls	Fish	Greens, collards or spinach	Watermelon	Orange juice	Banana split	Bacon, lettuce, and tomato
Doughnuts	Macaroni and cheese	Potatoes	Pear	Lemonade	Brownie	Roast beef

Modified from survey data of Lamme AJ, Lamme LL: Children's food preferences, *J Sch Health* 50(7):397, 1980.

know or accept. Some traditional favorite foods of American children are listed in Table 12.5.

The school-age child has increasing exposure to influences on food habits. Television becomes a strong source of food selection. There are positive learning opportunities in the classroom, particularly when parents provide support and reinforcement at home and nutrition education is integrated into other activities. Child athletes particularly need nutritional guidance.[12,13] Children aged 6 to 12 engaged in athletic competitions must have guidance of parents and coaches, with assistance of a qualified registered dietitian, to support sound nutrition practices to make healthful food choices to support exercise, training, and competition.

ADOLESCENT

Physical characteristics and growth

During the adolescent period, with the onset of puberty, the final growth spurt of childhood occurs. Maturation during this time varies so widely that chronologic age as a reference point for discussing growth ceases to be useful. **Physiologic age** becomes more important in dealing with individual boys and girls. It accounts for wide fluctuations in metabolic rates, food needs, scholastic capacity, and even illness. These capacities can be more realistically viewed only in physiologic growth terms.

The profound body changes in the adolescent period result from hormonal effects regulating the development of the sex characteristics. The rate at which these changes occur varies widely and is particularly distinct in growth patterns that emerge between the sexes. In girls the amount of subcutaneous fat deposit increases, particularly in the abdominal area. The hip breadth increases, and the bony pelvis widens in preparation for reproduction. A pelvic girdle of subcutaneous fat results. This is often a source of anxiety to many figure-conscious young

girls. In boys physical growth is manifested more by an increased muscle mass and long-bone growth. His growth spurt is slower than that of the girl, but he soon passes her in weight and height.

 ### Psychosocial development

Adolescence is an ambivalent period full of stresses and strains. On the one hand, teenagers look back to the securities of earlier childhood; on the other, they reach for the maturity of adulthood. The core psychosocial developmental problem adolescents struggle with is that of identity versus role diffusion. The search for self begun in early childhood reaches its climax in the identity crisis of the teen years. The profound body changes associated with sexual development cause changes in body image and resulting tensions in maturing girls and boys. Individual variance is great in response to these tensions, depending on the resources that have been provided for them in earlier developmental years.

The identity crisis of the adolescent years, largely revolving around sexual development and preparation for an adult role in a complex industrialized and technologic society, produces many psychologic, emotional, and social tensions. The actual period of rapid physical growth is relatively short, only 2 or 3 years. However, the attendant psychosocial development continues over a much longer period. The pressure for peer-group acceptance is strong, and fads in dress and food habits are common. Also, in a technically developed society such as in

---

physiologic age Rate of biologic maturation in individual adolescents that varies widely and accounts more for wide and changing differences in their metabolic rates, nutritional needs, and food requirements than does chronologic age.

the United States, where high values are placed on education and achievement, prolonged preparation for careers often delays marriage and family far beyond the initiation of the reproductive years. Social tensions and family conflicts are created. These conflicts may have nutritional consequences as teenagers eat away from home more often and develop a snacking pattern of personal and peer-group food choices.

Food and feeding

With the rapid growth of adolescence come increased demands for energy, protein, vitamins, and minerals.

1. *Energy.* Kcaloric needs increase with the metabolic demands of growth and energy expenditure. Although individual needs vary, girls require fewer kcalories than boys, or about 2200 kcal/day; boys need 2500 to 3000 kcal/day. Sometimes the large appetite characteristic of this rapid growth period leads adolescents to satisfy their hunger with snack foods that are high in sugar and fat and low in essential protein.
2. *Protein.* Adolescent growth needs for protein are increased, especially during the pubertal changes in both sexes and for the developing muscle mass in boys. Girls require 44 to 46 g/day; boys need 45 to 59 g/day to sustain daily need and maintain nitrogen reserves.
3. *Minerals.* The calcium requirement for all adolescents is increased to 1200 mg/day to meet the demands of bone growth. In fact, adolescence is a crucial time for the development of bone mass, under the influence of increasing sexual hormones, especially of estrogen in girls. New insight is developing into possible genetic mechanisms that determine peak bone density. Menstrual iron losses in the adolescent girl predispose her to simple iron-deficiency anemia. Young female athletes, such as gymnasts and runners, who begin their training before menarche, develop secondary amenorrhea and, in turn, reduced bone mineral density.[14] For all young athletes fluid replacement in any exercise or performance period is essential.[15,16]
4. *Vitamins.* The B vitamins are needed in increased amounts, especially by boys, to meet the extra demands of energy metabolism and muscle tissue development. Intakes of needed vitamins C and A may be low because of erratic food intake, especially in vegetables and fruits. A high incidence of folate deficiency has been found among adolescent girls, with a positive relation to megaloblastic anemia— low red blood cell folate and hemoglobin levels—all of which responded to supplemental folate therapy.

Eating habits

Physical and psychosocial pressures influence adolescent eating habits (see *To Probe Further* box). By and large, boys fare better than girls. Their large appetites and the sheer volumes of food they consume usually ensure intake of adequate nutrients. But the adolescent girl may be less fortunate. Two factors combine to place her under pressures concerning body weight:

1. *Physiologic sex differences.* Because of the girl's physiologic sex differences associated with fat deposits during this growth period and her comparative lack of physical activity, she may gain excess weight easily.
2. *Social and personal tensions.* Social pressures and tensions concerning figure control sometimes cause adolescent girls to follow unwise, self-imposed crash diets for weight loss. In some cases actual self-starvation regimens may result in complex and far-reaching eating disorders such as anorexia nervosa and bulimia (see Chapter 6). Usually these problems, which may assume severe proportions, involve a distorted self-image and a morbid, irrational pursuit of thinness, even when the actual body weight is normal or below age norms. Even in less clinical situations, constant dieting among teenage girls can bring varying degrees of poor nutrition at the very time in life when their bodies need to be building reserves for potential reproduction. The harmful effects that bad eating habits can have on the future course of a pregnancy are clearly indicated in many studies relating preconception nutritional status to the outcome of gestation (see Chapter 11).

TO SUM UP

Growth and development depend on nutrition to support heightened physiologic and metabolic processes. Nutrition, in turn, depends on a multitude of social, psychosocial, cultural, and environmental influences that affect individual growth potential throughout the life cycle.

Four types of growth are usually measured during each phase of development: physical, mental, emotional, and sociocultural. Each type of growth is evaluated in assessing the child's nutritional status and planning an effective counseling approach. Nutritional needs change with each growth period.

Infants experience rapid growth. They have relatively immature digestive systems and limited ability to absorb and excrete metabolites efficiently. Breast-feeding is preferred during the first 6 months of life. Solid foods are not needed, nor can they be adequately tolerated, until about 4 to 6 months of age.

Toddlers (ages 1 to 3 years), preschoolers (ages 3 to 6 years), and school-age children (ages 6 to 12 years) experience a slowed and erratic latent growth of childhood. Their energy requirements per unit of body weight are not as great as the infant's needs. Their nutritional needs center on protein for growth with attendant minerals and vitamins. Social and cultural factors influence the development of food habits.

To Probe Further

Food habits of adolescents

Teenagers have gained the reputation of having the worst eating habits in the world. Is this justified? Here's a closer look at the actual eating habits of American adolescents during the last 15 years.

Skipping meals

A study of California teenagers revealed that lunch—not breakfast, as most people assume—was the meal most frequently skipped. Breakfast was skipped most frequently by obese children, however. In all cases the frequency of regular meals increased with income and social status.

Snacking

Another study indicated that 12- to 16-year-olds met or exceeded their RDA per 100 kcalories for protein, riboflavin, and vitamin C through between-meal foods. Vitamin A, calcium, and iron levels fell considerably below the standard.

Fast-foods

Having a limited range of items, fast-food restaurant menus are more likely to be lacking one or more essential nutrients. They are generally considered to be inadequate in calcium and vitamin A and too high in kcalories, saturated fats, and sodium. Current marketing practices will continue to attract the young, who often consider fast-food restaurants as popular hangouts to escape the demands of an ever-encroaching adult world. Thus it is likely that these places will influence the nutritional quality of adolescent meals for some time.

Unusual food choices

Teenagers are likely to eat any type of food at any time of the day. Studies have shown that they are as likely to have barbecued chicken for breakfast as pancakes for dinner. These food choices are only unusual in terms of the time of day at which they are consumed, however, and usually present no threat to health or nutritional status.

Alcohol consumption

As adolescents approach the drinking age in their locale, alcohol begins to provide a more significant portion of their total caloric intake. As they begin to drink at younger and younger ages, even a mild form of abuse coupled with the elevated nutritional requirements of adolescence may compromise their nutritional status, especially in terms of folic acid, which is destroyed by excessive amounts of alcohol. Subclinical damage to the intestinal mucosa caused by chronic alcohol use could also influence the absorption of other nutrients.

In general the adolescent diet may be no worse than the average adult diet, although intakes of calcium, vitamin A, iron, and ascorbic acid are usually seriously inadequate during these years, especially among girls. In addition, eating habits and social pressures have made this age group susceptible to at least two important nutritional problems: obesity and anorexia nervosa.

Obesity

Obesity affects approximately 10% to 20% of the adolescent population. As in adults, an excessive intake of kcalories is less often the cause than lack of exercise. Concern about personal appearance could make the adolescent more reluctant than an adult to participate in activities (team sports, dance classes) that are popular ways of controlling weight.

Anorexia nervosa

This serious eating disorder is considered the flip side of the weight-management coin. It usually affects achievement-oriented, affluent girls, although the problem now crosses socioeconomic and sexual barriers. The self-induced starvation is often attributed to an obsession with attaining a slim figure—a desire that goes as far as to result in self-starvation, emaciation, and serious health problems, including amenorrhea.

The food habits of adolescents reflect a reduced influence of parents on eating habits, increased peer pressure or desire to conform, extrasensitvity to appearance, and elevated needs for energy. The nutrition counselor must remember these influences when helping adolescents and their families plan food patterns that will enhance health and meet growth requirements during the teenage years.

References

Cameron JL: Nutritional determinants of puberty, *Nutr Rev* 54(2):S17, 1996.

Nash M: Conferences, symposia, and reports: conference on adolescent nutritional disorders: prevention and treatment, *Nutr Today* 31(2): 68, 1996.

Witschi JC et al: Sources of fat, fatty acids, and cholesterol in the diets of adolescents, *J Am Diet Assoc* 90(10):1429, 1990.

Adolescents (ages 12 to 18 years) experience a second large growth spurt before reaching adulthood. This rapid growth is accompanied by sexual maturation as well as physical growth. Increased kcaloric and nutrient needs on the average are easier for boys to achieve than for girls, who frequently feel social and peer pressures to restrict food intake for weight control. This pressure may inhibit their ability to acquire the nutritional reserves necessary for later reproduction.

■ QUESTIONS FOR REVIEW

1. How is physical growth measured? What signs are used to measure mental, emotional, and sociocultural growth?

2. What factors are responsible for the major differences in nutritional and feeding needs of the preterm and full-term infant?

3. Why is breast-feeding the preferred method for feeding infants? Outline some dietary needs for the new breast-feeding mother and techniques for feeding the baby. Describe techniques for teaching a new bottle-feeding mother. Describe some types of commercial formulas that would provide appropriate alternative feeding.

4. Outline a general schedule for a new mother to use as a guide for adding solid foods to her infant's diet during the first year of life.

5. What changes in physical growth and psychosocial development influence eating habits in the toddler, preschool child, and school-age child? How do these factors influence the nutritional needs of each age group?

6. What factors influence the changing nutritional needs of adolescents? Who is usually at greater nutritional risk during this phase—boys or girls? Why? What nutritional deficiencies may be associated with this vulnerable age?

■ REFERENCES

1. Reed DB: Focus groups identify desirable features of nutrition programs for low-income mothers of preschool children, *J Am Diet Assoc* 96(5):501, 1996.

2. McKenzie J et al: Change in nutrient intakes, number of servings, and contributions of total fat from food groups in 4- to 10-year-old children enrolled in a nutrition education study, *J Am Diet Assoc* 96(9):865, 1996.

3. Erikson E: *Childhood and society*, New York, 1963, WW Norton.

4. Glinsmann WH et al: Dietary guidelines for infants: a timely reminder, *Nutr Rev* 54(2):50, 1996.

5. Skinner JD et al: Transitions in infant feeding during the first year of life, *J Am Coll Nutr* 16(3):209, 1997.

6. Nevling W et al: How do socioeconomic status and age influence infant food patterns? *J Am Diet Assoc* 97(4):418, 1997.

7. Birch LL: Children's food acceptance patterns, *Nutr Today* 31(6):234, 1996.

8. Borja ME et al: New lower-fat dessert recipes for the school lunch program are well accepted by children, *J Am Diet Assoc* 96(9):908, 1996.

9. Nahikian-Nelms M: Influential factors in behavior at mealtime: a study of 24 child-care programs, *J Am Diet Assoc* 97(5):505, 1997.

10. Hurd SL et al: Evaluation of implementation of the US Dietary Guidelines into the child nutrition programs in Texas, *J Am Diet Assoc* 96(9):904, 1996.

11. Getlinger MJ et al: Food waste is reduced when elementary-school children have recess before lunch, *J Am Diet Assoc* 96(9):906, 1996.

12. Jennings DS, Steen SN: *Play hard; eat right: a parents' guide to sports nutrition for children*, Minnetonka, Minn, 1995, American Dietetic Association and Chronimed Publishing.

13. Steen SN: Timely statement of the American Dietetic Association: nutrition guidance for child athletes in organized sports, *J Am Diet Assoc* 96(6):610, 1996.

14. Baer JT, Taper LJ: Amenorrheic and eumenorrheic adolescent runners: dietary intake and exercise training status, *J Am Diet Assoc* 92(1):89, 1992.

15. Steen SN: Nutrition for the competitive athlete. In Richert V, ed: *Adolescent nutrition*, New York, 1996, Chapman & Hall.

16. Steen SN: Timely statement of the American Dietetic Association: nutrition guidance for adolescent athletes in organized sports, *J Am Diet Assoc* 96(6):611, 1996.

17. American College of Sports Medicine: Position of the American College of Sports Medicine: exercise and fluid replacement, *Med Sci Sports Exerc* 28:i-vi, 1996.

■ FURTHER READING

Bronner YL: Nutritional status outcomes for children: ethnic, cultural, and environmental contexts, *J Am Diet Assoc* 96(9):891, 1996.

This excellent literature review explores relationships between nutritional status outcomes among ethnically diverse children and their cultural environments.

Kenedy E, Goldberg J: What are American children eating? Implications for public policy, *Nutr Rev* 53(5):111, 1995.

These authors review the changing health and demographic profile of the United States population with resulting changes in children's food patterns, and the impact of these changes on children's health.

McConnell PE, Shaw JB: Position of the American Dietetic Association: child nutrition services, *J Am Diet Assoc* 93(3):334, 1993.

Newman V: Position of the American Dietetic Association: promotion and support of breast-feeding, *J Am Diet Assoc* 93(4):466, 1993.

These two reports provide background for the supportive positions of ADA concerning the important contribution of breast-feeding to the nutritional well-being of infants, and the nutritional support of various child nutrition services to the growth and development of young children. In each case, the basis of the position is made clear and recommendations are made for actions to implement it.

Nutrition program for adolescents

Amanda Spencer is a graduate student of clinical nutrition assigned to the "Save Our Senior High" Project in Oakdale, a metropolitan community of 300,000 located in the northwestern United States. A representative of the city's educational advisory board approached her institution for assistance in developing a program that addresses three major problems faced by the majority of high school students: (1) popularity of fad diets among athletes, (2) obesity, and (3) iron-deficiency anemia.

Amanda and other members of her class met with students learning other health professions (medicine, dentistry, nutrition, nursing, social work), as well as several student representatives from the high school, to plan the program. After they developed goals and objectives, they decided that the nutrition topics would be addressed in a series of workshops entitled "Nutrition and Physical Fitness," "Food for the Teen Years," and "Snack Facts."

The program was introduced to the students through an advanced bulletin distributed at the largest high school in the city, where the project was to begin. The bulletin included an article written by Amanda, "Teenage Nutrition: A Seeming Paradox." This article responded to a common concern expressed by adolescents: the apparent preoccupation of school officials with the students' food habits when they, as a group, looked and usually felt very healthy.

Her article stirred a tremendous interest in the student population. Attendance at each session was high, and the discussions were lively. The evaluation results were positive. In reviewing the evaluative data and low cost of the project, the city council asked Amanda and her classmates to repeat the program at two other high schools where these problems were also prevalent. The council approached the school board about the possibility of including the project in the citywide high school curriculum for the coming year.

Questions for analysis

1. Outline the content of Amanda's article to reflect major points that you would have included.
2. Write a class outline for each workshop, including objectives, major topics, and questions you would expect from the students. What teaching methods and materials would you expect to be most effective in each workshop?
3. What outside influences on eating habits would you expect in this student population? How effective would you expect this educational program to be in influencing a change of behavior in eating habits?
4. Aside from in-school nutrition education programs, describe possible tactics for influencing the eating habits of teenagers.

Issues Answers

Feeding the premature infant

Babies born too soon or too small are surviving longer and with fewer serious physical and psychologic problems than before. Despite improvements in health, however, premature infants still present a number of problems that affect the feeding process: a poor sucking reflex; difficulty in swallowing, sucking, and breathing; small gastric capacity; reduced intestinal motility; tiring easily from eating and being handled; and increased nutrient requirements for catch-up growth. Thus the health team involved in the care of premature and small-for-gestational age infants is faced with a myriad of decisions to be made to overcome these feeding difficulties.

Should the infant be tube-fed?

Infants born before the thirty-fourth week of gestation are routinely given human milk or formula by tube (nasogastric, transpyloric) for up to several weeks after birth. Even older babies, born between 34 and 37 weeks of gestation, may receive some tube-feedings. This is believed to overcome sucking and swallowing difficulties, to slow gastric motility, and to prevent fatigue. Even in the hands of the most skilled nursing personnel, however, this method creates grave potential hazards. These dangers include irritation of the stomach and esophagus, gastric perforation, and excessive vagal stimulation, reflux, and aspiration, which may outweigh any problems caused by bottle-feeding.

In an attempt to minimize the potential complications in very low–birth weight (VLBW) infants weighing less than 1500 g (3⅓ lb) at birth, some medical centers have established nutritional care protocols based on tube-feedings. Once infants are medially stable, usually 3 to 4 days after admission, they are given half-strength formula, which is gradually increased as tolerated for 7 to 10 days or until weight gain begins. Criteria for beginning oral feedings are based on the absence of complications associated with enteral feedings—abdominal distention, reflux, diarrhea, and gastric residue. Infants treated in this manner in various studies have done well, although they tend to lose more weight at first and take a bit longer to regain their birth weights than anticipated.

Other workers have tried to avoid the complications of enteral feeding completely by initiating bottle-feedings as soon after birth as possible. Researchers have found that small-for-gestational age (SGA) infants could sustain appropriate weight gain through bottle-feeding,

even when bottles were given on demand. This response, however, has been observed in infants who were larger and healthier, weighing 1800 to 2500 g (4 to 5½ lb) at birth, than those treated by the previous tube-feeding protocol.

The advantages of one method over the other cannot be calculated in terms of weight gain because of the lack of standard growth rates established for different states of prematurity. However, since both methods have been successful, clinical practitioners should consider the patient's degree of illness, gestational age, and potential for imitating intrauterine growth from that age, without imposing stress on the metabolism and excretory system, when weighing the decision to recommend tube feedings or oral feedings for premature or SGA infants.

Should the infant's feeding be by schedule or on demand?

The trend toward on-demand feeding of full-term infants has grown with evidence of their ability to control caloric intake and avoid the effects of overfeeding or underfeeding. Premature infants, as indicated, have similar skills. Workers have even found that feeding on demand results in an adequate fluid and nutrient intake in less time than scheduled feedings among infants over 7 days old with birth weights of 1500 to 1800 g (3⅓ to 4 lb).

A modified-demand feeding method has been effective in infants with eating-related central nervous system disorders, lethargy, hyperbilirubinemia, and heart problems.

The resistance to on-demand feedings in premature or full-term infants during the hospital stay has often come from staff and administrators who think it would disrupt hospital routine. Cost-saving studies may make some administrators seriously reconsider the practicality of rigidly schedules routines, despite the effectiveness of such feedings for babies with special needs.

Should the infant be breast-fed or bottle-fed?

A variety of formulas reflect the estimated nutrient needs of low–birth weight babies (Table 12.6). These have been used safely, promoting weight gain similar to that expected in utero. Human milk was previously not considered for preterm infants because nutrient levels in mature milk were thought to be too low to meet the infant's needs. More recently studies have found that preterm milk is higher in protein, sodium chloride, mag-

Table

12.6 Nutritional value of special formulas and human milk for the preterm infant

Nutritional component	Advisable intake Birth weight		Human milk content		Standard formulas	Spec emature formulas		
	1.0 kg (2.2 lb)	1.5 kg (3.3 lb)	Preterm	Mature	Enfamil Similac[†] SMA[‡]	Enfamil* Premature with whey*	Similac Special Care[†]	"Preemie" SMA[‡]
Kilocalories/dl			73	73.0	67.0	81.0	81.0	81.0
Protein (g/200 kcal)	3.1	2.7	2.6[§]	1.5	2.2	3.0	2.7	2.5
Vitamins, fat-soluble								
D (IU/120 kcal/kg/day)	600.0	600.0	—	4.0	70-75	75.0	180.0	76.0
E (IU/120 kcal/kg/day)	30.0	30.0	—	0.3	2-3	2.0	4.0	2.0
Vitamins, water-soluble								
Folic acid (μg/120 kcal/day)	60.0	60.0	—	8.0	9-19	36.0	45.0	14.0
Vitamin C (mg/120 kcal/day)	60.0	60.0	—	7.0	10.0	10.0	45.0	10.0
Minerals								
Calcium (mg/100 kcal)	160.0	140.0	40.0	43.0	66-68	117.0	178.0	92.0
Phosphorus (mg/100 kcal)	108.0	95.0	18.0	20.0	49-66	58.0	89.0	49.0
Sodium (mEq/100 kcal)	2.7	2.3	1.5[‖]	0.8	1.0-1.8	1.78	1.9	1.7

*Mead Johnson Nutritional Division, Evansville, Indiana.
[†]Ross Laboratories, Columbus, Ohio.
[‡]Wyeth Laboratories, Philadelphia.
[§]Range: 1.9-2.8 g/100 kcal.
[‖]Range: 0.9-2.3 mEq/100 kcal.

nesium, and iron than mature milk and may be uniquely developed for preterm infants. Breast milk also offers immunologic protection as well as easy digestibility. However, the preterm infant relying solely on breast milk will require supplements of calcium and phosphorus to ensure adequate bone growth. Although requirements are not known, vitamins D and C and folic acid supplements are also recommended. Sodium supplements may also become necessary for infants weighing less than 1200 g (2.8 lb) because they are susceptible to hyponatremia.

What feeding practices should be followed during the infant's first year?

The most common feeding mistakes practiced by parents of full-term infants include introducing solid food before 4 months of age, introducing cow's milk before 6 to 12 months of age, serving solids in the nursing bottle, and serving low-fat milk before 2 years of age. Parents of premature infants may be more anxious to follow these practices to encourage growth. Unfortunately their negative effects on the health of full-term infants are exaggerated in the preterm child.

Parents must be reminded that their 4-month-old who was born 2 months prematurely is physiologically a 2 month-old and will present the same tongue-thrust reflex that is a sign of lack of preparedness for spoon feedings in a full-term 2-month-old. Parents should be encouraged to follow recommended infant feeding practices (see pp. 256-260) on the basis of the child's physiologic, or corrected, age rather than on the chronologic age.

In summary, current trends in feeding premature infants include:

- More bottle-feeding and breast-feeding to avoid the potential hazards of tube feeding.
- More on-demand feeding to prevent overfeeding or underfeeding and reduce health care costs.
- At-home feeding practices based on corrected chronologic age rather than birth age, using the preferred practice of delaying the start of solid foods until corrected age of 4 months, cow's milk until corrected age of 12 months, and low-fat milk until at least corrected age of 2 years.

In other words, premature babies are given more credit for their abilities to handle foods in ways similar to those of full-term infants.

References

Bhatia J, Rassin DK: Feeding the premature infant after hospital discharge: growth and biochemical responses, *J Pediatr* 118:515, 1991.

Bryson SR et al: Primary follow-up care in a multidisciplinary setting enhances catch-up growth of very low–birth weight infants, *J Am Diet Assoc* 97(4):386, 1997.

Fenton TR et al: Nutrition and growth analysis of very low–birth weight infants, *Pediatrics* 86(3):378,

Chapter

13

Nutrition for Adults: Early, Middle, and Later Years

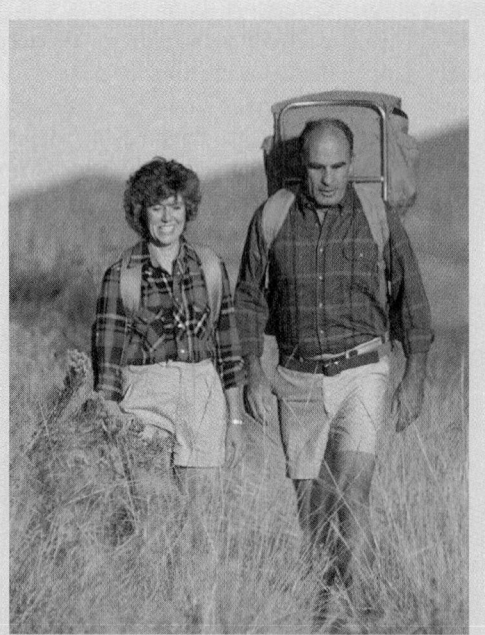

Chapter Outline

Adulthood: Continuing Human Growth and Development

Adult Age Group Needs: Health Promotion and Disease Prevention

The Aging Process

Individuality in Nutritional Needs of Elderly Persons

Health Care and Clinical Needs

In this chapter, we complete our three-chapter sequence on nutrition through the life cycle. Following the tumultuous adolescent years come the challenges, problems, and opportunities of maturity during adulthood.

Today when adolescents come of age, they have lived only about a quarter of their potential life span. They face a changing world of accelerated pace and complexity. America reflects these changes in its aging and increasingly diverse population.

Here we review adulthood—its early, middle, and later years. We look at each stage in terms of maturing needs and the role of nutrition in health concerns.

ADULTHOOD: CONTINUING HUMAN GROWTH AND DEVELOPMENT

AGING THROUGHOUT THE LIFE CYCLE

Aging is a positive concept. It starts at conception and ends at death. It encompasses the whole of life, not merely its latter stages. Indeed, every stage has its unique potential and fulfillment, and the periods of adulthood— young, middle, and older—are no exception. Basic human needs continue, although in changing patterns, as persons mature and grow older.

Throughout your study, it is important to view continuing adult growth as a positive changing period of maturing human life. Two important concepts are significant parts of the whole process:

- *The individual.* Although gradual aging throughout the adult years has group influences in a society, it is at the core an *individual* process.
- *The total life.* Although it changes at each stage of the life span, aging is a *total life* process.

These two basic concepts govern the needs of these years—physiologic, psychosocial, socioeconomic, and nutritional.

COMING OF AGE IN AMERICA

Young adults coming of age in America are experiencing extensive population and technology changes during this decade that affect their personal and working lives. The population explosion of "baby boomers" of the World War II era are now in their early 50s, facing a rapidly changing world.[1] And with our increasing life span and the growing number of older adults in our population, the personal, social, and health care needs are being felt in all our lives.

The report of the United States Department of Health and Human Services (USDHHS), *Healthy People 2000: National Health Promotion and Disease Prevention Objectives*, projects **demographic** changes we can expect in our society over the 1990s that will affect all adults and families.[2] The report summarizes these changes in terms of our total population and households, age distribution, racial and ethnic composition, economic expansion, and immigration by the year 2000:

- *Population and households.* The United States population will have grown about 7% to nearly 270 million. Average size of households will decline from 2.68 to 2.49, and two-parent households, from 58% to 53%.
- *Age distribution.* The United States. population will be older with average age more than 36; 35 million people (13%) will be over age 65. The fastest growing group, the "oldest-old"—those over age 85, will increase 30% to a total of 4.6 million. The number of

children under age 5 will decline from more than 18 million to fewer than 17 million.

- *Racial and ethnic composition.* Proportion of whites, not including Hispanic Americans, will decline from 76% to 72%, and the fastest growing group, the Hispanics, will rise from 8% to 11.3%, representing more than 31 million. Proportion of blacks will increase from 12.4% to 13.1%, and other racial groups—Native Americans and Alaska Natives, Asians and Pacific Islanders—will increase from 3.5% to 4.3%.
- *Economic expansion.* A shift in birth rates will decrease the number of young job seekers, and more jobs will require technical skills. Work force entry rates will be highest among women of all racial and ethnic backgrounds, making them almost half (48%) of the total work force. Occupations most likely to grow include service, technical, sales, professional, and management.
- *Immigration.* Up to 6 million people will probably be added to the American population by immigration, with the East and West coasts receiving most of them.

SHAPING INFLUENCES ON ADULT GROWTH AND DEVELOPMENT

Within this broader, rapidly changing world, today's adults are growing and developing in many divergent ways. In terms of our interest in nutrition and health at each life stage, however, four basic areas of adult life shape its general path: physical, psychosocial, socioeconomic, and nutritional.

Physical

Overall physical growth of the human body, governed by its genetic potential, levels off with physical maturity in the late teens and early adult years. Now physical growth is no longer marked by increasing numbers of cells and body size. Rather, it is the vital process of **replication**, growing new cells constantly to replace old ones to main-

---

demographic The statistical data of a population, especially those showing average age, income, education, births, deaths, and so on.

replicate To make an extract copy; to repeat, duplicate, or reproduce. In genetics, replication is the process by which double-stranded DNA makes copies of itself, each separating strand synthesizing a complementary strand. Cell replication is the process by which living cells, under gene control, make exact copies of themselves a programmed number of times during the life span of the organism. The process can be reproduced in the laboratory with cultured cell lines for special studies in cell biology.

tain body structure and function, increasing learning and strengthening mental capacities. Then at older ages, physical growth gradually declines. Individual vigor reflects the health status of preceding years.

Psychosocial

Here we pick up the threads of Erikson's eight stages of human personality development introduced in Chapter 12 at the beginning of the life cycle (see p. 255). Three remaining developmental tasks of personal psychosocial growth characterize the adult years: (1) young adults—intimacy versus isolation; (2) middle adults—generativity versus self-absorption; and (3) older adults—integrity versus despair. Individual adults at each age experience these struggles in some way, including their influence on lifestyle and health.

Socioeconomic status

We all grow up and live our lives in a social and cultural context. Our world is rapidly changing; we are experiencing major social and economic shifts, and most adults and their families are feeling the strain in some way. These pressures directly influence food security and health.

Nutritional needs

Basic energy and nutrient needs of individual adults in each age group, of course, vary according to living and working situations. However, current RDA standards for healthy adults, as shown in Table 13.1, reflect general needs and serve as a point of ready reference for comparing these needs in our discussion.

ADULT AGE GROUP NEEDS: HEALTH PROMOTION AND DISEASE PREVENTION

EARLY ADULT: 18 TO 40 YEARS

Physical characteristics

After the turbulent physical growth and sexual development of the preceding adolescent years, the young adult's body growth pattern levels off into a state of adult *homeostasis*. Finely regulated gene control of neural and hormonal activity and feedback maintain a stable internal environment of "body wisdom." The body functions are fully developed, including sexual maturation and reproductive capacity.

Psychosocial development

In the early adult years, every person is launched, for better or worse, as a socially mature individual. The core psychosocial growth task each young adult must resolve is the problem of *intimacy versus isolation* (Figure 13.1). It

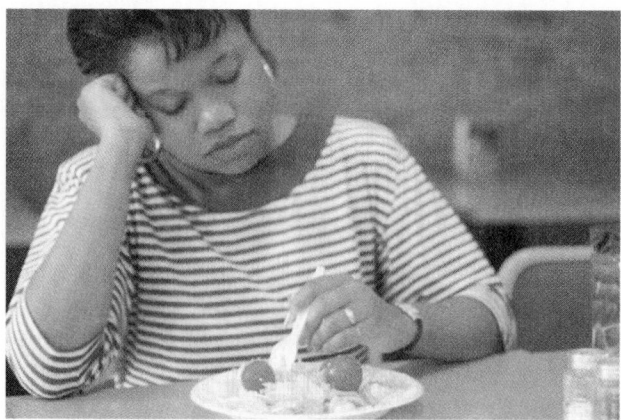

Figure 13.1   The early adult years center on the core problem of intimacy versus isolation.

is a time of physical maturity, of becoming comfortable with the physical self generally, and of increasing adult role demands. If positive development is achieved, the person can build intimate relationships leading to self-fulfillment, either in marriage or in other personal relationships. If these psychosocial strengths have not been developed in the previous years of growing up, the person may become increasingly isolated from others.

Socioeconomic status

The early adult years reflect the social and economic pressures of continued education to prepare for adult responsibilities and career beginnings, of establishing one's own home, of parenthood and starting young children on their way through the same life stages, and of early struggles to make one's way in the world. Given the changing economic environment in today's world, many young adults face difficulties in meeting these basic goals of education, work, and family.

Nutritional needs

All of these physical, psychosocial, and socioeconomic factors influence nutritional needs. Distinct differences in growth patterns that emerged between males and females during adolescence are strengthened in adult bodies. The young man's larger muscle mass and long bone growth are established. The young woman's wider hip breadth and pelvic girdle of subcutaneous fat, genetically designed to support reproduction, continue to prompt concerns and sometimes unwise actions in relation to social pressures for thinness that contribute to insufficient nutritional support. Nutritional needs of this period center on energy, protein, and the micronutrients.

1. *Energy.* The RDA energy standard for young men is 2900 kcal/day, and for young women, 2200 kcal/day (Table 13.1). The larger male body size and muscle mass require more energy to maintain, especially

because the lean muscle mass is the most metabolically active tissue in the body composition. The adult resting energy expenditure (REE) per unit of body weight, a measure of metabolic rate, differs by about 10% between the genders.[3] The remainder of the energy need is for physical activities (Figure 13.2), which is much smaller than that for metabolic needs. The height and weight reference figures in Table 13.1 are not meant to imply ideal ratios. They are actual **medians** for the designated age group reported by a large national nutrition and health survey. Women require additional energy to support pregnancy and lactation (see Chapter 11).

2. *Protein.* The RDA standard for protein during the early adult years is 58 g/day for men and 46 g/day for women. These allowances are based on a daily protein intake of approximately 0.8 g/kg body weight for both genders, which many American adults exceed. By the age of 25 years, protein needs are 63 g/day for men and 50 g/day for women. An additional 10 g/day of protein is needed for pregnancy; an added 15 g/day is needed for lactation.

3. *Minerals.* The RDAs for adults are sufficient if provided on a regular basis by a well-balanced diet. Two minerals, calcium and iron, need emphasis. In the current RDAs the calcium allowance has been increased from 800 to 1200 mg/day for young adults to ensure peak skeletal bone mass, which is attained by approximately the age of 35 years. Population groups of most concern for adequate bone mass are adolescents, women, and older adults.[4-6] Iron is another mineral often lacking in poor diets, resulting in iron-deficiency anemia. Women require more iron intake to offset iron loss from menstrual blood loss, so their RDA for iron is 15 mg/day; for men, it is 10 mg/day. Iron requirements for pregnancy are doubled, 30 mg/day, which is difficult to attain by diet, so a supplement is usually needed. No increase is needed during lactation.

4. *Vitamins.* The vitamin needs of young adults are usually met by regular, well-balanced diets. Problems in some individuals may relate more to inadequate regular intake rather than to increased need. A well-selected, mixed diet usually supplies all the vitamins in normally needed quantities.

MIDDLE ADULT: 40 TO 65 YEARS

Physical characteristics

Physical maintenance established during the early adult years continues into the middle adult years. However, the cell replication rate begins to decline slowly and a gradual cell loss starts. From their thirties and forties onward, both men and women show a decline in skeletal muscle mass and strength, a condition called *sarcopenia*, which means "vanishing flesh."[7,8] Depending on the

Figure 13.2   Energy needs vary according to degree of activity. (Tom McCarthy, The Stock Market.)

degree of physical activity, which may be less during these years, the body fat proportion may begin to increase. This is especially seen in postmenopausal women, which increases weight concerns. Also, periodic physical examinations and laboratory tests showing increased blood lipid levels may indicate early risks of chronic heart disease.

Psychosocial development

The psychosocial problem persons in the middle adult years face is that of *generativity*—active involvement in some way, usually with family and grandchildren or in community groups—*versus self-absorption*. The children are now adults themselves, grown and gone to make their own lives. For some, these years have been called the "empty nest." For many, however, it is an opportunity to

---

median In statistics, the middle number in a sequence of numbers.

Table 13.1	RDA for adults (National Research Council, 1989 version)

	Age (yr)	Weight		Height		Energy (kcal)	Protein (g)	Vit. A (µg RE)	Vit. D (µg)	Vit. E (mg α-TE)	Vit. K (µg)
		(kg)	(lb)	(cm)	(in)						
Males	19-24	72	160	177	70	2900	58	1000	10	10	70
	25-50	79	174	176	70	2900	63	1000	5	10	80
	51 +	77	170	173	68	2300	63	1000	5	10	80
Females	19-24	58	128	164	65	2200	46	800	10	8	60
	25-50	63	138	163	64	2200	50	800	5	8	65
	51 +	65	143	160	63	1900	50	800	5	8	65

expand personal growth—"it's my turn now" (Figure 13.3). There is a realistic coming-to-terms with what life is all about, together with a sharing of stored learnings by passing on life's teachings to younger persons. It is a regeneration of one's life in the lives of young people following in the same way. To the degree that these inner struggles are not won, there is an increasing self-absorption, a turning in on oneself, and a withering rather than a regenerating spirit of life.

Socioeconomic status

With a changing economy in the marketplace and increasing technology in business and manufacturing, shifts in the nature of employment bring increased job loss for workers or "outplacement" for executives and managers. No longer can employees expect job security with the same company all their working lives to retirement with a hefty pension at age 65 years. For adults in the middle of their working lives, supporting families and planning for the future, such financial problems can be devastating. Also, the numbers of "new poor" families only increase the poverty problem.

Nutritional needs

The energy and protein needs of earlier adult years continue, but calcium allowances return to 800 mg/day (Table 13.1). There is increasing evidence, however, that postmenopausal women need an increased intake of calcium to prevent bone mass calcium loss that follows the loss of protective estrogens in menopause, when osteoporosis risk is increased. Physical activity tends to decrease, adding to weight problems and increased vulnerability to fads that promise youth and vigor.

Figure 13.3   Middle adult years can often be a time to expand personal growth. (CLG Photographs, Inc.)

LATER ADULT: 65 TO 85 YEARS

Physical characteristics

The later adult years generally bring a gradual waning of physical vigor, work capacity, and strength. Usually physical activity decreases, along with overall energy bal-ance needs and metabolic requirements. With increasing age the body composition changes. Total body water, bone mass, and lean body mass decrease and body fat mass increases. Weight gain commonly occurs in postmenopausal women, a pattern that continues into later

Water-soluble vitamins							Minerals						
Vit. C (mg)	Thiamin (mg)	Riboflavin (mg)	Niacin (mg NE)	Vit. B$_6$ (mg)	Folate (μg)	Vit. B$_{12}$ (μg)	Calcium (mg)	Phosphorus (mg)	Magnesium (mg)	Iron (μg)	Zinc (mg)	Iodine (μg)	Selenium (μg)
60	1.5	1.7	19	2.0	200	2.0	1200	1200	350	10	15	150	70
60	1.5	1.7	19	2.0	200	2.0	800	800	350	10	15	150	70
60	1.2	1.4	15	2.0	200	2.0	800	800	350	10	15	150	70
60	1.1	1.3	15	1.6	180	2.0	1200	1200	280	15	12	150	55
60	1.1	1.3	15	1.6	180	2.0	800	800	280	15	12	150	55
60	1.0	1.2	13	1.6	180	2.0	800	800	280	10	12	150	55

years and frustrates many. Older persons are "fatter" in body composition for any given relative weight when compared with younger persons of the same weight, and the fat distribution, especially in men, centers mainly in the central abdominal area.

Psychosocial development

The final core psychosocial development problem between *integrity versus despair* is resolved in the later adult years. Depending on a person's resources at this point, a sense of wholeness and completeness predominates or a sense of bitterness and revulsion and of wondering what life was all about deepens. If the outcome of life's basic experiences has been positive, the individual arrives at older age a rich person—rich in the wisdom of the years. Building on each previous level, psychosocial growth now reaches its personal positive resolution.

But some of our older patients will not have resolved each of the core developmental problems along the way. They still struggle with those same problems that they have wrestled with in previous stages of life. Thus they arrive at middle and older years poorly equipped to deal with the adjustments of aging and health problems, and suffer from depression and failure to thrive.[9,10] On the other hand, many will have been enriched by life's human experiences in their maturing process. In turn they bring enrichment to our lives, and the resulting relationship is rewarding.

Socioeconomic status

Older adults often face retirement with a limited fixed income in a changing economy. Others may have no stable income source and lack economic security. As a result, studies consistently show significant differences in nutritional intake between older persons with low and high socioeconomic status, with those in low-economic circumstances having poorer diets. Living alone may also influence food intake, if social isolation causes depression and lack of incentive or ability to procure and prepare food. This is true of inner-city elderly persons and homebound rural older adults. Many of them experience economic and social deprivation.

Nutritional needs

The current RDAs for older adults generally remain the same as those for all adults above the age of 50 years, with some distinctions:

1. *Energy.* The basic energy allowance for all adults beyond 50 years of age is calculated at one-and-a-half times the REE. This makes the average need of men (weighing 77 kg) 2300 kcal/day and of women (weighing 65 kg) 1900 kcal/day, with a normal variation of ± 20%.[3] Energy needs of older adults beyond the age of 75 years are likely to be somewhat less because of reduced body size, REE, and activity. Light to moderate activity is encouraged to maintain muscle mass and well-being. The sharp decline in activity frequently seen in elderly persons is not inevitable and certainly not desirable.

2. *Protein.* The daily protein allowance remains the same beyond 50 years of age, based on approximately 0.75 to 0.8 g/kg of body weight for both sexes. This makes the average allowance for men 63 g/day and for women 50 g/day.[3] The older adult body has a gradually decreasing lean body mass. Thus this continuing basic protein allowance is higher per unit of lean body mass for older adults and should allow for some decrease in utilization deficiency.

3. *Minerals.* Daily mineral allowances remain the same as for middle adults.[3] However, some evidence indicates that older adults—especially postmenopausal women—may need increased amounts of calcium to continue protection against bone calcium loss and the development of osteoporosis.[5,6]

4. *Vitamins.* Daily vitamin allowances also remain essentially the same as those for middle adults. Basic needs are met with regular, well-balanced diets. Individual problems may occur with inadequate intake or during illness.

OLDEST-OLD: 85 YEARS AND OLDER

United States Census Bureau projections

All projections and our personal experiences indicate that as a population we are growing older. The oldest adult group among us is the fastest growing, but because this is so recent and rapid a phenomenon historically, this "oldest-old" group is the least understood. To distinguish the changing nature of the older adult population, the United States Census Bureau is now using three classifications instead of one: (1) the *young-old*—ages 65 through 74 years; (2) the *old-old*—ages 75 through 84 years; and (3) the *oldest-old*—ages 85 years and beyond. In projecting life expectancies for men and women in the United States, the Census Bureau issues estimates based on three levels of predicted mortality: low, middle, and high.[11] These estimates for low and middle predicted mortality by the years 2020 and 2040 are given in Table 13.2. The Census Bureau also projects over 1 million Americans 100 years or older in the year 2040. Given the rapid pace of biomedical research, many scientists working in this field think it is more likely that the actual numbers will surpass all of the Census Bureau projections.[14]

Nutritional needs

A growing consensus among clinicians and nutritionists caring for these older persons is that the current RDAs for adults at age 50 years, which actually include little change from those for younger adults, do not necessarily meet the highly individual and differing needs of persons ages 85 years and beyond. Elderly persons differ from younger adults in the way they absorb some nutrients, in gastric acidity, overall nutrient utilization, exercise response, body composition changes with age, and how these changes influence nutritional needs. For example, in comparison with needs of younger adults, they probably need more or less of several nutrients:

- Less *vitamin A* because they store more and use it less efficiently
- More *vitamin D* because they make it less efficiently and have less sun exposure
- More *pyridoxine (B_6)* because their increased sensitivity to depletion affects function of the nervous system and immune system
- More *cobalamin (B_{12})* because their decreased ability to make stomach acid limits its absorption

In addition, some elderly persons—often women, with small bodies and low daily energy intakes of about 1000 to 1200 kcal—may require prudent supplementation to the diet to help meet their overall nutritional needs.

POSITIVE HEALTH PROMOTION: DIETARY PATTERN FOR ADULT HEALTH

Two basic food guides, issued by the USDA and the USDHHS, can serve as patterns for planning healthy diets for adults of any age group. These are the Food Guide Pyramid, which provides a visual pattern for food choices from five basic food groups, and the United States Dietary Guidelines, which provides a general set of seven simple statements that summarize a sound approach to reducing risks for America's leading health problems. Both of these guides are described in Chapter 1. They emphasize the two basic keys to healthy diet planning and food behavior at any age—moderation and variety.

THE AGING PROCESS

BASIC GERONTOLOGY RESEARCH

Basic research in **gerontology** is moving rapidly to better understand the physical aging process, in terms of length and quality.

Length of life

Over the past century, general life expectancy of Americans has almost doubled from 40 years to nearly 80 years. Scientists agree that most of the advance thus far has resulted from the "easier" gains in reducing deaths of infants and young children and mothers in childbirth and that the "harder" work of increasing life expectancy lies ahead in more knowledge of the normal aging process, apart from the diseases of aging. Currently, the new tools of molecular biology of cells allow basic biomedical research to focus on the difficult task of separating out the many factors that cause cells to grow old. Studies thus far clearly support the theories that oxidative cell damage by free cell radicals has an influence in the aging process and that this damage may also be responsible for behavior deficits in aging. Ongoing research suggests a critical

Table 13.2	U.S. Census Bureau population projections for adults over age 85 years, for the years 2020 and 2040 (based on low and middle estimates of predicted mortality)	

Level of predicted mortality	Number of Americans age 85 years and over (millions)	
	2020	2040
Middle mortality	6.7	12.2
Low mortality	8.6	17.8

From Spencer G: *Projection of the population of the United States by age, sex, and race: 1988 to 2080,* Bureau of the Census, Current Population Reports, Series P-25, No 1018, Washington, DC, 1989, US Government Printing Office.

connection between the general functional decline of **senescence** and the "growing old" of human cells, which involves gene control and a biologic limit to cell replication rather than a chronologic age. Studies such as these are beginning to separate the diseases of age from the normal process of aging and lay the groundwork for a lengthened and improved ending of the human life span.

Quality of life

The United States demographic reports of a lengthened life span and a rapidly growing older population have forced a primary attention to the quality of that extended life. We are looking at a phenomenal future of increased numbers of elderly and elevated health care costs. The first of the World War II "baby boomers" turn 85 years old in the year 2031. By 2040, when the average baby boomer will be 85 years old, Medicare spending for the population 65 years and older could reach from $147 to $212 billion (in 1987 dollars).[11] Overall, the number of persons in the United States age 85 years and older is now growing six times faster than the rest of the population, and the cost of caring for the disabled in that group is expected to double in the next decade.

As a result of these projected needs, medical research has shifted its agenda for the 1990s to a revitalized study of aging, so that gerontology is reported to be a "growth industry." Top priorities of National Institutes of Health basic research center on the study of abnormal cell proliferation, and the neurosciences related to brain aging. A related top priority in clinical **geriatrics** research targets preventing and treating disabilities in older persons. This means a focus on nonfatal but highly disabling age-dependent conditions of frailty—arthritis, osteoporosis, sensory impairments such as blindness, and Alzheimer's disease.

GENERAL BIOLOGIC CHANGES IN AGING

The general biologic process of growth and gradual decline extends over the entire life span. It is conditioned by all previous life experiences and the imprint of these experiences on individual genetic heritage.

Nature of biologic change

During middle and older adulthood, there is a gradual cell loss and reduced cell metabolism, with a related gradual reduction in the performance capacity of most organ systems. These changes— both physical and mental—may occur rapidly in one organ system and slowly in others, and individuals vary widely in the rate and order in which these changes occur. But in general, lean body mass continues an age-related decline that accelerates in later life. For example, by the age of 70 years the kidneys and the lungs lose about 10% of their weight in comparison with values in young adults, the liver loses 18% of its weight, and skeletal muscle diminishes by 40%. Also, an important, overall reduction in the body's reserve capacities takes place. An important cause is the gradual reduction in cellular units. For example, functioning units of the kidney—the nephrons—are lost as the aging Western kidney, which evolved in prior ages of vastly different food intake needs, now responds to our modern high-protein diet (see Chapter 21).

Effect of biologic change on food patterns

Some resulting physiologic factors may affect food patterns. For example, secretion of digestive juices is diminished, and motility of the gastrointestinal tract is decreased. This contributes to decreased absorption and the use of nutrients. Sensory perceptions of taste, smell, hearing, and vision also diminish, although these responses are highly individual.[16] These senses influence appetite and the amount of food consumed, so food for older adults generally needs more—not less—enhancement in seasoning. Also, along with these biologic changes often comes an increased concern about body functions, increasing social stress, personal losses, and diminished social opportunities to maintain self-esteem. All of these responses can affect food intake.

INDIVIDUALITY OF THE AGING PROCESS

The biologic changes in aging are general. But in reality persons in the advancing years of life will display a wide variety of individual reactions. We all get old at different rates. Every person bears the imprint of individual trauma and accumulation of disease experience, and we grow older at our own individual and unique gene-controlled nature and rate of the process of aging. All of these factors directly affect individual aging. We can discuss aging and its nutritional needs in general terms, but individual situations and needs vary widely and must always be individually assessed. Actually, as we increasingly realize, the greatest influence of nutrition on the aging process takes place in earlier growth years when resources for later times are being built. Thus nutrition's most effective role is in growth and middle years, which prepare each one of us to meet the gradually declining metabolic processes of older age.

---

geriatrics Branch of medicine specializing in medical problems associated with old age.

gerontology Study of the aging process and its remarkable progressive events.

senescence The process of growing old; a consequence of advancing age or a premature aging process from disease.

INDIVIDUALITY IN NUTRITIONAL NEEDS OF ELDERLY PERSONS

ENERGY

The reduced basal metabolic requirements caused by losses in functioning cells and reduced physical activity combine to create less energy demand as age advances. Some studies have indicated that the concept of a limited, less rich diet—"undernutrition without malnutrition"—may actually lengthen life.[15,16] Individual needs vary with body size and physical activities, but an average estimate of energy need is about 1800 kcal/day, more or less.

There are major gaps in our knowledge of energy and nutrient needs of the elderly. For example, nutrient uptake by cells may decline with aging, so that older persons may need higher plasma levels to maintain optimal tissue concentrations. Also, because living situations vary widely among older adults, much more information is needed on their daily life activities and the degree of energy they may be capable of expending. Kcalorie requirements are highly individual, according to activity. Primary consideration must be given to the living situation of the person and the degree of activity in various phases of life. Perhaps the simplest criterion for judging adequacy of kcaloric intake is the maintenance of *normal* weight. However, there is current rethinking of traditional standards for appropriate weight based in life insurance weight-for-height tables (see Chapter 6). Recent assessment of these and other data has raised the possibility that the greatest longevity is not associated with the conventional "desirable" weight but with levels 10% to 25% greater. This view has obvious nutritional implications in terms of optimal energy intake for adults of all ages. To meet these energy needs, adults need ample carbohydrates but limited fats.

1. *Carbohydrates.* The optimal need for energy from carbohydrate is unknown, but it is usually recommended that at least 50% to 55% of daily kcalories in the diet come from carbohydrate foods, mostly complex carbohydrates such as starches. Easily absorbable sugars are used, and generally carbohydrate metabolism is not disturbed. The fasting blood sugar level is essentially normal in the elderly. They can choose freely among carbohydrate foods, according to individual needs, desires, and physical responses. Current findings indicate that much of the observed carbohydrate intolerance of older persons may be caused by factors other than biologic aging per se and that diet and exercise modifications can substantially curtail age-related glucose intolerance and insulin resistance.

2. *Fats.* Generally, Americans eat too much fat, sometimes amounting to as much as 40% of their diet's kcalories. Fat intake is best limited to about 20% of the total kcalories. Some fat is needed as a source of energy, important fat-soluble vitamins, and essential fatty acids. A reasonable goal is to avoid large quantities of fat, with more emphasis on the quality of the smaller amount of fat consumed, using mostly plant sources rather than animal fats. Digestion and absorption of fats may be somewhat delayed in elderly persons, but these functions are not greatly disturbed with age. There is no need to be unduly restrictive. Sufficient fat for food palatability aids appetite. Excessive fat, however, should be avoided because of the delayed absorption capacity of elderly persons.

3. *Protein.* There is a basic need for quality protein, although not in excessive amounts, to meet the needs of adults in our society:
   - *Basic needs.* The usual daily adult protein intake continues to meet the aging individual's need—about 0.8 g/kg of body weight. Even this amount provides an allowance for wide variation in individual needs. Also, although protein may be increased during illness or convalescence or during a wasting disease, the overall mass of actively metabolizing tissue decreases with age. There is inadequate research information on what levels of dietary protein can best preserve the lean body mass and tissue function of the aging adult. We need to know whether populations receiving 0.8 g/kg of body weight or less show any accelerated losses of lean body mass. It is possible that to maintain nitrogen balance, elderly persons need relatively more protein as their total energy intake is reduced.
   - *Protein quality.* Protein needs are influenced by two basic factors: (1) the biologic value of the protein based on the quantity and ratio of its essential amino acids, and (2) adequate kcaloric value of the diet. It is estimated that about 25% to 50% of the protein intake should come from animal sources, the only foods that are "complete" proteins with all the essential amino acids, with the remainder coming from plant protein sources. In a vegetarian diet, plant proteins—with additions of acceptable milk and egg protein—ensure adequate protein intake. Protein should supply from 15% to 20% of the day's total kcalories. Healthy older adults do not need supplemental amino acid preparations. They are an expensive and inefficient source of nitrogen.

Vitamins

Traditionally, nutrient standards have indicated that additional vitamin intake in the healthy adult is unnecessary, and that although tissue stores may gradually decrease with normal aging, there is no difference in requirement from that for normal adults. However, a growing concern among geriatric family physicians and researchers studying nutritional needs in elderly persons is that these older adults have different nutrient needs from those of their younger counterparts. Some individual problems may stem from inadequate normal intake rather than from an increased need. In most cases, a mixed diet of moderation and variety usually supplies needs. Increased therapeutic needs in illness should be evaluated on an individual basis.

Minerals

Usually increased minerals are not needed in normal aging. The same adult allowances are sufficient if provided on a continuing basis by a well-balanced diet. However, several essential minerals need emphasis in diets for the elderly, including calcium and iron, because of their relation to osteoporosis and anemia. Some individuals may need increased attention and encouragement to ensure adequate dietary sources of these minerals among their daily food choices.

Water

Too often the vital need for water in older adults is overlooked. The normal thirst mechanism sometimes diminishes with age, and dehydration can easily occur. About 1 in 5 elderly persons suffer from *xerostomia*, dry mouth caused by a severe reduction in the flow of saliva, which in turn affects their food intake. This condition may be associated with the use of certain medications, autoimmune diseases, or radiation therapy to the head and neck. Conscious attention to adequate fluid intake, not less than the recommended 1500 to 2000 ml daily and not dependent on normal thirst, is an important aspect of health maintenance and care.[12]

NUTRIENT SUPPLEMENTATION

Healthy adults of any age regularly consuming healthful diets rarely need added nutrient supplementation. However, elderly persons are at greater nutritional risk and often benefit from prudent, individually assessed supplementation—especially women, the oldest-old, persons in poor health, those having inadequate energy intake, those living alone or lacking social support or mobility, or those having insufficient money for food. There is some indication, however, that certain specific nutrient supplementation might be a rational approach to improve **cognitive** function in disoriented older adults (see *To Probe Further* box, p. 285). And in illness or debilitated states supplementation may well be needed to replenish losses.

HEALTH CARE AND CLINICAL NEEDS

SUCCESSFUL AGING

Many older Americans are not only living longer but also aging well. They have vigor and vitality and are often involved in positive health maintenance programs. Even

80% of individuals over the age of 85 years with disabilities and infirmities and with an average age of nearly 90 years are not in nursing homes but are able to live in the community, alone or with friends or family, in residential settings, or in adult foster care in private homes. Most urban elderly impaired or disabled persons are cared for in the community rather than in institutions. However, for many older individuals in nursing homes or hospitals and in the community, malnutrition is too often present and requires personal care and prevention.

MALNUTRITION

Incidence

Protein-energy malnutrition occurs among many elderly persons, especially among those in hospitals and outpatients, as well as those in nursing homes. Often there is a severe anorexia of aging.[14] Health care providers can and must communicate with these older adults whatever their situation may be.[17] It is not uncommon that some of these malnourished persons weigh less than 45.5 kg (100 lb). Wide experience has indicated that as many as half of these older clients have had no physician-recorded diagnosis of malnutrition or weight loss or any physician-prescribed nutrition supplement or nutrition assessment referral. Thus malnutrition, with or without a contributory disease, is all too common among elderly persons living in the community, and often a specific nutritional diagnosis is not made.

Warning signs and preventive care

Warning signs can alert us to early malnutrition in elderly persons. If heeded, they are crucial to preventing unnecessary and sometimes irreversible weight loss.[14,17]

1. *Physical signs.* Recent unintended weight loss, perhaps associated with eating problems, such as tooth loss or poorly fitting dentures; dry mouth from decreased salivary secretions; diminished sensory perceptions such as taste, smell, or sight; difficulty swallowing; mental confusion

2. *Multiple medications.* Long-term use of multiple medications, often termed "polypharmacy," with actions and side effects that are often unexplained to patient and family and that interact with food or nutrients or reduce appetite

3. *Psychosocial signs.* Grief from loss of spouse or family and friends; depression; loneliness or living alone; homebound with lack of sunlight; increased use or abuse of alcohol, which often displaces food intake

---

cognitive Pertaining to the mental processes of perceptions, memory, judgment, and reasoning, as contrasted with emotional and volitional processes.

4. *Economic problems.* Low socioeconomic status, lack of sufficient money for food, inadequate housing, homelessness
5. *Food-related difficulties.* Disability affecting food shopping or preparation and eating, missed meals and snacks or fluids, food wasted or rejected, insufficient food stores at home, lack of fruits and vegetables or fortified whole-grain products, poor nutrition knowledge, lack of ethnic "comfort foods" that increase interest in eating

NUTRITION SCREENING INITIATIVE

The recent Nutrition Screening Initiative (NSI) was a 5-year program to promote routine nutrition screening in all United States community health and medical care settings, working through a network of registered dietitians, public health and clinical nutritionists, physicians, other health care professionals, the public, and policy makers.[18] This initial multidisciplinary project of the American Dietetic Association, the American Academy of Family Physicians, and the National Council on the Aging first targeted the warning signs of malnutrition in older Americans because of their large burden of poor nutritional status in the United States population. Based on an initial comprehensive survey of research in gerontology and geriatrics and a consensus of leaders to establish goals, the working groups identified warning signs of malnutrition within a framework of the following seven basic risk factors:

- Inappropriate food intake
- Poverty
- Social isolation
- Dependency or disability
- Acute or chronic diseases or conditions
- Chronic medication use
- Advanced age

NSI developed a public awareness checklist for warning signs of poor nutritional health, "Determine Your Nutritional Health," including a nutrition information sheet based on the word *DETERMINE* as a mnemonic device to convey the basic nutrition information in a way that can be easily remembered.

CLINICAL PROBLEMS

Chronic diseases

Physicians specializing in geriatrics and clinical nutritionists working with older adults increasingly relax their strict "medically indicated" diets, especially for elderly patients in long-term care facilities. At these older ages the finer points of diets for lowering cholesterol or managing non-insulin-dependent diabetes mellitus are not the caring physician's and dietitian's major concern. In many older individuals, such highly restrictive diets lead to decreased food intake and serious weight loss and are thus inappropriate. Instead the general practice is to follow a regular diet—well-balanced nutritionally with a variety of food choices and some moderation in fats and sweets, as indicated for us all (see Chapter 1).

Disability

Currently, major attention in research and clinical practice has turned to improving the functional disabilities and infirmities that some elderly persons experience. The goal is to add quality of life to these extended years. For example, increased work in the field of musculoskeletal problems, such as arthritis and osteoporosis, relates malnutrition to increased falls and fractures by measures of many nutritional markers.[18-20] Programs for patients with osteoporosis and arthritis based on extensive knowledge about the disease and its management can make a difference in these patients' lives. Both individual and group sessions—including nutrition assessment and counseling, physical therapy, medical evaluation, and treatment—have a positive impact on patients' general physical and psychologic well-being, helping them to cope with the pain and chronic nature of the condition.

COMMUNITY RESOURCES

Government programs for older Americans

The regular government food assistance programs for individuals and families also provide support for older Americans. These include the Food Stamp Program (Figure 13.4) and the surplus agricultural commodities distribution program (see Chapter 10). These programs provide needed foods and food-buying extension for many older adults. However, the single greatest impact on the growing field of nutritional gerontology has been the Older Americans Act that created the National Nutrition Program for Older Americans.[21]

Older Americans Act—Title VII and Title III

In 1972, the Nutrition Program for Older Americans, Title VII of the Older Americans Act, was authorized by Public Law 92-258. The program was developed to meet the nutritional and social needs of persons 60 years of age and older who (1) could not afford adequate diets, (2) were unable to prepare adequate meals at home, (3) had limited mobility, or (4) were isolated and lacked incentive to prepare and eat food alone. The original program provided services such as outreach, escort and transportation, health services, information and referral, health and welfare counseling, and nutrition and consumer education. In 1978 amendments were authorized by Public Law 95-478, which coordinated nutrition services with other services for older people. Under this amended Act, Title III-C, the services funded after 1980 included the provision of meals, congregate and home-delivered, and related nutrition services and education.

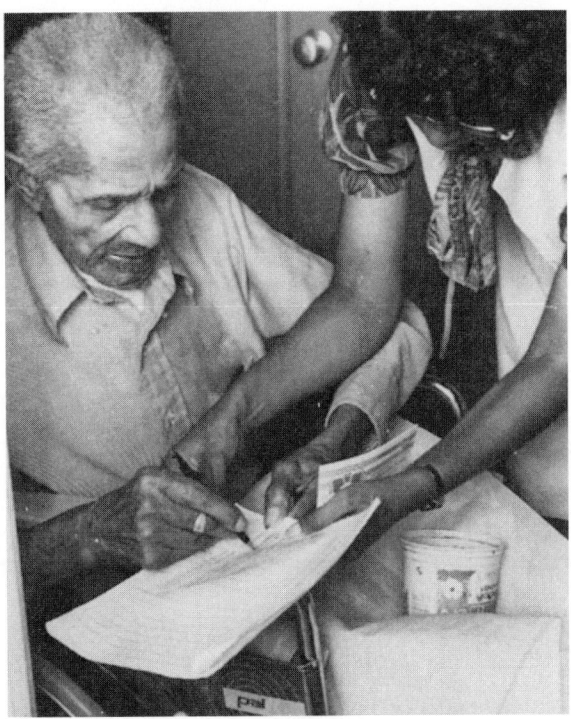

Figure 13.4   Elderly disabled man assisted by the Food Stamp Program to obtain needed food.

1. *Congregate meals.* The program provides older Americans, particularly those with low incomes, nutritionally sound meals at low cost in senior centers and other public or private community facilities. Older adults can gather for a hot noon meal and receive not only food but also social support. They also receive sound food and nutrition information to help dispel nutrition myths and misinformation, to which elderly persons are often vulnerable.[21]
2. *Home-delivered meals.* For those persons who are homebound by illness or disability, meals are delivered by couriers to the home. This service provides nutritional needs and human contact and support. Often the courier is the only person the homebound individual may contact during the day. For urban and rural elderly homebound participants, many of whom have poor diets, this single hot meal 5 days a week provides their main source of food intake.

United States Department of Agriculture research centers

The United Stated Department of Agriculture (USDA), in collaboration with universities, is establishing human nutrition research centers on aging, which are authorized by Congress to study nutrition's role in aging. Current investigations include such areas as protein needs in aged persons, the nutritional status of elderly men and women, and the prevention and slowing of osteoporosis.

United States Department of Agriculture extension services

The USDA operates agricultural extension services in state universities and county agencies. Through these agencies, county home advisors provide communities with much practical nutrition material and counseling for older adults and community workers.

Public health departments

Skilled health professionals work in the community through local and state public health departments. Health guidance for elderly persons is available through their resources. The public health nutritionist is a significant member of the health care team and provides counseling and nutrition education services, community program planning, and oversight of food service facilities in nursing homes licensed by the state (see *Practical Application* box, p. 284). Counseling is also provided concerning the various food assistance programs available (see Chapter 10).

PROFESSIONAL ORGANIZATIONS AND RESOURCES

National Council on the Aging

The National Council on the Aging, established in 1950, is located in Washington, DC. It is an organization for professionals and volunteers that works on many fronts to improve the quality of life for older Americans. It maintains a nonprofit central national resource for research, planning, training, information, technical assistance, advocacy, program and standards development, and publications that relate to all aspects of aging, including nutrition. This organization works with the American Dietetic Association and the American Academy of Family Physicians to identify and assist older Americans at risk for malnutrition.

American Geriatric Society

This professional organization of physicians engaged in medical care of elderly patients promotes research in geriatrics to advance scientific knowledge of the aging process and the treatment of its diseases. A number of nurses and other health professionals are associate members. The society publishes the *Journal of the American Geriatrics Society*.

The Gerontological Society

This society's membership includes a wide number of interested health professionals. Its committee on aging has stimulated increased interest among other related organizations and community and government agencies in gerontology and the problems of aging persons in our society. This organization publishes the *Journal of Gerontology*.

Improving the nutritional status of the elderly in long-term care facilities

Over the past three decades the number of nursing home beds has increased from about 880,000 to 1.5 million, and the need by the year 2000 is expected to exceed 3.5 million. Take a look at the following statistics on those who reside in long-term care facilities:

- 80% are 75 years of age or older
- 50% cannot feed themselves
- 85% have moderate to severe protein-energy malnutrition, which decreases their response to rehabilitative efforts

Residents of long-term care facilities have a wide spectrum of needs, and food is a critical issue. Daily meals become particularly significant to residents, a fact that some facilities with otherwise excellent care in nursing and imaginative cultural programs sometimes fail to realize in their food service. The use of full-time dietitians can often change this situation.

Improvements in the nutritional status of residents as a result of professional nutrition services by qualified nutrition specialists has been documented many times. These skilled and sensitive persons address the following factors in quality care that must be present to ensure the optimal nutritional status of their clients:

Administrative activities

- Developing cyclic menus based on nutritional requirements and reflecting the needs and desires of that population
- Training staff to ensure proper food preparation including appetizing seasonings and creative uses for foods that require changes in consistency from thin liquids to ground foods
- Working with nursing staff, speech therapists, and food service staff regarding the nutritional needs of patients suffering from dysphagia

Clinical activities

- Conducting nutritional assessments of residents on admission and at regularly scheduled intervals thereafter
- Encouraging use of appropriate consistency and texture of foods (e.g., not using pureed foods when ground foods can be used and not using ground foods when chopped foods can be used)
- Making accurate calculations of diets for persons with insulin-dependent diabetes mellitus (IDDM) and renal failure
- Discouraging abuse of alcohol, nicotine, drugs
- Developing resident education programs, such as appropriate physical activity to increase a sense of well-being
- Encouraging eating by recognizing cultural diversity in ethnic food patterns; considering individual food preferences; satisfying the desire for "something sweet" with products made from appropriate sweeteners; occasionally planning special events, such as picnics, which may include family members; creating a homelike atmosphere in the dining hall with appealing menus and regular food in the more current move away from "special diets"; preparing meals in the residential area to "entice" residents with the aroma; using color schemes and china patterns in soothing tones; planning special menus for festive events and special parties such as Octoberfest, luaus, monthly birthday parties with live music and a party menu, or a family dinner party with special orders from a "Touch of Class" menu

The overall goal of such quality food management is simple— "to get people to eat." The most nutritious meal in the world is no good unless it is eaten.

References

Endres J et al: Acceptance and consumption of crystalline fructose menu items by institutionalized elderly persons, *J Am Diet Assoc* 90(3):431, 1990.

Gallagher FA: Elegance adds appeal to nursing home food service, *J Am Diet Assoc* 90(12):1632, 1990.

Herbelin K: Techniques for supporting food choices of residents in long-term care facilities, *J Am Diet Assoc* 92(6):718, 1992.

Samolsky S et al: Feeding the Hispanic hospital patient: cultural considerations, *J Am Diet Assoc* 90(12):1707, 1990.

To Probe Further

Food for thought among the elderly

Among elderly persons, as well as others, it is a common observation that poor mental function and malnutrition go hand in hand. Although scientists have not yet figured out the precise connections, they find a strong correlation between nutritional deficiencies and poor cognitive performance and memory among elderly persons. A study of 260 noninstitutionalized adults over the age of 60 years reveals that those with poor nutritional food intakes scored poorly on special tests that measure nonverbal abstract thinking ability and memory. Protein, vitamin C, and various B vitamins—folate, niacin, pyridoxine, riboflavin, thiamin, and B$_{12}$—emerged as the nutrients of particular significance to the subjects' ability to think and remember.

Researchers are reluctant at this point to say on the basis of such studies that poor nutritional status causes poor thinking abilities and memory loss because a number of factors may intervene:

- Persons with poor memories may forget to take a vitamin pill. Those who don't recognize objects or shapes may have such difficulties preparing meals that they often fail to eat, leading to a poor nutritional status.
- Educated persons may be more inclined to take nutritional supplements and because of their experience in taking tests, score better than average.
- In a population of basically healthy elderly persons, a subgroup may have undetected clinical problems that contribute to poor mental performances.

There is no doubt that mental problems in elderly persons, including mental retardation, affect diet practices in residents of intermediate- or long-term care facilities and group homes and require regular developmental disability consultation with trained professionals. Less clear is just how poor nutritional status may precipitate, aggravate, or prolong mental problems in elderly persons. Some more obvious nutrient candidates involved are precursors for neurotransmitters: the amino acids tyrosine, tryptophan, threonine, and histidine, as well as choline. Other candidates are nutrients affecting the metabolism of neurotransmitters: pyridoxine, vitamin C, thiamin, copper, and iron. Still other candidates are nutrients with general effects on brain metabolism: glucose, folate, cobalamin, nicotinic acid, riboflavin, zinc, potassium, and magnesium.

Thus we can make a strong presumptive case for the potential importance of nutritional status in the mental abilities of older adults. But what we lack is precise knowledge of the possible mechanisms involved, which probably act in concert with many other contributory factors.

References

Bernard MA et al: Common health problems among minority elders, *J Am Diet Assoc* 97(7):771, 1997.

Klein GL et al: Nutrition and health for older persons in rural America: a managed care model, *J Am Diet Assoc* 97(8):885, 1997.

Mercer KC, Ekvall SW: Comparing the diets of adults with mental retardation who live in intermediate care facilities and in group homes, *J Am Diet Assoc* 92(3):356, 1992.

Russell RM: New views on the RDAs for older adults, *J Am Diet Assoc* 97(5):515, 1997.

Community groups

Local community groups representing health professions—such as the medical society, nursing organizations, and dietetic associations—sponsor a variety of programs to help meet the needs of elderly persons in their communities. In addition, qualified nutritionists and registered dietitians in private practice are available in most communities for individual counseling and community program support. Senior citizens centers in local communities also provide a broad range of services and available nutrition education and counseling.

Volunteer health organizations

Many activities of volunteer health organizations such as the American Heart Association and the American Diabetes Association relate to the health and nutrition needs of older persons. These organizations include professional and public members. They operate at national and community levels to fund and conduct research and education.

TO SUM UP

The challenge of meeting the nutritional needs of the older populations is compounded by the lack of needed research in this area; the interaction of current and past social, economic, and psychologic factors; and the wide range of individual differences in the biologic process of aging.

Nutritional requirements should, at least in part, be based on biologic changes caused by aging—reduced speed of conduction for nerve impulses, reduced blood flow and pulmonary function, reduced tissue mass in several organs, and so on. Current nutrient and energy standards, however, lack specific research on older adult needs and thus are based mainly on extrapolations of data available for younger adult populations, as well as requirements to counteract chronic disease processes prevalent in aging, such as cardiovascular disease.

Major illnesses found in elderly persons are often associated with malnutrition and weight loss. Malnutrition may be associated with a number of factors such as underlying illness, fad diets, poverty, or various conditions affecting food intake, such as oral problems (dry mouth, infections, lack of teeth, poorly fitting dentures, and swallowing difficulty), psychosocial problems resulting from isolation, and other personal factors contributing to boredom or apathy. The Nutrition Screening Initiative (NSI), a national project conducted by The American Dietetic Association, the American Academy of Family Physicians, and the American Council on the Aging, works in many communities to identify those elderly persons at risk for malnutrition and helps educate individuals and communities in preventive care.

QUESTIONS FOR REVIEW

1. Briefly describe five main ways the United States population is changing. Illustrate how these changes may have touched your own life or the life of someone you know. How do you think these changes may influence persons' diets or their nutrition and health status?

2. Describe the influence of physical, psychosocial, socioeconomic, and nutritional factors on adult growth and development. Give examples from the experience of any adult you may know.

3. Select any one of the adult age groups and describe the basic needs of this group in the adult life span in terms of physical growth, psychosocial development, socioeconomic status, and related nutritional needs.

4. Describe two basic United States food guides developed as patterns for planning healthful diets. How might you use them in helping a middle-aged couple on a limited income to improve their poor food intake pattern?

5. Distinguish between the two terms *gerontology* and *geriatrics*. Describe current research goals and activities in these fields in relation to length and quality of life.

6. Describe some of the general biologic changes in aging. How may these changes affect eating, food choices, and nutritional status?

7. Identify five basic warning signs of malnutrition in older adults. Give examples describing how each of these situations leads to poor nutrition. Give some ways that each situation might be improved to prevent malnutrition.

8. Describe the government programs for older Americans and other community resources for nutrition and health needs.

REFERENCES

1. Chernoff R: Baby boomers come of age: nutrition in the 21st century, *J Am Diet Assoc* 95(6):650, 1995.

2. US Department of Health and Human Services, Public Health Services: *Healthy people 2000: National health promotion and disease prevention objectives,* Pub No 91-50212, Washington, DC, 1990, US Government Printing Office.

3. Food and Nutrition Board, National Academy of Science—National Research Council: *Recommended dietary allowances,* ed 10, Washington, DC, 1989, National Academy Press.

4. Miller GD et al: Age consideration in nutrient needs for bone health, *J Am Coll Nutr* 15(6):553, 1996.

5. Anderson JJB, Rondona PA: Peak bone mass development of females: Can young adult women improve their peak bone mass? *J Am Coll Nutr* 15(6):570, 1996.

6. Heaney RP: Age considerations in nutrient needs for bone health: older adults, *J Am Coll Nutr* 15(6):575, 1996.

7. Raloff J: Vanishing flesh—muscle loss in the elderly finally gets some respect, *Sci News* 150(6):90, 1996.

8. Evans WJ: Effects of aging and exercise on nutritional needs of the elderly, *Nutr Rev* 54(1):S35, 1996.

9. Cass R, Shea ME: Recognizing depression in older adults: the role of the dietitian, *JAMA* 96(10):1042, 1996.

10. Egbert AM: The dwindles: failure to thrive in older patients, *Nutr Rev* 54(1):S25, 1996.

11. Spencer G: *Projections of the population of the United States by age, sex and race: 1988 to 2080,* Bureau of the Census, Current Population Reports, Series P-25, No 1018, Washington, DC, 1989, US Government Printing Office.

12. Chidester JC, Spangler AA: Fluid intake in the institutionalized elderly, *J Am Diet Assoc* 97(1):23, 1997.

13. Drewnowski A et al: Salt taste perceptions and preferences are unrelated to sodium consumption in healthy older adults, *J Am Diet Assoc* 96(5):471, 1996.

14. Morley JE: Anorexia of aging: physiologic and pathologic, *Am J Clin Nutr* 66:760, 1997.

15. Weindruch R: Caloric restriction and aging, *Sci Am* 274(1):46, 1996.

16. Sohal RS, Weindruch R: Oxidative stress, caloric restriction, and aging, *Science* 273(5271):59, 1996.

17. Wright KJ et al: Dietitians can and should communicate with older adults with hearing and vision impairments and communication disorders, *J Am Diet Assoc* 97(2):174, 1997.

18. Sahyoun NR et al: Nutrition Screening Initiative checklist may be a better awareness/educational tool than a screening one, *J Am Diet Assoc* 97(7):760, 1997.

19. Packard PT, Heaney RP: Medical nutrition therapy for patients with osteoporosis, *J Am Diet Assoc* 97(4):414, 1997.

20. Evans WJ, Cyr-Campbell D: Nutrition, exercise, and healthy aging, *J Am Diet Assoc* 97(6):632, 1997.

21. Hutchings LL, Tinsley AM: Nutrition education for older adults: how Title III-C Program participants perceive their needs, *J Nutr Ed* 23(2):53, 1991.

▃▃ FURTHER READING

Bernard MA et al: Common health problems among minority elders, *J Am Diet Assoc* 97(7):771, 1997.

This article reviews the primary health problems of elders in four of our most prominent minority population groups: African Americans, Hispanic Americans, Asian/Pacific Islander Americans and Native Americans, to assist health workers in decision-making in dietary counseling.

Chidester JC, Spangler AA: Fluid intake in the institutionalized elderly, *J Am Diet Assoc* 97(1):23, 1997.

Gloth FM et al: Nutrient intakes in a frail homebound elderly population in the community vs a nursing home population, *J Am Diet Assoc* 96(6):605, 1996.

These two articles provide background for assessing the vital need for adequate fluid and nutrient intakes of elderly persons being cared for at home or in a nursing home.

Egbert AM: The dwindles: failure to thrive in older patients, *Nutr Rev* 54(1):S25, 1996.

Evans WJ: Effects of aging and exercise on nutrition needs of the elderly, *Nutr Rev* 54(1):S35, 1996.

Guigoz Y et al: Assessing the nutritional status of the elderly: the Mini Nutritional Assessment as part of the geriatric evaluation, *Nutr Rev* 54(1):S59, 1996.

This single issue of *Nutrition Reviews* provides a number of excellent articles on nutritional needs of elderly persons. These three deal with failure to thrive, exercise needs, and a brief nutrition assessment, including a copy of the Mini Nutritional Assessment form for a simple and rapid tool to assess the risk of malnutrition in the elderly.

Issues & Answers

Can we eat to live forever?

The world is getting older. Our life span has extended from age 45 at the turn of the century to nearly 80 years today. It is expected to climb even higher.

We owe this lengthening of life to the conquest of infectious disease, the provision of safer work settings, and the development of more effective medical technology. In short, we have largely conquered our external environment. It's time we conquered our *inner* environment—through proper nutrition.

Scientists are beginning to consider the importance of nutrition in combating the physical deterioration that accompanies old age: a 10% loss of kidney and lung tissue, 18% loss of liver tissue, 40% loss of skeletal tissue, and as much as 25% (12% in men) loss of bone by the seventh decade of life. You would think that scientists could simply make biochemical calculations to find optimal blood levels for nutrients that could retard these losses and make recommendations for dietary intake. However, achieving an optimal diet among elderly persons is much more complex than that.

Sensory deprivation

Elderly persons tend to live alone. Such physical and emotional isolation tends to diminish the desire to eat. When this is combined with the progressive deterioration in sight, smell, touch, and hearing that occurs in some older adults, attempts to prepare meals are not only frustrating, they are dangerous.

Taste and smell

Oral infections, poor hygiene, and a reduced salivary flow rate contribute to the increased difficulty in taste and smell. To what extent does this affect the desire to eat? No one knows. Some scientists say the effect is little, suspecting poor research techniques in studies of this problem. Others believe it is serious enough to warrant further research to arrest ongoing losses.

Bone and tooth loss

Approximately half of all adults have lost their teeth by the age of 65 years. The main culprit is periodontal disease. Researchers are beginning to look at this problem as a possible manifestation of osteoporosis, or weakened

bone. They are focusing the study of calcium on the following:

- *Calcium RDAs.* Some suggest that 1200 to 1500 mg/day of calcium may be necessary to prevent calcium loss, rather than the current RDA of 800 mg.
- *Phosphate.* Calcium and phosphorus maintain an inverse ratio in the blood. Processed foods contribute heavily to phosphate levels in the American diet and are suspected of promoting calcium resorption from bone.
- *Megavitamins.* Excessive vitamin A levels have been associated with a greater loss of bone in elderly persons. Studies of elderly subjects usually reveal that many use vitamin supplements, with some adding additional amounts of vitamin A. This warrants further study.
- *Protein.* America's obsession with meat may harm aging bones, as a high-protein intake results in increased loss of calcium in the urine.

Kcaloric needs

It has repeatedly been reported that elderly persons fail to consume recommended amounts of kcalories. However, based on animal studies, some researchers claim that a restricted diet also makes people live longer, but this has not been proved and is still controversial. An even more recent reassessment of the effect of body weight suggests that we should all weigh 10% to 25% more than we do to live longer. Because the reassessment does not associate body size with detrimental habits such as smoking, it is also controversial.

Gastrointestinal problems

Reduced production of digestive juices, less peristaltic activity, and reduced mucosal surface area all work to inhibit nutrient absorption and promote such digestive disorders as constipation.

Drugs

The prevalence of chronic disease means a prevalence of prescription and over-the-counter drug use. Drugs, either individually or in combination with each other, can alter taste, appetite, and other factors and affect nutritional status.

Poverty

Many elderly persons either cannot work or are coerced into retirement. For these reasons they tend to be among the poorest citizens in the United States. As a result, even those individuals in good health often lack the money to shop, the transportation to reach a shopping area, or adequate food preparation and storage equipment to maintain a reasonably healthful diet.

Based on the information available thus far, the most nutritionally supportive environment for elderly persons is one in which they do the following:

- Have company for meals, such as at congregate meal sites, as well as family support and friends.
- Have foods with pleasant but distinctive aromas and flavors.
- Consume meals that are lower in protein-rich and processed foods, higher in fiber-rich foods (complex carbohydrates and a variety of fresh fruits and vegetables) and calcium (from nonbovine as well as bovine sources, to avoid excessive protein levels), and provide a moderate amount of kcalories.
- Avoid supplements, especially of vitamin A, unless medically indicated.
- Avoid unnecessary drugs and be informed of the action and side effects of every drug they take.

- Are subsidized financially or placed in living situations (senior centers or private homes with roommates) that provide some financial, emotional, and nutritional support.

Although these may seem like reasonable recommendations for any age group, elderly persons present such a myriad of long-standing compounding factors that a wide variety of service and professional assistance may be needed to avoid nutritional deficits. Thus counselors who hope to promote a nutritionally supportive environment for elderly clients must themselves maintain a network of professional sources available for referrals and must work together as a team to meet the unique needs of older persons.

References

Chidester JC, Spangler AA: Fluid intake in the institutionalized elderly, *J Am Diet Assoc* 97(1):23, 1997.

Heaney RP: Age considerations in nutrient needs for bone health: older adults, *J Am Coll Nutr* 15(6):575, 1996.

Morley JE: Anorexia of aging: physiologic and pathologic, *Am J Clin Nutr* 66:760, 1997.

Rhodus NL, Brown J: The association of xerostomia and inadequate intake in older adults, *J Am Diet Assoc* 90(12):1688, 1990.

Rolls BJ, McDermott TM: Effects of age on sensory-specific satiety, *Am J Clin Nutr* 54:988, 1991.

Chapter

14

Nutrition, Physical Fitness, and Stress

This chapter relates the three basic factors of nutrition, physical fitness, and stress to health maintenance throughout the life cycle. In an increasingly technologic society, building physical activity into our busy lives, as well as dealing with stress, requires commitment and effort. However, it is a vital cornerstone in the preventive approach to controlling our modern "chronic diseases of civilization."

First, we examine how nutrition works in energy fuels and muscle action. Then we apply these principles to athletic performance and building a reasonable and appropriate personal exercise program. Finally, we relate stress management to our overall health goals.

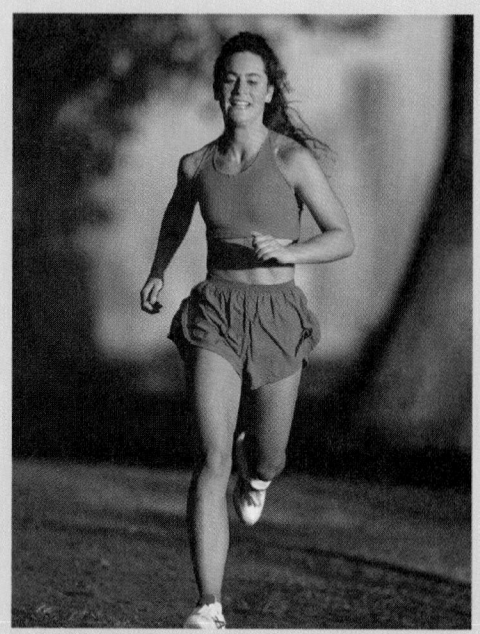

MODERN CIVILIZATION, CHRONIC DISEASE, AND PHYSICAL ACTIVITY

MODERN DEVELOPED NATIONS AND DISEASES OF CIVILIZATION

Over thousands of years our marvelous human bodies have developed from earlier ages of human history when survival depended on constant exercise and energy expenditure. Now, over only a few past generations, the developed nations of the world have come to live in very different circumstances. Our high-technology societies demand little if any physical activity in our work and in our lifestyle. As a result, our health has been paying a price. Our inactivity contributes to a host of modern ills, so-called diseases of civilization, including coronary heart disease, diabetes, hypertension, osteoporosis, and obesity.[1,2]

HEALTH TOLL OF INACTIVITY

American workers and leaders, students and teachers, and parents and children seem to be increasingly aware of the health toll of our inactivity. According to some estimates, 100 million Americans now practice some form of regular exercise, a twofold increase over the past two decades. Walking and swimming are our most popular outdoor activities, with bicycling and jogging close behind. In relation to the big business of athletics, we have seen the new specialty of sports medicine develop.

In everyday life, the need for exercise is serious. The modern health care approach of preventive medicine, as well as the necessity of dealing with chronic disease, demands positive attention to the related roles of nutrition and physical fitness in health care. Exercise has currently emerged as an effective therapy, along with nutritional care and weight management, in the control of hypertension, diabetes, cancer risk, and elevated blood lipids.[4-6] Whatever level of exercise or active pursuits a person is able to do, even a limited beginning builds into consistent habits. For many, it is a matter of life and health.

ENERGY SOURCES FOR PHYSICAL ACTIVITY

THE NATURE OF ENERGY

You will recall from Chapter 6 that the term *energy* refers to the body's ability, or power, to do work. The energy required to do body work takes several different forms: mechanical, chemical, electric, light, radiant, and heat. Energy, like matter, can neither be created nor destroyed. It can only be changed into another form and constantly cycled in the body and environment. We also speak of energy as being **potential** (stored) or **kinetic** (active). Potential energy is stored energy, ready to be used. Kinetic energy is active energy, being used to do work. Energy balance in physical activity requires a base of sound nutrition to supply the **substrate** fuels, which along with oxygen and water meet widely varying levels of energy demand for body action.

MUSCLE ACTION: FUELS, FLUIDS, AND NUTRIENTS

Muscle structures

The synchronized action of millions of specialized cells and structures that make up our skeletal muscle mass make possible all forms of physical activity. A finely coordinated series of small bundles within the muscle fibers (Figure 14.1), triggered by nerve endings, produce a smooth symphony of action through simultaneous and alternating contraction and relaxation. These successively smaller muscle structures include:

1. **Skeletal muscle.** The largest bundle in the series is the complete muscle. Each particular muscle is composed of muscle fibers called **fasciculi.**
2. **Muscle fiber.** Each muscle fiber is composed of bundles of still smaller strands called **myofibrils.**
3. **Myofibril.** Each single myofibril strand of the muscle fiber is made up of the smallest of all the fiber bundles, called **myofilaments.** Contraction occurs here.
4. **Myosin** and **actin.** Within each myofilament are the contractile proteins, **myosin** and **actin,** which are the smallest moving parts of every muscle.

---

actin Myofibril protein whose synchronized meshing action in conjunction with **myosin** causes muscles to contract and relax.

fasciculi A general term for a small bundle or cluster of muscle, tendon, or nerve fibers.

kinetic Energy released from body fuels by cell metabolism and now active in moving muscles and energizing all body activities.

myofibril Slender thread of muscle; runs parallel to the muscle fiber's long axis.

myofilaments Threadlike filaments of actin or myosin, which are components of myofibrils.

myosin Myofibril protein whose synchronized meshing action in conjunction with **actin** causes muscles to contract and relax.

potential Energy existing in stored fuels and ready for action, but not yet released and active.

substrate The specific organic substance on which a particular enzyme acts to produce new metabolic products.

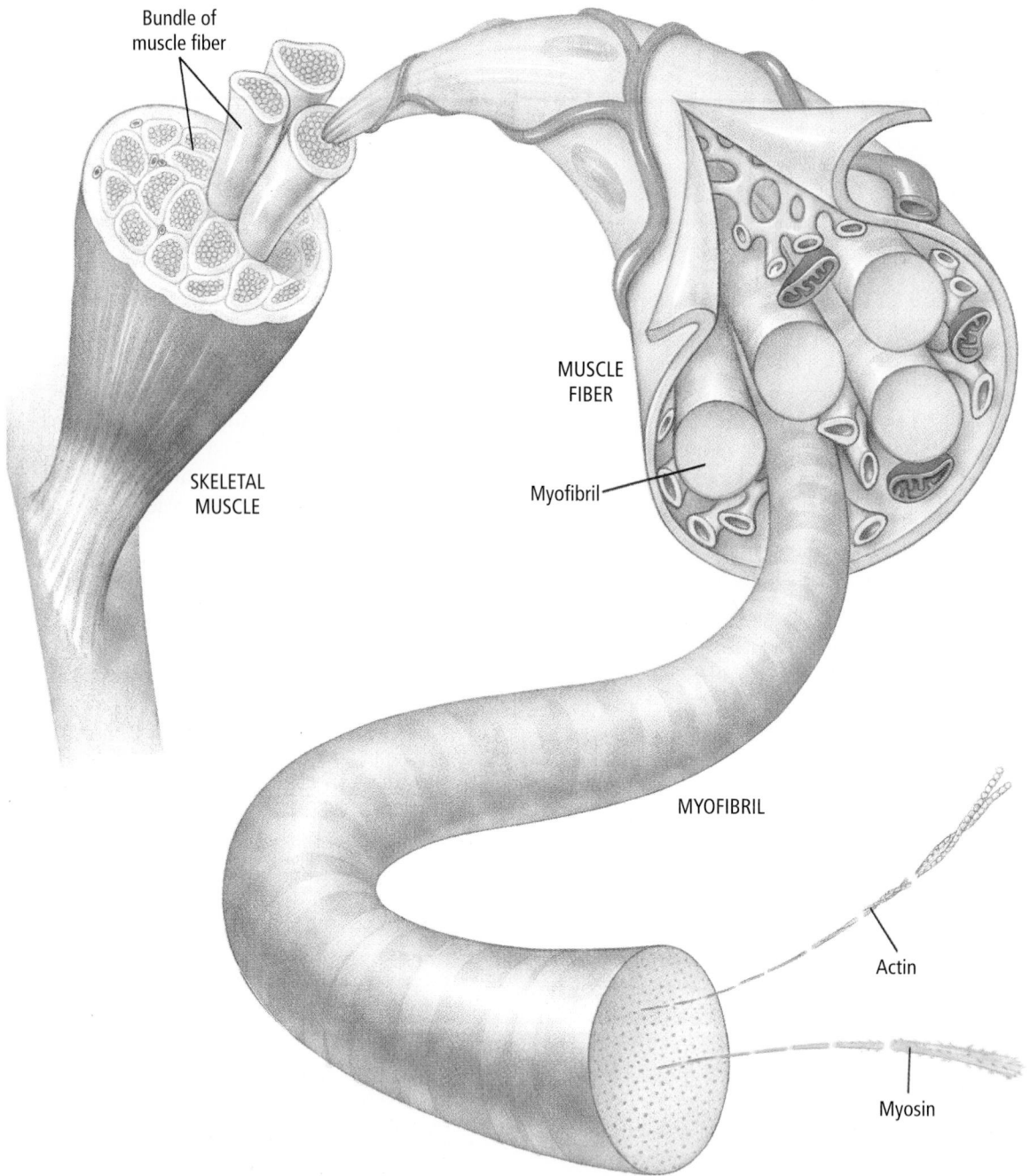

Figure 14.1   Skeletal muscle, showing the progressively smaller bundles within bundles. (Modified from Barbara Cousins; from Seeley RR, Stephens TD, Tate P: *Anatomy and physiology,* ed 2, New York, 1992, McGraw-Hill.)

Muscle action

Inside the cell membrane these contractile proteins, myosin and actin, are arranged in long parallel rows. These parallel rows slide together and mesh tightly when the muscle contracts and then pull apart when the muscle relaxes, allowing the muscle to shorten or lengthen as needed. When a specific motor nerve impulse excites these molecules of myosin and actin in a myofilament, they mesh together and thereby shorten the muscle. This contraction of the muscle bundles occurs instantly and simultaneously. Periods of relaxation occur between contractions. This alternating process continues until muscle fatigue builds up and the muscle can no longer respond. Muscle fatigue occurs for two reasons: (1) the supply of *glycogen,* the immediate muscle fuel, is exhausted and thus insufficient to sustain the required chemical reaction, and (2) *lactic acid,* the metabolic product of this chemical muscle reaction, accumulates during sustained high levels of exercise and cannot be removed fast enough.

Fuel sources

Phosphate bonds form high-energy compounds in body metabolism (see Chapter 8). The main high-energy compound of the body cells is *adenosine triphosphate (ATP)*. It has rightly been called the "energy currency" of the cell. Various forms of energy are called on for successive energy needs:

1. *Immediate energy.* High-power or immediate energy demands over a short time depend on ATP being readily available within the muscle tissue. This amount is used up rapidly and a backup compound, *creatine phosphate (CP)*, is made available. These high-energy phosphate compounds, however, will sustain exercise only for about 5 to 8 seconds.
2. *Short-term energy.* If an activity lasts longer than between 30 seconds and 2 minutes, *muscle glycogen* supplies the continuing need. Although the amount of available glycogen is small, it is an important rapid source of energy for brief muscular effort.
3. *Long-term energy.* Exercise continuing more than 2 minutes requires an oxygen-dependent or *aerobic* energy system. A constant supply of oxygen in the blood is necessary for continued exercise. Special cell organelles, the *mitochondria*, located within each cell, produce large amounts of ATP. The ATP is produced mainly from glucose and fatty acids and supplies continued energy needs of the body.

Fluids

An increased intake of water is essential in the course of exercise. A deficiency can be dangerous and limits capacity greatly. As exercise continues, the body temperature increases as part of the energy produced is released as heat. To control this temperature increase, the body shunts as much heat as possible to the skin, where it is released in sweat, which should be replaced with 4 ounces of water every 15 minutes. Over time, and especially in hot weather, excessive sweating can lead to *dehydration.* This is a serious complication.

Nutrients

The fuel nutrients also become depleted during continued exercise. As energy demands increase, the body burns blood glucose and muscle glycogen to provide energy. With prolonged exercise, levels of these nutrients fall too low to sustain the body's continued demands. Fatigue follows and exhaustion threatens.

OXYGEN USE AND PHYSICAL CAPACITY

Oxygen consumption

The most profound limit to exercise is the person's ability to deliver oxygen to the tissues and use it for the production of energy. This vital ability depends on the fitness of the pulmonary and cardiovascular systems. Because the heart is a muscle, exercise strength-

ens and enlarges it, enabling it to pump more blood per beat, a capacity called **stroke volume**. The **cardiac output**, how much the heart pumps out in a given period, depends on the amount of blood per contraction and on the cardiac rate, the number of contractions in a given time. In general, then, a person's **aerobic capacity** depends on the degree of fitness and body composition.

1. *Body fitness.* Physical fitness is defined in terms of aerobic capacity, which depends on the body's ability to deliver and use oxygen in sufficient quantities to meet the demands of increasing levels of exercise. Oxygen uptake increases with exercise intensity until either the demand is met or the ability to supply it is exceeded. This maximal oxygen (O_2) uptake, or aerobic capacity, is called the **VO$_2$max**—maximum uptake volume of oxygen.[7] This capacity determines the intensity and duration of exercise that a person can perform. From the resting level, there is a steep rise in oxygen consumption during the first 3 minutes of exercise. In about 6 minutes the rate levels off into a steady state, indicating an equilibrium between the energy required by the exercising muscles and the aerobic energy-producing system. This aerobic capacity of an individual is measured in terms of milliliters of oxygen consumed per kilogram of body weight per minute. Thus persons of differing sizes can be compared equally.
2. *Recovery period.* During exercise, to accommodate the body's increased energy demands, the heart rate increases and breathing becomes deeper and more rapid. After exercise stops these functions do not immediately return to their preexercise levels, especially if the exercise has been strenuous. This recovery takes time because the body must replenish its "oxygen debt."
3. *Body composition.* Sex differences in aerobic capacity reflect the sex differences in body composition. In general, men have a higher aerobic capacity because

---

aerobic capacity Milliters of oxygen consumed per kilogram of body weight per minute; influenced by body composition.

cardiac output Total volume of blood propelled from the heart with each contraction; equal to the stroke output multiplied by the number of beats per the time unit used in the calculation.

stroke volume The amount of blood pumped from a ventricle (chamber of the heart releasing blood to body circulations) with each beat of the heart.

VO$_2$max Maximal uptake volume of oxygen during exercise; used to measure the intensity and duration of exercise a person can perform.

of their larger lean body mass, the active metabolic body tissue. These highly metabolic tissues of the body thus use more oxygen than other tissues such as fat. When oxygen consumption is expressed only in terms of lean body mass instead of body weight, however, men and women have the same aerobic capacity. Women carry more body fat, a sex difference in body composition that serves critical biologic functions. Apart from stored adipose fat fuel, essential structural and functional body fat in women is about 12% of their body weight; in men it is only 3%. And since women must, of course, carry their entire body weight as part of their total workload, their performance will be affected accordingly.

4. *Genetic influence.* A person's aerobic capacity is mainly genetically determined. But the genetic heritage is influenced, as indicated, by body composition, which is associated with sex, and by aerobic training and age. Before puberty, lean body mass is about equal in boys and girls of comparable body size, but it increases rapidly in boys at puberty under the anabolic effect of testosterone. Maximal aerobic capacity then peaks at 18 to 20 years of age and declines gradually thereafter, largely as a result of age-related losses in lean body mass.[7]

DIET AND EXERCISE: FLUIDS AND NUTRIENTS

ROLE OF WATER AND NUTRIENTS IN EXERCISE

Along with oxygen, an increased intake of water and nutrients is necessary in the course of exercise. Water is essential in any exercise, but especially in prolonged exercise. A deficiency of water is dangerous and limits exercise capacity greatly. As exercise continues, the body temperature increases dramatically because part of the energy produced by the processes of glycolysis is released as heat. To control this increased heat, the body shunts as much water as possible to the skin, where it escapes in perspiration. Over time, and especially in hot weather, this excessive water loss from perspiration leads to dehydration. This is a serious complication limiting the intensity and duration of exercise.

Nutrients also become depleted during continued exercise as the body draws on its stored energy. As demands for cell ATP increase, the body metabolizes blood glucose and muscle glycogen to provide energy via anaerobic glycolysis. With prolonged exercise of greater intensity, however, the levels of these nutrients fall too low to sustain the body's demands. Fatigue follows, muscle failure occurs because of lactic acid buildup, and exercise cannot continue.

ENERGY-YIELDING MACRONUTRIENTS

Our diet supplies the necessary fuel substrate from the three energy-yielding macronutrients for meeting our energy needs. We need carbohydrate and fat as basic fuels but depend little on protein. General needs apply to all individuals, but the young person, especially the growing child, has some special needs.

PROTEIN

Protein as a fuel substrate

Protein is usually discounted as a fuel substrate in energy production during exercise. Although some amino acids can feed into the cell's basic energy cycle, the extent of this input during exercise is minimal. There is evidence that some amino acid breakdown occurs during exercise, and there is some nitrogen loss in sweat. But authorities agree that under normal circumstances protein makes a relatively insignificant contribution to energy during exercise. In endurance events, however, somewhat more protein may be used, especially when carbohydrate resources are exhausted.[7]

Protein in the diet

Most experts recommend 0.8 to 1 g protein/kg body weight to meet general needs of the active person. This amounts to the general RDA standard for adults, which contributes about 10% to 12% of the kcalories in the diet. Most Americans eat about twice this amount of protein, putting a taxing metabolic load on the kidneys and the liver. Unwise athletes who purchase and use excess protein supplements in various forms are subjecting their bodies to an even greater taxing load and dangers of abnormal metabolic stress. Nitrogen consumed in excess of need must be excreted. This requires an increased production of urea, which contributes to dehydration, a serious factor during strenuous exercise. High-protein diets and supplements can also lead to increased excretion of calcium in the urine.

FAT

Fat as fuel substrate

In the presence of oxygen, fatty acids are oxidized to provide energy. The rate at which this can occur is determined in part by the rate of mobilization of fatty acids from storage. But all stored fat is not alike. Actually, the body stores fat in two ways: (1) *depot* fat in adipose tissue, which is destined for transport back and forth to other tissues as needed for energy; and (2) *essential* fat in metabolically active tissue, such as bone marrow, heart, lungs, liver, spleen, kidneys, intestines, muscles, and nervous system, which is reserved in these places for necessary structural and functional use only. Although storage depot fat in men and women is roughly comparable, essential fat reserves make the big difference-they are about four times greater in women.

Free fatty acids, the fat fuel, are stored with glycerol as triglycerides in the body's adipose tissue. The enzyme *lipoprotein lipase* mobilizes these stores of fatty acids. This lipase is stimulated by exercise. Its activity is affected by levels of hormones also involved in exercise, especially growth hormone and epinephrine.

Fat in the diet

It is important to recognize that fat as a fuel substrate is not drawn from the diet directly, but from the body's stored adipose fat. Dietary fat is not necessary to maintain these body fat stores, since excess kcalories in the diet will be stored as fat regardless of their dietary source. We do not need to eat in excess of our dietary needs to burn fat, and there is no danger of depleting our fat stores before exercise has proceeded to exhaustion. Thus there is little basis for increased levels of fat in the diet. On the other hand, some fat in the diet is needed, especially as a source of the essential fatty acid, linoleic acid. In an apparent attempt to imitate the low-fat diet of the now-famous runners, the Tarahumara Indians of the mountains of Mexico, some compulsive runners in other countries have virtually eliminated fat from their diets, inducing a dangerous linoleic acid deficiency. Since the heart muscle prefers fatty acids, especially linoleic acid, as an energy source, there have been reports of deaths from cardiac arrest in some of these cases. Although some dietary fat is necessary, it should not exceed 25% to 30% of the total daily kcaloric intake.

CARBOHYDRATES

Carbohydrates as fuel substrate

Although fat and protein have their special roles to play in maintaining general health, the major nutrient for energy support in exercise is carbohydrate. Carbohydrate fuels come from two sources, the circulating blood glucose and glycogen stored in muscle and liver.

Carbohydrates in the diet

Because carbohydrates are the major energy nutrient, they should contribute about 60% of the daily kcaloric intake. Complex carbohydrates (starches) are preferable to simple carbohydrates (sugars). Starches provide a sustained source of blood glucose as well as glycogen storage. Simple sugars supply important daily energy, especially for athletes who may require as much as 5000 kcal/day, and also contribute to glycogen storage. However, in some persons, simple carbohydrates may contribute to the danger of subsequent hypoglycemia.

In repeated bouts of intense exercise, diets low in carbohydrate have proved to be incapable of restoring tissue glycogen levels.[7,8] A low-carbohydrate diet decreases capacity for work, which intensifies over time. Con-

versely, a high-carbohydrate diet restores glycogen concentrations to their regular levels. Numerous studies have shown poor exercise performance on low-carbohydrate diets. Athletes especially experience fatigue, ketoacidosis, dehydration, and hypoglycemia. However, athletes given carbohydrate feedings before and during exercise maintain glucose concentrations and rates of glucose oxidation necessary to exercise strenuously and thus are able to delay fatigue.[8]

Sometimes athletes use a classic glycogen-loading food plan, as shown in Table 14.1, to build up glycogen reserves for endurance events, but this diet manipulation carries potential side effects such as extra water storage in the muscles. A more modern, less taxing approach, now used more often, consists of a depletion-tapering sequence, such as the general pattern shown in Table 14.2. This modern depletion-tapering plan extends fuel reserves, and avoids the potential side effects such as extra water storage in muscles caused by the formerly used classic glycogen-loading program. In general, during the 3 days before the competition, athletes need to consume about 65% of their energy intake as complex carbohydrates or 550 g/day of carbohydrates, whichever is greater.[8]

REGULATING MICRONUTRIENTS

Vitamins and minerals as fuel substrate

Vitamins and minerals cannot be used as fuel substrates. They are not oxidized or used up in the process of energy production. They are essential in the energy production process but only as catalytic cofactors in enzyme reactions.

Vitamins and minerals in the diet

Increased exercise levels are not correlated with increased dietary needs for vitamins or minerals beyond the RDAs. A well-balanced diet will supply adequate amounts of vitamins and minerals, and exercise may well improve

Table 14.1	Modified depletion-taper precompetition program for glycogen loading	
Day	Exercise	Diet
1	90-minute period at 70%-75% VO$_2$ max	Mixed diet, 50% carbohydrate (350 g)
2-3	Gradual tapering of time and intensity	Diet above continued
4-5	Tapering of exercise time and intensity continues	Mixed diet, 70% carbohydrate (550 g)
6	Complete rest	Diet above continued
7	Day of competition	High-carbohydrate preevent diet

From Wright ED: Carbohydrate nutrition and exercise, *Clin Nutr* 7(1):18, 1988.

the body's efficient use of them. Because athletes, for example, have a dietary need for energy, their larger kcaloric intake from good food sources would automatically increase their general intake of vitamins and minerals. Multivitamin and mineral supplementation does not improve physical performance in healthy athletes eating a well-balanced diet; and the potential side effects from megavitamin supplements are well known (see Chapters 7 and 8). However, *therapeutic* iron supplements may be necessary for some athletes who experience anemia (see *Practical Application* box, p. 298). Also, special assessment of nutrient-energy status is needed for young adolescent amenorrheic athletes such as gymnasts and ballet dancers, who may be experiencing eating disorders such as anorexia nervosa.[9]

EXERCISE AND ENERGY

Physically active persons, especially athletes, need more fuel. The building of glycogen reserves is particularly important for athletes such as long distance runners who compete in endurance events. Exercise raises the body's kcaloric need. Also, exercise has the benefit of helping to regulate appetite to meet these needs. At mild to moderate levels of exercise, persons have actually been shown to eat less than inactive persons do. This may relate to an internal "set point" regulating the amount of body fat the person will carry. According to this theory (see Chapter 6), the set point is raised—that is, more body fat is stored—when the individual becomes inactive. In any case, when exercise levels rise above mild or moderate amounts to strenuous levels, kcaloric needs also rise to supply needed fuel.

Even for the athlete, however, there is no significantly greater need for protein or fat than for a nonactive person. Carbohydrate is the preferred fuel and critical foodstuff for the active person. Carbohydrates, both complex and simple, should be used at an intake that not only meets increased energy needs but also supplies added vitamins and minerals. Thus the recommended dietary composition for support of physical activity is approximately the following ratio:

Protein: 10% to 15% of total kcalories (1 to 1.5 g/kg)

Fat: 30% of total kcalories

Carbohydrate: 55% to 60% of total kcalories (or remainder of kcalories to meet energy needs)

Table 14.2					
Grams of carbohydrates in typical foods					

Food group	Carbohydrates per serving (g)	Food item	Food group	Carbohydrates per serving (g)	Food item
Starchy vegetables, breads, cereals	15	*One serving:* ½ cup dry breakfast cereal ½ cup cooked breakfast cereal ½ cup cooked grits ½ cup cooked rice ½ cup cooked pasta ½ cup baked beans ½ cup corn ½ cup beans 1 small baked potato ½ bagel ½ English muffin 1 slice bread ¾ oz pretzels 6 saltine crackers 2 four-inch diameter pancakes 2 taco shells	Fruits	15	*One serving:* ½ cup fresh fruit ½ cup fruit juice ¼ cup dried fruit 1 small apple 4 apricots ½ banana 12 cherries or grapes ½ grapefruit 1 nectarine 1 orange 1 peach 1¼ cups watermelon
			Milk	12	*One serving:* 1 cup milk 8 oz plain low-fat yogurt
			Sweets*	15	*One serving:* ½ slice plain cake 2 small cookies 3 gingersnaps ½ cup ice cream ¼ cup sherbet
Vegetables (carrots, green beans, broccoli, cauliflower, onions, spinach, tomatoes, vegetable juice)	5	*One serving:* ½ cup cooked vegetables 1 cup raw vegetables ½ cup vegetable juice			

From American Diabetes Association, American Dietetic Association: *Exchange lists for meal planning,* Chicago, 1995, The Association.
*NOTE: Also high in fat.

NUTRITION AND ATHLETIC PERFORMANCE

ATHLETES, COACHES, AND NUTRITIONAL PRACTICES

Misinformation

Athletes and their coaches are particularly susceptible to myths and claims about foods and dietary supplements. They search relentlessly for the competitive edge (see *Issues & Answers* box, p. 309). Knowing this, marketers unremittingly exploit this search, making this group particularly vulnerable. Manufacturers sometimes make distorted and false claims for products. For example, pangamic acid, marketed a few years ago as "vitamin B_{15}" but not a vitamin at all, carried claims about its ability to enhance oxygen transport during exercise. Naturally, if there were such a compound, it would be of interest to athletes and their trainers. However, scientific research has exposed these claims as unfounded.

Myths

In addition to specific fraud, the world of athletics is beset with superstitions and misconceptions. Some of these myths include the following:
- Athletes need protein for energy.
- Extra protein is needed to build bigger and stronger muscles.
- Muscle tissue is broken down during exercise, and protein supplements are needed to replace this breakdown.
- Vitamin supplements are needed to enable athletes to use more energy.
- Vitamins and minerals are burned up in workouts and training sessions.
- Electrolyte solutions are needed during exercise to replace sweat losses.
- A pregame meal of steak and eggs ensures maximal performance.
- Sugar is needed before and during performance to enhance energy levels.
- Drinking water during exercise will cause cramps.

Pregame meal

Traditionally, steak and eggs have been the ritual foods for the precompetition meal. However, if such a meal is eaten less than 6 hours before the athletic event, it will still be in the stomach during the event. Protein and fat delay the emptying of the stomach, and neither contributes to the glycogen stores needed during exercise. On the contrary, the ideal pregame meal is now known to be a light, low-fat, low-protein meal high in complex carbohydrate (starches) and eaten 2 to 4 hours before competition. This allows the body time to digest, absorb, and transform it into stored glycogen. Such a high-car-

bohydrate pregame meal is illustrated in Table 14.1. A high-carbohydrate diet with a minimum of 500 g/day is recommended throughout training. For competition days, a diet containing about 600 g/day is needed. Tables 14.2 and 14.3 may be used to calculate these diets. Small amounts of carbohydrate-containing foods or drinks may be taken up to a brief time before the event without affecting the performance. A total carbohydrate intake of 1 to 5 g/kg body weight taken from 5 minutes to 4 hours before the exercise is sufficient to enhance performance.

Table 14.3 A 600-g carbohydrate diet*	
Menu	**Carbohydrates (g)**
Breakfast	
1 orange	14
2 cups oatmeal	50
1 cup skin milk	12
2 bran muffins	48
Snack	
¾ cup chopped dates	98
Lunch	
Lettuce salad:	
1 cup romaine lettuce	2
1 cup garbanzo beans	45
½ cup alfalfa sprouts	5.5
2 tbsp French dressing	2
3 cups macaroni and cheese	80
1 cup apple juice	28
Snack	
2 slices whole wheat toast	26
1 tsp margarine	—
2 tbsp jam	14
Dinner	
2 oz turkey breast (no skin)	—
2 cups mashed potatoes	74
1 cup peas and onions	23
1 banana	27
1 cup skim milk	12
Snack	
1 cup pasta	33
2 tsp margarine	—
2 tbsp Parmesan cheese	—
1 cup cranberry juice	36
TOTAL	628

*This diet provides 4000 kcal, of which 61% are from carbohydrates (628 g), 14% are from protein (139 g), and 26% are from fat (118 g). A carbohydrate/protein/fat ratio of 60:15:25 is a good goal when planning a diet to aid athletic performance.

Women athletes: sports anemia and amenorrhea

Some women athletes, especially runners and gymnasts who enter their highly competitive and demanding sport in young adolescent and preadolescent years, experience anemia and amenorrhea during times of heavy training and endurance events. Reduced hemoglobin in an athlete's blood means reduced oxygen carrying capacity, with obvious implications for aerobic capacity and ability to sustain an exercise work load. Absence of menses or delayed puberty in young girls means less protective estrogen and higher risk of low bone density and stress fractures. A similar group of women at risk are those in the performing arts, especially highly skilled dancers, who spend arduous hours perfecting and performing strenuous routines. Many of these artists are anemic, at nutritional risk, and some suffer from eating disorders.

The definition of anemia has been set at a hemoglobin (Hb) value of less than 12 g/dl for women (normal is 14 g/dl). (For men, anemia is less than 14 g/dl and normal is 16 g/dl.) We know little, however, about the relative influence on athletic performance of Hb levels *within* the normal range. Some suggest that athletes' Hb levels should be higher for optimal performance, although excessive concentrations of Hb lead to increased blood viscosity and a decreased rate of flow. Maintenance of normal Hb levels at least of women has been proposed.

Although frank anemia is rare among competitive athletes, low normal values are typical. Heavy exercise may include transient anemia during the initial weeks of training, with the Hb level stabilizing in the long run at the low end of normal. Strenuous continued exercise is also associated with low iron stores in athletes, which pose long-term problems.

Possible causes of so-called sports anemia include (1) a diet inadequate in iron, (2) decreased iron absorption, and (3) increased iron losses. Current studies of athletes have revealed that some diets are low in iron. Decreased iron absorption and increased loss are additional causes that add to the problem. Women athletes have cyclic menstrual loss of iron unless they experience amenorrhea. Recent studies have also shown significant amounts of iron lost in profuse sweating. Another possibility is occasional *intravascular hemolysis*, the rupture of red blood cells (RBD) caused by the stresses of heavy exercise. This effect may be transient or chronic. It is manifested as free Hb in the urine but has not been reported often.

Another factor in athletes' low-normal Hb levels may be *hemodilution.* Strenuous training leads to an increase in plasma volume and absolute quantity of Hb, but the increases may not be proportional—plasma volume increases more than the Hb level. Hemodilution with increased iron loss and increased RBC turnover may account for the prevalence of low-normal values among athletes. Obviously this situation is complicated if the diet is inadequate in bioavailable iron, as is sometimes found.

Amenorrhea is defined in studies as absence of menses entirely, or less than two periods in a year. The normal hormonal functioning of estrogen initiates and controls the female reproductive cycle at puberty around the age of 12 years. When athletic training begins at an early age before normal menarche, this normal growth and development pattern is delayed, along with the secondary sex characteristics shaping the female figure, as evidenced in the small, flat bodies of young gymnasts. Older amenorrheic adolescent runners have usually entered training after menarche, then stopped menstruating after beginning their running program. Menstrual abnormalities in athletic women are usually associated with (1) reduced body fat, (2) age of menarche, (3) intensity of the training and competing program, and (4) nutritional inadequacies from weight loss efforts. Most dietary studies indicate an inadequate intake of two key nutrients—iron and calcium.

In either case, delayed or interrupted menses, normal estrogen levels are depressed. Estrogens cause increased osteoblastic activity (bone growth) to help ensure rapid adolescent bone development and mature bone maintenance. Thus the young amenorrheic athlete is faced with a constant juggling act. On one hand, she may lack sufficient estrogen activity to stimulate the usual bone growth pattern. On the other hand, she often lacks adequate dietary calcium and iron as she restricts her diet in a constant struggle with growth, strength, weight, optimal body fat, and intense exercise. As a result, she may be doubly at risk for low bone density and stress fractures, as well as for "sports anemia."

Perhaps the journalist's poignant question after covering young women athletes in Olympic competition may well echo our own: "Old too soon, wise too late?"

References

Baer JT, Tapir LJ: Amenorrheic and eumenorrheic adolescent runners: dietary intake and exercise training status, *J Am Diet Assoc* 92(1):89, 1992.

Dox LW, Dwyer J: Lifestyle and nutrition in musical performing arts, *Nutr Today* 31(5):203, 1996.

Myburgh KH: Low bone density is an etiologic factor for stress fractures in athletes, *Ann Intern Med* 113:754, 1990.

Press A: Old too soon, wise too late? *Newsweek* CXX(6):22, 1992.

Weaver CM, Rajram S: Exercise and iron status, *J Nutr* 122:782, 1992.

HYDRATION: WATER AND ELECTROLYTES

Water

Dehydration can be a serious problem for athletes. Its extent depends on the intensity and duration of the exercise, the surrounding temperature, the level of fitness, and the preexercise or pregame state of hydration. It is most severe in endurance events. For example, marathon runners sometimes collapse from dehydration. They may also have other problems such as cramps, delirium, vomiting, hypothermia, or hyperthermia—all caused by dehydration. With careful planning ahead of the event and providing fluid replacement along the way, many of these problems can be prevented. Mandatory weighing before and after the event is done, and each pound (2.2 kg) of weight lost is replaced by 16 ounces (480 to 500 ml) of fluid.

1. *Cause.* About 60% of the energy from the breakdown of glucose is released as heat. In minimal physical exercise this heat production maintains desirable body temperature. During heavier exercise it exceeds the body's needs and sometimes its heat tolerance. Sweating is our main mechanism for dissipating body heat. The major source of fluid loss in sweat is plasma fluid. Endurance events can cause the loss of several liters of water as sweat, which is pulled from the plasma fluid to control body heat. Unless this amount is replaced, serious consequences can follow.
2. *Prevention.* The thirst mechanism fails to keep pace with the body's increased need for fluid during exercise. The dehydrated person, therefore, must push fluids. To prevent dehydration, athletes are advised to drink more water than they think is needed, without dependence on the normal thirst mechanism. Cold water, about the temperature inside a refrigerator, is absorbed more quickly from the stomach. It is important to speed rehydration and to minimize the discomfort that a full stomach gives the athlete. Small cups of cold water, or mild solutions of saline and glucose during longer ultraevents such as 50-mile runs, 100-mile cycling, or triathlons, should be drunk frequently. Until quite recently it was thought that drinking water immediately before or during an athletic event would cause cramps. There is no basis for this claim.

Electrolytes

A number of special "sports drinks" are now being marketed with the indication that the electrolytes lost in sweat must be replaced (*To Probe Further* box, p. 306). This is true, but how? Sweat is more dilute than our internal fluids, and thus we lose proportionately, not just absolutely, much more water than anything else. Adding electrolytes and sugar to water simply delays its emptying from the stomach. In most instances, water is the rehydration fluid of choice. Electrolytes are replaced with the athlete's next meal. However, during longer and more demanding endurance events, especially in a warm environment, one of the newer mild saline and glucose (6% solution) sports drinks that has a rapid gastric emptying and intestinal absorption time may be used. Several studies now suggest that a carbohydrate-electrolyte beverage may improve moderate- to high-intensity exercise that lasts about 60 minutes.[10]

TRAINING AND PRECOMPETITION ABUSES AMONG ATHLETES

Weight control measures

The sport of wrestling has a long history of widely fluctuating weight patterns among its athletes. Wrestlers often restrict food and fluid intake to certify for a weight classification that is below their off-season weight, seeking to gain advantages in strength, speed, and leverage over a smaller opponent. This practice of "making weight" still seems to be an ingrained tradition that produces large, frequent, and rapid weight loss and regain cycles, with methods such as dehydration, severe food restriction, and loss of food and fluid through induced vomiting and use of laxatives and diuretic drugs. Such disordered eating affects normal growth, and progressive dehydration impairs regulation of body temperature and cardiovascular function. Other sports such as bodybuilding and gymnastics often follow similar routines, especially before competition. Young preadolescent girls in gymnastics, for example, forced to maintain a small body size in the face of advancing age, increasingly reduce food intake and body fat, sometimes developing eating disorders. As a result, a cascade of events may follow—impaired growth, delayed puberty, induced amenorrhea from low estrogen levels, a complicating factor in bone development and later osteoporosis. A similar pattern has been observed among young runners.

Drug abuse

From ancient Greek runners and discus throwers in the first Olympian contests to top competitors from world nations in today's Olympic events, athletes have experimented with various **ergogenic** aids in their eternal search for the competitive edge or the perfect body. Modern athletes—from national league football players to their aspiring high school counterparts—are doing the same thing, trying to find the magic potion in everything from bee pollen and seaweed to freeze-dried liver flakes, gelatin, amino acid supplements, and ginseng. Such efforts have been worthless in most cases, but fortunately not particularly harmful. However, in the case of the group of drugs called anabolic-androgenic steroids, which are now epidemic in the sporting world, great danger and even death lie ahead for the user.[11,12] These illegal drugs must be obtained through a black market network, which adds legal jeopardy and street preparation impurities to the drug's inherent dangers to personal health. These dangers have included reported death from fatal cardiac arrest, acute heart attack, and cancer of the liver and prostate. Abuse of steroids in the United States has now moved from early use among bodybuilders and has invaded almost all areas of athletics, becoming epidemic among football players, significantly among young junior and senior high school boys. In addition, other abuses amplify the dangers of steroids. For example, a large dosage of a diuretic such as furosemide (Lasix, 80 to 120 mg) is taken on the day of drug testing to dilute the urine and decrease the risk of detection. Also, large megadoses of vitamins and minerals become abused drugs and as such are used as ergogenic aids in all areas and levels of sports. Such megadoses of nutrients alter normal metabolic processes and cause severe disturbances.

BUILDING A PERSONAL EXERCISE PROGRAM

HEALTH BENEFITS

In various chapters we discuss physical activity in relation to different health problems. These chapters may be referred to for questions about particular conditions. Here we summarize health benefits of aerobic exercise.

Weight management

Exercise is extremely beneficial in weight management because it helps to regulate appetite, increases the basal metabolic rate, and reduces the fat deposit "set point" level. Together with a well-planned diet, physical exercise corrects the energy balance in favor of increased energy output and decreased energy intake (see Chapter 6). Exercise by itself has a significant effect on reducing fat and increasing lean body content.

Stress management

Exercise is a positive alternative activity to reduce excess stress-related eating. It also provides a physical outlet for working off the hormonal physiologic events produced in the body by stress, thus helping to reduce a major risk factor in the development of chronic disease (see p. 304).

Bone disease

Exercise helps increase bone mineralization, thus reducing the risk of bone weakness and of potential osteoporosis.

Mental health

Exercise stimulates the production of *endorphins*, brain proteins, which are also called the brain's natural opiates, that are associated with a decreased susceptibility to pain.

ASSESSMENT OF PERSONAL HEALTH AND EXERCISE NEEDS

There are many kinds of exercise. Choosing those kinds that are best depends on individual health and personal needs, the aerobic benefits involved, and personal enjoyment.

Health and personal needs

In planning an exercise program, it is important to assess individual health status, personal needs, present level of fitness, and resources required. What do you want to gain from your exercise? How much time can you commit to it? How much, if anything, does it cost? Perhaps it is even more important to ask yourself what you like to do. If the exercise you choose isn't fun, you will soon stop doing it, and it will be of no benefit. Also, it is wise to start slowly and build gradually rather than risk injury and discouragement. Moderation and regularity are key guides in planning.

Beneficial level of exercise

To build aerobic capacity, the level of exercise must raise the pulse rate to within 70% of maximal heart rate. Unless you have had an exercise tolerance or stress test and know precisely what your maximal exercising heart rate is, a rule of thumb is to determine your cardiac rate by subtracting your age from 220 (Table 14.4). This calculation estimates your maximal heart rate, and 70% of this figure tells you the rate to which you want to raise

Table 14.4	Target zone heart rate according to age to achieve aerobic physical effect of exercise		

Age	Maximal attainable heart rate (pulse: 220 minus age)	Target zone	
		70% Maximal rate	85% Maximal rate
20	200	140	170
25	195	136	166
30	190	133	161
35	185	129	157
40	180	126	153
45	175	122	149
50	170	119	144
55	165	115	140
60	160	112	136
65	155	108	132
70	150	105	127
75	145	101	124

Table 14.5	Aerobic exercises for physical fitness (maintained at aerobic level for at least 20 minutes)
Type of exercise	Aerobic forms
Ball playing	Handball
	Racquetball
	Squash
Bicycling	Stationary
	Touring
Dancing	Aerobic routines
	Ballet
	Disco
Jumping rope	Brisk pace
Running or jogging	Brisk pace
Skating	Ice-skating
	Roller-skating
Skiing	Cross-country
Swimming	Steady pace
Walking	Brisk pace

your pulse in the course of exercise. This rate should then be maintained for an uninterrupted period of at least 20 minutes and be practiced at least three times per week to have aerobic benefits. Check your resting pulse before starting the exercise period, then again during and immediately afterward, to monitor your progress in developing your maximal exercising heart rate and aerobic capacity.

TYPES OF PHYSICAL ACTIVITY

General exercise

There are many exercises from which you may choose. Many of them are enjoyable and healthful but do not reach aerobic levels. For example, golf is a passion for many and gets them outdoors, but it is far too slow and sporadic to be aerobic. Also, most sports in the hands of amateurs, rather than those with fast-paced extraordinary skill to provide sustained exercise, are too slow-paced to be aerobic. These include tennis, football, baseball, and basketball. Weight-lifting develops and strengthens muscles but is not an aerobic exercise.

Aerobic exercise

Forms of exercise that can be sustained at a necessary level of intensity to provide aerobic benefits include such activities as swimming, running, jogging, bicycling, and the recently popular aerobic dancing routines and workouts (Table 14.5). Perhaps the simplest and most popular form of stimulating exercise is *walking*. If the pace is fast enough to elevate your pulse and it is maintained for the

required 20 minutes at least, walking can be an excellent form of aerobic exercise. It is convenient and requires no equipment other than good walking shoes. It is appropriate for and available to many persons.

STRESS MANAGEMENT IN PHYSICAL FITNESS

Beyond planning a manageable program of physical activity, the search for physical fitness means that persons in our fast-paced society must learn to deal with physiologic responses to stress triggered through the neuroendocrine system. Successful management of stress is based in part on an awareness of the relationship among stress, disease, and nutrition.

STRESS AS A HEALTH-DISEASE RISK FACTOR

Automatic physiologic responses sweep through the body as adaptions to stress. Throughout human history these physiologic reactions have readied the body to confront or escape danger—the familiar "fight or flight" response. But this response is not well adapted to today's

---

ergogenic   Tendency to increase work output; various substances that increase work or exercise capacity and output.

high-pressured and sedentary modern society and lifestyle. Often we can neither fight nor flee. These simple options are usually not appropriate in our relatively high-pressure but unphysical modern lifestyle. These repeated physiologic reactions have been linked to reduced immune function and the emergence of many of the "diseases of civilization"—coronary heart disease, hypertension, diabetes, and cancer.

STRESS AND NUTRITIONAL CARE PLANNING

The classic work of Canadian physician Hans Selye shows the close relationship of stress to the risk and incidence of disease. Selye called stress "the rate of wear and tear in the human machinery that accompanies any vital activity."[13,14]

Over the years of his monumental work, Selye established the pattern of individual physiologic response to a given stress agent. Different reactions in different persons depend on *conditioning factors*, which can inhibit or enhance one or more stress effects. These factors may be internal, such as genetic predisposition, age, or sex. Or they may be external, such as poor diet or alcohol or other drug abuse. Other investigators have validated Selye's early foundation work with applications in many areas of health and disease. Stress management has thus become a necessary part of nutrition assessment and care planning as well as an essential component of health promotion programs.

HUMAN NEEDS AND LIFE CHANGES

Change and balance are essential to continued life. The dynamic interior metabolism of the human body must interface with a changing exterior environment. Normal physiologic stress is an integral part of this interface. For example, the physiologic stress of pregnancy adapts the maternal body to sustain fetal growth and prepare for birth. Also, the normal stress of skeletal muscles pulling on bones helps maintain calcium balance between bone and blood calcium levels. And the general stress of pain warns of injury or illness.

However, severe, prolonged, uncontrolled stress, whether physical and psychosocial hunger or pain, exhausts resources and can lead to illness or death. Health team members in any situation must seek to provide care based on identified human needs in the basic areas of (1) growth and development, (2) health or disease status, and (3) stress and coping balance. All of these areas include nutritional concerns.

NATURE OF STRESS

Perception of stress

Individual response to stress varies according to how it is perceived. Our perception of each life experience is influenced by three factors: (1) the stimulus of external reality, (2) the message of that stimulus conveyed by the nervous system to the brain's integrative centers, where stimuli are evaluated, and (3) the interpretation we put on each experience. Subjective elements—hunger, thirst, love, fear, self-interest, personal values—influence our responses.

Common life stressors

Three characteristics of stress influence its effect: (1) its strength, whether it is relatively mild or severe, (2) its duration, whether it is fairly transient or long-term, and (3) the strength of personal coping resources. Life stressors are (1) physical or physiologic and (2) psychologic, social, or economic. Emotional tension from multiple causes is the most common agent of human stress. It contributes to serious conditions such as cardiac and gastrointestinal diseases, especially if the body is already stressed by faulty diet or poor housing, as is often the case for high-risk families in the grip of poverty.

PHYSIOLOGIC-METABOLIC RESPONSE TO STRESS

The body automatically responds to defend itself from harm. Selye called this common physiologic response to stress the general adaptive syndrome.[13] An understanding of this automatic cascade of physiologic events is essential for (1) identifying needs and resources, (2) planning nutritional support, both immediate and long-term, and (3) rebuilding metabolic reserves. This immediate reaction of the body to stress involves actions of the combined neuroendocrine systems through three progressive stages of physiologic response (Figure 14.2).

COMBINED ACTIONS OF THE NEUROENDOCRINE SYSTEM

Both parts of the nervous system, the central nervous system and the automatic or sympathetic nervous system, constantly control and modulate reactions of the body to sensory stimuli and stress. Together with a large array of hormones and other chemical messengers, the overall neuroendocrine system provides a vast network of conscious and unconscious reactions to protect the body.[7]

Conscious response: central nervous system

Certain processes in the body are under conscious direction. In response to conscious direction the brain and central nervous system send messages to the muscles, which in turn carry out the specific actions involved, such as studying, eating, taking a walk, reading a book, or calling a friend.

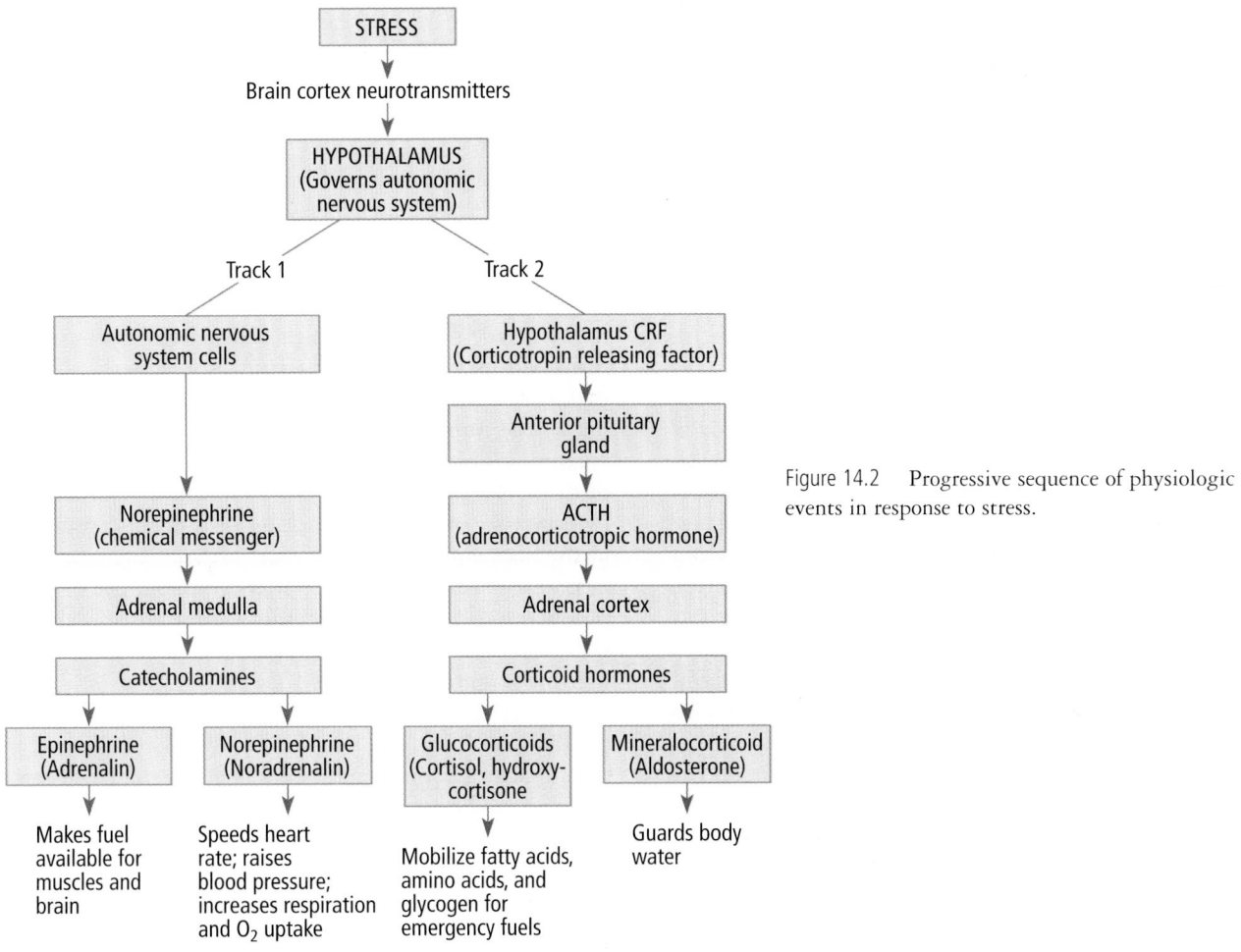

Figure 14.2 Progressive sequence of physiologic events in response to stress.

Unconsious response: autonomic nervous system

Other processes, such as breathing or contraction of the heart muscle, are essential to life and thus are automatically programmed and regulated. This essential control is managed by the autonomic, or sympathetic, nervous system.

Combined neuroendocrine response

In response to stress the autonomic nervous system and its hormones and other chemical messengers mobilize the body's reserves for protection. From his research, Selye identified three stages of the generalized response process: (1) the initial alarm reaction, in which the body's forces are mobilized for action; (2) the adaptation-resistance stage, in which energy reserves are adjusted or rebuilt; and (3) the exhaustion stage, in which resources give out if severe stress continues. In the body's response to daily life stresses these stages overlap, reflecting the intensity of the person's life situation. The automatic physiologic response to stress increases during nervous tension, physical injury, infections, muscular work, or any other strenuous activity.

STAGE I: INITIAL ALARM REACTION

Brain signals

In this first stage, the body's forces are mobilized for action. In response to a perceived threat, the brain instantly triggers the release of chemical messengers, *neurotransmitters*, in the brain cortex. These messengers then relay impulses along neuron tracks in the brain's outer edge to the *hypothalamus*, the "primitive" brain at the head of the brainstem that governs autonomic body functions, such as breathing, heart rate, blood pressure, digestion, hormonal balance, and many other vital activities. This part of the brain, the hypothalamus, has been called the "automatic pilot" or the "brain's brain." On receipt of the stress message, the hypothalamus instantly triggers other chemical messengers and hormones along two separate, yet integrated, tracks to adapt the body's normal physiology to changes needed to combat the danger. In Figure 14.2, you can trace these brain signals and message relays along their two tracks and note the body's important protective physiologic effects. Some liken this chain of events to a train switching freight at different stations. Others compare it to a symphony. No human creation is sufficiently well-orchestrated, complex, and efficient enough to compare with this remarkable system of control as the body readies for crisis.

STAGE II: ADAPTATION-RESISTANCE

Following the initial alarm reaction, if the particular stress does not overwhelm the person's coping resources, a second stage of resistance and adaptation follows. Here energy reserves are adjusted and rebuilt, allowing a certain tolerance to build up.

Hormonal feedback

The body's normal hormonal feedback mechanism now comes into play to shut off continued output of the initiating hormonal agent and thus return blood levels of hormones from various target glands back to their normal levels. For example, during the initial alarm reaction, thyroid hormone and adrenal cortex corticoids—which manage massive immediate metabolic needs—flood the circulation and raise blood levels of these substances. Then, in this second stage of response, these high levels in turn feed back to the controlling master gland-the pituitary—to now shut off or lower its triggering hormones—thyroid stimulating hormone (TSH) to the thyroid and adrenocorticotropic hormone (ACTH) to the adrenal gland-for a period of automatic adjustment back to normal balance.

Rebuilding reserves

As a result of the massive alarm reaction, normal body reserves are rapidly depleted. The blood becomes concentrated with metabolic materials, and there is marked loss of body weight. A period of restoration must eventually follow. This period allows the glands and other body tissue reserves to rebuild, the blood dilution to resume normal levels, and the body weight to return toward normal. This vital rebuilding process obviously requires positive nutrition support.

Adaptive homeostasis

The level of this adaptation to the initial or chronic stress depends on the extent of the stress and the person's coping powers. The stress reaction is generalized throughout the body, always resulting in this general adaptive syndrome identified by Selye. When stress is superimposed on persons made vulnerable by nutritional deficiency, disorder, or disease, the effect is to make a bad situation worse. Often this is the case—for example, in high-risk populations suffering chronic stress of poverty and malnutrition, or the malnutrition seen in some hospitalized patients.

STAGE III: EXHAUSTION

After prolonged exposure to stress, the body's adaptive powers weaken and a final stage of exhaustion follows. Under severe, prolonged stress, particularly when weakened immune capacity and disease compound it, the body's adaptive energy must be restored if the person is to survive.

Immunity

Persons under stress of life events experience depressed immune function and increased vulnerability to disease. This is true of both physiologic disease and psychosocial pressure, which can bring crises both large and small. Renewed research activity in nutritional immunology has resulted.[15] The stress of protein-energy malnutrition brings atrophy to lymphoid tissue, especially the thymus gland. The stress of malnutrition particularly depresses one of the immune functions, that of the activity of the "natural killer cells." These important cells are members of the T cell population of lymphoid cells, the **lymphocytes**, a type of white cell making up a major component of the body's remarkable defense system.[7] Together with a companion B cell population of lymphoid cells, which produce **antibodies** for defense against disease agents, these lymphocytes come from precursor cells in the bone marrow (Figure 14.3).

The T cells make up the majority of the circulating pool of small lymphocytes in blood and lymph and in certain areas of the lymph nodes and spleen. T cells recognize invading foreign substances such as viruses by means of specific special receptors on its surface. On contact with an **antigen**—any foreign intruder or "nonself," an alien substance such as a virus—the T cells immediately multiply and initiate specific cellular immune responses: (1) they activate the **phagocytes**, special cells that have intracellular killing and degrading mechanisms for destroying invaders, and (2) they release chemical mediators that start the inflammatory process. Some T cells can do even more by becoming "killer cells" themselves and attacking antigens directly. These special double-duty cells have been called "helper cell independent cytotoxic T lymphocytes," abbreviated more graphically to the name HIT cells. Also, during emergencies, cells in general produce stress proteins that repair cell damage.

Disease

Researchers studying crisis-related immunity have concluded that heightened and sustained stress can suppress immune function. But whether or not this condition leads to disease depends on individual conditioning factors, such as poor health and nutrition (see *To Probe Further* box, p. 306), exposure to infectious disease, and general physiologic and psychologic resources. Stress-related immunosuppression has its most significant consequences in elderly persons and others who have preexisting deficiencies in the immune system.

Death

The exhaustion stage of response to stress cannot be maintained for long periods because body systems begin

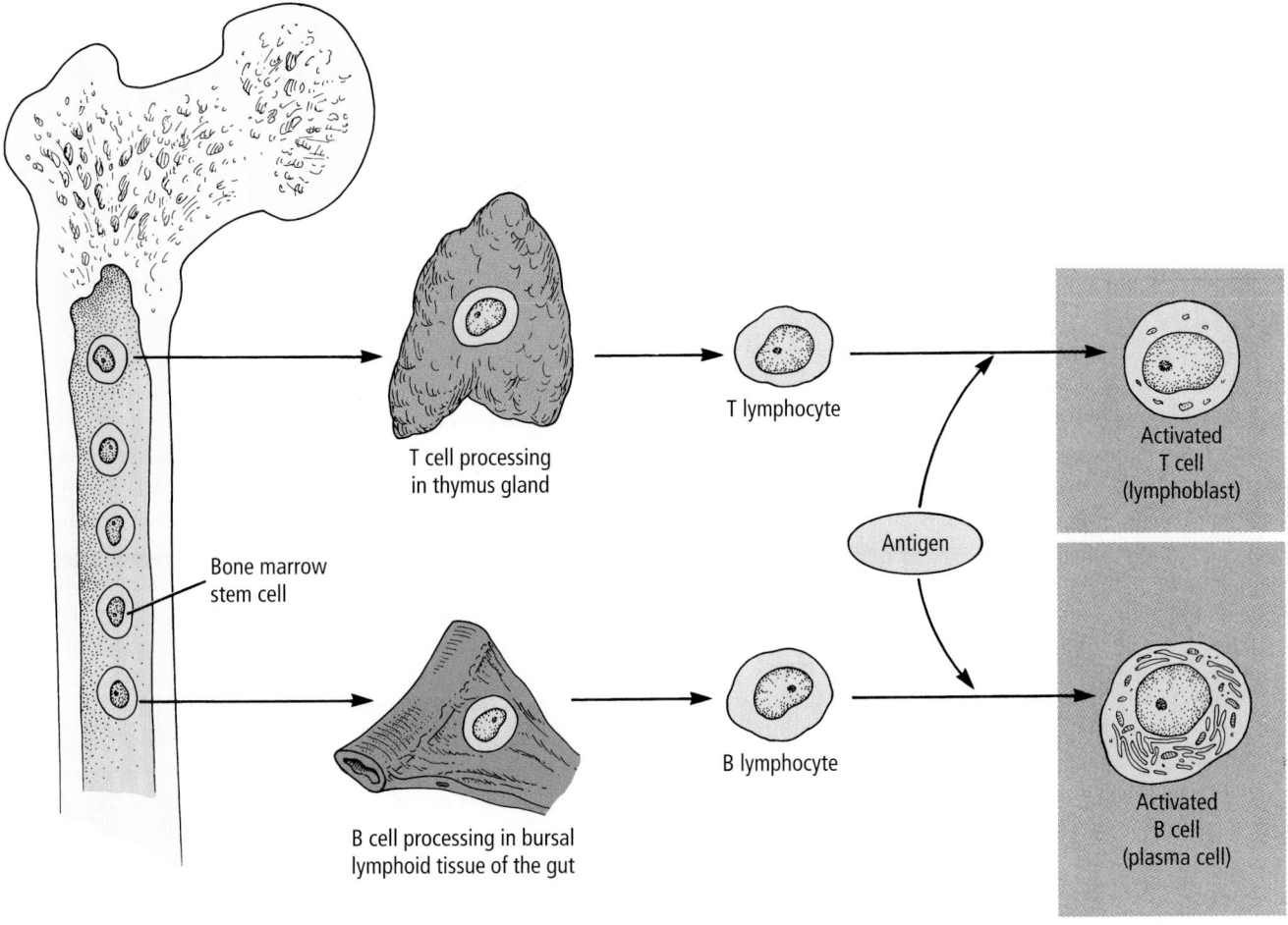

Figure 14.3   Development of the T and B cells, lymphocyte components of the body's immune system.

to wear out in their ability to cope. If resources are not restored and the stress is relentless and prolonged, finally the body's energy sources are depleted and death follows. Intervention must occur earlier to reduce stress, prevent disease, and promote health. A vital part of such intervention is nutrition support.

To sum up

The energy molecule of the body is adenosine triphosphate (ATP), and the powerhouse of the cell is the mitochondrion. The cell's storehouse of energy is creatine phosphate (CP). These two high-energy phosphate compounds are in limited supply. They can produce energy for only a brief initial period and need to be replenished for exercise to continue. This added supply is made available by anaerobic glycolysis, with added energy made available for continued exercise by the body's aerobic system of energy production. The process of glycolysis metabolizes only carbohydrate substrate, furnished either by blood glucose or stored glycogen. Dietary carbohydrate is necessary to replenish these fuel sources. Protein contributes little to

total energy production for exercise, whereas the body's ability to burn fat as fuel depends on the level of fitness. The higher the body's efficiency in using oxygen, the more fatty acids will contribute to the energy supply. Even in the best-trained athletes, fatty acid oxidation must be accompanied by glucose metabolism.

antibody   Any of numerous protein molecules produced by B cells as a primary immune defense for attaching to specific related **antigens;** animal protein made up of a specific sequence of amino acids that is designed to interact with its specific antigen during an allergic response or to prevent infection.

antigen   Any foreign or "non-self" substances—such as toxins, viruses, bacteria, and foreign proteins—that stimulate the production of **antibodies** specifically designed to interact with them.

lymphocytes   Special white cells from lymphoid tissue that participate in humeral and cell-mediated immunity.

phagocytes   Cells that ingest microorganisms, other cells, or foreign particles; macrophages.

To Probe Further

Sort out the sports drinks saga

The first of the so-called sports drinks hit the market about 25 years ago, and now, with all its followers, these beverages have spawned a multimillion dollar industry. Their claims abound, and sorting them out is not always easy for athletes and their coaches who forever seek that prize of the competitive edge.

The current saga of the sports drinks began with a solution called Gatorade, a beverage its developers named for their university's football team. They reasoned that if they analyzed the sweat of their players, they could replace the lost minerals and water in a drink containing some flavoring, coloring, and sugars to make it acceptable, and it would taste better and do a better job than plain water. Although it has been highly profitable for the university and for the manufacturer, most athletes do not need it. Physically fit athletes engaged in regular nonendurance exercise generally do as well on plain water as on a solution such as this product and get their minerals from their regular diets.

However, what long-term endurance athletes do need, especially in hot weather, is water and fuel, that is, carbohydrates. For example, so much water is lost by a runner in a long-distance marathon, when the body sweats 2% to 6% of its weight, that it cannot keep cool enough and the overall system overheats, leading to heatstroke and collapse. Also, without adequate carbohydrate replacement, the muscles soon run out of glycogen stores and slow down. But simply adding sugar to water holds it in the stomach longer where it does the body tissues no good for immediate needs.

To meet the body's dual need during such marathon events, a second category of sports drinks has now developed, using glucose polymers instead of sugar and adding less sodium. These short chains of about 5 glucose molecules—maltodextrins—are produced in the breakdown of starch. These drinks are less concentrated, are only slightly sweetened and flavored, and they leave the stomach rapidly, thus making them ideal as a continuing fuel source for the endurance athlete. Two such products in this category, marketed in powdered mix form, are Ross Laboratory's Exceed and Coca-Cola's Max. But these products cannot be found in supermarkets. They are provided mainly through pharmacies to professionals working with serious athletes.

Other sports drinks to enter the market have been Gatorade clones such as the product Recharge, which claims to add no sugar yet supplies an ample amount of it as fructose and glucose in its fruit juice base. And still another category has emerged in products such as Gear Up, which adds to its base of 10 fruit juices 10 vitamins in amounts yielding 137% of the RDAs in a single 10-ounce bottle but which contains no minerals. All of these extra vitamins do not help an athlete's performance at all, and on a hot day a perspiring athlete could easily down a megadose in four or five bottles. However, recent studies indicate that controlled use in intermittent moderate- to high-intensity exercise improves the athlete's performance.

So sort out the costs and claims of sports drinks. They are not for everyone. For the long run, special ones may meet the needs of the athlete in endurance events. But for nonendurance activities most persons don't need them. After all, water is the best solution for regular needs—and it costs far less.

References

Ball TC et al: Periodic carbohydrate replacement during 50 minutes of high-intensity cycling improves subsequent sprint performance, *Int J Sport Nutr* 5:151, 1995.

Below PR et al: Fluid and carbohydrate ingestion independently improve performance during 1 hour of intense exercise, *Med Sci Sports Exerc* 27:200, 1995.

Jackson DA et al: Effects of carbohydrate feedings on fatigue during intermittent high-intensity exercise in males and females, *Med Sci Sports Exerc* 27:S223, 1995.

Ryan M: Sports drinks: research asks for reevaluation of current recommendations, *J Am Diet Assoc* 97(suppl 2):S197, 1997.

Contrary to popular belief, the protein needs of the diet are not increased by exercise and neither is the body's need for vitamins and minerals. Exercise does increase the body's need for kcalories and water. Cold water taken in small, frequent amounts is the best way to prevent dehydration in endurance events. Electrolytes lost in sweat are replaced by a continuing diet of adequate quality and quantity. Depending on the amount added, electrolytes or sugar in water delays its emptying from the stomach and thus delays rehydration. A mild saline and glucose solution (6%) may supply fluid and fuel to sustain energy during endurance events. Some highly competitive athletes use harmful practices such as food and fluid deprivation for controlling weight and such ergogenic aids as illegal steroid drugs for bulking muscles.

The optimal diet for the athlete is 10% to 15% of the kcalories from protein, 30% or less from fat, and 55% to 60% from carbohydrates. The pregame meal should be small, having little or no protein and relying mainly on complex carbohydrates (starches).

The health benefits of general and aerobic exercise are many and increase with practice up to the point of overdoing. Excellent aerobic exercises include sustained fast walking, swimming, jogging, running, and aerobic dancing or workouts. Approach any exercise sensibly and choose those activities that are enjoyable.

Stress is a major risk factor for health. It triggers a physiologic "fight or flight" mechanism to protect the body, but in a modern stress-filled world this can only compound problems and contribute to illness. At any age, additional stress factors may increase health risks for vulnerable persons. These stress factors include physical trauma and disease, disability, and the multiple problems of poverty and general economic stress. High-stress management involves personal and social approaches based on identified individual and family needs, goals, and expectations. Methods of reducing stress and managing health risks focus on positive health and nutrition promotion, helping to build greater effective coping capacity through sound diet, relaxation, and physical activity, with a strengthened personal support system.

■ QUESTIONS FOR REVIEW

1. What are the component muscle structures, and how do they produce muscle action?

2. What type of substrate fuel does the body use for immediate energy needs? Short-term needs? Long-term needs?

3. How does oxygen relate to physical activity capacity and aerobic effect?

4. Outline the nutrition and physical fitness principles you would discuss with a client who is an athlete. Plan a diet for this client that would meet nutrient and energy needs.

5. Why is fluid balance vital during exercise periods? How is water and electrolyte balance achieved?

6. Describe the dangers of anabolic steroids used by some athletes for bulking muscles and gaining an edge in strength over an opponent.

7. Describe the general adaptive syndrome identified by Selye, which the body activates in response to stress, in terms of the physiologic events in each of its three stages. Why does this response create problems in today's modern society?

■ REFERENCES

1. Lee I-M et al: Exercise intensity and longevity in men, the Harvard Alumni Health Study, *JAMA* 273 (15):1179, 1995.

2. Paffenbarger RS et al: Changes in physical activity and other lifeway patterns influencing longevity, *Med Sci Sports Exerc* 26(7):857, 1994.

3. Wilmore JH: Increasing physical activity: alterations in body mass and composition, *Am J Clin Nutr* 63(suppl): 456S, 1996.

4. Williams PT: High-density lipoprotein cholesterol and other risk factors for coronary heart disease in female runners, *N Engl J Med* 334(6):1298, 1996.

5. Fluckey VA et al: Effects of resistance exercise on glucose intolerant subjects, *J Appl Physiol* 77(3):1087, 1994.

6. Lee I-M, Paffenbarger RS: Physical activity and its relation to cancer risk: a prospective study of college alumni, *Med Sci Sports Exerc* 26(7):831, 1994.

7. Guyton AC, Hall JE: *Textbook of medical physiology*, ed 9, Philadelphia, 1996, WB Saunders.

8. Butterfield GE: Dietary requirements of the athlete. In Shephard R, ed: *Current therapy in sports medicine*, ed 3, St Louis, 1994, Mosby.

9. Dox LW, Dwyer J: Lifestyle and nutrition in musical performing arts, *Nutr Today* 31(5):203, 1996.

10. Ryan M: Sports drinks: research asks for reevaluation of current recommendations, *J Am Diet Assoc* 16(1):S197, 1997.

11. Nnakwe N: Anabolic steroids and cardiovascular risk in athletes, *Nutr Today* 31(5):206, 1996.

12. Yesalis CE, Michael SB: Anabolic-androgenic steroids: current issues, *Sports Med* 19:326, 1995.

13. Selye H: *The stress of life,* New York, 1956, McGraw-Hill.

14. Selye H: Hunger and stress, *Nutr Today* 5(1):2, 1970.

15. Abbas AK et al: *Cellular and molecular immunology*, ed 2, Philadelphia, 1994, WB Saunders.

■ FURTHER READING

Barr SI, Costill DL: Water: can the endurance athlete get too much of a good thing? *J Am Diet Assoc* 89(11):1629, 1989.

Hoffman CJ, Coleman E: An eating plan and update on recommended dietary practices for the endurance athlete, *J Am Diet Assoc* 91(3):325, 1991.

Moses K, Manore MM: Development and testing of a carbohydrate monitoring tool for athletes, *J Am Diet Assoc* 91(8):962, 1991.

These three articles provide important information concerning water intake for the athlete, as well as an excellent eating plan and monitoring tool.

Hickson JF et al: Nutrition and the precontest preparations of a male bodybuilder, *J Am Diet Assoc* 90(2):264, 1990.

Kleiner SM et al: Metabolic profiles, diet, and health practices of championship male and female bodybuilders, *J Am Diet Assoc* 90(7):962, 1990.

These authors take us backstage in the world of body-builders to learn of their myths and practices in relation to diet, weight control, and drug use.

Steen SN: Timely statement of the American Dietetic Association: nutrition guidance for child athletes in organized sports, *J Am Diet Assoc* 96(6):610, 1996.

Steen SN: Timely statement of the American Dietetic Association: nutrition guidance for adolescent athletes in organized sports, *J Am Diet Assoc* 96(6):611, 1996.

These brief professional statements provide excellent guidelines for anyone, for example, coaches and parents, involved with young growing athletes.

Issues Answers

The winning edge—or over the edge?

Athletes, their coaches, and our entire culture have become increasingly aware that the percentage of body fat versus the percentage of lean body mass is a major influence on athletic performance. Each extra pound of body fat an athlete carries into competition is nonproductive weight. It is the muscles, the lean body mass, that provide the strength, agility, and endurance required to win.

Because of this, athletes strive to achieve as low a percentage of body fat as possible while still maintaining good health. In reaching for such a goal, however, many young athletes develop an abhorrence of body fat, resulting in food aversion and the undertaking of excessive weight-loss regimens. These self-generated excesses are commonly reinforced by those surrounding the young athletes: coaches, teammates, and perhaps the most demanding of all, parents.

Such an all-consuming focus results in compulsive behaviors, leading the young person to set unrealistic goals and resulting in abusive weight losses. The fear of failure—failure to make the team, failure in competition, and failure to live up to others' expectations—pushes young athletes in their campaign to beat the opponent, have a low level of body fat, and to win a particular contest by a large, decisive amount.

Fortunately, such excessive voluntary weight losses in young athletes are not usually caused by chronic emotional problems. The reasons typically are more superficial, resulting from an accumulation of immediate, short-term goals and concerns. These athletes usually respond well to counseling and can reverse the excessive behavior with the support of concerned friends and teammates.

Yet for some individuals excessive, compulsive fixation on lean body mass and the loss of body fat becomes obsessive and enduring. For example, a compulsive runner's ideal of 5% body fat is regularly found only in ballet dancers, gymnasts, fashion models, and victims of anorexia nervosa. Our culture reinforces this "positive" attribute of beauty: slimness in women, physical prowess in men. When a susceptible individual enters a time of stress in search for a firm identity, however, he or she may turn toward our cultural stereotypes to provide this self-concept. For women this stress is usually encountered in adolescence, when being physically attractive becomes important in dating. For men the sense of self is more closely tied to their vocational and sexual effectiveness, both of which are related to their physical abilities. Thus the test of a man's abilities tends to occur more often in adulthood, which may result in his preoccupation with physical fitness as a way to deny any decline in strength or ability. This may be why the majority of compulsive runners, those who feel they must run despite everything, including injury or ill health, are men. Often, resulting eating disorders require extensive counseling.

Although our culture views compulsive dieting, as in anorexia nervosa, as a serious emotional disorder, compulsive training is seen as a positive personality trait showing dedication. In reality, both may be symptomatic of unstable self-concepts and attempts to establish a firm sense of identity. They are perceptual disorders: whereas the anorexia victim always sees herself as fat, the compulsive runner always sees himself as out of shape. Such compulsive training becomes the whole life, although it is unnatural to be pushed by whatever means possible, legal or sometimes illegal and dangerous, as is the case of anabolic steroids and cardiovascular risk. No goal, once attained, is sufficiently satisfying. If 5% body fat is achieved, the person strives for 4%. Such striving, often despite physical indications against it, has even resulted in permanent disabilities and death, sometimes from cardiac arrest caused by a linoleic acid deficiency, as seen when a young American Olympic gymnast died recently from an eating disorder. These driven individuals have a strict sense of self-denial and are unable to enjoy any of life's more passive, receptive pleasures.

Although physical fitness and athletic accomplishments may be admirable goals, the thrill of victory for a small percentage of participants may be a hollow one if the victory is at the expense of their health and peace of mind. The ability to slow down, stop, and enjoy smelling the roses may mean more in the long run to the quality and quantity of a person's life span than the color of a coveted ribbon or medal that may be won.

References

Clark N: How to approach eating disorders among athletes, *Top Clin Nutr* 5(3):41, 1990.

Clark N: Counseling the athlete with an eating disorder: a case study, *J Am Diet Assoc* 94(6):656, 1994.

Kantrowitz B et al: Living with training, *Newsweek* CXX(6):24, 1992.

Nnakwe N: Anabolic steroids and cardiovascular risk in athletes, *Nutr Today* 31(5):206, 1996.

Introduction
to Clinical
Nutrition

Part 3

Chapter

15

Nutritional Assessment and Therapy in Patient Care

With this chapter we begin our final study sequence on clinical nutrition. In this concluding section we apply the principles of nutritional science and community nutrition already discussed to nutritional needs in disease.

Here we focus on the essential first step in comprehensive nutritional care—assessing nutritional needs and developing goals as the first step in planning sensitive and valid patient care. Wherever the place of care and whatever the need, the health care team of practitioners, patient, and family work together to support the healing process and promote health.

THE THERAPEUTIC PROCESS

ROLE OF NUTRITION IN CLINICAL CARE

Persons face acute illness or chronic disease and its treatment in a variety of settings: the acute care hospital, the long-term rehabilitation center, the extended care facility, the clinic, the private office, and the home. In all instances nutritional care is fundamental. Frequently it is the primary therapy in itself. About 2500 years have passed since Hippocrates admonished us to pay closer attention to this significant connection between nutrition and disease, but we are only now, in more modern scientific times, beginning to catch a glimmer of the real depth of his valuable instruction.

Comprehensive nutritional assessment provides the necessary basis for appropriate nutritional therapy based on identified needs. Clinical nutritionists, all registered dietitians (RDs), many with advanced degrees in nutritional science, use their expertise and skills to make sound clinical judgments and work effectively with the clinical care team. Together these professionals provide an essential component for successful medical treatment. They assist the patient in recovery from illness or injury, help the person maintain follow-up care to promote health, and also help to control health care costs.[1]

 STRESS OF THE THERAPEUTIC ENCOUNTER

In the modern hospital setting, the patient experiences a great deal of stress because he or she is sick, upset, or scared. The therapeutic encounter between health care providers and their patients occurs under stressful conditions at best.[2] Several factors can contribute to added nutritional toll.

Bed rest

Even though the reason for the hospitalization may indicate the need for bed rest, at the same time the bed rest itself can bring detrimental effects on the body's physiology.[3] For example, after just three days of lying supine in bed, the body begins to lose its resistance to the pull of gravity and continuing inactivity diminishes muscle tone, bone calcium, plasma volume, and gastric secretions, bringing some impairment of glucose tolerance and shifts in body fluids and electrolytes.

Hospital malnutrition

Hospital, or **iatrogenic**, malnutrition has been widely documented. First, hospitalized patients with hypermetabolic and physiologic stress of illness or injury are at particular risk for malnutrition from their increased needs for nutritional support. In addition, a fundamental problem is lack of adequate admission nutrition screening or follow-up monitoring to identify patients at malnutrition risk and to provide essential medical nutrition

therapy immediately, as indicated by malnutrition codes listed in the *International Classification of Diseases, Ninth Revision, Clinical Modification* (ICD-9-CM).[4,5] Other problems of hospital routine also contributing to lack of adequate nourishment include (1) highly restricted diets remaining on order and unsupplemented too long; (2) unserved meals because of interference of medical procedures and clinical tests, and (3) unmonitored patient appetite.

Hospital setting and system

Each injured or ill patient is a unique person and requires special treatment and care. At the same time, a formidable array of staff persons seek to determine needs and implement what each perceives to be appropriate care. It is no surprise that the course does not always run smoothly or that patients often feel intimidated and powerless. Sometimes our complex system and highly specialized technology get in the way and we lose sight of our reason for being-to meet individual human needs with personal care.[6,7]

Constant open and validating communication is essential, both among the health team members and between the health care provider and the patient and family. It is at such times we need to remind ourselves of the time tested fundamental ethical principles guiding all our patient care.[8-10] These principles should ensure that all we do must:
- *Benefit* the patient
- Do no *harm*
- Preserve the patient's *autonomy*
- *Disclose* full and truthful information for patient decisions concerning personal care
- Provide *social justice*

Such ethical behavior is based on the overriding fundamental principles of right action found within Anglo-American law, which emphasizes the basic rights of privacy and free choice.[9] Continuing open communication provides the basis for such ethical practices among the health team members and between the health care providers and the patient and family. It is especially important for many stressed elderly patients who fail to thrive. In this team effort for quality nutritional care, the clinical dietitian (RD; a clinical nutrition specialist with advanced degree and clinical training), with the physician, carries the primary responsibility.[11,12] The nurse and other primary care practitioners provide essential support.

FOCUS OF CARE: THE PATIENT

Patient-centered care

The primary principle of nutritional practice, too often overlooked in the many routine procedures of the hospital setting, is evident: to be valid, nutritional care must be person centered. In this renewed partnership **paradigm** for patient-centered health care, the patient must always be a senior partner. It must be based on initial identified needs, updated constantly with the patient, with continuing results monitored in relation to therapy goals. This is necessary, of course, to provide essential physical care. But it is also necessary to support the patient's personal needs for maintaining self-esteem and control as much as possible. In addition, a second fundamental fact needs emphasis: despite all methods, tools, and technologies described here or elsewhere, the most therapeutic instrument of such person-centered care is yourself. It is to this seemingly simple yet profoundly personal healing encounter that you bring yourself and your skills.

Health care team

In the setting of the individual medical center, with its strengths and its shortcomings and within the essential team care provided in a managed care system, the clinical dietitian must care for the patient's fundamental nutritional needs in close relationship to the medical care and nursing support.[13,14] Sensitive communication skills are essential for all ages and degrees of health problems. Determining the patient's initial nutritional status and ongoing medical nutrition therapy needs is a primary responsibility to support healing and avoid malnutrition.[15-17]

PHASES OF THE CARE PROCESS

Five distinct yet constantly interacting phases are essential in the therapeutic care process.
1. *Assessment: database.* A broad base of relative information about the patient's nutritional status, food habits, and life situation is necessary for making accurate initial assessments. Useful background information may come from a variety of sources, such as the patient, the patient's chart, family or other relatives and friends, oral and written communication with other hospital personnel or staff, and related research. A number of valuable assessment tools have been developed, some of which are described here.
2. *Analysis: problem list.* A careful analysis of all data collected determines specific patient needs. Some needs will be immediately evident. Others will develop as the situation unfolds. On the basis of this analysis, a list of problems may be formed to guide continuing care activities.
3. *Planning care: needs and goals.* Valid care is based on identified problems. The plan must always be based on personal needs and goals of the individual patient, as well as the identified medical care requirements or options discussed with the patient and family.
4. *Implementing care: actions.* The patient care plan is put into action according to realistic and appropriate activities within each situation. For example, nutritional care and education will involve decisions and actions concerning an appropriate food plan and mode of feeding, as well as the training and education needs of the patient, staff, and family who will carry it out.
5. *Evaluating and recording care: actions.* As every care activity is carried out, results are carefully evaluated to see if the identified needs have been met. Appropriate revisions of the care plan can be made as needed for continuing care. These results are carefully recorded in the patient's medical record. Clear documentation of all activities is essential.

In our discussion here, we look at each of these phases in terms of quality nutritional care. We focus on methods and tools of nutrition assessment, practical management of nutritional therapy and care, maintenance of effective medical records, and ways of ensuring quality standards of nutritional care.

NUTRITIONAL ASSESSMENT AND ANALYSIS

THE PURPOSE AND PROCESS OF COLLECTING NUTRITIONAL DATA

The fundamental purpose of nutritional assessment in general clinical practice is to determine (1) the overall nutritional status of the patient; (2) current health care needs, both physical and psychosocial as well as personal; and (3) related factors influencing these needs in the person's current life situation. The first step in nutritional assessment, as with assessing any situation to determine needs and actions, is to collect pertinent information—a database—for use in identifying needs. The clinical dietitian, assisted by other health team members as needed, uses several basic types of activities for nutritional assessment of patients' needs.
1. Diet evaluation and personal histories
2. Clinical observations
3. Biochemical tests
4. Anthropometrics

Each part of this approach is important because no single parameter alone directly measures individual nutritional status or determines problems or needs. Fur-

---

iatrogenic   Describes a medical disorder caused by physician diagnosis, manner, or treatment.

paradigm   A pattern or model serving as an example; a standard or ideal for practice or behavior based on a fundamental value or theme.

ther, the overall resulting picture must be interpreted within the context of personal social and health factors that may alter nutritional requirements. Only with this type of comprehensive evaluation can nutrition assessment become the real index to the quality of life that it should be. Since such a comprehensive history is a fundamental tool for planning health care, history-taking is a primary skill for all health professionals. A broad number of tests may be used for research purposes in a large facility with access to highly sophisticated equipment. However, the procedures outlined here provide a good base in general practice.

DIET EVALUATION AND PERSONAL HISTORIES

A careful nutrition history, including nutritional information related to living situation and other personal, psychosocial, and economic problems, is a fundamental part of nutrition assessment. But obtaining accurate information about basic food patterns and actual dietary intake is not a simple matter. However, a sensitive practitioner may obtain useful information by using one or more of the basic tools described here.

Specific 24-hour food record

For hospitalized patients, a record of food intake over a specific 24-hour period may be needed for tests such as a nitrogen balance study or for monitoring energy and nutrient intake. A careful explanation of purpose and procedure for the patient and staff is needed. However, such a brief recall or record in general practice has limited value in determining overall basic food habits.

Diet history

General knowledge of the patient's basic eating habits is needed to determine any possible nutritional deficiencies. In conjunction with the patient's usual living situation and related food attitudes and behaviors, social and family history, and medical history with current status and treatment, the nutrition interview provides an essential base for further personal nutrition counseling and planning of care (Figure 15.1). For example, an activity-associated day's food intake pattern, using guides discussed in Chapter 10 (Figure 10.1), can provide a useful tool for obtaining a fairly valid picture of food habits and eating behaviors. In addition to food and nutrition information, drug therapy data from the medical record or the patient and family is important to determine any possible drug-nutrient interaction involved or any teaching needed by the patient (see Chapter 17). Research carefully all prescriptions and over-the-counter drugs the patient is using.

Periodic food records

At various times, a 3- to 7-day food record is a helpful tool for assessing food patterns, especially when used to follow up a comprehensive initial diet history or counseling instructions for a special therapeutic diet required. A 3-day record is generally sufficient for determining overall food, energy, and nutrient intake. A number of appropriate software programs are available that make final computer analysis a simple matter (see *Issues & Answers*, p. 327). But, of course, the accuracy of the computer analysis depends entirely on the accuracy of the food record. Sometimes a food frequency questionnaire is helpful to determine food use over an extended period of time, and it provides useful data, especially in combination with specific food records.[18]

CLINICAL OBSERVATIONS

Keen observation is made of possible malnutrition signs as well as those evident through vital signs and physical examination.

Clinical signs of malnutrition

Careful attention to physical signs of possible malnutrition provides an added dimension to the overall assessment of general nutritional status (see *To Probe Further* box, p. 324). A guide for a general examination of such signs is given in Table 15.1. A careful description of any such observations is documented in the patient's medical record.

Figure 15.1 Interviewing patient to plan personal care. (Tom Tracy, Medichrome.)

Table

15.1 Clinical signs of nutritional status

Body area	Signs of good nutrition	Signs of poor nutrition
General appearance	Alert, responsive	Listless, apathetic, cachectic
Weight	Normal for height, age, body build	Overweight or underweight (special concern for underweight)
Posture	Erect, arms and legs straight	Sagging shoulders, sunken chest, humped back
Muscles	Well-developed, firm, good tone, some fat under skin	Flaccid, poor tone, undeveloped, tender, "wasted" appearance, cannot walk properly
Nervous control	Good attention span, not irritable or restless, normal reflexes, psychologic stability	Inattentive, irritable, confused, burning and tingling of hands and feet (paresthesia), loss of position and vibratory sense, weakness and tenderness of muscles (may result in inability to walk), decrease or loss of ankle and knee reflexes
Gastrointestinal function	Good appetite and digestion, normal regular elimination, no palpable (perceptible to touch) organs or masses	Anorexia, indigestion, constipation or diarrhea, liver or spleen enlargement
Cardiovascular function	Normal heart rate and rhythm, no murmurs, normal blood pressure for age	Rapid heart rate (above 100 beats/min tachycardia), enlarged heart, abnormal rhythm, elevated blood pressure
General vitality	Endurance, energetic, sleeps well, vigorous	Easily fatigued, no energy, falls asleep easily, looks tired, apathetic
Hair	Shiny, lustrous, firm, not easily plucked, healthy scalp	Stringy, dull, brittle, dry, thin and sparse, depigmented, easily plucked
Skin (general)	Smooth, slightly moist, good color	Rough, dry, scaly, pale, pigmented, irritated, bruises, petechiae
Face and neck	Skin color uniform, smooth, healthy appearance, not swollen	Greasy, discolored, scaly, swollen, skin dark over cheeks and under eyes, lumpiness or flakiness of skin around nose and mouth
Lips	Smooth, good color, moist, not chapped or swollen	Dry, scaly, swollen, redness and swelling (cheilosis), or angular lesions at corners of the mouth or fissures or scars (stomatitis)
Mouth, oral membranes	Reddish pink mucous membranes in oral cavity	Swollen, boggy oral mucous membranes
Gums	Good pink color, healthy, red, no swelling or bleeding	Spongy, bleed easily, marginal redness, inflamed, gums receding
Tongue	Good pink color or deep reddish in appearance, not swollen or smooth, surface papillae present, no lesions	Swelling, scarlet and raw, magenta color, beefy (glossitis), hyperemic and hypertrophic papillae, atrophic papillae
Teeth	No cavities, no pain, bright, straight, no crowding, well-shaped jaw, clean, no discoloration	Unfilled caries, absent teeth, worn surfaces, mottled (fluorosis), malpositioned
Eyes	Bright, clear, shiny, no sores at corner of eyelids, membranes moist and healthy pink color, no prominent blood vessels or mound of tissue or sclera, no fatigue circles beneath	Eye membranes pale (pale conjunctivae), redness of membrane (conjunctivae), redness of membrane (conjunctival infection), dryness, signs of infection, Bitot's spots, redness and fissuring of eyelid corners (angular palpebritis), dryness of eye membrane (conjunctival xerosis), dull appearance of cornea (corneal xerosis), soft cornea (keratomalacia)
Neck (glands)	No enlargement	Thyroid enlarged
Nails	Firm, pink	Spoon-shaped (koilonychia), brittle, ridged
Legs, feet	No tenderness, weakness, or swelling; good color	Edema, tender calf, tingling, weakness
Skeleton	No malformations	Bowlegs, knock-knees, chest deformity at diaphragm, beaded ribs, prominent scapulas

Modified from Williams SR: Nutrition assessment and guidance in prenatal care. In Worthington-Roberts BS, Williams SR: *Nutrition in pregnancy and lactation*, ed 5, St Louis, 1993, Mosby.

Vital signs and physical examination

Other physical data may include pulse rate, respiration, temperature, and blood pressure. A study of the common procedures of a normal physical examination will provide useful background orientation.

BIOCHEMICAL TESTS

A number of laboratory tests are available for studying nutritional status. The most commonly used ones for assessing and monitoring nutritional status and planning nutritional care in clinical practice are listed here. General ranges for normal values are given in standard texts.

Measures of plasma protein

Basic measures include serum albumin, hemoglobin, and hematocrit. Additional ones may include prealbumin (PAB), a thyroxin-binding protein, serum transferrin, or total iron-binding capacity (TIBC) and ferritin.

Measures of protein metabolism

Basic 24-hour urine tests are used to measure urinary creatinine and urea nitrogen levels. These materials are products of protein metabolism. The patient's 24-hour excretion of creatinine is interpreted in terms of ideal creatinine excretion for height—the creatinine-height index (CHI) (Table 15.2). Comparison is made with standard values for this index. The patient's 24-hour urea nitrogen excretion is used with the calculated dietary nitrogen intake over the same 24-hour period to calculate nitrogen balance:

N balance =
$$(\text{protein intake} \div 6.25) - (\text{urinary urea N} + 4)$$

The formula factor of 4 represents additional nitrogen loss through the feces and skin. Urinary urea nitrogen excretion reflects metabolism of dietary nitrogen, as the nitrogen balance formula indicates, and is a measure of the adequacy of protein nutrition.

Measures of immune system integrity: anergy

Basic measures are made of the lymphocyte count. Additional measures may be made by skin testing, observing delayed sensitivity to common recall antigens such as mumps or purified protein derivative of tuberculin (PPD). Skin tests are read at 24 and 48 hours, with greater than 5 mm considered positive and the presence of one positive test indicating intact immunity.

ANTHROPOMETRICS

Skill gained through careful practice is necessary to minimize the margin of error in making body measurements. Selection and maintenance of proper procedures and equipment, as well as attention to careful technique, are essential in securing accurate data.

Table 15.2	Ideal weight and urinary creatinine values for height (adults)*			
	Females		**Males**	
Height (cm)	Weight (kg)	Creatinine (mg)	Weight (kg)	Creatinine (mg)
140	44.9			
141	45.4			
142	45.9			
143	46.4			
144	47.0			
145	47.5		51.9	
146	48.0		52.4	
147	48.6	828	52.9	
148	49.2		53.5	
149	49.8		54.0	
150	50.4	852	54.5	
151	51.0		55.0	
152	51.5		55.6	
153	52.0	878	56.1	
154	52.5		56.6	
155	53.1	901	57.2	
156	53.7		57.9	
157	54.3	922	58.6	1284
158	54.9		59.3	
159	55.5		59.9	
160	56.2	949	60.5	1325
161	56.9		61.1	
162	57.6		61.7	
163	58.3	979	62.3	1362
164	58.9		62.9	
165	59.5	1005	63.5	1387
166	60.1		64.0	
167	60.7	1040	64.6	1421
168	61.4		65.2	
169	62.1		65.9	
170		1075	66.6	1465
171			67.3	
172			68.0	
173		1111	68.7	1516
174			69.4	
175		1139	70.1	1552
176			70.8	
177		1169	71.6	1589
178			72.4	
179			73.3	
180		1204	74.2	1639
181			75.0	
182			75.8	
183		1241	76.5	1692
184			77.3	
185			78.1	1735
186			78.9	
187				1776
188				
189				
190				1826

*1959 Metropolitan Life Insurance Company Standards corrected for nude weight without shoe heels.
Data from Jeffe DB: *The assessment of the nutritional status of the community,* Geneva, 1966, World Health Organization.

Weight

Hospitalized patients should be weighed at consistent times, for example, before breakfast after the bladder has been emptied. Clinic patients should be weighed without shoes in light, indoor clothing or an examining gown. For accuracy, use regular clinic beam scales with nondetachable weights. An additional weight attachment is available for use with very obese persons. Metric scales with readings to the nearest 20 g provide specific data; however, the standard clinic scale is satisfactory. Check all scales frequently and have them calibrated every 3 or 4 months for continued accuracy.

After careful reading and recording of the patient's weight, ask about the usual body weight and compare it with standard height-weight tables (see Chapter 6 and inside back covers), remembering that these tables are general guidelines and that underweight persons are at a greater health risk than are moderately overweight persons.[18-20] Interpret present weight in terms of percentage of usual and standard body weight for height. Check for any recent weight loss: 1% to 2% in the past week, 5% over the past month, 7.5% during the previous 3 months, or 10% in the past 6 months is significant. More than this rate can be severe. A check of unexplained weight loss in elderly persons is particularly important, since it may be a clue to depression or a wasting disease such as cancer, and needs to be on record and followed up. Values charted in the patient's record should indicate percentage of weight change.

Height

If possible, use a fixed measuring stick or tape on a true vertical flat surface. If such is not available, the moveable measuring rod on the platform clinic scales may be used with reasonable accuracy. Have the patient stand as straight as possible, without shoes or cap, heels together, and looking straight ahead. The heels, buttocks, shoulders, and head should be touching the wall or vertical surface of the measuring rod. Read the measure carefully and compare it with previous recordings. Note the growth of children or the diminishing height of adults. Metric measures of height in centimeters provide accurate data.

Body mass index (BMI)

The weight and height measures are used to calculate the patient's body mass index: weight (kilograms) divided by height (meters)^2. This ratio is commonly used in evaluating obesity states in relation to risk factors. Details of this calculation, conversion factors, and reference values are described in Chapter 6.

Body frame

Two added measures have recently been developed to answer questions about the arbitrary categories of body frame size for height and weight used in the current tables of the Metropolitan Life Insurance Company.

1. *Elbow breadth.* Standards of weight and body composition by frame size and height have been developed with frame size based on measurement of elbow breadth.[21] With the patient's arm extended and forearm bent upward to form a 90° angle, elbow breadth is measured with a specially developed instrument such as the Frameter, which measures the distance in centimeters between the two outer bony landmarks (medial and lateral epicondyles of the humerus).
2. *Wrist circumference.* This is a measure of height divided by wrist circumference (in centimeters).[22] With the patient's right hand extended and using a nonstretchable metric tape, measure the wrist circumference at the joint just distal (toward the fingers) to the bony wristbone protrusion (the styloid process). Interpret results by the following standard:

Frame size	Male ratio values	Female ratio values
Small	10.4	11
Medium	9.6 - 10.4	10.1 - 11
Large	9.6	10.1

Body measures

In general clinical practice, the clinician uses two basic body measurements—the mid-upper-arm circumference and the triceps skinfold thickness—and from these calculates a third measure, the mid-upper-arm muscle circumference. First, using a nonstretchable centimeter tape, locate the midpoint of the upper arm on the nondominant arm, unless it is affected by edema. The midarm circumference (MAC) is measured at this midpoint and read accurately to the nearest tenth of a centimeter and recorded. The resulting measure is compared with previous measurements to note possible changes. Second, using a standard millimeter skinfold caliper, take a measure of the triceps skinfold thickness (TSF) at this same midpoint of the upper arm. This measure provides an estimate of the subcutaneous fat reserves. Then, together with the midpoint circumference value at this same point, the midarm muscle circumference (MAMC) is calculated by the following formula:

$$\text{MAMC (cm)} = \text{MAC (cm)} - [3.14 \times \text{TSF (cm)}]$$

If desired, the TSF may be left in millimeters, as measured with the calipers, and the value of the factor (pi; π) in the formula changed to 0.314.

This final derived value gives an indirect measure of the body's skeletal muscle mass, a good indicator of body composition. Finally, to interpret the patient's measurements for monitoring nutritional status, these values are compared as percentages of standards in reference tables (Appendix J, *Assessment of Nutritional Status: Percentiles*).

Alternative measures for nonambulatory patients

Several alternative measures can provide values for estimating height and weight of persons confined to bed:

1. *Total arm length.* With the patient holding the arm straight down by the side of the body, and using a nonstretchable metric tape, measure the arm length from attachment at the shoulder to the end of the arm at the wrist. Reference standards indicate relation of this measure to height equivalents.[23] This is also a useful alternative to standing body height when body conditions distort usual standing height of ambulatory patients. For example, this measure is helpful with older persons, in whom a general thinning of weight-bearing cartilages, the bent-knee gait, and a possible **kyphosis** of the spine may make standing height measurement inaccurate.

2. *Arm span.* The full arm span measure is an alternate to height in adults, especially practical for elderly persons. Tests indicate that it may give a more accurate result than height in calculating BMI in elderly patients.[24] Using a flexible metric tape, measure the full arm span from fingertip to fingertip in centimeters, passing the tape in front of the clavicles. A recumbent half span measure from finger tip to body midline at the sternal notch may be used with patients having limited movement in one arm, then doubled to achieve the same result.

3. *Knee height.* With the patient lying in the supine position and the left knee and ankle each bent at a 90-degree angle, the knee height is measured with a special caliper.[25] A simple comparative measure of knee to floor height in the sitting position, from the outside bony point just under the kneecap, indicating the head of the tibia, down to the floor surface, may also be used.[26] The knee height (KH) measurement is then used to calculate the value for deriving body height equivalent:

$$\text{Height (women)} = [(1.83 \times KH) - (0.24 \times age)] + 84.88$$
$$\text{Height (men)} = [(2.02 \times KH) - (0.04 \times age)] + 64.19$$

4. *Calf circumference.* With the patient in the same supine position and the left knee bent at a 90-degree angle, and using nonstretchable metric tape, measure the calf circumference (CC) at the largest point. This measurement is then used with three other values—knee height (KH), midarm circumference (MAC), and subscapular skinfold (SSF)—to derive body weight value:[25,27]

$$\text{Weight (women)} = (1.27 \times CC) + (0.87 \times KH) + (0.98 \times MAC) + (0.4 \times SSF) - 62.35$$
$$\text{Weight (men)} = (0.98 \times CC) + (1.16 \times KH) + (1.73 \times MAC) + (0.37 \times SSF) - 81.69$$

Valid patient care planning requires analysis of all nutritional data collected. On this basis problems requiring solutions can be identified. A detailed analysis of the nutrition information helps determine nutritional diagnosis, any primary or secondary nutritional disease, and any underlying nutrition-related conditions.

Nutritional diagnosis

All the various nutritional data for each patient, collected by the clinical nutritionist and other team members through the broad assessment activities described, must be carefully analyzed to reach a valid nutritional diagnosis and plan of care. Every health team member participates in this analysis through various communications, discussions, case conferences, records, and reports (Figure 15.2). The nutritional diagnosis requires information about all aspects related to the patient's needs: nutrient deficiencies, underlying disease requiring a modified nutrient or food plan, any personal cultural and ethnic needs, or economic needs, as well as the mode of feeding and dietary mangement.

Primary and secondary nutritional disease

The clinical dietitian nutritionist coordinates these nutrition activities and carries a major responsibility on the health care team for interpreting nutrition-related data and making decisions and recommendations concerning any primary or secondary nutritional states. Primary deficiency disease results from a lack of essential nutrient in the diet, for whatever reason. Secondary deficiency disease results from one or more barriers to the use of the nutrients after they are consumed in food. This inability to use a given nutrient may stem from digestive or malabsorption problems or from lack of specific cell enzymes. Such problems may be caused by conditions such as lactose intolerance, celiac disease, inflammatory bowel disease, cell metabolism defects in genetic disease, chemotherapy, or radiation treatments.

Nutrition-related conditions

Related chronic disease problems with nutrition involvement will also be considered. These include such conditions as heart disease, hypertension, cancer, diabetes, liver and renal disease. Surgery also imposes nutrition demands and modifications. Any quantifiable data collected can be analyzed by computer. Two major nutritional tasks in which the computer excels are (1) baseline screening to identify persons at risk of malnutrition because of their disease, injury, or lifestyle; and (2) analysis of intake to monitor effectiveness of ongoing treatment. Laboratory data may be handled in a similar manner, with general patterns of change monitored over time. Careful appraisal of medical and personal data from histories, records, reports, and interviews will help focus on various needs and problems and provide a realistic picture of nutritional and eating difficulties.

Figure 15.2 The health team conference for planning patient care. Physician, nurse, clinical nutritionist, and social worker review patient's progress and needs. (R. Brady, Medichrome.)

Problem list

On the basis of this careful analysis, a problem list is usually developed. Around such a list, realistic and relevant personal care may be planned. Every aspect of the patient's needs is considered. In ongoing conferences with the health care team, the patient, family, and any other significant persons, personal goals are determined for care. These goals help establish priorities for immediate as well as long-term care.

NUTRITION INTERVENTION: FOOD PLAN AND MANAGEMENT

BASIC CONCEPTS OF DIET THERAPY

Normal nutrition base

A therapeutic diet is always based on the normal nutritional requirements and personal needs for each particular patient. It is modified only as the specific disease in the specific individual necessitates. In planning and counseling for nutritional care this is an important initial fact to grasp and impart to patients and clients. For example, it is a great source of encouragement to the parents of a newly diagnosed diabetic child to know that the food plan will be based on individual growth and development needs and will make use of regular foods.

Disease application

The principles of a special therapeutic diet will be based on modifications of the nutritional components of the normal diet as a particular disease condition may require. These changes may include the following types of modifications: (1) *nutrients*: modification of one or more of the basic nutrients—protein, carbohydrate, fat, minerals, and vitamins; (2) *energy*: modification in energy value as expressed in kcalories; (3) *texture*: modification in texture or seasoning, such as liquid or low residue.

Individual adaptation

A therapeutic diet may be theoretically correct and have well-balanced food plans, but if these plans are unacceptable to the patient, they will not be followed. A workable plan for a specific person must be based on individual food habits within the specific personal life situation. This can be achieved only through careful planning with the patient, or with the parents of a child requiring a special diet, based on an initial interview to obtain a diet history, knowledge of personal food habits, living conditions, and related factors. In this way, diet

---

kyphosis Increased, abnormal convexity of the upper part of the spine; hunchback.

principles can be understood and motivation secured to follow through. Whatever the problems, nutritional care is valid only to the extent that it involves this kind of knowledge, skills, and insights. Individual adaptations of the diet to meet individual needs are imperative for successful therapy.

ROUTINE HOUSE DIETS

A schedule of routine "house" diets, based on some type of cycle menu plan, is usually followed in hospitals for those patients not requiring a special diet modification. According to general patient need and tolerance, the diet order may be liquid (clear liquid or full liquid, with milk used on the full liquid diet), soft (no raw foods, generally somewhat bland in seasoning), and regular (a full, normal-for-age diet). Occasionally an interval step between soft and regular may be used (a light diet). Sample menus from hospital staff dietitians may be compared with note differences.

MANAGING THE MODE OF FEEDING

Depending on the patient's condition, the clinical dietitian may manage the diet by using any one of four feeding modes.

Enteral: oral diet

As long as possible, of course, regular oral feeding is preferred. Supplements are added if needed. According to the patient's condition, there may also be need for assistance in eating.

Enteral: tube feeding

If a patient is unable to eat but the gastrointestinal tract can be used, tube feeding may provide needed nutritional support. A number of commercial formulas are available or a blended formula may be calculated and prepared.

Parenteral: peripheral vein feeding

If the patient cannot take in food or formula via the gastrointestinal tract, intravenous feeding will be needed. Solutions of dextrose, amino acids, vitamins, and minerals, with intermittent lipid formula, can be fed through peripheral veins when the need is not extensive or long-term.

Parenteral: total parenteral nutrition (TPN)

If the patient's nutritional need is great and support therapy may be required for a longer time, feeding through a large central vein is needed. Placement of this tube is a special surgical procedure. More concentrated special solutions can be used and monitored by a nutrition support team. The formulas are determined by the dietitian and the physician, prepared by trained pharmacists, and administered by specially trained nurses.

This skilled nutritional support team is essential for successful therapy.

Details of these various modes of feeding are given in Chapter 18, as they apply to different conditions.

EVALUATION: QUALITY PATIENT CARE

GENERAL CONSIDERATIONS

When the nutritional care plan is carried out, patient care activities need to be considered in terms of the nutritional diagnosis and treatment objectives, and the extent to which each of the care activities helps to meet the particular goals of the patient and the family. This evaluation is both continuous and terminal and requires careful, objective documentation (see *Practical Application* box). It seeks to validate care while it is being given as well as to determine the effectiveness of a particular course of care. Various areas need to be investigated.

- *Estimate the achievement of nutritional therapy goals.* What is the effect of the diet or mode of feeding on the illness or the patient's situation? Is there need for any change in the nutrient ratios of the diet or formula as originally calculated, in the meal-distribution pattern, or in the feeding mode?
- *Judge the accuracy of intervention actions.* Is there need to change any of the nutritional care plan components? For example, is there need for a change in the type of food or feeding equipment, environment for meals, procedures for counseling, or types of learning activities for nutrition education and self-care procedures?
- *Determine patient's ability to follow the prescribed nutrition therapy.* Are there any hindrances or disabilities that prevent the patient from following the treatment plan? What is the impact of the nutrition therapy on the patient, the family, or the staff? Were the necessary nutrition assessment procedures for collecting nutrition data carried out correctly? Do the patient and family understand the information given for self-care? Have the community resources required by the patient and family been available and convenient for use? Has any needed food assistance program been sufficient to meet needs for the patient's ongoing care?

QUALITY PATIENT CARE

The current increased focus on cost control in managed health care reforms is leading to mechanisms for effectively evaluating patient care programs on the basis of: (1) cost effectiveness and (2) provision of nutritional services by the most qualified personnel. Also, health care legislation concerning quality care assessment and assur-

practical application

Nutritional assessment and therapy for a patient with cancer

Esther Landau is a 160 cm (5 ft, 4 in) tall, medium-frame, 43-year-old patient recovering from a *gastrectomy* performed 8 days ago to treat gastric cancer. Her weight has dropped gradually for the past 4 months from an average of 59 kg (130 lb) before her illness began. She continues to follow a full-liquid diet, consuming 60 to 120 ml (2 to 4 oz) of milk every few hours, plus 1 or 2 soft-boiled eggs each day. Today she informed the nutritionist that she consumed a total of 721 ml (24 oz) of milk and 2 eggs.

In reviewing Mrs. Landau's records, the nutritionist found the following nutritional assessment data: weight 47.3 kg (103 lb); triceps skinfold, 10 mm; and midarm circumference, 17 cm. Laboratory values include serum albumin, 3 g/dl; total iron-binding capacity (TIBC), 230 μg/dl; lymphocytes, 1200 cells/m^3 (23%); hematocrit, 35%, and hemoglobin, 10.5 g/dl. Urinalysis (24 hours) included urea nitrogen, 16 g; and creatinine, 1.75 g. Skin tests were pending.

After reviewing the data, the nutritionist calculated nitrogen balance, transferrin, and creatinine-height index, which were recorded on the patient chart. Basal energy expenditure needs and kcalories and protein needed to overcome catabolism were also calculated, along with estimates for additional vitamin and mineral requirements.

The clinical nutritionist noted that the physician had ordered chemotherapy for the patient, continuing after discharge, and recommended the use of TPN, also to be continued after discharge, as a means of meeting Mrs. Landau's nutritional needs. In addition, the nutritionist planned ways of meeting any feeding problems that often accompany chemotherapy, such as sore mouth, nausea, and food intolerances. Following a carefully prepared protocol developed by the hospital nutritional support team, both Mrs. Landau and her husband were instructed in procuring and using the home TPN treatment. The nutritionist also provided follow-up counseling for Mrs. Landau and her husband at the office and in the group sessions for cancer patients and their families.

Questions for analysis

1. Use a nutritional assessment data summary sheet from your hospital (or design your own) to record pertinent data given in this case study. What additional data would you collect? How would it be obtained?

2. For each test listed on your data sheet, explain what it measures and how that information contributes to an understanding of Mrs. Landau's status.

3. What specific nutritional needs can you identify in this case? List them in order of priority.

4. Calculate Mrs. Landau's nitrogen balance and transferrin for day 8. Why are these indices important to assessing her nutritional status?

5. What is Mrs. Landau's creatinine-height index? How does it reflect her nutritional status?

6. Interpret Mrs. Landau's anthropometric data, including your calculations of her midarm muscle circumference.

7. What skin tests were probably ordered? How would the results contribute to the assessment of her nutritional status?

8. What nutritional problems do you expect Mrs. Landau to encounter after discharge? How could they be resolved? What community agencies might contribute to her sense of well-being after discharge?

---

ance monitoring, as well as health care accreditation agencies such as the Joint Commission on Accreditation of Healthcare Organizations (JCAHO) to add the high standards professional seal of approval, are all increasingly mandating that such care be accurately recorded in an organized manner.[28-31]

enteral A mode of feeding that uses the gastrointestinal tract; oral or tube feeding.

parenteral A mode of feeding that does not use the gastrointestinal tract, but instead provides nutrition by intravenous delivery of nutrient solutions.

To Probe Further

Nutritional assessment: when being objective does not always mean being objective

Nutritionists and other health professionals like numbers. To identify malnutrition, they monitor serum levels of liver-secreted plasma proteins, such as albumin and transferrin, take anthropometric measurements, and determine creatinine-height indexes and cell-mediated immunity response. One study now suggests that these numbers do not add up to the accuracy of the clinical examination in determining a patient's nutritional status.

Researchers from the University of Toronto and Toronto General Hospital suggest that objective measurements may sometimes be inaccurate because they are influenced by several factors: (1) the effects of the disease process itself (rather than the distinct issue of malnutrition) on changes in nutrient levels, (2) delayed response to nutritional depletion (or repletion) because of the relatively long half-lives of such indexes as serum albumin and transferrin, and (3) the wide range of confidence limits in nutritional measurements.

These workers found that two physician clinical evaluators were able to agree on the nutritional status of 81% of 59 surgical patients examined independently. The history—emphasizing weight loss, edema, anorexia, unusual food intakes, and so on— and physical examination—stressing jaundice, muscle wasting, edema, conditions of oral structures, and similar findings—provided enough information for them to come to conclusions that agreed with objective evaluations.

Does this mean that laboratory tests should be placed in "semiretirement," limited to use in epidemiologic surveys instead of evaluating individuals? These researchers think they should, but they do acknowledge that accurate assessment tests do exist, such as total body nitrogen and total body potassium, although these are not generally available. They also suggest the possibility of combining several known indices to make a more sensitive one, even though this lends itself to the possibility of leaving out one measurement that could have an important effect on the calculations.

However, they do emphasize an important point: nutritional status is as dependent on what you *see* as on what you read on a laboratory sheet.

References

Baker JP et al: Nutritional assessment: a comparison of clinical judgment and objective measurements, *N Engl J Med* 306(16):969, 1982.

Detsky AS et al: What is subjective global assessment of nutritional status? *J Parenter Enter Nutr* 11:8, 1987.

COLLABORATIVE ROLES OF THE DIETITIAN AND NURSE

The clinical dietitian works closely with the nurse in managing the nutritional care of patients. At varying times, depending on need, the nurse may provide valuable nutrition assistance as coordinator, interpreter, or teacher. Skills in consultation and referral are therefore essential.

Coordinator

Nurses can coordinate special services or treatment required because of their close relationship to patients and their constant attendance. The nurse may help schedule activities to prevent conflicts or secure needed consultation for the patient with the dietitian, social worker, or other health team member. Sometimes hospital malnutrition exists simply because meals are constantly being interrupted by various procedures, staff interviews, or medical rounds.

Interpreter

Because of a close relationship with the patient, the nurse may often reduce tension by helping the patient understand explanations concerning various treatments and plans of care. This will include basic interpretation of the therapeutic diet from the clinical nutritionist and of the resulting food selections on the tray. The nurse may sometimes assist the patient in making appropriate selections from the menus provided.

Teacher or counselor

One of the nurse's most significant roles is that of health care educator and counselor. There will be innumerable informal opportunities during daily nursing care for planned conversation about sound nutrition principles, reinforcing the counseling of the clinical nutritionist. In addition, according to patient situations, the nurse may work with the clinical nutritionist during periods of instruction about principles of the patient's diet therapy in relation to the disease process. The nurse will work in close cooperation with the clinical nutritionist and the physician to coordinate nutritional and medical management of the patient's illness into overall nursing care. At all times the nurse will work closely with the hospital's clinical nutrition staff to support and reinforce primary nutrition education, as well as discharge planning for follow-up care. These clinical staff nutrition experts will always be excellent resources for needed nutrition consultation and referral.

Clearly, learning about the hospitalized patient's nutritional needs is a continuing activity beginning with admission. It should follow through and include plans for continuing application in the home environment. Follow-up care may be provided by the hospital's clinic dietitian, by consultation with clinical dietitians in community private practice, by public health nutritionists and nurses, or by referrals to community agencies and resources.

To sum up

The basis for an accurate assessment of the patient's nutritional needs begins with the individual patient and family. Physical as well as psychologic, social, economic, and cultural factors in and out of the clinical setting all play a role in evaluating the patient's health status and any possible problems with the nutritional care plan.

Nutritional assessment is based on a broad foundation of pertinent data, including food and drug uses and values. The effectiveness of an assessment based on analysis of these data depends in turn on effective communication with the patient, family members, and significant others in the development of an appropriate care plan, as well as with other members of the health care team. The patient's medical record is a basic means of communication among health care team members.

Nutritional therapy, based on a combination of the personal and physiologic needs of the patient, requires a close working relationship among nutrition, medical, and nursing staff in the health care facility. The nurse's schedule offers many opportunities to reinforce nutritional principles of the diet. Nutritional therapy doesn't end with the patient's discharge. Outpatient nutrition services, appropriate social services, and food resources in the community help meet continuing needs of patients and their families.

Questions for Review

1. Identify and discuss the possible effects of various psychologic factors on the outcome of nutritional therapy.
2. Outline a general procedure for assessing nutritional needs and building a care plan for a 65-year-old widower hospitalized with coronary heart disease (see Chapter 20). Include appropriate community agencies to refer the patient for follow-up care, services, and information.
3. Describe commonly used anthropometric procedures, blood tests, and urine tests for nutritional status information in terms of significance of the measure or test—what is being measured and what the results tell you.
4. Select several clinical signs used to assess nutritional status and describe what each sign shows in a malnourished person and why.
5. Describe the nature and purpose of quality assurance plans for standards of nutritional care.

References

1. Tucker HN, Miguel SG: Cost containment through nutrition intervention, *Nutr Rev* 54(4):111, 1996.
2. Bélanger M-C, Dubé L: The emotional experience of hospitalization: its moderators and its role in patient satisfaction with food services, *J Am Diet Assoc* 96(4):354, 1996.
3. Rubin M: The physiology of bed rest, *Am J Nurs* 88(1):50, 1988.
4. Gallacher-Allred CR et al: Malnutrition and clinical outcomes: the case for medical nutrition therapy, *J Am Diet Assoc* 96(4):361, 1996.
5. Swails WS et al: A proposed revision of current ICD-9-CM malnutrition code definitions, *J Am Diet Assoc* 96(4):370, 1996.
6. Dabhauser A et al: Preoperative nutritional status and prognostic nutritional index in patients with benign disease undergoing abdominal operations—part 1, *J Am Coll Nutr* 14:8, 1995.
7. Egbert AM: The dwindles: failure to thrive in older patients, *Nutr Rev* 54(1):S25, 1996.
8. Bone RC: Ethical principles in critical care, *JAMA* 263(5):696, 1990.
9. Monsen ER et al: Ethics: responsible scientific conduct, *Am J Clin Nutr* 54:1, 1991.
10. Posthauer ME et al, Council of Practice (COP) Quality Management Committee: Identifying patients at risk: ADA's definitions for nutrition screening and nutrition assessment, *J Am Diet Assoc* 94(8)838, 1994.
11. Young EA: The physician-dietitian roles in advancing medical nutrition therapy, *Perspect Appl Nutr* 2(3):25, 1995.
12. Williams SR: Our professional imperative as nutrition experts. In Helm KK, Klawitter B: *Nutrition therapy*, 1995, Helm Seminars.
13. Laramee SH: Nutrition services in managed care, *J Am Diet Assoc* 96(4):335, 1996.
14. Laramee SH: Position of the American Dietetic Association: nutrition services in managed care, *J Am Diet Assoc* 96(4):391, 1996.
15. Gallacher-Alred CR et al: Malnutrition and clinical outcomes: case for medical nutrition therapy, *J Am Diet Assoc* 96(4):361, 1996.

16. Elmore MF et al: Developing an effective adult screening tool for a community hospital, *J Am Diet Assoc* 94(10):1113, 1994.

17. Carey M, Gillesoie S: Position of the American Dietetic Association: cost effectiveness of medical nutrition therapy, *J Am Diet Assoc* 95(1):88, 1995.

18. Dwyer JT: Policy and healthy weight, *Am J Clin Nutr* 63(suppl):415S, 1996.

19. Abernathy RP, Black DR: Healthy body weights: an alternative perspective, *Am J Clin Nutr* 63(suppl):448S, 1996.

20. Meisler JG, St Joer S: Summary and recommendations from the American Health Foundation's Expert Panel on Healthy Weights, *Am J Clin Nutr* 63(suppl):474S, 1996.

21. Frisancho AR: Nutritional anthropometry, *J Am Diet Assoc* 88(5):553, 1988.

22. Nowak RK, Schultz LO: A comparison of two methods for the determination of body frame size, *J Am Diet Assoc* 87(3):339, 1987.

23. Mitchell CO, Lipschitz DA: Arm length measurement as an alternative to height in the nutritional assessment of the elderly, *J Am Geriatr Soc* 39:492, 1991.

24. Kwok T, Whitelaw MN: The use of armspan in nutritional assessment of the elderly, *J Am Geriatr Soc* 39:492, 1991.

25. Chumlea WC et al: *Nutrition assessment of the elderly through anthropometry,* Columbus, Ohio, 1987, Ross Laboratories.

26. Haboubi NY et al: Measurement of height in the elderly, *J Am Geriatr Soc* 8:1008, 1990.

27. Chumlea WC et al: Prediction of body weight for the non-ambulatory elderly from anthropometry, *J Am Diet Assoc* 88(5):564, 1988.

28. Robinson GE: Applying the 1996 JCAHO nutrition care standards in long-term care setting, *J Am Diet Assoc* 96(4):400, 1996.

29. Foiles RA: The 1995 JCAHO mental health manual—an overview for dietetics professionals, *J Am Diet Assoc* 96(4):403, 1996.

30. Westbrook NH: Applying the JCAHO standards to dietetics practice in home care, *J Am Diet Assoc* 96(4):404, 1996.

31. Charles EJ: Charting by exception: a solution to the challenge of the 1996 JCAHO's nutrition care standards, *J Am Diet Assoc* 97(suppl 2):S131, 1997.

▬ FURTHER READING

Arensberg MBF, Schiller MR: Dietitians in home care: a survey of current practice, *J Am Diet Assoc* 96(4):347, 1996.

These authors report the results of their survey of registered dietitians working as consultants in home care. The majority worked with patients receiving enteral tube feedings and total parenteral nutrition, with primary diagnoses of diabetes and cancer.

Beyer K et al: Nutrition screening among rural older persons, *Nutr Today* 31(1):24, 1996.

Guigoz Y et al: Assessing the nutritional status of the elderly: the Mini Nutritional Assessment as part of the geriatric evaluation, *Nutr Rev* 54(1):59, 1996.

Roubenoff R et al: Nutrition assessment in long-term care facilities, *Nutr Rev* 54(1):S40, 1996.

These three articles provide guidance for assessing nutritional needs of older adults; the first two include excellent examples of brief, easily administered tools for use in screening and assessing nutritional status and risk of malnutrition.

Licavoli L, Hahn N: Dietetics goes into therapy, *J Am Diet Assoc* 95(7):751, 1995.

This nutrition therapist describes to her interviewer her clinical practice, in which combining her additional study in counseling with her nutrition degree and registration (RD) has led her to establish a private practice firm focused on nutrition therapy. In this brief article, she explains why extended client-centered nutrition therapy counseling, as compared with the traditional brief nutrition education visit, is the necessary model for the future of dietetics practice.

Issues Answers

Selecting computer nutrient-calculation software

In our modern age of electronics, the computer has become a standard tool for rapid calculation procedures. In clinical and community nutrition practices as well as population studies, it saves valuable time and provides a precise nutrient analysis of an individual's reported food intake.

Certainly computerized nutrient analyses are time savers from the previous tedious manual calculations using published food value tables. But just how precise are the results? This depends on the heart of any nutrient-analysis software program—its nutrient database.

Over the past few years of computer use by clinicians, researchers, and educators, it has become increasingly evident that the quality of the nutrient database on which all calculations are based determines the quality of the resulting output. Experts in this field at the University of Minnesota's Nutrition Coordinating Center have provided important questions that may be used in evaluating the nutrient database in any software package being considered for purchase.

Does the database contain all foods and nutrients of interest?

Most databases contain the most common foods, but you may require particular foods such as ethnic, vegetarian, or fast-food items, brand-name products, and infant or nontraditional foods. The number of food items in a database does not necessarily indicate how comprehensive the system is. And adding your own foods to the database requires considerable effort.

Is the database complete for nutrients of interest?

Missing values are common in available software packages and often are not flagged, so you may be unaware of this source of error. Inappropriate patient counseling may result. Such missing value errors in small items such as spices or other condiments may not matter, but a missing value for total saturated fatty acids in a fast-food hamburger because the food manufacturers have not supplied it is not acceptable.

Do foods included in the database provide sufficient specific data to accurately assess nutrients of interest?

For example, if total fat and fatty acids are of concern, separate database entries must be included for such items as regular, low-fat, and nonfat dairy products and brand name high-fat items such as margarines and salad dressings. In other cases, inclusion of food items according to preparation method, or of any dietary supplements for vitamin-mineral calculations, may be required.

Is the nutrient database current with the changing marketplace and availability of new nutrient data?

The USDA routinely releases updates of the *Agricultural Handbook No. 8*, the common source of data for nutrient-calculation systems, as new information is available. Information from food manufacturers is also available. A well-maintained software product's database should include all such data updates, and the vendor should supply information about frequency of updating and sources of data.

Are manufacturers contacted routinely for new information or reformulations of existing products?

This question extends the previous question to emphasize the still too frequent neglect of brand-name product updating practices of software developers. Routine contact with food manufacturers is essential to maintaining an acceptable quality standard.

What quality control procedures are used to ensure database accuracy?

Because there are thousands of values for nutrients and nonnutrient information, for example, food-specific serving sizes, the margin for error is great and built-in maintenance procedures for checking such errors should be present.

Vendors of nutrient-calculation software packages should be able to give answers to these important questions. Ask before you buy!

References

Buzzard IM et al: Considerations for selecting nutrient-calculation software: evaluation of the nutrient database, *Am J Clin Nutr* 54:7, 1991.

Schakel SF et al: Sources of data for developing and maintaining a nutrient database, *J Am Diet Assoc* 88:1268, 1988.

Chapter

16

Drug-Nutrient Interactions

Chapter Outline

Drug-Nutrient Problems in Modern Medicine
Drug Effects on Food and Nutrients
Food and Nutrient Effects on Drugs
Nutrition-Pharmacy Team

In this chapter, continuing our clinical nutrition sequence, we look briefly at some main effects of combining food and nutrients with drugs. We will see how these interactions affect nutrition therapy.

Today consumers are generally better informed about drug misuse. However, many are dangerously uninformed or misinformed about the specific drugs they may be taking, especially in relation to the food they eat.

All members of the health care team must have a basic knowledge of drug actions and nutrition to make the wisest and most effective use of drugs and nutritional therapy. Here we examine some of these drug-nutrient effects and how these interactions affect our nutritional therapy and education.

DRUG-NUTRIENT PROBLEMS IN MODERN MEDICINE

PROBLEM SIGNIFICANCE: CAUSES, EXTENT, EFFECTS

Increasing complexity and specialization mark our modern medical world. Every medical specialty field easily becomes isolated from many other interacting factors in the care of clients and patients that fall outside its primary area of expertise. The medical specialists who prescribe medications, pharmacists who fill prescriptions, or nurses who administer medications may not be fully aware of the impact of a particular drug on an individual patient's nutritional state. They are often unaware of the patient's diet and how it may influence the drug's effects. Similarly, a clinical dietitian may provide a diet description and food plan and not be fully aware of the client's medication program and its implications for sound nutritional care (see *Practical Application* box, p. 330).

In general, people today know more about misuse of drugs, both prescription and over-the-counter nonprescription ones. Despite this general awareness, however, our society is overmedicated, and many persons know relatively little about the relation of the drugs they take, if any, to the food they eat.

The field of nutrient-drug interaction is complex and confusing. We face a drug-oriented medical environment and a bewildering array of drug items. Every year American physicians prescribe and pharmacists dispense a total amount of drugs sufficient to provide seven individual medications for each woman, man, and child in the United States. To this amount we can then add the large volume of nonprescription drugs that Americans purchase over the counter.

Some concerned persons have come to view the proliferation of pills in our society with alarm. For example, epidemiologic studies in America and Europe indicate that cycles of repeated antibiotic prescriptions may increase the patient's risk of contracting an antibiotic-resistant disease organism.[1] Knowledgeable and concerned pharmacologists indicate that outside of extremely serious illness, most general medical problems can be treated with less than 25 drugs. The World Health Organization (WHO) has estimated that only some 150 to 200 drugs are actually needed to take care of almost all ordinary illnesses around the world. Yet on our American market there are about 54,000 drugs, many of them only slight variations of other drugs, the "me too" drugs.

DRUG USE AND NUTRITIONAL STATUS

Elderly persons at risk

All of us, at any age, risk harmful drug or drug-nutrient interactions. However, elderly persons are particularly vulnerable.[2-4] Several things contribute to this increased risk among the elderly:

- They are likely to be taking more drugs for longer periods of time to control chronic diseases.
- Their drugs are likely to be more toxic.
- They respond to drugs with greater variability.
- They have less capability to handle drugs efficiently.
- Their nutritional status is more likely to be deficient.
- They are more likely to make increased errors in self-care because of illness, mental confusion, or lack of drug information.

As a result of these problems, concerned physicians, nutritionists, pharmacists, and nurses are increasingly working together as a team to provide drug and nutritional education and therapy on a sounder basis.[5,6] A number of drug-nutrient interactions demand this type of team work in patient care.

General hospital malnutrition

Studies of hospital malnutrition have revealed a number of possible mechanisms of nutrient-drug interaction that cause nutrition problems. Results of these studies give us information on contributing causes to this general malnutrition. Such causes are especially prevalent in hospitalized patients and require informed therapy.[7] These nutrient-drug mechanisms that influence nutritional status include those affecting the following:

- Decreased intestinal absorption
- Increased renal excretion
- Competition or displacement of nutrients for carrier protein sites
- Interference with synthesis of necessary enzyme, coenzyme, or carrier
- Hormonal effects on genetic systems
- The drug delivery system
- Components in drug formulation

In general, drugs are usually grouped according to primary action. Here we review briefly various effects of drugs on food and nutrients and effects of food and nutrients on drugs. In each case we give some examples for your reference in patient care.

DRUG EFFECTS ON FOOD AND NUTRIENTS

DRUG EFFECTS ON FOOD INTAKE

Increased appetite

The following drugs have an effect of increasing the appetite.[2-4,8]

1. *Antihistamines.* These drugs can lead to marked increase in appetite and subsequent weight gain. One of these agents, both an antihistamine and a serotonin antagonist, is cyproheptadine hydrochloride (Periactin).

practical application

The proof of the pudding...

The senses of taste and smell greatly affect our responses to various foods. The loss of these senses may drive persons to constantly seek elusive satisfaction by overeating, or it may stop them from eating entirely. In either case the pleasure of eating is gone, and nutritional status suffers. Patients taking drugs that affect taste and smell need counseling concerning food choices, combinations, and seasonings that can help overcome this difficulty.

Some drugs affecting taste and smell include the following:

Anesthetics, local—benzocaine, cocaine, procaine

Antibiotics—amphotericin B, ampicillin, griseofulvin, lincomycin, streptomycin, tetracyclines

Anticoagulant—phenindione

Antihistamine—chlorpheniramine maleate

Antihypertensive agents—captopril, diazoxide, ethacrynic acid

Antiinfectious agent—metronidazole

Cholesterol—lowering agent—clofibrate

Hypoglycemic agent—glipizide

Psychoactive agents—carbamazepine, lithium carbonate, phenytoin, amphetamines

Toothpaste ingredient—sodium lauryl sulfate

The proof of the pudding—our food—is in the tasting, which is easily affected by a variety of drugs, resulting in diminished appetite and necessary food intake. Patients on these drugs benefit from counseling about these taste effects, along with other effects, and ways of counteracting them in food selection, seasoning, and serving.

References

Roe DA: *Diet and drug interactions,* ed 2, New York, 1989, AVI Books.

Powers D, Moore A: *Food-medication interactions,* ed 6, Phoenix, AZ, 1988, Food-Medication Interactions.

Thomas JA: Drug-nutrient interactions, *Nutr Rev* 53(10):271, 1995.

Trovato A et al: Drug-nutrient interactions, *Am Fam Physician* 44(5):1651, 1991.

2. *Psychotropic drugs.* Some of the tranquilizers may lead to *hyperphagia,* or excessive eating (see *Issues & Answers,* p. 340). Those that lead to weight gain when given to psychotic patients may have the opposite effect on geriatric patients. Some of these drugs include chlordiazepoxide hydrochloride (Librium), diazepam (Valium), chlorpromazine hydrochloride (Thorazine), and meprobamate (Equanil). As with the tranquilizers, tricyclic antidepressants such as amitriptyline hydrochloride (Elavil) may promote appetite and lead to significant weight gain.

3. *Steroids.* Anabolic steroids, including testosterone, promote nitrogen retention, increased lean body mass, and subsequent weight gain. Some athletes and body builders form habits of drug abuse with steroids to obtain these characteristic effects, but harm their bodies in the process.

Decreased appetite

The following drugs have the effect of depressing the appetite[2-4,8]:

1. *Amphetamines.* These drugs act as stimulants to the central nervous system and have the effect of depressing the desire for food, thus leading to marked loss of weight. For this reason they have been used in the past as appetite-depressant drugs in the treatment of obesity. However, long-term use of these drugs in such treatment has caused problems, including addiction, since in most cases appetite itself is not the primary cause of the excess weight. For this reason, amphetamines are rarely used now for this purpose. Children taking amphetamines show dose-dependent growth retardation.

2. *Insulin.* A rapid drop in blood sugar, hypoglycemia, can occur in persons with insulin-dependent (type I) diabetes if food is not taken immediately after their scheduled insulin injection to balance with the rapid effect of the insulin (see Chapter 20). If some source of sugar is not readily available to counteract the rapid progression of the unrelieved severe hypoglycemia, coma and death occur. Nondiabetic persons who do not have regular meals may sometimes experience a rapid drop in blood sugar induced by their normal insulin production unrelieved by food. This effect is not marked by hunger but often causes nausea, weakness, headache, and aversion to foods.

3. *Alcohol.* Abuse of alcohol can lead to loss of appetite, reduced food intake, and malnutrition. Alcoholism

requires health-risk screening and significant nutritional support in rehabilitation efforts.[9,10] The anorexia, or loss of appetite, can stem from various effects of alcoholism, such as gastritis, lactose intolerance, hepatitis, cirrhosis, ketosis, pancreatitis, alcoholic brain syndrome, drunkenness, and withdrawal symptoms. The resulting reduced food intake can then lead to malnutrition, which further complicates the anorexia by causing deficiencies of thiamin, zinc, or protein. However, the interaction between alcohol and food appears to go both ways, with the intake of different foods also influencing alcohol use. For example, a high-carbohydrate, low-protein diet depresses alcohol intake, whereas a low-carbohydrate, high-protein food increases it. If such specific diets can help to depress alcohol intake, nutritional therapy might be useful in the treatment of alcohol abusers, probably not as a primary treatment, but as an adjunct to other forms of treatment.[11]

Taste changes

A loss of taste, or dysgeusia, may be caused by a number of drugs. For example, the chelating agent D-penicillamine is used in the treatment of conditions such as heavy metal poisoning, rheumatoid arthritis, or cystinuria. The side effect of taste loss occurs as the agent also binds zinc and causes a drug-induced zinc deficiency. Other drugs affecting taste acuity include diuretics and anticancer agents such as methotrexate and doxorubicin hydrochloride (Adriamycin), as well as agents used to treat Parkinson's disease. Even a 1-g dose of aspirin increases perception of a bitter taste. Sodium lauryl sulfate, a substance often used in toothpaste to make it clean teeth better, can make orange juice taste bitter. A number of other drugs can also affect taste and smell. Thus when any of these drugs are used, discussion of these sensory effects with the patient and use of food seasonings to enhance taste and smell is useful.

Nausea

Many drugs have the effect of decreasing appetite because they contribute to nausea and vomiting. For example, cardiac glycosides, digitalis, and related drugs can produce nausea if used in relatively large amounts. A number of drugs used in cancer chemotherapy (see Chapter 24) have similar effects and can contribute to malnutrition and weight loss.

Bulking effects

Various agents, such as methyl cellulose and other dietary fiber products, can interfere with absorption of nutrients and contribute to their loss. These bulking agents can also contribute to decreased intake of food by creating a sense of fullness and lack of desire for food intake. For this reason they have sometimes been used as adjunct therapy in weight management.

DRUG EFFECTS ON NUTRIENT ABSORPTION AND METABOLISM

Increased absorption

A number of drugs can increase nutrient absorption and thus benefit nutritional status. For example, cimetidine (Tagamet), a gastric antisecretory agent, helps patients with bowel resection in several ways. For example, the drug reduces gastric acid and volume output; it also lowers duodenal acid load and volume and reduces jejunal flow. It maintains pH of secretions, and it decreases fecal fat, nitrogen, and volume, thus improving absorption of protein and carbohydrates. This drug is therefore helpful in the treatment of various gastrointestinal disorders, including peptic ulcer disease (see Chapter 18).

Decreased absorption

A number of drugs contribute to primary malabsorption. Colchicine, for example, a drug used in the treatment of gout, leads to vitamin B_{12} deficiency, causing megaloblastic anemia. Alcohol abuse provokes malabsorption of thiamin and folic acid, causing peripheral neuritis and anemia. Laxatives produce severe malabsorption, leading to conditions such as osteomalacia. Secondary malabsorption may also be drug-induced. Some drugs inhibit vitamin D absorption, leading to malabsorption and consequent deficiency of calcium. For example, the antibiotic neomycin causes tissue changes in the intestinal villi, precipitates bile salts, prevents fat breakdown by inhibiting pancreatic lipase, and decreases bile acid absorption. These effects lead to steatorrhea and failure to absorb the fat-soluble vitamins A, D, E, and K. Malabsorption of vitamin D in turn leads to a calcium deficiency. Other drugs cause malabsorption of folic acid or impair its utilization, causing malabsorption of still other nutrients. Methotrexate, for example, used in cancer chemotherapy, is a folic acid antagonist that impairs the intestinal absorption of calcium.

Summaries of the drugs causing primary and secondary nutrient malabsorption are given in Tables 16.1 and 16.2.

Mineral depletion

Certain drugs can lead to mineral depletion through induced gastrointestinal losses or renal excretion.[12]

1. *Diuretics.* Diuretic drugs are intentionally used to reduce levels of excess tissue water and sodium. But they may also result in loss of other minerals, such as potassium, magnesium, and zinc. Potassium deficiency brings weakness, anorexia, nausea, vomiting, listlessness, apprehension, and sometimes diffuse pain, drowsiness, stupor, and irrational behavior. On the contrary, potassium-retaining diuretics, such as spironolactone, as well as overuse of potassium supplementation, cause the opposite effect of hyperkalemia.

Table

16.1   Drugs causing primary nutrient malabsorption

Drug	Use	Nutrients lost	Action
Cholestyramine	Holds bile acid; hypocho-lesterolemic agent	Fat; fat-soluble vitamins A, D, E, and K; vitamin B_{12}; iron	Binding agent for bile salts and nutrients
Colchicine	Antigout agent	Fat; vitamin B_{12}; provitamin A (carotene); lactose; sodium, potassium	Enzyme damage; inhibits cell division; structural defect
Methyldopa	Antihypertensive agent	Vitamin B_{12}, folic acid; iron	Unclear; possible autoimmune action
Mineral oil	Laxative	Fat; fat-soluble vitamins A, D, and K; provitamin A (carotene)	Nutrients dissolve in oil and are lost in feces
Neomycin	Antibiotic	Fat; vitamin B_{12}; nitrogen; lactose, sucrose; sodium, potassium, iron, calcium	Binds bile salts; lowers pancreatic lipase; structural defect
Paraaminosalicyclic acid	Antituberculosis agent	Fat; folic acid; vitamin B_{12}	Blocks mucosal uptake of vitamin B_{12}
Phenolphthalein	Laxative	Calcium, potassium; vitamin D	Rapid intestinal transit; loss of structural tissue integrity
Potassium chloride	Potassium replacement	Vitamin B_{12}	Lowered ileal pH
Salicylazosulfapyridine (Azulfidine)	Antiinflammatory agent (ulcerative colitis)	Folic acid	Blocks mucosal uptake of folic acid

Modified from Roe DA: Interactions between drugs and nutrients, *Med Clin North Am* 63:985, 1979; and Roe DA: *Diet and drug interactions,* ed 2, New York, 1989, AVI Books.

Table

16.2   Drugs causing secondary malabsorption of calcium

Drug	Use	Action
Phenytoin, phenobarbital, primidone	Anticonvulsant agents	Accelerated vitamin D metabolism
Diphosphonates	Paget's disease (increased bone resorption and deformity)	Vitamin D hormone ($[1,25[OH]_2D_2]$) formation decreased
Glucocorticoids, such as prednisone	Collagen disease; allergies	Calcium transport decreased
Glutehimide	Sedative	Impaired calcium transport
Methotrexate	Leukemia	Folic acid antagonist—acute deficiency of the vitamin

Modified from Roe DA: Interactions between drugs and nutrients, *Med Clin North Am* 63:985, 1979; and Roe DA: *Diet and drug interactions,* ed 2, New York, 1989, AVI Books.

2. *Chelating agents.* Penicillamine attaches to metals and leads to deficiency of such key trace elements as zinc and copper.
3. *Alcohol.* The abuse of alcohol can lead to diminished levels of potassium, magnesium, and zinc.
4. *Antacids.* These commonly used over-the-counter medications are of concern because they can produce phosphate deficiency, with symptoms of anorexia, malaise, **paresthesia**, profound muscle weakness, and convulsions as well as calcification of soft tissues from the prolonged hypercalcemia.

5. *Aspirin.* Salicylates such as aspirin (acetylsalicylic acid-ASA) can induce iron deficiency by causing low-level blood loss from erosions in the stomach or intestinal tissue when taken incorrectly (see *To Probe Further* box).

Vitamin depletion

Certain drugs act as metabolic antagonists and cause deficiencies of the vitamins involved.

1. *Vitamin antagonists.* Various drugs have been used successfully to treat disease because they are antago-

To Probe Further

The pain reliever doctors recommend most

Aspirin has a venerable history. Being a buffered form of salicylic acid, it is a modified version of an ancient folk-remedy of willow bark that had been used for many hundreds of years for fever, aches, and pain. The acetyl group in acetylsalicylic acid makes aspirin easier on the stomach than willow bark.

Aspirin is an analgesic agent, an effect enhanced in combination with caffeine, that is used for relief of minor aches and pains. Its mechanism of action is through inhibition of certain **prostaglandins** (see Chapter 4), which have a profound influence on a spectrum of physiologic functions, including blood clotting, blood pressure, the inflammatory process, contraction of voluntary muscles, and transmission of nerve impulses.

Studies implicate aspirin in alleviating many disorders, dangers, and discomforts, including the following:

- The risk of repeated transient ischemic attacks (TIAs), or little strokes, is reduced by 50% in men (but not women) who have already had one.
- Many studies indicate that aspirin is effective in reducing risk for myocardial infarction, that is, a heart attack.
- Aspirin is one of the most effective antiinflammatory drugs and is effective in the long-term treatment of arthritis.
- Aspirin may play a role in inhibiting the spread of some cancers through its action of inhibiting production of prostaglandin E_2.
- Aspirin's effect as an anticoagulant is important in the treatment of phlebitis and other clot-related disorders.
- Aspirin may be effective in promoting sleep. Many scientists now believe aspirin is as effective as most prescription sedatives, and it has far fewer and less serious side effects.
- Diabetic patients who take aspirin may have lower risk of developing retinopathy.

It is important to remember that aspirin is a drug. Many of the benefits of aspirin stem from its systemic, wide-reaching effects on metabolism, which may have unforeseen short- and long-term detrimental results. We do know that aspirin is to be strictly avoided by persons with hemophilia. Also, allergic reactions to aspirin can be severe. Aspirin seems to be implicated in asthma. Children are especially vulnerable to side effects and should not be given aspirin without a physician's instructions.

Aspirin is an irritant to the stomach and intestine. Its continuous use is associated with low-level chronic loss of iron caused by mucosal erosion. This can lead to iron-deficiency anemia.

Aspirin has been linked to birth defects, especially when it is taken later in the course of pregnancy. It increases risk of infant and neonatal mortality, low birth weight, and intracranial hemorrhage.

The best way to take aspirin is on an empty stomach with a full glass of water. This is important: the absorption of aspirin is facilitated by a large volume of liquid and inhibited by the presence of food. In addition, taking aspirin—especially on an empty stomach—without a large fluid intake invites erosion of the stomach lining. But aspirin should never be taken when using alcohol because it increases the bioavailability of alcohol, raising the blood concentration and thus the effect of alcohol on brain centers.

References

Koch PA et al: Influence of food and fluid ingestion on aspirin bioavailability, *J Pharm Sci* 67(11):1533, 1978.

Roine R et al: Aspirin increases blood alcohol concentrations in humans after ingestion of ethanol, *JAMA* 264(18):2406, 1990.

Schachtel BP et al: Caffeine as an aspirin adjuvant, *Arch Intern Med* 151:733, 1991.

nists of certain vitamins and thus can control key metabolic reactions in which that vitamin is involved. For example, coumarin anticoagulants inhibit regeneration of vitamin K, which is necessary for blood clotting. Also, some cancer chemotherapy drugs such as methotrexate have multiple antagonist effects on folate metabolism, thus inhibiting the synthesis of cell reproduction substances—deoxyribonucleic acid and ribonucleic acid (DNA and RNA)—and protein. In a similar manner, the anti-

parasthesia Abnormal sensations such as prickling, burning, and crawling of skin.

malaria drug, pyrimethamine, inhibits the action of folate in protein synthesis. A list of vitamin-antagonist drugs is given in Table 16.3.

2. *Hypovitaminosis from use of oral contraceptives.* Some women using oral contraceptive agents (OCA) have developed subclinical deficiencies of the vitamins folate, riboflavin, pyridoxine (B_6), cobalamin (B_{12}), and ascorbic acid (C). Apparently OCAs induce a greater demand for these vitamins.[13] However, a recent Canadian-United States study has shown that this effect does not hold true with folate.[14] Table 16.4 includes a list of some of these effects on nutritional status.

Special adverse reactions

Several reactions are related to specific drug interactions with particular nutrients.

1. *Monoamine oxidase inhibitors (MAOIs).* These antidepressant drugs increase the vascular effect of simple **vasoactive** amines, such as tyramine and dopamine, from food.[15] The resulting tyramine syndrome is marked by headache, pallor, nausea, and restlessness. With increased absorption, symptoms may escalate to apprehension, sweating, palpitations, chest pain, fever, and increased blood pressure, at times, although rarely, to the extent of hypertensive crisis and stroke. A low-tyramine food list (see Table 24.2) is provided for use by any patient taking one of these antidepressant drugs.

2. *Flushing reaction.* A number of drugs react with alcohol to produce a **flushing reaction** along with **dyspnea** and headache (Table 16.5). Central nervous system depressants, including hypnotic sedatives, antihistamines, phenothiazines, and narcotic analgesics, may cause a loss of consciousness if taken in combination with alcohol. Extreme caution must be exercised with these medications, and patients should be alerted to the dangers of mixing them with alcohol.

3. *Hypoglycemia.* Drugs such as chlorpropamide (Diabinese) and similar oral medications used to control non-insulin-dependent diabetes mellitus (NIDDM) (see Chapter 20) are hypoglycemic agents. They precipitate a rapid release of insulin, which may provoke a hypoglycemic reaction. This response of a rapidly reduced blood glucose level is especially

Table 16.3	Examples of drugs that act as vitamin antagonists
Target vitamin	**Drug**
Vitamin K	Coumarin anticoagulants
Folic acid	Methotrexate
	Pyrimethamine
	Triamterene
	Trimethoprim
Vitamin B_6	Cycloserine
	Hydralazine
	Isoniazid
	Levodopa

Modified from Roe DA: Interactions between drugs and nutrients, *Med Clin North Am* 63:985, 1979; and Roe DA: *Diet and drug interactions,* ed 2, New York, 1989, AVI Books.

Table 16.4	Interactions between oral contraceptive agents (OCA) and vitamins and minerals affecting nutritional status

Nutrient affected by OCA	Effect	Clinical result
Vitamins		
Retinol (vitamin A)	Impairs liver storage; increases plasma binding	Unclear
Pyridoxine (vitamin B_6)	Alters metabolism of tryptophan and vitamin B_6	Abnormal protein metabolism; mood changes
Cobalamin (vitamin B_{12})	Reduces vitamin B_{12} serum levels	Unclear
Folic acid	Reduces red cell concentration; increases folate-binding protein	Megaloblastic anemia
Minerals		
Copper	Increases plasma levels of ceruloplasmin	Unclear
Iron	Increases serum levels of transferrin	Unclear
Zinc	Reduces serum levels of zinc	Unclear

Data modified from Butterworth CE Jr, Weinsier RL: *Malnutrition in hospital patients: assessment and treatment.* In Goodhart RS, Shills ME, eds: *Modern nutrition in health and disease,* ed 6, Philadelphia, 1980, Lea & Febiger.

strong when the drugs are used with alcohol. The symptoms of hypoglycemia include weakness, mental confusion, and irrational behavior. If not treated, loss of consciousness can follow.

4. *Disulfiram reaction*. The drug **disulfiram**, commonly called Antabuse, is used in the treatment of alcoholism. It combats alcohol consumption by producing extremely unpleasant side effects when taken with alcohol. Within 15 minutes flushing ensues, followed by headache, nausea, vomiting, and chest or abdominal pain. Other drugs, including aldehyde dehydrogenase inhibitors, may have this similar disulfiram effect.

FOOD AND NUTRIENT EFFECTS ON DRUGS

PHYSIOLOGIC FACTORS IN DRUG ABSORPTION

The absorption of drugs is a complex matter. Physiologic events are important in a number of ways.

Solution

Before an orally administered tablet or capsule can dissolve, it must first disintegrate. The drug's absorption, either from solution in acid gastric secretions or in the more alkaline medium of the intestine, may be more or less complete depending on its degree of solubility. The drug then passes through the intestinal mucosa and liver circulation before entering systemic circulation. In the systemic blood circulation system, it may be subject to metabolism, deactivation, and elimination through the so-called first-pass mechanism. Food may affect eventual drug absorption at any of these points.

Stomach-emptying rate

The composition of the diet affects the rate at which the food enters the small intestine from the stomach. Slow emptying of food from the stomach has the effect of doling out small portions of a drug, creating more optimal

---

disulfiram White to off-white crystalline antioxidant; inhibits oxidation of the acetaldehyde metabolized from alcohol. It is used in the treatment of alcoholism, producing extremely uncomfortable symptoms when alcohol is ingested following oral administration of the drug.

dyspnea Labored, difficult breathing.

flushing reaction Short-term reaction resulting in redness of neck and face.

vasoactive Having an effect on the diameter of blood vessels

Table 16.5 Adverse drug reactions caused by alcohol and specific foods

Type of reaction	Drugs	Alcohol/foods	Effects
Flushing	Chlorpropamide (diabetes) Griseofulvin Tetrachlorethylene	Alcohol	Dyspnea, headache, flushing
Disulfiram reaction	Aldehyde dehydrogenase inhibitors: Disulfiram (Antabuse) Calcium carbamide Metronidazole Nitrofurantoin Sulfonylureas	Alcohol Foods containing alcohol	Abdominal and chest pain, flushing, headache, nausea and vomiting
Hypoglycemia	Insulin-releasing agents: Oral hypoglycemic drugs	Alcohol Sugar, sweets	Mental confusion, weakness, irrational behavior, unconsciousness
Tyramine reaction	Monoamine oxidase inhibitors (MAOIs): Antidepressants such as phenelzine Procarbazine Isoniazid (isonicotinic acid hydrazide)	Food containing large amounts of tyramine Cheese Red wines Chicken liver Broad beans Yeast	Cerebrovascular accident (CVA), flushing, hypertension

Modified from Roe DA: Interactions between drugs and nutrients, *Med Clin North Am* 63:985, 1979; and Roe DA: *Diet and drug interactions,* ed 2, New York, 1979, AVI Books.

saturation rates on the absorptive sites in the small intestine. Fats, high temperatures, and solid meals prolong the time the food stays in the stomach. Food usually increases secretion of bile, acid, and gut enzymes. It also enhances intestinal motility and splanchnic blood flow. Drugs may adsorb to certain food particles.

Clinical significance

Whether these physiologic events have clinical significance depends on the extent of the effect and the nature of the drug. A small change in absorption is critical for a drug with a steep dose-response curve but perhaps unnoticeable for a drug with a wide range of effective concentrations. In general, the amount of absorption is clinically more important than the rate, since it has more impact on the steady-state plasma concentration of the drug after multiple doses. Table 16.6 gives some examples of drugs that are better utilized when taken without food and those that should be taken with food.

EFFECTS OF FOOD ON DRUG ABSORPTION

Increased drug absorption

In summary, five basic circumstances contribute to the increased absorption of a drug.

1. *Dissolving characteristics.* When a drug does not dissolve rapidly after it has been taken, the time it remains in the stomach with food is prolonged. This increased time in the stomach may increase its effective dissolution and consequent absorption. In some instances the drug may not dissolve properly, due either to the drug or the gastric pH, and is excreted.
2. *Gastric-emptying time.* Delayed emptying of food from the stomach can have the effect of doling out small portions of a drug, creating more optimal saturation rates on the absorption sites in the small intestine.
3. *Nutrients.* Some nutrients promote absorption of certain drugs. For example, high-fat diets increase absorption of the antifungal drug griseofulvin. This drug is fat soluble, and high-fat diets stimulate the secretion of bile acids, which aid in absorption of the drug. Vitamin C, as well as gastric acid, enhances iron absorption. Recent studies indicate that citrus fruit reduced lipoprotein oxidation in persons consuming a high-saturated fat diet.[16] Anticoagulant drugs interact with dietary factors, and a consistent dietary intake of vitamin K is important.[17,18] Folic acid supplementation is needed when phenytoin is used for seizure control in epileptic patients.[19]
4. *Blood flow.* Food intake increases splanchnic blood flow carrying any ingested drugs. This direct circulation to the abdominal visceral organs stimulates absorption and results in an increased availability of the accompanying drugs.
5. *Nutritional status.* In addition to the presence of specific nutrients, nutritional status may also affect

Table	
16.6	Food effect on drug absorption

Absorption reduced by food	Absorption delayed by food
Amoxicillin	Acetaminophen
Ampicillin	Amoxicillin
Aspirin	Aspirin
Demethylchlortetracycline	Cephalexin
Doxycycline	Cephradine
Isoniazide	Digoxin
Levodopa	Furosemide
Methacycline	Sulfadiazine
Oxytetracycline	Sulfamethoxazole
Penicillin G, V(K)	Sulfamethoxypyridazine
Phenethicillin	Sulfanilamide
Phenobarbital	Sulfisoxazole
Propantheline	
Rifampin	
Tetracycline	

Modified from Roe DA: Interactions between drugs and nutrients, *Med Clin North Am* 63:985, 1979; and Roe DA: *Diet and drug interactions,* ed 2, New York, 1989, AVI Books.

bioavailability of certain drugs in different ways. For example, the antibiotic chloramphenicol is absorbed more slowly in children with protein-energy malnutrition, but elimination of the drug is slower in well-nourished children. In both cases the effect is a net increased bioavailability of the drug.

Decreased drug absorption

The absorption of some drugs is delayed or reduced by the presence of food.

1. *Aspirin.* The absorption of aspirin is reduced or delayed by food. It should be taken on an empty stomach with ample water, preferably cold (see *To Probe Further* box, p. 333). Because aspirin increases the effect of alcohol, however, it should not be taken with alcohol.[20] In addition, caffeine enhances the analgesic effect of aspirin.[21]
2. *Tetracycline.* Nutritional status may also have an impact on drug absorption. For example, tetracycline absorption is impaired in malnourished individuals. Absorption of this commonly used antibiotic is also hindered when it is taken with milk, as well as with antacids or iron supplements. The drug combines with these materials to form new insoluble compounds that the body cannot absorb, causing loss of the minerals involved, that is, calcium or iron.[15]
3. *Phenytoin.* The presence of protein inhibits the absorption of phenytoin. Carbohydrate increases its absorption, but fat has no impact.

FOOD EFFECTS ON DRUG DISTRIBUTION AND METABOLISM

Carbohydrate and fat

Dietary carbohydrate and fat, especially their relative quantities, influence liver enzymes that metabolize drugs. For example, the presence of fat increases the activity of diazepam (Valium). Fat increases the concentration of the unbound active drug by displacing it from binding sites in plasma and tissue protein.

Licorice

Licorice, a sweet-tasting plant extract used in making chewing tobacco, candy, and certain drugs, causes sodium retention and increased hypertension.[22] A person being treated for hypertension needs to avoid any licorice-containing product. The active ingredient in licorice is glycyrrhizic acid from the name of its natural plant source, *Glycyrrhiza glabra*, meaning "sweet root," a member of the legume family. An analog of this active part of licorice is marketed under the trade names Biogastrone and Duogastrone, which are widely used, especially in Europe, for healing gastric ulcers, but hypertension is a side effect.

Indoles

The **indoles** in **cruciferous** vegetables (cabbage, Brussels sprouts, broccoli, cauliflower) can speed up the rate of drug metabolism. They apparently induce mixed-function oxidase enzyme systems in the liver.

Cooking methods

The method of cooking foods may alter the rate of drug metabolism. Charcoal broiling, for example, increases hepatic drug metabolism through enzyme induction.

Changes in intestinal microflora

Changes in intestinal microflora related to the amount of dietary protein or fiber, for example, may influence intestinal drug metabolism.

VITAMIN EFFECTS ON DRUG ACTION

Vitamin effects on drug effectiveness

Pharmacologic doses, that is, large megadoses beyond nutritional need, of vitamins decrease blood levels of drugs when vitamins interact with the drugs. For example, large doses of folate or pyridoxine can reduce the blood level and effectiveness of such anticonvulsive drugs as phenytoin (Dilantin) or phenobarbital that are used for seizure control. Unwise self-medication with large drug-level doses of vitamins can cause severe toxic complications. On the other hand, vitamins themselves may become important medications when used as part of the medical treatment for a secondary deficiency induced by a childhood genetic or metabolic disease. Such is the case with biotin in treating certain organic acidemias, or riboflavin in treating certain defects in fatty acid metabolism.

Control of drug intoxication

Riboflavin is useful in treating boric acid poisoning. Boric acid combines with the ribityl side-chain of riboflavin and is excreted in the urine. Also, vitamin E combats pulmonary oxygen toxicity. Premature human infants at risk for development of bronchopulmonary dysplasia by oxygen treatment have been protected by vitamin E administration during the acute phase of respiratory distress requiring oxygen treatment.

NUTRITION-PHARMACY TEAM

DECADES OF CHANGE

A decade or so ago hospitalized patients as a whole were less severely ill than they are today. Now, however, reflecting our more complex medical system and economic reform efforts, patients that are hospitalized are more acutely ill. They are more at risk for nutritional deficits and more likely to develop malnutrition, which leads to increased lengths of stay and higher costs. In the 1960s and 1970s hospitals were beginning to develop multidisciplinary nutrition support committees to administer special enteral and parenteral feeding plans for more seriously ill persons. This was a form of nutritional care that required key roles of the clinical pharmacist and the clinical dietitian.[23] At the same time, the body of scientific knowledge advanced and more drugs were developed to match the advance. Thus the task of monitoring food and drug interactions also became more complex and required team responsibilities. It was soon recognized that coordinating pharmacy, food service, and clinical nutrition minimized adverse drug-nutrient interactions.

CURRENT TRENDS

The movement in hospitals and other health care facilities today is a shift in focus toward key processes and functions, such as drug-nutrient interactions in this case,

---

cruciferous Bearing a cross; botanical term for plants belonging to the botanical family *Cruciferae* or *Brassicaceae*, the mustard family, so-called because of cross-like four-petaled flowers; name given to certain vegetables of this family, such as broccoli, cabbage, Brussels sprouts, and cauliflower.

indole A compound produced in the intestines by the decomposition of tryptophan; also found in the oil of jasmine and clove.

rather than the traditional strictly compartmentalized tasks of departments. Current standards focus still on departmental or service roles. But this is changing because of economic necessity as well as philosophy of care. This changing focus is being shaped, for example, in the work of the Joint Commission on the Accreditation of Healthcare Organizations (JCAHO).[24]

By 1994 JCAHO's accreditation manual reflected the philosophy that key functions often involve different disciplines coming together, partners with clearly defined responsibilities. The team of clinical nutritionist and clinical pharmacologist is clearly one of these partnerships. The current JCAHO guideline mandates the monitoring of drug therapy by clinical dietitians responsible for diet therapy and counseling with patients about adverse drug-nutrient interactions.[25]

In fact, programs are already being developed in medical centers such as the comprehensive program initiated by the clinical nutrition staff at the University of Maryland Medical System in Baltimore.[26] In this program the departments of clinical nutrition, pharmacy, and nursing have coordinated responsibilities in the process of monitoring and counseling on potential drug-food-nutrient interactions. As computer capabilities are expanded, computer-generated flagging, monitoring systems, and printouts provide more commonly used tools for rapid communication. Then, as the Baltimore group has shown, partnerships of clinical nutrition—pharmacy—nursing professions and their patients in relation to drug-nutrient interactions will become routine. Further JCAHO directives will require such specific responsibilities.

To sum up

The field of nutrient-drug interaction is in its infancy. More research is needed to sort out complicated relationships and possible effects. Drugs can have multiple effects on the body's absorption, metabolism, retention, and nutrient status. They can provoke adverse reactions in combination with certain foods and can influence appetite, either repressing it or artificially stimulating it. Drugs can either increase an individual's absorption of nutrients, or, more commonly, decrease absorption, sometimes leading to clinical deficiencies. Drugs can also induce mineral and vitamin deficiencies by their mode of action.

Just as drugs affect our use of food, food affects our use of drugs. Food can affect the absorption of drugs in a variety of ways. Foods also have an effect on subsequent distribution and metabolism of drugs. Vitamins may interfere with drug effectiveness, especially if they are taken in large doses. On the other hand, large doses of specific vitamins can be effective in countering certain toxicity conditions or a specific secondary deficiency induced by a genetic disease.

■ QUESTIONS FOR REVIEW

1. Name four ways food may affect drug use and give examples of each.
2. If your patient were using a prescribed MAOI such as tranylcypromine sulfate (Parnate), what foods would you instruct him to avoid?
3. What is the most effective way to take aspirin? With what type of liquid? With or without food? Why?
4. What foods would you suggest to a hypertensive patient on the diuretic drug hydrochlorothiazide (HCTZ) as good sources of potassium replacement?
5. Outline suggestions you would discuss with a patient experiencing a drug-induced taste loss. How would you explain the cause of the taste loss?
6. How does cimetidine (Tagamet) help improve the nutritional status of persons with gastrointestinal disease?

■ REFERENCES

1. Smaglik P: Proliferation of pills, *Sci News* 151(20):310, 1997.
2. Roe DA: Diet, nutrition and drug reaction. In Shils ME, Olson JA, Shike M, eds: *Modern nutrition in health and disease,* ed 8, vol 2, Philadelphia, 1994, Lea & Febiger.
3. Roe DA: Medications and nutrition in the elderly, *Prim Care* 21(1):135, 1994.
4. Thomas JA: Drug-nutrient interactions, *Nutr Rev* 53(10):271, 1995.
5. Williams L: Mixing food and drugs, *Dietary Currents* 22(3):1, 1995.
6. Wix AR et al: Drug-food interaction counseling programs in teaching hospitals, *Am J Hosp Pharm* 49:855, 1992.
7. Torun B, Chew F: Protein-energy malnutrition. In Shils ME, Olson JA, Shike M, eds: *Modern nutrition in health and disease,* ed 8, vol 2, Philadelphia, 1994, Lea & Febiger.
8. Olin BR et al: *Professional's guide to patient drug facts for improved patient counseling,* St Louis, 1995, Facts and Comparisons, Wolters Kluwer.
9. Lieber CS: Mechanisms of ethanol-drug-nutrition interactions, *Clin Toxicol* 32:631, 1994.
10. Lieber CS: Medical disorders of alcoholism, *N Engl J Med* 333(16):1058, 1995.
11. Forsander OA: Dietary influences on alcohol intake: a review, *J Stud Alcohol* 59(1): 1998.
12. Murray JJ, Healy MD: Drug-mineral interactions: a new responsibility for the hospital dietitian, *J Am Diet Assoc* 91(1):66, 1991.
13. Masse PG: Nutrient intakes of women who use oral contraceptives, *J Am Diet Assoc* 91(9):1118, 1991.
14. Green TJ et al: Oral contraceptions did not affect biochemical folate indexes and homocysteine concentrations in adolescent females, *J Am Diet Assoc* 98(1):50, 1998.
15. Trovato A et al: Drug-nutrient interactions, *Am Fam Physician* 44(5):1651, 1991.

16. Harats D et al: Citrus fruit supplementation reduces lipoprotein oxidation in young men ingesting a diet high in saturated fat: vitamin E presumptive evidence for an interaction between vitamins C and E in vivo, *Am J Clin Nutr* 67(2):240, 1998.

17. Harris JE: Interaction of dietary factors with oral anticoagulates: review and applications, *J Am Diet Assoc* 95(5):1995.

18. Booth SL et al: Dietary vitamin K and stability of oral anticoagulation: proposal of a diet with constant vitamin K content, *Thromb Haemost* 77(3):408, 1997.

19. Lewis DP et al: Phenytoin–folic acid interaction, *Ann Pharmacother* 29(7/8);726, 1995.

20. Roine R et al: Aspirin increases blood alcohol concentration in humans after ingestion of ethanol, *JAMA* 264(18):2406, 1990.

21. Schachtel BP et al: Caffeine as an analgesic adjuvant, *Arch Intern Med* 151:733, 1991.

22. Morris DJ et al: Licorice, chewing tobacco, and hypertension, *N Engl J Med* 151:733, 1991.

23. Hard R: Food service, pharmacy team up for nutrition, *Hospitals* 65:46, 1991.

24. Kessler DA: Communicating with patients about their medications, *N Engl J Med* 325(23):1650, 1991.

25. Joint Commission on the Accreditation of Healthcare Organizations: *Accreditation manual for hospitals,* Oakbrook, Ill, 1990, JCAHO.

26. Lasswell AB, Loreck ES: Development of a program in accord with JCAHO standards for counseling on potential drug-food interactions, *J Am Diet Assoc* 92(9):1124, 1992.

■ FURTHER READING

Ahmed FE: Effects of nutrition on the health of the elderly, *J Am Diet Assoc* 92(9):1102, 1992.

Kerstetter JE et al: Malnutrition in the institutionalized adult, *J Am Diet Assoc* 92(9):1109, 1992.

These excellent companion articles speak to the twin problems of malnutrition and polypharmacy—multiple drug use—among elderly persons.

Clayman CB, ed: *The American Medical Association guide to prescription and over-the-counter drugs,* New York, 1988, Random House.

Clayman CB, ed: *Know your drugs and medications,* The American Medical Association Home Medical Library Series, Pleasantville, New York, 1991, Dorling Kindersley and Reader's Digest.

These two resources, prepared for public education and patient-professional reference, provide useful information about effects and interactions of drugs in common use.

Thomas JA: Drug-nutrient interactions, *Nutr Rev* 53(10):271, 1995.

This is an excellent review with numerous tables. It is a "must read" for all persons taking care of patients and clients.

I s s u e s Answers

The calming of America?

American medicine has many names for its psychoactive drugs that act on the mind to dull its reactions. These drugs interact dangerously with alcohol and in some cases with common foods. Perhaps the name that best fits the effect of these drugs is tranquilizer, from a Latin root meaning "calm, quiet, stillness." This meaning signifies the escape many persons seek from a turbulent, confusing world.

We live in an age of stress, often called the "Era of Anxiety." We also live in a culture committed to instant cures and the avoidance of discomfort. Often instead of probing the causes of our problems and striving to alter the conditions that develop them, we believe that we must never feel uncomfortable. If we do, we take something for it. We seek the magic potion to ease the pain and often the symptoms.

To what extent do we actually use such antianxiety drugs in our search for relief? According to the National Academy of Sciences, some 8.5 million Americans take prescription sleeping pills at least once a year. Two million Americans take them every night for at least 2 months at a time. A study conducted by the National Institute on Drug Abuse indicated that 17 million Americans have used stimulants, 28 million have taken sedatives, and 51 million, nearly one out of every four Americans, have taken tranquilizers.

America's single most widely prescribed tranquilizer drug is diazepam (Valium). For example, in one recent year, 3.2 billion pills were sold legally, up 50% from the year before and enough to provide every man, woman, and child in the United States with 145 pills a year. It is still widely prescribed for depression, along with others such as chlorpromazine and lithium. It is difficult to explain why Valium has been such a frequently prescribed psychoactive drug in the United States. Certainly from a scientific or a pharmacologic viewpoint, no superior effectiveness has been proved. Its popularity can probably be explained by an aggressive marketing program, leading increased numbers of physicians to prescribe it and increased quantities of the drug to be manufactured. In turn the increased amount of the drug available has led to increased black market exposure and easy street usage.

Valium belongs to a group of psychoactive drugs, first introduced in 1960, called benzodiazepines. These antianxiety drugs bind to specific receptor sites in the brain. Their clinical effects are mediated through the central nervous system. For some time scientists have sought the identity of the body's natural compound that occupies these receptor sites in the brain. Now pharmacologists report purification of this natural substance. Paradoxically they have discovered that this new 104–amino acid brain peptide not only blocks the receptor binding action of the antianxiety drugs but also appears to induce anxiety, indicating that it is not a natural tranquilizer but has just the opposite effect. This newly identified compound has been named diazepam-binding inhibitor (DBI) peptide. These scientists suggest that the naturally occurring DBI acts to trigger anxiety-associated behavior. Apparently drugs such as Valium achieve their antianxiety effect by getting in the way of this naturally occurring, anxiety-producing brain peptide.

Along with its desired effect a drug usually causes some unwanted side effects. In the case of antianxiety drugs such as Valium, several interactions and side effects relate to nutrition counseling needs.

Alcohol

Tranquilizers and alcohol do not mix. These drugs enhance the effects of alcohol and other central nervous system (CNS) depressant drugs that slow down the nervous system. In addition to alcohol, other CNS depressant drugs include over-the-counter antihistamines or medicine for hay fever, other allergies, or colds, as well as prescribed anticonvulsants such as Dilantin, pain medications, and narcotics. Long-term use of alcohol also induces liver enzyme changes, leading to more rapid metabolism and reducing the effect of drugs that are detoxified by the liver. Thus in the alcoholic person benzodiazepines may be metabolized more rapidly, and the person may use increasingly larger doses to achieve the desired effect.

Weight gain

Persons taking these antianxiety drugs often experience a great increase in appetite, with subsequent weight gain. This may bring added concern and require general weight management counseling.

Gastrointestinal problems

Some general side effects interfere with food intake and utilization. These problems range from heartburn, nausea, and vomiting to constipation and diarrhea. Individual counseling relating to food choice, combinations, and forms may be needed.

Pregnancy and lactation

Some cases of birth defects from benzodiazepine use during the first 3 months of pregnancy have been reported. In addition, continued use during pregnancy may cause fetal dependency with withdrawal side effects after birth. During lactation these drugs may pass into the breast milk and cause unwanted side effects in the infant.

A more recently introduced antidepressant drug with the trade name Prozac has widespread positive use, primarily because it is relatively free of side effects. However, such widespread use of tranquilizers means that we frequently encounter them in clinical practice and that nutrition counseling must cover their interactions with food and other drugs, including alcohol.

Current research at the National Institute of Mental Health is encouraging. The studies of psychiatrist Robert Post seem to indicate that repeated severe depressive episodes affect gene-modulated brain changes more permanently so that preventive drug therapy should be used more in recurrent illness. Early maintenance therapy may provide the double service of preventing not only the painful recurrences but also the more lasting brain cell changes. Post indicates that the key thing is to match the patient with the right type of medication, and in the long run there will be better medications to match with patients.

References

Griffith HW: *Complete guide to prescription and nonprescription drugs,* ed 5, Los Angeles, 1988, The Body Press, Price Stern Sloan.

Holden C: Depression: the news isn't depressing, *Science* 254:1450, 1991.

Olin BR et al: *Professional's guide to patient drug facts for improved patient counseling,* St Louis, 1995, Facts and Comparisons, Wolters Kluwer.

Chapter

17

Feeding Methods: Enteral and Parenteral Nutrition

In this chapter we look at alternate modes of feeding to provide nutrition support for patients with special needs. We examine ways of feeding when the gastrointestinal tract can still be used—enteral nutrition. Then we review the alternative of nutrient feeding directly into a vein when the gastrointestinal tract cannot be used—parenteral nutrition.

Protein-energy malnutrition is a serious concern in hospitalized patients, especially those with hypermetabolic illness or injury. Often a highly personalized aggressive nutritional program provided by the skilled hospital nutrition support team is life saving.

Here we compare these two special feeding methods. We see their various formulas, solutions, and delivery systems for use in hospital and home.

From Potter PA, Perry AG: *Fundamentals of nursing: concepts, process, and practice,* ed 4, St Louis, 1997, Mosby.

ENTERAL FEEDING IN CLINICAL NUTRITION

NUTRITIONAL SUPPORT NEEDS

The lack of adequate nutrition to meet metabolic demands is increasingly recognized as a serious concern in medical and surgical patients. A number of surveys have shown that as many as 50% of surgical patients and 44% of medical patients suffer significant protein-energy malnutrition.[1] Persons with underlying chronic disease or traumatic injury are particularly at risk. Elderly persons are especially vulnerable. These patients range widely from those with sudden severe burns or other critical injury to those developing alcoholic hepatitis or with a malignant cancer. In all such cases with the gastrointestinal tract functioning, **enteral** nutrition support provides a front line to restore or, in the case of sudden injury, to maintain an optimal state of nutrition.

Questions do not center on the effectiveness of enteral nutrition support, even feeding by tube if needed, for this has been proved. Rather, current questions center on the most appropriate formula for each patient's specific disease state, the preferred method of formula delivery, and in the case of tube-feeding, the causes and extent of possible tube-related complications, such as diarrhea or respiratory problems.[2,3] The hospital's official interdisciplinary Nutrition Support Committee has the responsibility for providing enteral and parental nutrition through its team members from the departments of Medicine, Surgery, Dietary or Clinical Nutrition (nutrition support specialist), Nursing, and Pharmacy.[4] The new standards of the Joint Commission on Accreditation of Healthcare Organizations (JCAHO) and the Accreditation Manual for Hospitals (AMH) have focused on key functions of the multidisciplinary nutrition support team that ensure quality patient outcomes.[5]

MODES OF ENTERAL NUTRITION SUPPORT

Even though they have a functioning gastrointestinal tract, some patients cannot restore or maintain a good nutritional status because they cannot eat enough regular food to sustain themselves. They need to take in more nutrient-dense nourishment. Two routes of enteral nutrition support are possible-oral or tube.

Oral supplements

Depending on the patient's condition the initial option may be to add an oral general energy-nutrient food supplement such as Ensure (Ross) with or between meals. In addition, the energy value of foods in the regular diet may be increased as tolerated with added sauces, seasonings, and dressings. More frequent, less bulky, concentrated small meals may be helpful, making every bite count.

Tube feeding

If sufficient oral intake of food and supplemental formula is not possible, then the second option is enteral nutrition by tube feeding, either as a supplement or as the complete meal.

ASSESSMENT AND PATIENT SELECTION

Clinical experience has shown that underlying malnutrition carries its own substantial risk of illness and death above and beyond that associated with the patient's primary disease. Thus a general assessment program at hospital admission should be routine procedure to identify those already in states of malnutrition as well as those at risk of potential malnutrition because of their underlying disease or injury.[6,7] Metabolic activity factors (MAFs) (see Chapter 22) have been recognized and coded according to their added stress on the clinical state—disease, trauma, surgery, or sepsis. In the hospital the attending nurse may discover eating problems or disorders in a patient and confer with the nutrition support dietitian, who can evaluate any malnutrition risks in the current hospitalization.[8,9] In some instances, the nutrition support dietitian with specialty training writes the enteral-parenteral orders for treatment.[10] Conference with the attending physician may lead to medical referral of the patient to the nutrition support team for full assessment and follow-up care.

Basic factors indicating need of nutritional support for medical-surgical patients are the inability to eat for more than 7 to 10 days or maintenance on low-kcalorie intravenous fluids for 10 days or more. Box 17.1 provides guidelines the nutrition support team uses for making decisions concerning the choice of feeding mode required.

After patients in need of nutritional support have been identified and the indicated mode of feeding is enteral nutrition, the choices of formula and delivery system follow.

ENTERAL FORMULAS

COMPLETE ENTERAL FORMULAS

Blender mixed or commercial

Our current age of advanced nutritional science and technology has brought a variety of commercial formulas and smaller, safer feeding tubes. The question of a blender-mixed formula seldom arises. However, in some instances of home enteral feeding, the patient or family may want to explore the possible use of a home blender-mixed diet.

---

enteral   A mode of feeding that uses the gastrointestinal tract, that is, oral, or tube feeding.

Can the gastrointestinal tract be used safely?
 No   Use parenteral nutrition.
 Yes   Proceed with enteral nutrition.
Is there adequate intestinal absorption?
 No   Use defined formula diet.
 Yes   Use protein isolate diet.
Will nutritional support last longer than 4 to 6 weeks?
 No   Use nasoenteric tube feeding.
 Yes   Use enterostomy tube feeding.
Is the patient at risk for aspiration?
 No   Use shorter nasogastric or gastrostomy tube.
 Yes   Use longer duodenal or jejunal tube.
Is nutritional support providing adequate nutrient delivery?
 No   Add small vein peripheral parenteral nutrition.
 Yes   Continue present formula tube feeding and route.

Starch—polysaccharides

Modified food starch
Hydrolyzed cereal solids
Tapioca starch
Pureed vegetables: green beans, peas, carrots

Glucose polymers*

Glucose polysaccharides
Glucose polymers
Glucose oligosaccharides
Maltodextrins
Corn syrup, corn syrup solids

Disaccharides

Sucrose—from starch hydrolysis
Lactose—from milk
Maltose—from starch and oligosaccharide hydrolysis

Monosaccharides

Glucose (dextrose)
Fructose

*From partial hydrolysis of cornstarch

Although there may be emotional comfort in the use of home-prepared food, they need to know the problems involved. These problems involve its physical form, safety, and digestion and absorption:

1. *Physical form.* Foods broken down and mixed in a blender generally yield a **viscous** solution that is difficult to feed through a tube. Thus because of particle size and tendency to stick to the tube, a large-bore feeding tube that is more uncomfortable is required.

2. *Safety.* Such blender-mixed formulas carry problems of bacterial growth and inconsistent nutrient composition from settling out of solid components.

3. *Digestion and absorption.* The blended food formula requires a fully functioning digestion and absorption system to digest the food and absorb its released nutrients. Some patients have gastrointestinal deficits that require nutrients with varying degrees of predigestion (hydrolysis) or smaller molecular structure.

In overall comparison, commercial formulas provide a sterile, homogenized solution suitable for more comfortable small-bore feeding tubes and ensure a fixed profile of nutrients in intact or predigested form.

NUTRIENT COMPONENTS

Carbohydrates

About half of the kcalories in the American diet come from carbohydrates, starches and sugars, the body's primary energy source. Although the large starch molecules are well tolerated and easily digested by most patients, their relative insolubility creates problems in most formulas. Thus the smaller saccharides formed by partial or complete hydrolysis of corn starch are common formula components. In addition to the simple sugars glucose and sucrose, the carbohydrate components include intermediate glucose polymers of varying chain lengths. These intermediate products of hydrolysis may be glucose polysaccharides of more than 10 glucose units or glucose oligosaccharides of only a few, about 2 to 10 glucose units, as shown in Box 17.2.

The disaccharide lactose is often deleted in the manufacture of nutrition support formulas because of primary (inherited lactase deficiency) and secondary (mucosal damage, enzyme deficiency) lactose intolerance in may malnourished individuals, as well as a relative deficiency following gastrointestinal surgeries. Some of these causes of lactase deficiency indicate use of a lactose-free formula are shown in Box 17.3.

Protein

The protein content of standard enteral formulas is most critical because it maintains the body cell mass and its major functions (see Chapter 4). The biologic quality of dietary protein depends on its amino acid profile, especially its relative proportions of essential amino acids (see Table 5.1, p. 70). Traumatized, catabolic, or seriously undernourished patients require at least 40% of the total amino acid intake as essential amino acids to restore and maintain desired nutritional status.[11] To supply these needs, three major forms of protein are used in nutrition support enteral formulas: intact proteins, hydrolyzed pro-

Primary: inherited

Racial, ethnic
Genetic

Secondary: enzyme deficiency, mucosal damage

Fasting
Malnutrition
Inflammatory bowel disease
Infections (gastroenteritis, cholera)
Medications (colchicine, neomycin)
Radiation

Relative deficiency

Gastric surgery
Short bowel syndrome

teins, and crystalline amino acids. Table 17.1 shows some common sources of protein in standard commercial formulas and examples of conditions for which they are used.

1. *Intact proteins.* Intact proteins are the complete and original forms as found in foods, although protein isolates such as lactalbumin and casein from milk are intact proteins that have been separated from their original food source.
2. *Hydrolyzed proteins.* Hydrolyzed proteins are those protein sources that have been broken down by enzymes into smaller protein fragments and amino acids. These smaller products—tripeptides, dipeptides, and free amino acids—are absorbed more easily into the blood circulation, but the larger peptides must be broken down further before they can be absorbed.
3. *Crystalline amino acids.* Pure crystalline amino acids are easily absorbed, but because of their small size they increase the osmotic effect of the formula. Also, they adversely affect the formula taste and, if used as an oral supplement, require flavoring aids or different forms to improve palatability, for example, liquid beverage, pudding, frozen slush, or popsicle.

Fat

The major role of fat in a nutrition support enteral formula is to supply a concentrated energy source. The major forms of fat used in standard formulas are butterfat in milk-based mixtures; vegetable oils from corn, soy, safflower, or sunflower; the specially produced medium-chain triglycerides (MCT), monoglycerides, and diglycerides; and lecithin. The vegetable oils supply a rich source of essential fatty acids, especially linoleic acid. Current research is leading to the development of alternate structured lipids from various combinations of

Table

17.1 Common protein forms in commercial enteral nutrition formulas and examples of use

Protein forms	Examples of use
Intact protein	*Use intact protein with:*
Milk protein: casein isolates, lactalbumin, whey	Normal small intestine absorption capacity
Sodium and calcium caseinates	Normal pancreatic enzymes
Soy protein isolates	
Pureed beef	
Egg white solids	
Hydrolyzed protein	*Use hydrolyzed protein with:*
Casein, lactalbumin, whey	Reduced absorbing surface
Soy protein	Disorders of amino acid transport
Meat protein, collagen	Pancreatic insufficiency
Crystalline amino acids	*Use crystalline amino acids with:*
L-Amino acids	Liver failure
	Kidney failure

short-chain fatty acids, medium-chain fatty acids, and omega-3 fatty acids (see Chapter 3).[12,13]

Vitamins and minerals

To provide complete nutrition, standard whole diet commercial formulas include sufficient vitamins and minerals for nutrient requirements when energy needs are fully met. However, low-kcaloric intakes and use of diluted formulas require evaluation and supplementation of deficient formulas with liquid vitamin and mineral preparations.

PHYSICAL PROPERTIES

After the initial choice of a formula according to nutritional requirements and individual gastrointestinal function, attention is given to certain physical properties of formulas that may affect tolerance. A main physical property is **osmolality**, which is based on the concentration of the formula and defined as the number of osmotic particles per kilogram of solvent (water), the kcalorie-nutrient density, and residue. Individual intolerance is reflected in

---

viscous (viscid) Physical property of a substance dependent on the friction of its component molecules as they slide by one another; viscosity.

gastric retention with abdominal distention and pain, diarrhea, or constipation. These problems, of which diarrhea is the most common, are often unrelated to the formula itself but may result from inappropriate tube-feeding techniques or drug interactions (see *Issues & Answers,* p. 360).

MEDICAL FOODS FOR SPECIAL NEEDS

Certain formulas designed for special nutritional therapy are called medical foods. The United States Food and Drug Administration (FDA) first recognized the concept of medical foods as distinct from drugs in 1972, when the first such special formula was developed for treatment of the genetic disease phenylketonuria (PKU) in newborns (see Chapter 18). During these early years as medical research developed an increasing number of special formulas, the definition of "**medical foods**" remained rather murky between labels of food or drug. In 1988 Congress amended the Orphan Drug Act to include medical foods, defining them as food specifically formulated for use under medical supervision for primary treatment of metabolic-genetic disease having distinctive nutritional requirements based on recognized scientific principles.[14] Specific regulatory statutes for medical foods are being defined by the FDA. The Orphan Drug Act Amendment to include and define medical foods has now been incorporated into the reformed Nutrition Labeling and Education Act of 1990. In addition to metabolic-genetic medical foods, four other categories of special medical food formulas have been developed: (1) end-stage renal disease, (2) hepatic disease, (3) pulmonary disease, and (4) hypermetabolic stress states.[15]

MODULAR ENTERAL FORMULAS

The commercial complete enteral formula products for tube feeding are designed with a fixed ratio of nutrients to meet general standards for nutritional needs. However, some patients' particular needs are not met by these standard fixed-ratio formulas, and they require an individualized modular formula. Such an individual formula is planned, calculated, prepared, and administered with the combined expertise of the nutrition support team, with the clinical nutrition support dietitian on the team having a major responsibility. The modules vary from a single nutrient to a combination of several nutrients. For example they may be single modules of carbohydrate, fat, and protein or either combined or single vitamins and minerals.

The advances in modular formula products for planning and calculating nutrition support have made possible more specific nutrient-energy combinations. Using these modules, the nutrition support dietitian can tailor an individual formula to meet underlying disease needs in conditions such as diabetes, congestive heart failure, renal failure, or liver disease.

ENTERAL NUTRITION DELIVERY SYSTEMS

FEEDING EQUIPMENT

Feeding tubes

Recent advances in science and technology have made possible the enteral nutrition delivery systems used today. Modern small-bore nasoenteric feeding tubes made of softer, more flexible polyurethane and silicone materials have replaced former large-bore stiff tubing. These modern feeding tubes are more comfortable for patients and easily carry the variety of nutrient materials now available in enteral nutrition support formulas. Also, these nasoenteric tubes can be inserted not only into the stomach (Figure 17.1, *A*) but also beyond the pyloric valve into the small intestine, duodenum or jejunum (Figure 17.1, *B*). These lower placements are used to avoid dangers of vomiting and aspiration by patients on ventilators or for those who are restrained, have a depressed gag reflex, or are comatose. These longer tubes have weighted tips to hold them in place. Insertion and correct placement are guided by radiographic visualization.[16-18]

Containers and pumps

Additional parts of the enteric tube-feeding system are the formula container and often an infusion pump. A number of containers and feeding sets are available. Clinical dietitians and nurses working with patients on tube feedings need to know details of their comparative advantages and limitations. For example, containers that hold a large volume of formula, as much as 1 L, may be convenient for the nursing staff, but if they are not used within a limited time they are subject to bacterial contamination. Sets that attach to the manufacturer's container reduce contamination. Also, an accurate flow rate must be controlled. A pump may be needed for more accurate control, which is essential for feedings that that go directly into the small intestine or for more viscous formulas.

In the final analysis, whatever the type of formula and equipment used, microbiologic quality control programs maintained by enteral nutrition support services at all institutions are essential.[19,20] Such quality standards of practice reduce bacterial counts significantly, thus improving patient tolerance to enteral feeding and reducing complications of infection, diarrhea, and sepsis.

ALTERNATE ROUTES OF FORMULA DELIVERY

The nasoenteric route described is usually indicated for short-term therapy in many clinical situations. However, for long-term feedings, enterostomies-surgical placement of the tube at progressive points along the gastrointestinal tract-are the preferred route[16,17]:

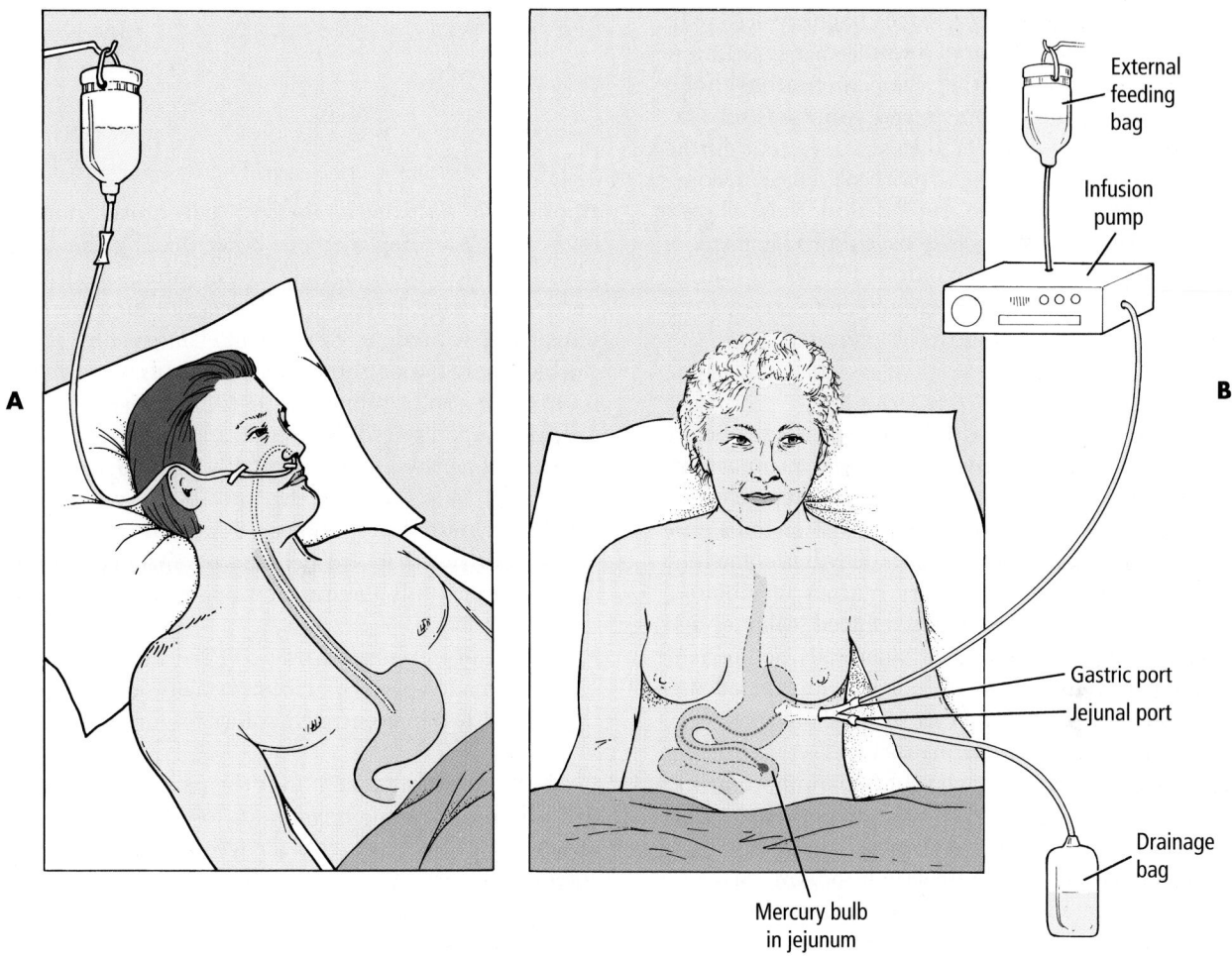

Figure 17.1   Types of tube feeding. **A,** Common nasogastric feeding tube. **B,** Gastrostomy-jejunal enteral feeding tube.

- **Esophagostomy.** A cervical esophagostomy is often placed at the level of the cervical spine to the side of the neck after head and neck surgeries for cancer or traumatic injury. This removes the discomfort of the nasal route and the entry point can be concealed easily under clothing.
- **Gastrostomy.** A gastrostomy tube may be surgically placed in the stomach if the patient is not at risk for aspiration.
- **Jejunostomy.** A jejunostomy tube is surgically placed in the duodenum, the middle section of the small intestine, if the patient is at risk for aspiration. This procedure is indicated for patients who lack a competent gag reflex or who have gastric cancer or gastric ulcerative disease.

MONITORING THE TUBE-FED PATIENT

The nutrition support team carefully monitors all patients who are being nourished by tube-feeding.[21] The nursing staff administering the formula to the patient checks for gastric residuals or gastric emptying rate, noting any signs of abdominal distention or bloating, and

monitors usual vital signs—temperature, pulse, and respiration. Attending nurses also monitor the flow rate and record the intake and output of formula and fluid, as well as observe and report any individual patient responses to the formula.

The nutrition support team clinical dietitian monitors tolerance for the formula, state of hydration, and nutritional status response following laboratory test panels commonly included in nutrition support assessment protocols (see p. 351). Also monitored are any other special test results related to the patient's disease status or metabolic complications, such as insulin-dependent diabetes mellitus (IDDM), traumatic injury, or sepsis.

Formula tolerance

Gastrointestinal signs of vomiting, abdominal distention or bloating, and frequency and consistency of bowel move-

---

medical foods   Specially formulated nutrient mixtures for use under medical supervision to treat various metabolic diseases.

ments are noted. If these occur, the feeding may need to be adjusted to a less concentrated formula that is fed more slowly with continuous rather than intermittent bolus feeding until tolerance improves and symptoms subside. Daily blood and urine tests for glucose and acetone during the first week or so, according to protocol, reflect carbohydrate tolerance. Patients who are diabetic or those who are severely stressed with sepsis may have difficulty metabolizing carbohydrate and are monitored closely.[21] Rather than reducing the formula carbohydrate needed for energy, sometimes insulin is given as indicated.

Hydration status

Daily weights, compared with a baseline weight before starting the formula, along with daily *separate* input-output measures and records of formula and water are essential. Sudden weight changes indicate hydration imbalance and need to be investigated. Signs of dehydration include weight loss; poor skin turgor; dry mucous membranes; low blood pressure from decreased blood volume; and increased levels of serum protein, blood cells, and hematocrit. Signs of overhydration include weight gain, edema, jugular vein distension, and elevated blood pressure.

Regular protocol monitoring includes serum tests for glucose, potassium, sodium, chloride, albumin, complete blood cell counts, and blood urea nitrogen along with periodic tests for urine specific gravity. Dehydration indicators include elevated blood levels of sodium, chloride, glucose, and urea and elevated levels of hematocrit and urine specific gravity. Severe dehydration is critical and life-threatening. It can be prevented by careful monitoring and supplying the patient's daily fluid requirements with needed water given through the tube. If it does occur, the feeding is stopped and intravenous rehydration with a 5% glucose solution usually follows. The nutrition support clinical dietitian monitors the patient's nutritional response with regular assessments according to the hospital's established protocol.

DOCUMENTATION OF THE ENTERAL NUTRITION TUBE-FEEDING

The patient's medical record is always one of the most essential means of careful communication among the members of any health care team. It is especially necessary for nutrition support teams in monitoring each tube-fed patient and responding rapidly to individual reactions and needs. Divisions of team responsibilities vary, but the team clinical dietitian, usually a certified nutrition support specialist with advanced academic and clinical preparation, is involved in actions and documentation related to (1) all ongoing nutritional analyses of the actual formula intake, (2) tolerance of the formula and any complications, (3) recommendations for corrective actions in formula changes, tubing, method and rate of delivery, and (4) education for patient and family.

PARENTERAL FEEDING IN CLINICAL NUTRITION

BASIC TECHNIQUE

Applied to nutritional therapy, **parenteral** nutrition refers to any feeding methods other than by the normal gastrointestinal route. Specifically, in current medical and nutritional usage, it refers to the special feeding method of infusing basic predigested nutrient elements directly into the blood circulation through certain veins when the gastrointestinal tract cannot be used. Depending on the nutrition support need, two routes are available:

- *Central parenteral nutrition (CPN).* The use of a large central vein, usually the subclavian vein leading directly into the rapid blood flow of the superior vena cava to the heart, to deliver concentrated solutions that supply full nutritional support for longer periods (Figure 17.2).
- *Peripheral parenteral nutrition (PPN).* The alternate use of a smaller peripheral vein, usually in the arm, to deliver less concentrated solutions for brief periods (Figure 17.3).

Since the development over the past three decades of these basic surgical techniques of inserting venous catheters into specific veins for feeding basic nutrients, enteral and parenteral nutrition have provided major advances in critical patient care.[22] They serve the needs of patients with major illness from traumatic injury or extensive debilitating disease. They combat actual or potential malnutrition and meet hypermetabolic nutritional demands. When the patient's condition is further complicated by inability to eat or take enteral tube feeding, nutritional status can be improved and maintained over extended periods solely through intravenous feeding. Hypertonic solutions of essential nutrients can be fed into the greater, rapid blood flow of a large central vein, avoiding the vascular inflammation and thrombosis potential of such concentrated solutions in smaller vessels. Thus individually required amounts of life-sustaining nourishment, which is otherwise not available, are delivered. This complete sustaining of individual nutritional requirements through intravenous feeding has been termed *total parenteral nutrition (TPN)*.

TOTAL PARENTERAL NUTRITION DEVELOPMENT

Largely through the pioneering work of American surgeon Stanley Dudrick and his associates, the current era of parenteral nutrition found its direction in the early 1970s.[23,24] In following years, development of the surgical technique, equipment, and solutions to meet the increased nutritional requirements of catabolic illness and injury has led to its current widespread use and future directions.[22]

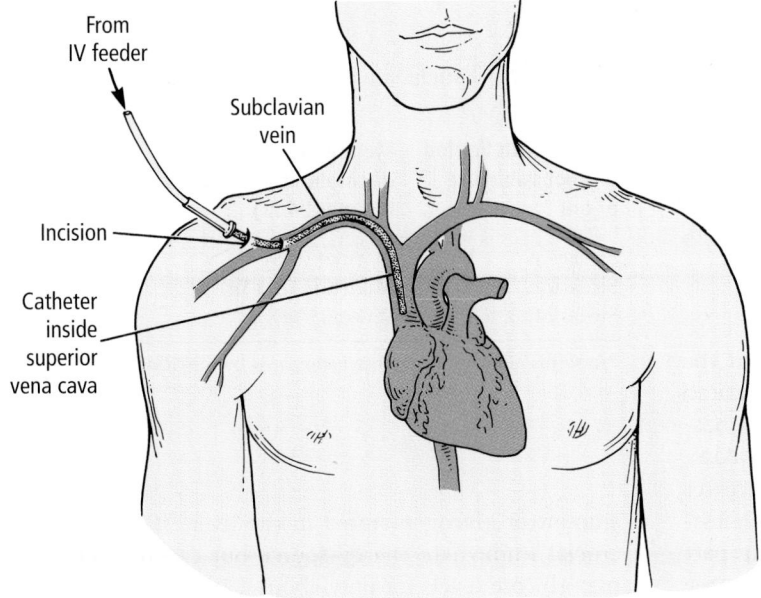

Figure 17.2   Catheter placement for total parenteral nutrition (TPN) made for feeding via subclavian vein to superior vena cava.

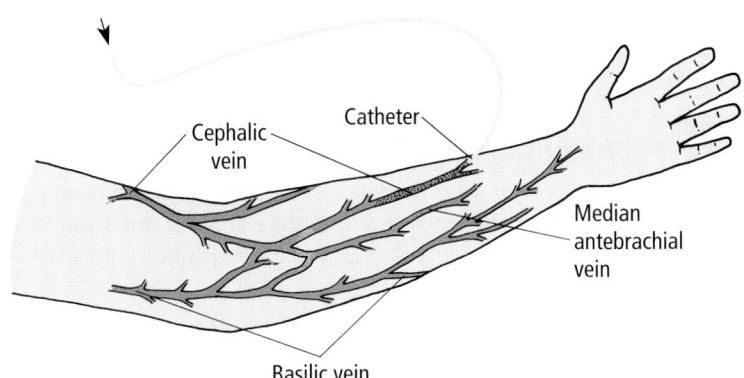

Figure 17.3   Peripheral parenteral nutrition feeding into small veins in the arm.

Over the past two decades since its early development, TPN has provided not only brief periods of concentrated nutrition rehabilitation but also an ongoing life support system for some individuals on a continuing basis for at least 10 years. Many studies in the past few years have demonstrated the effectiveness of carefully administered TPN by a highly skilled nutrition support team to wisely selected patients. Also, clinical experience has shown that PPN can be used in many cases as a viable alternative for brief periods, or it may be used in conjunction with oral intake or tube feeding. This is frequently the case in transition feeding. The nutritional support team's clinical dietitian assesses the patient's nutritional status, calculates the nutritional needs, and then designs an appropriate parenteral solution to be recommended to the team physician. Currently, a wide spectrum of nutrient solutions and delivery systems exist from which individual nutritional therapy can be planned to meet the clinical problems presented. Nutrition support team pharmacists mix each individual patient solution, and after surgical placement of the indwelling venous catheter, nutrition support nurses administer the individualized solution to the patient.

INDICATIONS FOR PARENTERAL NUTRITION SUPPORT

Three basic factors govern decisions about the use of parenteral nutrition: availability of the gastrointestinal tract, degree of malnutrition, and degree of hypermetabolism or catabolism.[25] Risks are involved as well as considerable increase in costs. Thus careful assessment of each of these considerations is imperative.

---

parenteral   A mode of feeding that does not use the gastrointestinal tract, but instead provides nutrition by intravenous delivery of nutrient solutions.

Availability of the gastrointestinal tract

If major abdominal injury, for example, has made the natural gastrointestinal pathway totally unusable, an alternate means of sustaining nutrition and life is an obvious necessity. In other cases the gastrointestinal tract may be unavailable because of obstruction, **fistulas**, or malignant disease. In still other cases the patient may be unable to eat because of coma, severe anorexia and self-starvation, or mental disturbance.

Degree of malnutrition

Any medical treatment has less chance of success if the patient is malnourished. Many studies have indicated that far more general malnutrition exists among hospitalized patients than was previously assumed. Also, it is now clear that disease imposes an even greater threat to positive nutritional status. Thus the assessment of nutritional status becomes an important part of overall care, especially for hospitalized patients (see Chapter 15). For the severely malnourished patient, especially those facing problems such as major organ failure or extensive surgery, serious consideration of TPN is indicated (Table 17.2).

Degree of hypermetabolism or catabolism

When a patient is suffering from major trauma or severe sepsis from radiation or chemotherapy enteritis in treatment for malignant disease (see Chapter 24), the rate of catabolism, or the inability to absorb nutrients, may take a devastating toll on the body's resources. This toll as measured by nitrogen balance studies may range up to 15 g of nitrogen over 24 hours. The loss may be even more severe in some patients such as athletes with large lean body masses and extensive injuries. Catabolic periods seem inevitable following extensive surgery and large losses of body resources. The extent of these increased demands is seen in the increased nutritional requirements, especially in energy demand.

BASIC RULES FOR TOTAL PARENTERAL NUTRITION USE

With these three basic considerations in mind, most clinicians have formed general rules to guide TPN decisions as the preferred means of therapy. Some combinations of these factors are illustrated in Table 17.2. Two basic rules have evolved that form the basis for choice of TPN.

The "rule of five"

If a patient has had no food for 5 days and is likely not to be able to eat for another 5 days, TPN must be considered then rather than waiting until malnutrition has developed. It is an easier task to maintain positive nutrition than to replenish body stores from malnutrition losses. Starvation effects on the body, even during relatively brief periods, are well documented. The small

Table 17.2	Patient situations imposing need for TPN	
Patient with limited or impossible use of gut	**Metabolic rate, degree of catabolism (nitrogen loss per 24 hr)**	**Degree of malnutrition***
Situation 1	Normal (0.8g)	Normal
Situation 2	Moderate (8-15g)	Moderate
Situation 3	Severe (15g)	Severe

*In terms of percent of normal standards by nutritional assessment.

amount of glycogen stored in the liver, 50 to 75 g, is a crucial immediate energy source but can maintain normal glucose levels for only about 12 hours. Amino acids from body tissue proteins are then deaminated to provide blood glucose for needed metabolic functions with a urinary nitrogen loss of 10 to 15 g/day. Also, fatty acids are mobilized from the body's adipose tissues to provide keto acids as the principle fuel for the heart, brain, and other vital organs.

Weight loss rule

Any patient who has lost 7% of their usual body weight over 2 months and who is deprived of oral nutrition for 5 to 7 days or longer is a candidate for TPN.

PATIENT CANDIDATES FOR PARENTERAL NUTRITION

Total parenteral nutrition

On the basis of these general considerations, a number of patient situation examples suggest a need for vigorous TPN support[26]:

- *Preoperative preparation of severely malnourished patients:* Congenital anomalies causing gastrointestinal disorders, stricture or cancer of the esophagus and swallowing difficulty, cancer of the stomach, severe peptic ulcer disease, or gastric obstruction
- *Postoperative surgical complications:* Prolonged ileus and obstruction; stomal dysfunction; short bowel syndrome; enterocutaneous, biliary, or pancreatic fistulas; and peritoneal sepsis
- *Inflammatory bowel disease:* Intractable gastroenteritis, regional enteritis (for example, acute Crohn's disease; see Chapter 18), ulcerative colitis, extensive diverticulitis, and radiation enteritis
- *Inadequate oral intake or malabsorption:* Malignant neoplasms and chemotherapy or radiation therapy; acute and relapsing pancreatitis; hypermetabolic states, major trauma, and massive burns; coma, hepatic insufficiency, or encephalopathy; and chronic malnutrition or anorexia nervosa

Peripheral parenteral nutrition

Generally, decisions to use peripheral parenteral nutrition (PPN) instead of TPN are based on comparative energy demands and anticipated time of use. PPN is usually the choice in the following situations:

- *Energy needs:* No more than 2000 kcal/day required
- *Time of use:* No more than 10 days of therapy needed

NUTRITION ASSESSMENT

The nutrition support team clinical dietitian provides initial nutritional assessment and ongoing monitoring of nutritional status. Initial assessment data supply the necessary basis for (1) identifying patients requiring special therapy, (2) calculating their nutritional requirements, and (3) determining the specific nutrient formulas to meet these requirements. Once therapy begins, careful monitoring helps maintain optimal therapy and avoid metabolic complications.

Guidelines for nutrition assessment

Necessary nutrition assessment is done by the standard approach: (1) dietary evaluations, (2) clinical observations, (3) biochemical laboratory data, (4) anthropometrics—together with comprehensive detailed histories.[27] These methods are described in detail in Chapter 15. Specific guidelines for parenteral nutrition support, depending on individual needs and clinical situations, include the following six procedures.

1. *Classify degree of weight loss.* Use measures of current body weight and height. Interpret actual body weight (ABW) in terms of desirable body weight for height (DBW), usual body weight (UBW), and amount of recent weight change:

   Percent desirable weight = ABW ÷ DBW × 100
   Percent usual body weight = ABW ÷ UBW × 100
   Percent weight change =
   [(UBW − ABW) ÷ UBW] × 100

   Compare the patient's amount of recent weight change with the values indicating malnutrition given in Table 17.3.

2. *Estimate body fat stores and skeletal muscle mass.* Use measure of triceps skinfold (TSF) and standard reference tables (Appendix I) for TSF data. Estimate body fat stores using measures of mid-upper arm circumference to derive value for mid-upper arm muscle circumference (MAMC) and compare with standard reference tables. This gives an estimate of the patient's muscle mass interpreted as a percentage of the standard:

   MAMC (cm) = MAC (cm) − [0.314 × TSF (mm)]

3. *Estimate lean body mass.* Use the creatinine-height index (CHI) as an estimate of overall lean body mass. Compute the patient's CHI by using the daily urinary creatinine excretion value determined by laboratory analysis of a 24-hour urine collection. Compare this value with the ideal creatinine value for the patient's height in centimeters from standard tables (see Chapter 15). This gives an effective index of the patient's overall muscle mass and total lean body mass.

4. *Calculate degree of catabolism.* Measure the degree of catabolism by calculating the daily nitrogen balance, using the patient's protein intake for the day (food or formula) and the laboratory analysis of the urinary urea nitrogen output in a 24-hour urine collection for the same day:

   N balance = N intake (protein intake ÷ 6.25)
   − N loss (urinary urea N + 4)

5. *Estimate immune function.* Use the total lymphocyte count or the percentage of lymphocytes in the total white blood cell (WBC) count to determine general function of the patient's immune system. Compare this with the values in Table 17.4.

   Total lymphocyte count = Percent lymphocytes
   × WBC ÷ 100

   Delayed sensitivity skin testing is occasionally used with hospitalized patients at risk for **anergy** as a means of detecting cellular immune status (see Chapter 15).

6. *Measure plasma protein compartment.* Measure serum transferrin directly, or using laboratory analysis of total iron-binding capacity (TIBC), calculate the value for transferrin, the body's iron transport protein compound:

   Transferrin (mg/dl) = [TIBC (μg/dl) × 0.8] − 43

   The serum albumin measure (half-life of 21 days) provides additional long-term data concerning the body's visceral protein mass. However, a decreased transferrin value (half-life of 10 days) is a more sensitive marker of recent malnutrition. Prealbumin (half-life of 2 days) is the most sensitive marker of current status. Compare these serum values obtained for the patient with values in Table 17.4.

Baseline and monitoring assessment for total parenteral nutrition

Baseline nutritional data before starting TPN provide a means of measuring effectiveness of treatment. At designated periods during therapy, certain tests are repeated to

---

anergy Diminished immunologic reactivity to specific antigens.

fistula Abnormal passageway, usually between two internal organs or leading from an internal organ to the surface of the body.

Table 17.3	Indication of severe protein-kcalorie malnutrition according to percentage of recent weight loss	
Body weight loss (%)		**Time period**
2		1 week
5		1 month
7.5		3 months
10		6 months

Table 17.4	Determination of protein-kcalorie malnutrition by plasma values			
			Degree of malnutrition	
Laboratory data	**Normal values**		**Moderate**	**Severe**
Serum albumin (g/dl)	3.5		2.1-3	<2.1
Serum transferrin (mg/dl)	180-260		100-150	<100
Total lymphocyte count per mm^3	1500-4000		800-1200	<800
% WBC	20-53			

monitor the patient's course and avoid metabolic complications. Specific protocols vary in different medical centers. However, a general guide for such standard monitoring data is summarized in Box 17.4. All baseline and monitoring data are recorded in the patient's chart, along with all TPN solution orders.

Clinical recommendations

Generally, clinicians give primary importance to two major monitoring procedures: (1) constant evaluation of kcalorie intake to ensure adequacy of the energy base to meet metabolic demands and (2) regular measure of protein—nitrogen adequacy to meet tissue rebuilding needs. Nutrition support teams are increasingly using the laboratory test for **prealbumin (PAB)**—normal value 15.7 to 29.6 mg/dl-as the most sensitive rapid plasma protein marker of current malnutrition status and response to nutritional support because of its rapid turnover and half-life of only 2 days.[21,27]

PARENTERAL SOLUTIONS

THE TOTAL PARERNTERAL NUTRITION PRESCRIPTION

The TPN prescription and plan of care are based on the calculation of basic nutritional requirements plus additional needs resulting from the patient's degree of catabolism, malnutrition, and any activity. An example of a basic TPN formula plan is shown in Table 17.5. This same principle guides nutritional therapy in any feeding mode. Nutritional needs are fundamental—energy (kcalories), protein, electrolytes, minerals, and vitamins.

ENERGY REQUIREMENTS

The energy needs of critically ill patients are great, even as high as twice the normal basal rates in the case of major trauma such as massive burns.[28] Energy require-

ments from three sources must be met: basal energy expenditures (BEE), added energy cost of catabolism, fever, and malnutrition—the metabolic activity factor (MAF) (see Chapter 22), and any physical activity.

Basal energy expenditure

An estimate of the adult patient's energy needs for basal tissue metabolism is commonly calculated by the classic Harris-Benedict equations, which involve measures of weight in kilograms, height in centimeters, and age in years:[29]

Women: BEE = 655 + [9.6 × weight(kg)] + [1.7 × height(cm)] − [4.7 × age(yr)]

Men: BEE = 66 + [13.7 × weight(kg)] + [5 × height(cm)] − [6.8 × age(yr)]

The term *resting energy expenditure (REE)* is often used interchangeably with BEE in discussing basal energy needs. For practical purposes they are synonymous and are calculated by the same equations. Recent studies of the effect of age on response to TPN reinforce the fact that depleted body composition in malnourished older patients over the age of 65 years is restored more slowly than in younger adults and requires a greater kcaloric intake.[30]

Additional energy requirements

In addition to basal energy needs, total kcalorie requirements reflect the large energy drain of the illness or injury, including the additional metabolic injury factor (MAF) (see Chapter 22). Physiologic stress demands sufficient kcalories to combat the hypermetabolism and its resulting catabolic state and weight loss. If any large degree of malnutrition exists, even more kcalories are needed. Total energy requirements must also include any muscular or physical activity. This need varies considerably depending on the patient's condition, respiratory status, fever or sepsis, and extent of mobility.

Box
17.4 Monitoring protocol for TPN

Baseline tests

CBC: Hb   Nitrogen balance   SGOT
      Hct   Fe and TIBC   Alkaline phos-
                          phatase
      RBC indexes   FBS   Serum osmolality
      WBC differ-   BUN   Cholesterol
        ential count
      Platelets   Creatinine   Triglycerides
Na^+ Ca^{++} Uric acid   Urinalysis
K^+ PO_4 PT   Chest x-ray film
Cl^- Mg^{++} PTT   ECG
CO_2 Prealbumin   Body weight (kg)
               Albumin   Height (cm)
Skin tests (PPD,   Total protein
   mumps, cocci)   Bilirubin

Stabilization tests (daily for first 5-7 days)

Fractional urine (sugar and acetone) every 6 hours; simulta-
   neous blood sugar first and second days
Body weight
Intake and output record
Nitrogen balance
Serum electrolytes
Blood glucose
Prealbumin

Follow-up routine

Daily   Fractional urine (sugar and acetone)
                Body weight
                Intake and output
                Electrolytes (Na+, K+, Cl^-, CO_2)
                Prealbumin
Once a week   CBC: Platelets   PT Mg^{++}
                    RBC indexes   Ca++
                Creatinine PO_4
                BUN
Once a month   Repeat baseline tests
                Add serum vitamin B_{12}, folate, Zn^{++}

CBC, Complete blood cell count: *Hb,* hemoglobin; *Hct,* hematocrit; *RBC,* red blood cell; *WBC,* white blood cell; *PPD,* purified protein derivative of tuberculin; *TIBC,* total iron-binding capacity; *FBS,* fasting blood sugar; *BUN,* blood urea nitrogen; *PT,* prothrombin time; *PTT,* partial thromboplastin time; *SGOT,* serum glutamic oxaloacetic transaminase; *ECG,* electrocardiogram.

In comparison with normal needs, the general range of energy requirements for hospitalized patients on parenteral nutrition support varies with the degree of added metabolic stress:

- Normal needs—25 to 30 kcal/kg/day
- Elective surgery—28 to 30 kcal/kg/day
- Severe injury—30 to 40 kcal/kg/day
- Extensive trauma or burns—45 to 55 kcal/kg/day

Table
17.5 Example of basic TPN formula components

Components	Amounts
Basic solution	
Crystalline amino acids	2.75%
Dextrose	25%
Additives	
Electrolytes	
Na	50 mEq/L
Cl	50 mEq/L
K	40 mEq/L
HPO_4	25 mEq/L
Ca	5 mEq/L
Mg	8 mEq/L
Vitamins	
Multiple (MV)	1.7 ml conc./L
Vitamin C (per day)	500 mg
Trace elements solution (per day)	
Zn	3 mg
Cu	1.6 mg
Cr	2 μg
Se	120 μg
Mn	2 μg
I	120 μg
Fe	1.5 μg
Other additives (as needed)	
Regular insulin	0-25 U/L
Heparin	1000 U/L

PROTEIN REQUIREMENTS

Nitrogen balance

The function of protein in health is to sustain tissue growth and maintenance. In healthy adults this ideal state is reflected in nitrogen equilibrium. In illness, however, catabolism is reflected by negative nitrogen balance, that is, more nitrogen loss than intake, indicating wasting of tissue protein. Thus the goal of nutritional therapy in illness is to maintain positive nitrogen balance, constantly monitored by accurate nitrogen balance studies, to counteract the catabolic deterioration.[31]

Essential amino acids

The quality of the protein intake in terms of equivalent essential amino acids is fundamental to tissue synthesis (see *To Probe Further* box, p. 354). The essential amino acids must be present in the optimal ratio for best use of

prealbumin (PAB) Plasma protein with short life used a biochemical measure for assessing current nutritional status.

To Probe Further

General comfort tips for patients on nasoenteric tube feedings

- *Thirst, oral dryness.* Lubricate lips, chew sugarless gum, brush teeth, rinse mouth frequently with water, suck lemon drops occasionally.
- *Tube discomfort.* Gargle with a mixture of warm water and mouth wash, gently blow nose, and clean tube regularly with water-soluble lubricant. If persistent, pull tube out gently, clean it, and reinsert the tube. (Many long-term users of tube feeding have learned to pass their own nasogastric tubes.)

- *Tension, fullness.* Relax and breathe deeply after each feeding.
- *Loud stomach noises.* Take feedings in private.
- *Limited mobility.* Change positions in bed or chair, and walk around the house or hospital corridor.
- *General gustatory distress with feeding.* Warm or chill feedings, but avoid having formula too cold because that causes diarrhea, and check about occasional use of blender-mixed "regular" foods.
- *Persistent hunger.* Chew a favorite food, then spit it out; chew gum, or suck lemon drops.
- *Inability to drink.* Rinse mouth frequently with water or other liquids.

---

individual amino acids. Two additional protein substances recently found to be "conditionally essential" in TPN use: (1) *glutamine*, the most abundant amino acid in the blood, and (2) *choline*, an amine that is everywhere throughout the body. During prolonged TPN, glutamine protects the epithelial tissue lining the gastrointestinal tract.[32-34] Choline helps protect the liver from hepatic fat deposits that hinder its function.[35]

Ratio of nitrogen to nonprotein kcalories

To protect the nitrogen sources (the amino acids) and make them available for tissue synthesis, sufficient nonprotein (fat and carbohydrate) energy sources must be present to meet the increased kcaloric need. Carbohydrates are necessary to promote incorporation of plasma amino acids into muscle tissue protein. For optimal use, the normal adult diet sustains a ratio of 150 nonprotein kcal/1 g of nitrogen. To meet the metabolic stress of critical illness with minimal activity, this ratio should be 150 to 200 kcal/1 g of nitrogen. In terms of protein, the requirements in illness reflect these increased needs:

Catabolic state: Weight (kg) × 1.2 to 1.5 g protein

Healthy state: Weight (kg) × 0.8 to 1 g protein

ELECTROLYTE REQUIREMENTS

Special electrolyte profiles are required in intracellular and extracellular fluid for all tissues to maintain normal water balances throughout the body (see Chapter 8). These balances must be maintained during illness in the face of metabolic imbalances. For example, active tissue synthesis requires phosphate and potassium and is also influenced by available sodium and chloride ions. Moni-

toring of individual electrolyte status supplies the data needed to determine daily electrolyte requirements.

In general, the basic electrolyte needs for a 3000 kcalorie intake (3 L solution) are approximately the following:

Chloride (Cl)	150 mEq
Potassium (K)	120 mEq
Sodium (Na)	120 to 150 mEq
Phosphate (HPO_4)	60 to 75 mEq
Magnesium (Mg)	24 to 36 mEq
Calcium (Ca)	6 to 15 mEq

VITAMIN AND MINERAL REQUIREMENTS

Vitamin and mineral needs are based on normal standards (see current RDAs listed inside front cover of this book), with increases according to metabolic states. Individual nutrients may be added as needed to cover increased metabolism and depletion states. Attention to necessary trace elements is especially important. Patients on long-term TPN have shown deficiencies of iron, zinc, and copper, and more recently significant deficiencies of selenium, chromium, and molybdenum have occurred. Trace element supplements of zinc and copper are needed especially by patients with severe burns because of their essential roles in wound healing during the acute recovery period.[36] The prescribed TPN solution reflects these needs and additions.

PREPARATION OF THE TOTAL PARERNTERAL NUTRITION SOLUTION

A number of differing strength solutions of the basic nutrients are available for use by the TPN team in formulating individual nutritional needs, including protein, nonprotein energy, electrolytes, vitamins, and minerals.

Protein-nitrogen source

In the TPN solution, protein-nitrogen need is supplied by essential and nonessential crystalline amino acids. Standard commercial amino acid solutions produced by various manufacturers range in concentration from 3% to 11.4%, but the general standard product is the 8.5% solution.

In addition, two types of specialized amino acid solutions have been formulated, although they are more expensive than standard solutions and their superiority remains unclear. One type is enriched with the three branched-chain amino acids (BCAAs)-isoleucine, leucine, and valine-and designed for patients with extensive trauma and severe catabolic stress, or with liver failure, who have shown low plasma levels of these three amino acids. The other type is enriched with essential amino acids and designed to prevent development of hyperuremia in patients with acute renal failure. For most TPN patients, a usual amino acid need is supplied by a 4.25% dilution achieved by the use of 1 L of standard 8.5% amino acid solution mixed with 1 L of dextrose solution.

Nonprotein energy source (kcalories)

Nonprotein kcalories in TPN solutions protect protein (amino acids) for tissues synthesis demands. The major energy needs are supplied by glucose and lipid solutions.

1 *Glucose (dextrose).* Glucose is the most common and least expensive source of kcalories used for parenteral nutrition support. Hypertonic 50% to 70% solutions are available for use in TPN formulations. The most commonly used standard is the 50% solution. Glucose used in parenteral nutrition support is commercially available as dextrose monohydrate ($C_6H_{12}O_6H_2O$), which has an energy value of 3.4 kcal/g, not the energy value of 4 kcal/g of the regular dietary glucose form ($C_6H_{12}O_6$).

2. *Lipids.* Lipid emulsions provide a concentrated energy source, 9 kcal/g, as well as the essential fatty acid, linoleic acid. Lipids also have practical values associated with their effects on respiratory gas (carbon dioxide and oxygen) exchange, autoimmune disease, and vascular disease. About 4% to 10% of the daily kcaloric intake should consist of fat emulsion to prevent fatty acid deficiency. A 500-ml bottle of 10% or 20% fat emulsion provides 555 kcalories (1.1 kcal/ml) or 1000 kcalories (2 kcal/ml), respectively. Available commercial products use lipid emulsions of soybean oil and safflower combined or soybean oil alone.

Traditionally, lipid emulsions were fed separately. More recently, however, with improved solutions and equipment, in some cases lipids have been combined with the dextrose and amino acid base and called a 3-in-1 **admixture**.[36-37] With the additional modules of electrolytes and vitamins and adequate fluid, the whole feeding is identified as a *total nutrient admixture (TNA)*. Stable TNAs have also been prepared successfully for pediatric use.[38] Current refinements in products and technique have allowed various admixtures of lipids, carbohydrates, and protein in a common bag, complete with adequate fluid and electrolytes and either single or multiple forms of vitamins and trace elements. Newer alternative lipid sources include forms such as short-chain fatty acids, medium-chain fatty acids, omega-3 fatty acids, and blended or structured lipids.

Electrolytes

Electrolytes in TPN formulas are based on the usual requirements for normal electrolyte balance with adjustments according to individual patient monitoring. Commercial amino acid formulations are available with or without added electrolytes. If electrolytes are present in the amino acid solution, they must be taken into account when calculating additions for a specific patient requirement. Three actions are basic in managing individual needs: (1) correct any preexisting deficits immediately, (2) recognize and replace excessive fluid and electrolyte losses to prevent chronic deficits, and (3) monitor and determine electrolyte needs daily.

Vitamins

The Nutrition Advisory Group of the American Medical Association has established guidelines for parenteral administration of 12 vitamins: A, D, E, thiamin, riboflavin, niacin, pantothenic acid, pyridoxine, folate, biotin, cobalamin, and ascorbic acid. Multivitamin preparations based on these guidelines are available. Vitamin K is not a component of any formulation for adults. If it is needed for individual maintenance, it is added to the solution. Any larger deficit is treated by periodic intramuscular injection as needed.

Trace elements

The American Medical Association has also set guidelines for the addition of four trace elements in TPN solutions: zinc, copper, manganese, and chromium. To these four elements, some manufacturers add selenium in a separate product. Single mineral products are also available for each of these trace elements. Iron is not routinely added. If it is needed by an individual patient, it is administered apart from the TPN admixture. Caution is needed in

---

admixture A mixture resulting from adding or mingling another ingredient; a combination of two or more substances that are not chemically united or that exist in no fixed proportion to each other.

adding minerals to the TPN solution. Incompatibilities of certain electrolytes and other components may form insoluble substances that separate out, depending on ion concentration and solution pH.

PARENTERAL NUTRITION DELIVERY SYSTEM

EQUIPMENT

Strict aseptic technique throughout the entire TPN administration by all the special nutrition support team members involved is absolutely essential. This includes: (1) the solution preparation by the pharmacist, (2) the surgical placement of the venous catheter by the physician, and (3) the care of the catheter site and all external equipment and administration of the solution by the nurse. At every step of the TPN process, strict infection control is one of the primary team responsibilities.

Venous catheter

Surgical placement of the venous catheter is done by the physician (a surgeon) at the bedside, using local anesthesia. Commercially prepared sterile kits contain all the necessary equipment items for gaining access to a large central vein for feeding the nutrition support solution directly into the central blood circulation. Flexible silicone catheters are available in different lengths and calibers.[39,40] Smaller, shorter catheters (15 to 25 cm) are designed for use in the hospital. Larger, longer catheters such as the 1.6 mm caliber Hickman catheter are designed for long-term intermediate or home use. The catheter is passed through the outer vein, usually the subclavian vein, into the central superior vena cava, which leads directly into the heart (Figure 17.2). In the vena cava the catheter tip lies so that concentrated solutions, five times the concentration of blood plasma, can be infused at a rate of 2 to 3 ml/min and can be immediately diluted by a large blood flow of 2 to 5 L/min, a dilution factor of at least a thousand.[39,40] The continuing development of TPN has led to new catheters and insertion techniques that have greatly reduced catheter-related complications. Commercial sterile dressing kits for continuing nursing care have also aided aseptic technique and infection control.

Infusion devices

Various infusion devices control the solution flow rate and maintain an accurate flow range. Infusion pumps may be used to deliver the solution at a constant rate to prevent metabolic complication. Protocols for external delivery system tubing changes guided by infection control monitoring include maintenance of sterility of the catheter hub and tubing junction.[39,40]

SOLUTION ADMINISTRATION

During the administration of the TPN solution, each patient has individual responses and needs for adjustments, according to fluctuations and changes in the illness or injury and the concentrated feeding. The skilled nutrition support nurse checks frequently to see that the entire TPN delivery system is operating accurately according to the support team protocol (see *Practical Application* box).

MONITORING

In the hands of a well-trained TPN team, risks have been minimized and complications controlled by constant team effort. Specific protocols, updated periodically as needed, guide continuing assessment and monitoring. Related solution adjustments by the nutrition support team are made according to metabolic and nutritional needs.

HOME NUTRITION SUPPORT

HOME ENTERAL NUTRITION

Patient selection

Home enteral nutrition tube-feeding is not useful to all patients. But for those who require continued tube-feeding to meet their clinical and nutritional needs, it provides a safe, and relatively simple method of replenishing and maintaining nutrition support. Recent rapid developments in enteral formulas and tube-feeding equipment have now simplified home feeding and made it easier to manage.[41] As a result, the number of patients using tube-feeding for home enteral nutrition continues to grow as a means of cutting hospital costs and allowing earlier family support at home. Home care requires training of both patient and family. A recent survey of dietitians in home care indicated that 55% of their patients were receiving enteral tube feedings, 29% received TPN, or a combination of tube feedings and TPN, 17%.[42]

Teaching plan

Educating the patient and family for home care is usually a team responsibility of the nutrition support clinical dietitian and nurse. First, the clinical dietitian determines the patient's current nutrient and fluid requirements, selects the formula, complete or modular, computes formula amounts to be used, and outlines the feeding schedule. Then the dietitian and the nurse develop and carry out a teaching plan together, which includes the following topics and related tasks in preparing patients and families for discharge on home enteral feeding:[41,42]

- The nature of the formula, its rationale and preparation
- The feeding process, equipment, and function
- How to flush the tube and care for the tube site

practical application

Total parenteral nutrition administration

Of all the various ways of nourishing the human body-normal eating, liquid diets, enteral nutrition, parenteral nutrition-total parenteral nutrition (TPN) requires the highest degree of skilled and precise administration. The risk of potentially life-threatening complication and infection is ever present. The role of the trained nutrition support nurse is central in successful TPN. The nutrition support nurse administers the TPN solution according to the nutrition support team protocol, monitoring the entire TPN system frequently to see that it is operating accurately.

Specific clinical protocols will vary somewhat, but they usually include the following points:
- **Start slowly.** Give the patient time to adapt to the increased glucose concentration and osmolality of the solution.
- **Schedule carefully.** During the first 24 hours give 1 to 2 L by continuous drip. The slow rate is usually regulated by an infusion pump.
- **Monitor closely.** Note metabolic effects of glucose (blood glucose levels not to exceed 200 mg/dl) and electrolytes.

- **Increase volume gradually.** After the first day, increase by 1 L/day to reach desired daily volume.
- **Make changes cautiously.** Watch the effect of all changes and proceed slowly.
- **Maintain a constant rate.** Keep to the correct hourly infusion rate, with no "catch-up" or "slow-down" effort to meet the original volume order.
- **Discontinue slowly.** Discontinue TPN feeding gradually, reducing rate and daily volume about 1 L/day.

- How to recognize formula intolerance
- How to avoid complications
- How to give medications with the feeding

The nutrition support clinical dietitian is responsible for the tasks that assess needs and determine the formula components and their preparation. The nurse is usually responsible for tasks related to feeding process and equipment. Then the dietitian and the nurse share the teaching tasks related to formula intolerance, complications, and medications. In reality, it is team teaching throughout. The nutrition support team clinical pharmacist may share the final topic on medications.

The hospital's nutrition support team develops a teaching manual with illustrations to guide the teaching-learning process and for continuing reference at home. The teaching plan should start as soon as the decision for home feeding is made. A social worker should join the team to (1) schedule a separate counseling visit to determine any personal, psychosocial, or economic problems with the care, and (2) confer with the nutrition support team to help work through these problems.

Finally, the teaching plan should allow 2 full days before discharge for the patient and family to practice with the support nurse and for the clinical dietitian to observe the patient (1) administering the formula and (2) recording all necessary information about formula and fluid intake, formula tolerance, and complications. Direc-

tions for this record are included in the home care manual. Records are reviewed regularly by home support team specialists providing follow-up care at home and in the clinic.

Follow-up monitoring

The plan for follow-up monitoring should be guided by the specific protocol schedule developed by the nutrition support team for laboratory, clinical, and nutritional assessments. In early home visits the clinical dietitian-nurse team checks progress. Together with the patient and family they troubleshoot any problems that need to be worked out or that require adjustments in the formula or feeding plan.

HOME PARENTERAL NUTRITION

Experience from home use of other long-term medical care equipment, such as that for renal dialysis, has led to the concept of self-infusion of parenteral nutrients at home. Following the pattern given for home enteral nutrition, a full patient and family TPN education plan with supervised practice is essential. In the hands of selected, well-trained patients and their families, home TPN allows mobility and travel. It has offered special promise in long-term management of conditions such as severe abdominal injury or chronic severe inflammatory bowel disease. Special equipment, solutions, and guidelines for training selected patients and families have been developed and are successfully being used in a number of cases.

TO SUM UP

For patients with functioning gastrointestinal tracts, enteral nutrition support has proved to be a potent tool against present or potential malnutrition. This nutritional support is achieved by a regular oral diet with nutrient-energy supplementation or alternately by tube-feeding when the patient cannot, will not, or should not eat. Modern commercial products provide complete formulas or separate nutrient modules for individualizing a formula mixture to meet special needs. Companion advances in tube-feeding technology have provided extended tube-feeding systems of two types: (1) longer nasoenteric tubes reaching the duodenum and jejunum of the small intestine, and (2) surgical enterostomies in which tubes are placed at progressively extended positions along the gastrointestinal tract. New systems of formulas, tubing and container systems, and electric pumps, together with a comprehensive teaching plan for patient and family and follow-up monitoring by the clinical team, have allowed home enteral feeding to increase rapidly.

For patients with critical hypermetabolic injury or illness or obstruction that makes the gastrointestinal tract unavailable, parenteral nutrition support acts as an artificial gut, an alternate lifeline. This feeding method depends heavily on biomedical technology for the development of tubes, bags, pumps, and other equipment for feeding nutrients directly into veins for blood circulation to the cells. The route of entry may be a large central vein for full feeding over a long period of time or a smaller peripheral vein for feeding less concentrated solutions for a shorter period of time. Home parenteral nutrition support is being successfully used by selected well-trained patients, with the support of equally well-trained families and constant clinical back-up.

■ QUESTIONS FOR REVIEW

1. Describe several types of patient situations in which enteral nutrition support may be indicated. What nutrition assessment procedures may help to identify these individuals?
2. Describe the nutrient components of a typical complete enteral formula. How does it differ from a modular formula?
3. What are medical foods? In what types of cases are they used?
4. Define parenteral nutrition and identify examples of conditions in which it would be used.

The following questions apply to the case of a man referred to nutrition support services. Imagine you are caring for this patient:

1. A previously healthy 45-year-old man, while on a long transport haul as a truck driver, suffered an accident in which he sustained a severe abdominal injury requiring extensive surgical repair and leaving the gastrointestinal tract unavailable for use for an undetermined period of time. He is referred to the nutritional support team for follow-up TPN. Early in this care he asks you how this feeding works. How would you describe and explain the TPN feeding process?
2. What nutritional status assessment procedures would be done and how would you explain to him the nature and purpose of each measure?
3. From your study of this chapter, outline your estimate of his basic nutritional needs to serve as a basis for determining his TPN therapy.
4. List the typical components of a basic TPN formula that he may require, and describe the purpose of each to help reassure him of its adequacy and importance.
5. Sufficient energy (kcalories) intake is essential to immediately meet his metabolic needs after surgery. Assume a normal preinjury weight and height and an added metabolic activity factor (MAF) for stress of one and a half times his basal energy expenditure (BEE). Calculate his total kcalorie need, using the Harris-Benedict equation for BEE and adding the MAF stress need.
6. Define *prealbumin* and describe why it is a primary test for monitoring the effectiveness of the TPN formula in meeting his nutritional support needs for recovery.

■ REFERENCES

1. Benya R, Morbarham S: Enteral alimentation: administration and complications, *J Am Coll Nutr* 10(3):209, 1991.
2. Mobarhan S, DeMeo M: Diarrhea induced by enteral feeding, *Nutr Rev* 53(3):67, 1995.
3. Kazi N, Mobarhan S: Enteral feeding associated gastroesophageal reflux and aspiration pneumonia: a review, *Nutr Rev* 54(10):324, 1996.
4. Fisher GG, Opper FH: An interdisciplinary nutrition support team improves quality of care in a teaching hospital, *J Am Diet Assoc* 96(2):176, 1996.
5. Dougherty D et al: Nutrition care given new importance in JCAHO standards, *Nutr Clin Prac* 10(1):26, 1995.
6. Rombeau JL, Caldwell MD: *Enteral and tube feeding,* Philadelphia, 1990, WB Saunders.
7. Hill GL: The clinical assessment of adult patients with protein energy malnutrition, *Nutr Clin Prac* 10(4):129, 1995.
8. Olree K, Skipper A: The role of nutrition support dietitians as viewed by chief clinical and nutrition support dietitians: implications for training, *J Am Diet Assoc* 97(11):1255, 1997.

9. Mueller C, Shronts EP: Position of the American Dietetic Association: the role of registered dietitians in enteral and parenteral nutrition support, *J Am Diet Assoc* 97(3):302, 1997.

10. Schwartz DB: Enhanced enteral and parenteral nutrition practice and outcomes in an intensive care unit with a hospital-wide performance improvement process, *J Am Diet Assoc* 96(5):484, 1996.

11. Bell SJ et al: A chemical score to evaluate the protein quality of commercial parenteral and enteral formulas: emphasis on formulas for patients with liver failure, *J Am Diet Assoc* 91(5):586, 1991.

12. Bell SJ et al: Alternate lipid sources for enteral and parenteral nutrition: emphasis on formulas for patients with liver failure, *J Am Diet Assoc* 91(1):74, 1991.

13. Gottschlich MM: Selection of optimal lipid sources in enteral and parenteral nutrition, *Nutr Clin Prac* 7(4):152, 1992.

14. Talbot JM: Guidelines for the scientific review of enteral food products for special medical purposes, *J Parenter Enter Nutr* 15(suppl 3):100S, 1991.

15. Mueller C, Nestle M: Regulation of medical foods: toward a rational policy, *Nutr Clin Prac* 10(1):8, 1995.

16. Caulfield KA et al: Technique for intraduodenal placement of transnasal enteral feeding catheters, *Nutr Clin Prac* 6(1):23, 1991.

17. Gore DC et al: Surgically placed gastro-jejunostomy tubes have fewer complications compared with feeding jejunostomy tubes, *Am Coll Nutr* 15(2):144, 1996.

18. Clevenger FW, Rodriguez DJ: Decision-making for enteral feeding administration: the why behind where and how, *Nutr Clin Prac* 10(3):104, 1995.

19. McClave SA et al: Comparison of the safety of early enteral vs parenteral nutrition in mild acute pancreatitis, *J Parenter Enter Nutr* 21(1):14, 1997.

20. Fagerman KE: Microbiologic standards for enteral nutrient solutions overdue in the United States, *J Am Diet Assoc* 92(3):336, 1992.

21. Bernstein LH: Monitoring quality of nutrition support, *Diet Currents* 19(2):1, 1992.

22. Klein S et al: Nutrition support in clinical practice: review of published date on recommendations for future directions, *J Parenter Enter Nutr* 21(3):133, 1997.

23. Dudrick SJ et al: Can intravenous feeding as the sole means of nutrition support growth in the child and restore weight loss in an adult? *Ann Surg* 169:974, 1969.

24. Dudrick SJ: A clinical review of nutritional support of the patient, *Am J Clin Nutr* 33(suppl):1191, 1982.

25. De Chicco RS, Matarese LE: Selection of nutrition support regimens, *Nutr Clin Prac* 7(5):239, 1992.

26. Hester DD et al: Evaluation of the appropriate use of parenteral nutrition in an acute care setting, *J Am Diet Assoc* 96(6):602, 1996.

27. Sawicky CP et al: Adequate energy intake and improved prealbumin concentration as indicators of the response to total parenteral nutrition, *J Am Diet Assoc* 92(10):1266, 1992.

28. Ireton-Jones CS, Baxter CR: Nutrition for adult burn patients: a review, *Nutr Clin Prac* 6(1):3, 1991.

29. Harris JA, Benedict FG: *A biometric study of basal metabolism,* Washington, DC, 1919, Carnegie Institution of Washington.

30. Shizzal HM et al: The effect of age on the caloric requirements of malnourished individuals, *Am J Clin Nutr* 55:783, 1992.

31. Konstantinides FN: Nitrogen balance studies in clinical nutrition, *Nutr Clin Prac* 7(5):231, 1992.

32. Shipley SG: Glutamine in total parenteral nutrition, *Nutr Today* 31(2):74, 1996.

33. van der Hulst R et al: Glutamine and intestinal immune cells in humans, *J Parenter Enter Nutr* 21(6):310, 1997.

34. Lacey JM et al: The effects of glutamine-supplemented parenteral nutrition in premature infants, *J Parenter Enter Nutr* 20(1):74, 1996.

35. Shronts EP: Essential nature of choline with implications for total parenteral nutrition, *J Am Diet Assoc* 97(6):639, 1997.

36. Cunningham JJ et al: Zinc and copper status of severely burned children, *J Am Coll Nutr* 10(1):57, 1991.

37. Warshawsky KY: Intravenous fat emulsions in clinical practice, *Nutr Clin Prac* 7(4):187, 1992.

38. Bullock L et al: Emulsion stability in total nutrient admixtures containing a pediatric amino acid formulation, *J Parenter Enter Nutr* 16(1):64, 1992.

39. Flowers JF et al: Catheter-related complications of total parenteral nutrition. In Fischer JE, ed: *Total parenteral nutrition,* ed 2, Boston, 1991, Little, Brown.

40. Shils ME: Parenteral nutrition. In Shils ME, Olson JA, Shike M, eds: *Modern nutrition in health and disease,* ed 8, vol 2, Philadelphia, 1994, Lea & Febiger.

41. Ireton-Jones C et al: Clinical pathways in home nutrition support, *J Am Diet Assoc* 97(9):1003, 1997.

42. Arensberg MBF, Schiller MR: Dietitians in home care: a survey of current practice, *J Am Diet Assoc* 96(4):347, 1996.

■ FURTHER READING

Fisher GG, Opper FH: An interdisciplinary nutrition support team improves quality of care in a teaching hospital, *J Am Diet Assoc* 96(2):176, 1996.

Hester DD et al: Evaluation of the appropriate use of parenteral nutrition in an acute care setting, *J Am Diet Assoc* 96(6):602, 1996.

Schwartz DB: Enhanced enteral and parenteral nutrition practice and outcomes in an intensive care unit with a hospital-wide performance improvement process, *J Am Diet Assoc* 96(5):484, 1996.

These three articles report clear examples of positive associations between nutrition support team management of enteral and parenteral feeding of hospitalized patients in both financial and humanitarian benefits.

Schauster H, Dwyer J: Transition from tube feedings to feedings by mouth in children: preventing eating dysfunction, *J Am Diet Assoc* 96(3):277, 1996.

This article describes the transition period from tube feeding to regular eating for a child's development and the importance of careful planning ahead for this vital developmental process.

Issues Answers

Troubleshooting diarrhea in tube-fed patients: a costly chase

Clinicians seem to agree generally that diarrhea is one of the most common complications associated with tube feeding, yet the reported incidence ranges widely from as little as 2% to as much as 63% in general patient populations and as high as 68% in intensive care patients. Questions that relate to this wide variance and that plague investigators apparently center on definition and cause. But the ultimate bottom line for patient and family and their health insurers is the price of the clinical search for the culprit. As we shall see, it is a costly chase.

Problem of definition

It would appear on the surface that the question of what diarrhea is, is easy to answer. We've all had some experience, more or less. However, a valid clinical research study demands more-a precise operational definition on which to establish a research design and evaluate results. Judging from reports, investigators have not been able to agree on a definition, methods of reporting the extent of the diarrhea, the length of time tube-fed patients were monitored, and the patients who were studied.

In fact, a current report of a 3-month study clearly indicates that the messy state of defining and reporting diarrhea in tube-fed patients resembles that of the disorder itself. These investigators-using the usual diarrhea criteria of frequency, consistency, and quantity-found as many as 14 different definitions in their review of studies in the scientific literature, no doubt accounting for the varying incidence reported. Of course, the tube-fed patients, if asked, could have easily defined their diarrhea in terms of the psychologic problem and physical discomfort involved, as could their nurses in terms of increased cleanup work and concern for the patient.

Problem of cause

Reported causes of diarrhea in tube-fed patients also vary. These concerns usually center first on the formula itself, often followed by numerous adjustments in components and concentrations that only cloud the picture further and make the search for the actual culprit more difficult. A variety of conflicting causes associated with the complication of diarrhea have been reported, including not only the formula itself but also medications or some aspect of the patient's condition.

Formula. Possible formula factors relate to osmolality or concentration and to rate of delivery. However, conflicting reports have shown no increase in the incidence of diarrhea when the formula concentration varied widely from 145 to 430 mOsm, and no significant association has been made between malabsorption and formula osmolality or rate of delivery. Formulas providing 30% or more of total kcalories as fat have been associated with a higher incidence of diarrhea, whereas those providing 20% fat rarely were involved. Further study of fat composition is needed, specifically comparing medium-chain versus long-chain triglycerides and omega-3 versus omega-6 fatty acids. Studies of the role of fiber in tube feedings have also been conflicting. Reviewers have found that the studies thus far have been few, the models used variable, the limitations substantial, and the conclusions of the investigators mixed.

Bacterial contamination. Studies have demonstrated that the problem of diarrhea does not lie in the quick assumption that the formula as such was at fault but in the reality that bacterial contamination, frequently *Clostridium difficile* toxin, of the formula or feeding equipment was the cause. This problem may result from lack of careful aseptic technique in handling the formula and equipment. Or it may relate to neglect in following the manufacturers' guidelines for appropriate hang times for formulas. This time is usually no longer than 8 hours for systems set up by the nursing staff and 24 hours for systems prefilled with formula by the manufacturer and attached by connections. The less any system is handled and opened, the less chance there is for contamination. Bacteria are easily introduced where the delivery tubing connects with the patient's feeding tube and whenever the system is open.

Patient's condition. Malnourished or critically ill patients are more susceptible to mucosal tissue breakdown, depressed serum albumin levels, and malabsorption leading to diarrhea. The hypoalbuminemia contributes to reduced colloidal osmotic pressure within blood vessels (see Chapter 8). This loss of osmotic pressure in turn, leads to edema of the intestinal mucosa, malabsorption, and diarrhea. Use of an easily absorbed elemental enteral formula is probably helpful, at least until the nutritional status improves sufficiently to progress to a standard intact-protein formula. Albumin may be given intravenously, but unless there is adequate nutritional support the body uses the infused albumin for energy rather than tissue rebuilding. In addition, periods of stress, including sepsis and central nervous system insults, can result in decreased motility of the gastrointestinal tract, including ileus. Such decreased motility contributes to bacterial overgrowth.

Medications. Multiple medications routinely given to hospitalized patients have been related to diarrhea. Antibiotics are most often associated, but this practice coexists with poor patient condition, multiple organ failure, and therefore with diarrhea. In general, drug reactions may relate to the metabolically active agent or to another ingredient added for its physical properties in the form of the drug, for example, tablet or liquid as the following case illustrates.

The case of the costly chase

A recently reported case of unexplained diarrhea in a tube-fed patient illustrates the difficult, and often costly, search for the cause. Max was a 55-year-old man who had suffered an aortic aneurysm and had emergency surgery to repair it. In the intensive care unit, the postoperative course was complicated by respiratory problems requiring ventilator assistance. He was given a bronchodilator drug, theophylline, in tablet form, crushed and given by nasogastric tube with water. When Max was able to take nourishment, an isotonic formula given by enteral tube feeding was started and the crushed theophylline tablets were changed to a sugar-free theophylline solution. Within a day, Max began to have progressive abdominal distention and continuous liquid diarrhea. To rule out an abdominal catastrophe related to the aneurysm or surgery, a computed abdominal tomography scan, an aortogram, and a colonoscopy were done, but all of these studies were normal.

Despite stopping the enteral feeding, the distention and diarrhea continued. Stool specimens were tested for fecal leukocytes, parasites, and *Clostridium difficile* toxin, and an enteric pathogen culture was prepared. All were nondiagnostic. Extensive additional serum and urine tests, as well as a sigmoidoscopy with rectal biopsy, gave no clue. Then stool electrolytes and osmolality measures suggested an osmotic diarrhea. Because Max was not receiving enteral feedings, his physicians thought a secretory bacterial toxin was probably causing the continuing diarrhea, so the previous studies were repeated to confirm the osmotic nature of the diarrhea. In addition, all the medications were reviewed, but none appeared to be the cause.

Because the continued diarrhea prohibited enteral feeding, and Max needed nourishment, total parenteral nutrition (TPN) was ordered. This move immediately brought an automatic Nutrition Support Service consultation, which included further assessment of medications. This evaluation revealed that the sugar-free theophylline solution was 65% *sorbitol.*

Sorbitol is a polyhydric alcohol used as a sweetener in many sugar-free products such as dietetic foods and chewing gum. There was no information about sorbitol on the label or package insert of the drug for the physicians to know these facts, and because sorbitol was not thought to be an active agent, this information could be obtained only by contacting the manufacturer.

Fortunately for Max, however, the nutrition support team did know the components of the medication and found the hidden culprit. The nutritionist knew that sorbitol in larger doses is a laxative! After calculations of the regular daily amount of the theophylline Max was taking, he was receiving nearly 300 g of sorbitol daily when the usual laxative dose was only 20 to 50 g. The nutritional support team immediately recommended that this sorbitol-sweetened solution of theophylline be discontinued and that a sorbitol-free form of the medication be used instead. Almost immediately the diarrhea began to decrease, and in 3 days it was gone.

The extent of this costly chase was revealed in Max's hospital bill. He had continued to receive the faulty drug for almost half of his 3-month hospital stay, during which time the diarrhea prevented enteral feeding and he had to have the more expensive TPN. The TPN cost $4860 more than the enteral feedings would have cost for the same period. In addition, all the extensive investigations to find the cause of the diarrhea cost $4250, which together with the indirect costs for extra days of care and supplies made a total hospital bill of about $170,000.

The causes of diarrhea in tube-fed patients are many, but in the hands of a skilled nutritional support team, the formula is seldom one of them. It is often found in the medications. Just remember what this medication's hidden ingredient—sorbitol—cost Max.

References

Bliss DZ et al: Defining and reporting diarrhea in tube-fed patients—what a mess! *Am J Clin Nutr* 55:753, 1992.

Bokus S: Troubleshooting your tube feedings, *Am J Nurs* 91:24, May, 1991.

Hill DB et al: Osmotic diarrhea induced by sugar-free theophylline solution in critically ill patients, *J Parenter Enter Nutr* 15(3):332, 1991.

Mobarham S, DeMeo M: Diarrhea induced by enteral feeding, *Nutr Rev* 53(3):67, 1995.

Chapter

18

Gastrointestinal Diseases

Chapter Outline

Nutritional Management

Problems of the Mouth and Esophagus

Problems of the Stomach and Duodenum: Peptic
Ulcer Disease

Small Intestine Diseases

Large Intestine Diseases

Food Allergies and Sensitivities

Food Intolerances from Genetic-Metabolic Disease

Diseases of the Gastrointestinal Accessory Organs

In this chapter, we consider diseases of the gastrointestinal tract and its surrounding accessory organs—the liver, gallbladder, and pancreas. In health, the digestion and absorption of our food is accomplished by a series of intimately interrelated actions among these organ systems. To the extent that disease or malfunction at any point interferes with this finely meshed process, nutritional therapy must modify food intake.

The gastrointestinal tract is a sensitive mirror of the individual human condition. It often reflects both physical and emotional conditioning. Its physiologic function reflects physical and psychologic conditioning. In this chapter we relate these basic functions and the healing process not only to the nutritional therapy indicated but also to the individual's personal needs.

NUTRITIONAL MANAGEMENT

When food is taken into the mouth, the act of eating stimulates the gastrointestinal tract into accelerated action. Throughout the digestive process, highly coordinated systems and interactive functions respond (see Chapter 2, Figure 2.1, p. 19). Secretory functions provide the necessary environment and agents for chemical digestion, and peristalsis moves the food mass along. Nutrients are absorbed into the blood circulation and carried to the cells, which take up what is needed to nourish the body. Emotional factors influence the overall individual response pattern. This highly individual and interrelated functional network forms the basis for nutritional therapy in disease.

After food is taken into the mouth, masticated, and swallowed, the esophagus conducts the food mass to the stomach by peristalsis and gravity. The gastroesophageal sphincter muscle at the entry to the stomach forms a controlling valve. It relaxes to receive the food, then closes to hold each bolus for some initial digestive action of enzymes in the gastric acid mix. After leaving the stomach, food moves to the small intestine, where most digestion occurs. A number of small intestine and accessory organ conditions may interfere with normal food passage and create malabsorption problems. These overall conditions vary widely from brief periods of functional discomfort to serious disease and complete obstruction. Medical nutrition therapy is adapted to the degree of dysfunction in food choice and feeding mode.

PROBLEMS OF THE MOUTH AND ESOPHAGUS

MOUTH PROBLEMS

Tissue inflammation

The tissues of the mouth often reflect a person's basic nutritional status. In malnutrition these tissues deteriorate and become inflamed and more vulnerable to local infection or injury, causing pain and difficulty with eating. These conditions in the oral cavity include (1) gingivitis, inflammation of the gums, involving the mucous membrane with its supporting fibrous tissue circling the base of the teeth; (2) stomatitis, inflammation of the oral mucosa lining the mouth; (3) glossitis, inflammation of the tongue; and (4) cheilosis, a cracking and dry scaling process at the corners of the mouth affecting the lips and corner angles, making opening the mouth to receive food difficult.

These oral tissue problems may also be nonspecific and unrelated to nutritional factors. In some cases, gingivitis and stomatitis occur in mild form in relation to another disease or stress. Occasionally a severe form of acute necrotizing ulcerative gingivitis occurs. It is caused by a specific infectious bacterium *Fusobacterium nucleatum*, often in conjunction with the spirochete *Treponema vincentii*; it is also known as Vincent's disease, from the Paris physician Henri Vincent (1862-1950), who first identified the disease process. The gums around the bases of the teeth become puffy, shiny, and tender, overlapping the teeth margins. Affected gums often bleed, especially during tooth brushing. This serious condition destroys gum tissue and the supporting tissues of the teeth, and requires a course of antibiotic treatment.

Mouth pain in these conditions often causes decreased food intake. Maintaining adequate nutrition then becomes a major problem. Generally, patients are given high-protein, high-kcalorie liquids and then soft foods, usually nonacidic and without strong spices in order to avoid irritation. Temperature extremes may also be avoided if they cause pain. Gradually foods are increased according to toleration, and foods are often supplemented with vitamins. In severe disease, the use of a mouthwash containing a mild topical local anesthetic before meals helps relieve the pain of eating.

Dental problems

The incidence of dental caries has recently been reduced in children and young adults. However, it is still present in many older adults, especially those unable to afford regular dental care, and causes tooth loss and chewing problems. In older adults, some 65 million in the United States alone, periodontal disease is a major cause of tooth loss. Especially if dental caries is untreated or if dental hygiene is poor, gum tissue at the base of the teeth becomes damaged and pockets form between the gums and the teeth. Dental plaque forms from a sticky deposit of mucus, food particles, and bacteria. The plaque hardens into calculus, a mineralized coating developed from the plaque and saliva. These hardened particles then collect in the pocket openings at the base of the teeth, where the bacteria attack the periodontal tissue. The result is bacterial erosion of bone tissue surrounding affected teeth and subsequent tooth loss. Preventive care through daily dental care with fluoridated toothpaste, careful flossing, and periodic plaque removal by the dentist and dental hygienist is the best approach. Extensive tooth loss leads to the need for tooth replacement with dentures. In many elderly people these dentures become ill-fitting and hinder adequate chewing. All of these dental problems need to be reviewed in any patient's nutritional history so that food textures and forms can be adjusted to individual needs.

Salivary glands and salivation

Disorders of the salivary glands affect eating because saliva carries an amylase that begins starch breakdown and is vital in moistening the food to facilitate chewing. Problems may arise from infection, such as infection with the mumps virus, which attacks the parotid gland. Other problems come from excessive salivation, which occurs in numerous disorders affecting the nervous system, such as Parkinson's disease, and from local disorders such as mouth infections or injury. Problems may arise from any disease or drug that causes overactivity of the parasympathetic division of the autonomic nervous system, which controls the salivary glands.

Conversely, lack of salivation, which causes dry mouth, may be a temporary condition caused by fear, salivary gland infection, or action of anticholinergic drugs that hinder the normal action of neurotransmitters. Permanent dry mouth is rare but does occur in Sjögren's syndrome, a symptom complex of unknown cause that is thought to be an abnormal immune response. It occurs in middle-aged or older women and is marked by xerostomia (dry mouth) and enlargement of the parotid glands, and it is often associated with rheumatoid arthritis. It may also result from radiation therapy. There is difficulty in swallowing and speaking, interference with taste, and tooth decay. The extreme mouth dryness may be partially relieved by spraying the inside of the mouth with an artificial saliva solution. If dental problems occur, dietary fiber may be decreased to soft or liquid food texture according to need.

Swallowing disorders

The process of swallowing involves highly integrated actions of the mouth, pharynx, and esophagus (Figure 18.1). Swallowing difficulty, known medically as dysphagia, is a fairly common problem with a wide variety of conditions, including stroke or neurologic deficits as major causes. It may be only temporary, as a piece of food lodged in the back of the throat, for which the **Heimlich maneuver** is appropriate first aid, or it may be involved with insufficient production of saliva and xerostomia. Such dysfunctional swallowing often causes children and adults alike to aspirate food particles, in turn causing coughing and choking episodes. The problem is usually referred to a special interdisciplinary team providing care. The team includes physician, nurse, clinical dietitian, physical therapist, and an occupational therapist,

who has special training in swallowing problems. Thin liquids are the most difficult food form to swallow, so various foods, such as baby rice cereal, and commercial agents are used for thickening liquids for individuals with dysphagia.[1,2]

Central problems

The esophagus is a long, muscular tube lined with mucous membranes that extends from the pharynx, or throat, to the stomach (Figure 18.1). It is bounded on both ends by circular muscles, or sphincters, that act as valves to control food passage. The upper sphincter remains closed except during swallowing, thus preventing airflow into the esophagus and stomach. Disorders along the tube that may disrupt normal swallowing and food passage include esophageal spasm (uncoordinated contractions of the esophagus), esophageal stricture (a narrowing caused by a scar from previous inflammation, ingestion of caustic chemicals, or a tumor), and esophagitis (an inflammation). These problems hinder eating and require medical attention through dilation, stretching procedures, or surgery to widen the tube or drug therapy.

Lower esophageal sphincter problems

Defects in the operation of the lower esophageal sphincter (LES) muscles may come from changes in the smooth muscle itself or from the nerve-muscle hormonal control. In general, these LES problems arise from spasm, stricture, or incompetence.

Achalasia

Spasms occur when the LES muscles maintain an excessively high muscle tone, even while resting, and thus fail to open normally when the person swallows. This condition is called **achalasia**, from its unrelaxed muscle state. It is also known as cardiospasm, from the proximity of the heart, although it has no relation to heart action. Patient symptoms include swallowing problems and frequent intractable nausea and vomiting.[3] There may be a feeling of fullness in the chest, weight loss from eating

Figure 18.1 Parts of mouth, pharynx, and esophagus involved in the swallowing process. (From Wardlaw GM, Insel PM: *Perspectives in Nutrition,* ed 2, New York, 1993, McGraw-Hill.)

difficulty, serious malnutrition, and pulmonary complications and infection caused by aspiration of food particles, especially during sleep hours.

Surgical treatment involves dilating the LES or slitting the muscle, an esophagomyotomy, which improves the stricture but not the peristalsis. Postoperative course starts with oral liquids and progresses to a regular diet within a few days according to toleration. General guidelines for nutritional management are given in Table 18.1. To achieve similar results for some elderly patients with comorbid disease, in whom surgery presents considerable risk, gastrologists are using intermittent botulism toxin as drug therapy to reduce smooth muscle tone in the gastrointestinal tract.[4]

Gastroesophageal reflux disease

Ongoing lower LES problems lead to chronic esophageal reflux disease (GERD). Clinicians view this situation of "acid setting up shop in the esophagus" as serious and difficult for both the patient and the physician as a peptic ulcer disease in the stomach and duodenum.[5] The true incidence of GERD is uncertain because many cases go undetected, and it is estimated that only the tip of the iceberg of chronic sufferers are seen clinically.[6] Regurgitation of the acid gastric contents into the lower part of the esophagus creates constant tissue irritation. The acid and pepsin cause tissue erosion with symptoms of substernal burning, cramping, pressure sensation, or severe pain. Symptoms are aggravated by lying down or by any increase of abdominal pressure, such as that caused by tight clothing. The condition is related to (1) a nonfunctioning gastroesophageal sphincter, (2) frequency and duration of the acid reflux, and (3) inability of the esophagus to produce normal secondary peristaltic waves to prevent prolonged contact of the mucosa with the acid pepsin. A hiatal hernia may or may not be present.

Clinical symptoms

The most common symptom is **pyrosis**—a frequently severe heartburn, occurring 30 to 60 minutes after eating. United States surveys report that this common symptom occurs in 33% of persons with GERD at least once a month and in 7% of persons with GERD daily.[6] Sometimes substernal pain radiates into the neck and jaw or down the arms. In addition to hiatal hernia, the acid reflux may be caused by pregnancy, obesity, pernicious vomiting, or nasogastric tubes. Other symptoms include iron deficiency anemia with chronic bleeding and aspiration, which may cause cough, dyspnea, or pneumonitis.

Complications

The most common complications are *stenosis* and esophageal ulcer. Also, significant **gastritis** in the herniated portion of the stomach may cause **occult bleeding**.

Treatment

Obesity is often a precipitating factor; thus weight reduction is essential. The patient must avoid lying down immediately after eating and must sleep with the head of the bed elevated. Frequent use of antacids help control the symptoms. From 85% to 90% of the patients respond to weight reduction and conservative measures. Table 18.2 summarizes these management principles.

Hiatal hernia

The esophagus normally enters the chest cavity at the hiatus, an opening in the diaphragm membrane and immediately joins the upper portion of the stomach. A hiatal hernia occurs when a portion of the upper part of

Table 18.1	Dietary principles for care of achalasia
Principles	**Foods included**
Energy nutrients	Modified protein and carbohydrates and increased fat to help reduce LES pressure and gastric section
Texture	Liquid or semisolid food as tolerated
	Moderate to low fiber if it aids swallowing
Temperature	No very hot or very cold foods
Irritants	No citrus juices to injure mucosa if retained
	No highly spiced foods to irritate if retained
Meal pattern	Frequent, small meals as tolerated
Eating pace	Eat slowly in small bites and swallows

Modified from Zeman FJ: *Clinical nutrition and dietetics,* ed 2, Englewood Cliffs, NJ, 1991, Prentice Hall.

achalasia Failure to relax the smooth muscle fibers of the gastrointestinal tract at any point of juncture of its parts; especially failure of the esophagogastric sphincter to relax when swallowing, as a result of degeneration of ganglion cells in the wall of the organ. The lower esophagus also loses its normal peristaltic activity. Also called cardiospasm.

gastritis Inflammation of the stomach.

Heimlich maneuver A first-aid maneuver to relieve a person who is choking from blockage of the breathing of the breathing passageway by a swallowed foreign object or food particle. Standing behind the person, clasp the victim around the waist, placing one fist under the sternum (breastbone) and grasping the fist with the other hand. Then make a quick, hard, thrusting movement inward and upward.

occult bleeding Obscure, difficult to detect, concealed from observation; such a small blood loss that it can be detected only by a microscope or chemical test.

pyrosis Heartburn.

the stomach at this entry point of the esophagus protrudes through the hiatus alongside the lower portion of the esophagus (Figure 18.2). Food is easily held in this herniated area of the stomach and mixed with acid and pepsin, then it is regurgitated back up into the lower part of the esophagus. Gastritis can occur in this herniated portion of the stomach and cause bleeding and anemia. The reflux of gastric acid contents causes symptoms similar to those described above.

A regular diet of choice is used as tolerated, usually in frequent small feedings for comfort. Also, because obesity is often associated with hiatal hernia, weight reduction is a primary need. Avoiding tight clothing helps relieve discomfort. Patients will need to avoid leaning over or lying down immediately after meals and should sleep with the head of the bed elevated. Antacids help relieve the burning sensation. Large hiatal hernias or smaller sliding hernias may require surgical repair.

Table 18.2	Dietary care of gastroesophageal reflux
Outcome	**Action**
Decrease esophageal irritation	Avoid common irritants such as coffee, carbonated beverages, tomato and citrus juices, and spicy foods
Increase lower esophageal sphincter pressure	Increase protein foods
	Decrease fat to about 45 g/day or less; use nonfat milk
	Avoid strong tea, coffee, and chocolate if poorly treated
	Avoid peppermint and spearmint
Decrease reflux frequency and volume	Eat small, frequent meals
	Sip only a small amount of liquid with meal; drink mostly between meals
	Avoid constipation; straining increases abdominal pressure reflux
Clear food materials from the esophagus	Sit upright at the table or elevate the head of bed
	Do not recline for 2 hours or more after eating

Modified from Zeman FJ: *Clinical nutrition and dietetics,* ed 2, Englewood Cliffs, NJ, 1991, Prentice Hall.

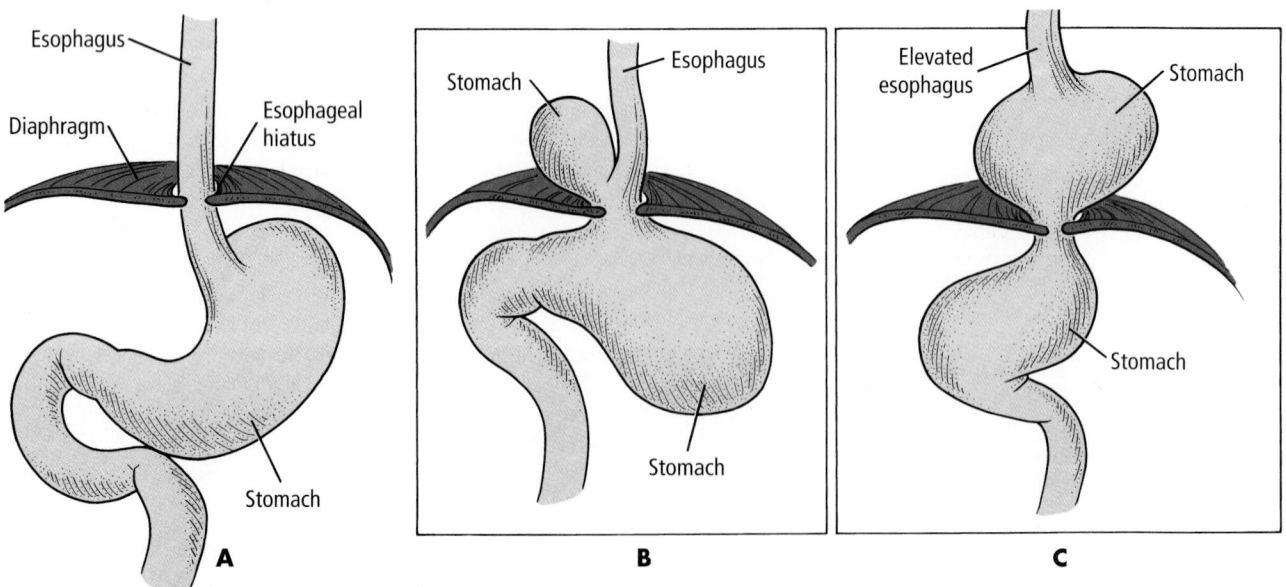

Figure 18.2   Hiatal hernia compared with normal stomach placement. **A,** Normal stomach; **B,** paraesophageal hernia (esophagus in normal position); **C,** esophageal hiatal hernia (elevated esophagus).

PROBLEMS OF THE STOMACH AND DUODENUM: PEPTIC ULCER DISEASE

INCIDENCE

Peptic ulcer disease was uncommon in the previous century, but it began to increase greatly during the early part of the 1990s. The increase seems to have peaked about the mid-1950s, as a result of increased knowledge of the disease process and rapid progress in its medical management. In spite of the remarkable progress in knowledge and care, peptic ulcer disease remains a common, chronic, and recurring disease, still one of the most prevalent of the gastrointestinal disorders. Now with an aging population, an increasing number of older adult patients have the disease. Major complications are bleeding, perforation, and obstruction, but these are rare with modern management. Fewer than 2% of the patients under treatment experience such a complication in any given year.[7]

GENERAL NATURE

Peptic ulcer is the general term for an eroded mucosal lesion in the central portion of the gastrointestinal tract. The areas affected include the lower portion of the esophagus, the stomach, and the first portion of the duodenum, called the duodenal bulb. Esophageal and gastric ulcers are less common. Most ulcers occur in the duodenal bulb, where gastric contents emptying into the duodenum through the pyloric valve are most concentrated. Gastric ulcers occur usually along the lesser curvature of the stomach. Peptic ulcer itself is a **benign** disease. Gastric ulcers, however, are more prone to develop into **malignant** disease.

DISCOVERY OF THE CAUSATIVE MICROBE

An Australian team of pathologists working at the Royal Perth Hospital finally discovered the causative microbe, a corkscrew-shaped bacterium, later named *Helicobacter pylori* because of its coiled helix structure ("helico") and its major infection site surrounding the pyloric valve area between the lower stomach and the first section of the small intestine, the duodenal bulb ("pylori").[8-10] They published their first report early in 1983 and followed with a more definitive study in 1984.[8]

INCIDENCE

As with other infectious processes, *H. pylori* grows vigorously in poor, crowded living conditions. For example, in developing countries the infection occurs early in life, usually at 6 to 8 months of age, and persists as a chronic condition infecting 80% of the population by the age of 20 years.[10] In contrast, in developed countries the infection rate increases slowly with age and 50% of the persons 60 years old are infected, but only a small minority of these people develop gastric pathology, peptic ulcers or gastric cancer.[10,11]

ETIOLOGY

The causative role of *H. pylori* is now clearly established. The United States National Institutes of Health (NIH) has officially approved these findings in a report by an NIH Consensus Development Conference, which has been endorsed by the American Medical Association.[12] Reported risk factors among United States adults include older age, short education, low family income, and smoking.[13]

MEDICAL TREATMENT

In the past few years, with the discovery and knowledge of *H. pylori* infection as the direct cause of peptic ulcer disease and gastric acidity as the indirect supporting factor, we have seen a revolution in our understanding of the pathophysiology of peptic ulcer disease. Three components of the disease and its medical management form the basis of clinical therapy.[14]

Gastric acid and pepsin

There is hypersecretion of gastric hydrochloric acid and pepsinogen, which the acid quickly converts to the strong active protein enzyme pepsin. The amount of acid varies, but the classic medical dictum—"no acid, no ulcer"—still holds.

Nonsteroidal antiinflammatory drugs

Widely used nonsteroidal antiinflammatory drugs (NSAIDs), the most commonly known of which is ibuprofen (Advil, Motrin), as well as the common analgesic aspirin (acetylsalicylic acid—ASA), irritate the gastric mucosa and cause bleeding, erosion, and ulceration, especially with prolonged or excessive use. The NSAID group of drugs are so named to distinguish them from the corticosteroids, synthetic variants of the natural adrenal hormones. The NSAIDs include a dozen antiinflammatory drugs.

Helicobacter pylori infection

H. pylori are common spiraling, rod-shaped bacteria inhabiting the gastrointestinal area around the pyloric valve, the lower gastric antrum, and the upper duodenal

---

benign Not malignant or recurrent; favorable for recovery.

malignant An abnormal condition, such as a tumor, that tends to become progressively worse and results in death.

bulb. Infection by this organism causes peptic ulcer disease. Evidence has indicated that it is the necessary infectious agent in the ulcerative process, aided by the tissue irritation of acid and pepsin.

Clinical symptoms

Basic symptoms of peptic ulcer are increased gastric tone and painful hunger contractions when the stomach is empty. In duodenal ulcer, the amount and concentration of hydrochloric acid is increased. In gastric ulcer it may be normal. Nutritional deficiencies are evident in low plasma protein levels, anemia, and loss of weight. Hemorrhage may be the first sign in some patients. Diagnosis is based on clinical findings, x-ray tests, or visualization by fiberoptic gastroscopy.

MEDICAL MANAGEMENT

In treating patients with peptic ulcer disease, the physician has five basic goals: (1) to kill the causative bacteria, (2) to alleviate the symptoms, (3) to promote healing, (4) to prevent recurrences, and (5) to prevent complications. In addition to general traditional measures, the rapidly expanding knowledge base and development of a number of new drugs have increased the physician's available management tools.

General therapeutic measures

Adequate rest, relaxation, and sleep have long been a foundation for general care of peptic ulcer disease to enhance the body's natural healing process. Positive stress coping and relaxation skills, which help patients deal with personal psychosocial stressors, can be learned and practiced. Simple encouragement to talk about anxieties, anger, and frustrations helps to make patients feel better, and as soon as they are able, appropriate physical activity helps work out tensions. Habits that contribute to ulcer development, such as smoking and alcohol use, should be eliminated. Common drugs such as aspirin and NSAIDS should be avoided.

Drug therapy

Current medical management of peptic ulcer disease has a wider choice of drugs to control underlying physiologic causes and clinical symptoms and to support healing. In various ways, five types of drugs now suppress gastric acid and pepsin secretion, protect mucosal tissue, buffer acid, and eliminate infection.

1. *Histamine H₂-receptor antagonists.* These agents, commonly called *H₂-blockers,* are popular drugs for controlling gastric acid secretin. They competitively block the cell entry and function of histamine. Normally, histamine attaches to its specific cellular **receptors** (type H_2) on the acid-producing parietal cells of the gastric mucosa and mediate their secretion of hydrochloric acid. Thus their blocking action effectively controls acid and pepsin because the inactive pepsinogen requires the acid for activation. Four of these drugs have now been reclassified for over-the-counter purchase: (1) cimetidine (Tagamet), (2) ranitidine (Zantac), (3) famotidine (Pepcid), and (4) nizatidine (Axid).

2. *Proton pump inhibitors.* This newer class of drugs, more potent than the H_2-blockers, also suppresses gastric acid, but by a different action. Without competition, they irreversibly prevent action of a key enzyme that actively secretes hydrogen ions needed for hydrochloric acid (HCl) production. Without available H^+ ions, the HCl cannot be made. Then without the acid, ulcers heal rapidly. An example of this type drug is omeprazole.

3. *Mucosal protectors.* Drugs of this type act as cytoprotective agents by helping the stomach heal itself. They produce a gel-like suspension that binds to the ulcer base and covers it and the surrounding normal mucosal tissue to protect the involved tissue from harm while it heals. This drug also forms complexes with pepsin that inactivates the pepsin. An example of this type drug is sucralfate.

4. *Antacids.* These well-known substances counteract or neutralize acidity. The two main types are (1) magnesium-aluminum compounds (Maalox TC or Mylanta II) and (2) aluminum hydroxide (Basaljel, Amphojel).

5. *Antibiotics.* Drugs of this type are used to control the *H. pylori* infection associated with peptic ulcer disease. Although the organism is easily suppressed, it seems to be more difficult to eradicate. However, combinations being used by investigators and clinicians include the following bacterial or suppressant agents:
   - Bismuth (Pepto-Bismol), bismuth subsalicylate, or colloid bismuth subcitrate
   - Metronidazole (Flagyl), a bacterial and protozoan killer
   - Amoxicillin (Amoxil, Polymox), a penicillin derivative, or tetracycline (Achromycin-V, Panmycin) a frequently used wide-spectrum antibody.

Other drugs for general needs include acetaminophen (Tylenol) to replace aspirin or NSAIDs. Also, if needed briefly for mild sedation to aid the initial need for relaxation and sleep, a tricyclic antidepressant such as amitriptyline (Elavil) may be prescribed.

The main challenge now is to develop a maintenance therapy that prevents recurrence of the disease.[15,16] Currently the best approach seems to include continuous low-dose drug therapy, intermittent full-dose treatment, or symptomatic self-care with the same agents used to heal the ulcer. Success rates hinge on the relative strengths of risk factors that influence recurrence (Table 18.3).

Nutritional management

The revolutionary advance in knowledge of peptic ulcer disease and development of drugs for its medical management have also brought welcome reevaluation of the role of nutrition in its basic care. There is now both medical and nutritional agreement that the old restrictive bland milk-based diet routines of the past, long since known to be ineffective and potentially harmful, have no role in the modern management of peptic ulcer disease.[11,12,16-18] Instead, a positive nutrition approach and basic dietary principles guide our current practice.

1. *Current positive nutrition approach.* The current nutritional practice is that of basic health maintenance or preventive approach in overall health care today.[15] As with any disease process involving tissue injury, the prime nutritional requirement is clear: sufficient energy-nutrient intake supplied by a regular well-balanced diet to support the primary medical management of (1) tissue healing and (2) tissue maintenance of structural and functional integrity. Initial and periodic nutritional assessment is needed to determine energy-nutrient status and any area of individual need.

2. *Dietary principles.* The basic nutrition principles of a well-balanced diet are found in the regular guidelines of the RDA energy-nutrient standards and the United States Dietary Guidelines for health promotion (see Chapter 1). In addition to the major goal of optimal nutritional support, a second dietary goal is to avoid stimulating excess acid secretion and directly irritating the gastric mucosa. Only a few related food factors or habits have been shown to cause excess acid secretion and irritation:

   - *Meal pattern.* Eat three regular meals a day without frequent snacks, especially at bedtime. Any food intake stimulates more acid output.

   - *Food quantity.* Avoid stomach distention with large quantities of food at a meal.

   - *Milk intake.* Avoid drinking milk frequently. It stimulates significant gastric acid secretion, has only a transient buffering effect, and its animal fat content is undesirable. Also, the milk sugar lactose creates problems of abdominal cramping, gas, and diarrhea for many persons with lactose intolerance caused by a deficiency of the enzyme lactase.

   - *Seasonings.* Individual tolerance is the rule. However, several agents have caused variable results and may need to be watched: hot chili peppers, black pepper, and chili powder.

   - *Dietary fiber.* There is no evidence for restricting dietary fiber. Some fibers, especially soluble forms, are beneficial.

   - *Coffee.* Avoid regular and decaffeinated coffee. Coffee stimulates acid secretion and may cause dyspepsia. The comparative effect of regular tea and colas may be milder with some persons, but these beverages also stimulate acid secretion.

   - *Citric acid juices.* These juices may induce gastric reflux and discomfort in some persons.

   - *Alcohol.* Avoid alcohol in concentrated forms, such as 40% (80 proof) alcohol. Other less concentrated forms of wine, taken with food in moderate amounts, are tolerated well by some patients. Avoid beer; it has been shown to be a potent stimulant of gastric acid. For patients who find it particularly difficult to avoid alcohol and coffee completely, some physicians have suggested they may try a small serving of wine with dinner occasionally, or a small cup (*demitasse*) of coffee at the close of the meal to minimize the acid secretion.

   - *Smoking.* The habit of smoking is often associated with food intake. It is best eliminated completely at any time. It not only affects gastric acid secretion but also influences the effectiveness of drug therapy.

   - *Food environment.* Finally, consider the food environment. Eat slowly and savor the food in a calm environment. Respect individual responses or tolerances to specific foods experienced at any time. Remember that the same food may evoke different responses at different times depending on the stress factor.

Table 18.3 Recurrent peptic ulcer risk factors	
Chance of recurrence	**Risk factors**
Possible	Positive family history
	Emotional stress
	Continued use of concentrated alcohol
Good	History of recurrences and complications
	Continued use of aspirin and other NSAIDs
	Increased *Helicobacter pylori* infection
Strong	Poor compliance with maintenance diet or drug plan
	Continued smoking (10 or more cigarettes/day)
	Gastric acid hypersecretion

Modified from Earnest DL: Maintenance therapy in peptic ulcer disease, *Med Clin North Am* 75(4):1013, 1991.

receptor Any one of various specific protein molecules in surface membranes of cells and cell organelles, to which complementary molecules, such as hormones, neurotransmitters, drugs, viruses, or other antigens or antibodies, may become bound.

Personal focus

Sound nutritional management plays an important supportive role in the total medical care of persons with peptic ulcer disease. The individual must be the focus of treatment. The patient is not "an ulcer," but a person with an ulcer. The course of the disease is conditioned by the individuality of the patient and his or her life situation. The presence of the ulcer affects the patient's life. In the long run, a wide range of foods, attractive to the eye and the taste, and regular, unhurried eating habits provide the best course of action.

SMALL INTESTINE DISEASES

CONDITIONS OF MALABSORPTION AND DIARRHEA

General diarrhea

General diarrhea may result from basic dietary excesses. There may be fermentation of sugars involved or excess fiber stimulation of intestinal muscle function. In other cases it may result from a specific foodborne infectious organism or from acute food poisoning with bacterial toxin. In the case of lactose intolerance, the accumulated concentration of undigested lactose in the intestine, resulting from the lack of the enzyme lactase, creates increased osmotic pressure. This pressure effectively draws water into the gut and stimulates hypermotility, abdominal cramping, and diarrhea. Milk treated with lactase enzyme is tolerated by these persons without the difficulty encountered with regular milk. Secretory, osmotic, and inflammatory processes in the intestine result in increased losses of fluid and electrolytes from diarrhea (see *Issues & Answer* box, p. 392).[19]

Malabsorption

There are multiple causes of a malabsorption condition.[19] Some of these causes include the following:

- *Maldigestion problems*: pancreatic disorders, biliary disease, bacterial overgrowth, ileal disease (inflammatory bowel disease)
- *Intestinal mucosal changes:* mucosal surface alterations, intestinal surgery such as resections that shorten the bowel, lymphatic obstruction, intestinal stasis
- *Genetic disease*: cystic fibrosis with its complications of pancreatic insufficiency and lack of the pancreatic enzymes lipase, trypsin, and amylase
- *Intestinal enzyme deficiency*: lactose intolerance caused by lactase deficiency
- *Cancer and its treatment*: absorbing surface effect of radiation and chemotherapy
- *Metabolic biochemical defects:* absorbing surface effects of pernicious anemia or gluten-induced enteropathy (celiac sprue)

Here we briefly review four of these malabsorptive conditions-celiac sprue, cystic fibrosis, inflammatory bowel disease, and short-bowel syndrome.

CELIAC SPRUE

Metabolic defect

In 1889 a London physician named Gee observed a number of malnourished children having extensive fatty diarrhea, steatorrhea, and distended abdomens. He gave the name "celiac" to the general clinical condition from the Greek word *kolia*, meaning "belly" or "abdomen." It was not until the mid 1950s that the Dutch pediatrician Willem-Karel Dicke and his associates discovered the causative agent. Their tissue studies confirmed that the gliadin fraction of the protein gluten in wheat produced the fat malabsorption, and further that what had been called celiac disease in children and nontropical sprue in adults was a single disease, which came to be called celiac sprue.[20] As currently used, the alternate terms *celiac disease* and *gluten-sensitive enteropathy* are synonymous with celiac sprue. In all cases, such diseased tissues consistently show an eroded mucosal surface lacking the number and form of normal villi and having few microvilli. This erosion effectively reduces the absorbing surface by as much as 95%.

Clearly, gluten somehow interacts with and damages the intestinal mucosa, but the primary mechanism remains obscure.[19,20] Studies indicate a biochemical metabolic defect probably involving an enzyme deficiency and a genetic base. It is now apparent that the steatorrhea (about 80% of the ingested fat appears in the stools) and the progressive malnutrition are secondary effects caused by the primary biochemical reaction to gliadin in sensitive persons.

Nutritional management

The goal of nutritional management is to control the dietary gluten and prevent malnutrition. The diet is better defined as low-gluten rather than gluten-free, since it is impossible to remove all the gluten completely. Usually a small amount is tolerated by most patients, except in the prolonged use of newer products labeled "gluten-free," but containing wheat starch as a thickening agent, which cannot be recommended.[21] Wheat and rye are the main sources of gluten; it is also present in oats and barley. Thus these four grains have always been eliminated from the diet. However, a growing body of evidence now suggests that moderate amounts of oats may be safely used in the diets of most adults with celiac disease.[22] Corn and rice are the substitute grains used. Parents of celiac children need special instructions about food products to avoid, what constitutes a basic meal pattern, and recipes for food preparation. Careful label-reading habits must be discussed, since many commercial products use the offending grains as thickeners or fillers, and parents' knowledge of gluten-containing food products is highly variable and influences the child's attitudes toward dietary compliance. With an increasing number of processed foods being marketed, as well as increasing use of ethnic foods in Western society, it is difficult to detect all foods containing gluten, so a home test kit for gluten has been developed.[23] Good dietary management varies according to the child's age, pathologic conditions, and clinical status. Generally, a dietary program based on the low-gluten diet given in Table 18.4 may be followed. In a small subgroup of patients, the symptoms persist despite strict adherence to the diet. In rare instances, persons with such a refractory form of the disease respond only to parenteral nutrition support.[20]

CYSTIC FIBROSIS

Genetic-metabolic defect

Cystic fibrosis is inherited as an autosomal recessive trait mainly in Caucasian populations in which 1 in 20 is a carrier and now 1 in 2500 newborns is affected.[24] It occurs rarely in other populations, for example, 1 in 17,000 black live births and 1 in 90,000 Oriental live births. It is the most common fatal genetic disease in North America. In past years, children carrying the disease have generally lived to about the age of 10 years, dying from complications such as chronic obstructive pulmonary disease with progressive damage to airway epithelial cells and pancreatic insufficiency from fibrosis and resulting lack of pancreatic enzymes. Improved man-

---

Table 18.4   Low-gluten diet for children with celiac disease

Dietary principles

Kcalories—high, usually about 20% above normal requirement to compensate for fecal loss
Protein—high, usually 6 to 8 g/kg weight
Fat—low, but not fat-free, because of impaired absorption
Carbohydrates—simple, easily digested sugars (fruits, vegetables) should provide about one half of the kcalories
Feedings—small, frequent feedings during ill periods; afternoon snack for older children
Texture—smooth, soft, avoiding irritating roughage initially, using strained foods longer than usual for age, adding whole foods as tolerated and according to age of child
Vitamins—supplements of B vitamins, vitamins A and B in water-miscible forms, and vitamin C
Minerals—iron supplements if anemia is present

Food groups	Foods included	Foods excluded
Milk	Milk (plain or flavored with chocolate or cocoa) Buttermilk	Malted milk; preparations such as Cocomalt, Hemo, Postum, Nestle's chocolate
Meat or substitute	Lean meat, trimmed well of fat Eggs, cheese Poultry, fish Creamy peanut butter (if tolerated)	Fat meats (sausage, pork) Luncheon meats, corned beef frankfurters, all common prepared meat products with any possible wheat filler Duck, goose Smoked salmon Meat prepared with bread, crackers, or flour
Fruits and juices	All cooked and canned fruits and juices Frozen or fresh fruits as tolerated, avoiding skins and seeds	Prunes, plums (unless tolerated)
Vegetables	All cooked, frozen, canned as tolerated (prepared *without* wheat, rye, oat, or barley products); raw as tolerated	Any causing individual discomfort All prepared with wheat, rye, oat, or barley products
Cereals	Corn or rice	Wheat, rye, oat, barley; any product containing these cereals
Breads, flours, cereal products	Breads, pancakes, or waffles made with suggested flours (cornmeal, cornstarch; rice, soybean, lima bean, potato, buckwheat)	All bread or cracker products made with gluten; wheat, rye, oat, barley, macaroni, noodles, spaghetti; any sauces, soups, or gravies prepared with gluten flour, wheat, rye, oat, or barley
Soups	Broth, bouillon (no fat or cream; no thickening with wheat, rye, oat, or barley products); soups and sauces may be thickened with cornstarch	All soups containing wheat, rye, oat, or barley products

agement of the disease based on increasing scientific knowledge has helped push the life expectancy up into the third decade of life. Currently, a screening test for newborns helps detect the disease early. Then early intervention and support of a skilled cystic fibrosis team of health care specialists can accurately assess individual needs, help families cope, and develop an appropriate therapeutic plan.[24]

In the summer of 1989, the cystic fibrosis gene was discovered, and shortly after that, continuing studies disclosed the underlying biochemical defect.[25] The normal gene's large protein product, composed of 1480 amino acids in 5 domains (see Chapter 5), controls the opening and closing of ion channels that actively transport chloride ions across epithelial cell membranes. Scientists have named this large protein for its function, cystic fibrosis transmembrane conductance regulator (CFTR).[25] The mutant cystic fibrosis gene cannot produce this controlling protein product called CFTR. Thus because of the resulting defective epithelial ion transport, chloride is trapped in the cells and excess sodium is also absorbed. This imbalance leads to the thickened mucus formation and clinical effects in the various organ systems involved.

Clinical symptoms

The classic clinical symptoms of cystic fibrosis include the following effects in body organ systems:[26,27]

1. *Thick mucus in the lungs* that accumulates and clogs air passages, damages the epithelial tissue of these airways, and leads to chronic obstructive pulmonary disease (COPD) and frequent respiratory infections, both contributing to increased metabolism and increased energy-nutrient needs
2. *Pancreatic insufficiency* caused by progressive clogging of pancreatic ducts and functional tissue degeneration, resulting in lack of normal pancreatic enzymes: protein-splitting trypsin, chymotrypsin, carboxypeptidase; fat-splitting lipase; and starch-splitting amylase. Progressive loss of functional insulin-producing beta cells in the Islets of Langerhans, resulting in insulin-dependent diabetes mellitus (IDDM)
3. *Malabsorption* of undigested food nutrients and extensive malnutrition and stunted growth
4. *Biliary cirrhosis* caused by progressive clogging of bile ducts producing biliary obstruction and functional liver tissue degeneration
5. *Salt (NaCl) concentration* increased in the body perspiration, resulting in salt depletion

Nutritional management

Current nutritional management of cystic fibrosis follows guidelines developed by a consensus committee of the United States Cystic Fibrosis Foundation (CFF).[26] This more aggressive nutritional management program, used in all the CFF centers throughout the United States,

results from three factors: (1) increased knowledge of the disease process, (2) early diagnosis and intervention, and (3) improved therapeutic products such as replacement pancreatic enzymes in the form of capsule encased enteric coated microspheres—"beads"—that correct the maldigestion and help support energy-nutrient growth needs.[28] With this pancreatic enzyme replacement therapy, commonly called "PERT," it is now recommended that persons with cystic fibrosis consume a high-energy, high-protein diet with no fat restriction. However, some persons continue to follow the low-fat advice given to them before the development of the enteric-coated enzymes preparations.[29] Treatment with PERT is very individualized. Even with maximum use, 10% to 20% of the ingested energy will usually be malabsorbed. The overall goal is to support normal nutrition and growth for all ages.

This PERT management program is based on an initial and ongoing schedule for assessment, including anthropometrics, laboratory studies, and nutrition evaluation (Table 18.5). Related therapy is then outlined in five levels according to individual assessment results and nutritional care needs and actions (Table 18.6).

Directions for calculating energy needs for cystic fibrosis patients, basal metabolic rate (BMR) and daily energy requirements (DER), physical activity and disease status, are included in Appendix N, *Guidelines for Nutritional Assessment in Care of Cystic Fibrosis Patients.*

IRRITABLE BOWEL SYNDROME

Nature and incidence

Irritable bowel syndrome, first described by the British physician Frederick Osler in 1892, has confounded physicians for over a century.[30] The general term *irritable bowel syndrome (IBS)* is now used to apply to two intestinal conditions having similar symptoms but different underlying clinical problems—Crohn's disease and ulcerative colitis.[31,32] Both of these conditions produce extended mucosal tissue lesions, although these lesions differ in extent and nature. However, they have been classed medically in a single group because they are similar in their clinical symptoms and management. The incidence of these diseases, especially Crohn's disease, has increased worldwide. Crohn's disease is particularly prevalent in industrialized areas of the world. It also appears among otherwise low-risk persons who move from rural to urban centers. These factors suggest a role for pathogenic agents in the environment. Its incidence is highest among teenagers, with a secondary peak at ages 55 to 60 years. Although epidemiologic and clinical studies continue to increase knowledge of the disease processes involved, the causes of these two inflammatory bowel diseases remain unknown. Sensitive or specific serologic or genetic markers have yet to be identified.[33,34]

Table				

18.5 Basic nutritional assessment for nutritional management of cystic fibrosis

Key assessments	Monitoring schedule and indications			
Anthropometry		**Biochemical data**	
Weight	Every 3 months or as needed for growth evaluation and routine care	CBC[†]	Yearly routine care, interim as needed to detect deficiencies, iron status
Height (length)		TIBC,[†] serum iron, ferritin	
Head circumference (until age 2 yr)		Plasma/serum retinol, alpha-tocopherol	As indicated, weight loss, growth failure, clinical deterioration
Midarm circumference		Albumin, prealbumin	
Triceps skin fold		Electrolytes, acid-base balance	Summer heat, prolonged fever
Midarm muscle circum-ference (derived)*			
		Dietary evaluation	
		Dietary intake	As indicated, history and food records, full energy-nutrient analysis
		3-day fat balance study‡	As indicated, weight loss, growth failure, clinical deterioration
		Anticipatory guidance	Yearly, interim as needed according to growth or situational needs

*See Chapter 16 for equations
†*CBC,* Complete blood count; *TIBC,* total iron-binding capacity.
‡Three-day food records for analysis of fat intake; stool collections for analysis of fat content and degree of malabsorption.
Modified from CFF consensus report; Ramsey B et al: Nutrition assessment and management in cystic fibrosis; a consensus report, *Am J Clin Nutr* 55:108, 1992.

Ulcerative colitis and Crohn's disease have severe, often devastating tissue effects and nutritional consequences. But they can be distinguished by two main differences: (1) anatomic distribution of the inflammatory process, and (2) the nature of tissue changes involved. Crohn's disease occurs in any part of the intestinal tract; in contrast, ulcerative colitis is confined to the colon and rectum. In Crohn's disease, the inflammatory tissue changes become chronic and can involve any part of the intestinal wall and may penetrate the entire wall. Often this extensive tissue involvement leads to partial or complete obstruction and to fistula formation.[34] In contrast, the tissue changes in ulcerative colitis are usually acute, lasting brief periods, and are limited to the mucosal and submucosal tissue layers of the intestinal wall.

Clinical symptoms

A chronic bloody diarrhea is the most common clinical symptom, occurring at night as well as during the day. Ulceration of the mucous membrane of the intestine leads to various associated nutritional problems such as anorexia, nutritional edema, anemia, avitaminosis, protein losses, negative nitrogen balance, dehydration, and electrolyte disturbances. Clinicians have observed evidence of specific deficiencies of zinc and vitamin E, with improvement occurring when supplements of the particular nutrients involved are taken. There is general weight loss, often general malnutrition, fever, skin lesions, and arthritic joint involvement. In Crohn's disease, the overall malnutrition resembles kwashiorkor and is an important cause of abnormal immunologic function.

Medical management

Over the years, the precise nature and cause of irritable bowel syndrome (IBS) has continued to puzzle practitioners. Gastroenterologists have aptly called it "a dilemma within a dilemma surrounded by dilemmas."[35] Medical management of IBS has centered on drug therapy to control the inflammatory process and promote healing, as well as moderate use of antidepressants for reactions to situational stress factors. Ongoing development of new agents in addition to mainstays of the past hold promise for future therapy.[34-36] The physician has available three types of drugs to use in developing individual therapy for IBD: (1) a corticosteroid—prednisone; (2) an antiinflammatory agent—sulfasalazine, which is a

Table 18.6	Levels of nutritional care for management of cystic fibrosis	
Levels of care	**Patient groups**	**Nutrition actions**
Level I—Routine care	All	Diet counseling, food plans, enzyme replacement, vitamin supplements, nutrition education, exploration of problems
Level II—Anticipatory guidance	Above 90% ideal weight-height index, but at risk of energy imbalance; severe pancreatic insufficiency, frequent pulmonary infections, normal periods of rapid growth	Increased monitoring of dietary intake, complete energy-nutrient analysis, increased kcaloric density as needed; assess behavioral needs; provide counseling, nutrition education
Level III—Supportive intervention	85%-90% ideal weight-height index, decreased weight-growth velocity	Reinforce all the above actions, add energy-nutrient–dense oral supplements
Level IV—Rehabilitative care	Consistently below 85% ideal weight-height index, nutritional and growth failure	All of the above plus enteral nutrition support by nasoenteric or enterostomy tube feeding (see Chapter 18)
Level V—Resuscitative or palliative care	Below 75% ideal weight-height index, progressive nutritional failure	All of the above plus continuous enteral tube feedings or TPN (see Chapter 18)

Modified from CFF consensus report: Ramsey B et al: Nutrition assessment and management in cystic fibrosis: a consensus report, *Am J Clin Nutr* 55:108, 1992.

combination of sulfapyridine and 5-aminosalicylic acid; and (3) an immunosuppressant agent especially for Crohn's disease—mercaptopurine.[34,36]

In general, after comprehensive tests and examinations to rule out organic disease, drug therapy consists largely of (1) moderate use of *antidepressant agents* for transient reactions to situational stress factors seen in the larger patient group in general medical care, with referrals as needed to counseling or psychiatric services, and (2) frequent use of *anticholinergic agents* for reducing the impact of neurotransmitters of the enteric nervous system on smooth muscles of the intestine causing spastic contractions.[35] Other drugs used include stool bulk formers and antidiarrheal agents. Effects of these drugs become important aspects of planning supportive nutritional care. Optimal treatment of patients with irritable bowel syndrome focuses on symptom severity and degree of disability.[31]

Nutritional management

Nutrition therapy centers on supporting the healing process and avoiding nutritional deficiency states. In general, a high-fiber, low-fat diet is used, with individual adjustments as needed. In serious conditions, enteral nutrition support includes elemental formulas of absorbable isotonic preparations of amino acids, glucose, fat, minerals and vitamins. In patients who tolerate these feedings, there is diminished gastrointestinal protein loss and improved nutrition, accompanied by clinical remission. In cases where the small bowel has been shortened or the disease process is extensive, as in Crohn's disease, total parenteral nutrition support (TPN) is most effective.[37] Such vigorous nutritional therapy is particularly impor-

tant in childhood to prevent severe growth retardation. Nutritional repletion improves symptoms dramatically. There is diminished gastrointestinal secretion and motility, decreased disease activity, relief of partial intestinal obstruction, occasional closure of enteric fistulas, and renewed immunocompetence. Nutritional supplements are usually necessary to avoid deficiencies in agents such as zinc, copper, chromium, selenium, and other nutrients.

General continuing nutritional management

With a careful history as a base, a reasonable and appropriate food plan may be developed with the patient and family. Periodic food records and related symptoms provide the basis for continued counseling and adjustments. In general, the food plan gives attention to the following basic principles:

1. *Increase dietary fiber.* Increased dietary fiber aids functions of the of the large intestine mainly by: (1) increasing and softening the fecal output, (2) regulating transit time of the final food mass through the colon, and (3) lowering segmental pressures in the final section of the colon, especially the sigmoid area. A regular diet with optimal energy-nutrient composition and dietary fiber food sources-such as whole grains, fruits, and vegetables-should provide the basic therapy (Table 18.7). Then moderate supplemental dietary fiber may be used if needed, with controlled additions of bran, often better tolerated in cooked forms, or more soluble forms of bulking agents such as psyllium seed products (Metamucil).

2. *Recognize gas formers.* Some foods are recognized gas formers for many people because of known constituents such as certain oligosaccharides, as in the

Figure 18.3   Phenylketonuria (PKU). This child is a perfectly developed 3-year-old. With her condition screened and diagnosed at birth, she has eaten a carefully controlled low-phenylalanine diet and is growing normally.

from other food sources. Parents quickly learn to check labels carefully on all commercial products to detect any lactose or lactose-containing substances.

DISEASES OF THE GASTROINTESTINAL ACCESSORY ORGANS

Three major accessory organs lie adjacent to the gastrointestinal tract and produce important digestive agents that enter the intestine and aid in the processing of food substances. Specific enzymes are produced for each of the major nutrients, and bile is added to assist in the enzymatic digestion of fats. These three major organs are the liver, gallbladder, and pancreas. Diseases of these organs can easily affect gastrointestinal function and cause problems in the normal handling of specific types of food.

VIRAL HEPATITIS

Structural scheme of the liver lobules

The unique structural design of these basic functional units of the liver enable this vital organ to do its life-sustaining work. Each liver lobule is constructed around a central vein that empties into the hepatic veins which flow into the vena cava. From this central vein many hepatic cellular plates radiate outward like spokes in a wheel (Figure 18.4).

Etiology

Viral hepatitis, inflammation of the liver, is a major public health problem throughout the world, affecting hundreds of millions of people. It causes considerable illness and death in human populations from the acute infection or its effects, which may include chronic active hepatitis,

cirrhosis, and primary liver cancer. During the past few years, knowledge of the viruses causing different types of hepatitis has grown rapidly. Currently, six unrelated human hepatitis viruses, A, B, C, D, E, and the newly discovered hepatitis virus G, have been isolated and described.[44-46] The two most common and well known are A and B, which serve as examples:

- *Hepatitis A virus (HAV)*. HAV, the infectious agent of hepatitis type A, was formerly called infectious hepatitis. It was discovered in the early 1970s in the feces of infected patients and is transmitted by the classic oral-fecal route by contaminated food and water. It is a prevalent infection worldwide, especially where there is overcrowding and poor hygiene or sanitation. An HAV vaccine has recently been developed that is far more effective than the former large and painful injection of gamma globulins, antibodies isolated from the blood. This vaccine protects travelers to developing countries, where the virus is **endemic** and may easily contaminate water and food.
- *Hepatitis B virus (HBV)*. HBV, the infectious agent of hepatitis type B, was formerly called serum hepatitis. It was discovered in the late 1960s, mainly spread sexually and by sharing of contaminated needles among drug abusers. It has now been implicated worldwide as the major causative factor in chronic liver disease and associated liver cancer. The HBV infection is closely related to the body's immune system. The estimate of carriers is about 300 million worldwide, 75% of whom are Asians. The WHO indicates that about 40% of these infected persons will die of chronic active hepatitis or liver cancer. An

---

endemic   Characterizing a disease of low morbidity that remains constantly in a human community but is clinically recognizable in only a few.

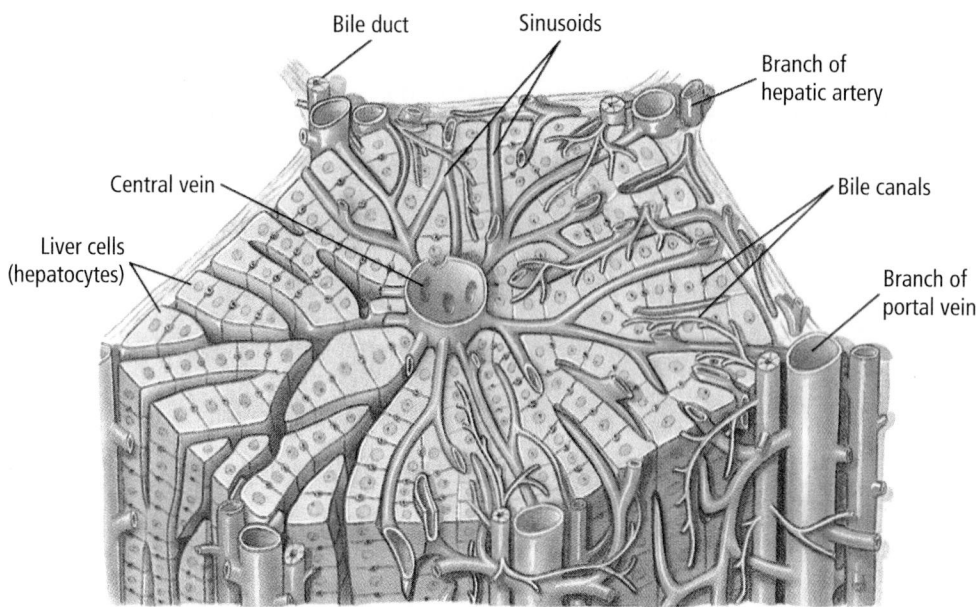

Figure 18.4   Liver structure showing hepatic lobule and hepatic cell.

improved vaccine was developed in 1986 and is now being used with high-risk groups such as health care personnel and babies of antibody-carrier mothers in most developed countries.[47] In some endemic areas, all newborns are routinely vaccinated.

Clinical symptoms

The viral agents of hepatitis produce diffuse injury to liver cells, especially the **parenchymal cells**. In milder cases the liver injury is largely reversible, but with increasing severity, more extensive **necrosis** occurs. In some cases massive necrosis may lead to liver failure and death. A cardinal symptom of hepatitis is anorexia, contributing to the risk of malnutrition. Varying clinical symptoms appear depending on the degree of liver injury. **Jaundice**, a major symptom, may be obvious or not, depending on the severity of the disease, and can have both nutritional and psychologic effects (see *Practical Application* box, p. 382). In an outbreak of hepatitis, many infected persons may be **nonicteric** and thus go undiagnosed and untreated because jaundice has not developed enough to be seen. Malnutrition and impaired **immunocompetence** contribute to spontaneous infections and continuing liver disease. General symptoms, in addition to the main sign of anorexia, include malaise, weakness, nausea and vomiting, diarrhea, headache, fever, enlarged and tender liver, and enlarged spleen. When jaundice develops, it usually occurs for a **preicteric** period of 5 to 10 days, deepens for 1 to 2 weeks, then levels off and decreases. After this crisis point there is a sufficient recovery of injured cells and a convalescence of 3 weeks to 3 months follows. Optimal care during this time is essential to avoid relapse.

General treatment

Bedrest is essential. Physical exercise increases both severity and duration of the disease. A daily intake of 3000 to 3500 ml of fluid guards against dehydration and gives a general sense of well-being and improved appetite. However, optimal nutrition is the major therapy. It provides the essential foundation for recovery of the injured liver cells and overall return of strength.

Nutritional therapy

Full nutrition assessment and initial personal histories provide the basis for planning care. Nutritional therapy principles relate to the liver's function in metabolizing each of the nutrients:

1. *Adequate protein.* Protein is essential for liver cell regeneration, as well as for maintaining all of the body's essential functions. It also provides lipotropic agents such as methionine and choline for the conversion of fats to lipoproteins and removal from the liver, thus preventing fatty infiltration. The daily diet should supply 1.5 to 2 g/kg of actual body weight, or about 100 to 150 g, of high-quality protein. This amount is usually enough to achieve a positive nitrogen balance.

2. *High carbohydrate.* Sufficient available glucose must be provided to restore protective glycogen reserves and meet the energy demands of the disease process. Also, adequate glucose for energy ensures the use of protein for vital tissue regeneration. The diet should supply about 50% to 55% of the total kcalories as carbohydrates, or about 300 to 400 g/day.

3. *Moderate fat.* An moderate amount of fat makes the food more palatable and therefore encourages the anorexic patient to eat. If steatorrhea is present, a more easily absorbed medium-chain triglyceride product such as MCT oil may be used for a brief time. Then regular vegetable oil products and small amounts of butterfat may be resumed to ensure adequate amounts of essential linoleic acid. The diet should supply about 30% to 35% of the total kcalories as fat, or about 80 to 100 g/day.

4. *Increased energy.* The classic Harris-Benedict equations are used to estimate basal energy expenditure (BEE). For total energy needs, malnourished patients should receive 150% of these calculated BEE values. Ambulatory patients require more energy intake to cover any physical activity, or a total of about 2500 to 3000 kcal/day. This increased energy intake is needed to furnish energy demands of the tissue regeneration process, to compensate for losses from fever and general debilitation, and to renew strength and recuperative powers.

5. *Micronutrients.* Fat-soluble vitamins in water-soluble form should be provided in amounts twice the normal RDAs. Other water-soluble vitamins also require supplementation.

Meals and feedings

The problem of supplying a diet adequate to meet the increased nutritive demands for a patient whose illness makes food almost repellent calls for creativity and supportive encouragement. The food may need to be in liquid form at first, using concentrated commercial or blended formulas for frequent feedings (Table 18.8). As the patient improves, appetizing and attractive food is needed. Since nutritional therapy is the key to recovery, a major nutrition and nursing responsibility requires devising ways to encourage the increased amounts of food intake needed, as suggested in Table 18.9. The clinical dietitian and the nurse work together closely to achieve this goal. All staff attendants follow appropriate precautions in handling the patient's tray to prevent spread of the infection.

CIRRHOSIS

Cirrhosis is the general term used for advanced stages of liver disease, whatever the initial cause of the disease may be. Among all digestive diseases, cirrhosis of the liver is the leading nonmalignant cause of death in the United States and most of the developed world. These deaths occur largely among young and middle-aged adults. The French physician René Laënnec (1781-1826) first used the term **cirrhosis** (from the Greek word *kirrhos*, meaning "orange yellow") to describe the diseased liver's abnormal color and rough surface. The cirrhotic liver is a firm, fibrous, dull yellowish mass with orange nodules projecting from its surface (Figure 18.5).

Table 18.8 High-protein, high-kilocalorie formula for patient with hepatitis			
Ingredients	Amount	Approximate food value	
Milk	1 cup	Protein	40 g
Egg substitute	Equivalent of 2 eggs	Fat	30 g
Skimmed milk powder or Casec	6 to 8 tbsp	Carbohydrates	70 g
	2 tbsp	Kilocalories	710
Sugar	2 tbsp		
Ice cream	2.5 cm (1 in) slice or 1 scoop		
Cocoa or other flavoring	2 tbsp		
Vanilla	Few drops, as desired		

Etiology

Some forms of cirrhosis result from biliary obstruction, with blockage of the biliary ducts and accumulation of bile in the liver.[48] Other cases may result from liver necrosis from undetermined causes or in some cases from previous viral hepatitis. A common problem is fatty cirrhosis, associated with the complicating factor of malnutrition. Continuing fatty infiltration causes cellular destruction and fibrotic tissue changes.

Clinical symptoms

Early signs of cirrhosis include gastrointestinal disturbances such as nausea, vomiting, loss of appetite, disten-

---

cirrhosis Chronic liver disease, characterized by loss of functional cells, with fibrous and nodular regeneration.

icterus Alternate term for jaundice: **nonicteric** indicates absence of jaundice; **preicteric** indicates a state before development of icterus, or jaundice.

immunocompetence The ability or capacity to develop an immune response, that is, antibody production and/or cell-mediated immunity, following exposure to antigen.

jaundice A syndrome characterized by hyperbilirubinemia and deposits of bile pigment in the skin, mucous membranes, and sclera giving a yellow appearance to the patient.

necrosis Cell death caused by progressive enzyme breakdown.

parenchymal cells Functional cells of an organ as distinguished from the cells comprising its structure or framework.

Jaundice: when to expect it and what to do about it

Since jaundice is not usually a life-threatening condition, it is easy for the health care professional to take it lightly. The resulting yellow-to-orange skin color seems harmless, only reflecting an accumulation of excessive bile pigments in the blood that results from a rise in *bilirubin*, a product of heme released when red blood cells are destroyed. The underlying condition resulting in hemolysis, not the jaundice itself, is the major issue.

This may be true in a biologic sense. However, in a psychologic sense, jaundice can be devastating. The embarrassment of an altered body image, with accompanying depression and withdrawal, can affect the appetite and willingness to comply with the therapy that is recommended for the illness. To promote a healthy recovery, health workers must treat jaundice as seriously as these effects dictate. Several actions would be helpful:

1. Explain to the patient the reason for jaundice.
   - *Prehepatic jaundice*. Prehepatic jaundice most often is caused by a massive breakdown in red blood cells. It is seen most often in Rh factor sensitization, hemolytic anemias, sickle cell anemia, massive lung infarctions, transfusion reactions, and septicemia. The result is an excessive amount of bilirubin in a form that cannot be excreted, that is, fat-soluble. The body's bilirubin transport system, based on albumin, then deposits the excess in the patient's skin and in a few other tissues.
   - *Hepatic jaundice*. In hepatic jaundice the liver cannot convert fat-soluble bilirubin into the water-soluble form required for its removal from the blood. This condition is seen in hepatitis, cirrhosis, metastatic cancer, and prolonged drug use, especially of drugs broken down by the liver.
   - *Posthepatic jaundice*. Posthepatic jaundice occurs when the flow of bile into the duodenum is blocked. Since bile carries water-soluble excretable bilirubin, this blockage backs up the bile, resulting in a backlog of bilirubin in the blood. Blockage often occurs with inflammation, scar tissue, stones, or tumors in the liver, bile, or pancreatic systems.

2. Explain to the patient assessment procedures and tests. A careful and comprehensive assessment process involving members of the health care team provides vital information for medical, nutritional, and nursing care plans.
   - *Include a careful history and anthropometry*. A full personal, family, psychosocial, medical, and nutritional history will help detect any possible hepatic virus sources and current nutritional status and needs.
   - *Check anthropometric data*. Routine body measures including skinfold thicknesses help determine nutritional status.
   - *Evaluate results of routine biochemical tests*. Relate these tests to medical diagnosis and nutritional status and needs.

   - *Explain each procedure*. A clear explanation of each procedure will help the patient participate more meaningfully in diagnostic and care-planning processes and will allay anxieties about the jaundice.

3. Identify nutrition-related problems. Jaundice is often associated with anorexia, indigestion, nausea, and vomiting.
   - *Help resolve nutrition-related problems*. To overcome indigestion or anorexia, recommend small meals that offer some of the patient's favorite foods. To overcome nausea or vomiting, simple foods may be necessary. Also, foods rich in fat and caffeine should also be avoided.
   - *Encourage the patient to discuss personal feelings and concerns*. Such information is essential for the nurse and nutritionist to develop a treatment plan. Also, this counseling may help the patient feel psychologically stronger and ready to contribute to the health care process.
   - *Discuss pertinent needs with the patient's family and friends*. Often other significant persons avoid the patient out of embarrassment or lack of understanding. A discussion of the patient's need for support may help other persons accept the patient socially and support any other efforts made to resolve the underlying health problem.

References
Sherlock S: *Diseases of the liver and biliary system,* ed 8, Cambridge, Mass, 1989, Blackwell Scientific Publications.
Vail BA: Management of chronic viral hepatitis, *Am Fam Physician* 55(8): 2749, 1997.

- *Make appropriate referrals as needed.* If jaundice was caused by alcohol or drug abuse, the patient and possibly the patient's family may require special counseling. Referral to community programs after hospital discharge may help provide needed follow-up therapy.

tion, and epigastric pain. In time, jaundice may appear, with increasing weakness, edema, ascites, and anemia from gastrointestinal bleeding, iron deficiency, or hemorrhage. A specific **macrocytic anemia** from folic acid deficiency is also frequently observed. Steatorrhea is a common symptom. Essentially, the major symptoms are caused by a basic protein deficiency and its multiple metabolic problems: (1) plasma protein levels fall leading to failure of the capillary fluid shift mechanism (see Chapter 8), causing ascites, (2) lipotropic agents are not supplied for fat conversion to lipoproteins and damaging fat accumulates in the liver tissue, (3) blood clotting mechanisms are impaired because factors such as prothrombin and fibrinogen are not adequately produced, and (4) general tissue catabolism and negative nitrogen balance continue the overall degenerative process.

As the disease progresses, the increasing fibrotic scar tissue impairs blood circulation through the liver, and portal hypertension follows.[49] Contributing further to the problem is the continuing ascites. The impaired portal circulation with increasing venous pressure may lead to esophageal **varices**, with danger of rupture and fatal massive hemorrhage.

Nutritional therapy

When alcoholism is an added underlying problem, treatment is difficult. Each patient requires supportive care. Therapy is usually aimed at correcting fluid and electrolyte problems and providing nutritional support for hepatic repair as much as possible. In any case, guidelines for nutritional therapy for cirrhosis of the liver should include the following principles:
1. *Protein according to tolerance.* In the absence of impending hepatic encephalopathy (see the following discussion about hepatic encephalopathy), the protein intake should be continued at the level indicated for hepatitis, about 1.5 to 2 g/kg of actual body weight, or about 100 to 150 g/day. The protein is needed to correct severe undernutrition, regenerate functional liver tissue, and replenish plasma protein. However, if signs of hepatic encephalopathy appear, protein must be decreased to individual tolerance.
2. *Low sodium.* Sodium is usually restricted to about 1000 mg/day to help reduce fluid retention.

3. *Texture.* If esophageal varices develop, it may be necessary to give soft foods that are smooth in texture to prevent danger of rupture and hemorrhage.
4. *Optimal general nutrition.* The remaining overall diet principles outlined for hepatitis are continued for cirrhosis for the same reasons. Kcalories, carbohydrates, and vitamins are supplied according to individual need and deficiency. Moderate fat is used. Alcohol is strictly forbidden.

Table 18.9 High-protein, high-carbohydrate, moderate-fat daily diet

Food	Amount
Milk	1 L (1 qt)
Egg substitute	Equal to 1-2 eggs
Lean meat, fish, or poultry	224 g (8 oz)
Vegetables (4 servings)	
Potato or substitute	2 servings
Green leafy or yellow	1 serving
Other vegetables (including 1 raw)	1-2 servings
Fruit (3-4 servings, includes juices often)	
Citrus (or other good source of ascorbic acid)	1-2 servings
Other fruit	2 servings
Bread and cereal (whole grain or enriched	6-8 servings
Cereal	1 serving
Sliced bread or crackers	5-6 servings
Butter or fortified margarine	2-4 tbsp
Jam, jelly, honey, and other carbohydrates	As patient desires and is able to eat them
Sweetened fruit juices	To increase carbohydrates and fluids

macrocytic anemia An anemia (deficiency of normal red cells) characterized by abnormally large red cells.

varices (plural) Varicose veins; enlarged and tortuous veins, full of twists, curves, or windings.

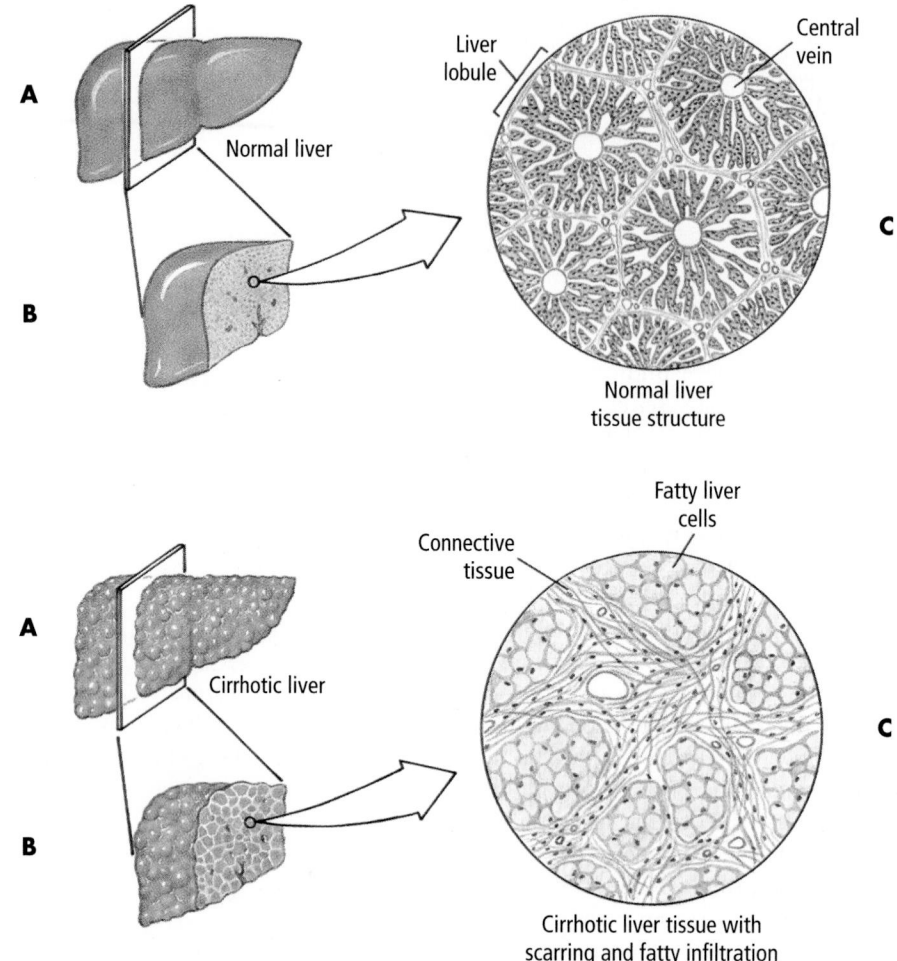

Figure 18.5 Comparison of normal liver and liver with cirrhotic tissue changes. **A,** Anterior view of organ; **B,** cross-section; **C,** tissue structure.

HEPATIC ENCEPHALOPATHY

The term **encephalopathy** refers to any disease or disorder that affects the brain, especially chronic degenerative conditions. The brain effect in hepatic encephalopathy is a major serious complication of end-stage liver disease. The accumulation of toxic substances in the blood as a result of liver failure impairs consciousness and contributes to memory loss, personality change, tremors, seizures, stupor, and coma.

Etiology

As cirrhotic changes continue in the liver, the portal blood circulation diminishes and liver functions begin to fail. The normal liver has a major function of removing ammonia from the blood by converting it to urea for excretion. The failing liver can no longer inac-tivate or detoxify substances or metabolize others. A key factor involved in the progressive disease process is an elevated blood level of ammonia, although it is by no means the sole agent. The resulting hepatic encephalopathy brings changes in consciousness, behavior, and neurologic status.

Clinical symptoms

Typical response involves disorders of consciousness and alterations in motor function. There is apathy, confusion, inappropriate behavior, and drowsiness, progressing to coma. The speech may be slurred or monotonous. A coarse, flapping tremor known as **asterixis**, is observed in the outstretched hands, caused by a sustained contraction of a group of muscles. The breath may have a fecal odor, **fetor hepaticus.**

Basic treatment objectives

The fundamental objective of treatment is twofold: (1) removal of the sources of excess ammonia, and (2) provision of nutritional support. Medical and nutritional therapy are involved. Parenteral fluid and electrolytes are used to restore normal balances. Two drugs may be used to control ammonia-lactulose and neomycin. Lactulose is a nonabsorbable synthetic disaccharide that reduces the absorption of intestinal ammonia. Neomycin is an antibiotic that reduces the population of urea-splitting organisms within the bowel that produce ammonia. To stop bleeding into the intestine as another source of intestinal ammonia, a Sengstaken-Blakemore tube may be used.

Nutritional therapy

General nutritional support for hepatic encephalopathy is based on the following principles of dietary management.

1. *Low protein.* General protein intake is reduced individually as necessary to restrict the dietary sources of nitrogen in amino acids. The amount of restriction varies with the circumstances, but the usual amounts range from 30 to 50 g/day, depending on whether symptoms are severe or mild. A simple method for controlling dietary protein uses a base meal pattern containing approximately 15 g protein and then adds small items of protein foods according to the level of protein desired (Table 18.10).
2. *Branched-chain amino acids.* The three branched-chain amino acids (BCAAs)—leucine, isoleucine, and valine—are not catabolized by the liver but are taken up by other tissues. Thus they can be metabolized without depending on healthy liver tissue, as is the case with the other amino acids. They provide a useful energy source, as well as a better tolerated source of needed protein that may be utilized directly by the muscles, heart, liver, and brain. Oral BCAA formula has been used, with the patients becoming neurologically normal. The clinical use of BCAA supplementation in enteral and parenteral nutrition support formulas is an important part of standard therapy in liver failure and may improve chance of survival.
3. *Kcalories and vitamins.* Adequate energy intake is crucial to the patient's recovery, especially through the impact of kcaloric intake on liver glycogen reserves and their protective role in the healing process. The amounts of kcalories and vitamins are prescribed according to need. About 2000 kcal/day is needed to prevent tissue catabolism, with sufficient carbohydrate as the primary energy source and some fat as tolerated. Vitamin K is usually given parenterally, along with other vitamins and minerals, especially zinc, that may be deficient.
4. *Fluid intake.* Fluid intake-output balance is carefully controlled.

LIVER TRANSPLANTATION

The development of liver transplantation as an acceptable therapy for end-stage liver disease has been an important medical advance. Candidates for transplant include patients with end-stage chronic liver disease or acute liver failure, progressive liver disease for which conventional treatment has failed, and the prognosis of which indicates a survival of less than 10%.[50] In such cases, **orthotopic** (normal placement) liver transplacement remains the best chance of prolonged survival, especially with end-stage disease in children.[51] Liver transplantation is indicated for patients, mostly women, with intractable symptoms of primary biliary cirrhosis.[52] Less suitable cases include problems such as alcoholic cirrhosis and malignant tumors, and those complicated by sepsis or advanced lung and kidney disease. As with all major surgery, aggressive nutritional support reduces risks. Careful pretransplant nutritional assessment and support helps prepare the patient for the surgery. Enteral or parenteral nutritional support may be required for optimal postoperative nutritional status. A number of posttransplant young women, with the new healthy liver and good nutrition support, have experienced return of fertility and been able to conceive and maintain the high-risk pregnancy to a successful conclusion with closely monitored medical and nutritional management.[53] In such cases, immediate follow-up contraception with a barrier method is recommended because birth control pills may interfere with accurate **cyclosporine** dosing for maintaining the transplant.

GALLBLADDER DISEASE

Metabolic function

The basic function of the gallbladder is to concentrate and store the bile produced in its initial watery solution by the liver. The liver secretes about 600 to 800 ml/day of bile, which the gallbladder normally concentrates five-

---

asterixis Neuromotor disturbance marked by an inability to hold outstretched hands in a steady position, resulting in an intermittent flapping of the hands, characteristic of hepatic coma.

cyclosporine An immunosuppressant drug used following organ transplants to control the immune system and prevent rejection of the new tissue.

encephalopathy Any degenerative disease of the brain.

fetor hepaticas The peculiar odor of the breath that is characteristic of advanced liver disease.

orthotopic Occurring at the normal place in the body; placement of a transplanted organ in the position formerly occupied by tissue of the same kind.

fold to tenfold to accommodate this daily bile production in its small capacity of 40 to 70 ml. Through the cholecystokinin (CCK) mechanism, the presence of fat in the duodenum stimulates contraction of the gallbladder with the release of concentrated bile into the common duct and then into the small intestine.

Cholecystitis and cholelithiasis

The prefix *chole-* of the two terms *cholecystitis* and *cholelithiasis* comes from the Greek word *chole*, which means "bile." Thus cholecystitis is an inflammation of the gallbladder, and cholelithiasis is the formation of gallstones.

Inflammation of the gallbladder usually results from a low-grade chronic infection and may occur with or without gallstones. However, in 90% to 95% of patients, acute cholecystitis is associated with gallstones and is caused by the obstruction of the cystic duct by stones, resulting in acute inflammation of the organ. Gallstones can be classified into two main groups: cholesterol and pigment stones.

1. *Cholesterol stones.* In the United States and most Western countries, more than 75% of the gallstones are cholesterol stones. The infectious process produces changes in the gallbladder mucosa, which affects its absorptive powers. Normally bile's main ingredient cholesterol, which is insoluble in water, is kept in solution by the other bile ingredients. However, when the absorbing mucosal tissue of the gallbladder is inflamed or infected, changes occur in the tissue. The absorptive powers of the gallbladder may be altered, affecting the solubility of the bile ingredients. Excess water or excess bile acid may be absorbed. Under these abnormal absorptive conditions cholesterol may precipitate, forming gallstones of almost pure cholesterol. Excessive use of dietary fat over a long period of time predisposes persons to gallstone formation because of the constant stimulus to produce more cholesterol as a necessary bile ingredient to metabolize fat.[54,55]

2. *Pigment stones.* Both black and brown pigment gallstones, although they differ in chemical composition and clinical features, are colored by the presence of bilirubin, the pigment in red blood cells. They are associated with chronic hemolysis in conditions such as sickle cell disease, thalassemia, cirrhosis, long-

---

Table

18.10　Low-protein diets (15 g, 30 g, 40 g, and 50 g protein)

General description

The following diets are used when dietary protein is to be restricted
The patterns limit foods containing a large percentage of protein, such as milk, eggs, cheese, meat, fish, fowl, and legumes.
Avoid meat extractives, soups, broth, bouillon, gravies, and gelatin desserts.

Basic meal patterns (contains approximately 15 g of protein)

Breakfast	Lunch	Dinner
½ cup fruit or fruit juice	1 small potato	1 small potato
½ cup cereal	½ cup vegetable	½ cup vegetable
1 slice toast	Salad (vegetable or fruit)	Salad (vegetable or fruit)
Butter	1 slice bread	1 slice bread
Jelly	Butter	Butter
Sugar	1 serving fruit	1 serving fruit
2 tbsp cream	Sugar	Sugar
Coffee	Coffee or tea	Coffee or tea

For 30 g protein	Examples of meat portions
Add: 1 cup milk	28 g (1 oz) meat = 1 thin slice roast, 4 × 5 cm (1½ × 2 in)
28 g (1 oz) meat, 1 egg, or equivalent	1 rounded tbsp cottage cheese
	1 slice American cheese

For 40 g protein	
Add: 1 cup milk	70 g (2½ oz) meat = Ground beef patty (5 can be made from
70 g (2½ oz) meat, or 1 egg and 42 g (1½ oz) meat	448g [1 lb])
	1 slice roast

For 50 g protein	
Add: 1 cup milk	112 g (4 oz) meat = 2 lamb chops
112 g (4 oz) meat, or 2 eggs and 56 g (2 oz) meat	1 average steak

term TPN, and advancing age.[56] Pigment stones are often found in the bile ducts and may be related to a bacterial infection with *Escherichia coli.*

Clinical symptoms

When inflammation, stones, or both are present in the gallbladder, contraction from the cholecystokinin-pancreozymin (CCK-PZ) mechanism causes pain. Sometimes the pain is severe. There is fullness and distention after eating and particular difficulty with fatty foods.

General treatment

Surgical removal of the gallbladder, a cholecystectomy, is usually indicated. If the patient is obese, some weight loss before surgery is advisable if surgery can be delayed. Supportive therapy is largely nutritional. Several new nonsurgical treatments for removing the stones, using chemical dissolution or mechanical stone fragmentation, have been developed (see *To Probe Further* box below). These methods provide effective alternatives to surgery in some cases.

Nutritional therapy

Basic principles of nutritional therapy for gallbladder disease include the following:

1. *Fat.* Because dietary fat is the principal cause of contraction of the diseased organ and subsequent pain, it is poorly tolerated. Energy should come primarily from carbohydrate foods, especially during acute phases. Control of fat will also contribute to weight control, a primary goal because obesity and excess food intake have been repeatedly associated with the development of gallstones.

To Probe Further

Dissolution and fragmentation: alternate solutions to the problem of gallstones

The 25 million Americans with gallstones may be able to have relief without surgery. Chemical dissolution by use of a drug, alone or combined with mechanical fragmentation by ultrasound waves, offers possible alternatives.

Chenodiol (chenodeoxycholic acid), and its companion *ursodiol* (ursodeoxycholic acid) are two natural bile acids that reduce the concentration of cholesterol in bile and dissolve cholesterol stones harmlessly, thus sparing many persons the discomfort, risk, and cost of major surgery. Their biologic activity prevents excessive cholesterol from separating out of bile to form the most common type of gallstone. Other stones consisting of combinations of calcium carbonate, bilirubin, and other compounds make up only 15% to 20% of all gallstones.

These two naturally occurring bile acids, CDCA and UDCA, have been studied for a number of years and are now used to treat gallstones in more than 40 countries. Clinically, they appear to be effective at dissolving "floating" gallstones less than 1.25 cm ($\frac{1}{2}$ in) in diameter with few side effects (such as diarrhea) and only temporary reversible changes in some liver enzymes. This makes it potentially beneficial to patients who are surgical risks because of other medical problems.

Other nonsurgical methods of removing gallstones are also now in experimental stages of development and may expand these alternatives still further. An additional chemical dissolution method is the instillation of liquid solvents such as methyl tert-butyl ether (MTBE) directly into the gallbladder or the common bile duct. Additional mechanical fragmentation by pulsed lasers is being studied.

These alternate means may help patients avoid gallbladder surgery, but they do not eliminate the need for a diet emphasizing carbohydrates and fiber and controlling fat with an eye to weight management. Further, most of these alternatives work mainly on small stones rather than on larger clumps of cholesterol. Also, they are not recommended for everyone. Chronic liver disease or a bile duct obstruction may rule them out, as does pregnancy. For many persons however, these alternatives may provide successful treatments. Those who suffer from gallstones may be able to say good-bye to pain, indigestion, nausea, and jaundice without fear of surgery.

References

Albert MB, Fromm H: Nonsurgical alternatives in the management of gallstones, *J Intensive Care Med* 4(1):3, 1989.

Editorial: Bile acid therapy in the 1990s, *Lancet* 340:1260, Nov 21, 1992.

Hochberger J et al: Lithotripsy of gallstones by means of a quality-switched giant-pulse neodymium:yttrium-aluminum-garnet laser, *Gastroenterology* 101(5):1391, 1991.

2. *Kcalories.* If weight loss is indicated, kcalories will be reduced according to need. Principles of weight management are discussed in Chapter 6. Usually such a diet will have a relatively low fat ratio and meet the needs of the patient for fat moderation.

3. *Cholesterol and "gas formers."* Two additional modifications usually found in traditional diets for gallbladder disease concern restriction of foods containing cholesterol and foods labeled "gas formers." Neither modification has a valid rationale. The body daily synthesizes more cholesterol than is present in an average diet. Thus restriction of dietary cholesterol has little effect in reducing gallstone formation. Total dietary fat reduction is more important. As for the use of "gas-formers," such as legumes, cabbage, or fiber, blanket restriction seems unwarranted, since food tolerances in any circumstances are highly individual.

DISEASES OF THE PANCREAS

Pancreatitis

Acute inflammation of the pancreas, that is, pancreatitis, is caused by the digestion of the organ tissues by the enzymes it produces, principally trypsin. Normally, enzymes remain in the inactive form until the pancreatic secretions reach the duodenum through the common duct. However, gallbladder disease may cause a gallstone to enter the common bile duct and obstruct the flow from the pancreas or cause a reflux of these secretions and bile from the common duct back into the pancreatic duct. This mixing of digestive materials activates the powerful pancreatic enzymes within the gland. In such activated form, they begin their damaging effects on the pancreatic tissue itself, causing acute pain. Sometimes infectious pancreatitis may occur as a complication of mumps or a bacterial disease. Mild or moderate pancreatitis may subside completely, but it has a tendency to recur.

General treatment

Initial care consists of measures recommended for acute disease involving shock. These measures include intravenous feeding at first, replacement therapy of fluid and electrolytes, blood transfusions, antibiotics and pain medications, and gastric suction.

Nutritional therapy

In early stages, nutritional support is maintained by parenteral feeding and oral feedings are withheld because entry of food into the intestines stimulates pancreatic secretions. As healing progresses and oral feedings are resumed, a light diet is used to avoid excessive stimulation of pancreatic secretions. Alcohol and caffeine should be avoided to decrease pancreatic stimulation. Alcohol in Western societies and malnutrition worldwide are the major causes of chronic pancreatitis. Persons with this disease are usually thin and have low serum lipid concentrations, suggesting that they have latent digestion disorders or malabsorption.[56]

TO SUM UP

The nutritional therapy of gastrointestinal disease is based on careful consideration of four major factors: (1) *secretory functions*, providing the chemical agents and environment necessary for digestion to occur; (2) *neuromuscular functions*, required for motility and mechanical digestion; (3) *absorptive functions*, enhancing the entry of nutrients into the circulatory system; and (4) *psychologic factors*, reflected by changes in gastrointestinal function.

Esophageal problems vary widely from simple dysphagia to serious disease or obstruction. Nutritional therapy and mode of intake vary according to degree of dysfunction.

Peptic ulcer disease is a common gastrointestinal problem affecting millions of Americans. It is an erosion of the mucosal lining, mainly in the duodenal bulb and less commonly in the lower antrum portion of the stomach. It results in increased gastric tone and painful hunger contractions on an empty stomach, as well as nutritional problems such as low plasma protein levels, anemia, and weight loss. Current medical management consists of acid and infection control with a coordinated system of drugs, rest, and a regular diet with few food and drink considerations to supply the essential nutritional support for tissue healing.

Intestinal diseases are classified as (1) *anatomic changes*, such as the development of small tubular sacs branching off the main alimentary canal in *diverticular disease*; (2) *malabsorption*, from multiple maldigestive and malabsorptive conditions; and (3) *Inflammatory bowel disease (IBD)*, resulting from mucosal changes and infectious processes, as seen in *ulcerative colitis* and *Crohn's disease*, or (4) *short-bowel syndrome*, resulting from surgical resection of parts of the intestine. Nutritional therapy involves fluid and electrolyte replacement, modifications in the diet's protein and energy content and food texture, and increased vitamins and minerals, with continuous adjustment of the diet according to changes in toleration for specific foods. Allergic responses to common food allergens, as well as missing cell enzymes in genetic disease, may also contribute to gastrointestinal and metabolic problems from related food intolerances.

Accessory organs to the gastrointestinal tract-liver, gallbladder, and pancreas-have important functions related to nutrient digestion, absorption, and metabolism, and their diseases interfere with these normal functions. Common liver disorders include hepatitis, usually caused by viral infection, and cirrhosis, an advanced liver disease leading to hepatic encephalopathy and progressive liver failure. Nutrient and energy levels required vary with each condition.

Diseases of the gallbladder include cholecystitis, inflammation that interferes with the absorption of water and bile acids, and cholelithiasis, or gallstone formation. Treatment involves a generally reduced-fat diet and surgical removal of the gallbladder. Diseases of the pancreas include acute and chronic forms of pancreatitis, in which alcohol abuse can be a primary cause. Other causes include biliary disease, malnutrition, drug reactions, abdominal injury, and genetic predisposition. In acute pancreatitis, pain is severe because of pancreatic enzyme reflux with self-digestion of pancreatic tissue by its own enzymes. Parenteral nutrition support is used to avoid enzyme stimulus, with gradual return to small, frequent meals as the attack subsides. In chronic pancreatitis, which is caused by alcoholism in Western societies and malnutrition worldwide, maldigestion from lack of enzymes because of pancreatic insufficiency creates nutritional problems. Nutritional care focuses on a nourishing diet with enzyme replacement and vitamin-mineral supplementation.

QUESTIONS FOR REVIEW

1. What is the basic principle of diet planning for patients with esophageal problems? Outline a general nutritional care plan for a patient with gastroesophageal reflux disease (GERD) complicated by a hiatal hernia.

2. In current practice, what are the basic principles of diet planning for patients with peptic ulcer disease? How do these principles differ from former traditional therapy?

3. Outline a course of nutritional management for a person with peptic ulcer disease, based on the current approaches to medical management. How would you plan nutrition education for continuing self-care and avoidance of recurrence?

4. Describe the etiology, clinical signs, and treatment of each of the following intestinal diseases: malabsorption and diarrhea, inflammatory bowel disease, diverticular disease, irritable bowel disease, and constipation.

5. Compare the basis of food intolerances resulting from food allergy and a specific genetic disease such as PKU.

6. How are the major metabolic functions of the liver affected in liver disease? Give some examples.

7. What is the rationale for treatment in the spectrum of liver disease-hepatitis, cirrhosis, and hepatic encephalopathy?

8. Develop a 1-day food plan for a 45-year-old man, 183 cm (6 ft, 1 in) tall, weighing 90 kg (200 lb), with infectious hepatitis; another plan for a similar patient with cirrhosis of the liver; and another for a patient with hepatic encephalopathy. What principles of diet therapy apply for each?

9. What are the principles of nutritional therapy for gallbladder disease? Write a 1-day meal plan for a 30-year-old woman, 165 cm (5 ft, 6 in) tall, weighing 81 kg (180 lb), who has an inflamed gallbladder with stones and is awaiting a cholecystectomy.

10. Compare acute and chronic forms of pancreatitis in terms of etiology, symptoms, and nutritional therapy. What role does special enteral and parenteral nutrition support play in this therapy?

REFERENCES

1. Stanek K et al: Factors affecting use of food and commercial agents to thicken liquids for individuals with swallowing disorders, *J Am Diet Assoc* 92(4):488, 1992.

2. Mann LL, Wong K: Development of an objective method for assessing viscosity of formulated foods and beverages for the dysphagic diet, *J Am Diet Assoc* 96(6):585, 1996.

3. Pasricha PJ et al: Botulinum toxin for achalasia: long-term toxin for achalasia: long-term outcome and predictors of response, *Gastroenterology* 110:1410, 1996.

4. Brzana PJ, Koch KL: Gastroesophageal reflux disease presenting with intractable nausea, *Ann Intern Med* 26(9):704, 1997.

5. Gelfans MD: Gastroesophageal reflux disease, *Med Clin North Am* 75(4):923, 1991.

6. Kitchin LI, Castell DO: Rationale and efficiency of conservative therapy for gastroesophageal reflux disease, *Arch Intern Med* 151:448, 1991.

7. Katz J: The course of peptic ulcer disease, *Med Clin North Am* 75(4):1013, 1991.

8. Marshall BJ, Warren JR: Unidentified curved bacilli in the stomach of patients with gastritis and peptic ulceration, *Lancet* 8390:1311, 1984.

9. Blaser MJ: The bacteria behind ulcers, *Sci Am* 274(2):104, 1996.

10. Marchetti M et al: Development of a mouse model of *Helicobacter pylori* infection that mimics human disease, *Science* 267(5204):1655, 1995.

11. Megraud F: Epidemiology of *Helicobacter pylori* infection, *Gasteroenterol Clin North Am* 22(1):73, 1993.

12. HIH Consensus Development Panel on *Helicobacter pylori* in peptic ulcer disease, *JAMA* 65:272, 1994.

13. Sonnenberg A, Everhart JE: The prevalence of self-reported peptic ulcer in the United States, *Am J Pub Health* 86(2):200, 1996.

14. Walsh JH, Peterson WL: The treatment of *H. pylori* in the management of peptic ulcer disease, *N Engl J Med* 333(15):984, 1995.

15. Hentschel E et al: Effect of ranitidine and amoxicillin plus metronidazole on the eradication of *Helicobacter pylori* and the recurrence of duodenal ulcer, *N Engl J Med* 328(5):308, 1993.

16. Damianos AJ, McGarrity TJ: Treatment strategies for *Helicobacter pylori* infection, *Am Fam Physician* 55(8):2765, 1997.

17. Tompkins LS, Falkow S: The new path to preventing ulcers, *Science* 267(5204):1621, 1995.

18. Nowak R: The gold bug: *Helicobacter pylori, Science* 267(5195):173, 1995.

19. Caspary WF: Physiology and pathophysiology of intestinal absorption, *Am J Clin Nutr* 55(suppl):299S, 1992.

20. Trier JS: Celiac sprue, *N Engl J Med* 325(24):1709, 1991.

21. Chartrand LJ et al: Wheat starch intolerance in patients with celiac disease, *JADA* 97(6):612, 1997.

22. Thompson T: Do oats belong in a gluten-free diet? *J Am Diet Assoc* 97(12):1413, 1997.

23. Skerritt JH, Hill AS: Self-management of dietary compliance in celiac disease by means of ELISA "home test" to detect gluten, *Lancet* 337:379, 1991.

24. Marcus MS et al: Nutritional status of infants with cystic fibrosis associated with early diagnosis and intervention, *Am J Clin Nutr* 54:578, 1991.

25. Thomas PJ et al: Cystic fibrosis transmembrane conductance regulator: nucleotide binding to a synthetic peptide, *Science* 251:553, 1991.

26. Cystic Fibrosis Foundation: Guidelines for patient services, evaluation, and monitoring in cystic fibrosis centers, *Am J Dis Child* 144:1311, 1990.

27. Moran A et al: Pancreatic endocrine function in cystic fibrosis, *J Pediatr* 118:715, 1991.

28. Brady MS et al: Effectiveness of enteric coated pancreatic enzymes given before meals in reducing steatorrhea in children with cystic fibrosis, *J Am Diet Assoc* 92(7):813, 1992.

29. Dowsett J: Nutrition in the management of cystic fibrosis, *Nutr Rev* 54(1):31, 1996.

30. Maxwell PR et al: Irritable bowel syndrome, *Lancet* 350:1691, 1997.

31. Dalton CB, Drossman DA: Diagnosis and treatment of irritable bowel syndrome, *Am Fam Physician* 55(3):875, 1997.

32. Fackelman K: Gastrointestinal blues, *Sci News* 150(19):302, 1996.

33. Hoffenberg EF et al: Circulating antioxidant concentrations in children with inflammatory bowel disease, *Am J Clin Nutr* 65:1482, 1997.

34. Hanauer SB: Inflammatory bowel disease, *N Engl J Med* 334(13):841, 1996.

35. Friedman G: Treatment of the irritable bowel syndrome, *Gastroenterol Clin North Am* 20(2):325, 1991.

36. Rosenberg IH, Mason JB: Intestinal disorders: inflammatory bowel disease. In Shils ME, Olson JA, Shike M, eds: *Modern nutrition in health and disease,* ed 8, vol 2, Philadelphia, 1994, Lea & Febiger.

37. Jeejeebhoy KN: Intestinal disorders: short-bowel syndrome. In Shils ME, Olson JA, Shike M, eds: *Modern nutrition in health and disease,* ed 8, vol 2, Philadelphia, 1994, Lea & Febiger.

38. Parker SL et al: Foods perceived by adults as causing adverse reactions, *J Am Diet Assoc* 93(1):40, 1993.

39. Bishop JM et al: Natural history of cow milk allergy: clinical outcome, *J Pediatr* 116:862, 1990.

40. Sampson HA et al: Safety of casein hydrolysate formula in children with cow milk allergy, *J Pediatr* 118:520, 1991.

41. Björkstén B: Dietary management of food allergy, *Semin Pediatr Gastroenteral Nutr* 3(2):13, 1992.

42. Nash JM et al: *Allergies, Time* 139(25):54, 1992.

43. Elsas LJ II, Acosta PB: Nutritional support of inherited metabolic disease. In Shils ME, Olson JA, Shike M, eds: *Modern nutrition in health and disease,* ed 8, vol 2, Philadelphia, 1994, Lea & Febiger.

41. Lau JYN et al: Viral hepatitis, *Gut* 32(suppl 9):47, 1991.

42. Hoffman M: Hepatitis A vaccine shows promise, *Science* 254:1581, 1991.

43. *Bull World Health Organ* 66:443, 1988.

44. Vail BA: Management of chronic viral hepatitis, *Am Fam Physician* 55(8):2749, 1997.

45. Martinot M et al: Influence of hepatitis G virus infection on the severity of liver disease and response to interferon-α in patients with chronic hepatitis C, *Ann Intern Med* 126(11):874, 1997.

46. Koff RS: Interferon-α for chronic hepatitis C: reducing the uncertainties, *Ann Intern Med* 127(10):1997.

47. Lee WM: Hepatitis B virus infection, *N Engl J Med* 337(24):1733, 1997.

48. Silk DBA et al: Nutritional support in liver disease, *Gut* 32(suppl 9):29, 1991.

49. Everhart JE, Hoofnagle JH: Hepatitis B-related end-stage liver disease, *Gastroenterology* 103(5):1692, 1992.

50. Poterucha JJ, Wiesner RH: Liver transplantation and hepatitis B, *Ann Intern Med* 126(8):805, 1997.

51. Holt RIG et al: Orthotopic liver transplantation reverses the adverse nutritional changes of end-stage liver disease in children, *Am J Clin Nutr* 65:534, 1997.

52. Neuberger J: Primary biliary cirrhosis, *Lancet* 350(Sept 20):875, 1997.

53. Laifer SA et al: Pregnancy in liver transplant patients—and vice versa, *Gastroenterology* 10(5):1443, 1991.

54. Ortega RM et al: Differences in diet and food habits between patients with gallstones and controls, *J Am Coll Nutr* 16(1):88, 1997.

55. Lee SP, Sekijima J: Gallstones. In Yamada T, ed: *Textbook of gasteroenterology,* vol 2, New York, 1991, JB Lippincott.

56. Vaona B et al: Food intake of patients with chronic pancreatitis after onset of the disease, *Am J Clin Nutr* 65:851, 1997.

▰ FURTHER READING

Anderson JA: Milk, eggs, and peanuts: food allergies in children: *Am Fam Physician* 56(5):1365, 1997.

Lallè JP, Peltre G: Biochemical features of grain-legume allergens in humans and animals, *Nutr Rev* 54(4):101, 1996.

These two articles will aid in counseling with patients who have allergies to commonly used foods.

Chartrand LJ et al: Wheat starch intolerance in patients with celiac disease, *J Am Diet Assoc* 97(6):612, 1997.

Thompson T: Do oats belong in a gluten-free diet? *J Am Diet Assoc* 97(12):1413, 1997.

These two articles provide a helpful resource for practical ways of providing food for special diets.

Dalton CB, Drossman DA: Diagnosis and treatment of irritable bowel syndrome, *Am Fam Physician* 55(3):875, 1997.

The authors present a sensitive article about this common but frustrating condition in elderly persons, providing helpful background for all those who care for these patients.

Mann LL, Wong K: Development of an objective method for assessing viscosity of formulated foods and beverages for the dysphagic diet, *J Am Diet Assoc* 96(6):585, 1996.

Here are practical ways of providing soft foods for persons with a range of swallowing disorders, a real need especially when the disorder is long-term or permanent and economy is a problem.

Case study

The patient with peptic ulcer disease

Lowell Randolph is a 40-year-old businessman who was admitted to the city hospital 3 weeks ago after an incidence of vomiting bright-red blood. A medical history revealed that a dull, gnawing pain in the upper abdomen began several months ago and has increased in severity during that time. It became more severe after his most recent out-of-state trip to one of his stores. Because the pain was usually accompanied by headaches, he took aspirin to help relieve it.

Initial hospital treatment consisted of blood transfusions, intravenous fluids and electrolytes, and vitamin C. Mr. Randolph continued to feel nauseous and weak, but he stopped vomiting. However, he passed several large, tarry stools during the first 24 hours. His initial nutritional assessment results included: weight 68 kg (150 lb); height 179 cm (70 in); albumin 2.8 g/dl; prealbumin 14 mg/dl; transferrin 18% saturation value; hemoglobin 11 g/dl; and hematocrit 35%. His medications included cimetidine, sucralfate, magnesium-aluminum hydroxide, and triple antibiotic therapy.

The patient began slowly to tolerate sips of clear liquids, then advanced to a regular diet as tolerated, showing continued improvement. Before he was discharged at the end of the second week, the nutritionist and the nurse discussed general nutritional needs with Mr. Randolph and his wife. They advised him to eat his meals regularly in as relaxed a setting and manner as possible, eliminate his frequent between-meal snacks, and take his multivitamin supplement daily with his meals. Also, they reviewed his general guidelines sheet, listing a few food-related items or habits to avoid. They also advised him to stop smoking and to rest as much as possible before returning to work. His physician had also advised him to reduce his work load and scheduled a follow-up appointment in 1 week.

Mrs. Randolph accompanied her husband to the next appointment and reported that she was pleased with his ability to put aside business duties and take more time to enjoy his family. Mr. Randolph stated that his two teenage sons had been surprisingly supportive in assisting him in following the prescribed regimen and that he plans to make it his general habit.

Questions for analysis

1. The x-ray diagnosis of Mr. Randolph's illness was a gastric ulcer in the antrum lesser curvature. What does this mean? Where do most ulcers occur? Why?
2. What factors contributed to Mr. Randolph's ulcer? What effect did each of them have?
3. Evaluate the results of Mr. Randolph's initial nutritional assessment data. How would you use this information in nutrition counseling?
4. Identify Mr. Randolph's basic nutritional needs. Outline a teaching plan based on these needs that you would use to help him with his new diet plan. How would you include his wife in formulating and implementing his nutritional care plan?
5. What role does vitamin C play in Mr. Randolph's therapy? What other vitamins and minerals play a significant role in his care? Describe each role.
6. Why should Mr. Randolph give up coffee, cigarettes, and alcohol? What problems do you think he may encounter in trying to change these habits?

Issues Answers

Nutritional aspects of diarrhea

Gastrointestinal disease so often presents barriers to efficient nutrient absorption that nutritional deficiencies are planned for automatically. Ironically many of these conditions also frequently lead to diarrhea, which results in further loss of fluids and electrolytes. As expected, their replacement is the initial and primary concern of therapy. However, different types of diarrhea also present other differences; the control of type-specific problems requires different modes of treatment coordinated with the treatment of the disease it accompanies. Before looking into possible treatment modes, examine first three of the most common types of diarrhea: watery, fatty, and small volume.

Watery diarrhea occurs when the amount of water and electrolytes moving into the intestinal mucosa exceeds that amount absorbed into the bloodstream. This movement of water and electrolytes into the mucosa may be secretive or osmotic.

If this movement of water and electrolytes into the mucosa is *secretive*, it may be active or passive. *Active movement* occurs with excessive gastric hydrochloric acid secretion or enterotoxin-induced infections such as cholera. *Passive movement* occurs with a rise in hydrostatic pressure that accompanies such infectious diseases as salmonellosis or tuberculosis, nonbacterial infections, fungal infections, renal failure, irradiation enteritis, and inflammatory bowel disease. Other conditions associated with watery diarrhea include hyperthyroidism, thyroid carcinoma, and hypermotility of the gastrointestinal tract.

If this movement of water and electrolytes into the mucosa is osmotic, it will occur when these nutrients are not absorbed because of intolerable levels of nonabsorbable particles present in the intestinal chyme. Such particles include lactose (milk sugar) in lactase-deficient individuals or gluten (grain protein) in persons with a reduced gastrointestinal transit time caused by the removal of part of the intestinal tract.

Fatty diarrhea, or steatorrhea, occurs with maldigestion or malabsorption. *Maldigestion* involves a lack of enzymatic activity required to completely digest food, such as reduced pancreatic exocrine activity (release of intestinal enzymes from the pancreas) caused by pancreatic insufficiency. *Malabsorption* means that digested materials do not make it across the intestinal mucosa to enter the bloodstream. This fail-

ure occurs in conditions in which the intestinal villi are destroyed, such as celiac disease.

Small-volume diarrhea occurs mainly when the rectosigmoid area of the colon is irritated, such as in inflammatory bowel disease (Crohn's disease or ulcerative colitis). It also occurs when inflammatory conditions affect areas adjacent to the colon, as in pelvic inflammatory disease, diverticulitis, appendicitis, or hemorrhagic ovarian cysts.

The metabolic consequences of each type of diarrhea are similar. Uncontrolled, they result in *syncope, hypokalemia, acid-base imbalances,* and *hypovolemia,* with resulting *renal failure.* They may also be accompanied by low levels of fat-soluble vitamins, B_{12}, or folic acid, or eventually lead to protein-energy malnutrition. In addition to these conditions, each type also manifests problems associated with the disorder they accompany. Workers with the Memorial Sloan-Kettering Cancer Center in New York and the Department of Medicine at Brooke Army Medical Center in Texas have developed recommendations for treating gastrointestinal diseases associated with each type of diarrhea. These are summarized here, with the focus on the diarrheal aspects of disease.

Watery diarrhea often accompanies inflammatory bowel conditions, such as Crohn's disease, for which diet therapy involves (1) increased protein and kcalories, (2) low fats and lactose, and (3) avoidance of foods that stimulate peristalsis. Thus secretive diarrhea is reduced by eliminating foods that may stimulate gastric acid secretion, and all types of watery diarrhea are avoided by reducing the motility of the gastrointestinal tract. In other conditions in which osmotic diarrhea occurs, such as *dumping syndrome,* this problem is avoided by giving fluids *between* meals to avoid any extreme difference in osmotic pressures on either side of the intestinal wall. Small, frequent meals also help prevent this problem as well as the problem of painful distention.

Fatty diarrhea frequently accompanies conditions associated with maldigestion, such as chronic pancreatitis. The dietary management of this disease involves (1) frequent meals, high in protein and carbohydrates and low in fat; (2) use of medium-chain triglycerides, which are more easily absorbed under adverse conditions; and, (3) avoiding gastric stimulants, especially caffeine and alcohol. Fatty diarrhea also accompanies conditions of malabsorption, such as gluten-sensitive enteropathy. In addition to diet management strategies listed, treating this type of diarrhea also requires the removal of products that damage the mucosal villi, including lactose and gluten, which is found in wheat, rye, barley, and oats, and food products and fillers such as hydrolyzed vegetable protein products. It sometimes requires restricting fat as well. In both cases the primary concern is to monitor fats that would otherwise appear in the feces. As the therapy progresses, the fat content of the meal can be increased as tolerated to normal levels to improve palatability.

Small-volume diarrhea may accompany diverticulosis of the colon. A high-residue diet is recommended to increase fecal bulk, thereby preventing diarrhea. To prevent flatulence and distention, however, the fiber—such as wheat bran, fruits, and vegetables—should be added to the diet gradually.

All types of diarrhea can result in malnutrition, primarily because of electrolyte and fluid losses. It is important to identify the *type* of diarrhea occurring with each patient. Only then can an effective nutritional management strategy be designed to replace those losses, as well as to eliminate or prevent other nutrition-related problems that are possible for each case.

References

Banwell JG: Pathophysiology of diarrheal disorders, *Rev Infect Dis* 12(suppl 1):30, 1990.

Barrett KE, Dharmsathaphorn K: Secretion and absorption: small intestine and colon. In Yamada T, ed: *Textbook of gastroenterology,* Philadelphia, 1991, JB Lippincott.

Gorbach SL: Efficacy of lactobacillus in treatment of acute diarrhea, *Nutr Today* 31(suppl 6):19S, 1996.

Kaaila M, Isolauri E: Nutritional management of acute diarrhea, *Nutr Today* 31(suppl 6):16S, 1996.

Diseases of the Heart, Blood Vessels, and Lungs

In this chapter, we consider interrelated diseases of the circulatory system—the heart, blood vessels, and lungs. In recent decades these diseases of modern civilization have become the major causes of death in the United States and most other Western societies. The magnitude of this overall health care problem is enormous.

Here we examine the health problems relating to the blood circulation and the vital organs that maintain it. We see how nutritional therapy focuses on modification of key nutrients involved.

INTERACTIONS
OF THE CIRCULATORY SYSTEM

Efficient interaction of three major organ systems is essential for normal operation of the body's life-sustaining blood circulation to service cell metabolism. First, a healthy heart muscle must provide a never-ceasing pump to keep the lifeblood constantly flowing. Second, a vast network of healthy blood vessels, from large arteries to minute capillaries, must transport multiple nutrients and metabolites to nourish every single microscopic body cell. And third, healthy lungs must provide the necessary oxygen–carbon dioxide gas exchange to sustain continuing metabolic life.

HEART: THE CENTRAL PUMP

The human heart has been called "a marvel of inspired engineering." It faithfully contracts over three billion times in a lifetime to provide a constant supply of blood and nutrients to the entire body.[1]

The heart lies in the center of the chest with its right edge directly underneath the right side of the *sternum* (breastbone). The remaining body leans to the left, and its lowest point, the apex, lies directly underneath the left nipple. Throughout life, this muscular pump beats rhythmically and continuously to send blood to the lungs and the rest of the body. At an average rate of 75 heartbeats per minute, your heart beats about 108,000 times every 24 hours.

Structure and function

The heart muscle, the *myocardium*, is a thick interconnecting network of muscle fibers. A smooth inner membrane, the *endocardium*, lines its interior surface. A tough outer membrane, the *epicardium*, covers and protects its exterior surface. Together these three layers comprise the strong wall of the heart. In its interior layout, the heart is actually two separate pumps. The *right heart* pumps blood through the lungs to get rid of carbon dioxide and take on needed oxygen, and the *left heart* pumps the returning freshly oxygenated blood through the body. A thick central muscular wall, the *septum*, divides the heart's interior into these two separate halves. The separate pump in each half has an upper chamber, the **atrium**, and a lower larger one, the **ventricle**, joined by special one-way valves to prevent backflow. In both of the separate pumps, the atrium serves mainly as a receiving blood reservoir and a primer pump. The larger ventricle supplies the major force that drives the blood forward into circulation. This functional design that routes blood through the heart can be traced in Figure 19.1. The broad overall scheme of the body's blood circulation and the central control position of the heart is outlined in Figure 19.2.

Cardiac cycle

The period of time from the beginning of one heartbeat to the beginning of the next is called the *cardiac cycle*. The pumping action of the heart in one beat has three phases regulated by electrical waves that spread from the heart's own pacemaker, the *sinoatrial node*, and are clearly seen in an electrocardiogram tracing (Figure 19.3).[2]

1. *Diastole.* In diastole, the resting phase, the heart fills with blood as deoxygenated blood from the body flows into the right side and at the same time oxygenated blood from the lungs flows into the left side. The heart muscle is at rest, and the electrical impulse begins to spread from the sinoatrial node (Figure 19.3, *diastole*).

2. *Atrial systole.* In the second phase, atrial systole, both atria (upper heart chambers) contract simultaneously and squeeze more blood into the ventricles (lower heart chambers), completely filling them. The electrical impulse reaches the atrioventricular node (Figure 19.3, *atrial systole*).

3. *Ventricular systole.* In the final phase, ventricular systole, both ventricles contract, producing two simultaneous actions:

   - *Deoxygenated blood* from the right ventricle is pumped into the pulmonary artery going to the lungs for more oxygen.

   - *Oxygenated blood* from the left ventricle is pumped into the *aorta*, the body's major central artery that serves the network of smaller branching blood vessels throughout body tissues.

By these two simultaneous actions both lower heart chambers are emptied. During this final phase, waves of electrical activity cover the ventricles and stimulate this forceful emptying, and then the cycle begins again (Figure 19.3, *ventricular systole*).

---

atrium   An anatomic chamber; usually used alone to designate one of the pair of smaller upper chambers of the heart within thin muscular walls, which receives blood from the body's inflowing circulation via the superior and inferior vena cava and delivers it to the thicker-walled ventricles.

ventricle   A small cavity; one of the pair of lower chambers of the heart with thick muscular walls, which makes up the bulk of the heart. The ventricles receive blood from the atria and in turn force blood out into body circulation to the lungs for oxygenation and then into systemic body circulation to service the cells.

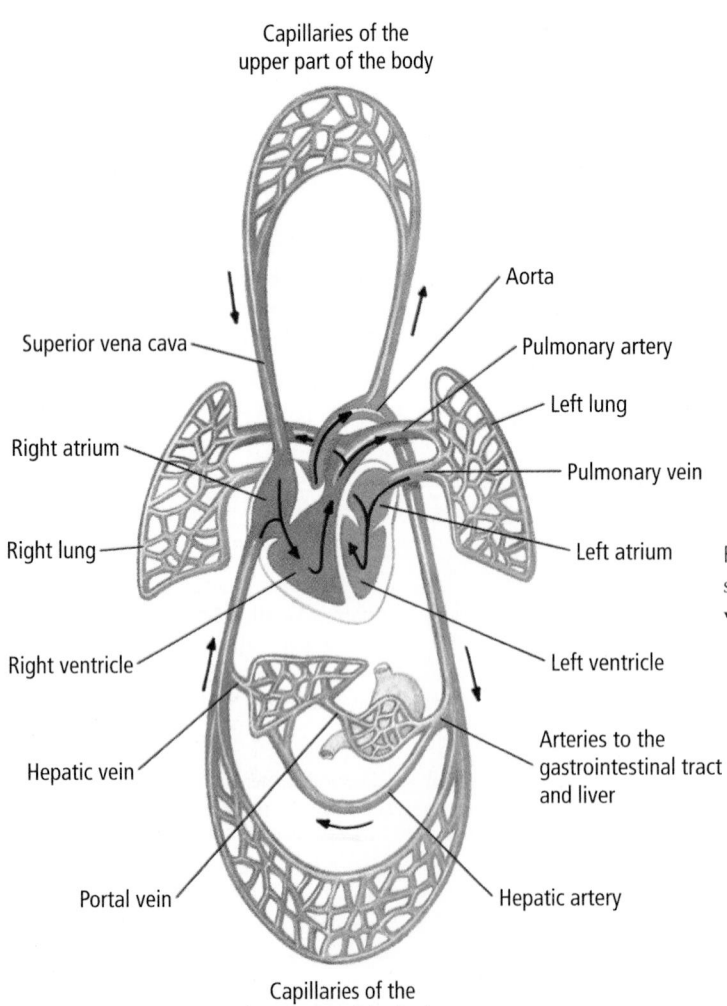

Figure 19.1   The normal human heart. Anterior internal view showing cardiac circulation. (From Seeley RR, Stephens TD, Tate P: *Anatomy and physiology,* ed 2, New York, 1992, McGraw-Hill.)

Aorta

Left pulmonary arteries

Pulmonary veins

Left atrium

Left ventricle

Right atrium

Inferior vena cava

Right ventricle

Capillaries of the upper part of the body

Superior vena cava

Aorta

Pulmonary artery

Left lung

Right atrium

Pulmonary vein

Right lung

Left atrium

Right ventricle

Left ventricle

Hepatic vein

Arteries to the gastrointestinal tract and liver

Portal vein

Hepatic artery

Capillaries of the lower part of the body

Figure 19.2   General scheme of the human circulatory system showing relative arrangement of heart, blood vessels, and lungs.

Diastole   Atrial systole   Ventricular systole

A

B

C

Sinoatrial node

Atrio-ventricular node

Figure 19.3   Three phases of the heartbeat that comprise the cardiac cycle. **A,** Heart action and blood flow at each phase as incoming blood is received and efficiently pumped out with heart muscle contraction. **B,** Electrocardiogram tracing of each phase. **C,** Action of the heart's own pacemaker, the sinoatrial node, sending electric waves that are picked up by the atrioventricular node and passed on to both ventricles, the major strong muscular pumps, signaling strong contractions that empty the heart.

BLOOD VESSELS: TRANSPORT AND REGULATORY SYSTEMS

General structure and function

Blood vessels are uniquely structured to meet their functional needs as a transport system to convey a smooth, steady blood supply to working body cells. Basically the arteries and veins are pliable tubes with relatively thick walls composed of three layers: (1) a smooth inner lining, (2) a muscular elastic middle layer, and (3) a fibrous outer layer (Figure 19.4). The arteries have a thicker muscle layer, a tough outer layer, plus an extra thin elastic layer, enabling them to control surges of pulsing pressure from the heartbeat. Thus they are effectively able to provide a tissue blood flow that is hardly affected by the pulsating nature of heart pumping and allows the blood to efficiently nourish the cells. Conversely, the thinner walls of veins allow them to distend and provide blood reservoirs as needed.

Specific endothelial regulation

Traditionally, blood vessels have been viewed solely as described above—mere "plumbing," that is, as conduits for a constant blood supply, as the term *circulation* implies. Now, however, researchers are discovering that blood vessels play a far more dynamic role in regulating blood pressure and blood clotting as well as their own growth. The key to these regulatory functions, according to the new research findings, lies in the *endothelial cells.* These thin, flat, elongated cells form the inner cell layer of blood vessels and provide an essential interface between the vessel and the blood. They constitute a major line of defense for the cardiovascular system. Endothelial injury is now recognized as a major underlying link to cardiovascular disease and hypertension.[2,3] A functionally intact **endothelium** and the release of its key substance, now known to be *nitrous oxide (NO)*, which affects vascular tone and can dilate blood vessels, are necessary to maintain appropriate blood pressure. Although scientists are just now beginning to discover some of the extraordinarily beneficial roles that NO has in human physiology and health, this clearly demonstrated role in cardiovascular health was sufficient for these scientists to give it their 1992 "Molecule of the Year" award.[3,4]

LUNGS: OXYGEN STATION

The lungs lie in the chest within the rib cage behind the heart, immediately connected with a network of blood vessels that comprise the pulmonary circulation (Figure 19.5). They provide a constant supply of oxygen through the *respiratory system.* Oxygen-laden air inhaled through the nose or mouth travels down a central tube—the *trachea*, which branches in the chest into two main air passages—the *bronchi*. These passages supply the right and left lungs. Each of the bronchi in turn forms a bronchial tree, branching out into smaller bronchi and then into still smaller *bronchioles*, which open out into tiny grape-like clusters of air sacs—the *alveoli*. Through the thin walls of the tiny alveoli the blood gases oxygen (O_2) and carbon dioxide (CO_2) diffuse into and out of the blood. An extensive capillary network, often called a capillary

---

endothelium   Layer of epithelial cells that line the cavities of the heart, the blood and lymph vessels, and the serous cavities of the body, originating from the mesoderm.

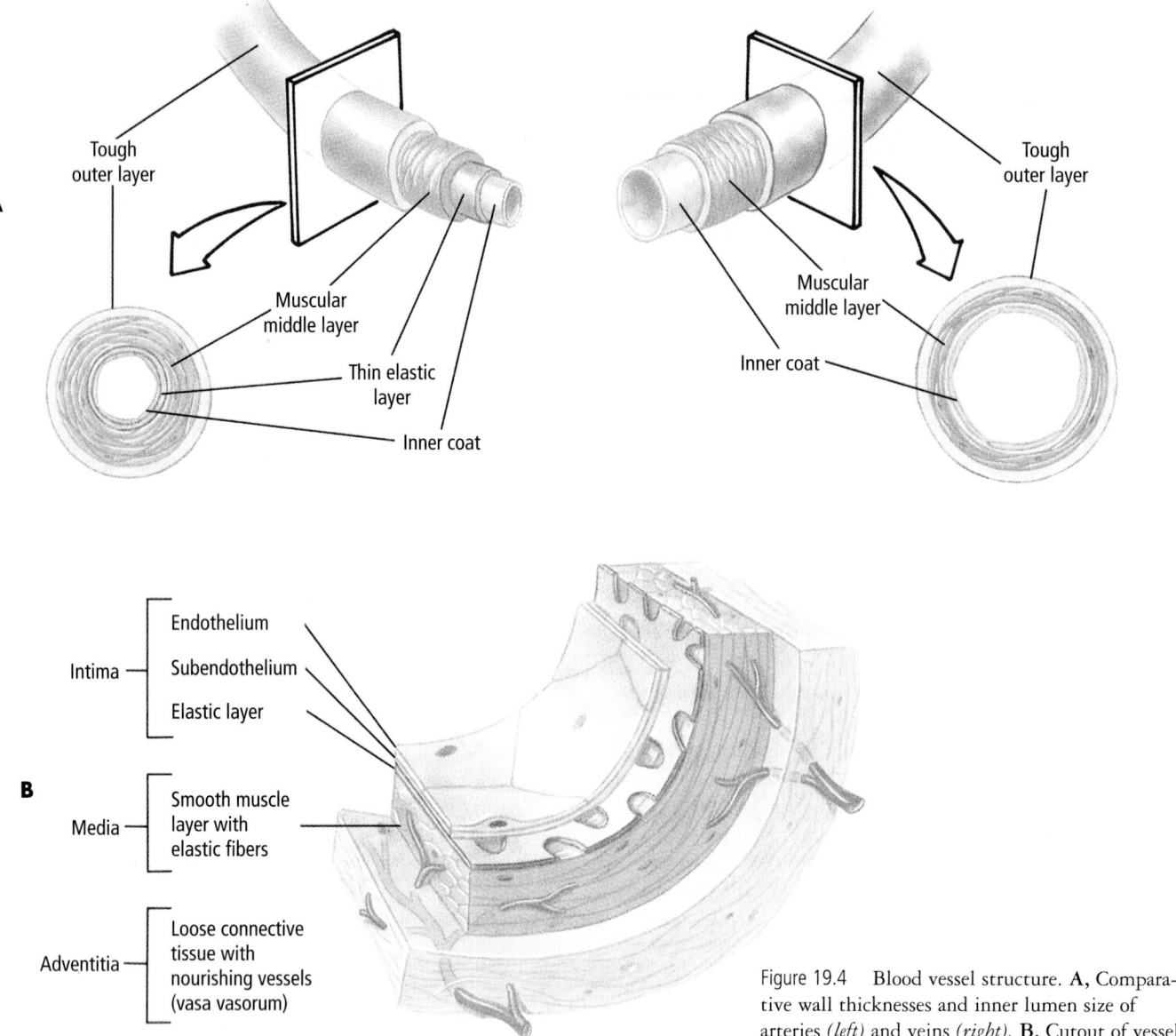

A

Tough
outer layer

Muscular
middle layer

Thin elastic
layer

Inner coat

Tough
outer layer

Muscular
middle layer

Inner coat

B

Intima —
Endothelium
Subendothelium
Elastic layer

Media —
Smooth muscle
layer with
elastic fibers

Adventitia —
Loose connective
tissue with
nourishing vessels
(vasa vasorum)

Figure 19.4   Blood vessel structure. **A,** Comparative wall thicknesses and inner lumen size of arteries *(left)* and veins *(right).* **B,** Cutout of vessel wall showing three basic layers of tissue involved: intima, media, and adventitia.

bed, fans out through each lung and surrounds each tiny twig of the bronchial tree. Here the oxygen is absorbed and carbon dioxide is released and exhaled into the air (Figure 19.6). To facilitate this task of respiration, each lung is covered with a double membrane called the *pleura.* This unique membrane allows the lungs to slide freely as they expand and contract during breathing.

OXYGEN UPTAKE

Oxygen diffuses from the alveoli into the pulmonary blood where it combines with hemoglobin in red blood cells to form oxyhemoglobin. The oxygenated blood then returns through the pulmonary circulation to the heart. Here the heart pumps the oxygenated blood throughout the body network of main arteries and smaller branching arterioles. Finally it reaches the feathery network of tissue capillaries, whose thin membrane is a single layer of thin, elongated epithelial cells to facilitate passage of blood gases, fluids and electrolytes, and nutrients. Here the oxygen is released to the cells for use in cell metabolism of the nutrients. These metabolic cell actions form large quantities of carbon dioxide, which in turn enters the tissue capillaries and is transported back via the heart to the lungs for expiration and exchange for more oxygen.

Diseases in any of these vital organs that form the body's circulatory system—heart, blood vessels, and lungs—have devastating effects. We consider now such disorders in each of the organ systems involved.

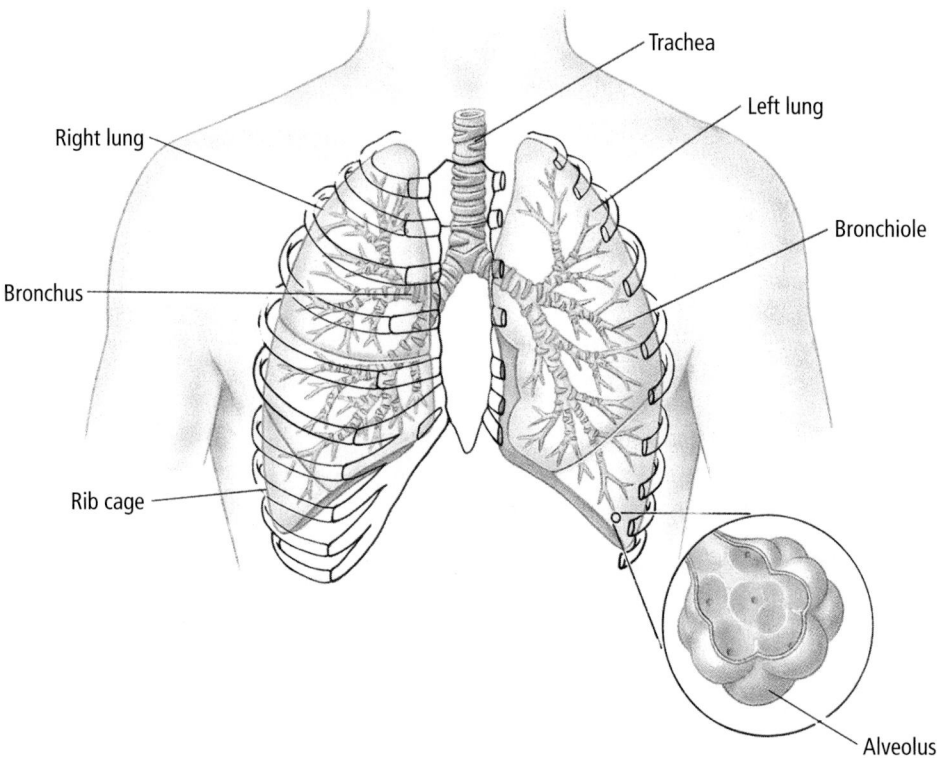

Figure 19.5   Structure and placement of lungs.

CORONARY HEART DISEASE: THE PROBLEM OF ATHEROSCLEROSIS

THE UNDERLYING DISEASE PROCESS

Atherosclerosis, the major **arteriosclerosis** disease and the underlying pathologic process in coronary heart disease, is paramount in ongoing study in modern medicine. The characteristic lesions involved, as observed at autopsy, are raised fibrous **plaques** (Figure 19.7). They appear on the interior surface, the **intima**, of the blood vessel as discrete lumps, elevated above the unaffected surrounding tissue and ranging in color from pearly gray to yellowish gray. The main cellular component of the plaque is a smooth muscle cell similar to the major cell of the normal artery wall. The plaque usually contains fatty material, such as lipoproteins, the carriers of cholesterol in the blood. Deep in the lesions is debris from dead and dying cells, as well as various amounts of lipids. Crystals of cholesterol can be seen with the unaided eye in the softened cheesy debris of advanced lesions.

It is this fatty debris that suggested the original name **atherosclerosis**, from the Greek words *athera* (gruel) and *sclerosis* (hardening). This fatty degeneration and thickening narrows the vessel lumen and may allow

a blood clot, an *embolus*, to develop from its irritating presence. Eventually the clot may cut off blood flow in the involved artery. If the artery is a critical one, such as a major coronary vessel, a heart attack occurs. The tissue

---

arteriosclerosis   Blood vessel disease characterized by thickening and hardening of artery walls, with loss of functional elasticity, mainly affecting the intima (inner lining) of the arteries.

artherosclerosis   Common form of arteriosclerosis, characterized by the gradual formation—beginning in childhood in genetically predisposed individuals—of yellow cheese-like streaks of cholesterol and fatty material that develop into hardened plaques in the intima or inner lining of major blood vessels, such as coronary arteries, eventually in adulthood cutting off blood supply to the tissue served by the vessels; the underlying pathology of coronary heart disease.

intima   General term indicating an innermost part of a structure or vessel; inner layer of the blood vessel wall.

plaque   Thickened deposits of fatty material, largely cholesterol, within the arterial wall that eventually may fill the lumen and cut off blood supply to the tissue served by the damaged vessel.

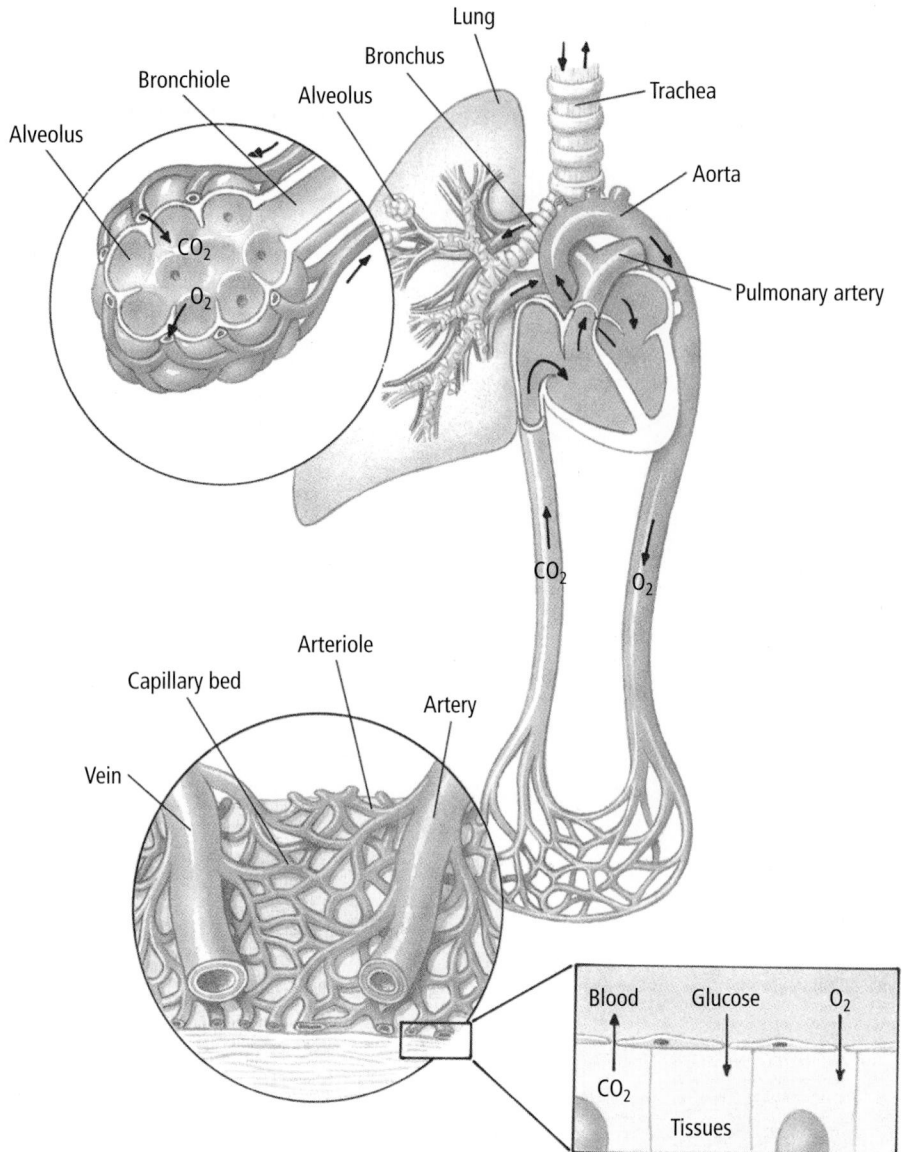

Figure 19.6   Interacting pulmonary and systemic circulatory systems, showing oxygenation of blood in the lungs and metabolic transfers in body tissues.

area serviced by the involved artery is deprived of its vital oxygen and nutrient supply, a condition called **ischemia**, and the cells die. The localized area of dying or dead tissue is called an **infarct**. Because the artery involved supplies the cardiac muscle, the *myocardium*, the result is called an acute *myocardial infarction (MI)*. The two major *coronary arteries*, with their many branches, are so named because they lie across the brow of the heart muscle and resemble a crown (Figure 19.7).

Thus the focus of the problem in coronary heart disease is the development of these characteristic fatty plaques called **atheromas**. Injury to the important inner *endothelial lining* of the blood vessel wall leads to a thickening thrombosis and lipid deposits, with the develop-

ment of *atherosclerosis*. A growing mass of evidence from large clinical trials relates lipids, especially cholesterol, and other lifestyle risk factors to incidence of the disease process in numerous population groups (Table 19.1).

ETIOLOGY: RELATIONSHIP TO GENERAL LIPID METABOLISM

Over the past few years, large-scale studies have indicated an association between types of dietary fat and elevated blood lipid levels, especially cholesterol. Dietary substitution of plant foods high in *polyunsaturated* fatty acids for animal foods high in *saturated* fatty acids, as well as total dietary fat reduction, produced a lowering of blood

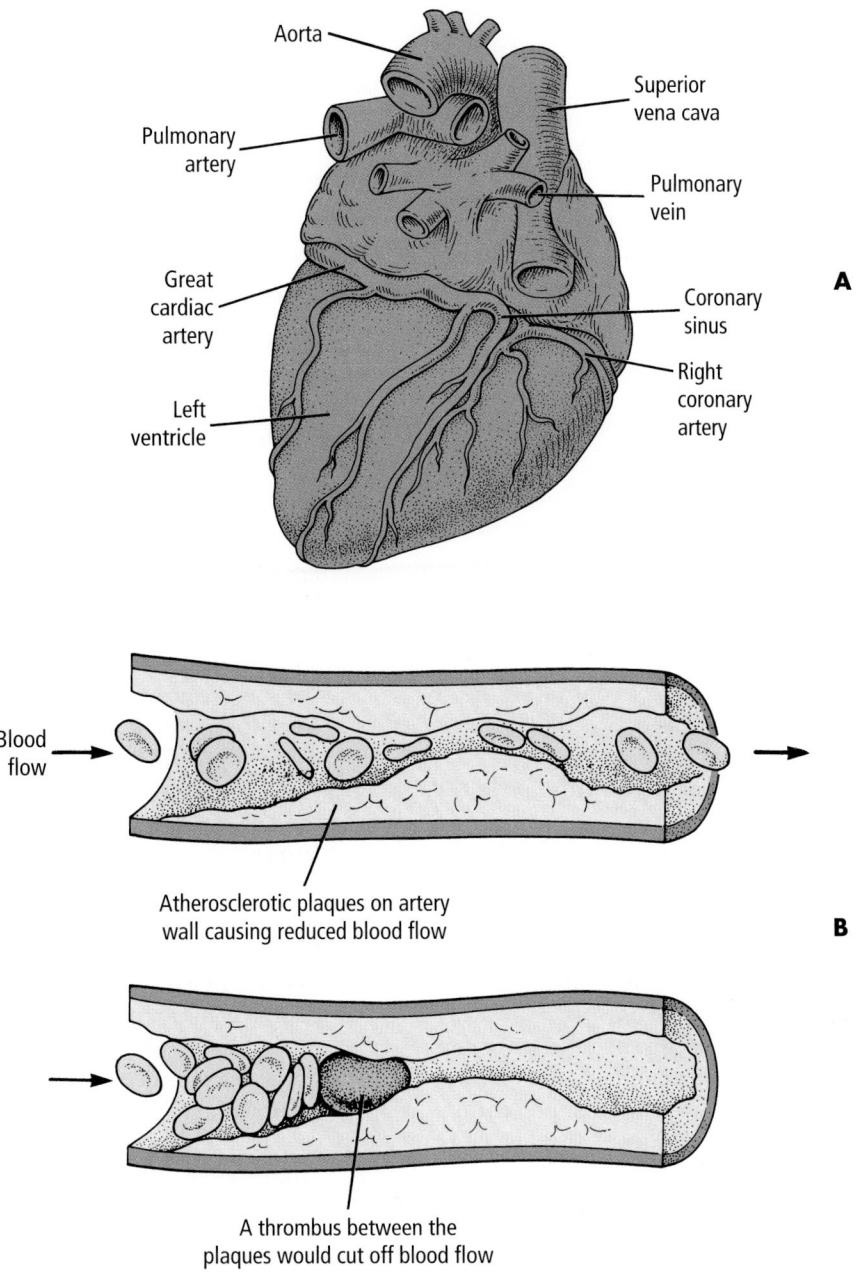

Figure 19.7   Coronary blood circulation and diseased arteries. **A,** Posterior external view showing coronary arteries; **B,** atherosclerotic plaque in artery.

cholesterol. The work of many investigators provided an increasing understanding about the mechanisms, transport, and metabolism of cholesterol, thus control of blood cholesterol levels. This knowledge contributed to our present dietary practices and future directions.[5]

A broad international consensus emerged, which the cholesterol-lowering guidelines of the United States Consensus Conference (NIH, 1985) and the follow-up National Cholesterol Education Program reflect.[6-8] A concerted effort has been made to control

atheroma   A mass of fatty plaque formed in inner arterial walls in atherosclerosis.

infarct   An area of tissue necrosis caused by local ischemia, resulting from obstruction of blood circulation to that area.

ischemia   Deficiency of blood to a particular tissue, resulting from functional blood vessel constriction or actual obstruction walls in atherosclerosis.

Table 19.1	Multiple risk factors in cardiovascular disease		
Personal characteristics (no control)	**Learned behaviors (intervene and change)**	**Background conditions (screen and treat)**	
Gender	Stress and coping	Hypertension	
Age	Smoking	Diabetes mellitus	
Family history	cigarettes	Hyperlipidemia (especially hypercholesterolemia)	
	Sedentary		
	lifestyle		
	Obesity		
	Food habits		
	Excess fat		
	Excess sugar		
	Excess salt		

cholesterol levels as a major means of controlling heart disease. Advancing research indicated two things about atherosclerosis:

- *Elevated serum cholesterol* is a major contributor to the heart disease process.
- *Dietary fat intake*, especially saturated fat, affects serum cholesterol levels.

Current status

These efforts, incorporated in the National Research Council's recent review, *Diet and health: implications for reducing chronic disease risks*, have given impetus to our ongoing nutrition intervention efforts.[9] This work, together with advances in treatment and prevention, brought a decline in heart disease deaths.[10] In addition to medical advances in treatment, credit for the decline also goes to two preventive measures: (1) avoiding heart disease in the first place by not smoking, losing excess weight, and lowering blood pressure and cholesterol; and (2) reducing risk of a second heart attack through changes in diet and lifestyle. Even with the decline in mortality rates over the past two decades, experts indicate that heart attacks still strike some 700,000 in an average year, killing 10% and leaving survivors with weakened hearts.[10] Thus these preventive measures are essential if we are to stem this tide of death and heart injury.

Lipoproteinemia

Two cholesterol-carrying *lipoproteins*, in increased blood concentrations, are without question atherogenic. These are the low-density lipoproteins (LDL) and the very low–density lipoproteins (VLDL), which are derived from chylomicrons or VLDLs by the action of lipoprotein lipase. Lipoproteins are the major transport form of lipids, especially cholesterol, in the blood (see Chapter 3).

An increase in one or more of these plasma lipoproteins creates the condition called **hyperlipoproteinemia**. A more general term referring to elevated blood lipids is *hyperlipidemia*.

Classes of lipoproteins

The lipoproteins in the blood are produced mainly in two places: (1) the intestinal wall after initial ingestion, digestion, and absorption of exogenous fat from a meal; and (2) the liver, from endogenous fat sources in the body. These endogenous lipoproteins carry fat and cholesterol to the tissues for use in energy production and for interchange with other products in cell metabolism. The five types of lipoproteins are classified according to their fat content and thus their density, with those having the highest fat content possessing the lowest density:

1. **Chylomicrons** have the highest lipid content and lowest density and are composed mostly of dietary triglycerides (TGs), with a small amount of carrier protein. They accumulate in portal blood following a meal and are efficiently cleared from the blood by the specific enzyme *lipoprotein lipase*.
2. **Very low–density lipoproteins (VLDL)** still carry a large lipid (TG) content but include about 10% to 15% cholesterol. These lipoproteins are formed in the liver from endogenous fat sources.
3. **Intermediate-density lipoproteins (IDL)** continue the delivery of endogenous TGs to cells and carry about 30% cholesterol.
4. **Low-density lipoproteins (LDL)** carry, in addition to other lipids, about two thirds or more of the total plasma cholesterol; formed in the blood serum from catabolism of VLDL. Because LDL carries cholesterol to the cells for deposit in the tissues, it is considered the main agent in elevated serum cholesterol levels, the "bad" cholesterol.
5. **High-density lipoproteins (HDL)** carry less total lipid and more carrier protein. They are formed in the liver from endogenous fat sources. Because HDL carries cholesterol from the tissues to the liver for catabolism and excretion, higher serum levels of this "good" cholesterol form are considered protective against cardiovascular disease. The "normal" (statistical) range for HDL-cholesterol is 30 to 80 mg/dl, and a value of 75 mg/dl or above contributes definite protection and decreased risk.

The characteristics of these classes of lipoproteins are summarized in Table 19.2. Note the comparative functions of LDL and HDL. Because LDL carries cholesterol to the peripheral cells, for example, it contributes the "cholesterol of concern" in familial hypercholesterolemia and is a more valid measure of risk status than is the total cholesterol value.[11] The LDL value may be calculated by the following formula:

$$LDL = \text{Total cholesterol} - (20\% \ TG + HDL)$$

Table **19.2** Characteristics of the classes of lipoproteins					
Characteristic	**Chylomicrons**	**Very low–density (VLDL)**	**Intermediate-density (IDL)**	**Low-density (LDL)**	**High-density (HDL)**
Composition					
Triglycerides (TGs)	80%-95%; diet, exogenous	60%-80%; endo-genous	40%; endogenous	10%-30%; endogenous	5%-10%; endogenous
Cholesterol	2%-7%	10%-15%	30%	45%-50%	20%
Phospholipid	3%-6%	15%-20%	20%	15%-22%	25%-30%
Protein	1%-2%	5%-10%	10%	20%-25%	45%-50%
Function	Transport dietary TGs to plasma and tissues, cells	Transport endogenous TGs to cells	Continue transport of endogenous TGs to cells	Transport choles-terol to peripheral cells	Transport free cholesterol from membranes to liver for catabolism
Place of synthesis	Intestinal wall	Liver	Liver	Liver	Liver
Size, density					
Description	Largest, lightest	Next largest, next lightest	Intermediate size, lighter	Smaller, heavier	Smaller, densest, heaviest
Density	0.095	0.095-1.006	1.00-1.03	1.019-1.063	1.063-1.210
Size in nano-meters (nm)	75-100	30-80	25-40	10-20	7.5-10

FUNCTIONAL CLASSIFICATION OF LIPID DISORDERS

Current clinical practice is based on a useful functional classification that reveals two important factors: (1) recognition of the genetic factors involved; and (2) focus on the role of *apoproteins* in the course of lipoprotein formation, transport, or destruction. Both of these factors will be encountered in readings and in clinical work with patients. Thus the outline provided in this discussion and the summaries in Table 19.3 of apoproteins and in Table 19.4 of the functional classification of lipid disorders are useful in understanding the clinical problems involved and in counseling patients.

Apoproteins

The term **apoprotein** refers to a major protein part of a combined metabolic product, in this case a specific protein part of a combined lipid-protein molecule (Figure 19.8). These apoproteins are increasingly recognized as important parts of the lipoprotein molecule as more of them are identified, analyzed, and classified by letter and number. For example, apoprotein B is a common attachment to LDLs and serves two basic functions: (1) aids transport of lipids in a water medium, the blood, and (2) transports lipids into cells for metabolic purposes. When apoprotein B-100, a single large protein molecule, attaches to one pole of the LDL (Figure 19.8), it provides a recognition site for the LDL receptors on the cell, causing the entire LDL to be transported by pinocytosis into the cell for use in cell metabolism.[2] Various types of LDLs have specific receptor sites for particular apopro-

teins to which the apoprotein is attracted and which in large measure determine function.

Function

When lipoproteins are synthesized in the intestinal wall, liver, and blood serum, the protein component is made up of varying kinds of apoprotein parts. These genetically determined components influence the structure, receptor binding, and metabolism of lipoproteins. It is an apoprotein component that helps to form the special spherical droplets of lipid material for transport in the bloodstream (see Chapter 3). Apoprotein determination is currently a useful laboratory tool for identifying persons at high risk for coronary heart disease.[12,13]

Classes

A number of apoproteins and their corresponding *apolipoproteins* have been identified. The class designations in common use are apoprotein A, B, C, and E.

---

apoprotein A separate protein compound that attaches to its specific receptor site on a particular lipoprotein and activates certain functions, such as protein synthesis of a related enzyme. For example, apoprotein C II is an apoprotein of HDL and VLDL that functions to activate the enzyme lipoprotein lipase.

hyperlipoproteinemia Elevated level of lipoproteins in the blood.

Table

19.3   Apoproteins in the structure of human plasma lipoproteins

Apoprotein	Related lipoprotein	Tissue origin	Function
A-I	CM, VLDL, HDL	Intestine, liver	Activates LCAT
A-II	CM, VLDL, HDL	Intestine, liver	Unclear
A-III	Subfraction of HDL		Catalyzes transfer of cholesterol esters among lipoproteins
A-IV	CM, VLDL, HDL, free in plasma	Intestine, liver	May activate LCAT
B-48	CM	Intestine	Secretes CM; transports cholesterol and TGs
B-100	VLDL, IDL, LDL	Liver	Secretes VLDL; recognizes LDL receptor
C-I	CM, VLDL, HDL	Liver	Inhibits hepatic uptake of lipoproteins
C-II	CM, VLDL, HDL	Liver	Activates lipoprotein lipase
C-III	CM, VLDL, HDL	Liver	Inhibits lipoprotein lipase and premature remnant clearance
D	HDL	Spleen, liver, intestine, and adrenal glands	Functions in cholesterol ester transfer complex
E	CM, VLDL, IDL, trace amounts in LDL and HDL	Liver, macrophages, and body tissues except the intestine	Recognizes remnant and LDL receptor; acts as regulator in immune system; modulates cell growth

CM, Chylomicron; *HDL,* high-density lipoprotein; *IDL,* intermediate-density lipoprotein; *LDL,* low-density lipoprotein; *VLDL,* very low–density lipoprotein; *LCAT,* lecithin-cholesterol acyltransferase; *TG,* triglyceride.

Table

19.4   Functional classification of lipid disorders

Type of defect or lipid disorder	Abnormal lipid pattern	Clinical characteristics	Nutritional therapy
Defective synthesis of apolipoproteins			
Apolipoprotein A deficiency	Decreased HDL level Increased tissue cholesterol level Decreased serum cholesterol level Increased serum TG level	Rare Genetic Tangier disease	Low cholesterol Low fat
Apolipoprotein B deficiency	High mucosal tissue fat No lipoprotein synthesis possible	Rare Genetic Serious prognosis for child Malabsorption Steatorrhea	Very low fat
Apolipoprotein C deficiency	Increased TG level Increased chylomicron level	Rare Genetic Early childhood Abdominal pain (pancreatitis) Lipedemia, retinalis Xanthomas Hepatosplenomegaly	Very low fat (20 g) High carbohydrate Medium-chain triglycerides (MCTs)
Apolipoprotein E deficiency	Increased chylomicron remnants Decreased serum LDL level Increased cholesterol level Increased TG level	Relatively uncommon Genetic Xanthomas Premature atherosclerosis	Low cholesterol (<300 mg) Low saturated fat Increased substitution of polyunsaturated fat Weight reduction
Enzyme deficiency			
Lipoprotein lipase deficiency	Increased chylomicron level	Rare Genetic Early childhood	Very low fat (20 g) High carbohydrate MCTs

Table

19.4   Functional classification of lipid disorders—cont'd

Type of defect or lipid disorder	Abnormal lipid pattern	Clinical characteristics	Nutritional therapy
Lecithin-cholesterol acyltransferase deficiency	Overall abnormal lipid pattern: all lipoproteins have low amounts of cholesterol esters and high concentrations of free cholesterol and lecithin Accumulation of large LDL particles rich in unesterified cholesterol	Abdominal pain (pancreatitis) Lipidemia, retinalis Xanthomas Hepatosplenomegaly Rare Genetic Abnormal cornea Anemia Kidney damage	Low cholesterol Low fat
LDL-receptor deficiency			
Familial hypercholesterolemia	Increased LDL level Increased total cholesterol level Increased VLDL level	Common Genetic Increased atherosclerosis All ages Xanthomas	Low cholesterol level (<300 mg) Low saturated fat Substitution of polyunsaturated fat
Other inherited hyperlipidemias			
Familial hypertriglyceridemia	Increased VLDL level Increased TG level Increased cholesterol level Sometimes increased blood sugar	Common Genetic Glucose intolerance Possible type II (non-insulin-dependent) diabetes mellitus Obesity Accelerated atherosclerosis	Weight reduction Low simple carbohydrates Low saturated fat Low cholesterol
Familial multiple hyperlipoproteinemia	Increased VLDL level Increased LDL level	Fairly common Genetic Adult Xanthomas; vascular disease	Low cholesterol level (<300 mg) Low saturated fat Substitution of polyunsaturated fat Weight reduction
Familial type V hyperlipoproteinemia	Increased chylomicron level Increased VLDL level Increased cholesterol level Increased TG level	Rare Glucose intolerance Obesity Abdominal pain (pancreatitis) Hepatosplenomegaly	Weight reduction Controlled carbohydrate and fat intake High protein

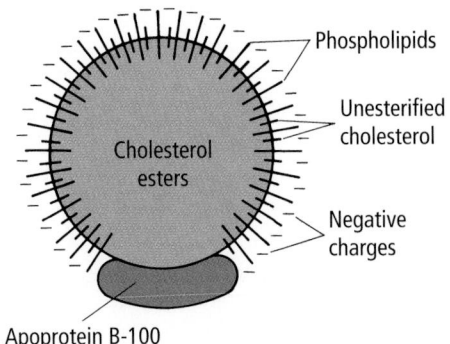

Figure 19.8   Composition and structure of low-density lipoprotein (LDL), primary transporter of cholesterol in human plasma. Apoprotein B-100 binds to LDL and provides recognition site for transport into cells. (Modified from Guyton AC: *Textbook of medical physiology,* ed 8, Philadelphia, 1991, WB Saunders.)

Figure 19.9   Classification spectrum by total and low-density lipoprotein (LDL) cholesterol levels. Initial classification by plasma total cholesterol followed by LDL cholesterol evaluation for persons with high levels. National Cholesterol Education Program, adult treatment panel guidelines. *Report of the Expert Panel on Detection, Evaluation, and Treatment of High Blood Cholesterol in Adults,* US Department of Health and Human Services (Public Health Services), National Institutes of Health, National Heart, Lung, and Blood Institute, NIH Pub No 88-2925, Washington, DC, 1988, Government Printing Office.

In turn, each class consists of several different proteins, for example, A-I, A-II, A-III, and A-IV and C-I, C-II, and C-III. All of these classes of apoproteins are made by the liver, and the intestinal mucosa makes A and B apoproteins. Table 19.3 lists these various classes of apoproteins with their related lipoproteins and functions.

Defects in synthesis of apolipoproteins

The current functional approach classifies lipid disorders in four major groups based on the underlying functional problem: (1) defects in apoprotein synthesis, (2) enzyme deficiencies, (3) LDL-receptor deficiency, and (4) other inherited hyperlipidemias. The summary of these lipid disorders in Table 19.4 provides a review of these basic related conditions and nutritional therapies.

GENERAL PRINCIPLES OF NUTRITIONAL THERAPY: FAT-MODIFIED DIETS

Basic guidelines

The two major lipid factors of concern in a fat-controlled diet are (1) the total amount of fat in the diet, and (2) the kind of fat used in terms of cholesterol and saturated fats. These two principles were first applied in the generally used approach of the "prudent" food pattern, as originally proposed a decade ago by the American Heart Association (AHA)[5] (see Appendix R, p. 689). The initial AHA prudent diet has been revised to meet current lipid-lowering recommendations[6] (see Appendix S, p. 690). The reports of the Expert Panel on Detection, Evaluation, and Treatment of High Blood Cholesterol in Adults issued in 1988 and the Expert Panel on Population Strategies issued in 1990 further refined these dietary principles with specific guidelines for practitioners.[10,11] These current dietary recommendations for adults are shown in Table 19.5, and the related food guide for adults is given in Table 19.6. The related National Cholesterol Education Program treatment criteria for adults is shown in Table 19.7 and Figure 19.9. This stepwise approach calls first for a vigorous dietary effort to lower serum cholesterol before drugs are added.

Recent recommendations have also been made for children and adolescents, especially for those in high-risk families.[12,13] Food guides focus on helping children and

Table 19.5	Step 1 and Step 2 diets for treating high plasma cholesterol levels in adults (NCEP)*	
Nutrient	**Step 1 % total kcalories**	**Step 2 % total kcalories**
Total fat	30	30
Saturated	10	7
Monounsaturated	10-15	10-15
Polyunsaturated	10	10
Carbohydrates	50-60	50-60
Protein	10-20	10-20
Cholesterol	300	200
Total kcalories	Sufficient to achieve and maintain desirable weight	Sufficient to achieve and maintain desirable weight

*National Cholesterol Education Program, adult treatment panel guidelines. *Report of the Expert Panel on Detection, Evaluation, and Treatment of High Blood Cholesterol in Adults,* US Department of Health and Human Services (Public Health Services), National Institutes of Health, National Heart, Lung, and Blood Institute, NIH Pub No 88-2925, Washington, DC, 1988, Government Printing Office.

adolescents develop early food habits on a healthy, less rich, and less excessive basis. Recommendations have been made for public health (population) needs, especially for children from high-risk families, and for individual needs of children and adolescents with identified high serum levels of total cholesterol and LDL-C (Tables 19.8 through 19.10).[12,13] A general population (Steps 1 and 2) food guide for children and adolescents is provided in Table 19-11.

Amount of fat

Almost half of the kcalories of the average American adult's diet is contributed by fat. It is recommended that this excess be moderated to at most 30% of the total kcalories or lowered further to 20% for higher levels of serum cholesterol. Limiting the total amount of fat is, of course, especially indicated when weight management is needed.

Kind of fat

Because of the high status of meat and dairy products in

Table 19.6	Step 1 diet guide: modifications to lower plasma cholesterol levels in adults (NCEP)*	
Food groups	**Choose**	**Decrease**
Fish, chicken, turkey, and lean meats (3-oz cooked portions)	Fish; poultry without skin; lean cuts of beef, lamb, pork, or veal; shellfish	Fatty cuts of beef, lamb, or pork; spare ribs; organ meats; regular cold cuts; sausages; hot dogs; bacon; sardines; roe
Skimmed and low-fat milk, cheese, yogurt, and dairy substitutes	Skimmed or 1%-fat milk (liquid, powdered, evaporated), buttermilk	Whole milk (4% fat): regular, evaporated, condensed; cream; half & half; 2% milk; imitation milk products; most nondairy creamers; whipped toppings
	Nonfat (0% fat) or low-fat yogurt	Whole milk yogurt
	Low-fat cottage cheese (1% or 2% fat)	Whole milk cottage cheese (4% fat)
	Low-fat cheeses, farmer or pot cheeses (all of these should be labeled no more than 2 to 6 g fat per oz)	All natural cheeses (e.g., blue, Roquefort, Camembert, cheddar, Swiss)
		Low-fat or "light" cream cheese, low-fat or "light" sour cream
		Cream cheeses, sour cream
	Sherbet, sorbet	Ice cream
Eggs	Egg whites (2 whites = 1 whole egg in recipes), cholesterol-free egg substitutes	Egg yolks
Fruits and vegetables	Fresh, frozen, canned, or dried fruits and vegetables	Vegetables prepared in butter, cream, or other sauces
Breads and cereals	Homemade baked goods using unsaturated oils sparingly, angel food cake, low-fat crackers, low-fat cookies	Commercially baked goods: pies, cakes, doughnuts, crossants, pastries, muffins, biscuits, high-fat crackers, high-fat cookies
	Rice, pasta	Egg noodles
	Whole-grain breads and cereals (e.g., oatmeal, whole wheat, rye, bran, multigrain)	Breads in which eggs are major ingredient
Fats and oils	Baking cocoa	Chocolate
	Unsaturated vegetable oils: corn, olive, rapeseed, safflower, sesame, soybean, sunflower	Butter, coconut oil, palm oil, palm kernel oil, lard, bacon fat
	Margarine or shortenings made from one of the unsaturated oils listed above	
	Diet margarine	
	Mayonnaise, salad dressings made with unsaturated oils listed above	Dressings made with egg yolk
	Low-fat dressings	
	Seeds and nuts	Coconut

*National Cholesterol Education Program, Adult treatment panel guidelines. *Report of the Expert Panel on Detection, Evaluation, and Treatment of High Blood Cholesterol in Adults,* US Department of Health and Human Services (Public Health Services), National Institutes of Health, National Heart, Lung, and Blood Institute, NIH Pub No 88-2925, Washington, DC, 1988, Government Printing Office.

the traditional American diet, about two thirds of the total fat in the American diet has been of animal origin and therefore mainly saturated fat. The remaining one third has come from vegetable sources and is mainly unsaturated fat. However, this ratio has gradually been changing over the past few years with the use of less animal and more plant fat. This has been the general goal of the prudent diet, illustrated by its breakdown of total fat according to degree of saturation with emphasis on unsaturated fats reflected in the **polyunsaturated/saturated (P/S) ratio.**

Cholesterol

The current stepwise guidelines place greater emphasis on the control of cholesterol and total fat and the degrees

of fat saturation, according to blood serum levels of LDL cholesterol and presence of heart disease history and other risk factors (Table 19.5). Blood serum cholesterol values used in the program as guidelines for testing and monitoring are shown in Table 19.7 for adults and Table 19.9 for children.

Additional dietary factors

Several additional dietary factors are involved in nutritional therapy for heart disease. These include dietary

---

P/S ratio Ratio of polyunsaturated to saturated fats in the diet.

Table

19.7   Evaluation criteria for screening and monitoring adults for treatment of elevated blood cholesterol (NCEP)*

Type of test	Blood level classifications (mg/dl)
Total plasma cholesterol	
Desirable level	<200
Borderline-high level	200-239
High level	≥240
LDL-cholesterol	
Borderline-high risk	130-159
High risk	≥160

*National Cholesterol Education Program, adult treatment panel guidelines.Adult treatment panel guidelines. *Report of the Expert Panel on Detection, Evaluation, and Treatment of High Blood Cholesterol in Adults,* US Department of Health and Human Services (Public Health Services), National Institutes of Health, National Heart, Lung, and Blood Institute, NIH Pub No 88-2925, Washington, DC, 1988, Government Printing Office.

Table

19.8   Current versus recommended nutrient intake in children and adolescents

	Current	Recommended
Saturated fatty acids (% of kcalories)	14	<10
Total fat (% of kcalories)	35-36	Average no more than 30
Polyunsaturated	6	Up to 10
Monounsaturated	13-14	10-15
Cholesterol (mg/day)	193-296	<300

From preliminary data from USDA's 1987-1988 Nationwide Food Consumption Survey and National Cholesterol Education Program; *Report of the expert panel on blood cholesterol in children and adolescents,* USDHHS (PHS), National Institutes of Health, Washington, DC, 1991, US Government Printing Office.

Table

19.9   Cutpoints of total and LDL-cholesterol for dietary intervention in children and adolescents with a family history of hypercholesterolemia or premature cardiovascular disease

Category	Total cholesterol (mg/dl)	LDL (mg/dl)	Dietary intervention
Acceptable	<170	<110	Recommended population eating pattern
Borderline	170-199	110-129	Step 1 diet prescribed, other risk factor intervention
High	≥200	≥130	Step 1 diet prescribed, then Step 2 diet if necessary

From National Cholesterol Education Program: *Report of the expert panel on blood cholesterol levels in children and adolescents,* USDHHS (PHS), National Institutes of Health, Washington, DC, 1991, US Government Printing Office.

Table

19.10   Characteristics of Step 1 and Step 2 diets for lowering blood cholesterol in children and adolescents

	Recommended intake	
Nutrient	Step 1 diet	Step 2 diet
Total fat	Average of no more than 30% of total kcalories	Same
Saturated fatty acids	Less than 10% of total kcalories	Less than 7% of total kcalories
Polyunsaturated fatty acids	Up to 10% of total kcalories	Same
Monounsaturated fatty acids	Remaining total fat kcalories	Same
Cholesterol	Less than 300 mg/day	Less than 200 mg/day
Carbohydrates	About 55% of total kcalories	Same
Protein	About 15%-20% of total kcalories	Same
Kcalories	To promote normal growth and development and to reach or maintain desirable body weight	Same

From National Cholesterol Education Program: *Report of the expert panel on blood cholesterol levels in children and adolescents,* USDHHS (PHS), National Institutes of Health, Washington, DC, 1991, US Government Printing Office.

Food group	Choose	Decrease
Meat, poultry, fish	Beef, pork, lamb; lean cuts trimmed well before cooking	Beef, pork, lamb, regular ground beef, fatty cuts, spare ribs, organ meats, sausage, regular luncheon meats, wieners, bacon
	Poultry without skin	Poultry with skin, fried chicken
	Fish, shellfish	Fried fish, fried shellfish
	Processed meat prepared from lean meat (e.g., turkey ham, tuna, wieners)	Regular luncheon meat (e.g., bologna, salami, sausage, wieners)
Eggs	Egg whites (2 whites = 1 whole egg in recipes), cholesterol-free egg substitute	Egg yolks (if more than 4 per week on Step 1 or if more than 2 per week on Step 2; includes egg used in cooking)
Dairy products	Milk: skim or 1% fat (fluid, powdered, evaporated), buttermilk	Whole milk (fluid, evaporated, condensed), 2% low-fat milk, imitation milk
	Yogurt: nonfat or low-fat yogurt or yogurt beverages	Whole milk yogurt, whole milk yogurt beverages
	Cheese: low-fat natural or processed cheese (part-skim mozzarella, ricotta) with no more than 6 g fat per oz on Step 1, or 2 g fat per oz on Step 2	Regular cheeses (American, blue, Brie, cheddar, Colby, Edam, Monterey Jack, whole milk mozzarella, Parmesan, Swiss), cream cheese, Neufchâtel cheese
	Cottage cheese: low-fat, nonfat, or dry curd (0% to 2% fat)	Cottage cheese (4% fat)
	Frozen dairy dessert: ice milk, frozen yogurt (low-fat or nonfat)	Ice cream
		Cream, half & half, whipping cream, nondairy creamer, whipped topping, sour cream
Fats and oils	Unsaturated oils: safflower, sunflower, corn, soybean, cottonseed, canola, olive, peanut	Coconut oil, palm kernel oil, palm oil
	Margarine made from unsaturated oils listed above, light or diet margarine	Butter, lard, shortening, bacon fat
	Salad dressings made with unsaturated oils listed above, low-fat or oil-free	Dressings made with egg yolk, cheese, sour cream, whole milk
	Seeds and nuts: peanut butter, other nut butters	Coconut
	Cocoa powder	Chocolate
Breads and cereals	Breads: whole-grain bread, hamburger and hot dog bun, corn tortilla	Bread in which eggs are a major ingredient, crossants
	Cereals: oat, wheat, corn, multigrain	Granola made with coconut
	Pasta	Egg noodles and pasta containing egg yolk
	Rice	
	Dry beans and peas	
	Crackers, low-fat: animal-type, graham, saltine-type	High-fat crackers
	Homemade baked goods using unsaturated oil, skim or 1% milk, and egg substitute: quick breads, biscuits, cornbread muffins, bran muffins, pancakes, waffles	Commercial baked pastries, muffins, biscuits
	Soup: chicken or beef noodle, minestrone, tomato, vegetarian, potato	Soup containing whole milk, cream, meat fat, poultry fat, or poultry skin
Vegetables	Fresh, frozen, or canned	Vegetables prepared with butter, cheese, or cream sauce
Fruits	Fruit: fresh, frozen, canned, or dried	Fried fruit or fruit served with butter or cream sauce
	Fruit juice: fresh, frozen, or canned	
Sweets and modified fat desserts	Beverages: fruit-flavored drinks, lemonade, fruit punch	
	Sweets: sugar, syrup, honey, jam, preserves, candy made without fat (candy corn, gumdrops, hard candy), fruit-flavored gelatin	Candy made with chocolate, coconut oil, palm kernel oil, palm oil
	Frozen desserts: sherbet, sorbet, fruit ice, popsicles	Ice cream and frozen treats made with ice cream
	Cookies, cake, pie, pudding prepared with egg whites, egg substitute, skim milk or 1% milk, and unsaturated oil or margarine; gingersnaps; fig bar cookies; angel food cake	Commercial baked pies, cakes, doughnuts, high-fat cookies, cream pies

*Energy expenditure depends on the physical fitness (that is, amount of lean body mass) of the individual and continuing of exercise. Note that some of these activities can be used as aerobic activities to promote cardiovascular fitness.

From the National Cholesterol Education Program: *Report of the expert panel on blood cholesterol levels in children and adolescents,* USDHHS (PHS), National Institutes of Health, Washington, DC, 1991, US Government Printing Office.

fiber, currently recognized by FDA approval of a recent health claim on an oatmeal label for oat's soluble fiber—beta-glucan—which lowers blood cholesterol.[14] Other factors include omega-3 fatty acids (see *To Probe Further* box below), and sodium. Each of these factors may need consideration along with the primary focus on fat and cholesterol.

ACUTE CARDIOVASCULAR DISEASE: MYOCARDIAL INFARCTION

Medical management

Initial medical treatment of myocardial infarction (MI), or heart attack, usually includes strong analgesics for the severe unremitting pain, oxygen therapy, and intravenous fluids for shock. Drugs may include (1) lidocaine, an antiarrhythmic drug to reduce risk of *ventricular fibrilla-* *tion* (irregular heartbeat); (2) diuretics for heart failure to avoid accumulation of fluid in the lungs; and (3) beta-blockers that occupy the beta-receptors and prevent stimuli of norepinephrine to the muscles. In some hospitals patients who arrive shortly after the heart attack are treated with a fast-acting thrombolytic drug, *streptokinase*, an enzyme that dissolves blood clots, followed by *angioplasty*, a procedure used to widen the narrowed coronary arteries. In this procedure, done under local anesthesia and guided by x-ray imaging, a balloon at the tip of a catheter is inserted into the artery and positioned at the narrowed point. The balloon is then inflated and deflated a few times to widen the vessel and then withdrawn. Follow-up use of the cholesterol-lowering drug *pravastatin* has proved to be successful in maintaining a blood cholesterol level lower than the average of 210 mg/dl, which is too high.[15]

To Probe Further

Added food factors in coronary heart disease therapy

The primary focus of nutritional therapy for coronary heart disease focuses on control of lipid factors, including cholesterol and saturated fats. Two other food factors, however, play a different role. In varying ways they help to protect us from coronary heart disease development.

Dietary Fiber

Studies indicate that water-soluble types of dietary fiber have significant cholesterol-lowering effect. Soluble fiber includes gums, pectin, certain hemicelluloses, and the body's storage polysaccharide glycogen. Foods rich in soluble fiber include oat bran and dried beans, with additional amounts in barley and fruits. Oat bran, for example, contains a primary water-soluble gum, beta-glucan, which is a lipid-lowering agent. Soluble dietary fiber:

- Delays gastric emptying
- Slows intestinal transit time
- Slows glucose absorption
- Is fermented in the colon into short-chain fatty acids that may inhibit liver cholesterol synthesis and help clear LDL-cholesterol

On the other hand, insoluble dietary fiber—cellulose, lignin, and many hemicelluloses—found in vegetables, wheat, and most other grains does not have these lipid-lowering effects. Thus an increased use of soluble fiber food sources, especially oat bran and legumes, would have beneficial effects.

Omega-3 fatty acids

Studies indicate that the omega-3 fatty acids, *eicosapentaenoic acid (EPA)* and *docosahexaenoic acid (DHA)* (see Chapter 3), which are found mostly in seafood and marine oils, also have protective functions. They can:

- Change the pattern of plasma fatty acids to alter platelet activity and reduce platelet aggregation that causes blood clotting, thus lowering risk of coronary thrombosis
- Decrease synthesis of very low–density lipoproteins (VLDL)
- Increase antiinflammatory effects

It would seem, then, that factors in foods such as oats, dried beans, and fatty fish would provide valuable lipid-lowering additions to our diets.

References

Anderson JW, Gustafson NJ: Dietary fiber and heart disease: current management concepts and recommendations, *Top Clin Nutr* 3(2):21, 1988.

Simopoulos AP: Omega-3 fatty acids in growth and development, Part II: the role of omega-3 fatty acids in health and disease: dietary implications, *Nutr Today* 23(3):12, 1988.

Nutritional management

In the initial acute phase of cardiovascular disease, a myocardial infarction requires close attention to dietary modifications. The basic clinical objective is cardiac rest to allow the healing process to begin. All care is directed toward this basic need for cardiac rest so that the damaged heart can be restored to normal functioning. The diet is therefore modified in energy value and texture, as well as in fat and sodium.

1. *Energy (kcalories).* A brief period of undernutrition during the first few days after the attack is advisable. The metabolic demands for digestion, absorption, and metabolism of food require a generous cardiac output volume. Small intakes of food at a time, spread over the day, decrease the metabolic work load to a level that the weakened heart can accommodate. The patient progresses to more food as healing occurs. During the initial recovery stages the diet may be limited to about 1200 to 1500 kcalories to continue cardiac rest from metabolic work loads. If the patient is obese, as is frequently the case, this kcalorie level may be continued for a longer period to help the patient begin very gradually to lose some of the excess weight.

2. *Texture.* Early feedings generally include foods soft in texture or easily digested to avoid excess effort in eating. Smaller meals served more frequently may give needed nutrition without undue strain or pressure. Avoid temperature extremes in solid and liquid foods.

3. *Lipids.* The general prudent diet controls the amount and kind of fat, as well as cholesterol, for most patient needs. Individual modifications may be used to meet any additional needs.

4. *Sodium.* A moderately reduced sodium content in the foods selected is also emphasized. This will help control any tendency to fluid accumulation in the body tissues. Added tissue fluid causes more work for the heart to maintain an increased blood volume circulation.

Additional risk factors

Heavy coffee drinking has an effect on blood cholesterol levels and also disrupts heart rhythms. An abnormal heart rhythm is seen after only one or two cups of coffee in patients with a history of irregular heart rate. The best practice is to avoid caffeine or limit regular coffee to two cups per day.[16,17] Heavy use of alcohol also increases triglycerides and atherosclerotic risk. If alcohol is used, the amount should be moderate. In addition, stress and anxiety have been shown to increase risk of heart disease complications and management.[18,19] This is particularly true, for example, for persons who suffer long-term exposure to little or no control in their working situation.[20]

CHRONIC CORONARY HEART DISEASE: CONGESTIVE HEART FAILURE

In chronic coronary heart disease, a condition of congestive heart failure may develop over time. Each year in the United States, it causes over 700,000 hospitalizations.[21] The progressively weakened heart muscle, the myocardium, is unable to maintain an adequate cardiac output to sustain normal blood circulation. The resulting fluid imbalances cause edema, especially **pulmonary edema**, to develop. This condition brings added problems in breathing called respiratory distress or *dyspnea*, which places added stress on the laboring heart. Thus heart failure is now considered a disorder of circulation, not merely a disease of the heart.[22]

Etiology: relationship to sodium and water

The fluid congestion of chronic heart disease relates to imbalances in the body's capillary fluid shift mechanism and its resulting hormonal effects.

1. *Imbalance in capillary fluid shift mechanism.* As the heart fails to pump out the returning blood fast enough, the venous return is retarded. This causes a disproportionate amount of blood to accumulate in the vascular system working with the right side of the heart. The venous pressure rises, a sort of "backup" pressure effect, and overcomes the balance of filtration pressures necessary to maintain the normal capillary fluid shift mechanism (see Chapter 8). Fluid that would normally flow between interstitial spaces and blood vessels is held in the tissue spaces rather than recirculated.

2. *Hormonal mechanisms.* Two hormonal mechanisms are involved in fluid balance in the normal circulation. In this instance, both contribute to cardiac edema.
   - *Aldosterone mechanism.* This mechanism, described more completely by its full name *renin-angiotensin-aldosterone* mechanism, is normally a lifesaving sodium- and water-conserving mechanism to ensure essential fluid balances. In this case, however, it only compounds the edema problem. As the heart fails to propel the blood circulation forward, the deficient cardiac output effectively reduces the blood flow through the kidney nephrons. The decreased renal blood pressure triggers the renin-angiotensin system. Renin is an enzyme from the renal cortex that combines in the blood with its substrate, *angiotensinogen*, which is produced in the liver, to produce in turn *angiotensin* I and II. Angiotensin II acts as a stimulant to the adrenal glands to produce aldosterone. This hormone in turn

---

pulmonary edema Accumulation of fluid in tissues of the lung.

effects a reabsorption of sodium in an ion exchange with potassium in the distal tubules of the nephrons, and water reabsorption follows. Ordinarily this is a lifesaving mechanism to protect the body's vital water supply. In congestive heart failure, however, it only adds to the edema problem. The mechanism reacts as if the body's total fluid volume is reduced, when in truth the fluid is excessive; it is just that it is not in normal circulation but is being retained in the body's tissues.

- *ADH mechanism.* This water-conserving hormonal mechanism also adds to the edema. The cardiac stress and the reduced renal flow cause the release of the **antidiuretic hormone (ADH)**, also known as **vasopressin**, from the pituitary gland. ADH then stimulates still more water reabsorption in the nephrons of the kidney, further increasing the problem of edema.

Increased cellular free potassium

As the reduced blood circulation depresses cell metabolism, cell protein is broken down and releases its bound potassium in the cell. As a result, the amount of free potassium inside the cell is increased, which increases intracellular osmotic pressure. Sodium ions in the fluid surrounding the cell then also increase in number to balance the increased osmotic pressure within the cell and prevent cell dehydration. In time, the increased sodium outside the cell causes still more water retention.

Nutritional management

The basis for all care of the person with congestive heart disease is reduction of the work load of the heart. Medical treatment involves oxygen therapy, decreased physical activity, and drug therapy with (1) diuretic agents to control fluid congestion in the lungs, and (2) digitalis drugs to strengthen contractions of the heart muscle. Nutritional support involves the following:

- *Low sodium.* Sodium should be restricted to 500 to 1000 mg/day, with individual fluid restriction as needed to help reduce fluid retention, and amounts depending on the severity of the heart failure and tissue fluid accumulation.
- *Food texture and meal pattern.* Food should have relatively soft texture, require little physical effort to eat, and be divided into small feedings eaten slowly.
- *Kcalories.* Kcalories should be decreased to reduce any obesity, as well as to decrease the work of the heart to meet circulatory demands for digestion and absorption.
- *Vitamins and minerals.* The person with congestive heart disease should receive a full allowance of vitamins and minerals, with special attention to any drug-nutrient interactions causing losses. For example, potassium replacement is needed when potas-

sium-depleting diuretics are used, and added vitamin B_6 may be needed when the vasodilator *hydralazine* is used for hypertension control. This drug binds vitamin B_6 and increases its excretion.

CARDIAC CACHEXIA

Etiology

Sometimes with prolonged myocardial insufficiency and heart failure, an extreme clinical condition of *cardiac cachexia* develops. Progressive profound malnutrition results from an insufficient oxygen supply that cannot meet the demands of red blood cell formation by the bone marrow or energy needs for basic breathing. The enlarged, laboring heart is unable to maintain a sufficient blood supply to the body tissues, and nutrient delivery to cells is impaired. The edema, unpalatable sodium-restricted diets, drug reactions, and postoperative complications of cardiac surgery all worsen the anorexia and reduce food intake. In addition, the individual has probably become hypermetabolic and hypercatabolic. It should be no surprise that the incidence of *nosocomial* (hospital induced) cardiac cachexia is a common occurrence.

Nutritional therapy

The goal is to help restore heart-lung function as much as possible and rebuild body tissue. Team care involving the physician, clinical dietitian, nurse, patient, and family is essential. Nutrition support focuses on energy, nutrients, supplements, and feeding plan:

- *Energy.* Sufficient kcalories are needed to cover basal energy needs, as well as energy for minimal activity and the hypermetabolism of severe congestive heart failure; more kcalories may be needed if major surgery is planned. Depending on the extent of malnutrition indicated by the nutritional assessment, an increase of 30% to 50% of basal needs may be indicated.
- *Fluids.* Sufficient but not excessive fluid intake is needed, at a rate of about 0.5 ml/kcal/day or 1000 to 1500 ml/day.
- *Protein.* Approximately 0.8 to 1 g/kg body weight is needed to replace tissue losses and cover malabsorption.
- *Fat.* Using a medium-chain triglyceride (MCT) oil for part of the fat allowance modifies losses from malabsorption.
- *Sodium.* Sodium restriction varies with individual status, usually in a range of 500 to 2000 mg/day, with attention to multiple alternate seasonings to enhance palatability of food (see Appendix F).
- *Mineral-vitamin supplementation.* General supplementation at one and a half to two times the RDAs, with follow-up monitoring of blood concentrations, is usually provided to meet needs for tissue rebuilding, malabsorption losses, and hypermetabolic state.

- *Feeding plan.* Small, frequent feedings are better tolerated. Large meals add to the risk of carbon dioxide accumulation and respiratory failure.
- *Enteral and parenteral nutrition support.* Enteral feeding of high-density formula is needed if regular intake is less than 1500 kcal/day, and carefully monitored parenteral nutrition support is required if intake drops to less than 500 kcal/day (see Chapter 18).

ESSENTIAL HYPERTENSION AND VASCULAR DISEASE

THE PROBLEM OF HYPERTENSION

Incidence

High blood pressure is one of the most prevalent vascular diseases worldwide.[23] It is a common problem in the United States affecting the lives of approximately 43 million people.[24,25] It is a major factor in the half million strokes and 1.25 million heart attacks that occur each year. At least 95% of these persons have **essential hypertension**, meaning that its cause is unknown, although there is apparently a strong familial predisposition with its onset in young teen-aged years. It has become the fourth largest public health problem in America. It has often been called the "silent disease" because it carries no overt signs, but it can have serious implications if not treated and controlled. The large recently completed United States study—DASH (Dietary Approaches to Stop Hypertension)—has clearly indicated that a diet rich in fruits, vegetables, and low-fat dairy foods and with reduced saturated and total fat can substantially lower blood pressure.[24,25] Individual treatment uses the current antihypertensive drugs available today as needed. However, other sociocultural factors—such as stressors related to racial discrimination and environmental factors, access to medical care, health education, and lifestyle—influence mass *population* hypertension and stroke risk in the "high normal blood pressure and mild hypertensive" groups.[26,27]

Public awareness

During the past decade, the United States National Heart, Lung, and Blood Pressure Institute of the National Institutes of Health (NIH) has initiated a public education campaign about the serious problem of hypertension and the value of preventive care. As a result, public awareness of the successful treatment of hypertension with new drugs, as well as nondrug programs for mild elevations, has grown widely.[28]

Nondrug approaches

Within the broader current preventive move in health care, there is a renewed focus on nondrug approaches,

which have proved to be effective treatment for mild hypertension and an important adjunct in more severe cases. In any case, the goal of all treatment is to reduce the quantity of drugs required as much as possible. Numerous continuing studies have shown the value of nondrug nutritional therapy.[24-26] These therapies have included weight reduction, regular physical exercise, reduction of salt intake, reduction of dietary fat and cholesterol, and relaxation and stress management. Such nutrition and health therapies help to avoid some unwanted side effects and the considerable cost of lifetime drug treatment.[27-29]

BLOOD PRESSURE CONTROLS

Arterial pressure

As commonly measured, blood pressure is an indication of the arterial pressure in the vessels of the upper arm. This measure is obtained by an instrument for determining the force of the pulse (Figure 19.10). This instrument is called a *sphygmomanometer*, from the Greek words *sphygmos* (pulse), *manos* (thin), and *metron* (measure). The pulse pressure is measured in millimeters of mercury (mm Hg) rise in thin contained tubes, or in equivalent values read on gauges or digital indicators. The higher or upper value recorded is the *systolic* pressure from the contraction of the heart muscle. The lower value recorded is the *diastolic* pressure, produced during the relaxation phase of the cardiac cycle. Thus the upper limit of a normal adult blood pressure would be recorded 150/89 mm Hg.

Several factors contribute to maintaining the fluid dynamics of normal blood pressure: (1) increased pressure on the forward blood flow; (2) increased resistance from the containing blood vessels; and (3) increased viscosity of the blood itself, making movement through the vessels more difficult. Of these factors, increased viscosity is a rare event. Thus in discussing high blood pressure in general terms, we are dealing with the first two factors, the pumping pressure of the heart muscle propelling the blood forward, and the resistance to this forward flow presented by the blood vessel walls normally or by any abnormal added constriction or thickening.

---

antidiuretic hormone (ADH) Water-conserving hormone from posterior lobe of pituitary gland; causes resorption of water by kidney nephrons according to body need.

essential hypertension An inherent form of hypertension with no specific discoverable cause and considered to be familial; also called primary hypertension.

vasopressin Alternate name of ADH.

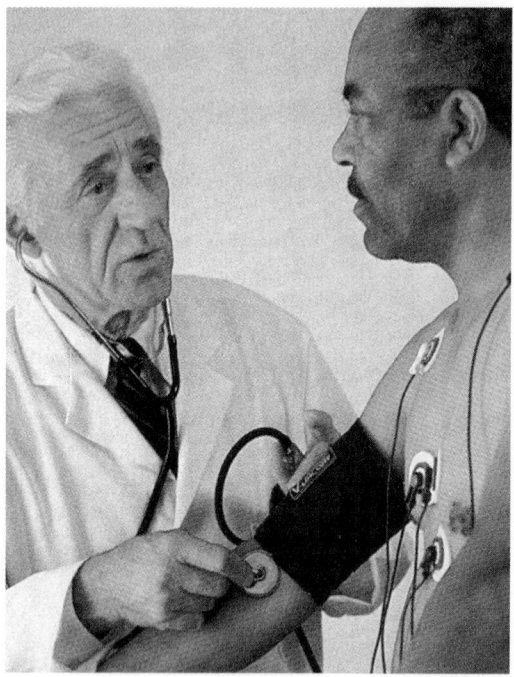

Figure 19.10   Monitoring blood pressure. This patient has successfully used nonpharmacologic therapy to control his hypertension.

Muscle tone of blood vessel walls

In hypertension the body's finely tuned mechanisms designed to maintain fluid dynamics are not operating effectively. Normally, these systems include several agents that act to variously dilate and constrict the blood vessels to meet whatever need is present at a given time. In a hypertensive person, however, the dilation or constriction of blood vessels does not occur in the normal manner. If not effectively treated, uncontrolled elevated blood pressure results. The body systems that operate to help maintain normal blood pressure include (1) neuroendocrine functions of the sympathetic nervous system, mainly mediated by chemical neurotransmitters, such as *norepinephrine*; (2) hormonal systems such as the renin-angiotensin-aldosterone mechanism and its *vasopressor* effect; and (3) enzyme systems such as the *kallikrein-kinin* mechanism (sometimes operating with *prostaglandins*), which controls substances that act to dilate or constrict smooth muscle as needed.

STEP-CARE TREATMENT APPROACH

Based on national studies and widespread community screening programs, current medical treatment focuses on an improved "step-care" method of identifying types of blood pressure levels and matching standard treatment programs to these diagnosed types. Increased emphasis is given to nondrug therapies, limited use of drugs, and "step-down" weaning from drugs as lifestyle habits

improve.[24,28,30] The identification of persons with hypertension according to degree of severity has improved the basic approach to care. These steps of care are termed mild, moderate, or severe.

Mild hypertension

Diastolic pressure (relaxed phase of the cardiac cycle; the lower value) is 90 to 104 mm Hg. Initial consideration is given to other risk factors such as excess weight, lack of exercise, or stress. Individual treatment is started with nondrug approaches and focuses on nutritional therapies of weight control, fat and sodium modification, regular physical activity, relaxation exercises, and behavioral techniques for habit changes.

Moderate hypertension

Diastolic pressure is 105 to 119 mm Hg. Prompt evaluation and treatment is indicated. A combination of drugs may be used: a diuretic agent to decrease the blood volume and a blocking agent to decrease muscle constriction of blood vessel walls. The basic nutritional therapy, exercise, and relaxation modes described previously continue as vital support, with the goal of reducing the amount of medication required.

Severe hypertension

Diastolic pressure is 120 to 130 mm Hg and above. Immediate evaluation and vigorous drug therapy are demanded. Diuretic and blocking agents are continued, and a third drug may be added, a peripheral vasodilator to assist in reducing arterial resistance to blood flow. In all cases the implications for diet therapy revolve around potassium replacement, the use of diuretics, and nutritional support for weight management, sodium modification, as well as physical exercise, stress-reduction activities, and cessation of smoking.

CEREBROVASCULAR ACCIDENT

Incidence

Arteriosclerotic vascular injury and hypertension may also affect blood vessels in the brain. In small vessels the result may be brief passing *transient ischemic attacks (TIAs)*. But in larger vessels serving more tissue the result is a *cerebrovascular accident (CVA)*. A CVA may vary in degree from a disabling stroke to major artery involvement causing massive hemorrhage and a fatal stroke. Over the past two decades, with the declining United States early death rate from heart disease, stroke stands in fourth place—following cancer, heart disease, and injuries—in the leading causes of death of adults ages 25 to 65 years.[31] Of the nearly 150,000 Americans who die annually of stroke, approximately 13% are ages 25 to 65. However, the large majority of stroke victims are older adults. Among all United States population groups, black men have the highest rate of stroke. Their resulting death rate is about twice that of white men and substantially higher than that of black women.[32-34]

Treatment

Treatment of TIAs includes an absolute ban on smoking, drug therapy for hypertension, and moderate dietary control of sodium, with the fat and cholesterol modification indicated for a prudent healthy diet. The proportion of elderly persons in the American population has been progressively increasing, and age appears to be the most important risk factor for stroke. Thus the number of elderly stroke patients is gradually increasing, and their evaluation and management requires particular attention. In the case of a CVA, a permanent disability may result that requires rehabilitation care (see Chapter 25).

PERIPHERAL VASCULAR DISEASE

Etiology

Peripheral vascular disease (PVD) is characterized by narrowing of blood vessels in the legs and sometimes in the arms. The blood flow is restricted and causes pain in the affected area. Contributory risk factors include hypertension and diabetes mellitus. However, the greatest risk factor is cigarette smoking, which constricts blood vessels. More than 90% of patients with PVD are or were moderate to heavy smokers.

Symptoms and complications

As the arteries gradually narrow because of atherosclerosis (the most common cause), an aching, tired feeling occurs in the leg muscles when walking. Resting the leg for a few minutes relieves the pain, but it recurs shortly when walking is resumed. For this reason the symptom is called **intermittent claudication**. Sometimes, a sudden arterial blockage occurs when a blood clot develops on the top of a plaque or a clot formed in the heart is carried to a peripheral artery and blocks it. The blockage causes sudden severe pain in the affected area, which becomes cold and either pale or blue and has no pulse. Movement and sensation are lost.

Treatment

By far the most important treatment for the patient is to stop smoking. As with coronary vessels, surgery on the diseased vessels is sometimes required: (1) *arterial reconstructive surgery* to bypass them, (2) *endarterectomy* to remove the obstructing fatty deposits on the inner linings, or (3) *balloon angioplasty* to widen the vessels. Drug therapy may include antiplatelet or anticoagulant agents to prevent blood clotting. Nutritional therapy consists of the regular fat and cholesterol modifications described for coronary heart disease. Exercise is also important. The person should walk every day, gradually increasing to about an hour, stopping whenever intermittent pain occurs and resuming when it stops. Regular inspection of the feet, daily washing and stocking change, good-fitting shoes to avoid pressure, and scrupulous foot care (ideally by a *podiatrist*) are essential to prevent infection.

CHRONIC OBSTRUCTIVE PULMONARY DISEASE

CLINICAL CHARACTERISTICS

Progressive congestive heart failure, as well as other respiratory problems, contributes to lung disease and the risk of respiratory failure. Malnutrition is common with the debilitating condition of *chronic obstructive pulmonary disease (COPD)*. This term describes a group of disorders in which the airflow in the lungs is limited and respiratory failure develops. The two main interrelated COPD conditions are chronic bronchitis and emphysema. Malnutrition usually accompanies COPD, and its presence increases the illness and death rates associated with the disease process. Anorexia and significant weight loss reflect a growing inability to maintain adequate nutritional status, which in turn severely compromises pulmonary function.[35] Progression of the disease process, with its increasing shortness of breath, prevents the person from living a normal life, and prognosis is poor. Eventually, in progressive respiratory failure, the patient becomes dependent on a mechanical respirator and controlled oxygen supply. Surveys have shown that a poor prognosis is associated with a compromised nutritional status in these patients.[35]

NUTRITIONAL MANAGEMENT

Ratio of fuel macronutrients

Respiratory failure is actually a failure of the pulmonary exchange of oxygen and carbon dioxide. Thus its common manifestations are **hypoxemia**, deficient oxygenation of the blood, and **hypercapnia**, excess carbon dioxide in the blood. Nutritional therapy is guided by the *respiratory quotient (RQ)*, the ratio of carbon dioxide pro-

---

hypercapnia Excess carbon dioxide in the blood.

hypoxemia Deficient oxygenation of the blood, resulting in hypoxia, reduced oxygen supply to tissue.

intermittent claudication A symptomatic pattern of peripheral vascular disease, characterized by the absence of pain or discomfort in a limb, usually the legs, when at rest, which is followed by pain and weakness when walking, intensifying until walking becomes impossible, and then disappearing again after a rest period; seen in occlusive arterial disease.

duced and oxygen consumed, per unit of time, by each of the fuel nutrients. This becomes apparent in the special diet nutrient proportions used[36]:

- *Fat*. Contrary to generally recommended diets, fat is the favored fuel source in COPD because of its lower oxidative RQ value (0.7 compared with 1 for carbohydrate). Also, fat is a concentrated source of needed kcalories. It is lower in osmolality than carbohydrate, and it does not contribute to the hyperglycemia often seen in critically ill patients fed formulas largely composed of dextrose and amino acids. Fat should provide about 30% to 50% of the nonprotein kcalories in the diet.
- *Carbohydrate*. A lower-than-usual amount of carbohydrate is recommended because of its less favorable RQ value. The metabolic effect of larger amounts of carbohydrate is to increase oxygen consumption and carbon dioxide production and retention. This is a critical imbalance for a patient with failing respiratory function. Carbohydrate should provide no more than about 50% of the nonprotein kcalories in the diet.
- *Protein*. The need for protein in ill persons' diets to counteract the catabolic stress on body tissue is well understood. The recommended amount for this person ranges from 1 to 2.5 g protein/kg/day. This amount is adjusted according to the degree of malnutrition and stress. However, in respiratory failure more is not better, and protein allowances must be carefully prescribed. In a prudent diet for failing pulmonary function, protein should provide about 15% of the total kcalories.

Energy needs

Adequate energy intake is based on extent of protein-energy malnutrition and loss of lean body mass. However, as with protein, kcalorie increases are approached with caution to avoid the dangers of hypercaloric feeding in a patient with limited respiratory reserve.[37,38] Individual needs are calculated to cover basal energy expenditure, with added amounts of metabolic activity factors according to the degree of disease activity and its physiologic stress. Based on body weight, energy needs are about 25 to 35 kcal/kg/day for maintenance and 45 kcal/kg/day for anabolic needs to restore lean body mass.[35,38]

Special enteral feeding

Enteral feeding is the preferred mode of feeding, orally for dietary supplementation if possible or by nasoenteric tube if needed (see Chapter 17). Appropriate commercial formulas based on the recommended nutrient ratios indicated, such as Pulmocare (Ross), are available.

General guidelines for dietary modification in chronic pulmonary disease for professional use based on these nutrition support principles are available.[39] Suggestions for use in counseling COPD clinical patients in menu planning and food preparation are included.

EDUCATION AND PREVENTION

PRACTICAL GUIDANCE: "WHY" AND "HOW"

Personal lifestyle habits, especially rich food and limited exercise, create risks for heart disease and hypertension problems. Thus a large part of the health team's work is to help individuals change longstanding habits rooted in the larger society's way of life. These lifestyle changes are important both in treating present disease and in preventing disease development. This is not an easy task, but it is a primary task. Persons want to know *why* such personal habit change is important, which requires a sound knowledge base for motivation. And they want to know *how* to achieve these desired changes in practical ways in their life situation. All the while, they need to feel a sense of being in control of their own lives and their own decision making. So a basic part of the healing process is a partnership with patients that empowers each one to achieve that degree of self-care to the best of their ability, with constant encouragement and support. This is the primary goal of our therapy.

In this final chapter section, we look at this important area of patient education and disease prevention in relation to our major health problems of cardiovascular disease and hypertension. Nutrient management focuses, for the most part, on fat, cholesterol, and sodium. The larger background and guidelines for fat and cholesterol control have been detailed in previous sections of the chapter. In this final section we provide general guides for sodium-restricted diets and practical approaches to planning nutritional intervention and disease prevention.

SODIUM IN GENERAL DIETS

The taste for a given amount of salt with food is an acquired one, not a physiologic necessity. Sufficient sodium for the body's need is provided as a natural mineral in foods consumed. Some persons salt their foods heavily and thus form high salt taste levels. Others form lighter tastes by using smaller amounts. Common daily adult intakes of sodium range widely from about 2 to 4 g with lighter tastes to as high as 10 to 12 g with heavier use. Salt (sodium chloride—NaCl) intakes are about twice these amounts, since sodium (Na) makes up about 40% of the NaCl molecule. The large amount of salt in the American diet, estimated to be about 6 to 15 g sodium/day (260 to 656 mEq), is largely a result of the increased use of many processed food products.

SODIUM-RESTRICTED DIETS

The main source of dietary sodium is common table salt. Sodium compounds that are used less often, such as baking powder and baking soda, contribute small amounts. Otherwise, the remaining dietary source is sodium occurring in some foods as a natural mineral. In general, three levels of dietary sodium restriction are used, as initially outlined by the American Heart Association—mild, moderate, and strict. For practical purposes, each of these levels of restriction can be achieved by a regular diet with the following basic food guides for deletion of higher salt/sodium foods:

- *Mild sodium restriction: 2 to 3 g sodium (70 to 130 mEq).* Salt may be used *lightly* in cooking, but *none* is added at the table. Salty processed foods, for example—pickles, olives, bacon, ham, chips—are avoided.
- *Moderate sodium restriction: 1 g sodium (43.5 mEq).* No salt is used in cooking, no salt is added at the table, and no salty foods are used. Some control of natural sodium foods begins at this level. Vegetables with higher sodium levels are somewhat limited in use (see the following list under strict guide). Salt-free canned vegetables are substituted for regular canned ones, salt-free baked products are used, and meat and milk are used in moderate portions.
- *Strict sodium restriction: 0.5 g sodium (22 mEq).* This strict level is used occasionally in more severe individual cases. In addition to the deletions thus far, foods with higher natural sodium content—meat, milk, and eggs—are allowed only in small portions, and higher sodium vegetables (artichoke, beet greens, beets, carrots, celery, kale, mustard greens, spinach, Swiss chard, and turnips) are generally avoided.

NUTRITIONAL MANAGEMENT OF HYPERTENSION

There is no question that nutritional therapy including sodium restriction plays a large role in the treatment of hypertension. Widespread studies conducted throughout the world in a variety of communities indicate that hypertensive persons respond to some degree of sodium restriction.[40,41] Adequate potassium relates to its electrolyte balance with sodium and its replacement need when potassium-depleting diuretics are used. Studies of the influence of calcium on hypertension have shown variable results and the mechanism involved remains unclear (see *Issues & Answers,* p. 423).

In general, the current focus of nutritional therapy is on (1) sodium restriction, (2) weight management following NCEP guidelines for fat and cholesterol control, and (3) an individualized food plan. A moderately reduced daily sodium intake of about 2 to 3 g (90 to 120 mEq) is a reasonable goal. Persons in a high-risk category for the development of hypertension should reduce their sodium intake as a preventive measure.

LOW-SODIUM FOOD PLAN

Food preparation

Public awareness of healthy diets is creating a new market for popular guides in cookbooks and magazines for preparation of primary foods with alternative seasonings to salt and fat. Many are available and full of good ideas. A variety of alternate seasonings can be used, such as herbs and spices, onions and garlic, and whole fruits and juices, especially lemon and lime juice. Such substitute seasonings create appetizing dishes and help train the taste for less salt (see *Practical Application,* p. 418). References related to sodium values of foods and a salt-free seasoning guide are provided in Appendixes D to F.

Food products

Close attention to the new food product labeling system is important. The new labeling regulations and format (see Chapters 9 and 10) provide additional information about product ingredients so that consumers can make wise choices for controlled use of or eliminating altogether salt, fat, and cholesterol or other food additives of concern.

Special needs

Individual adaptation is fundamental in all nutrition counseling. In this case, special attention needs to be given to those types of ethnic diets, such as Chinese, that are traditionally high in sodium. Some reduced-sodium products, such as soy sauce, are now being marketed. Also, a number of alternate nonsalty condiments are used in Chinese dishes.

PLANNING NUTRITION INTERVENTION AND EDUCATION

Coronary heart disease, hypertension, and their related vascular problems are chronic in nature. Thus an important responsibility of the health care team is educating the patient and family about self-care needs for maintaining health.

Start early for the hospitalized patient (Phase I)

Current hospital stays after a heart attack, as well as coronary bypass graft or coronary angioplasty, are brief. Opportunity for preparing patients and families, especially the spouse, for convalescence and recovery at home is limited.[42] During this period of hospitalization, or Phase I, the main concern of patient and family is survival. Attention span and information retention are limited. Forget about the old involved "discharge instructions" during the anxious preparation for departure. Instead, the clinical dietitian meets with the patient and family a day or so before discharge for brief follow-up planning:

- Provide a firm connection for continuing personal support.
- Supply written names and telephone numbers for communication.
- Briefly describe individual or group resources and programs.
- Plan appointment for initial follow-up contact at home, office, or clinic to provide counseling and education services.
- Respond to any immediate needs expressed.

practical | application

The spice of life: breaking up the salt monopoly

Human essential hypertension appears to be a salt-related disease; societies consuming low amounts of salt have no hypertension. Thus because a diet high in salt can raise blood pressure in susceptible people, the basic treatment is to help these individuals learn ways to reduce salt in their diets. This can be done.

If you counsel with persons on sodium-restricted diets, you probably spend a lot of time answering the question "Is there life without salt?" The standard reply is something like, "Of course there is. You'll just have to get used to the natural flavor of foods." This answer usually falls flat.

We learn to like the taste of salt; it's a taste that "accumulates" over the years. That's why it's unreasonable, for example, to expect a middle-aged man who has just discovered he has hypertension to suddenly give up his lifetime seasoning habits. It's overly optimistic to expect anyone raised on hot dogs, potato chips, and TV dinners to fall in love with the flavor of fresh broccoli overnight if it has never been a favorite food.

There is hope, however. Subjects in one study developed a lower tolerance for salty foods after following a low-sodium diet for 5 months. If you can convince clients to reduce their salt intake for a significant period, you might get them to fall out of love with the taste of salt.

There's still the problem of getting clients to use less salt to begin with. The solution is to introduce them to the world of salt-free seasonings. Some persons are already familiar with a variety of alternate seasonings and only need some recipes that show how to use them creatively. Those who think that gourmet cooking means just using pepper instead of salt need a little extra help in selecting and using salt-free seasonings successfully. The following are some suggestions for guidelines:

- Stop adding salt at the table; it's pure habit. Get rid of the shaker—throw it away, hide it, or get it out of sight—anything to remove the reminder.
- If foods taste too bland without added salt, sprinkle them with fresh lemon juice, not salt.
- When cooking, cut the amount of salt in the recipe in half and avoid other sodium-rich seasonings.
- If you're already a good cook, or even if you're not, refer to guides for hints on spicing up old favorites without salt.
- If you're not the world's greatest chef, enroll in a basic cooking class at a local adult education center or community college and use these guidelines when preparing meals at home. You may also want to check the foods section of your local newspaper for listings of special low-sodium cooking classes offered by local health organizations.
- Relax for a moment while dinner is simmering on the stove and enjoy the wonderful new aromas filling your kitchen. Sodium reduction introduces you to a flavorful new adventure with food.

References

Bertino M et al: Long-term reduction in dietary sodium alters the taste of salt, *Am J Clin Nutr* 36:1134, 1982.

Tobian L: Dietary sodium chloride and potassium have effects on the pathophysiology of hypertension in humans and animals, *Am J Clin Nutr* 65(suppl):606S, 1997.

Wylie-Rossett J: Spices to the rescue, *Prof Nutr* 14:4, 1982.

Use a variety of resources (Phase II)

After the patient returns home, Phase II rehabilitation begins. Many excellent resources are available for patient and family education. Practical discussions need to center on self-management development, spouse involvement, lifestyle risk factor changes, and food buying and preparation to make diets palatable and enjoyable.[43-46] Many helpful suggestions and recipes are included in the American Heart Association low fat, low cholesterol cookbook.[44] A survey trip to local markets helps identify commercial products and label information. Guidelines and food plans for general weight management (Chapter 6) can be modified as needed to control sodium, fat, and cholesterol.

Build family health habits

The wisest control of coronary heart disease and hypertension lies in prevention and positive health promotion. Real contributions begin in childhood, especially in families with strong histories of heart disease and hypertension. Sound health habits learned and practiced early within the family focus on good nutrition—including food behaviors related to fat, sugar, and salt—and a physically active life.

Target high-risk groups

The medical community is giving increased attention to preventing elevated blood cholesterol levels and hypertension in children of high-risk families. Along with meeting general growth needs, some preventive measures related to weight management through physical exercise and healthy food habits without excess fat and salt should be included.[47-49] Prevention in childhood is easier than trying to change strong adult habits. Also, certain high-risk groups for hypertension, including African Americans, should have access to family educational activities, counseling, and materials concerning the risks of hypertension.

Use community resources

A number of community agencies, programs, and materials provide resources on hypertension and heart disease.

- *Community health agencies.* In addition to local chapters of the American Heart Association, hypertension councils have been formed in many areas. A number of materials and active educational programs are available.
- *Nutrition resources.* A number of resource persons and programs may be found in most communities to assist persons and families in planning self-care. These include various weight-management programs, registered dietitians in private practice or in local health centers who provide nutritional counseling, or public health nutritionists and nurses in city and county Public Health Departments. Other outreach programs of the Cooperative Extension Service reach rural and urban communities through county-city networks.
- *Educational materials.* Cooking guides and informational material for diets low in fat, cholesterol, and salt may also be found in public bookstores and libraries. Community screening programs sponsored by industry and community agencies are sources for additional guidance. Through community health agencies, persons with heart disease or hypertension and their families may learn to make decisions about their own health, change food habits to reduce health risks, and take more control in managing their own health needs.

TO SUM UP

Coronary heart disease remains the leading cause of death in the United States. *Atherosclerosis*, its underlying pathology, involves the formation of plaque, a fatty substance that builds up along the interior surfaces of blood vessels, interfering with blood flow and damaging blood vessels. If this buildup becomes severe, it cuts off blood supplies of oxygen and nutrients to tissue cells, which in turn begin to die. When this occurs in a coronary artery, the result is a *myocardial infarction*, or heart attack. When it occurs in a brain vessel, the result is a *cerebrovascular accident*, or stroke.

The risk for atherosclerosis increases with the amount and type of blood lipids (lipoproteins) available. The *apoprotein* portion of lipoproteins is an important genetically determined part of the disease process. Elevated *serum cholesterol* is a primary factor in atherosclerosis development.

Initial dietary recommendations for *acute cardiovascular disease* (heart attack) include caloric restriction, soft-textured foods, and small, frequent meals to reduce the metabolic demands of digestion, absorption, and metabolism of foods and their nutrients. Maintenance of a lean body weight is important. Also, fat, saturated fat, cholesterol, and sodium should be restricted. Persons with *chronic coronary disease* (congestive heart failure) and those with *essential hypertension* benefit from weight management, exercise, and sodium restriction to overcome cardiac edema and help control elevated blood pressure.

Current dietary recommendations to help prevent coronary heart disease involve maintaining a healthy weight; limiting fats to 25% to 30% of all kcalories, with the majority being unsaturated food forms; limiting sodium intake to 2 to 3 g/day; and increasing exercise.

Concerted efforts are needed to combat the development of *cardiac cachexia* in progressive heart failure. Also, atherosclerotic plaques may occur in the extremities, usually the legs, causing *peripheral vascular disease* and the pain of *intermittent claudication* when walking. Progressive respiratory failure interferes with normal exchange of blood gases, oxygen and carbon dioxide, and results in *chronic obstructive pulmonary disease (COPD)*, for which changed ratios of the fuel macronutrients are required.

▄ QUESTIONS FOR REVIEW

1. Which types of hyperlipoproteinemia occur most often? Identify the lipids that are elevated in each case, as well as predisposing factors. Describe the types of diet recommended for each.
2. Identify four dietary recommendations that should be made for the person with a heart attack. Describe how each recommendation helps recovery.
3. Discuss the three levels of sodium restriction, describing general food choices and preparation methods.
4. What dietary changes can the average American make to reduce saturated fats and to substitute polyunsaturated fats?

5. What does the term *essential hypertension* mean? Why would weight management and sodium restriction contribute to its control?

6. Outline the nutritional therapy for cardiac cachexia and discuss the rationale for each aspect of the feeding plan.

7. Discuss the cause and treatment of peripheral vascular disease.

8. Outline the nutritional therapy for chronic obstructive pulmonary disease (COPD) and discuss the rationale for the fuel macronutrient adjustments.

■ REFERENCES

1. Yue DT: Quenching the spark in the heart, *Science* 276(5313):755, 1997.

2. Guyton AC: *Textbook of medical physical physiology,* ed 9, Philadelphia, 1996, WB Saunders.

3. Culotta E, Koshland DE: NO news is good news, *Science* 258:1862, 1992.

4. Koshland DE: The molecule of the year, *Science* 258:1861, 1992.

5. Havel RJ, Papaport E: Management of primary hyperlipidemia, *N Engl J Med* 332(22):1491, 1995.

6. Consensus Conference: Lowering blood cholesterol to prevent heart disease, *JAMA* 253:2080, 1985.

7. National Cholesterol Education Program: *Report of the expert panel on detection, evaluation, and treatment of high blood cholesterol in adults,* USDHHS (PHS), National Institutes of Health, National Heart, Lung, and Blood Institute, Pub No 88-2925, Washington, DC, 1988, US Government Printing Office.

8. National Cholesterol Education Program: *Report of the expert panel on population strategies for blood cholesterol reduction,* USDHHS (PHS), National Institutes of Health, National Heart, Lung, and Blood Institute, Pub No 90-3046, Washington, DC, 1990, US Government Printing Office.

9. Food and Nutrition Board, Committee on Diet and Health, National Academy of Science—National Research Council: *Diet and health: implications for reducing chronic disease risk,* Washington, DC, 1989, National Academy Press.

10. Hunink MGM et al: The recent decline in mortality from coronary heart disease, 1980-1990: the effect of secular trends in risk factors and treatment, *JAMA* 277(7):535, 1997.

11. Feldman EB: Nutrition and diet in the management of hyperlipidemia and atherosclerosis. In Shils ME, Olson JA, Shike M, eds: *Modern nutrition in health and disease,* ed 8, Philadelphia, 1994, Lea & Febiger.

12. Anding JD et al: Blood lipids, cardiovascular fitness, obesity, and blood pressure: the presence of potential coronary heart disease risk factors in adolescents, *J Am Diet Assoc* 96(3):238, 1996.

13. National Cholesterol Education Program: *Report of the expert panel on blood cholesterol levels in children and adolescents,*

USDHHS (PHS), National Institutes of Health, National Heart, Lung, and Blood Institute, Pub No 91-2732, Washington, DC, 1991, US Government Printing Office.

14. Raloff J: FDA allows heart health claims for oats, *Sci News* 151(5):71, 1997.

15. Sacks FM et al: The effect of pravastatin on coronary events after myocardial infarction in patients with average cholesterol levels, *N Engl J Med* 335(14):, 1996.

16. Soroko S et al: Reasons for changing caffeinated coffee consumption: the Rancho Bernardo Study, *J Am Coll Nutr* 15(1):97, 1996.

17. Nygård O et al: Coffee consumption and plasma total homocysteine: the Hordaland Homocysteine Study, *Am J Clin Nutr* 65:136, January 1997.

18. Moser D, Dracup K: Is anxiety early after myocardial infarction associated with subsequent ischemia and arrhythmic events? *Psychosom Med* 58:395, 1996.

19. Roush W: Profile: Herbert Benson: mind-body maverick pushes the envelope, *Science* 276(5311):357, 1997.

20. Johnson JV et al: Long-term psychosocial work environment and cardiovascular mortality among Swedish men, *Am J Public Health* 86(3):324, 1996.

21. Chin MH, Goldman L: Factors contributing to the hospitalization of patients with congestive heart failure, *Am J Public Health* 87(4):643, 1997.

22. Packer M: Pathophysiology of chronic heart failure, *Lancet* 340:88, July 11, 1992.

23. Kannel WB, Wolf PA: Inferences from secular trend analysis of hypertension control, *Am J Public Health* 82(12):1593, 1992.

24. Appel LJ et al: A clinical trial of the effects of dietary patterns on blood pressure, *N Engl J Med* 336(16):1117, 1997.

25. Taubes G: New study says low-fat diet can lower blood pressure, *Science* 276(5311):350, 1997.

26. Casper M et al: Antihypertensive treatment and US trends in stroke mortality, 1962 to 1980, *Am J Public Health* 82(12):1596, 1992.

27. Jacobs DR et al: The United States decline in stroke mortality: what does the ecological analysis tell us? *Am J Public Health* 82(12):1596, 1992.

28. National Institutes of Health, National Heart, Lung, and Blood Institute: *Nonpharmacological approaches to the control of high blood pressure, final report of the Subcommittee on Nonpharmacological Therapy of the 1984 Joint National Committee on Detection, Evaluation, and Treatment of High Blood Pressure,* USDHHS (PHS) Pub No 1986-491-292:41147, Washington, DC, 1986, US Government Printing Office.

29. Wylie-Rosett J et al: Trial of antihypertensive intervention and management: greater efficacy with weight reduction than with a sodium-potassium intervention, *J Am Diet Assoc* 93(4):408, 1993.

30. Schieder RE et al: Antihypertensive therapy: to stop or not to stop? *JAMA* 265(12):1566, 1991.

31. US Department of Health and Human Services, Public Health Service: *Healthy people 2000: national health promotion and disease prevention objectives,* Pub No 91-50212, Washington, DC, 1990, US Government Printing Office.

32. National Center for Health Statistics: *United States, 1989, and preventive profile,* USDHHS (PHS) Pub No 90-1232, Washington, DC, 1990, US Government Printing Office.

33. Saunders E: Hypertension in blacks, *Prim Care* 18(3):607, 1991.

34. Cooper R et al: The prevalence of hypertension in seven populations of West African origin, *Am J Public Health* 87(2):160. 1997.

35. Chin R, Jr., Haponik EF: Nutrition, respiratory function, and disease. In Shils ME, Olson JA, Shike M, eds: *Modern nutrition in health and disease,* ed 8, vol 2, Philadelphia, 1994, Lea & Febiger.

36. Miller MA: A practical approach to eating and breathing in respiratory failure, *Top Clin Nutr* 1(4):61, 1986.

37. DeMeo MT et al: The hazards of hypercaloric nutritional support in respiratory disease, *Nutr Rev* 49(4):112, 1991.

38 Schols A et al: Resting energy expenditure in patients with chronic obstructive pulmonary disease, *Am J Clin Nutr* 54:983, 1991.

39. Monograph: *Dietary modification in chronic pulmonary disease,* Columbus, OH, 1986, Ross Laboratories.

40. Kaplan NM: New evidence on the role of sodium in hypertension: the Intersalt Study, *Am J Hypertens* 3:168, 1990.

41. Law MR et al: By how much does dietary salt reduction lower blood pressure? *Br Med J* 302:811, 1991.

42. Montgomery DA, Amos RJ: Nutrition information needs during cardiac rehabilitation: perceptions of the cardiac patient and spouse, *J Am Diet Assoc* 91(9):1078, 1991.

43. Barnes MS, Terry RD: Adherence to the cardiac diet: attitudes of patients after myocardial infarction, *J Am Diet Assoc* 91(11):1435, 1991.

44. Grundy SM, Winston M: *American Heart Association Low Fat, Low Cholesterol Cookbook,* New York, 1992, Random House.

45. Sharlin J et al: Nutrition and behavioral characteristics and determinants of plasma cholesterol levels in men and women, *J Am Diet Assoc* 92(4):434, 1992.

46. Shenberger DM et al: Intense dietary counseling lowers LDL cholesterol in the recruitment phase of a clinical trial of men who had coronary artery bypass graft, *J Am Diet Assoc* 92(4):441, 1992.

47. Beresford SAA et al: A dietary intervention in primary care practice: the Eating Patterns Study, *Am J Public Health* 87(4):610, 1997.

48. McMurray MP et al: Family-oriented nutrition intervention for the lipid population, *J Am Diet Assoc* 91(1):57, 1991.

49. Shannon B et al: A dietary education program for hypercholesterolemic children and their parents, *J Am Diet Assoc* 91(2):208, 1991.

■ FURTHER READING

McNamara DJ: Cholesterol intake and plasma cholesterol: an update, *J Am Coll Nutr* 16(6):530, 1997.

This article is "must" reading for professionals and students in the field of nutrition and heart disease. It presents an alternate view, based on recent and ongoing studies, that dietary cholesterol itself is not related to either blood cholesterol or heart disease deaths. Consistent clinical and epidemiologic data seem to indicate increasingly that dietary cholesterol has little effect on plasma cholesterol in most individuals and raises a number of questions about the justification of population-wide restrictions on dietary cholesterol intake.

Connor WE, Connor SL: Should a low-fat, high-carbohydrate diet be recommended for everyone? The case for a low-fat, high-carbohydrate diet, *N Engl J Med* 337(Aug 21):562, 566, 1997.

Katan MB, Grundy SM, Willett WC: Should a low-fat, high-carbohydrate diet be recommended for everyone? Beyond low-fat diets, *N Engl J Med* 337(Aug 21):563, 567, 1997.

These well-known researchers in the field of heart disease also emphasize the role of obesity and little physical exercise as risk factors in heart disease.

Fortmann SP et al: Effect of long-term community health education on blood pressure and hypertension control: the Stanford Five-City Project, *Am J Epidemiol* 132(4):629, 1990.

This report provides ample evidence of the strong relation between elevated blood pressure and sodium, and the values of community health education in preventing and controlling essential hypertension.

Brownson RC et al: Preventing cardiovascular disease through community-based risk reduction: the Bootheel Heart Health Project, *Am J Public Health* 86(2):206, 1996.

This interesting heart disease risk reduction project in six southeastern Missouri counties—using community-based activities such as exercise groups, healthy cooking demonstrations, blood pressure and cholesterol screenings, and cardiovascular disease education—clearly shows how such a program can achieve positive results within a relatively brief period, even with modest resources.

Oster G, Thompson D: Estimated effects of reducing dietary saturated fat intake on the incidence and costs of coronary heart disease in the United States, *J Am Diet Assoc* 96(2):127, 1996.

Rhodes KS et al: Intensive nutrition counseling enhances outcomes of National Cholesterol Education Program dietary therapy, *J Am Diet Assoc* 96(10):1003, 1996.

These two brief reports focus on the cost of heart disease. They indicate how population-based interventions that encourage persons to reduce dietary intake of saturated fat can prevent tens of thousands of cases of coronary heart disease and save billions of dollars in related costs.

Case study

The patient with myocardial infarction

Edward Bennett is a 37-year-old sedentary executive seen for an annual physical examination 6 months ago. He had no complaints, other than feeling the "everyday pressures" of his job as a corporate attorney and head of the legal division. He admitted smoking two packs of cigarettes a day as a means of relieving stress.

Mr. Bennett is 175 cm (5 ft 10 in) tall and at the time of his examination weighed 83 kg (185 lb). His blood pressure was 148/90 and serum cholesterol was 285 mg/dl. He was advised to quit smoking, exercise daily at a moderate pace, and lose 9 kg (20 lb).

He arrived in the hospital emergency room 3 months later complaining of severe chest pains and difficulty breathing. His wife reported that he had appeared pale that evening, had broken out into a cold sweat, and had vomited shortly after arriving home from work. Once regular breathing was restored by the emergency medical team and his pain subsided, a number of laboratory tests were ordered. These tests included serum glutamic-oxaloacetic transaminase (SGOT), lactate dehydrogenase (LDH), prothrombin time, lipid panel plus HDL-cholesterol, sedimentation rate, coagulation times, fasting blood sugar (FBS), blood urea nitrogen (BUN), and complete blood count (CBC). An electrocardiogram (ECG) was also ordered. The patient was then transferred to the coronary care unit for closer monitoring.

The following tests results were elevated: SGOT, LDH, LDL and total cholesterol, triglycerides, glucose, prothrombin time, white blood cell count, and sedimentation rate. The HDL level was low. The ECG revealed an infarction of the posterior wall of the myocardium. The diagnosis was myocardial infarction, with underlying familial hypercholesterolemia.

In consultation with the clinical nutritionist the cardiologist ordered a liquid diet, increasing it to an 800 kcalorie soft diet with low saturated fats 2 days later. The nutritionist noted continued improvement in the patient's appetite accompanying recovery and recommended a full diet. A 1200-kcalorie, low-saturated fat, low-cholesterol full diet was ordered by the end of the week. The nutritionist specified that the cholesterol be limited to 300 mg or less and that the total dietary fat content be limited to 25% of total kcalories with emphasis on use of unsaturated fats.

Two weeks later Mr. Bennett was discharged. During his convalescence the nutritionist and the nurse met with him and his wife several times to discuss his continuing care at home. At each follow-up clinic visit with the physician and with the nutritionist, Mr. Bennett showed good general recovery and enjoyment of his new modified fat and cholesterol food habits.

Questions for Analysis

1. What predisposing factors in Mr. Bennett's lifestyle place him in the high-risk category for coronary heart disease?

2. Why was moderate, consistent exercise originally recommended?

3. Explain the causes for Mr. Bennett's initial symptoms.

4. How does each laboratory test ordered in the emergency room relate to cell metabolism? Why were the results elevated?

5. What were the reasons for modifications in texture, fat, and total caloric levels in each diet prescribed for Mr. Bennett? Explain the association between the final diet order and his lipid disorder.

6. Outline a 1-day menu for Mr. Bennett that complies with the final hospital diet order.

7. What nondietary needs might Mr. Bennett have while convalescing at home? What community agencies might be of assistance?

Issues & Answers

Is calcium a new risk factor in hypertension control?

If you had high blood pressure, what would you do—give up salt or drink more milk? This question may sound absurd to anyone familiar with traditional methods of hypertension control, which include a low-sodium diet. To them, giving up salt is the obvious reply. However, in the general public the question is being taken seriously, since a growing number of popular news articles state that persons with high blood pressure may need more calcium.

These reports are based on a number of studies showing that persons with hypertension drink less milk and also have lower serum calcium levels than those with normal blood pressure levels. These studies contradict the findings of earlier studies in which high serum calcium levels were observed in persons with high blood pressure. The latter results are to be expected because of calcium's known contracting effect on smooth muscle tissue such as blood vessels. Large amounts of calcium should cause blood vessels to contract, thus squeezing on the blood flow and bringing a buildup of pressure against arterial walls. The "new" research claims that persons with hypertension don't handle calcium normally. Some of these researchers believe that the sodium-calcium exchange system through which the calcium enters the cell when the sodium leaves it is defective. They tend to discredit the sodium theory because sodium reduction doesn't work for everyone with hypertension; even traditionalists realize that only about half of those with high blood pressure can control it through sodium reduction alone. Nonetheless there are problems with the calcium research:

- Most of the studies are based on a small number of subjects. For example, McCarron's study at the University of Oregon was based on only 23 subjects. Another study, which found a different correlation of high blood pressure with high serum calcium, was based on 9321 subjects.

- Although calcium researchers found low serum calcium levels in subjects with hypertension, total blood calcium levels did not vary with variable blood pressure readings in their study.
- In conditions characterized by high calcium levels, such as hyperparathyroidism, blood pressure levels are also high. As the condition improves and the serum calcium levels fall, blood pressure readings also fall.
- The calcium intake of subjects in the studies was based on oral 24-hour recall information on diet, which is not generally considered the most accurate method of determining nutrient intake.
- Assuming that the dietary information obtained is accurate, it indicated that subjects with hypertension may have consumed less milk but still obtained *adequate* amounts of calcium.

Another important point to remember is that most calcium-rich foods have higher-than-average sodium levels per serving. For example, 1½ ounces of American cheese may provide 250 to 300 mg of calcium, but it also provides more than 400 mg of sodium.

Newer studies in many parts of the world, modern and primitive, have demonstrated a strong relationship between sodium and blood pressure. Unanswered questions remain about the effects of calcium, potassium, and many other factors on blood pressure. In any event, the American Heart Association and other health organizations strongly advise the general public (1) to limit sodium intake and (2) to take in enough calcium to meet various needs for growth, bone and tooth maintenance, and muscle function.

References
Kaplan NM: New evidence on the role of sodium in hypertension: the Intersalt Study, *Am J Hypertens* 3:168, 1990.
Law MR et al: By how much does dietary salt reduction lower blood pressure? *Br Med J* 302:811, 1991.
McCarron DA et al: Dietary calcium and blood pressure: modifying factors in specific populations, *Am J Clin Nutr* 54:215S, 1991.
McGregor GA: Sodium is more important than calcium in essential hypertension, *Hypertension* 7:628, 1985.

In this chapter in our continuing clinical nutrition series, we look at the problem of diabetes. We seek to understand its nature and how it can be managed to maintain good health and avoid complications.

About 11 million Americans, or 1 in 20 persons, have diabetes. Of this total, 15% are insulin dependent and 85% are non–insulin dependent. In the North American population, diabetes complications have become the fifth ranking cause of death from disease.

Here, we see that sound nutritional therapy remains the fundamental base of management for all persons with diabetes. We focus on the vital tools of daily self-management: (1) a sound nutritional base, (2) newer forms of oral medications and insulin, and (3) self-monitoring of blood glucose.

NATURE OF DIABETES

HISTORY

The metabolic disease we know today as *diabetes mellitus* has been with us for a long time. Ancient records describe its devastating effects as observed by early healers. In the first century AD the Greek physician Aretaeus wrote of a malady in which the body "ate its own flesh" and gave off large quantities of urine. He gave it the name *diabetes*, from the Greek word meaning "siphon" or "to pass through." Much later, in the seventeenth century, the word *mellitus*, from the Latin word for "honey," was added because of the sweet nature of the urine. This addition also distinguished it from **diabetes insipidus** ("insipid," meaning tasteless, or *not* sweet), another disorder, although uncommon, in which the passage of copious amounts of urine had been observed. Today, use of the single name *diabetes* always means diabetes mellitus.

As medical knowledge began to grow, early clinicians—such as Rollo in England and Boushardat in France—observed that diabetes became less severe in overweight patients who lost weight. Later another French physician, Lancereaux, and his students described two kinds of diabetes: *diabete gras*—"fat diabetes," and *diabete maigre*—"thin diabetes."[1] All these observations preceded any knowledge about insulin or any relation to the pancreas. Throughout these times, which have aptly been called the "diabetic dark ages," persons with diabetes had short lives and were maintained on a variety of semistarvation diets.[2]

Later, evidence began to point to the pancreas as a primary organ involved in the disease process. Paul Langerhans (1847-1888), a young German medical student, found special clusters—or islets—of cells scattered throughout the human pancreas that were different from the rest of the tissue. Although their function was still unknown, these special islet cells were named for their young discoverer: the islets of Langerhans. Research at that time focused on the pancreas. Finally, in the years of 1921 and 1922 a University of Toronto team discovered and successfully used the controlling agent from the "island cells," naming it **insulin** for its source (see *To Probe Further* box, p. 426).[3]

CONTRIBUTING CAUSES

Genetics: insulin activity

For some time, the early insulin assay tests that were developed to measure the level of insulin activity in the blood found insulin-like activity in diabetes to be two or three times the normal insulin levels. Investigators postulated that the insulin was present but bound with a protein, making it unavailable. It is now evident that diabetes is a syndrome with multiple forms, resulting from (1) lack of insulin, as in *insulin-dependent diabetes mellitus (IDDM)—type I*, or (2) insulin resistance and subsequent beta cell dysfunction, as in *non–insulin-dependent diabetes mellitus (NIDDM)—type II*.[4-6]

Weight

Diabetes has long been associated with weight, since early observations of differences in "fat diabetes" and "thin diabetes."[1] Current research has reinforced the relation of the overweight state to NIDDM—type II. Apparently, the obesity interacts with an underlying genetic predisposition to trigger the non–insulin-dependent form of diabetes.

Heredity

Diabetes has usually been defined in terms of heredity. But increasing evidence indicates that there is considerable *genetic* variation between the two main types of diabetes, IDDM—type I and NIDDM—type II. Studies have shown that an autoimmune attack by the body's insulin-producing cells is at fault, and scientists express growing confidence that within this decade continuing research will lead to safe preventive therapies.[6] Presently, however, insulin resistance is common in Western societies and is associated with a variety of conditions, including obesity, hypertension, hyperlipidemia, and hyperuricemia, as well as a sedentary lifestyle.[7]

Environmental role: "thrifty gene"

Environmental factors apparently play a role in unmasking the underlying genetic susceptibility, a "thrifty" diabetic genotype that probably developed from primitive times for survival. This theory indicates that diabetes may be associated with past genetic modifications for survival during varying periods of food availability. In the past this state of diabetes was a saving—or "thrifty"—trait that provided better storage and metabolism of food during

---

diabetes insipidus A condition of the pituitary gland and insufficiency of one of its hormones, vasopressin or antidiuretic hormone; characterized by a copious output of a nonsweet urine, great thirst, and sometimes a large appetite. However, in diabetes insipidus these symptoms result from a specific injury to the pituitary gland, not a collection of metabolic disorders as in diabetes mellitus. The injured pituitary gland produces less vasopressin, a hormone that normally helps the kidneys reabsorb adequate water.

insulin Hormone formed in the B cells of the islets of Langerhans in the pancreas. It is secreted when blood glucose and amino acid levels rise and assists their entry into body cells. It also promotes glycogenesis and conversion of glucose into fat and inhibits lipolysis and gluconeogenesis (protein breakdown). Commercial insulin is manufactured from pigs and cows; new "artificial" human insulin products have recently been made available.

To Probe Further

Insulin: saga of a success story

Looking at numbers only, it would appear that the development of insulin was a causal factor in changing the status of diabetes mellitus from a rare disease to one that affects over 10 million Americans. Closer inspection of the facts, however, reveals that the disease was thought to be rare only because its victims died young—fewer persons were around who had the disease. Today insulin enables over 2 million insulin-dependent individuals to live longer and enjoy productive lives.

The success story behind insulin lies not only in its ability to extend the life span of the person with diabetes but also in its own resilience. Insulin was discovered during the summer of 1921 at the University of Toronto by Frederick Banting, a surgeon who, according to newspaper accounts of the day, solved the mystery of insulin in his sleep, and Charles Best, a college graduate who was not yet enrolled in medical school. Their insulin was derived from the pancreas of dogs by tying off pancreatic ducts, waiting for the organ to "die," and then making an extract of the remaining tissue.

The extract worked fairly well in their tests with dogs. An extract that worked in humans was not developed for another 6 months, partly because their extract was originally given by mouth. Even when injected, their formula failed, which indicated that faulty purification methods may have been involved.

Finally, in January of 1922, a successful extract was developed by a new member who joined the research team, J.B. Collip. Its effect on one patient's diabetic condition was not enough to counteract the effect of the treatment of the day—a diet that derived almost 71% of its kcalories from fat. The patient died at age 27 years with atherosclerosis and coronary heart disease. However, the team was successful with their third patient. The young girl, who was first diagnosed as having diabetes when she was 11 years old, lived to be 73 years of age. After insulin therapy was initiated, she was taken off the popular "starvation" diet of the day, gained weight, and led a normal life.

Ironically, despite Collip's successful extraction procedure, his subsequent actions almost stopped their project. Jealousies developed and, with the permission of the head of the university's physiology department, Collip refused to share his purification methods with Banting. Then, after his extraction product was a success, Collip conveniently "forgot" how to make it! As a result of this foolish battle, at least one patient died because the researchers ran out of the original extract.

Fortunately, Collip miraculously "remembered" how to make his extract the following May. Soon after, insulin was being mass-produced and made available to the growing number of persons who depended on it for their survival.

References

Altman, LK: The tumultuous discovery of insulin: finally, the hidden story is told, *New York Times,* September 14, 1982.

Bliss M: *The discovery of insulin,* Chicago, 1982, University of Chicago Press.

Nestle M et al: A case of diabetes mellitus, *N Engl J Med* 81:127, 1982.

times when our ancestors lived under more primitive and difficult survival conditions. As food supplies became more plentiful, the negative aspects of the diabetic trait began to appear. Such is indeed the case, for example, with the experience of the Pima Indians in Arizona, as earlier studies and recent archaeologic excavations there have indicated.[7-9] In earlier times this group ate a limited diet, mainly of carbohydrate foods harvested by heavy physical labor in a primitive agriculture. Now, however, with the "progress" of civilization, the Pimas have become obese, and half of the adults have NIDDM—type II , the highest reported rate of this type of diabetes in the world. This same pattern is seen among populations of now-urbanized Pacific Islanders, South Asians, Asian Indians, and Cre-

oles.[10,11] Thus evidence suggests that groups such as these have a genetic susceptibility to NIDDM—type II (diabetic genotype) and that the disease is triggered by environmental factors, including obesity. Just as obesity may result from more than one genetic error, so too may diabetes. As we commonly observe, diet can interact with genetics to develop adult-onset diabetes.

CLASSIFICATION

Increasing evidence indicates differences between non–insulin-dependent (type I) and insulin-dependent (type II) diabetes, and epidemiologic studies in various population groups have provided newer clinical and pathogenic information. With this growing evidence, an international work group sponsored by the National Institutes of Health (NIH) proposed a basic classification for the diabetes syndrome according to the need of insulin for control. This basis is now used to designate the two main types (Table 20.1):

1. Type I: Insulin-dependent diabetes mellitus (IDDM)
2. Type II : Non–insulin-dependent diabetes mellitus (NIDDM)

Insulin-dependent diabetes mellitus (IDDM—type I)

In its insulin-dependent form, diabetes develops very rapidly and is more severe and unstable. This form occurs mainly in children, and the child is usually underweight. Acidosis is fairly common. Peak ages of onset are between 6 and 11 years of age, affecting about 1 in every 600 school-age children.[12]

Table 20.1	Comparison of IDDM and NIDDM	
	IDDM	**NIDDM**
Other names	Type I Juvenile-onset Brittle diabetes Ketosis-prone	Type II Adult-onset Stable diabetes Ketosis-resistent Maturity-onset
Prevalence	5%-10%	80%-95%
Age of onset	Any age; usually less than 40 years	Any age; usually more than 40 years
Cause	Deficient or no insulin production, autoimmune disorder, viral infection	Insulin resistance; hyperinsulemia, obesity
Symptoms at onset	Polydipsia, polyuria, polyphagia, weight loss	Often none; can have polydipsia, fatigue, blurred vision, symptoms of vascular or neural complications
Usual medical treatment: Medication	Insulin	Sulfonylureas (insulin required by some)
Diet	Required (timing and consistency critical)	Required (may be the only form of treatment for some)
Exercise	Recommended (to be integrated with other treatments)	Recommended (to be integrated with other treatments)

Non–insulin-dependent diabetes mellitus (NIDDM—type II)

In this form, diabetes develops more slowly and is usually milder and more stable. This form occurs mainly in adults. The obesity-diabetes genetic base plays a strong role—80% to 90% of these adults are obese. Thus obesity and physical inactivity in adults are strong risk factors.[10-12] Because NIDDM—type II is a milder metabolic form, acidosis is infrequent. The majority of patients improve with weight loss and are maintained on diet therapy alone.[13] Sometimes there is a need for an oral hypoglycemic medication.

SYMPTOMS

Initial observations

Early signs of diabetes, or its uncontrolled state, include the following:
- Increased thirst (polydipsia)
- Increased urination (polyuria)
- Increased hunger (polyphagia)
- Weight loss with IDDM—type I or obesity with NIDDM—type II

Laboratory test results

Various clinical laboratory tests taken at this time reveal the following:
- Glycosuria (sugar in the urine)
- Hyperglycemia (elevated blood sugar)
- Abnormal glucose tolerance tests

Other possible symptoms

Additional signs may appear as the uncontrolled condition becomes more serious:
- Blurred vision
- Skin irritation or infection
- Weakness and loss of strength

Results of uncontrolled diabetes

Continued metabolic consequences may occur as the uncontrolled condition progresses:
- Fluid and electrolyte imbalance
- Acidosis (ketoacidosis)
- Coma

THE METABOLIC PATTERN OF DIABETES

OVERALL ENERGY BALANCE AND THE ENERGY NUTRIENTS

Because the initial symptoms of glycosuria and hyperglycemia are related to excess glucose, diabetes has been called a disease of carbohydrate metabolism. However, as

Figure 20.1   Sources of blood glucose (food and stored glycogen) and normal routes of control.

more becomes known about the intimate interrelationships of carbohydrate, fat, and protein metabolism, we now view it in more general terms. It is a metabolic disorder resulting from a lack of insulin (absolute, partial, or unavailable) affecting more or less each of the basic energy nutrients. It is especially related to the metabolism of the two fuels, carbohydrate and fat, in the body's overall energy system.

NORMAL BLOOD GLUCOSE CONTROLS

Control of the blood glucose level within its normal range of 70 to 120 mg/dl (3.9 to 6.7 mmol/L) is vital to life. A knowledge of these controls in maintaining a normal blood glucose level is essential to understanding the impairment of these controls in diabetes (see Chapters 3 and 4). An overview of these normal balancing controls is given in Figure 20.1.

Sources of blood glucose

Two sources of blood glucose ensure a constant supply of this primary body fuel: (1) *diet*—the energy nutrients in our food—dietary carbohydrate, protein, and fat, and (2) *glycogen*—the backup source from constant turnover of "stored" liver glycogen by a process called **glycogenolysis**.

Uses of blood glucose

To prevent a continued rise of blood glucose above normal limits, several basic uses for blood glucose are constantly available according to need. These include the following: (1) **glycogenesis**—conversion of glucose to glycogen for

"storage" in liver and muscle, (2) **lipogenesis**—conversion of glucose to fat and storage in adipose tissue, and (3) **glycolysis**—cell oxidation of glucose for energy.

Pancreatic hormonal controls

Three types of islet cells scattered in clusters throughout the pancreas (islets of Langerhans) provide hormones closely interbalanced in regulating blood glucose levels. This specific arrangement of human islet cells is illustrated in Figure 20.2.

1. **B cells**. The largest portion of the islets is occupied by B cells filling the central zone or about 60% of the gland. These primary cells synthesize *insulin*.
2. **A cells**. Arranged around the outer rim of the islets are the A cells, one to two cells thick, making up about 30% of the total cells. These cells synthesize *glucagon*.
3. **D cells**. Interspersed between the A and B cells—or occasionally between A cells alone—are the D cells, the remaining 10% of the total cells. These cells synthesize *somatostatin*.

Interrelated hormone functions

Juncture points of the three types of islet cells act as sensors of the blood glucose concentration and its rate of change. They constantly adjust and balance the rate of secretion of insulin, glucagon, and somatostatin to match whatever conditions prevail at any time. Each one of the three hormones has specific interbalanced functions.

1. **Insulin**. Although the precise mechanisms are not entirely clear in every case, insulin has a pro-

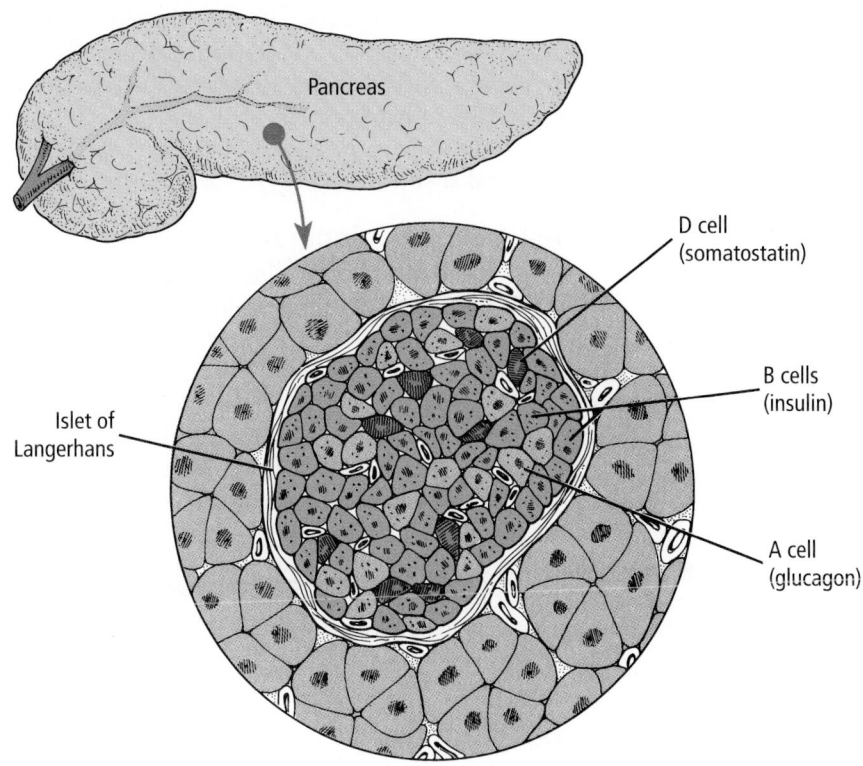

D cell
(somatostatin)

B cells
(insulin)

A cell
(glucagon)

Islet of
Langerhans

Pancreas

Figure 20.2   Islets of Langerhans, located in the pancreas.

found effect on glucose control. It functions extensively in the metabolism of all three of the energy nutrients:

- Insulin facilitates transport of glucose through cell membranes by way of special insulin receptors. These receptors are located on the membrane of insulin-sensitive cells, including those in adipose tissue, muscle tissue, and monocytes. Researchers are reaching a better understanding of these special receptors and how to treat the disease by studying insulin receptors.[14] These insulin receptors mediate all the metabolic effects of insulin. Research has shown that the cells of obese persons with diabetes have fewer than the normal number of insulin receptors. Weight loss in obese individuals and physical exercise increase the number of these receptors.
- Insulin enhances the conversion of glucose to glycogen and its consequent storage in the liver (glycogenesis).
- Insulin stimulates conversion of glucose to fat (lipogenesis) for storage as adipose tissue.
- Insulin inhibits fat breakdown (lipolysis) and the breakdown of protein.
- Insulin promotes the uptake of amino acids by skeletal muscles thus increasing protein synthesis.

- Insulin influences glucose oxidation through the main glycolytic pathway.
2. **Glucagon**. The hormone glucagon functions as a balancing antagonist to insulin. It rapidly causes the breakdown of liver glycogen, and—to a lesser extent—fatty acids from adipose tissue, to serve as body fuel. This action raises blood glucose levels to protect the brain and other body tissues. It helps maintain normal blood

glucagon   A polypeptide hormone secreted by the A cells of the pancreatic islets of Langerhans in response to hypoglycemia; has an opposite balancing effect to that of insulin, raising the blood sugar, and thus is used as a quick-acting antidote for the hypoglycemic reaction of insulin. It stimulates the breakdown of glycogen (glycogenolysis) in the liver by activating the liver enzyme phosphorylase, and thus raises blood sugar levels during fasting states to ensure adequate levels for normal nerve and brain function.

glycogenesis   Synthesis of glycogen from blood glucose.

glycogenolysis   Production of blood glucose from liver glycogen.

glycolysis   Cell oxidation of glucose for energy.

lipogenesis   Synthesis of fat from blood glucose.

glucose levels during fasting hours of sleep. A lowering of the blood glucose concentration, increased amino acid concentrations, or sympathetic nervous system stimulation triggers glucagon secretion.

3. **Somatostatin.** Although the pancreatic islet D cells are the major source of somatostatin, this hormone is also synthesized and secreted in different regions of the body, including the hypothalamus. It acts in balance with insulin and glucose to inhibit their interactions as needed to maintain normal blood glucose levels. It also helps regulate blood glucose levels by inhibiting the release of a number of other hormones as needed.

METABOLIC CHANGES IN DIABETES

In uncontrolled diabetes, insulin is lacking to facilitate the operation of normal blood glucose controls. Abnormal metabolic changes occur that affect glucose, fat, and protein and account for symptoms of diabetes.

Glucose

The blood glucose cannot be oxidized properly through the main glycolytic pathway in the cell to furnish energy (see Chapter 6). Therefore it builds up in the blood (hyperglycemia).

Fat

The formation of fat (lipogenesis) is curtailed, and fat breakdown (lipolysis) increases. This leads to excess formation and accumulation of ketones (ketoacidosis). The appearance of the major ketone, *acetone,* in the urine indicates the development of ketoacidosis.

Protein

Tissue protein is also broken down in an effort to secure energy. This causes weight loss and nitrogen excretion in the urine.

GENERAL MANAGEMENT OF DIABETES

DIAGNOSIS

Glucose-tolerance testing

The guiding principles for treating diabetes are early detection and prevention of complications. The traditional glucose tolerance test is no longer used in regular practice. Instead, a 75-g dose of glucose is used and two blood tests are taken: fasting and a 2-hour plasma glucose. Persons with 126 mg/dl (69.93 mmol/L) now qualify as diabetic (the former threshold was 140 mg/dl (77.7

mmol/L).[15] Any reading over 110 mg/dl (61 mmol/L) is now considered dangerous. This earlier diagnosis will identify persons with diabetes sooner so that treatment can be initiated to help prevent or delay common complications from damage to tissues of the eyes, nerve tissues, and renal tissues.

Glycosylated hemoglobin A$_{1c}$

This additional test, Hb A$_{1c}$, is used in diabetes screening and monitoring. Glycohemoglobins are relatively stable molecules within the red blood cell. During the 120-day life of the cell, glucose molecules attach themselves to the hemoglobin. This irreversible glycosylation of hemoglobin depends on the concentration of blood glucose. The higher the level of circulating glucose over the life of the red blood cells, the higher the concentration of glycohemoglobin. Thus the measurement of hemoglobin A$_{1c}$ relates to the level of blood glucose over a longer period of time. It provides an effective tool for evaluating long-term management of diabetes and degree of control.[16]

TREATMENT GOALS

Basic objectives

The diabetes health care team—physician, dietitian, nurse—is guided by three basic objectives in the care of each person with diabetes.

1. *Maintain optimal nutrition.* The first objective is to fulfill the basic nutritional requirement for health, growth and development, and a desirable body weight.

2. *Avoid hypoglycemia or hyperglycemia.* This second objective is designed to keep the person relatively free of hypoglycemia or insulin reaction, which requires immediate countermeasures, and hyperglycemia, which, if untreated, contributes to more serious ketoacidosis or diabetic coma.

3. *Prevent complications.* The third objective recognizes the increased risk a person with diabetes faces for developing complicating problems that reflect the damaging effects of chronic diabetes on tissues of small and large blood vessels and peripheral nerves.[17,18] These damages may occur in tissues such as eyes (**retinopathy**), nerve tissues (**neuropathy**), and renal tissues (**nephropathy**). In addition, coronary artery disease occurs in persons with diabetes about four times as often as in the general population. Peripheral vascular disease occurs about 40 times as often.

In all of these areas there is evidence that consistent, well-planned food habits and exercise, balanced as needed with early aggressive insulin therapy, can significantly reduce risks of these potentially serious complications.[17]

This aggressive insulin therapy consists of multiple daily injections or continuous subcutaneous infusion by pump and is constantly guided by self-monitoring of blood glucose levels. Current nutritional recommendations of the American Diabetes Association recognize the added risk of vascular disease for persons with diabetes and include revised lipid-lowering diet guidelines.

Self-care role of the person with diabetes

To control diabetes effectively, the person with diabetes must have a central position. Daily self-discipline and informed self-care, supported by a skilled and sensitive health care team, are required for sound diabetes management. Ultimately, all persons with diabetes must treat themselves. This is especially true with the tighter normal blood sugar control currently being used, with frequent self-monitoring of blood glucose and multiple insulin injections. Thus there is even greater need now for comprehensive diabetes education programs that encourage self-monitoring and self-care responsibility.

PRINCIPLES OF MEDICAL NUTRITION THERAPY FOR DIABETES

THE DIABETES CONTROL AND COMPLICATIONS TRIAL

Recognizing the need for a more comprehensive program of care of diabetes, based on the individual metabolic balance concept and designed to help delay or avoid the life-threatening complications of this chronic disease, a national United States clinical research study supported by the National Institutes of Health was organized. This large Diabetes Control and Complications Trial (DCCT) involved 1441 subjects in 29 clinical centers across the country for approximately 10 years.[19,20] The study was designed to compare effects of intensive insulin therapy aimed at achieving blood glucose levels as close as possible to the normal nondiabetic range with the effects of conventional therapy on early microvascular complications of IDDM—type I. The highly significant positive results of the trial were published in 1993. These results indicated the strength of the expanded role of the dietitian, assisted as needed by the diabetes team nurse, in individualizing medical nutrition therapy with various diet management tools and insulin balance.[21,22]

REVISED RECOMMEDATIONS OF THE AMERICAN DIABETES ASSOCIATION

Based on the remarkable DCCT results, the American Diabetes Association issued a new revised position paper in March 1994 on nutrition recommendations and principles for persons with diabetes mellitus, which was immediately endorsed by the American Dietetics Association House of Delegates the following month on April 17, 1994.[23] These guidelines outlined the goals of medical nutrition therapy to assist clients with diabetes in making changes in nutrition and exercise habits in balance with insulin (either internal or external source).[24-26]

CARE OF PERSONS WITH IDDM

The core problem in diabetes is energy balance or regulation of the body's primary fuel, glucose. Based on this concept of balance, three basic principles of nutrition therapy emerge: (1) total energy balance, (2) nutrient balance, and (3) food distribution. The fundamental underlying principle may be stated simply: *The diet for any person with diabetes is always based on the normal nutrition needs of that individual.* This optimal nutrition is illustrated and summarized, for example, in the food guides *Dietary Guidelines for Americans* and the *Food Guide Pyramid,* which can be used by people with diabetes and their families. Whatever particular food-planning tool is chosen by the individual with diabetes in collaboration with the diabetes care team dietitian, the personal diet is expressed in terms of basic nutritional needs: (1) total requirement of kcalories for energy; (2) ratio of kcalories in grams of carbohydrate, protein, and fat; and (3) a general food distribution pattern for the day.

---

nephropathy Disease of the kidneys; in diabetes, renal damage associated with functional and pathologic changes in the nephrons, which can lead to glomerulosclerosis and chronic renal failure.

neuropathy General term for functional and pathologic changes in the peripheral nervous system; in diabetes, a chronic sensory condition affecting mainly the nerves of the legs, marked by numbness from sensory impairment, loss of tendon reflexes, severe pain, weakness, and wasting of muscles involved.

retinopathy Noninflammatory disease of the retina—the visual tissue of the eye—characterized by microaneurysms, intraretinal hemorrhages, waxy yellow exudates, "cotton wool" patches, and macular edema; a complication of diabetes that may lead to proliferation of fibrous tissue, retinal detachment, and blindness.

somatostatin A hormone formed in the D cells of the pancreatic islets of Langerhans and the hypothalamus. It is a balancing factor in maintaining normal blood glucose levels by inhibiting insulin and glucogen production in the pancreas as needed.

Kilocalories

The total kcalorie specification of the diet prescription for IDDM-type I is based on needs for normal growth and development, physical activity, and maintenance of a desirable lean body weight.

Weight management

Because IDDM-type I usually begins during childhood (average age is 11 years), the weight-height measure for children is an index to adequate growth. For adults, the maintenance of a lean weight is a continuing goal (see Chapter 11).

Nutrient balance

The ratio of carbohydrates, protein, and fat in the diet is based on current recommendations of the American Diabetes Association and the American Dietetic Association concerning ideal glucose regulation and lower fat intake to reduce risks of complications such as cardiovascular disease.

Carbohydrates

A more liberal use of carbohydrates, spaced through the day, is needed for smoother blood sugar control. About 45% to 55% of the total kcalories is assigned to carbohydrates. However, several characteristics of carbohydrate foods must be remembered:

1. *Simple and complex carbohydrates.* Both simple (sugars, including sucrose), and complex (starches) carbohydrates are used in the diet. From a clinical standpoint, it is the total amount of carbohydrate eaten, not the source, that is the critical factor affecting blood glucose levels after meals.[27,28] Occasional sweets containing sucrose may be substituted for another carbohydrate in an individual meal plan.[28]

2. *Glycemic index.* Modification of carbohydrate food to take into account the glycemic index of single foods and food combinations, at least in the light of our current knowledge, provides little clinical assistance in designing meals for persons with diabetes. However, most individuals with IDDM—type I have developed their own personal "glycemic index" list based on their own personal experience of blood glucose response to specific foods and make insulin adjustments accordingly. Research on the glycemic index of various foods has indicated that a small amount of sucrose or fructose (see *Issues and Answers*) is not necessarily detrimental but must be controlled and used in mixed forms with other foods. Honey is a form of sugar (mainly fructose) and is not a sugar substitute, as some persons may believe.

3. *Fiber.* The revised American Diabetes Association recommendation for fiber intake for people with diabetes is the same as for the general population—20 to 35 g/day from a wide variety of food sources.[29] Additional intake beyond this reasonable amount is not justified by current conflicting research data; such increased amounts are often difficult to achieve, ineffective, and may divert attention and energy from more beneficial self-management efforts of the person with diabetes.[29,30]

4. *Sugar substitute sweeteners.* Nutritive and nonnutritive sweeteners are appropriate in the diet when used in moderation.[26,30,31] Various sugar substitutes are available. Approved noncaloric sweeteners include saccharin, aspartame, and acesulfame-K. The agent aspartame is made from two amino acids, phenylalanine and aspartic acid, and is metabolized as such. Caloric sweeteners such as small amounts of sucrose, fructose, and sorbitol must be accounted for in the meal. However, many persons are intolerant of sorbitol and experience significant diarrhea from its use. A summary of dietary sweeteners is given in Table 20.2.

Protein

Normal age requirements for protein govern the amount indicated for persons with diabetes. In general, protein intake among Americans is excessive and may accelerate the development of nephropathy in persons with diabetes. Thus for adults the 1994 American Diabetic Association recommends that a nutrition prescription should include approximately 10% to 20% of the total kcalories as protein, using the lower end of the range for those individuals with the onset of nephropathy.[33] Regular Recommended Dietary Allowances (RDAs) provide guidelines for children and pregnant or lactating women.

Fat

Fat is generally used in limited amounts, with greater attention given to the control of saturated fats and cholesterol (Table 20.3). The revised 1994 recommendations indicate that total fat intakes should be individualized based on personal eating habits and energy balance with total carbohydrate intake, according to blood glucose and lipid goals.[34] Thus percent of total energy from fat can vary from person to person, with goals of 10% of total energy from saturated fat and no more than 300 mg cholesterol per day.

Sodium and alcohol

In addition, it is recommended that sodium intake not exceed 3000 mg/day. Also, alcohol should be limited to occasional use or no use; only 1 or 2 drinks are allowed each day, with 1 drink considered 12 ounces of beer, 5 ounces of wine, or 1½ ounces of distilled spirits.[35]

Table

20.2 A summary of dietary sweeteners

Sweetener	Commercial use	Comparative sweetness*	Effectiveness in carbohydrate metabolism and diabetes control	Problems
Nutritive sweeteners (provide 4 kcal/g)				

Aspartame
  Combination of
    two amino acids:
    aspartic acid and
    a methyl ester
    of phenylalanine
	Soft drinks
	Chewing gum
	Powdered beverages
	Whipped toppings
	Puddings
	Gelatin
	Tabletop sweetener
		180-200	Does not contribute significant
			  amount of kcalories or
			  carbohydrates
				Possibly
				  tumorigenic†
				Possible source of
				  excess phenylala-
				  nine for children
				  with PKU

Fructose
  Naturally occuring
    monosaccharide
    found in honey,
    fruits, high-fructose
    corn syrup
	Baked products
	Frosting mixes
	Tabletop sweetener
	Home food preparation
		1.4
		
		Enhanced by:
		  Use in liquids
		  Low tempera-
		    ture
		  Acidity
		  Dilution
			Absorbed more slowly than
			  sucrose
			Does not require insulin for entry
			  into cells
			Achieves similar level of sweet-
			  ness with smaller amounts
			Contributes moderate amounts
			  of kcalories and carbohydrates
			  to prevent hypoglycemia
			Should not be used by poorly
			  controlled, obese diabetics
				Caloric, carbohy-
				  drate values must
				  be considered in
				  calculating diets
				  and recipes
				Intake of more than
				  75 g/day increases
				  risk of hyper-
				  glycemia

Sorbitol
  Sugar alcohol nat-
    urally occuring
    in fruits
    and vegetables
	Baked products
	Sugar-free gum
		0.67	Not generally recommended for
			  diabetes control, because large
			  amounts are needed to sweeten
			  foods
			Lack of insulin results in
			  increased conversion to glu-
			  cose‡
				Doses of more than
				  50-60 g/day
				  result in diarrhea

Xylitol
  "Wood sugar"
    found in straw,
    fruits, corncobs
	Banned for commercial
	  use in the United
	  States in 1982
		1.22		Tumorigenic

L-Glucose, L-fructose:
  mirror images (iso-
  mers) of D-glucose
  and D-fructose
	Currently under study
	  for possible com-
	  mercial use
		Same as D-glu-
		  cose (0.72)
		  and D-fructose
		  (1.4)
			Contributes no kcalories or carbo-
			  hydrates because isomeric con-
			  figuration prevents absorption	

Nonnutritive sweeteners (noncaloric)				

Saccharin	Baked products
	Soft drinks
	Tabletop sweetener
		300-600	Contributes no kcalories or carbo-
			  hydrates to the diet
				Bladder cancer in
				  test animals§

Cyclamate	Banned for commercial
	  use in the United
	  States in 1970
				Bladder cancer in
				  test animals

*The sweetness of sucrose is assigned the value of 1.

†A breakdown product of aspartame, diketopiperazine, is considered tumorigenic by some researchers.

‡Sorbitol is metabolized to fructose, then glucose.

§FDA plan to ban saccharin in 1977 failed because of saccharin's popularity.

Table 20.3	Comparison of AHA and ADA diet recommenddations*		
	AHA Step 1 (% total kcal)	AHA Step 2 (% total kcal)	ADA/ADA (% total kcal)
Total fat	30	30	30
Mono-unsaturated	10-15	10-15	12-14
Saturated	10	7	10
Poly-unsaturated	Up to 10	Up to 10	6-8
Carbohydrate	50-60	50-60	55-60
Protein	15-20	15-20	0.8 g/kg
Cholesterol	300 mg/day	200 mg/day	300 mg/day

*AHA, American Heart Association; ADA, American Diabetes Association and American Diatetic Association

Table 20.4	Meal-planning guide for active people with type I diabetes mellitus	
Exchange needs for		Sample menus
Moderate activity		
30 minutes		
1 bread or		1 bran muffin or
1 fruit		1 small orange
1 hour		
2 bread + 1 meat or		Tuna sandwich or
2 fruit + 1 milk		½ cup fruit salad + 1 cup milk
Strenuous activity		
30 minutes		
2 fruit or		1 small banana or
1 bread + 1 fat		½ bagel + 1 tsp cream cheese
1 hour		
2 bread + 1 meat + 1 milk or		Meat and cheese sandwich + + 1 cup milk or
2 bread + 2 meat + 2 fruit		hamburger + 1 cup orange juice

FOOD DISTRIBUTION BALANCE

General rule

In general, fairly even amounts of food should be spread throughout the day and adjusted to regular blood glucose self-monitoring. Increased meal-snack frequency also has metabolic advantages for persons with NIDDM—type II. In either case this spread helps avoid excessive intakes at some points and longer fasting between meals, eliminating the "peaks and valleys" in food intake and consequent blood sugar swings. This means that a regular schedule of meals at fairly consistent times throughout the day with interval snacks as needed is a basic pattern on which to build.

Daily activity pattern

Food distribution needs to be planned ahead and adjusted according to each day's scheduled activities. Practical consideration is given to work, school, social events, and stress periods.

Exercise

For persons with IDDM—type I , it is especially important that any exercise period or additional physical activity be accommodated in the food distribution plan (Table 20.4) as well as in insulin adjustment.[36] For obese adults with diabetes, regular exercise is an essential part of a successful weight management program.

Summary: diet prescription

In general, based on guidelines set by the recent Diabetes Control and Complications Trial (DCCT), the basic principle guiding daily energy needs is sufficient kcalories to meet growth and development needs, physical activities, and 90% to 120% maintenance of ideal body weight. The nutrient allocation of total kcalories recommended is as follows:

1. *Carbohydrate.* Approximately 50% of the total kcalories, with 45% to 55% as the acceptable range. Simple sugars should contribute no more than 25% of energy from carbohydrate. Encourage food choices with fiber; avoid pharmacologic fiber supplements.

2. *Protein.* About 10% to 25% of total daily energy intake but no less than 0.8 g/kg of body weight for nonpregnant, nonlactating adults and 0.84 g/kg for persons aged 11 to 14 years. Follow the general RDA standard for pregnant and lactating women.

3. *Fat.* About 30% to 35% of total energy intake; consistent with the National Cholesterol Education Program (NCEP) Step 1 guidelines:
   - Cholesterol, less than 300 mg/day
   - Total fat, less than 30% of total energy
   - Saturated fatty acids, up to 10% of total energy
   - Polyunsaturated fatty acids, up to 10% of total energy
   - Monounsaturated fatty acids, 10% to 15% of total energy

A general comparative summary of diet planning needs for both types of diabetes is given in Table 20.5.

INSULIN THERAPY

The management goal for persons with IDDM—type I is to maintain a normal blood glucose level as closely as possible. Strong evidence from the DCCT, as well as

Table

20.5 Dietary strategies for the two main types of diabetes mellitus

Dietary strategy	IDDM (nonobese)	NIDDM (usually obese)
Decrease energy intake (kcalories)	No	Yes
Increase frequency and number of feedings	Yes	Usually no
Have regular daily intake of kcalories, carbohydrates, protein, and fat	Very important	Not important if average kcaloric intake remains in low range
Plan consistent daily ratio of protein, carbohydrates, and fat for each feeding	Desirable	Not necessary
Use extra or planned-ahead food to treat or prevent hypoglycemia	Very important	Not necessary
Plan regular times for meals/snacks	Very important	Not important
Use extra food for unusual exercise	Yes	Usually not necessary
During illness use small, frequent feedings of carbohydrates to prevent starvation ketosis	Important	Usually not necessary because of resistence to ketosis

accumulating practice experience, indicates that maintaining such a "normoglycemic" state helps prevent the chronic complications of long-term uncontrolled hyperglycemia.[18,19] To achieve this goal, more aggressive insulin therapy with different types of insulin now available is being used.

Types of insulin

A number of insulin preparations are available for therapeutic use, and new ones are constantly being developed to meet medical care needs for individual patients and market changes. Individual responses to these insulins are highly variable. According to time of action, they are rapid-, intermediate-, and long-acting.

1. *Rapid-acting insulins.* These insulins have various names, depending on the manufacturer: for example, Humulin R, Regular, Semilente, and Velosulin R. A recently developed human insulin analogue, Humalog (generic name, insulin lispro), approved by the Food and Drug Administration in 1996, has the shortest time-action curve of any insulin currently available.[37,38] A number of variables influence absorption rate, such as site of injection, physical activity, skin temperature, and any circulating antiinsulin antibodies. Effect on blood glucose can be detected in about an hour, peaks at 4 to 6 hours, and lasts about 12 to 16 hours. In patients with type II diabetes, insulin may be used alone or in conjunction with oral agents such as sulfonylureas, acarbose, metformin, or troglitazone.[39]

2. *Intermediate-acting insulins.* These insulins include Humulin L, Lente, NPH, Insulatard N, and Insulatard. Effect is detected in about 2 hours, peaks at about 11 hours, and lasts about 20 to 29 hours.

3. *Long-acting insulins.* These insulins include Humulin U and Ultralente. Their duration is somewhat longer than the intermediate-acting insulins. They are seldom used, except for special needs, because their slow onset and extended action is more difficult to predict or control. Also, the tighter control being used today requires shorter-acting insulins with multiple injections according to self-monitoring of blood glucose levels, to meet variations in need during the day.

Sources of insulin

The commercial source of insulins has been beef and pork pancreases, which had been the main United States source until recently. But these animal-derived insulins are immunogenic to humans, beef more so than pork; in time they induce antiinsulin antibodies that delay or blunt their action. Now, however, human insulin is available from two sources: (1) biosynthesis by recombinant DNA technology through rapidly reproducing bacteria that have been given the human gene; and (2) chemical substitution of the terminal amino acid of the beta-chain of pork insulin. Because they carry the human insulin structure, these newer insulins are almost nonimmunogenic.

Insulin and exercise balance

Exercise benefits all persons with diabetes through its action in increasing the number of insulin receptors on muscle cells, thus increasing insulin efficiency.[36] However, physical activity must be regular to be effective.[40] A detailed history of personal activity and exercise habits provides the information needed to help a client plan a wise program of regular moderate exercise. Guidelines for extra food to cover periods of heavier exercise, athletic practice or competition can be included (Table 20.4). Gregory reports the experience of a college football player with diabetes and his carefully planned blood sugar control during games.[41] In general, exercise programs make persons feel better both physically and psychologically. This improved sense of well-being should not be underestimated in persons facing a chronic disease.

Insulin delivery systems

Intensive insulin therapy for maintaining more normal blood glucose control requires multiple injections of rapid-acting insulin, alone or in combination with basal intermediate-acting insulin. This is accomplished either by regular injection with disposal syringes or with an insulin pump. The pump is not for everyone, but for many it has made life easier with a steady control of blood sugar level. It is a small device, easily worn on the belt with a subcutaneous needle in the abdomen and buttons the wearer pushes to obtain a fixed programmed flow of insulin in balance with food intake.

Testing methods for monitoring results

Frequent testing of blood glucose levels is necessary for successful "tight" control of IDDM and its complications. Two of the following methods are regular tools; the third serves for occasional backup.

Self-monitoring of blood glucose. For insulin doses to be administered in sufficient time intervals and amounts to maintain normal blood glucose, close monitoring of immediate blood glucose levels is mandatory.[39] Small, lightweight, easy-to-use, hand-size meters, easily carried in pockets and handbags, are available for convenient use. A reagent test strip is inserted into the blood glucose meter, a drop of capillary blood from the finger obtained with an automatic lancer is placed on the reagent test strip, and a digital reading of the blood glucose level appears on the meter. The frequency of monitoring varies according to need for control and goal of care. More frequent self-monitoring is indicated for unstable forms of diabetes, persons using insulin pumps, and those who want close control and freedom of movement. Usually two to eight before- and after-meal tests are performed daily.

Glycosylated hemoglobin A_{1c}. The Hb A_{1c} test is also used for monitoring an intensive insulin therapy program. The physician uses this test every few weeks or monthly to measure blood glucose response over time. Because glucose attaches to the hemoglobin over the life of the red blood cell, the test gives an accumulated history of glucose levels over a period of time, providing an effective management tool for evaluating progress and making decisions about treatment changes.

Physical activity habits

In counseling clients with diabetes, a detailed history of personal activity and physical exercise habits should be discussed. This information is then used as a basis for planning together a wise program of *regular* moderate exercise. Guidelines for extra food to cover periods of heavier exercise or athletic practice and competition are included (Table 20.4).[42] Self-monitoring is a regular procedure now used by most persons with IDDM—type I. It is a helpful means of determining the balance needed at any point in time between exercise, insulin, and food.

CARE OF PERSONS WITH NIDDM

By far the greater number of persons with diabetes, approximately 85% of the total, have non–insulin-dependent diabetes mellitus (NIDDM)-type II. This usually milder form of diabetes differs from IDDM-type I in that insulin is being produced by the beta cells in the islets of Langerhans, but the body cells are resistant to its action. It has been called a genetically programmed failure of the beta cell to compensate for insulin resistance.[7]

Contributing factors

A number of factors contribute to the development of NIDDM—type II, including age, obesity, little physical activity, diet, toxins, and stress. It usually appears in later adult years after the age of 40 years, and 60% to 90% of the individuals are obese and sedentary.

Treatment goals

Goals for treating NIDDM—type II focus on achieving improved medical outcomes. These results include optimal blood glucose control, normal blood lipids, managing hypertension, and minimizing complications such as neuropathy and nephropathy.[42]

Nutrition therapy

Similar medical nutrition therapy for NIDDM—type II helps to achieve overall treatment goals, especially in cost-effectiveness. The basic nutrition therapy principles described for treatment of IDDM—type I carry over to the practice guidelines for NIDDM—type II. However, because the two conditions differ in nature, there are some differences in individualized therapy, as follows:

1. *Energy balance.* Because the large majority of persons with NIDDM—type II are obese, the major focus for determining kcalorie requirements is that of weight reduction. Specific caloric requirements to facilitate weight are calculated for each person to account for individual differences. Generally, a diet of about 1200 kcalories for women and 1500 kcalories for men brings about successful weight reduction.
2. *Nutrient balance.* Therapy for both types of diabetes is the same. The current nutrition recommendations

Table 18.7 Dietary fiber and kilocalorie values for selected foods

Foods	Serving	Dietary fiber (g)	Kcalories
Breads and cereals			
All Bran	1/3 cup	8.5	70
Bran (100%)	1/2 cup	8.4	75
Bran Buds	1/3 cup	7.9	75
Corn Bran	2/3 cup	5.4	100
Bran Chex	2/3 cup	4.6	90
Cracklin' Oat Bran	1/3 cup	4.3	110
Bran Flakes	3/4 cup	4.0	90
Air-popped popcorn	1 cup	2.5	25
Oatmeal	1 cup	2.2	144
Grapenuts	1/4 cup	1.4	100
Whole-wheat bread	1 slice	1.4	60
Legumes, cooked			
Kidney beans	1/2 cup	7.3	110
Lima beans	1/2 cup	4.5	130
Vegetables, cooked			
Green peas	1/2 cup	3.6	55
Corn	1/2 cup	2.9	70
Parsnip	1/2 cup	2.7	50
Potato, with skin	1 medium	2.5	95
Brussels sprouts	1/2 cup	2.3	30
Carrots	1/2 cup	2.3	25
Broccoli	1/2 cup	2.2	20
Beans, green	1/2 cup	1.6	15
Tomato, chopped	1/2 cup	1.5	17
Cabbage, red and white	1/2 cup	1.4	15
Kale	1/2 cup	1.4	20
Cauliflower	1/2 cup	1.1	15
Lettuce (fresh)	1 cup	0.8	7
Fruits			
Apple	1 medium	3.5	80
Raisins	1/4 cup	3.1	110
Prunes, dried	3	3.0	60
Strawberries	1 cup	3.0	45
Orange	1 medium	2.6	60
Banana	1 medium	2.4	105
Blueberries	1/2 cup	2.0	40
Dates, dried	3	1.9	70
Peach	1 medium	1.9	35
Apricot, fresh	3 medium	1.8	50
Grapefruit	1/2 cup	1.6	40
Apricot, dried	5 halves	1.4	40
Cherries	10	1.2	50
Pineapple	1/2 cup	1.1	40

Modified from Lanza E. Butrum RR: A critical review of food fiber analysis and data, *J Am Diet Assoc* 86:732, 1986.

case of legumes (see Chapter 3). Others provide gaseous discomfort on an individual basis, such as the cruciferous family of vegetables, including cabbage, Brussels sprouts, broccoli, turnips, and radishes. Several brands of needed enzyme for use in a few drops with such foods are being marketed for persons with this deficiency, allowing them to enjoy using these foods.

3. *Respect food intolerances*. Lactose intolerance, caused by a deficiency of the digestive enzyme, is a well-known disorder resulting in intestinal cramping, bloating, and diarrhea after drinking milk or eating dairy products. However, preparations of lactase enzyme such as Lactaid allow lactose-intolerant persons to use dairy products.

4. *Reduce total fat intake*. Excess fat delays gastric emptying and contributes to malabsorption problems in the intestine and subsequent diarrhea. For healthier diets in general, moderation in total dietary fat also helps reduce risks of fatty buildup in major blood vessels that leads to heart disease problems.

5. *Avoid large meals*. Large amounts of food in one meal create discomfort from gastric distention and gas generated in the stomach, especially when the meals are of high caloric content. Smaller, more frequent meals may reduce these symptoms.

6. *Decrease air-swallowing habits*. Certain habits of eating contribute to gas swallowed or generated in the stomach. These include eating rapidly, eating large amounts, and excessive fluid intake, especially carbonated beverages. Habits of chewing gum and smoking also contribute to gas formation.

SHORT-BOWEL SYNDROME

Etiology

Short-bowel syndrome (SBS) is a pattern of varying metabolic and physiologic consequences of surgical removal of parts of the intestine with extensive dysfunction of the remaining portion of the organ.[36] These resections result from intrinsic disease such as Crohn's disease or radiation enteritis, surgical bypass, or massive abdominal injury and trauma. They may also be required for vascular problems such as blood clots leading to death of involved tissue, or for extensive fistula formation, radiation injury, congenital abnormalities, or cancer.

Nutritional management

Degrees of surgical resection create different problems and nutrition therapy must be tailored to individual functional capacity remaining. Early enteral or parenteral nutrition support usually supplies initial needs. Frequent monitoring of nutritional responses, especially fluid and electrolyte balances and malnutrition signs, is essential. Later weaning to an oral diet with vitamin and mineral supplementation follows as tolerated, with continued nutrition assessment. As adaptation progresses, the early restriction of fat may be liberalized somewhat with moderate use of the more easily absorbed medium-chain triglycerides (MCT oil) to obtain needed kcalories.

Large intestine diseases

Diverticular disease

Nature and etiology

A diverticulum is a small tubular sac protruding off from a main canal or cavity in the body. The formation and presence of these small diverticula protruding from the intestinal lumen, usually the colon, produces the condition diverticulosis. More often diverticulosis occurs in older adults. It develops at points of weakened musculature in the bowel wall, along the track of blood vessels entering the bowel from without. The direct cause is a progressive increase in pressure within the bowel from segmental circular muscle contractions that normally move the remaining food mass along and form the feces for elimination. When pressures become sufficiently high in one of these segments, and dietary fiber is insufficient to maintain the necessary bulk for preventing high internal pressures within the colon, diverticula, small protrusions of the muscle layer, develop at that point. The condition causes no problem unless the small diverticula become infected and inflamed from fecal irritation and colon bacteria. This diseased state is called **diverticulitis**. The commonly used collective term covering diverticulosis and diverticulitis is *diverticular disease.*

Clinical symptoms

As the inflammatory process grows, increased hypermotility and pressures from luminal segmentation cause pain. The pain and tenderness are usually localized in the lower left side of the abdomen and are accompanied by nausea, vomiting, distension, diarrhea, intestinal spasm, and fever. If the process continues, intestinal obstruction or perforation may necessitate surgical intervention.

Nutritional management

Diverticular disease is a common gastrointestinal disorder among middle-aged and elderly persons. It may often be accompanied by malnutrition. Aggressive nutritional therapy hastens recovery from an attack, shortens the hospital stay, and reduces costs. Numerous studies and extensive clinical practice have demonstrated better management of chronic diverticular disease with an increased amount of dietary fiber than with old practices of restricting fiber. In acute episodes of active disease, however, the amount of dietary fiber may need to be moderately reduced. The relationship of dietary fiber and diverticu-

lar disease has been further reinforced by studies of populations, such as those in Japan, that have recently experienced the Westernization of their culture. Chapter 2 provides an extended discussion of dietary fiber and its relation to health and disease.

Constipation

A common disorder, usually of short duration, constipation is characterized by retention of feces in the colon beyond the normal emptying time. It is a problem for which Americans spend a quarter of a billion dollars for laxatives each year. However, the "regularity" of elimination is highly individual, and it is not necessary for health to have a bowel movement every day. Usually, this common short-term problem results from various sources of nervous tension, worry, and changes in social setting. Such situations include vacations and travel, with alterations in usual routines. Also, it may be caused by prolonged use of laxatives or cathartics, low-fiber diets, or lack of exercise, all of which can contribute to a decreased intestinal muscle tone. Improved exercise, dietary, and bowel habits are usually sufficient to remedy the situation. The diet should include increased dietary fiber and naturally laxative fruits, such as dried prunes and figs, as well as increased fluid. If chronic constipation persists, however, agents that increase stool bulk may be necessary. These bulking agents include bran or more soluble forms of fiber. Taking laxatives or enemas on a regular basis should be avoided. The problem of constipation occurs in all age groups, but is almost epidemic in elderly people. In all cases a personalized approach to management of constipation is fundamental.

Food allergies and sensitivities

Underlying etiology

The word *allergy* comes from the Greek *allos* (other) and *ergon* (work). Thus the name implies an unusual or inappropriate response to a stimulus, usually an environmental factor. An allergic condition results from a disorder of the immune system. It is immunity gone wrong.

The term *food allergy* should be used only for hypersensitivity that is caused by immunoglobulin E-mediated food reaction to specific food constituents or their digestive products.[38] The term *food sensitivity* is a general nonspecific term often used incorrectly as synonymous with food allergies. However, in tests many of these claimed sensitivities are unconfirmed. Food allergy is distinct from food intolerances, which are caused by nonimmunologic mechanisms, for example, cow's milk intolerance resulting from lactase deficiency. In general, the process of diagnosis and treatment of adverse reactions to foods includes clinical assessment, dietary manipulation, and laboratory tests. Appropriate dietary counseling is essential.

COMMON FOOD ALLERGENS

The care of an allergic child presents many problems. A wide variety of environmental, emotional, and physical factors influence reaction, and a suitable regimen is sometimes difficult to find. Since sensitivity to protein substances is a common basis for food allergy, the early foods of infants and children are frequent offenders. Fortunately, however, children tend to become less allergic to food sources as they become older.

Milk

Cow's milk has long been a common cause of allergic response in infants.[38,39] In sensitive children it causes gastrointestinal difficulties such as vomiting, diarrhea, and colic, or it may cause respiratory and skin problems. The problem is generally identified by clinical symptoms, family history, and a trial on a milk-free diet, using an appropriate substitute hypoallergenic formula such as the casein hydrolysate formulas Nutramigen and Pregestimil (both from Mead Johnson) or the special hydrolysate formula Alimentum (Ross).[40] Freedom from symptoms on a milk-free diet is then followed by a retrial on milk to determine if it causes the symptoms to reappear. Only then is the diagnosis of milk allergy established. Often symptoms appear and disappear spontaneously, regardless of dietary changes. But they tend to be more often caused by food if gastrointestinal problems are present.

Eggs, wheat, and other foods

Among the dominant food allergens in infants are chicken eggs, cow's milk, and wheat. The specific biochemical sensitivity to gluten (a protein found in wheat) in the child with gluten-induced celiac sprue is caused by a specific biochemical defect in the mucosal cells in celiac disease and represents a different sensitivity mechanism from the immunophysiology causing a true food allergy. Other true food allergens among children, some continuing through adulthood, include peanuts, soy, tree nuts, other cereal grains, and shellfish.[41]

NUTRITIONAL MANAGEMENT

In an allergic child's diet, solid foods are usually added slowly to the original formula, with common offenders excluded in early feedings. The following basic list of most frequently offending food allergens must be avoided [41,42]:
- Chicken eggs
- Cow's milk
- Wheat
- Peanuts
- Tree nuts
- Soy products
- Shellfish, fish

Citrus fruits, berries, and tomatoes may cause skin rash, but this is a local reaction. It is not the immunologic response that identifies true allergy.[41]

In some cases a series of diagnostic food elimination diets may be used to identify offending food allergens. A core of less-often offending foods is used initially, with gradual addition of other single foods one at a time to test the response. If a given food causes return of the allergy, the food is then identified as an allergen and eliminated from use. It may be retested later to determine if it is still an allergen. Guidance in the substitution of special food products and in the use of special recipes can be provided for the child's parents. Most food allergies tend to weaken as the child grows older. However, serious allergy to a few key foods, especially peanuts, may continue into adulthood and require constant monitoring of food products and dishes to avoid severe attacks.[42] These attacks of severe anaphylactic shock are marked by sudden bronchial spasms, vomiting, dropping blood pressure, and irregular heart rhythm.

FAMILY EDUCATION AND COUNSELING

The education of the parents and family of an allergic child must include a knowledge and understanding of the allergic state and the many factors that may influence it. If specific foods have been definitely identified as offenders, careful guidance to eliminate these from the diet is needed. Common uses of the offending food in daily meal patterns and its occurrence in a number of commercial products and other hidden sources should be discussed. Label reading and recipe adaptation are important. As an allergic child grows older, reaction to a given food may wane, and it can gradually be added to the diet.

FOOD INTOLERANCES FROM GENETIC-METABOLIC DISEASE

Certain food intolerances may also stem from underlying genetic disease that affects the metabolism of one or more specific nutrients. Genetic disease results from the individual's specific gene inheritance. Genes in each cell control the metabolic functions of the cell. They regulate the synthesis of some 1000 or more specific cell enzymes that control metabolism within the cell. When a specific gene is abnormal (mutant), the enzyme whose synthesis that

---

diverticulitis Inflammation of pockets of tissue (diverticuli) in the lining of the mucous membrane of the colon.

gene controls cannot be made. In turn, then, the specific metabolic reaction controlled by that specific missing enzyme cannot take place. The specific genetic disease caused by this metabolic block then manifests clinical symptoms connected with resulting abnormal metabolic products. As primary examples here, we look briefly at two such genetic diseases affecting food-nutrient intolerances: (1) phenylketonuria, which affects amino acid metabolism and hence protein foods; (2) galactosemia, which affects carbohydrate metabolism, specifically food sources of lactose. Both are detected by newborn screening procedures, now mandatory by law.

PHENYLKETONURIA

Metabolic defect and clinical symptoms

Phenylketonuria (PKU) results from the missing cell enzyme, phenylalanine hydroxylase, which metabolizes one of the essential amino acids, phenylalanine, to tyrosine, another nonessential amino acid. Phenylalanine then accumulates in the blood, and its alternate metabolites, the phenyl acids, are excreted in the urine. One of these urinary acids, phenylpyruvic acid, is a phenylketone; hence the name of the disease. Untreated PKU can produce devastating effects, but present nutritional therapy can avoid these results.[43] In past years, before current newborn screening laws and dietary treatment practices from birth, the most profound effect observed in persons with untreated PKU was severe mental retardation. The IQ of affected persons was usually below 50 and frequently less than 20. Central nervous system damage caused irritability, hyperactivity, convulsive seizures, and bizarre behavior.

Nutritional therapy

PKU can now be well controlled by special diet therapy. After screening at birth, a special low-phenylalanine diet effectively controls the serum phenylalanine levels so they are maintained at appropriate amounts to prevent clinical symptoms and promote normal growth and development.[43] Since phenylalanine is an essential amino acid necessary for growth, it cannot be totally removed from the diet. Blood levels of phenylalanine are constantly monitored, and the metabolic team nutritionist calculates the special diet for each infant and child to allow only the limited amount of phenylalanine tolerated. Based on extensive studies, guidelines for dietary management of PKU are currently being used effectively to build lifetime habits, since research now indicates that there is no safe age at which a child may discontinue the diet.[43] This dietary management is built on two basic components: (1) a substitute for milk, a special medical food continued past infancy and childhood into adolescence and adulthood; and (2) guidelines for adding solid foods, both regular and special low-protein products, and then building continuing food habits.

Family education and counseling

Initial education and continuing support of parents is essential, since dietary management of PKU is the only known effective method of treatment and maintaining the diet becomes more difficult as the child grows older. But parents must understand and accept the necessity of the diet, and this requires patience, understanding, and continued reinforcement. The PKU team, together with parents, provides initial and continuing care so that the PKU child will grow and develop normally (Figure 18.3). Such a child, diagnosed at birth by widespread screening programs, can have a healthy and happy life, instead of the profound disease consequences experienced in the past. This current practice of long-term dietary management is especially critical for young women who are reaching the age of potential high-risk pregnancies with maternal PKU.

GALACTOSEMIA

Metabolic defect and clinical symptoms

This genetic disease, also caused by a missing cell enzyme, affects carbohydrate metabolism. The missing enzyme controls the conversion of galactose, which is derived from lactose, to glucose. Milk, the infant's first food, contains a large amount of the precursor lactose (milk sugar). After galactose is initially combined with phosphate to begin the metabolic conversion to glucose, it cannot proceed further in the galactosemic infant. Galactose rapidly accumulates in the blood and in various body tissues. In the past the excess tissue accumulations of galactose caused rapid damage to the untreated infant. The child failed to thrive, and clinical symptoms appeared soon after birth. Continued liver damage brought jaundice, an enlarged liver with cirrhosis, enlarged spleen, and ascites. Without treatment, death usually resulted from liver failure. If the infant survived, continuing tissue damage and hypoglycemia in the optic lens and the brain caused cataracts and mental retardation. Now, however, with newborn screening programs, these infants are diagnosed at birth and started on special dietary management. With this vital nutritional therapy, they continue to grow and develop normally.

Nutritional therapy

The main indirect source of dietary galactose is the lactose in milk. Therefore, all forms of milk and lactose must be removed from the diet. In this instance a galactose-free diet is used. Any needed amount of galactose for certain body structures can be synthesized by the body. A soy-base formula is used. Breast-feeding, of course, cannot be used. Later, as solid foods are added to the infant's diet at about 6 months of age, careful attention must be given to avoiding lactose are based on principles of blood glucose and blood lipid controls.

3. *Food distribution balance.* Because NIDDM—type II does not require insulin, the timing of meals or interval snacks is not so important that it needs to be balanced with activity. A summary of the two types of diabetes is provided in Table 20.5.

Oral antidiabetic drugs

Oral antidiabetic drugs are sometimes used to treat hyperglycemia in NIDDM—type II because they lower the elevated blood glucose level. In general, they act in various ways to stimulate the pancrease to produce more endogenous insulin or by inhibiting some phase of metabolism or absorption. Some of these antidiabetic drugs include such agents as tolbutamide and glipizide, which effectively lower blood glucose levels at significantly lower doses than most of the sulfonylurea compounds. Two newer oral antidiabetic drugs are (1) metformin (Glucophage), a biguanide that inhibits hepatic glucose and enhances peripheral glucose uptake, and (2) acarbose (Precose), a glucosidase inhibitor that interferes with the digestion of dietary disaccharides and complex carbohydrates and delays glucose absorption.[42,43]

MANAGEMENT OF DIABETES MEDICAL NUTRITION THERAPY

THE NEW MODEL: MEDICAL NUTRITION THERAPY FOR DIABETES

Following the results of the DCCT and the new 1994 recommendations of the American Diabetes Association and the American Dietetics Association, the clinical practice of medical nutrition therapy in diabetes has been nothing short of revolutionary. The American Diabetes Association position paper clearly stated that there was now no one "diabetic" or "on the ADA" diet. Now the recommended diet is a dietary prescription based on individual nutritional assessment and treatment goals.[44,45] This new model, *medical nutrition therapy for diabetes*, emphasizes the actions of the diabetes team clinical dietitian in an individualized, integrated four-point approach: assessment, goal setting, intervention, and evaluation.

Assessment

The first step involves a comprehensive assessment of the client's background. It includes clinical information, medical and lifestyle data such as personal self-monitoring of blood glucose, and dietary history. Interview follow-up tools such as questionnaires and food records assess general food patterns and nutrient intake.

Goal setting

The second step guides the client in setting up personal goals in the self-care of diabetes. To be valid, these goals must be reasonable and negotiable as follow-up experience may indicate.

Nutrition intervention

The third step guides the client in selecting and using the most appropriate meal-planning guide from the number that are now available, based on individual needs for knowledge and skills to change or maintain eating habits and daily living practices.

Evaluation

Together the client and the dietitian evaluate the goals and nutrition intervention as well as ongoing clinical data, to help the client succeed at the individual program established. Then they make any desired adjustments, and the dietitian provides continuing counseling and education as needed.

DIABETES MEAL PLANNING TOOLS

The DCCT research dietitians developed a number of resources in addition to the familiar food exchange lists for use as meal-planning guides for broader variety in meeting individual needs related to literacy or education level. The American Dietetic Association has published a 1996 comprehensive guide to all these resources.[46] Whatever the diabetes medical nutrition therapy management tool, the first vital principle in working with persons who have diabetes is that you must start where they are. Any food-planning process must focus first on the unique individual rather than on the "case" or disease. Numerous planning approaches are used by skilled and sensitive clinical dietitians who tailor their actions to the person's learning needs and abilities, nutritional needs, personal needs, and lifestyle issues. Because of the wide use of the exchange lists as a dietary management tool, a review of this meal-planning tool is briefly discussed here.

THE EXCHANGE SYSTEM OF MEAL PLANNING

THE FOOD EXCHANGE SYSTEM

The exchange system for planning diabetic diets is based on the concept of food equivalents. It has been developed jointly by the American Diabetes Association and the American Dietetic Association. In most cases, initial instruction is provided by a professional diet counselor—a registered dietitian with extensive clinical experience. Since its introduction, the Food Exchange System as out-

Table 20.6	Exchange lists			
Food groups/lists	**Carbohydrate**	**Protein**	**Fat**	**Kcalories**
Carbohydrate group				
Starch	15	3	1 or less	80
Fruit	15	—	—	60
Milk				
Skim	12	8	0-3	90
Low-fat	12	8	5	120
Whole	12	8	8	150
Other carbohydrates	15	Varies	Varies	Varies
Vegetables	5	2	—	25
Meat and meat substitute group				
Very lean	—	7	0-1	35
Lean	—	7	3	55
Medium-fat	—	7	8	100
High-fat	—	7	8	100
Fat group	—	—	5	45

From American Dietetic Association and American Diabetes Association: *Exchange lists for meal planning,* Chicago, IL, 1995, ADA/ADA.

lined or in modified form has been widely used for nutritional care and teaching. Combined with professional counseling, it is a sound means of regulating the diet that is flexible enough to meet a variety of living situations. Three food groups are used in the newly revised lists (Table 20.6):

1. *Carbohydrates*, which include five subgroups: starch, fruit, milk (with three subgroups according to fat content), other carbohydrates including sweets, and vegetables.
2. *Meat and meat substitutes*, which include four subgroups: very lean, lean, medium-fat, and high-fat.
3. *Fats*, which include three subgroups: monounsaturated, polyunsaturated, and saturated fats.

Markers indicate foods higher in sodium. Additional lists include free foods, combination foods, and fast-foods. All information is provided in a well-written and colorfully illustrated booklet, *Exchange Lists for Meal Planning*, for the counselor and the client.[47] These completely revised food lists are given in Appendix L. A brief listing of these three food groups according to their general composition and characteristics is given in Table 20.6. In using the food groups as a guide, food items within any one group may be freely exchanged within that group because all foods in a particular group in the portion indicated have approximately the same food value. These three main food groups and their subgroups form the basis for calculating diet needs and for helping clients learn to make wide food selections and substitutions.

Developing an individual food plan

As with the use of any meal-planning tool, the clinical dietitian learns as much as possible about each client's food patterns and needs through a comprehensive history (see Chapter 15). A wide range of areas are included, such as personal and family needs, psychosocial development,

Table 20.7	Guidelines for estimating approximate daily energy need for persons with diabetes mellitus according to age, gender, and general physical activity		
		Daily energy intake	
Persons with diabetes		**kcal/lb**	**kcal/kg**
Children			
1 year		55	120
1-10 years (gradual decline with age)		45-36	100-80
Males			
11-15 years		20-36 (average, 30)	50-80 (average, 65)
16-20 years			
Very active		20-22	50
Average activity		18	30
Sedentary		15	30
Females			
11-15 years		17	35
15 years		15	30
Adults			
Men, active women		15 × DWB* (lb)	30
Sedentary men, most women, adults over age 55		15 × DWB (lb)	28
Sedentary women, obese persons, sedentary adults over age 55		10 × DWB (lb)	20
Pregnant women			
First trimester		13-15	28-32
Second and third trimesters; lactation		16-17	36-38

Data from Franz MJ: Diabetes and nutrition: state of the science and the art, *Top Clin Nutr* 3(1):1, 1988.
*DBW, desirable body weight (reasonable body weight).

social activities, school and work commitments, typical day's routine, and food habits defined and described. A full medical history is needed, with particular reference to the diabetes, its course, and the client's personal experience with it. Medical and nutritional status data include laboratory tests and measures of weight, height, and body composition.

Determining the nutrition prescription

Based on the information gathered through the comprehensive nutritional assessment, the clinical dietitian determines an appropriate nutrition prescription based on the individual's usual eating habits. The American Dietetic Association's recommendations and clinical practice guidelines are used to calculate general energy needs (Table 20.7).

Determining the individual meal pattern

The number of food exchanges the dietitian calculates for each food group is distributed as food units into the day's meal pattern to provide the overall food distribution balance according to the type of insulin therapy, basic food habits, home-school-work situations, and any specific exercise periods. A general individualized pattern fairly evenly spread throughout the day as indicated provides an initial guide with modification as experience suggests. The pattern resulting from the diet calculation in Table 20.8 follows this general distribution plan.

Planning a day's menu

The food exchange lists are used for meal planning according to the scheme developed with the client. The client and family are guided in using these food lists for making various appropriate food choices to fulfill the individual food pattern. Table 20.9 shows a sample food plan based on the this nutrition prescription.

Adjusting the plan to the individual

In follow-up sessions, the dietitian and the client discuss any needed adjustment of the original plan. The plan is tailored to fit practical individual needs, living situation, and general eating habits. Counseling continues to determine any further adjustments or changes that are needed.

PLANNING FOR SPECIAL NEEDS

Sick days

When general illness occurs, the food and insulin amounts must be adjusted accordingly. The texture may be modified as needed to use easily digested and absorbed liquid foods while still maintaining as much as possible the glucose equivalents of the usual food plan (Table 20.10).

Table 20.8 Calculation of diabetic diet using exchange system (2200 kcal)

Food group	Total day's exchanges	Carbohydrates: 275 g (50% kcal)	Protein: 110 g (20% kcal)	Fat 75 g (30% kcal)	Breakfast	Lunch	Dinner	Snacks After-noon	Snacks Bed-time
Carbohydrates									
Fruit	3	45			1	1		1	
Vegetable	4	20	8			2	2		
Other carbohydrates	1	15	Varies	Varies			1		
Milk									
Skim	2	24	16		1				1
Low-fat	—								
Whole	—								
SUBTOTAL		104							
Starch	11.5	172	34.5		3	3	3	1	1.5
Subtotal			58.5						
		276							
Meat and Meat Substitutes									
Very lean	2		14	0-1				1	1
Lean	3		21	9			3		
Medium-fat	2		14	10	1	1			
High-fat	—								
SUBTOTAL				20					
			107.5						
Fat	11			55	3	3	3	1	1
				75					
Total g		276	107.5	75					

Table 20.9	Sample menu prescription: 2200 kcal:

$$275 \text{ g carbohydrates } (50\% \text{ kcal})$$
$$+$$
$$110 \text{ g protein } (20\% \text{ kcal})$$
$$+$$
$$75 \text{ g fat } (30\% \text{ kcal})$$

Meal	Food item

Breakfast

1 medium, sliced fresh peach
Shredded Wheat cereal
1 poached egg on whole-grain toast
1 bran muffin
1 tsp margarine
1 cup low-fat milk
Coffee or tea

Lunch

Vegetable soup with wheat crackers
Tuna sandwich on whole wheat bread
Filling: Tuna (drained ½ cup)
Mayonnaise (2 tsp)
Chopped dill pickle
Chopped celery
Fresh pear

Afternoon snack

10 crackers with 2 tbsp peanut butter
Orange

Dinner

Pan-broiled pork chop (trimmed well)
1 cup brown rice
½-1 cup green beans
Tossed green salad with Italian dressing (1-2 tbsp)
½ cup applesauce
1 bran muffin

Evening snack

3 cups popped, plain popcorn
1 oz cheese
1 cup low-fat milk

Physical activity

For any unusual physical activity the IDDM client must make special plans ahead. This is particularly true of a young person with diabetes engaging in athletic practice or competition.[40] The energy demands of exercise are discussed in Chapter 14.

Travel

When a trip is planned, the clinical dietitian must confer with the client to guide food choices according to what will be available. Self-monitoring of blood glucose levels and insulin therapy equipment and making food plans are as important on vacation or a business trip as they are at home. The traveler always needs to plan ahead with the health care team (see the *Practical Application* box).

Table 20.10	How to modify a diabetic meal plan for sick days

Usual food intake	Exchange	Carbohydrates (g)
½ chicken breast, roasted	3 meat	0
1 tsp margarine	1 fat	0
½ cup rice	1 bread	15
Tossed green salad, lemon wedge	Free food	0
¾ cup strawberries	1 fruit	15
1 cup skim milk	1 milk	12
		TOTAL 42

Sick day intake*	Exchange	Carbohydrates (g)
2 cups broth	Free food	0
½ cup gelatin	1 fruit	15
1 cup ginger ale (regular)	2 fruit	30
2 cups herbal tea	Free food	0
		TOTAL 45

*The objective is to provide required amounts of carbohydrates for times when the person with diabetes does not feel like eating much.

Eating out

Provide similar guidelines and suggestions for various situations when the client eats meals away from home. As a general rule, the plan must be made ahead of time so that accommodations for what is eaten at home before and after the meal eaten away from home reflects continuing balance needs of the day.

Stress

Any form of emotional stress is reflected in variations of diabetes control.[47-49] These variations are caused by hormonal responses, which act as antagonists to insulin. The clinical dietitian must help the client learn and practice a variety of useful stress-reduction activities.

DIABETES EDUCATION PROGRAM

GOAL: PERSON-CENTERED SELF-CARE

In past years the traditional medical model has guided diabetes education in its methods, language, and respective roles assumed. The professionals have viewed themselves as having major authoritative roles and assigned to the person with diabetes the more passive role of "patient." With notable exceptions in certain places, this model has been followed in most cases. However, with the increasing movement toward changing roles of practitioners and consumers in the health care system, persons with diabetes are assuming a more active voice in planning and conducting their own care. Several barriers

Travel and illness: "real-life" diabetic situations

What do you do when your client with diabetes wants to travel or catches cold? In both cases, the client has too many distractions to concentrate fully on planning the most ideal menu. The fact remains, however, that diabetes management relies heavily on the food plan and, in the case of IDDM—type I, on a flexible meal and snack pattern that can be adjusted to meet changing demands.

The following are a few helpful hints you may want to offer clients for those common situations:

Travel
Promote confidence about meal-planning skills. Review the number and type of exchanges allowed at each meal. Encourage the client to practice measuring portion sizes. Review tips on eating out.

Learn about the foods that will be available. For a cruise, the client should get a copy of the menu in advance. For air travel, advise the client to order diabetic meals in advance. If foreign travel is involved, the client should ask the travel agent for information about foods commonly served to tourists.

Select appropriate snacks. Extra carbohydrate and caloric needs must be met during extra physical activities such as hiking, swimming, skiing, and mountain climbing.

Plan for time
Extending driving time should be avoided. The client should plan to include about 20 g of carbohydrates for every 2 hours of travel. For emergencies and unexpected delays, food for two meals and two snacks, including nonperishable items and liquids, should be on hand.

Plan for time zone changes. The schedule may need to be changed. If so, discuss any necessary meal schedule revisions to balance with insulin activity pattern.

Prepare companions. The client's companions must be able to recognize signs and symptoms of hypoglycemia and hyperglycemia and know their treatment. Remind the client to carry quick-acting carbohydrates at all times.

To support the medical regimen of insulin-dependent clients, remind them (1) to carry an identification bracelet, pendant, or card at all times; (2) to ask their physician for a letter explaining the need for syringes; (3) to carry adequate supplies and equipment for maintaining a schedule for self-testing blood; and (4) to take a prescription for insulin and secure brand names used for insulin in the country to which they are traveling.

Sick day survival
Nausea and diarrhea. Fluid and electrolyte replacement is crucial with nausea and diarrhea. Advise the client to use salted crackers, broth, or soups as tolerated to replace sodium. The client should use a cola drink such as Coca Cola (small amounts of high-sugar foods may be tolerated as replacement for short periods of time such as during illness), tea, broth, or orange juice to replace potassium. The client should drink something at least every 2 to 3 hours to replace liquids.

Gastrointestinal disturbances. The insulin dosage may have to be decreased. A clear liquid diet including fruit juices, fruit ices, and soups for adequate amounts of carbohydrates is recommended. Protein supplementation through elemental nutrition may be necessary if symptoms last longer than 72 hours. As food tolerance improves, the client should progress to a soft diet that includes milk drinks, custards, and eggs.

Colds and fever. These conditions are often treated with aspirin, which tends to lower the sugar level. The client must not skip meals. If necessary, regular meals may be subdivided into small, frequent snacks. Insulin must not be omitted. If the client is completely unable to eat, the physician should be contacted for advice regarding insulin dosage.

In summary, in all cases the client must be advised (1) to maintain a steady intake of food every day, (2) to replace the carbohydrate value of solid foods with that of liquid or soft foods as needed, (3) to monitor blood and urine frequently for sugar and acetone levels, and (4) to contact the physician if the illness lasts more than a day or so.

References
American Diabetes Association: *Medical management of type I diabetes,* ed 2, Alexandria, VA, 1994, American Diabetes Association.

Diabetes Day-by-Day Series: *Treating hypoglycemia* (18); *Illness* (31), American Diabetes Association, 1994 (pamphlets).

Franz MJ, Joynes JO: *Diabetes and brief illness,* Minnetonka, MI, 1993, Chronimed Publishing.

in our traditional system stem from three sources: (1) our culture, (2) our health care delivery system, and (3) our professional training habits. Essentially, much of the core problem focuses on *communication*. For example, a list of words we too commonly use that are objectionable to persons with diabetes, along with the preferred language, include the following:

1. *"Diabetic" used as a noun*. The word *diabetic* is an adjective and should not be used alone as a noun. Use instead the phrase *person with diabetes*.

2. *Compliance*. The word *compliance* raises red flags in the minds of persons with diabetes. It is a purely medical term and connotes an authoritative physician position. Instead the word *adherence* should be used, which has been adopted now by national committees and associations working in the field of diabetes. The word *adherence* indicates placement of more decision-making responsibility on the person with diabetes to determine courses of action in varying situations, which is, of course, the necessity.

3. *Patient*. Instead of "patient" the phrase *person with diabetes* should be used. Persons with diabetes, like any other person, are patients *only* when they are in the hospital or seeing a physician for an illness.

4. *Cheating*. A particularly abusive word in the minds of many persons with diabetes, especially parents of children and young people with diabetes, is the word *cheating*. This flagrant language abuse suggests dishonesty or failure to live up to an external code. By and large, persons with diabetes do not "cheat." They may kid themselves or they may be inaccurate in their reporting, but they do not cheat. Instead phrases such as *having difficulty* or *having a problem with* should be used.

CONTENTS: TOOLS FOR SELF-CARE

A plan for diabetes education must recognize the need for building self-sufficiency and responsibility within persons with diabetes and their families. It should provide practical guidelines that build on the necessary skills a person with diabetes must have for the best possible control, as well as additional surrounding factors related to life situations and psychosocial needs. Content areas include needs in relation to the nature of diabetes, nutrition and basic meal-planning, insulin (or oral medication) effects and how to regulate them, monitoring of blood glucose, urine sugar and acetone levels, hypoglycemia control, and how to deal with illness. These educational needs may be organized on three levels: (1) survival level, (2) home management level, and (3) lifestyle level. The Diabetes Care and Education dietetic practice group of the American Dietetic Association has

provided two such management guidelines, one for children and adolescents and one for adults.[12]

EDUCATIONAL MATERIALS: PERSON-CENTERED STANDARDS

A broad, confusing array of diabetes education materials is available. Some are excellent, and some should be discarded. Whatever we use should measure up to several basic person-centered requirements by doing the following:

1. Give the intended receiver credit for having some intelligence and wanting new information.

2. Inform persons fully and completely, giving both sides when experts disagree—as they surely do on occasion.

3. Appeal to various levels of audience, ranging from basic to sophisticated.

4. *Never* be patronizing, dehumanizing, or childish.

Whatever methods or materials we use, one central fact remains: the person who has diabetes is the *most important* and a *fully equal* member of the diabetes care team. Interdisciplinary approaches and strategies that involve this recognition can be developed.

TO SUM UP

Diabetes mellitus is a syndrome composed of many metabolic disorders collectively characterized by hyperglycemia and other symptoms. The treatment relies heavily on a basic type of therapy—a carefully controlled diet. Diabetes is classified in two main types: insulin-dependent diabetes mellitus (IDDM—type I) and non-insulin-dependent diabetes mellitus (NIDDM—type II).

Blood glucose levels are controlled primarily by the hormones of the pancreatic islet cells: *insulin*, which facilitates passage of glucose through cell membranes via special membrane receptors; *glucagon*, which ensures adequate levels of glucose to prevent hypoglycemia; and *somatostatin*, which controls the actions of insulin and glucagon to maintain normal blood glucose levels. The diabetic state results from inadequate insulin secretion or insulin resistance from too few receptor sites. Symptoms range from polydipsia, polyuria, polyphagia, and signs of abnormal energy metabolism to fluid and electrolyte imbalances, acidosis, and coma in seriously uncontrolled conditions.

IDDM—type I affects about 15% of all persons with diabetes. It occurs more often in children and is more severe and unstable. Its treatment involves blood glucose self-monitoring, insulin administration, and regular meals and exercise to balance insulin activity. NIDDM—type II occurs mostly in adults, particularly those who are overweight. Acidosis is rare. Its treatment consists of weight management and exercise. The food plan for both types of diabetes should be rich in complex carbohydrates and fiber; low in simple sugars and fat, especially in saturated fats and cholesterol; and moderate in protein. Moderate regular exercise increases the number of receptor sites on cell membranes and aids in weight management.

QUESTIONS FOR REVIEW

1. Describe the major characteristics of the two types of diabetes mellitus. Explain how these characteristics influence differences in nutrition therapy. List and describe medications used to control these conditions.

2. Identify and explain symptoms of uncontrolled chronic diabetes mellitus.

3. Describe the three major complications of uncontrolled chronic diabetes and the current DCCT program of intensive individual therapy designed to maintain normal blood glucose levels and help avoid these complications.

4. Mr. Smith just found out that that he has diabetes mellitus. He is a sedentary, 45-year-old man who is 170 cm (5 ft, 8 in) tall and weighs 94 kg (210 lb). No medications were prescribed for him. What is his desirable lean body weight? If a 1500-kcalorie diet is prescribed, how many grams of carbohydrate, protein, and fat should be included? If he decides to drink, how much alcohol could be allowed and how should he fit it into his diet? Should he purchase sugar substitutes or diet foods? Defend your answer. Mr. Smith wants to help his children reduce their chances of developing diabetes. What advice would you offer?

REFERENCES

1. Whitehous FW: Classification and pathogenesis of the diabetes syndrome: a historical perspective, *J Am Diet Assoc* 81(3):243, 1982.

2. Nestle et al: A case of diabetes mellitus, *N Engl J Med* 81:127, 1982.

3. Bliss M: *The discovery of insulin,* Chicago, 1982, University of Chicago Press.

4. Moller DE, Flier JS: Insulin resistance—mechanism, syndromes, and implications, *N Engl J Med* 325(13):938, 1991.

5. Berdanier CD: Genetic errors that result in diabetes mellitus, *Nutr Today* 29(1):17, 1994.

6. Olefsky JM, Nolan JJ: Insulin resistance and non-insulin-dependent diabetes mellitus: cellular and molecular mechanisms, *Am J Clin Nutr* 61(suppl):980S, 1995.

7. Polonsky KS et al: Non-insulin-dependent diabetes mellitus—a genetically programmed failure of the beta cell to compensate for insulin resistance, *N Engl J Med* 334(12):777, 1996.

8. Walston J et al: Time of onset of non-insulin-dependent diabetes mellitus and genetic variation in the β_3-adrenergic receptor gene, *N Engl J Med* 333(6):343, 1995.

9. Wendorf M, Goldfine ID: Archeology of NIDDM-excavation of the thrifty genotype, *Diabetes* 40:161, 1991.

10. McKeigue PM et al: Relation of central obesity and insulin resistance with high diabetes prevalence and cardiovascular risk in South Asians, *Lancet* 337:382, 1991.

11. Dowse GK et al: Abdominal obesity and physical inactivity as risk factors for NIDDM and impaired glucose tolerance in Indian, Creole, and Chinese Mauritians, *Diabetes Care* 14(4):271, 1991.

12. Connell JE, Thomas-Doberson D: Nutritional management of children with insulin-dependent diabetes mellitus: a review by the Diabetes Care and Education dietetic practice group, *J Am Diet Assoc* 91(12):1556, 1991.

13. Hayes C: Pattern management: a tool for improving blood glucose control with exercise, *J Am Diet Assoc* 97(10 suppl 2):S167, 1997.

14. Bell GI: Molecular defects in diabetes mellitus, *Diabetes* 40:413, 1991.

15. Fackelmann KA: Panel urges widespread testing for diabetes, *Sci News* 152(1):4, 1997.

16. Delahanty LM: Clinical significance of medical nutrition therapy in achieving diabetes outcomes and the importance of the process, *J Am Diet Assoc* 98(1):28, 1998.

17. Porte D Jr, Schwartz MW: Diabetes complications: why is glucose potentially toxic? *Science* 272(5262):699, 1996.

18. Clarke CM Jr, Lee DA: Prevention and treatment of the complications of diabetes mellitus, *N Engl J Med* 332(18):1210, 1995.

19. Anderson EJ et al: The DCCT Research Group: nutrition interventions for the intensive therapy in the Diabetes Control and Complications Trial, *J Am Diet Assoc* 93(7):768, 1993.

20. The Diabetes Control and Complications Trial Research Group: The effect of intensive treatment of diabetes on the development and progression of the long-term complications in insulin-dependent diabetes mellitus, *N Engl J Med* 329(14):977, 1993.

21. Delahanty L et al: Expanded role of the dietitian in the Diabetes Control and Complications Trial: implications for clinical practice, *J Am Diet Assoc* 93(7):758, 1993.

22. Lyon RB, Vinci DM: Nutrition management of insulin-dependent diabetes mellitus in adults: review by the Diabetes Care and Education dietetic practice group, *J Am Diet Assoc* 93(3):309, 1993.

23. American Diabetes Association, American Dietetic Association: Nutrition recommendations and principles for people with diabetes mellitus, *J Am Diet Assoc* 94(5):504, 1994.

24. Tinker LF, Heins JM, Holler HJ; Diabetes Care and Education Practice Group of The American Dietetic Association: Commentary and translation: 1994 nutrition recommendations for diabetes, *J Am Diet Assoc* 94(5):507, 1994.

25. Powers MA, Wheeler ML: Model for dietetics practice and research: the challenge is here, but the journey was not easy, *J Am Diet Assoc* 93(7):755, 1993.

26. Franz MJ: A new era in nutrition therapy for diabetes, *On The Cutting Edge* 16(2):5, 1995.

27. Franz MF, Maryniuk MD: Position of the American Dietetic Association: use of nutritive and nonnutritive sweeteners, *J Am Diet Assoc* 93(7):816, 1993.

28. Pratt R: Sucrose and other sweeteners: total carbohydrate is the name of the game, *On The Cutting Edge* 16(2):15, 1995.

29. Babione L: Fiber: how fabulous for diabetes management? *On The Cutting Edge* 16(2):16, 1995.

30. Nuttall F: Dietary fiber in the management of diabetes, *Diabetes* 42:503, 1993.

31. Uusitupa MIJ: Fructose in the diabetic diet, *Am J Clin Nutr* 59(suppl):753S, 1994.

32. Drewnowski A: Intense sweeteners and control of appetite, *Nutr Res* 53(1):1, 1995.

33. Murtaugh MA, Kerver J: Dietary protein and renal disease: impact of the 1994 nutrition recommendations, *On The Cutting Edge* 16(2):22, 1995.

34. Tinker LF: Dietary fat: is less or more better? *On The Cutting Edge* 16(2):17, 1995.

35. Kowisto VA et al: Alcohol with a meal has no adverse effects on postprandial glucose homeostasis in diabetic patients, *Diabetes Care* 16:1612, 1993.

36. Hayes C: Pattern management: a tool for improving blood glucose control with exercise, *On The Cutting Edge* 17(4):4, 1996.

37. Thom S: Humalog (insulin lispro): nutritional implications and educational considerations, *On The Cutting Edge* 17(4):8, 1996.

38. Trautmann ME et al: Intensive insulin therapy with insulin lispro in patients with type I diabetes reduces the frequency of hypoglycemia episodes, *Endocrinol Diabetes* 104:25, 1996.

39. Setter SM: New drug therapies for the treatment of diabetes, *On The Cutting Edge* 19(2):3, 1998.

40. Joyce M, King J: Consideration in selecting appropriate blood glucose monitoring devices, *On The Cutting Edge* 17(4):16, 1996.

41. Gregory RP et al: Nutrition management of a collegiate football player with insulin-dependent diabetes: guidelines and a case study, *J Am Diet Assoc* 94(4):775, 1994.

42. Beebe C: Implementation of the 1994 Nutrition Recommendations in Clinical Practice: NIDDM, *On The Cutting Edge* 16(2):11, 1995.

43. Flood TM: New oral therapy for type II diabetes, *On The Cutting Edge* 17(4):10, 1996.

44. Robbins DC: Acarbose: a new approach to the management of type II diabetes, *Practical Diabetol* 15:2, 1996.

45. American Diabetes Association, American Dietetics Association: Position paper: Nutrition recommendations and principles for people with diabetes mellitus, *J Am Diet Assoc* 94(5):504, 1994.

46. Tinker LF et al; Diabetes Care and Education Practice Group of the American Dietetic Association: Commentary and translation: 1994 nutrition recommendations for diabetes, *J Am Diet Assoc* 94(5):507, 1994.

47. Holler HJ, Pastors JG: *Diabetes medical nutrition therapy: a professional guide to management and nutrition education,* Chicago, 1996, American Dietetic Association.

48. Holler HJ et al: *Exchange lists for meal-planning,* Chicago, 1995, American Dietetic Association/American Diabetes Association.

49. Chapman KM et al: Applying behavioral models to dietary education of elderly diabetic patients, *J Nutr Ed* 27(2):75, 1995.

50. Schlundt DG et al: Situational obstacles to dietary adherence for adults with diabetes, *J Am Diet Assoc* 94(8):874, 1994.

51. Jacobson AM: The psychological care of patients with insulin-dependent diabetes mellitus, *N Engl J Med* 334(19):1249, 1996.

■ FURTHER READING

Gallagher AM, Crawley C, eds: Applying new technology in diabetes management to nutrition counseling: meters, insulin, and insulin delivery systems, *On The Cutting Edge* 13(4):1-33, 1992.

This resource from the Diabetes Care and Education (DCE) dietetic practice group of the American Dietetic Association provides an excellent reference for care of persons with insulin-dependent diabetes mellitus and use of the technologies developed for "tight" blood glucose control: meters for measuring blood glucose levels, types of insulin, and insulin delivery systems.

Hollerorth HJ, Kaplan D, Bertorelli AM: *Everyone likes to eat: how children can eat most of the foods they enjoy and still take care of their diabetes,* Minneapolis, 1993, Chronimed Publishing.

Holzmeister LE: Application of the 1994 nutrition recommendations to children and adolescents, *On The Cutting Edge* 16(2):31, 1995.

These helpful guidelines for nutrition management of children and adolescents with IDDM—type I with updates from the 1994 Recommendations of the American Diabetes Association/American Dietetic Association provide much practical support for the entire family.

Gregory RP et al: Nutrition management of a collegiate football player with insulin-dependent diabetes: guidelines and a case study, *J Am Diet Assoc* 94(7):775, 1994.

This interesting account of balancing insulin, high level of physical activity, and a daily training diet of 6200 kcalories relates a sample game day schedule of meals and interval blood tests with related amounts of a sports drink before the game, at half-time, and after the game. This college athlete had no problem finishing the 11-game season (his senior year) with excellent game performances.

Case study

The patient with insulin-dependent diabetes mellitus

Angela Delano is a 45-year-old woman diagnosed 2 years ago with insulin-dependent diabetes mellitus (IDDM)—type I. She has three children whose birth weights were in the range of 4.5 to 5 kg (10 to 11 lb). The children, now teenagers, show no signs of diabetes, and their weights are reported to be within normal limits, despite their mother's fondness for cooking. Her husband, an underpaid construction worker, is slightly overweight.

Six months ago, Mrs. Delano was seen with a complaint of a series of infections that lasted longer than usual during the past 2 months. At that time she was measured as 165 cm (5 ft 5 in) and 93 kg (205 lb). Her glucose tolerance test was positive. She was seen for follow-up twice during the following month, each time showing hyperglycemia and glycosuria. At the second follow-up, an oral hypoglycemic agent was prescribed, and she was referred to the Nutrition Clinic for weight management counseling.

Mrs. Delano did not keep this appointment or her subsequent medical appointment. She was not seen again until a month ago, when she was admitted with ketoacidosis. She responded well to treatment and was placed on a 1200-kcalorie diet and a mixture of intermediate- and rapid-acting insulin given in two injections a day. On discharge, she was again referred to the Nutrition Clinic for individual counseling and diabetes education classes.

Questions for analysis

1. What factors do you think contributed to the ketoacidosis? Why? What relation do these factors have to diabetes control?

2. What additional information about Mrs. Delano is necessary to understand her major nutritional problems? Why? How could this information be obtained?

3. Based on the information provided, what nutritional problems can be identified? What is the scientific basis for each problem?

4. Determine an appropriate diet prescription for Mrs. Delano and calculate her diet using the exchange system and short method. Using this diet calculation as a guide, outline a meal plan and a schedule of self-monitoring of blood glucose for Mrs. Delano. Assume that she administers the insulin before breakfast and before the evening meal.

5. Identify any personal factors that may affect Mrs. Delano's follow-through with her treatment plan. Do you anticipate any problems? If so, how would you attempt to help her solve them? Outline a diabetes education plan for Mrs. Delano.

Issues Answers

Questions from persons on diabetic diets

Persons with diabetes have many questions about their diets, especially when they are newly diagnosed and anxieties are high. They don't want just a "Yes" or "No" answer. For any item of concern, they want to know if it can be used at all and if use is limited, why and how much. Questions about alcohol and various sweeteners are common.

Alcohol and diabetes: do they mix?

Two shots of whiskey on an empty stomach lowers blood sugar dramatically. For this reason, alcohol has been a taboo for years for persons with diabetes. It definitely has some negative effects because of the following:

- Alcohol interferes with the body's ability to regulate insulin-induced hypoglycemia (persons in poor control are most susceptible to this effect).
- It increases serum cholesterol levels, although this effect is transient.
- Alcohol consumption leads to hyperlipoproteinemia in susceptible persons, including persons with diabetes, when it is excessive.
- Alcohol consumption leads to hyperglycemia when it is excessive, although this is a transient effect usually lasting only a few hours.
- Alcohol induces a diabetic condition when used in excess by a prediabetic individual (in such persons, however, the blood sugar returns to normal following total abstinence, without the patient's having to resort to the use of insulin or an oral hypoglycemic agent.)

Alcohol may not be quite as bad as most people think for the person with diabetes because it does the following:

- Alcohol does not require insulin for its metabolism.
- It enhances the glucose-lowering effect of hypoglycemic agents, including insulin, when used in *moderate* amounts.
- It raises the high-density lipoprotein–cholesterol (HDL-C) levels when used in *moderate* amounts, thus possibly providing some protection against cardiovascular disease.

In the light of this information, it appears that diabetes and alcohol can mix—*if* shaken gently. For your clients who choose to use alcohol, you want to discuss the following items with them:

1. Carry personal diabetes identification at all times in case of a hypoglycemic attack induced by alcohol.
2. Ask the physician if there are any contraindications to using alcohol such as hypertriglycerides, gastritis, pancreatitis, some types of cardiac and renal disease, and any drug interactions (such as that occurring with the use of barbiturates or tranquilizers).
3. Always sip alcoholic drinks slowly.
4. Never drink alcohol on an empty stomach.
5. Limit alcohol use to no more than one or two alcohol equivalents per day about 2 or 3 days a week. One equivalent is found in the following:
   - 1 1/2 ounces (a shot glass) of distilled alcoholic beverage (whiskey, Scotch, rye, vodka, brandy, cognac, rum)
   - 4 ounces dry wine
   - 2 ounces dry sherry
   - 12 ounces beer (preferably "light" or reduced-kcalorie)
6. Avoid sweet drinks (for example, liqueurs; sweet wines; drinks mixed with tonic, soda, or fruit juice; and other liquids that have a high concentration of sugar.

In addition, warn any clients taking oral hypoglycemic agents about some of the problems that may occur when they drink alcohol (for example, nausea, deep flushing, tachycardia, and impaired speech). The effect is slightly delayed, beginning 3 to 10 minutes after taking a drink, and lasting up to an hour or longer.

Warn clients receiving insulin that they should *not* reduce their food intake. Persons with NIDDM—type II must consider the caloric value of the alcohol and omit 2 fat exchanges for each drink. In contrast, persons with IDDM—type I should continue to eat their full diet as prescribed because of their susceptibility to hypoglycemia induced by alcohol.

Can I use fructose in my diabetic diet?

How would you answer this question from your diabetic client? Fructose has been touted as a sweetener for persons with diabetes because it is a naturally occurring sugar that is as much as one to one-and-a-half times as sweet as sucrose. But can the person with diabetes use it safely?

Although fructose as a sweetener is not for all persons with diabetes, generally you can reply, "Yes, but with qualifications."

Fructose must be calculated in the diabetic diet. Advertising claims promoting fructose are sometimes so misleading that many consumers mistakenly believe that it can be used as a "free" food. However, fructose has the same nutritive value as other sugars—4 kcal/g. Especially those persons with IDDM—type I should be instructed to use fructose as carefully as they use any other food with a caloric and carbohydrate value.

The quantity must be limited. If used, the maximum amount is 75 g a day.

Fructose should be used under specific conditions. Its sweetness varies with temperature, acidity, and dilution. It has been used satisfactorily in some cooked desserts. However, with high temperatures, a rise in pH, and increased concentration of solution, its sweetness is reduced. This leads to overconsumption, which affects blood sugar levels.

Refined fructose should be used. Natural sources of fructose such as honey also contain considerable amounts of glucose. Thus in comparison, if it is used at all, the person with diabetes is better off using a measured amount of refined fructose.

The American Diabetes Association emphasizes that until further studies show any clinical advantages for using fructose instead of sucrose, fructose should be used only in its pure form, in small amounts, and only by those persons with well-controlled diabetes who are not overweight.

References

Chitwood M, Welch CB: Alcohol, alcohol, everywhere—but not a drop to drink? *Diabetes Forecast* 46(11):38, 1992.

Franz MJ: Diabetes mellitus: considerations in the development of guidelines for the occasional use of alcohol, *J Am Diet Assoc* 83(2):147, 1983.

Laine DC: Are sucrose and fructose compatible with a diabetic diet? *Top Clin Nutr* 3(1):46, 1988.

Powers MA, Laine DC: Sweeteners. In Powers MA, ed: *Handbook of diabetes nutritional management,* Rockville, MD, 1987, Aspen.

In this chapter we look at the problems of renal disease. First, we examine the vital structure and function of the kidney and its vast array of minute functional units, the nephrons. Then we see how serious functional problems develop when disease attacks these tissues.

Kidney diseases affect the lives of more than 8 million Americans and kill 60,000 a year. The recent advent of renal dialysis technology and kidney transplant techniques prolongs life, but this survival is not without great human and monetary cost.

Here, we consider problems of infection, tissue breakdown, renal failure, and stone formation. In each case we relate nutritional therapy to the nature of the illness and the renal functions impaired.

PHYSIOLOGY OF THE KIDNEY

RENAL FUNCTIONS

Basic functional unit—the nephron

Knowledge of the normal functions of the kidney forms the essential background for understanding therapy in renal disorders based on the organ's impaired functioning in disease. The basic anatomical and functional unit of the kidney is the **nephron**. Major advances today in treating kidney disease are based on providing maximal support for these vital functions of the nephron (Figure 21.1).

We are provided at birth with about 2 million of these filtering-reabsorbing nephron units, far more than we need. But we begin to lose them gradually after the age of 30 years. Each nephron is an exquisite example of a highly complex, minute tissue unit. It is adapted in fine detail to its vital function—maintaining an internal fluid environment compatible with life. These small vital units of the kidney are the master chemists of our bodies. We have the kind of body fluids and tissues that we have not merely because of what the mouth takes in but because of what the kidneys keep. Only because they work in the way they do has it become possible for us to have specific tissues of a specific nature to do specific tasks.

Specific integrated nephron functions

Each kidney contains some 1 million nephrons. As the body fluid flows through these finely structured units, the nephrons perform four significant functions to support life:

1. *Filters* most constituents from the entering blood except red cells and proteins.
2. *Reabsorbs* needed substances as the filtrate continues along the winding tubules.
3. *Secretes* additional ions to maintain acid-base balance.
4. *Excretes* unneeded materials in a concentrated urine.

BASIC RENAL STRUCTURES AND FUNCTIONS: THE NEPHRONS

Specific nephron structures, as shown in Figure 21.1, perform unique metabolic tasks to maintain body balances. These key structures include the **glomerulus** and the tubules.[1]

Glomerulus

At the head of each nephron, blood enters in a single capillary and then branches into a group of collateral capillaries. This tuft of collateral capillaries is held closely together in a cup-shaped membrane. This cup-shaped capsule is named **Bowman's capsule**, for the young English physician, Sir William Bowman, who in 1843 first clearly established the basis of plasma filtration and consequent urine secretion based on this intimate relationship of the blood-filled glomeruli and the enveloping membrane. The filtrate formed here is cell free and virtually protein free. Otherwise it carries the same constituents as does the entering blood.

Tubules

Continuous with the base of Bowman's capsule, the nephron tubules wind in a series of convolutions toward their terminal in the renal pelvis. Specific reabsorption functions are performed by the four sections of the tubule:

1. *Proximal tubule.* In the first section nearest the glomerulus, major nutrient reabsorption occurs. Essentially 100% of the glucose and amino acids and 80% to 85% of the water, sodium, potassium, chloride, and most other substances are reabsorbed. Only 15% to 30% of the filtrate remains to enter the next section.
2. *Loop of Henle.* This narrowed midsection of the renal tubule is named for the celebrated German anatomist, Friedrich Henle, who in 1845 first demonstrated its unique structure and function in creating the necessary fluid pressures for ultimately forming a concentrated urine. At this narrowed midsection, the thin loop of the tubule dips into the central renal **medulla**. Here, through a balanced system of water and sodium exchange through sodium pumps in the limbs of the loop (the countercurrent system), important fluid density is created surrounding the loop. This area of increased density in the central part of the kidney is important to concentrate the urine by osmotic pressure as the lower collecting tubule later passes through this same area of the kidney.
3. *Distal tubule.* This latter portion of the tubule functions primarily in providing acid-base balance through secretion of ionized hydrogen. It

---

medulla   Inner-tissue substance of the kidney (see Figure 21-1).

nephron   Microscopic anatomic and functional unit of the kidney that selectively filters and resorbs essential blood factors, secretes hydrogen ions as needed for maintaining acid-base balance, then resorbs water to protect body fluids, and forms and excretes a concentrated urine for elimination of wastes. The nephron includes the renal corpuscle (glomerulus), the proximal convoluted tubule, the loop of Henle, the distal convoluted tubule, and the collecting tubule, which empties the urine into the renal medulla. The urine passes into the papilla and then to the pelvis of the kidney. Urine is formed by filtration of blood in the glomerulus and by the selective reabsorption and secretion of solutes by cells that comprise the walls of the renal tubes. There are approximately 1 million nephrons in each kidney.

A

B

Figure 21.1   **A,** Longitudinal section of the kidney. **B,** Nephron of the kidney. (From Lewis SM, Collier IC, Heitkemper MM: *Medical-surgical nursing: assessment and management of clinical problems,* ed 4, St. Louis, 1996, Mosby.)

also conserves sodium by reabsorbing it under the influence of the hormones aldosterone and vasopressin (also called antidiuretic hormone, or ADH).

4. *Collecting tubule.* In this final widened section of the tubule the filtrate is concentrated to save water and form urine for excretion. Water is absorbed under the influence of the pituitary hormone vasopressin (also called antidiuretic hormone [ADH]) and the osmotic pressure of the more dense surrounding fluid in this central part of the kidney. The resulting volume of urine, now concentrated and excreted, is only 0.5% to 1% of the original water and solutes filtered at the beginning in Bowman's capsule.

RENAL FUNCTION IN DISEASE

A number of agents or conditions may interfere with the normal functioning of the nephrons and cause renal disease.

Inflammatory and degenerative disease

Inflammation of the small blood vessels and membranes in the nephrons may be short term, as in acute forms of glomerulonephritis. In other cases it may diffusely involve entire nephrons or nephron segments, disrupting normal function. Nephrotic lesions develop, leading to progressive chronic renal failure. Nutritional disturbances in the metabolism of protein, electrolytes, and water follow.

Infection and obstruction

Bacterial infection of the urinary tract may range from occasional mild, uncomfortable bladder infection to more involved chronic recurrent disease and obstruction from kidney stones. This obstruction anywhere in the urinary tract blocks drainage, causing further infection and tissue damage.

Damage from other diseases

Circulatory disorders such as prolonged hypertension, often associated with the vasopressor effect of the renin-angiotensin-aldosterone mechanism, can cause degeneration of the small renal arteries and curtail efficient function.[1,2] A vicious cycle ensues as the demand on the kidney in turn causes more hypertension and still more damage. Other diseases, such as diabetes mellitus and gout, may also damage kidney function.[3,4] Abnormalities present from birth may lead to poor function, infection, or obstruction.

Damage from other agents

Environmental agents such as insecticides, solvents, and similar materials are poisons that can damage the kidneys.[5] Some toxic drugs may also harm renal tissue.[6]

In the treatment of renal disease, nutritional therapy is based on impaired renal function and resulting clinical symptoms. In this chapter we focus primarily on the more serious degenerative processes of glomerulonephritis, nephrotic syndrome, and renal failure. Then we briefly review the more common problems that occur in the urinary tract—obstructive kidney stones and urinary tract infection.

GLOMERULONEPHRITIS

DISEASE PROCESS

Glomerulonephritis is an inflammatory process affecting the glomeruli, the small blood vessels in the cup-shaped head of the nephron. It is most common in acute form in children 3 to 10 years of age, although 5% or more of the initial attacks occur in adults past the age of 50 years. The most common cause is a previous streptococcal infection. It has a more or less sudden onset, a brief course in its acute form, and is usually completely cleared in a year or two. In some cases it progresses to a chronic form, involving an increased amount of renal tissue and eventually requiring dialysis and other support treatments.

Immune complex disease

Immunologic studies and electron microscopy have demonstrated the underlying process as an immune complex disease. An *antigen* or "foreign invader" in the body excites responses from the defense system to combat potentially harmful effects. In glomerular disease the antigens are usually substances attacking the body from the outside: bacteria, viruses, and chemicals, including antibiotics and other drugs. In response, *antibodies* are produced by the body to ward off or neutralize the effect of the antigen. An excess of antigen and antibodies produced leads to the formation of *antigen-antibody complexes* in the circulation, which become trapped in the glomeruli. These complexes bind components of **complement**, a complex series of enzymatic proteins in the blood that serve as part of the body's immune system. The activated complement in turn provides active chemical factors that attract white blood cells, whose lysosomal enzymes incite the resulting injury to the glomerulus.

---

glomerulonephritis   A form of nephritis affecting the capillary loops in an acute short-term infection. It may progress to a more serious chronic condition leading to irreversible renal failure.

complement   A complex series of enzymatic proteins occuring in normal serum that interact to combine with and augment (fill out, complete) the antigen-antibody complex of the body's immune system, producing lysis when the antigen is an intact cell; composed of 11 discrete proteins or functioning components, activated by the immunoglobulin factors IgG and IgM.

These antigen-antibody complexes appear as lumpy deposits between the epithelial cells of the cupped nephron capsule and the basement membrane of the glomeruli. Lesions develop, leaving scar tissue that obstructs the circulation through the glomerulus. Fatty degeneration and necrosis of the conjoined tubules follow, and ultimate destruction of the nephron results. In time, if the disease becomes progressive, the net result is a reduction in the number of functioning nephrons available in the kidneys.[1,7-9]

CLINICAL SYMPTOMS

Classic symptoms include gross **hematuria** and **proteinuria**. Varying degrees of edema may occur with shortness of breath resulting from sodium and water retention and circulatory congestion. Also, moderate **tachycardia** and mild or marked elevation of blood pressure may occur. The patient is generally anorexic, which contributes to feeding problems. If the disease progresses to renal insufficiency, **oliguria** or **anuria** occurs, which signals development of acute renal failure.[7]

 ## MEDICAL NUTRITION THERAPY

General care in uncomplicated disease

The general treatment is symptomatic and designed to provide optimal nutritional support. In short-term acute cases in children, pediatricians and clinical nutritionists generally favor overall optimal nutrition with adequate protein, unless symptoms of oliguria or anuria develop. These complications usually last no more than 2 to 3 days and are managed by conservative treatment. Salt is usually not restricted unless complications of edema, hypertension, or oliguria become dangerous. Thus in most patients with acute uncomplicated disease, especially in children with poststreptococcal glomerulonephritis, diet modifications are not crucial. The main treatment focuses on bed rest and antibiotic drug therapy. The fluid intake will be adjusted to output as a rule, including losses in vomiting and diarrhea.

Specific therapy in progressive disease

If the disease process advances, however, more specific nutritional therapy measures are indicated. The nutrient factors most involved are protein, carbohydrate, sodium, potassium, and water:

1. *Protein.* If the **blood urea nitrogen (BUN)** is elevated and oliguria is present, dietary protein must be restricted. Usually the diet contains 0.5 g of protein/kg of ideal body weight. Some patients may use 1 g/kg as long as renal function is adequate to maintain a normal BUN level.
2. *Carbohydrate.* To provide sufficient kcalories to meet energy needs, carbohydrate should be given liberally. This will also reduce the catabolism of tissue protein and prevent starvation ketosis.
3. *Sodium.* The restriction of sodium varies with the degree of oliguria. If renal function is impaired, the sodium is restricted to 500 to 1000 mg/day. As recovery occurs, sodium intake can be increased.
4. *Potassium.* With severe oliguria, renal clearance of potassium is impaired. Potassium intoxication may occur, requiring dialysis. Thus potassium intake is monitored carefully according to disease progression.
5. *Water.* Fluids are restricted according to the kidney's ability to excrete urine. If restriction is not indicated, fluids can be consumed as desired.

NEPHROTIC SYNDROME

DISEASE PROCESS

Nephrotic syndrome, or **nephrosis**, is characterized by a group of symptoms resulting from kidney tissue damage and impaired nephron function. The most evident symptoms are massive *edema* and *proteinuria*. This condition may be caused by progressive glomerulonephritis or by *glomerulosclerosis* in which fibrosis and scarring result in degeneration of the renal glomeruli.[9] It may also be associated with other diseases, such as diabetes or connective tissue disorders **(collagen disease)**. In some cases, it may result from drug reactions, especially exposure to heavy metals, or even from reaction to toxic venom following a bee sting.

The primary degenerative lesion is in the capillary basement membrane of the glomerulus, permitting escape of large amounts of protein into the filtrate. The tubular changes that occur are a result of the high protein concentration in the filtrate, with some protein uptake from the tubular lumen. Both filtration and reabsorption functions are disrupted.

CLINICAL SYMPTOMS

The cardinal symptom of massive edema is evident. *Ascites* is common. The abdomen becomes increasingly distended as fluid collects in the serous cavities. Often *striae* (stretch marks) appear on the stretched skin of the abdomen and extremities.

The massive edema is largely caused by the gross loss of protein, principally albumin, in the urine, some 4 to 10 g/day or more. This means that the plasma protein is greatly reduced. The albumin fraction is largely responsible for maintaining the capillary fluid shift mechanism (see Chapter 8). Thus fluid balance between tissue fluid and circulating fluid is decreased to less than 3 to 4 g/dl. Serum lipid levels are elevated, with cholesterol being over 300 mg/dl. Free fat, oval fat bodies, or fatty droplets are found in the urine. Protein losses are also indicated by the presence of urinary globulins and specialized binding proteins for thyroxine and iron, producing signs of hypothyroidism and anemia. As serum protein loss continues, tissue proteins are broken down and general malnutrition ensues. Fatty tissue changes in the liver and general sodium retention further contribute to the edema. Severe ascites and pedal edema mask the gross tissue-wasting.

 ## MEDICAL NUTRITION THERAPY

Nutrition therapy is directed toward control of the major symptoms, edema and malnutrition, resulting from the massive protein losses.[8-12]

Protein

In the past the standard recommendation for patients with nephrotic syndrome was a high-protein diet, sometimes as high as 3 to 4 g/kg of body weight/day to restore the serum protein pool and prevent malnutrition. However, evidence has grown that high-protein diets may actually accelerate loss of renal function. Because of the increasing concern of investigators and clinicians that high-protein diets may accelerate progression of renal disease, patients with nephrotic syndrome are now being individually treated with a moderately restricted protein diet. Commonly used protein intakes are 0.6 to 0.8 g/kg of body weight/day (the adult RDA is 0.8 g/kg/day), plus 1 g/day of high biologic protein for each gram of urinary protein lost daily.[8,10]

Kilocalories

Sufficient kcalories must always be provided to ensure protein use for tissue synthesis. High daily intakes of 35 to 60 kcal/kg of ideal weight, depending on the patient's weight, are essential. Appetite is usually poor, so much encouragement and support are needed. The food must be as appetizing as possible and in a form most easily tolerated.

Sodium

With diuretic drugs to help reduce the edema, moderate sodium restriction in the diet supports this tissue fluid management. Usually a 500- to 1000-mg sodium diet (see Chapter 19) is sufficient to help initiate **diuresis**.

The general dietary management is similar to that given for hepatitis (see Chapter 18), with the additional need for sodium restriction. There is no need to restrict potassium. Iron and vitamin supplements may be indicated.

ACUTE RENAL FAILURE

DISEASE PROCESS

Renal failure may occur as an acute phase with sudden shutdown of renal function following some metabolic insult or traumatic injury to normal kidneys.[6] The situation is often life-threatening, and the mortality rate associated with renal failure is high. Survival is less than 50%, especially following surgery. In this medical emergency, the nutritionist and nurse play important supportive roles. Immediate and continuing nutritional support is essential.

Acute renal failure may have various causes: (1) severe injury such as extensive burns or crushing injuries that cause widespread tissue destruction; (2) infectious diseases such as peritonitis; (3) traumatic shock following surgery on the abdominal aorta; (4) toxic agents in the environment such as carbon tetrachloride or poisonous mushrooms; or (5) immunologic drug reactions in allergic or sensitive persons, such as penicillin reaction.

CLINICAL SYMPTOMS

The major sign of such an acute renal failure is oliguria, diminished urine output, often accompanied by proteinuria or hematuria. This diminished urine output is

---

blood urea nitrogen (BUN)   The nitrogen component of urea in the blood; a measure of kidney function; elevated levels of BUN indicate a disorder of kidney function.

collagen disease   Diseases attacking collagen tissues, the protein substance of the white fibers (collagenous fibers) of skin, tendon, bone, cartilage, and other connective tissue; any of a group of diseases that are clinically distinct but have in common widespread pathologic changes in the connective tissue, such as rheumatoid arthritis, lupus erythematosis, scleroderma, and rheumatic fever.

diuresis   Increased urine excretion.

hematuria   The abnormal presence of blood in the urine.

nephrosis   Nephrotic syndrome caused by degenerative epithelial lesions of the renal tubules of the nephrons, especially in the *mesangium,* the thin basement membrane that helps support the capillary loops in a renal glomerulus; marked by edema, albuminuria, and a decreased serum albumin level.

oliguria   Secretion of a very small amount of urine in relation to fluid intake.

proteinuria   The presence of an excess of serum proteins, such as albumin, in the urine.

tachycardia   Excessively rapid action of the heart; usually applied to a heart rate above 100 beats per minute.

brought on by the underlying tissue problems that characterize acute renal failure. Usually there is blockage of the tubules caused by cellular debris from tissue trauma or urinary failure with backup retention of filtrate materials.

Oliguria

Diminished urinary output is a cardinal symptom, often with proteinuria or hematuria accompanying the small output. Water balance becomes a crucial factor. The course of the disease is usually divided into an oliguric phase followed by a diuretic phase. The urinary output during the oliguric phase varies from as little as 20 to 200 ml/day.

Anorexia, nausea, and lethargy

During this initial phase of acute renal failure the patient may be lethargic and anorectic and may suffer nausea and vomiting. Blood pressure elevation and signs of uremia may be present. Oral intake is usually difficult in this catabolic period.

Increasing serum urea nitrogen and creatinine levels

During the initial catabolic period following injury, surgery, or some other metabolic dysfunction, the serum urea nitrogen level increases along with the creatinine level. These increases result from the tissue breakdown of muscle mass. Blood potassium, phosphate, and sulfate levels also increase, and sodium, calcium, and bicarbonate levels decrease.

General medical management

Usually after an initial conservative medical therapy, recovery occurs in a few days to 6 weeks. However, in more complicated cases in which the oliguria continues 4 to 5 days, more aggressive therapy, including **hemodialysis** and total parenteral nutrition (TPN), is used.

 MEDICAL NUTRITION THERAPY

Oliguric phase

The major goals of initial nutrition therapy are to support overall medical management. These include reestablishing fluid and electrolyte balance, stopping the catabolic response, supporting tissue healing, and preventing infection. Thus in nutrition therapy the clinical nutritionist and the nurse pay close attention to fluid, electrolyte, and nutrient balances. The major challenge for nutrition therapy is to improve the nutritional status, especially in patients with marked catabolism.

Fluids

Fluid intake is usually restricted to a basic allowance of 400 ml/day for the average adult. Any losses of fluids caused by vomiting, sweating, diarrhea, and other routes

may be replaced with additional fluid. Allowance must also be made for the "water of combustion" resulting from the metabolism of fat, carbohydrates, and protein and from the catabolism of tissues that provide intracellular water. Children with acute renal failure especially require prompt, carefully monitored fluid resuscitation.[7,11]

Electrolytes

Electrolyte replacement is provided only for observed deficits. Special caution should be taken to avoid potassium administration because serum potassium levels are usually elevated after massive tissue destruction.

Nutrition therapy

Depending on the patient's condition, nutrient intake may be oral or intravenous. In either case, *no protein should be given* in this acute phase to limit nitrogen sources and potassium, phosphate, and sulfate levels. Carbohydrate intake should be increased to supply kcalories to meet energy demands of the illness and to prevent ketoacidosis and further protein catabolism. A daily intake of 100 to 200 g or more is indicated. Additional kcalories may be obtained from fat, either through oral feedings or through lipid emulsions in intravenous feedings. Peripheral vein feeding of a 20% to 50% glucose solution may be administered continuously over 24 hours. B-complex vitamins and vitamin C should be provided to support the needed energy metabolism and tissue healing. If the patient is undergoing dialysis, TPN may be used as a feeding method (see Chapter 17).[6] In these cases, a mixture of essential and nonessential amino acids as tolerated, especially those that are partially synthesized in the kidney, supplemented by glucose and lipid emulsions, is used to prevent excessive catabolism of tissue and to support healing and recovery of renal function.

Monitoring

Daily records of fluid intake and output, as well as of weight, are essential to monitor fluid balance and tissue catabolism. Daily monitoring of serum electrolyte levels, particularly potassium, and creatinine is necessary.

Diuretic phase

After successful initial therapy a diuretic phase follows. This reflects the improved renal function and ability to excrete collections of the excess water and electrolytes that have gathered during the oliguric phase. At this time the fluid and dietary intake may be increased as the diuresis progresses until a normal intake is reached. However, protein should continue to be restricted until the BUN and the creatinine levels decline toward normal. If the diuresis is accompanied by retention of sodium, dietary sodium must be restricted accordingly. Sufficient amounts of water and glucose are also needed to correct **hypernatremia**.

With the skilled care of a trained team consisting of a physician, clinical dietitian, and nurse, the patient is supported until spontaneous healing occurs. After recovery there is usually little residual impairment of renal function.

CHRONIC RENAL FAILURE

Disease process

The course of renal failure may become chronic with progressive degenerative changes in renal tissues and marked depression of all renal functions.[1,8] At this stage, few functioning nephrons remain and these gradually deteriorate (see *To Probe Further* box, p. 456). The symptom complex of advanced renal insufficiency is commonly although imprecisely called by its old term *uremia*.

Chronic renal insufficiency may result from a variety of diseases that involve the nephrons: (1) primary glomerular disease; (2) metabolic disease with renal involvement, such as insulin-dependent diabetes mellitus (IDDM); (3) exposure to toxic substances; (4) infections; (5) renal vascular disease; (6) renal tubular disease; (7) chronic pyelonephritis; or (8) congenital abnormality of both kidneys. Depending on the nature of the predisposing renal disease, there is extensive scarring of renal tissue. This distorts the kidney structure and brings vascular changes from the prolonged hypertension involved.

Clinical symptoms

Symptoms result from the progressive loss of nephrons and the consequent decreased renal blood flow and glomerular filtration. As the nephrons are lost one by one, the remaining nephrons gradually lose their ability to maintain body water balance, concentration of solutes in body fluids (osmolality), and electrolyte and acid-base balance.[11-13] This continuing loss of nephrons brings many metabolic insults.

1. *Water balance.* The increased load of solutes causes an osmotic diuresis. Increasingly the kidney cannot excrete a normal concentrated urine. Dehydration follows and may become critical. On the other hand, water intoxication may occur if there is excess fluid intake.

2. *Electrolyte balance.* A number of imbalances among electrolytes result from the decreasing nephron function:
   - *Sodium.* With the osmotic diuresis, sodium loss contributes to a decreasing extracellular fluid volume. As the plasma volume decreases, renal filtration declines further, worsening the renal failure. In this state the kidney cannot respond appropriately to maintain sodium balance. Any sudden increase in sodium intake cannot be excreted readily and causes edema.
   - *Potassium.* The balance of potassium is usually not impaired as readily until the oliguria becomes severe or acidosis increases.
   - *Phosphate, sulfate, and organic acids.* With reduced nephron function there is reduced filtration and excretion of these materials produced by the metabolism of food nutrients. Thus these anions become concentrated in body fluids, with subsequent displacement of bicarbonate, causing metabolic acidosis.
   - *Calcium and phosphate.* Metabolism of these electrolytes is greatly disturbed as a consequence of renal tissue loss. Two metabolic functions of the kidney—(1) activation of vitamin D hormone, and (2) parathyroid hormone control of serum calcium-phosphorus levels—cannot proceed at normal levels. The impaired vitamin D hormone activation results in a bone disease called **osteodystrophy**. This disturbance causes bone pain, various bone deformities, awkward gait, and in children impaired growth. Also, there may be calcification of soft tissues, which further hinders renal function.

3. *Nitrogen retention.* Increasing loss of nephron function brings elevated amounts of nitrogenous metabolites such as urea and creatinine. The urea load results from dietary protein metabolism; the creatinine load results from increasing catabolism of muscle mass.

4. *Anemia.* The normal kidney participates in the production of red blood cells, through synthesis of erythrocytes. The damaged kidney cannot accomplish this task, and there is depressed red blood cell production. The red cells that are produced survive a shorter time but have a usual size and hemoglobin content.

5. *Hypertension.* When blood flow to renal tissue is increasingly impaired, the resulting ischemia brings increasing hypertension through the nephrons' close relationship to the renin-angiotensin-aldosterone mechanism. In turn hypertension causes cardiovascular damage and further deterioration of the kidney.

---

hemodialysis Removal of certain elements from the blood according to their rates of diffusion through a semipermeable membrane—e.g., by a hemodialysis machine.

hypernatremia Excessive levels of sodium in the blood.

osteodystrophy Defective bone formation.

To Probe Further

The aging Western kidney

Renal disease typically follows a progressively downhill course. Why should this be? The pivotal early work of Brenner's group at Harvard indicates that the stage may well have been set in our distant evolutionary past as an adaptation of the kidney to meet the nitrogenous excretion needs of our hunter/scavenger, meat-eating ancestors.

Because our ancestors were carnivores, their protein intake was transient and intermittent; they could only eat after a successful hunting expedition. Thus at these times of surfeit a large number of extra nephrons had to be available to meet their needs for the prompt excretion of waste products, largely urea, and the conservation of fluid and electrolytes until the next meal became available. They achieved this metabolic task mainly by *hyperfiltration* through increased use of their many extra superficial glomeruli, largely in the outer part (cortex) of the kidney, which normally maintains a resting state. It was only in the past 500 to 10,000 years, when population groups developed agriculture and herding, that a more continuous food intake pattern became possible. Now in many Western countries our adult diet averages approximately 3000 kcalories and more than 100 g of protein, largely meat, *daily*.

Thus the answers to our initial questions—Why do we have far more nephrons than we seem to need? Why do we begin losing some of these nephrons through a "normal aging process" of glomerular sclerosis after the age of 30 years? Why is renal disease so inexorably progressive?—lie in a fundamental mismatch between the evolutionary design of our kidneys and the functional burden we place on them by our modern eating habits. Our sustained excessive protein levels in the blood, along with other solutes, impose demands for sustained increases in renal blood flow and glomerular filtration rates. This requires that our reserve glomeruli of the outer renal cortex be in more or less continuous use and predisposes even healthy persons to the observed progressive glomerular sclerosis over time, with deterioration of normal kidney function. In health this deterioration poses no problem because we have so many extra nephrons. But when renal disease occurs, the burden is compounded. The disease accelerates the deterioration process and makes coping impossible. The downhill course inevitably ensues. The aging and vulnerable kidney of people living in the Western countries thus seems to be related inevitably to our lifetime of large protein meals.

References

Brenner BM et al: Dietary protein intake and the progressive nature of kidney disease, *N Engl J Med* 307(11):652, 1982.

Foreman JW et al: Nutritional intake in children with renal insufficiency: a report of growth failure in children with renal insufficiency: a report of Growth Failure in Children with Renal Diseases study, *J Am Coll Nutr* 15(6):579, 1996.

Kopple JD: Nutrition, diet, and the kidney. In Shiles ME, Olson JA, Shike M, eds: *Modern nutrition in health and disease*, ed 8, vol 2, Philadelphia, 1994, Lea & Febiger.

6. *Azotemia*. The elevated blood urea nitrogen (BUN), serum creatinine, and serum uric acid levels are reflected in the characteristic laboratory finding of **azotemia**.

General signs and symptoms

The increasing loss of renal function brings progressive weakness, shortness of breath, general lethargy, and fatigue. Thirst, anorexia, weight loss, and gastrointestinal irritability with diarrhea or vomiting result. Increased capillary fragility brings skin, nose, oral, and gastrointestinal bleeding. Nervous system involvement brings muscular twitching, burning sensations in the extremities, or uremic convulsions. Cheyne-Stokes respiration (irregular, cyclic type of breathing) indicates acidosis. There is ulceration of the mouth, a persistent bad or metallic taste, and fetid breath. Malnutrition lowers resistance to infection. Osteodystrophy continues with aching and pain in bone and joints.

THE MODIFICATION OF DIET IN RENAL DISEASE STUDY

In a similar approach to that used in the large Diabetes Control and Complications Study (DCCT), described in Chapter 20, the National Institutes of Health (NIH) recently conducted the full national United States clinical research study concerning a more comprehensive program of nutrition therapy in renal disease, the Modification of Diet in Renal Disease (MDRD), with a primary focus on protein management, to help delay or avoid the life-threatening complications of chronic renal disease.[11]

This large MDRD study involved 840 adult subjects aged 18 to 70 years with renal insufficiency at representative clinical centers across the country for approximately 10 years. The study was conducted in four phases: (1) planning and development, beginning with the administrative decision of the United States Department of Health and Human Services in 1985; (2) a 2-year feasibility study; (3) the full-scale trial covering 6 years; and (4) data analysis. The study was designed to test the effect of three levels of protein and phosphorous intake and two levels of blood pressure control on the progression of chronic renal disease, using participant self-management and dietitian support to promote long-term adherence. Primary reports cover the feasibility study and four main study areas: (1) a self-management approach to nutrition intervention strategies[12]; (2) adherence to the dietary protein intervention[13]; (3) dietary satisfaction and relation to psychosocial factors[14]; and (4) clinical and research activities of the highly trained dietitians involved.[15]

In a follow-up Dietary Satisfaction Questionnaire, study participants indicated that dietary satisfaction with their modified diets correlated with their adherence to their assigned study diet plan.[16]

ꙥ MEDICAL NUTRITION THERAPY

BASIC TREATMENT GOALS

Treatment must be individual, adjusted according to progression of the illness, the type of treatment being used, and the patient's response. In general, however, basic therapy objectives are as follows:

Reduce and minimize protein breakdown

- Prevent protein catabolism and minimize uremic toxicity
- Avoid dehydration or overhydration
- Correct acidosis carefully
- Correct electrolyte depletions and avoid excesses
- Control fluid and electrolyte losses from vomiting and diarrhea
- Maintain optimal nutritional status
- Maintain appetite, general morale, and sense of well-being
- Control complications—hypertension, bone pain, nervous system problems
- Retard progression of renal failure, postponing ultimate dialysis

Table 21.1	Protein and nitrogen needs for those in chronic renal failure		
Creatine clearance (ml/min)	**Nitrogen* (g/day)**	**Protein (g/day)**
40 and above	Unrestricted	Unrestricted
10-40	9.6	60
5-20	6.4	40†
2-10	2.5-3.0 (+1.3-2.6)	20 (+EAA/analogs)†
8 and below	Tranplantation Dialysis	
5 and below	Dialysis	

From Bergstrom J: *Proceedings of the Twelfth Annual Contractors Conference, Artificial Kidney—Chronic Uremic Program,* NIAMDD, National Institutes of Health, Bethesda, Md, NIH Pub No 81-1979, 1981.
*Total protein: 6.25.
†*EAA,* Essential amino acids; alpha-keto-acid and alpha-hydroxy-acid analogs of EAAs.

GENERAL MEASURES

Nutritional care plays a major role in many of these treatment objectives. The clinical nutritionist and the nurse are indispensable members of the renal care team. Principles of therapeutic nutrition for chronic renal failure include nutrient adjustments according to individual need.

1. *Protein.* The crucial problem is to provide sufficient protein to prevent protein breakdown, yet avoid an excess that would elevate urea levels. In general, limitation of protein to 0.5 g/kg of body weight/day helps reduce azotemia and hyperkalemia and control acidosis. Protein is usually adjusted according to creatinine clearance. Restriction of protein intake is not needed until the creatinine clearance falls below 40 ml/minute.[17] Thereafter the dietary protein must be regulated according to declining renal function (Table 21.1).

   If caloric requirements are liberally met, patients may be maintained in nitrogen balance for prolonged periods on as little as 35 to 40 g/day of protein. However, when blood urea levels rise, protein intake must be reduced to 20 g/day. Only essential amino acids are supplied by small amounts of milk and egg protein. Thus the patient is not burdened with nonessential amino acids that make demands on the body for

---

azotemia An excess of urea or other nitrogenous substances in the blood.

the disposal of their nitrogenous waste products and do little to counteract the tissue protein catabolism. In any event, protein must be closely controlled according to individual need, ranging in quantity from 20 to 60 g/day and having a high biologic value to supply essential amino acids.

2. *Amino acid supplements*. Promising approaches to protein replacement have been developed using mixtures of essential amino acids or of amino acid precursors such as alpha-keto-acid and alpha-hydroxy-acid analogs. Supplements have been developed containing nitrogen-free analogs of the branched-chain amino acids phenylalanine and methionine, which are metabolized in the liver, plus the remaining essential amino acids. Also, general nutrition supplements tailored for dialysis patients are available in products such as Nepro (Ross Laboratories).

3. *Kilocalories*. Adequate kcalories are mandatory. Carbohydrate and fat must supply sufficient nonprotein kcalories to spare dietary protein for tissue protein synthesis and energy supply. About 300 to 400 g carbohydrate is the average daily need. Sufficient fat, 75 to 90 g, is added to give the patient 2000 to 2500 total kcalories daily. Patients are encouraged to consume all the carbohydrates and fats they can because the end products of their metabolism, carbon dioxide and water, do not impose a burden on the progressive renal failure.[18] If the kcalorie intake is inadequate, body protein tissue catabolism to supply energy further aggravates the renal failure.

4. *Water*. Total fluid intake must be guarded to avoid water intoxication from overloading or dehydration from too little water. The capacity of the damaged kidney to handle water is limited, and in many cases solids are excreted better with a controlled amount of water. With predialysis patients, the fluid intake should be sufficient to maintain adequate urine volume. Sometimes the obligatory water loss may be high because of the large solute load in sodium and urea that must be excreted by an increasingly smaller number of nephrons.

5. *Sodium*. The need for sodium intake varies. Both severe restriction and excess are to be avoided. The dietary need is closely related to the patient's handling of water. If hypertension and edema are present, the sodium intake needs to be restricted. Usually, the sodium intake will vary between 500 to 2000 mg/day.

6. *Potassium*. Serum potassium levels may be depressed or elevated. Adjustment of intake is made accordingly to maintain normal levels. If significant losses occur with severe vomiting or diarrhea, *careful* supplementation may be needed. In general the damaged kidney cannot clear potassium adequately. Thus the dietary intake is kept at about 1500 mg/day.

7. *Phosphate and calcium*. Abnormal serum electrolyte levels of phosphate and calcium result from the secondary **hyperparathyroidism** caused by the damaged kidney function. Phosphate intake should be restricted early to retard or prevent this developing imbalance, which leads to the complicating bone disease osteodystrophy, before symptoms of bone pain or deformity occur.[19] Further control of phosphate levels is ensured by use of aluminum hydroxide gel to bind phosphate and prevent its intestinal absorption. A calcium supplement such as calcium lactate tablets relieves the hypocalcemia and its resulting tetany. In some cases, calcium carbonate is used because it also buffers the accompanying metabolic acidosis.

8. *Vitamins*. In more restricted protein diets, supplementary vitamins are usually advisable, since a diet supplying 40 g protein or less does not contribute the full daily spectrum of all vitamins. A multivitamin tablet or capsule is usually added to the diet of renal patients on protein restriction. To help correct the bone disease present, an activated form of vitamin D hormone may be used with caution.

MAINTENANCE KIDNEY DIALYSIS

Since the advent of the artificial kidney machine, a number of kidney **dialysis** centers have been established for the treatment of progressive chronic renal insufficiency (Figure 21.2). Home units are also available, although considerable skill is required to operate them. These treatments, however, are expensive. The combined costs of the dialysis machine, replacement materials, various drugs, and trained personnel in dialysis centers is from $20,000 to $35,000 per year or more. The home treatment runs between $5,000 to $15,000 per year. Much of the cost is now paid under a provision of Medicare. Some 18,000 to 20,000 patients receive this needed artificial kidney care, usually at dialysis centers. A patient with chronic renal failure usually requires 2 to 3 treatments per week, each treatment lasting 4 to 8 hours.

During each treatment the patient's blood circulates through the dialysis solution in the artificial kidney, maintaining normal blood levels of life-sustaining substances that the patient's own kidneys can no longer accomplish. In some selected cases, an alternative form of **peritoneal dialysis** is practical for long-term ambulatory therapy at home (see *Practical Application* box, p. 460).

The diet of a patient on kidney dialysis is a vital aspect of maintaining biochemical control. Several basic

Figure 21.2 The patient undergoing maintenance kidney dialysis must carefully follow an individualized diet plan.

objectives govern each individually tailored diet, designed to (1) maintain protein and kcalorie balance, (2) prevent dehydration or fluid overload, (3) maintain normal serum potassium and sodium blood levels, and (4) maintain acceptable phosphate and calcium levels. Control of infection is always an underlying goal. Nutritional therapy in most cases can be planned with more liberal nutrient allowances than indicated in the usual RDAs. An underlying zinc deficiency, shown in impaired taste acuity, is often reported in chronic dialysis patients and improved with a supplement of 25 mg/day of zinc, thus enabling them to eat a better diet.[20]

Protein

For most adult dialysis patients, a standard protein allowance of 1 g/kg lean body weight provides for nutritional needs, maintains positive nitrogen balance, does not produce excessive nitrogenous waste, and replaces the amino acids lost during each dialysis treatment. At least 75% of this daily protein allowance should consist of protein of high biologic value, such as eggs, meat, fish, and poultry, but little if any milk. Milk is restricted because it adds more fluid and has a high content of sodium, phosphate, and potassium.

Kilocalories

Carbohydrates and fats, depending on blood lipid levels, are supplied in generous amounts to provide the needed energy for daily activities and to prevent tissue protein breakdown. The usual need is 40 kcal/kg lean body weight. Most of the carbohydrate should be supplied by simple carbohydrate foods, with control of complex car-

dialysis Process of separating crystalloids and colloids in solution by the difference in their rates of diffusion through a semipermeable membrane; crystalloids pass through readily and colloids pass through only very slowly or not all.

hyperthyroidism Abnormally increased activity of the parathyroid gland, resulting in excessive secretion of parathyroid hormone, which usually helps regulate serum calcium levels in balance with vitamin D hormone; excess secretion occurs when the serum calcium level falls below normal, as in chronic renal disease or in vitamin D deficiency.

peritoneal dialysis Dialysis through the peritoneum into and out of the peritoneal cavity.

Continuous ambulatory peritoneal dialysis: nutritional needs of clients on portable dialysis machines

Persons with end-stage renal disease (ESRD) used to spend up to 18 hours a week on hemodialysis machines in a hospital or dialysis center. Now approximately 2800 Americans undergo dialysis 24 hours a day, 7 days a week, without spending 1 minute in a hospital room.

These individuals use Continuous Ambulatory Peritoneal Dialysis (CAPD), a home dialysis process that introduces dialysate directly into the peritoneal cavity, where it is exchanged for fluids that contain the metabolic waste products. This is done by attaching a disposable bag containing the dialysate to a catheter permanently inserted into the peritoneal cavity, waiting 20 to 30 minutes for the solution exchange, then lowering the bag to allow the force of gravity to cause the waste-containing fluid to drain into it. When the bag is empty, it can be folded around the waist or tucked into a pocket, allowing the user mobility.

The exchange takes place by osmosis and diffusion, the rate being determined by the amount of dextrose in the solution. The most common dialysates are 1.5%, 2.5%, or 4.25% dextrose in 1.5 to 2 L of solution. Most CAPD users require three to five exchanges each day. They are not only free to move, but with good self-care they are also free from some of the following extensive dietary restrictions placed on hemodialysis patients:

- Protein and amino acid losses are usually minimal and easily replaced by diet. High losses were more common in early CAPD systems because of peritonitis, a common problem associated with the need to replace bags frequently.
- Potassium requirements depend on the number of solution exchanges that take place each day. The fewer the number of exchanges, the greater the chance of developing high serum potassium levels. Also, patients who stop using CAPD must immediately reduce their potassium intake, since serum levels rise rapidly.
- Phosphorus-binding antacids are not needed as much because of improved control of phosphorus blood levels with CAPD use.
- Sodium restriction is not necessary. In patients susceptible to hypotension, high-sodium diets have even been recommended.
- Fluid restriction is unnecessary, since 2000 to 2200 ml fluid may be removed with two 1.5% plus two 4.25% dextrose solutions used in 1 day. Some CAPD users even become dehydrated easily.

CAPD does pose a few nutrition-related problems, mainly because of the amount of dextrose in the dialysate. A study of patients given three 1.5% and two 4.25% dextrose solutions in 1 day revealed an intake of more than 800 kcalories above the energy value of their regular diets. In addition to posing possible weight-management problems, the extra dextrose can lead to elevated triglycerides and low-density lipoprotein (LDL) levels, and depressed levels of protective high-density lipoproteins (HDL), thus increasing the risk of coronary heart disease in long-term users.

Nutritionists and nurses who counsel patients being transferred from hemodialysis to the CAPD regimen are faced with a special problem: patients are often reluctant to give up their special diets. To help the individual with ESRD make the transition to CAPD as trouble free as possible, you may find it useful to explain as clearly as possible some of the possible effects of a restricted diet while on CAPD: (1) **hypotension** and dizziness from sodium depletion; (2) **potassium depletion,** resulting in nausea, vomiting, muscle weakness, irregular heartbeat, or listlessness; and (3) **dehydration** caused by rapid fluid removal.

As a guide for patient counseling, you may find it helpful to use the dietary regimen followed by nutritionists at a number of clinics:

- Increase protein intake to provide 1.2 to 1.5 g/kg of body weight.
- Limit phosphorus intake to 1200 mg/day by restricting phosphorus-rich foods, such as nuts and legumes, to one serving a week, and dairy products, including eggs, to a half-cup portion or one egg or its equivalent each day.
- Increase potassium intake by eating a wide variety of

fruits and vegetables each day.

- Encourage liberal fluid intake to prevent dehydration.
- Avoid sweets and fats to control triglyceride and HDL levels.
- Maintain lean body weight by incorporating the kcalories provided by the dialysate into the total meal plan.

Another important factor to keep in mind is that hemodialysis patients often lose their appetite. Thus the most basic aspect of your efforts to help CAPD clients adjust to this new system is to encourage them to eat.

References

Meyer K et al: Quality of life in the HEMO study: an interim report, *L Am Soc Neph* 8:204, 1997.

Moore LW: Nutritional implications of the proposed clinical practice guidelines for peritoneal dialysis, *Ren Nutr Forum* 16(4):1, 1997.

Report—For your information: Meeting the challenge of the renal diet, *J Am Diet Assoc* 93(6):67, 1993.

Stover J, ed: *A clinical guide to nutrition care in end-stage renal disease,* Chicago, 1993, American Dietetic Association.

Wilkens KG, Schiro KB, eds: Suggested guidelines for nutrition care of renal patients, Chicago, 1992, American Dietetic Association.

---

bohydrates. The complex carbohydrate food forms such as grains and legumes contribute incomplete protein and should not take up large amounts of the limited protein allowance.

Water balance

Fluid is usually limited to 400 or 500 ml/day, plus an amount equal to urinary output, if any. The total intake must account for additional fluids in the foods consumed and in water derived from metabolism of the food nutrients, as well as in fecal fluid losses. Even with this restriction there may be a mild fluid retention between dialysis treatments, with a daily weight gain in that period of about 1 lb (0.45 kg).

Sodium

To control body fluid retention and hypertension, sodium should be limited to 1000 to 2000 mg/day of sodium. This restriction helps to prevent pulmonary edema or congestive heart failure from fluid overload.

Potassium

Potassium restriction is imperative to prevent hyperkalemia, which can become a problem. Potassium accumulation can easily cause cardiac arrhythmias or cardiac arrest. Thus a dietary allowance of 1500 to 2000 mg/day of potassium is usually followed.

Vitamins

During the dialysis treatments, water-soluble vitamins from the blood are lost in the dialysate filtered out of the circulating blood. A daily supplement of all the water-soluble vitamins is therefore usually given. However, the fat-soluble vitamins, especially vitamins A and D, may build up. Thus multivitamin preparations used usually exclude these vitamins.

Peritoneal dialysis

An alternate form of dialysis, **peritoneal dialysis,** allows dialysate solutions to flow directly through a catheter port established through the abdominal wall into the abdominal cavity. The presence of this concentrated solution causes the waste materials to diffuse across the saclike **peritoneum** lining the abdominal cavity (see *Practical Application* box). Then this dialysate collection of waste materials flows back into the dialysate bag for disposal. The peritoneal membrane serves and the filtering mechanism. This procedure may be used in cases such as the following: (1) short periods in acute renal failure or brief infections or (2) longer periods of home care, especially for elderly persons and children and for persons with diabetes or systemic diseases.

Any one of three procedures may be used for peritoneal dialysis: (1) *intermittent peritoneal dialysis (IPD)* that is given usually at night, 10 hours each time, four times a week; (2) *continuous ambulatory peritoneal dialysis (CAPD)* in which a dialysis solution in a plastic pouch is infused and drained by gravity each day (24 hours), five times at 4-hour intervals; and (3) *continuous cyclic peritoneal dialysis (CCPD)* in which three or four machine-delivered exchanges are given at night, about 3 hours each, leaving about 2 L of dialysate solution in the peritoneal cavity for 12 to 15 hours during the day. Dietary management in each case is based on nutritional requirements and protein intake sufficient to cover any losses, with individual monitoring of need.

---

peritoneum A strong smooth surface—a serous membrane—lining the abdominal/pelvic walls and the undersurface of the diaphragm, forming a sac enclosing the body's vital visceral organs within the peritoneal cavity.

Clearly, all of the dietary factors play a role in the progression of renal disease. Although the relative importance of each factor varies depending on the underlying cause of the disease and its stage of progression, studies do show that nutritional therapy helps decrease the rate of renal function deterioration.[21] For many appropriate candidates, this delayed progression provides the needed time and nutritional status to prepare for the alternative decision of possible kidney transplant.

POLYCYSTIC KIDNEY DISEASE

Another cause of renal failure and ultimate kidney transplant is the inherited disease, polycystic kidney disease (PKD). It affects about 1 in 1000 people world wide. The large underlying gene causing the most common form of PKD has just recently been discovered.[22,23] PKD is a major cause of chronic renal failure and accounts for about 10% of all patients who require long-term dialysis or kidney transplant. The disease is characterized by the formation of enlarged renal cysts and interstitial fibrosis, resulting in progressive loss of renal tissue.

PATIENT EDUCATION MATERIALS

The renal diet is complex and presents a challenge to practitioners and, even more so, to patients. A basic resource, the National Renal Diet educational series, provides valuable guides.[22] These standardized guidelines for nutrition intervention and patient education in renal disease have been developed by the collaborative work of renal dietitians from The American Dietetic Association Renal Dietitians dietetic practice group and the National Kidney Foundation Council on Renal Nutrition. The Professional Guide can be used in conjunction with ADA's other guides for care of renal disease patients.[24-26] Because dietary management must be tailored to the stage of the disease and method of treatment, the series of materials contains a professional guide and six client booklets, each designed with special food lists to meet specific needs of the various renal disease requirements. These ADA resources give the practitioner a comprehensive basis for individualizing dietary instructions and provide the patient and family with a practical guide for everyday decisions and plans for food choices. Also, the National Kidney Foundation (NKF) has developed a new series of 5 professional practice guidelines for quality care of dialysis patients: anemia, hemodialysis, peritoneal dialysis, vascular access, and nutrition.[27]

KIDNEY TRANSPLANT

Kidney transplantation has become a widely accepted treatment of chronic renal failure. With refined techniques and development of immunosuppressive drugs to prevent organ rejection, an increasing number of kidney transplants are performed each year in the United States and an estimated 30,000 Americans are awaiting transplants.[26-28] Nutritional support for the surgical procedures is an important adjunct to therapy. This care is complex and individual and best provided by a clinical dietitian specialist in renal disease. Consideration is given to optimal protein and energy intake, with relative restriction of simple sugars, total fat, cholesterol, and saturated fat.[29] Successful kidney transplantations have given new life to many patients.[30] The quality of this extended life becomes a part of patient and family counseling (see *Issues & Answers*, p. 470).

KIDNEY STONE DISEASE

DISEASE PROCESS

Kidney stone disease is an ancient medical problem. Since the days of Hippocrates, records of its incidence have appeared in medical documents. It continues to be a prevalent health problem. Multiple stone attacks affect 12% to 20% of American men and 5% to 10% of women during their lifetimes, with most of the stones today composed of calcium oxalate mixed with varying proportions of calcium phosphate.[31] Kidney stone disease appears to be chronic and recurrent. The basic cause is unknown, but many predisposing risk factors have been found to be involved with calcium as well as protein, as well as sodium—mostly in the form of dietary salt (NaCl)—receiving the most attention.[32] Although the basic cause of kidney stones remains unknown, many factors contribute directly or indirectly to their formation. These factors relate to the nature of the urine itself or to the conditions of the urinary tract environment. According to the concentration of urinary constituents, the major stones formed are calcium stones, struvite stones, uric acid stones, and cystine stones (Figure 21.3).

CALCIUM STONES

Most kidney stones are composed of calcium compounds, usually calcium oxalate or calcium oxalate mixed with calcium phosphate. In persons who form stones, which is a familial tendency, the urine produced is supersaturated with these crystalloid elements, and there is a lack of normal urine substances that prevent the crystals from forming stones.[33] Excessive urinary calcium may result from the following:

1. *Excess calcium intake.* Prolonged use of large amounts of milk, alkali therapy for peptic ulcer, and use of a hard water supply contribute to calcium loads. However, in the case of calcium stones, new research has indicated that the culprit is not so much dietary calcium but

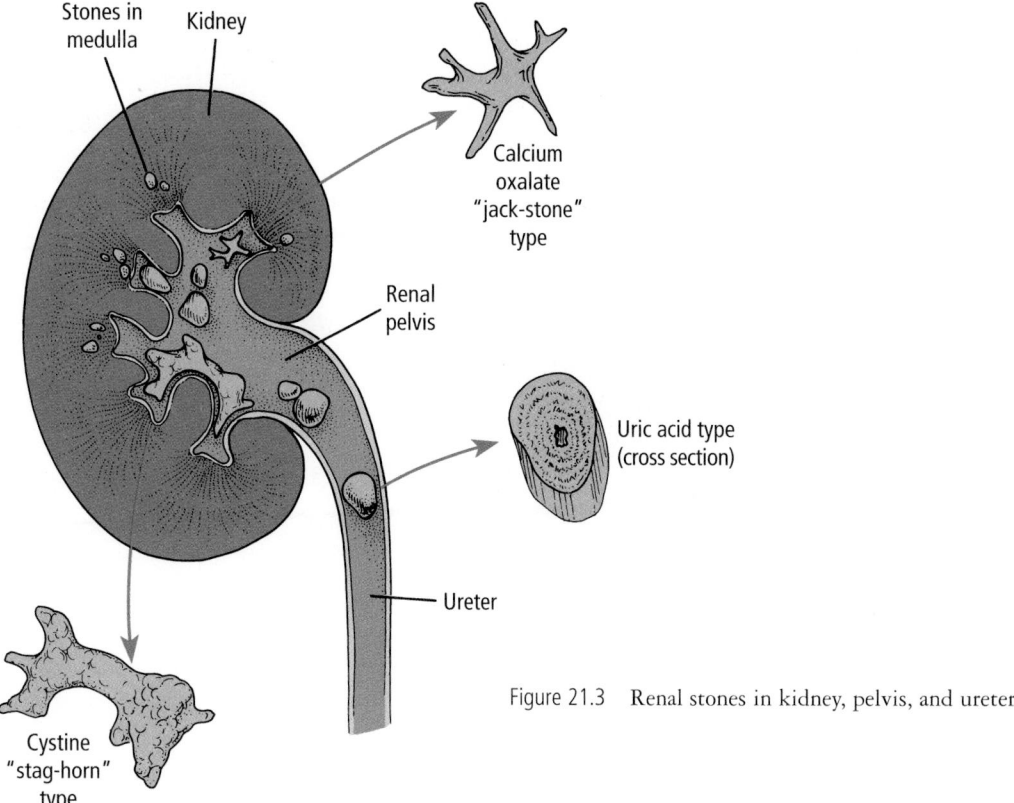

Stones in medulla

Kidney

Calcium oxalate "jack-stone" type

Renal pelvis

Uric acid type (cross section)

Ureter

Cystine "stag-horn" type

Figure 21.3   Renal stones in kidney, pelvis, and ureter.

supplemental calcium that increases the risk, causing some physicians to comment and question, "Diet and calcium—end of an era?" [34,35]

2. *Excess salt (NaCl) intake.* Recent research, both salt-loading studies and reports of free-living populations, confirms earlier observations that high intakes of NaCl result in hypercalciuria.[32]

3. *Excess vitamin D.* Hypervitaminosis D may cause increased calcium absorption from the intestine as well as increased withdrawal from bone.

4. *Prolonged immobilization.* Body casting or immobilization from illness or disability may lead to withdrawal of bone calcium and increased urinary concentration.

5. *Hyperparathyroidism.* Primary hyperparathyroidism causes excess calcium excretion. About two thirds of the persons with this endocrine disorder have kidney stones, but this disorder accounts for only about 5% of total calcium stones.

6. *Renal tubular acidosis.* Excess excretion of calcium is caused by defective ammonia formation.

7. *Idiopathic calcinuria.* Some persons, even those on a low-calcium diet, for unknown reasons may excrete as much as 500 mg of calcium daily.

8. *Oxalate.* Because of a metabolic error in handling oxalates, about half of the calcium stones are compounds with this material. Oxalates occur naturally only in a few food sources (Box 21.1), and individual absorption/excretion rates influence availability. Studies in normal volunteers consuming oxalate-rich foods have indicated that the increased urinary oxalate values were not proportional to the oxalate values of food.[33] Only eight foods caused a significant increase in urinary oxalate excretion: spinach, rhubarb, beets, nuts, chocolate, tea, wheat bran, and strawberries. Nutrition therapy for stone-forming individuals may be limited to restriction of these eight foods, with results monitored by laboratory analysis of urine composition.

9. *Animal protein.* A diet high in animal protein, for example, the typical American diet, has been linked to increased excretions of calcium, oxalate, and urate. A vegetarian-type diet has been recommended by some investigators as a wise choice for stone-forming persons.

10. *Dietary fiber.* Added dietary fiber has been found to reduce risk factors for stone formation, especially calcium stones.

Box

21.1   Food sources of oxalates

Fruits	Vegetables	Nuts	Beverages	Other
Berries, all	Baked beans	Almonds	Chocolate	Grits
Currants	Beans, green and wax	Cashews	Cocoa	Tofu
Concord grapes	Beets	Peanuts	Draft beer	Soy products
Figs	Beet greans	Peanut butter	Tea	Wheat germ
Fruit cocktail	Celery			
Plums	Chard, Swiss			
Rhubarb	Chives			
Tangerines	Collards			
	Eggplant			
	Endive			
	Kale			
	Leeks			
	Mustard greens			
	Okra			
	Peppers, green			
	Rutabagas			
	Spinach			
	Squash, summer			
	Sweet potatoes			
	Tomatoes			
	Tomato soup			
	Vegetable soup			

Struvite stones

Next to calcium stones in frequency are *struvite stones,* composed of a single compound—magnesium ammonium phosphate ($MgNH_4PO_4$). These are often called "infection stones" because they are associated with urinary tract infections. The offending organism in the infection is *Proteus mirabilis*. This is a urea-splitting bacterium that contains urease, an enzyme that hydrolyzes urea to ammonia. Thus the urinary pH becomes alkaline. In the ammonia-rich environment struvite precipitates and forms large, "stag-horn" stones. Surgical removal is usually indicated.

Uric acid stones

Excess uric acid excretion may be caused by an impairment in the intermediary metabolism of purine, as occurs in gout. It may also result from a rapid tissue breakdown in wasting disease.

Cystine stones

A heredity metabolic defect in renal tubular reabsorption of the amino acid cystine causes this substance to accumulate in the urine. This condition is called *cystinuria*. Since this is a genetic disorder, it is characterized by early onset age and a positive family history. This is one of the most common metabolic disorders associated with kidney stones in children before puberty.

URINARY TRACT CONDITIONS

The physical changes in the urine and the organic stone matrix provide urinary tract conditions that lead to the formation of kidney stones.

Physical changes in the urine

Susceptible persons form stones when physical changes in the urine predispose to such formation. Such physical conditions include:

1. *Urine concentration.* The concentration of the urine may result from a lower water intake or from excess water loss, as in prolonged sweating, fever, vomiting, or diarrhea.
2. *Urinary pH.* Changes in urinary pH from its mean 5.85 to 6 may be influenced by the diet or altered by the ingestion of acid or alkali medications.

Organic stone matrix

Formation of an organic stone matrix provides the necessary core or nucleus (nidus) around which crystals may precipitate and form a mucoprotein-carbohydrate complex. In this complex galactose and hexosamine are the principal carbohydrates. Some possible sources of these organic materials include (1) bacteria masses from recurrent urinary tract infections; (2) renal epithelial tissue of the urinary tract that has sloughed off, possibly because of vitamin A deficiency; and (3) calcified plaques (Randall's plaques) formed beneath the renal epithelium in hypercalciuria. Irritation and ulceration of overlying tissue cause the plaques to slough off into the collecting tubules.

CLINICAL SYMPTOMS

Severe pain and numerous urinary symptoms may result, with general weakness and sometimes fever. Laboratory examination of urine and chemical analysis of any stone that is passed help determine treatment.

GENERAL TREATMENT

Fluid intake

A large fluid intake produces a more dilute urine and is a foundation of therapy. The dilute urine helps to prevent concentration of stone constituents.

Urinary pH

An attempt to control the solubility factor is made by changing the urinary pH to an increased acidity or alkalinity, depending on the chemical composition of the stone formed. An exception is calcium oxalate stones, since the solubility of calcium oxalate in urine is not pH-dependent. Conversely, however, calcium phosphate is soluble in an acid urine.

Stone composition

When possible, dietary constituents of the stone are controlled to reduce the amount of the substance available for precipitation.

Binding agents

Materials that bind the stone elements and prevent their absorption in the intestine cause fecal excretion. For example, sodium phytate is used to bind calcium, and aluminum gels are used to bind phosphate. Glycine and calcium have a similar effect on oxalates.

 NUTRITION THERAPY

Nutrition therapy is directly related to the stone chemistry.

Calcium stones

A low-calcium diet of about 400 mg/day is usually given, although this practice is now being questioned.[24,35] Avoiding calcium supplements is the more effective action. The low-calcium diet amount is half of an average adult intake of about 800 mg/day. This lower level is achieved mainly by removal of milk and dairy products. Other calcium food sources that can be limited are leafy vegetables and whole grains. If the stone is calcium phosphate, phosphorous foods are also reduced. This is also

Box 21.2	Acid and alkaline ash food groups	
Acid ash	**Alkaline ash**	**Neutral**
Meat	Milk	Beverages (coffee, tea)
Whole grains	Vegetables	
Eggs	Fruits (except	
Cheese	cranberries, prunes,	
Cranberries	and plums)	
Prunes		
Plums		

accomplished mainly by removal of milk and dairy products. Sometimes a test diet of 200 mg of calcium may be used to rule out hyperparathyroidism as a causative factor.

Since calcium stones have an alkaline chemistry, an acid ash diet may also be used to help create a urinary environment less conducive to the precipitation of the basic stone elements. The classification of food groups is based on the pH of the metabolic ash produced (Box 21.2). An acid ash diet increases the amount of meat, grains, eggs, and cheese. It limits the amounts of vegetables, milk, and fruits. An alkaline ash diet outlines the opposite use of these foods. The use of cranberry juice has been promoted to assist in the acidification of urine. However, the commercially prepared cranberry juices on the consumer market are too dilute to be effective, since they contain only about 26% cranberry juice. Thus an inordinate volume would be required to achieve any consistent effectiveness as a urinary acidifying agent. Instead, to effect a sustained acidifying of urinary pH, most physicians rely on drugs.

Uric acid stones

About 4% of the total incidence of renal calculi are uric acid stones. Since uric acid is a metabolic product of purines, dietary control of this precursor is indicated. Purines are found in active tissue such as glandular meat, other lean meat, meat extractives, and in lesser amounts, in plant sources such as whole grains and legumes. An effort to produce an alkaline ash to help increase the urinary pH is indicated.

Cystine stones

About 1% of the total stones produced are cystine, since this condition is a relatively rare genetic disease. Cystine is a nonessential amino acid produced from the essential amino acid methionine. Thus a diet low in methionine is used. This diet is used with high fluid intake and alkaline diet therapy.

<table>
<thead>
<tr><th colspan="2">Table</th><th></th></tr>
<tr><th colspan="2">21.2   Summary of dietary principles in renal stone diseases</th><th></th></tr>
<tr><th>Stone chemistry</th><th>Nutrient modification</th><th>Dietary ash (urinary pH)</th></tr>
</thead>
<tbody>
<tr><td>Calcium</td><td>Low calcium (400 mg)</td><td>Acid ash</td></tr>
<tr><td>　Phosphate</td><td>　Low phosphorus (1000-1200 mg)</td><td></td></tr>
<tr><td>　Oxalate</td><td>　Low oxylate</td><td></td></tr>
<tr><td>Struvite (MgNH$_4$PO$_4$)</td><td>Low phosphorus (1000-1200 mg) (associated with urinary infections)</td><td>Acid ash</td></tr>
<tr><td>Uric acid</td><td>Low purine</td><td>Alkaline ash</td></tr>
<tr><td>Cystine</td><td>Low methionine</td><td>Alkaline ash</td></tr>
</tbody>
</table>

The nutrition therapy principles in renal stone disease are outlined in Table 21.2. Dietary guides for each of these kidney stone conditions are provided in Appendix O.

URINARY TRACT INFECTION

DISEASE PROCESS

The term *urinary tract infection (UTI)* refers to a wide variety of clinical infections in which a significant number of microorganisms are present in any portion of the urinary tract.[36] A common form is cystitis, an inflammation of the bladder very prevalent in young women. At least 20% of women experience a UTI during their lifetime, the vast majority of which are cases of uncomplicated cystitis.[36,37] The condition is called recurrent UTI if three or more bouts are experienced in a year.

The majority of cases are caused by aerobic members of the fecal flora, especially *Escherichia coli.*[38] The presence of these organisms in the urine is termed *bacteriuria*. Urine produced by the normal kidney is sterile and remains so as it travels to the bladder. In UTI, however, the normal urethra has microbial flora, so that any voided urine normally contains many bacteria. Bacteriuria is present when the quantity of organisms is more than 100,000 bacteria/ml of urine. The female anatomy is more conducive to entry of these bacteria into the urinary tract. Recurrent cystitis occurs mostly in young and otherwise healthy women who have infections that usually correspond with sexual activity and continued diaphragm use. In most cases, simply changing to another birth control method will solve the problem. Cystitis is characterized by frequent voiding and burning on urination.

Treatment

Currently antibiotic treatment of UTI has been cut back a great deal. Clinical experience indicates that a single dose of antibiotic is just as effective as the usual 7- to 10-day course treatment in 90% of all women who have uncomplicated cystitis. General nutritional measures include acidifying the urine by taking vitamin C, since cranberry juice is not effective, and drinking plenty of fluids to produce a dilute urine. Control of UTI is an important measure, since it is a risk factor in stone formation. Current medical research shows promise for development of new vaccines to prevent urinary tract infections.[38]

TO SUM UP

Through its unique functional units, the nephrons, the kidneys act as a filtration system, reabsorbing substances the body needs, secreting additional hydrogen ions to maintain a proper pH balance in the blood, and excreting unnecessary materials in a concentrated urine.

Renal function may be impaired by a variety of conditions. These include inflammatory and degenerative diseases, infection and obstruction, chronic diseases such as hypertension and diabetes, environmental agents such as insecticides and solvents and other toxic substances, as well as some medications and trauma. Some clinical conditions affecting structure and function include glomerulonephritis, nephrotic syndrome, acute and chronic renal failure, renal calculi, and urinary tract infection. In many cases, except nephrotic syndrome, dietary protein may need to be reduced as part of the nutritional care plan. Water, electrolytes, and kcalorie intake should also be closely monitored to match individual needs. The recent large United States research project, the Modification of Diet in Renal Disease (MDRD) study, indicated variable responses from study subjects according to their degree of adherence to their diet plan.

Chronic kidney disease and its result, end-stage renal disease (ESRD), is treated by *dialysis*—hemodialysis or peritoneal dialysis—and *kidney transplant*. Dialysis patients must be monitored closely for protein, water, and electrolyte balance. Nutritional support of transplant patients is needed primarily as support for the surgical procedure. A normal diet is often well tolerated after surgery and convalescence.

Renal diseases have predisposing factors. For example, untreated urinary tract infections may lead to kidney stones, and progressive glomerulonephritis may lead to nephrotic syndrome. The Western diet is suspect as a predisposing factor in the development of chronic renal failure. Excess protein intake may overtax human nephrons, which were not originally designed to handle a steady diet of protein-rich foods.

■ QUESTIONS FOR REVIEW

1. For each of the following conditions, outline the nutritional components of therapy, explaining the impact of each on kidney function: glomerulonephritis, nephrotic syndrome, acute renal failure (renal insufficiency), and chronic renal failure.

2. Identify four clinical conditions that impair renal function. Give an example of each, describing its effect on various structures in the kidney.

3. List the nutritional factors that must be monitored in individuals undergoing renal dialysis.

4. Describe the recent United States MDRD study of protein management of the diet to delay or avoid complications of chronic renal disease. In general terms, how would you evaluate its results?

5. Outline the medical and nutritional therapy used for patients with various types of kidney stones. Describe each type of stone and explain the rationale for each aspect of therapy.

6. For what condition is a urinary tract infection a predisposing factor? What general nutritional principles are recommended in the treatment of such infections?

■ REFERENCES

1. Guyton AC, Hall JE: *Textbook of medical physiology,* ed 9, Philadelphia, 1996, WB Saunders.

2. Guyton AC: Blood pressure control—special role of the kidneys and body fluids, *Science* 252(5014):1813, 1991.

3. Clark CM Jr, Lee DA: Prevention and treatment of the complications of diabetes mellitus, *N Engl J Med* 332(18):1210, 1995.

4. Porte D Jr, Schwartz MW: Diabetes complications: why is glucose potentially toxic? *Science* 272(5262):699, 1996.

5. Abuelo IG: Renal failure caused by chemicals, foods, plants, animal venom, and misuse of drugs: a review, *Arch Intern Med* 150:505, 1990.

6. Thadhani R et al: Acute renal failure, *N Engl J Med* 334(22):144, 1996.

7. Feld LG et al: Fluid needs in acute renal failure, *Pediatr Clin North Am* 37(2):337, 1990.

8. Macias WL et al: Impact of the nutritional balance in patients with acute renal failure, *J Parenter Enter Nutr* 20(1):56, 1996.

9. Kopple JD: Nutrition, diet, and the kidney. In Shils ME, Olsen JA, Shike M, eds: *Modern nutrition in health and disease,* ed 8, Philadelphia, 1993, Lea & Febiger.

10. Savin VJ et al: Circulating factor associated with increased glomerular permeability to albumin in recurrent focal segmental glomerulosclerosis, *N Engl J Med* 334(14):878, 1996.

11. Kopple JD: The nutrition management of the patient with acute renal failure, *J Parenter Enter Nutr* 20(1):3, 1996.

12. Foreman JW et al: Nutritional intake in children with renal insufficiency: a report of Growth Failure in Children with Renal Diseases Study, *J Am Coll Nutr* 15(6):579, 1996.

13. Snetselaar L et al: The MDRD Study Group: Reduction of dietary protein and phosphorus in the Modification in Diet in Renal Disease Feasibility Study, *J Am Diet Assoc* 94(9):986, 1994.

14. Coggins CH et al: Serum lipid changes associated with modified protein diets: results from the Feasibility Phase of the Modification of Diet in Renal Disease Study, *Am J Kidney* 23:514, 1994.

15. Gillis BP et al; The MDPD Study Group: Nutrition intervention program of the Modification of Diet in Renal Disease Study: a self-management approach, *J Am Diet Assoc* 95(11):1288, 1995.

16. Milas NC et al: The MDRD Study Group: factors associated with adherence to the dietary protein intervention in the Modification of Diet in Renal Disease Study, *J Am Diet Assoc* 95(11):1295, 1995.

17. Klahr S et al: The Modification of Diet in Renal Disease Study Group: the effects of dietary protein restrictions of chronic renal disease, *N Engl J Med* 330:877, 1994.

18. Coyne T et al; The MDRD study: Dietary satisfaction correlated with adherence in the Modification of Diet in Renal Disease Study, *J Am Diet Assoc* 95(11):1301, 1995.

19. Hruska KA, Teitebaum SL: Renal osteodystrophy, *N Engl J Med* 333(3):166, 1995.

20. Reid DJ et al: Effects of folate and zinc supplementation on patients undergoing chronic hemodialysis, *J Am Diet Assoc* 92(5):574, 1992.

21. Ahmed FE: Effect of diet on progression of chronic renal disease, *J Am Diet Assoc* 91(10):1266, 1991.

22. The International Polycystic Kidney Disease Consortium: Polycystic kidney disease: the complete structure of the PDK1 gene and its protein, *Cell* 81:289, 1995.

23. Fackelmann K: Megagene unmasked: huge gene leads to many tumors in the kidneys, *Sci News* 147(21):330, 1995.

24. Report—For Your Information: Meeting the challenge of the renal diet, *J Am Diet Assoc* 93(6):637, 1993.

25. Wilkens KG, Schiro KB, eds: *Suggested guidelines for nutrition care of renal patients,* ed 2, Chicago, 1992, American Dietetic Association.

26. Stover J, ed: *A clinical guide to nutrition care in end-stage renal disease,* Chicago, 1993, American Dietetic Association.

27. Moore LW: Nutritional implications of the proposed clinical practice guidelines for peritoneal dialysis, *Ren Nutr Forum* 16(4):1, 1997.

28. Lipsyte R: Transplant, *Am Health* 13(4):24, 1994.

29. Terasaki PI et al: High survival rates of kidney transplants from spousal and living unrelated donors, *N Engl J Med* 333(6):333, 1995.

30. Soulillou J-P: Kidney transplantation from spousal donors, *N Engl J Med* 333(6):379, 1995.

31. Burtis WJ et al: Dietary hypercalciuria in patients with calcium oxalate kidney stones, *Am J Clin Nutr* 60(3):1995.

32. Massy LK, Whiting SJ: Dietary salt, urinary calcium, and kidney stone risk, *Nutr Rev* 53(5):131, 1995.

33. Massey LK et al: Effect of dietary oxalate and calcium on urinary oxalate and risk of formation of calcium oxalate kidney stones, *J Am Diet Assoc* 93(8):901, 1993.

34. Curhan GC et al: Comparison of dietary calcium with supplemental calcium and other nutrients as factors affecting the risk for kidney stones, *Ann Intern Med* 126(7):497, 1997.

35. Coe FL et al: Diet and calcium: the end of an era? *Ann Intern Med* 126(7):553, 1997.

36. Dranov P: Urinary tract infection, *Am Health* 14(4):66, 1995.

37. Service RE: New vaccines may ward off urinary tract infections, *Science* 276(5312):533, 1997.

38. Langermann S et al: Prevention of mucosal *Escherichia coli* infection by FimH-adhesin-based system vaccination, *Science* 276(5312):607, 1997.

■ FURTHER READING

Ahmed FE: Effect of diet on progression of chronic renal disease, *J Am Diet Assoc* 91(10):1266, 1991.

Dr. Ahmed of the Food and Nutrition Board, National Research Council–National Academy of Sciences, provides a helpful review of the literature concerning the impact of diet on the course of chronic renal disease and how nutritional management is used as therapy for persons with renal insufficiency.

Beto JA: Which diet for which renal failure: making sense of the options, *J Am Diet Assoc* 95(8):898, 1995.

This excellent article from an experienced professor and clinician sorts out the various types of renal diseases and their modes of treatment, with a clear eye and heart for the needs of patients. It does indeed "make sense" of all the options.

Groot PJ et al: Optimizing dialysis: past, present, and future, *Nutr Today* 32(1):332(1):30, 1997.

Burrowes JD: The HEMO Study: rationale, design, and role of nutrition in a prospective hemodialysis study, *Ren Nutr Forum* 17(2):1, 1998, American Dietetic Association.

Degroot reviews the phenomenal growth of end-stage renal disease and the growing health care problem it has become in the United States. The author presents the history of dialysis and discusses the continuing research that will help assess and refine this treatment for end-stage renal disease for the over 300,000 persons who are expected to need it by the year 2000. Burrowes describes in detail the multicenter clinical trial that is investigating the effects of hemodialysis on patient morbidity and mortality, and also examines the role of nutrition and its implications.

Stover J, ed: *A clinical guide to nutrition care in end-stage renal disease,* ed 2, Chicago, 1993, American Dietetic Association.

Wilkins KG, Schiro KB, eds: *Suggested guidelines for nutrition care of renal patients,* ed 2, Chicago, 1992, American Dietetic Association.

The American Dietetic Association has provided definitive guidelines for practitioner and patient in its comprehensive patient education materials. The new National Renal Diet educational series, developed jointly with the National Kidney Foundation Council on Renal Nutrition, contains a professional guide and six client booklets, each with special food lists, to meet the various needs of renal disease patients. Copies of this new series of resource material are available from ADA; information on how to order can be found in current copies of the Journal of the American Dietetic Association.

Case study

The patient with chronic renal failure

Aaron Steinberg is 45 years old, married, and works as a city planner for a large municipal government. He cited a recent history of nausea, anorexia, hematuria, and swollen ankles during a physical examination. His wife reported that he had been tiring more easily than usual during the past year. A history of prior illnesses proved negative, except for a severe case of influenza with sore throat 10 years before during an epidemic when he was stationed with the Army overseas. Tests were ordered, and the patient was advised to return in a week for review of the test results and sooner if there were any changes in his symptoms.

Mr. Steinberg did return, with additional symptoms of headaches and occasionally blurred vision. At that time his blood pressure was 160/98, his temperature was 37.5° C (99.6° F), and he had lost 4 kg (8.75 lb). The laboratory tests showed albumin and red and white blood cells in the urine, with an elevated BUN; a PSP indicated a reduced filtration rate. The diagnosis was chronic renal failure.

The physician discussed the diagnosis and its serious prognosis with Mr. and Mrs. Steinberg, giving them the benefits and disadvantages of both hemodialysis and kidney transplantation. Antihypertensive medication was prescribed along with other drugs to minimize discomfort.

During the following weeks Mr. Steinberg continued to lose weight, had increasing joint pain, and became anemic. He found it increasingly difficult to maintain his hectic schedule of frequent meetings, conferences, and public speeches because of gastrointestinal bleeding, increasing nausea, and occasional muscle spasms. Small mouth sores made eating very difficult.

Finally the Steinbergs informed the physician of their decision to accept the kidney transplant as a means of controlling the disease process. They were referred to the clinical nutritionist for renal diet counseling to control protein, sodium, potassium, phosphate, and fluids, as well as to ensure adequate kcalories. After discussing these needs for nutritional maintenance before surgery, the nutritionist helped them develop a meal plan based on Mr. Steinberg's food preferences. Food selection and preparation were discussed in detail, with many ideas for building in as much variety and taste appeal as possible.

The Steinbergs' follow-up with the food plan was excellent. One month later the laboratory values were almost normal, blood pressures averaged 140/88, the headaches and blurred vision had virtually disappeared, and Mr. Steinberg had gained 3.2 kg (7 lb) of his lost weight. The nutrient supplements, including the amino acid analogues, were taken each day as instructed.

Fortunately a kidney donor was soon found, and with the aid of drug control of immune responses it was apparently a success. Mr. Steinberg convalesced well at home, kept all follow-up visits with the health care team, and has continued to be asymptomatic 1 year following surgery.

Questions for Analysis

1. Identify a metabolic imbalance caused by renal failure that may account for each symptom presented by Mr. Steinberg.
2. What would be the objectives in care of renal failure such as Mr. Steinberg was experiencing?
3. What factors affect the amount of protein needed by persons with chronic renal failure? What amounts are usually used? Why? What are the amino acid analogues used with the low-protein diet, and why are they used?
4. What factors affect the amount of sodium needed by persons with chronic renal failure? How much is usually recommended?
5. Why is it important to control potassium levels? How much is recommended? What clinical signs presented by Mr. Steinberg may indicate that he had not been getting enough potassium?
6. Why is control of phosphate important in the diet for chronic renal failure? What additional means may be used to control it?
7. What factors affect fluid balance in chronic renal failure? How much is usually allowed?
8. What is the basic principle of the low-protein dietary regimen? List and explain each factor in the diet and potential problems in its management.
9. Outline a general teaching plan you would use to instruct the Steinbergs about the presurgical and postsurgical dietary needs.

Issues Answers

Renal disease: technology versus the quality of life

Imagine spending up to 18 hours a week hooked up to a machine to which you literally owe your life. Imagine having a 40% chance of never being able to work outside the home again, leading a life of poverty and restricted mobility, all because of that machine.

This is probably hard for most of us to conceive. Yet for approximately 55,000 Americans on maintenance dialysis (the number of patients with end-stage renal disease [ESRD] requiring hemodialysis is increasing), this is the reality of their everyday lives. The medical-nutrition-nursing renal care team must also deal with this reality daily in work with these persons and their families. Sensitivity is especially needed in nutrition counseling and teaching. Food is tied up with so many personal values that when it must be drastically changed, or when choice is gone altogether, it's as if a part of the self has been diminished.

Researchers, physicians, and patients are becoming increasingly concerned with the *quality* of life rather than merely the *length* of life available to the person on dialysis. The only alternative currently available is kidney transplantation. On the surface, transplantation could be considered preferable to hemodialysis or even peritoneal dialysis because it frees the individual from any mechanical device. However, researchers are beginning to investigate the quality of life a transplant provides to determine whether either method is preferable to the other.

The first issue of greatest concern is the effect of the treatment on the person's life span. Mortality rates for individuals on dialysis, 8% to 15%, are in the same range as for those receiving their first kidney transplant, 10% to 15%. However, rates among young dialysis patients with no extrarenal disease can drop as low as 2%, in contrast with rates that can soar to 30% among individuals receiving kidneys from cadavers. Still, some persons believe that the benefits of increased mobility outweigh the drawbacks of a possible reduction in life span.

In one study life quality measures (sleep habits, food habits, energy level, sexual activity, changes in income and employment, satisfaction with marriage, and so on) were examined among individuals undergoing dialysis or with successful and unsuccessful transplant operations. As expected, subjects who had successful operations reported a near-normal quality of life; they were less tired, were less inconvenienced by frequent medical treatments, and had better incomes and/or more full-time employment following renal failure than other renal patients.

Also as expected, individuals whose transplant operations were not successful indicated that the quality of their lives was the lowest of all subjects. For example, none of these subjects reported full-time employment since renal failure. They were mainly recipients of kidneys from cadavers; thus this process is assumed to be the least desired of all possible alternatives.

A surprising result of this study was that dialysis patients who never received a transplant thought that the quality of their lives was also near normal. Researchers admit that the reason for this probably includes denial or accommodation. However, they also acknowledge that human response to life experiences is an extremely complex issue, one that is difficult to assess with current "immature" research methods available for evaluating the quality of life in general.

The health care team responsible for the patient with renal failure may have their own set of parameters for determining the quality of life each mode of treatment may provide. The results of this study suggest that the patient's own evaluation of life may involve factors much more complex than those to which the professional has been exposed. The study serves as a reminder that professionals must be open to the concerns and viewpoints of the individual faced with such major choices in treatment and must relate care planning in all areas to these personal concerns.

References

Collins AJ et al: Changing risk factor demographics in end-stage renal disease patients entering hemodialysis and impact on long-term mortality, *Am J Kidney Dis* 15:422, 1990.

Husbye DG et al: Psychosocial, social, and somatic prognostic indicators in old patients undergoing long-term dialysis, *Arch Int Med* 147:1921, Nov 1987.

Report—For your information: Meeting the challenge of the renal diet, *J Am Diet Assoc* 93(6):637, 1993.

Kutner NG et al: Continued survival of older hemodialysis patients: investigation of psychosocial predictors, *Am J Kidney Dis* 24:42, 1994.

Stover J: *A clinical guide to nutrition care in end-stage renal disease*, Chicago, 1993, American Dietetic Association.

Nutritional Care of Surgery Patients

In this chapter, we look at the needs of patients undergoing various surgical procedures. A major focus is gastrointestinal surgeries. The type and extent of the surgical procedure, as well as the nature of any preceding injury, influence special nutritional therapy requirements and the mode of feeding needed to meet these nutritional demands.

A primary underlying need is the prevention of malnutrition. Numerous American and European surveys of hospitalized patients indicate that nearly 50% of surgical patients have clinical evidence of protein-energy malnutrition.

Here we see how careful preoperative nutritional preparation, together with vigorous postoperative nutritional support, reduces complications and provides resources for better healing and more rapid recovery.

NUTRITIONAL NEEDS OF GENERAL SURGERY PATIENTS

PREOPERATIVE NUTRITION

Nutrient stores

A poor postoperative outcome is often the result of preoperative malnutrition. Thus when surgery is planned, a primary task is immediate attention to nutritional status.[1] Nutritional reserves fortify the patient for the demands of surgery. When time permits, nutritional preparation should correct any nutrient deficiencies. It should also provide resources for the surgery itself and for the immediate postoperative period until regular feedings can be resumed (see *Practical Application* box below).

1. *Protein.* The most common nutritional deficiency of surgery patients is that of protein. Tissue and plasma reserves are imperative to prepare the patient for blood losses during surgery and for tissue breakdown in the immediate postoperative period of catabolism.
2. *Energy.* Sufficient kcalories must be provided to build up any deficit. Carbohydrates are needed as the main energy source to help prevent progressive protein-energy malnutrition.
3. *Vitamins and minerals.* Normal tissue stores of vitamins are needed for the added metabolism of carbohydrates and protein. Any deficiency state such as anemia should be corrected. Electrolytes and fluids should be in balance and correction made of any dehydration, acidosis, or alkalosis.

---

practical application

Energy and protein requirements in general surgery patients

General surgery patients vary in their nutritional needs depending on two basic factors: (1) individual nutritional status and (2) the metabolic stress of the underlying illness or injury and the surgery. For example, compare the following patient situations.

Adequately nourished preoperative patient

For the patient with normal energy and nitrogen balance, approximately 40 kcal/kg/day and 1.5 g of protein/kg/day should maintain these balances for the surgery ahead.

Adequately nourished postoperative patient

After surgery, energy requirements remain about the same—40 kcal/kg/day. However, increased nitrogen losses, from decreased protein synthesis during surgery and the immediate postoperative period, increase protein needs to 1.8 to 1.9 g protein/kg/day.

Nutritionally depleted, nonstressed patient

The patient requires repletion of body fat stores and lean body mass. Nutrient needs are similar to those of the adequately nourished postoperative patient, with 40 kcal/kg/day and 1.8 to 1.9 g protein/kg/day producing moderate gains in fat and protein.

Nutritionally depleted, stressed patient

This patient has depleted energy and protein stores. These losses need to be matched, *and* extra protein (2 to 2.2 g/kg/day) is required for repletion. Part of the kcalorie load (45 kcal/kg/day) should be given as fat. A 50:50 glucose-fat mix is recommended.

Adequately nourished, stressed patient

This patient has the highest requirements for energy (50 kcal/kg/day) and protein (2.5 g/kg/day), although the aim is to prevent loss, not to replenish. Glucose is not utilized sufficiently to provide adequate energy intake, so some of the energy needs to be provided as fat (50:50 glucose-fat mix).

An analysis of published reports underscores the importance of nutritional status to surgery outcome. Reviewers conclude that when malnourished patients receive total parenteral nutrition in adequate amounts for 7 to 15 days preoperatively, significant improvements in both nutritional status and postoperative outcome occur.

References

Campos ACL, Meguid MM: A critical appraisal of the usefulness of perioperative nutritional support, *Am J Clin Nutr* 55:117, 1992.

Dickson TC: Clinical pathway nutrition management for outpatient bone marrow transplantation, *J Am Diet Assoc* 97(1):61, 1997.

Immediate preoperative period

In the usual preparation for surgery, nothing is given by mouth for at least 8 hours before surgery. This ensures that the stomach has no retained food at the time of the operation. In case of emergency surgery, if the patient has recently eaten a meal, gastric suction is used. Food in the stomach may be vomited or aspirated during surgery or recovery from anesthesia. Also, any food present may increase the possibility of postoperative gastric retention and dilation. It may also interfere with the procedure itself, especially in abdominal surgery. Before gastrointestinal surgery, a low-residue or residue-free diet may be followed for several days to clear the operative site of any food residue. Low-residue, chemically defined formulas, or *elemental formulas*, can provide a complete diet in liquid form. Such formulas, if palatable enough, can be taken orally in sufficient amounts to maintain nutritional resources. Otherwise they may be fed by tube (see Chapter 17).

POSTOPERATIVE NUTRITION

Healthy body tissues undergo continuous turnover, with small physiologic losses being constantly replenished by nutrients in the food eaten. In illness, however, especially surgical illnesses, losses are greatly increased. At the same time, replacement from food is diminished or even absent for a brief or extended period. Nutritional support, therefore, becomes all the more significant as a means of aiding recovery.

Protein

Adequate protein intake in the postoperative recovery period is of primary therapeutic concern to replace losses and supply increased demands. A catabolic period with progressively increasing protein deficiency is common in surgical patients. Negative nitrogen balances of as much as 20 g/day may occur. This amount of nitrogen loss represents an actual loss of tissue protein of more than 1 lb/day. If any degree of prior malnutrition or chronic infection has existed, the patient's protein deficit may become even more severe and cause serious complications. There are a number of reasons for this increased protein demand:

1. *Tissue synthesis in wound healing.* Tissue proteins can be synthesized only by essential amino acids brought to the tissue by the circulating blood. The necessary essential amino acids must come either from the diet protein or by intravenous feeding. Tissue protein deficiencies are best met by oral feeding. When appetite is poor, palatable concentrated liquid drinks or commercial drinks, such as Ensure (Ross), may be useful (see Chapter 17). During early feeding periods or with the extremely malnourished patient, only small amounts of protein may be tolerated.

However, increased intake is needed as early as possible to achieve the amount of protein required to restore lost protein tissues and to synthesize new tissue at the wound site. In addition to protein losses from tissue breakdown, added loss of plasma proteins can occur through hemorrhage, wound bleeding, and **exudates**. Increased metabolic losses of protein can also result from extensive tissue destruction and inflammation or from trauma and infection. Although tissue protein is broken down more rapidly during stress, it is also built up more rapidly, provided sufficient amino acids are present to supply the anabolic demand.

2. *Avoidance of shock.* Reduced blood volume—*hypovolemia*—from a loss of plasma proteins and a decrease in circulating red blood cell volume contributes to the potential danger of shock. When protein deficiencies exist, this danger is increased.

3. *Control of edema.* When the serum protein is low, edema develops as a result of the loss of colloidal osmotic pressure required to maintain the normal shift of fluid between the capillaries and the surrounding interstitial tissue spaces. This general edema may affect heart and lung action. Also, local edema at the surgical site delays closure of the wound and hinders normal healing.

4. *Bone healing.* In orthopedic surgery, extensive bone healing is involved. Protein is essential for proper **callus** formation and calcification. A sound protein matrix is mandatory for the anchoring of mineral matter in bone tissue. This is especially true with bone fractures among the growing United States population of elderly persons, particularly among older women.[2,3]

5. *Resistance to infection.* Amino acids are necessary constituents of the proteins involved in body defense mechanisms. These defense agents include antibodies, special blood cells, hormones, and enzymes. Tissue integrity itself is a first line of defense against infections.

6. *Lipid transport.* Proteins are necessary for the transport of lipids in the body's blood circulation. They provide essential material to form

---

callus Unorganized meshwork of newly grown, woven bone developed on pattern of original fibrin clot (formed after fracture or surgery) and normally replaced in the healing process by hard adult bone.

exudate Various materials (e.g., cells, cellular debris, fluids), usually resulting from inflammation, that have escaped from blood vessels and are deposited in or on surface tissues.

lipoproteins, the transport form of fat in the body. Proteins thus protect the liver, a main site of fat metabolism, from danger caused by fatty infiltration.

Multiple clinical problems may easily develop following surgery when protein deficiencies exist. There may be poor wound healing (**dehiscence**), delayed healing of fractures, anemia, failure of gastrointestinal stomas to function, depressed lung and heart function, reduced resistance to infection, extensive weight loss, liver damage, and increased mortality risks.

Water

Water balance is a vital concern after surgery. Adequate fluid therapy is necessary to prevent dehydration. Large water losses may occur from vomiting, hemorrhage, exudates, diuresis, or fever. When drainage is involved, as is common in many surgeries, still more fluid loss occurs. Table 22.1 indicates the general magnitude of water requirements for surgical patients. Intravenous therapy will supply initial needs, but oral intake should begin as soon as possible. Water intake must be maintained in sufficient quantity, according to individual needs, to avoid extremes of dehydration and water intoxication. Daily weight measurement of the patient provides a guideline for meeting fluid requirements.

Energy

As is always the case when increased protein is demanded for tissue rebuilding, sufficient nonprotein energy kcalories must be supplied to protect the amino acids for use in tissue synthesis. Adequate amounts of carbohydrate are essential to ensure the use of protein for building tissue and to supply the energy required for the increased metabolic demands. As protein is increased, the total kcalories must be increased as well because sufficient caloric intake is often crucial to the successful outcome of the surgical procedure. About 2800 kcal/day must be provided before protein can be used to repair tissue and not be diverted to help provide energy. In acute stress, as in extensive surgery or burns, when protein needs may be as high as 200 g/day, 4000 to 6000 kcalories may be required. In addition to its protein-sparing action, carbohydrates also help to avoid liver damage from depletion of glycogen reserves. Fat must be adequate to maintain body tissue fat reserves, but it must not be excessive.

Vitamins

All of the vitamins play important roles in the healing process. Vitamin C is imperative for wound healing. It is necessary for the formation of cementing material in the ground substance of connective tissue, in capillary walls, and in the building up of new tissue. Extensive tissue regeneration such as occurs in burns or radical surgeries may require vitamin C supplements. As kcalorie and protein intake are increased, the B vitamins must also be increased. They provide essential coenzyme factors for protein and energy metabolism. Vitamin K is essential in the blood clotting mechanism.

Minerals

Replacing mineral deficiencies and ensuring continued adequacy is essential. In tissue breakdown, potassium and phosphorus are lost. Electrolyte losses, especially sodium and chloride, accompany fluid losses. Iron-deficiency anemia may develop from blood loss or faulty iron absorption.

GENERAL DIETARY MANAGEMENT

Oral feeding

The majority of general surgical patients can and should progress to oral feeding as soon as possible to provide adequate nutrition. Remember that routine postoperative intravenous fluids are intended to supply hydration needs and electrolytes, not to sustain nutritional needs. Routine postoperative intravenous fluids cannot supply full nutrient needs or compete with oral feedings. For example, of a 5% dextrose solution, 1 L contains 50 g of glucose, with an energy value of only 200 kcalories. Thus 3 L/day supplies only 600 kcalories and no protein. The basal energy requirement alone is much more, without taking into consideration the increased metabolic stress demands of surgical illness. Wherever possible, a rapid return to regular eating should be encouraged and maintained.

Table 22.1	Daily water requirements of the surgical patient	
Type of case and fluid needs		**Average fluid required (ml)**
Uncomplicated cases		
For vaporization		1000-1500
For urine		1000-1500
TOTAL		2000-3000
Complicated cases (sepsis, elevation of temperature, humid weather, renal damage)		
For vaporization		2000-2500
For urine		1000-1500
TOTAL		3000-4000
Seriously ill patients with drainage		
For vaporization		2000
For urine		1000
For replacement of body fluid losses		
Bile drainage		1000
Wangensteen drainage		3000
TOTAL		7000

<table>
<tr><td>

B o x

22.1 Diet for postoperative gastric dumping syndrome

General description

- 5 or 6 small meals daily
- Relatively high fat content to retard passage of food and help maintain weight
- High protein content (meat, egg, cheese) to rebuild tissue and maintain weight
- Relatively low carbohydrate content to prevent rapid passage of quickly used foods
- No milk; no sugar, sweets, or desserts; no alcohol or sweet carbonated beverages
- Liquids between meals only; avoid fluids for at least 1 hour before and after meals
- Relatively low-roughage foods; raw foods as tolerated

Meal pattern

Breakfast
  2 scrambled eggs with 1 to 2 tbsp butter or margarine
  $\frac{1}{2}$ to 1 slice bread or small serving cereal with butter or margarine
  2 crisp bacon strips
  1 serving solid fruit*
Midmorning sandwich as follows:
  1 slice bread
  Butter or margarine
  56 g (2 oz) lean meat
Lunch
  112 g (4 oz) lean meat with 1 or 2 tbsp butter or margarine
  Green or colored vegetable† with butter or margarine
  $\frac{1}{2}$ to 1 slice bread with butter or margarine
  $\frac{1}{2}$ banana or other solid fruit*
Midafternoon
  Same snack as midmorning
Dinner
  112 g lean meat with 1 or 2 tbsp butter or margarine
  Green or colored vegetable† with butter or margarine
  $\frac{1}{2}$ to 1 slice bread with butter or margarine (or small serving starchy vegetable substitute)
  1 serving sliced fruit
Bedtime
  56 g meat or 2 eggs or 56 g cheese or cottage cheese
  1 slice bread or 5 crackers
  Butter or margarine

---

*Fruit choice: applesauce, baked apple, canned fruit (drained), banana, or orange or grapefruit sections.
†Vegetable choice: asparagus, spinach, green beans, squash, beets, carrots, or green peas.

</td></tr>
</table>

GALLBLADDER SURGERY

Surgical procedure

For patients suffering from acute *cholecystitis* or *cholelithiasis* (Figure 22.2), the treatment is usually surgical removal of the gallbladder—**cholecystectomy**. Now the "gold standard" for gallstone removal is minimal surgery involving only small skin punctures, thus the common name "key-hole" or "Band-Aid" surgery, rather than a long abdominal incision.[6,7] Through these small openings the surgeon can insert needed instruments and a laparoscope fitted with miniature camera and bright fiberoptic lighting. With only a single stitch and a small bandage closing each of the three openings, the patient can go home almost immediately and be fully recovered—and have a videotape of the whole procedure.

Nutrition problems

Following surgery, some control of the fat in the diet aids wound healing and comfort. The presence of fat in the duodenum continues to stimulate the *cholecystokinin* mechanism (see Chapter 18), which causes contraction and pain in the surgical area. There is also a period of readjustment to the more aqueous supply of liver bile available to assist fat digestion and absorption.

Dietary management

Depending on individual tolerance and response, a relatively low-fat diet may need to be followed for a brief time with moderate fat use thereafter, as recommended in the United States Dietary Guidelines for all healthy Americans.

ILEOSTOMY AND COLOSTOMY

In cases of intestinal lesion or obstruction or when inflammatory bowel disease (see Chapter 18) involves the entire colon, the treatment of choice is usually resection of the intestine to remove the diseased portion. An *ileostomy*, usually permanent but sometimes temporary, may also be established. In this procedure the end of the remaining small intestine, the ileum, is attached to an opening in the abdominal wall, and a **stoma** is formed to provide for discharge of the intestinal contents (Figure 22.3, *A*). In other cases, a temporary or permanent *colostomy* may be indicated with resection of only the final left side of the colon, and a stoma is made with the remaining sigmoid, or descending, colon (Figure 22.3, *B*). In other cases a *jejunoileostomy* may be performed (Figure 22.4).

---

cholecystectomy Surgical removal of the gallbladder.

gastrectomy Surgical removal of the whole (total gastrectomy) or part (partial gastrectomy) of the stomach.

postprandial Occurring after a meal.

stoma The opening established in the abdominal wall, connecting with the ileum or colon, for elimination of intestinal wastes after surgical removal of diseased portions of the intestinal tract.

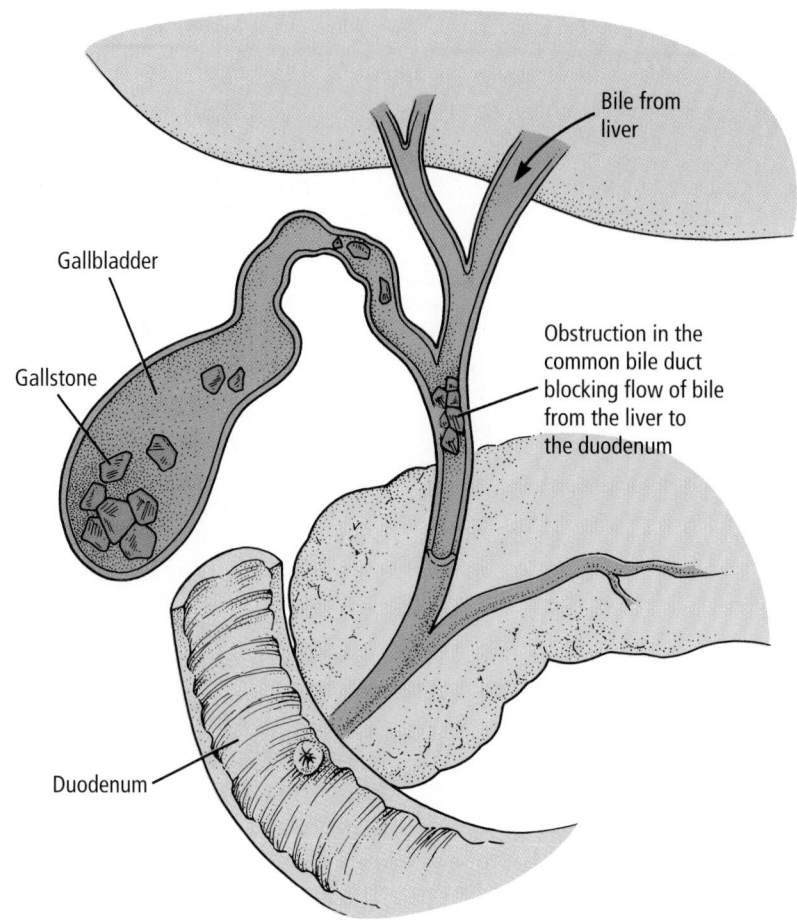

Figure 22.2   Gallbladder with stones (cholelithiasis).

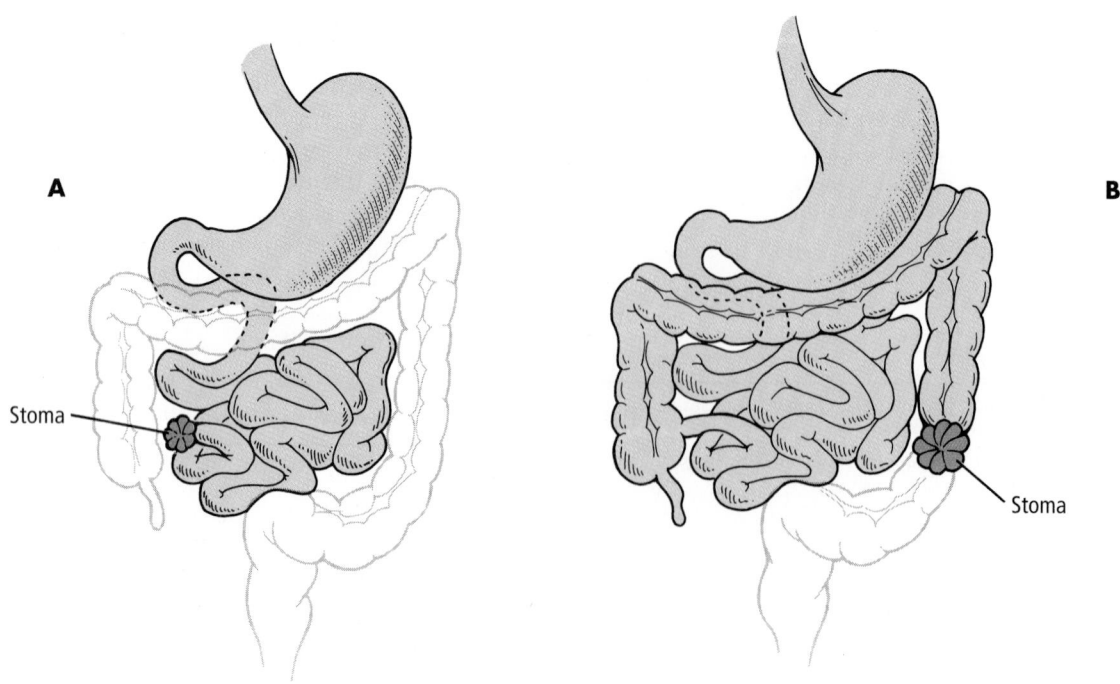

Figure 22.3   **A,** Ileostomy. **B,** Colostomy.

Jejunum

Ileum

Figure 22.4 Jejunoileostomy.

Nutrition problems

An ileostomy and a colostomy produce different problems in management. With an ileostomy, the intestinal contents at the point of the ileus are unformed, irritating, and even erosive to the skin. The standard Brooke ileostomy (Figure 22.3, *A*), with outside pouch, drains freely, almost continuously.[8] Also, bacterial fermentation of nondigestible carbohydrates such as resistant starch usually takes place in these pouches to an appreciable extent.[9] Thus establishment of controlled functioning is difficult. Many patients, however, do develop a reasonable degree of regularity in regard to meals. The modified Koch pouch, an internal abdominal reservoir, has served as an alternative procedure. The surgeon forms a reservoir inside the abdominal cavity out of intestinal tissue, and a one-way valve holds the collection until periodically the patient inserts a catheter to empty it.[8] A recently developed, more attractive alternate procedure, the *J-pouch–anal anastomosis*, done in connection with a total colectomy, provides an interior ileoanal reservoir and channel for elimination through the regular anal route.[8,9] The ileoanal reservoir is constructed in two stages. First, a total **proctocolectomy** is done, usually indicated by the progressive inflammatory disease or colon cancer. The ileoanal reservoir is formed from loops of ileum placed in the rectal vault, and a temporary loop ileostomy is created to allow healing of the new ileoanal reservoir.[8-10] Second, about 3 months later, the loop ileostomy is closed and the new ileoanal reservoir is used for bowel movements. Stool frequency, although greatly reduced to about eight bowel movements per day, remains a personal concern.

Dietary management

The diet therapy challenge focuses on management of bowel output. In general, patients with ostomies should eat regular diets of foods that agree with them. Their food should be sufficient in quantity and nutritive value to maintain proper weight and energy. Patients with ileoanal reservoirs can best achieve control by (1) consuming no more than three meals a day (every time food is eaten the gastrointestinal tract is stimulated); (2) eating the last meal at least 2 hours before bedtime; and (3) evaluating individual bowel pattern to determine how long after a meal one can safely leave home. The basis of the diet is a well-balanced regular plan of three meals, including a variety of foods and noting individual food tolerances. Despite its drawbacks, the ileoanal reservoir is an increasingly popular surgical alternative to stoma formation.[8] However, of the ostomies with external stomas, a colostomy is more manageable. The normal contents of the intestine at this point in the lower colon are solid or semisolid because more water and electrolytes have been absorbed by the first parts of the colon. The consistency of the discharge and its less irritating nature create fewer control problems. Often a sigmoid colostomy can be adequately controlled by simple dietary measures and periodic irrigation, so that in many cases no protective appliance is needed. Coping with any of these surgical

---

proctocolectomy Surgical removal of the rectum and colon.

procedures is difficult at best. Patients need much support and practical help, along with resources for learning about self-care.[8-10]

RECTAL SURGERY

Nutrition problems

For a brief period following rectal surgery, or a *hemorrhoidectomy*, there is pain on elimination. Thus bowel movements are delayed until initial healing is begun.

Dietary management

A clear fluid or nonresidue diet is indicated for brief initial use. The basic foods used are almost completely digested and nutrients absorbed in the small intestine, leaving minimal residue for elimination by the colon. An outline of foods used in such a diet is given in Table 22.2. In some cases a nonresidue commercial formula may be used during the initial postoperative period.

Table 22.2	Nonresidue diet for postsurgical nonresidue diet

General description—nonresidue diet

- This diet includes only those foods that are free from fiber, seeds, and skins and with the minimal amount of residue.
- Fruits and vegetables are omitted, except for strained fruit juices.
- Milk is omitted.
- The diet is adequate in protein and kcalories, containing approximately 75 g protein, 110 g fat, 250 g carbohydrates, and 2260 kcalories. It is likely to be inadequate in vitamin A, calcium, and riboflavin.
- If patients remain a long time on this diet, supplementary vitamins and minerals should be given.

	Allowed	Not allowed
Beverages	Carbonated beverages, coffee, tea	Milk and milk drinks
Bread	Crackers, melba, or rusks	Whole grain bread
Cereals	Refined, as Cream of Wheat, farina, fine cornmeal, Malt-o-Meal, pablum, rice, strained oatmeal, corn flakes, puffed rice, Rice Krispies	Whole grain and other cereals
Cheese		None allowed
Desserts	Plain cakes and cookies, gelatin desserts, water ices, angel food cake, arrowroot cookies, tapioca puddings made with fruit juice only	Pastries and all others
Eggs	As desired, preferably hard cooked	Fried eggs
Fats	Butter or substitute, small amount cream	None are restricted
Fruits	Strained fruit juices	All others
Meat, fish, poultry	Tender beef, chicken, fish, lamb, liver, veal, and crisp bacon	Fried or tough meat, pork
Potatoes or substitute	Only macaroni, noodles, spaghetti, refined rice	Potatoes, corn, hominy, unrefined rice
Soup	Bouillon and broth only	All others
Sweets	Hard candy, fondant, gumdrops, jelly, marshmallows, sugar, syrup, and honey	Other candy, jam, marmalade
Vegetables	Tomato juice	All others
Miscellaneous	Salt	Pepper

General description—postsurgical nonresidue diet

- This diet is slightly higher in residue but has greater variety, including potatoes, white bread products, processed cheese, sauces, desserts made with milk, and cream for coffee and cereal.
- The average daily menu contains 85 g protein and 2300 kcalories and is slightly higher in vitamins and minerals.

Selection of foods

To the list add the following:
   Cheese: processed cheese, mild cream cheeses
   Potatoes: prepared any way, no skin
   Bread: any kind without bran, white bread, rolls, pancakes, waffles
   Fats: 2 oz cream or half-and-half per meal, cream sauce, cream gravy
   Desserts: all desserts, except those containing fruit and nuts
   Condiments: as desired

SPECIAL NUTRITIONAL NEEDS FOR PATIENTS WITH BURNS

NUTRITIONAL SUPPORT BASE

A major concern of therapy for the patient with extensive burns is rigorous nutritional support. The clinical dietitian on the burn team is in a strategic position to assess, plan, implement, and monitor the nutritional care for these patients.[11,12] Strong assistance is needed in nursing care. Three important factors guide this vital nutritional therapy: (1) large catabolic losses, (2) essential anabolic healing demands, and (3) deep personal support needs.

Treatment and prognosis

The plan of care and its outcome depend on several factors:
1. *Age*—elderly persons and very young children are most vulnerable.
2. *Health condition*—the presence of any preexisting condition, such as diabetes, heart or renal disease, or any other associated injuries, complicates care.
3. *Burn severity*—the location and severity of the burn wounds and the time elapsed before treatment are significant.

Degree and extent of burns

The depth of the burn wound affects its healing process (Figure 22.5). Burns are usually classified by degree:
1. First-degree burns—**erythema** involving cell necrosis above the basal layer of the epidermis
2. Second-degree burns—erythema and blistering, and necrosis within the dermis
3. Third-degree burns—full-thickness skin loss, including the fat layer.

First-degree, or partial thickness, burns regenerate new skin tissue from the epithelial cells lining the skin appendages, such as hair follicle, sweat glands, and **sebaceous** glands. Second- and third-degree, or full thickness, burns do not leave sufficient skin for healing purposes. Thus they heal only from the skin margins. Small area burns heal in this manner, but extensive burns require skin grafting.

The body surface area injured by the burn is a basic factor in calculating nutritional support needs. Generally the burn team estimates body surface area involved by the "rule of nines" or by a more accurate calculation using prepared charts. Second- and third-degree burns covering 15% to 20% or more of the total body surface, or even 10% in children and elderly persons, usually cause extensive fluid loss and require intravenous fluid and electrolyte replacement therapy. Burns of severe depth covering more than 50% of the body surface area are often fatal, especially in infants and older persons. Patients with major burn injuries are usually transferred immediately to a specialized burn care facility.

STAGES OF NUTRITIONAL CARE

The nutritional care of the patient with massive burns is constantly adjusted to individual responses and needs. At all times attention to amino acid needs is vital, in addition to critical fluid-electrolyte balance and energy (kcalories) support. Generally, three stages of care may be identified: (1) immediate "ebb" or shock period and following "flow" or recovery response (see *To Probe Further* box, p. 483); (2) secondary critical recovery phase of vigorous feeding; and (3) the follow-up period of reconstructive surgery and rehabilitation.

Stage 1: Immediate shock period

Massive flooding edema occurs at the burn site during the first hours after injury and continues until about the second day. Loss of enveloping skin surface and exposure of tissue fluids lead to immediate loss of water and electrolytes, mainly sodium, and excessive protein depletion. In an effort to balance this loss, water shifts from the surrounding tissue spaces in the body, only adding to the continuous loss at the burn site. As a result, water circulating in the blood is withdrawn, thus decreasing the overall blood volume (*hypovolemia*) and blood pressure. Blood concentration and diminished urine output occur as a result. Cell dehydration follows as cell water is drawn out to balance the tissue fluid losses. Cell potassium is also withdrawn, and circulating serum potassium levels rise.

Immediate intravenous fluid therapy replaces water and electrolytes by use of a balanced salt solution such as **lactated Ringer's solution**, helping to correct the hypovolemia and prevent shock. Acute renal failure is a rare occurrence when resuscitation is started early. During the first part of this initial shock period (the first 12 to 14 hours after the injury) **colloid** solutions such as albumin or plasma are not effective because most of such solutions are lost in fluids at the burn site. Usually vascular endothelial permeability returns to normal after the first day, however, and colloid solutions can then be used to help restore plasma volume. During this initial period, no attempt is made to meet nutritional requirements in protein and kcalories because (1) glucose-free balanced electrolyte solutions are needed, since infusion of glucose at this time

---

colloid   Glutinous, glue like; a dispersion of matter throughout a liquid.

erythema   Redness of the skin produced by coagulation of the capillaries.

lactated Ringer's solution   Sterile solution of calcium chloride, potassium chloride, sodium chloride, and sodium lactate in water given to replenish fluid and electrolytes.

sebaceous   Secreting the fatty lubricating substance *sebum*.

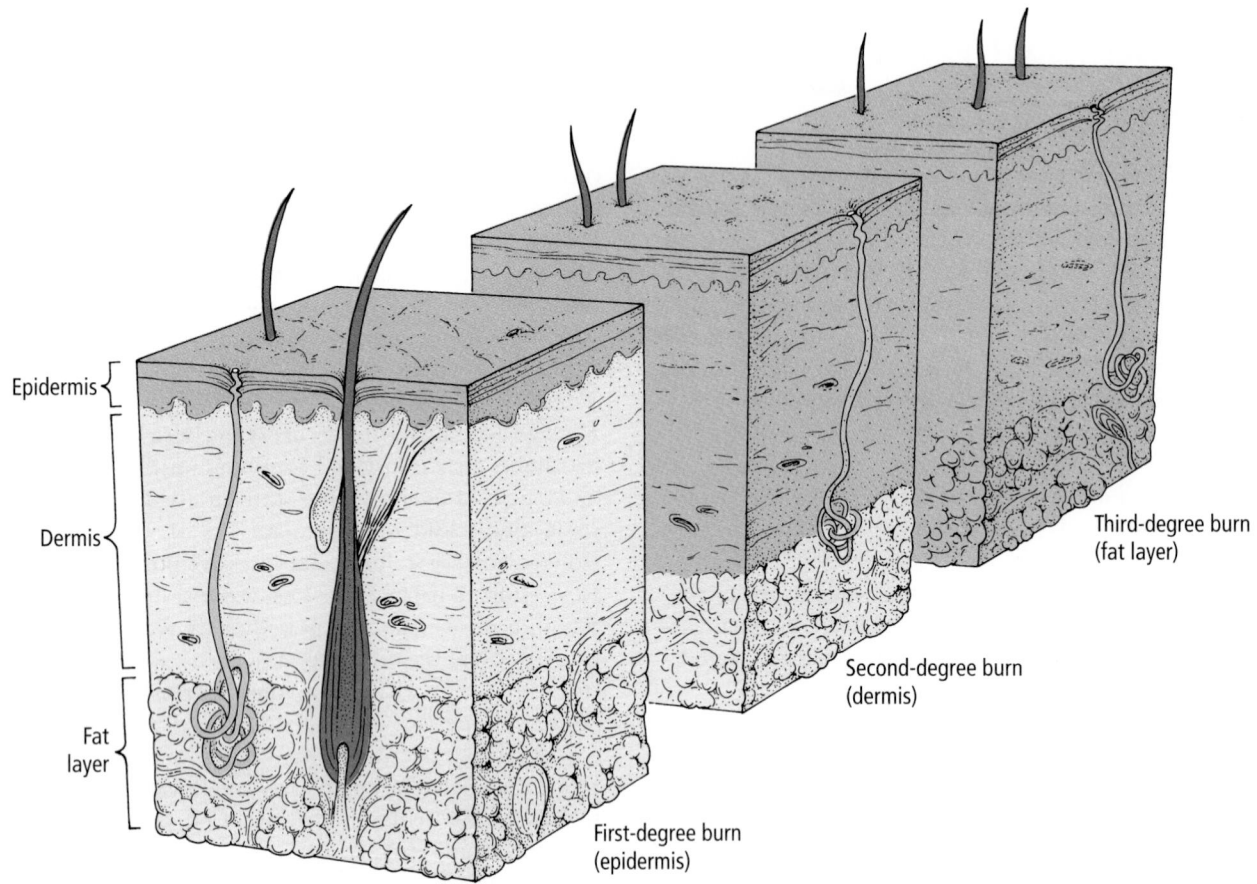

Figure 22.5   Depth of skin area involved in burns.

may result in hyperglycemia; and (2) an *adynamic ileus* (lack of usual functional powers of the lower portion of the small intestine) develops after the injury and precludes any use of the gastrointestinal tract at this time.

Stage 1: Recovery period

After about 48 to 72 hours, tissue fluids and electrolytes are gradually reabsorbed into the general circulation, balance is established, and the pattern of massive tissue loss is reversed. At this point a sudden *diuresis* occurs, indicating successful therapy. The patient returns to preinjury weight by about the end of the first week. A careful check of fluid intake and output is essential, with constant checks for signs of dehydration or overhydration.

Stage 2: Secondary feeding period

Toward the end of the first postburn week, adequate bowel function returns, and a vigorous feeding period must begin. At this point, despite the patient's depression and anorexia, life may depend on rigorous nutritional therapy. Several factors necessitate this increased intake:[12-14]

1. *Tissue destruction*. The massive burn injury has brought large losses of protein and electrolytes that must be replaced.

2. *Tissue catabolism*. Tissue protein breakdown has followed the injury, with consequent loss of lean body mass and nitrogen.

3. *Increased metabolism*. Increased metabolic demands arise from additional needs. **Sepsis** or fever requires extra kcalories for energy needs. Extra carbohydrate and B vitamins are needed for energy as the body resources mobilize to meet heightened basal metabolic requirements. Tissue regeneration requires extra protein and key vitamins such as ascorbic acid and minerals such as zinc. The success of follow-up skin grafting requires optimal tissue health.

Stage 2: Nutritional therapy

Successful nutritional therapy during this critical period is based on vigorous energy and protein therapy, which the burn team clinical dietitian calculates and updates regularly in collaboration with the team physician and nurse.[13-15] This burn protocol then guides therapy.[14]

1. *Energy*. From 3500 to 5000 kcalories, with a high percentage of carbohydrate, is necessary to spare protein for tissue regeneration and to supply the greatly increased metabolic demands for energy.[16] The amount of kcalories required depends on the patient's preburn body weight

To Probe Further

Metabolic response to injury

Two distinct phases of injury response may be identified—the "ebb" and the "flow." The initial ebb phase occurs immediately after the injury and is associated with shock. It is characterized by the following specific metabolic events:

- Decreased oxygen consumption and cardiac output
- Decreased body temperature
- Increased blood glucose accompanied by normal glucose production
- Increased lactate and free fatty acid production
- Increased catecholamine, glucagon, and cortisol levels
- Decreased insulin production and insulin resistance

If the injured patient survives, the ebb phase evolves into the flow phase. This recovery period is characterized by the following events:

- Increased oxygen consumption and cardiac output
- Increased body temperature
- Increased nitrogen excretion
- Mild elevation of blood glucose accompanied by increased glucose production
- Normal lactate level and mild increase of free fatty acid level
- Increased catecholamine, glucagon, and cortisol levels
- Increased insulin production and insulin resistance

Clinical efforts in the ebb phase are focused on maintaining heart action and blood circulation. The flow phase is a period of increased metabolism that demands appropriate nutritional support.

References

Mayes T et al: Evaluation of predicted and measured energy requirements of burned children, *J Am Diet Assoc* 96(1):24, 1996.

Persinger M: Burn protocol sets goals for protein and micronutrient intake, *J Am Diet Assoc* 97(5):489, 1997.

---

and the percent of body surface area burned. The classic Harris-Benedict equations (see Chapter 17, p. 352) may be used to determine basal energy expenditure (BEE) needs. This value is then multiplied by the appropriate metabolic stress activity factor (MAF) involved in such severe illness and trauma (Table 22.3). Adjustment of kcalories is necessary on an individual basis in relation to weight changes or complications such as infection, which change energy requirements.[13,14]

2. *Protein.* Aggressive supplementation of protein is crucial to promote early wound healing and to support immune function.[13] Depending on the extent of the burn injury and catabolic losses, individual needs for protein vary from 150 g to as high as 400 g. Children require two to four times the normal RDAs of protein for age. In general, most adults require an increased amount of protein, 2 to 3 g/kg of body weight, to achieve nitrogen balance.

3. *Vitamins and minerals.* These micronutrients are essential in nutrition support of burn patients because of their roles in immune functions and increased needs for wound healing.[13] From 1 to 2 g of vitamin C may be needed for tissue regeneration. Increased thiamin, riboflavin, and niacin are necessary to metabolize the extra carbohydrate and protein. Special attention is also given to zinc, iron, and vitamin A.

Stage 2: Dietary management

To meet these crucial nutrient demands, either enteral or parenteral modes of feeding may be required.

1. *Enteral feeding.* To achieve the necessary intake of increased nutrient density indicated, a careful intake record must be maintained. Oral feedings are desirable if at all tolerated by the patient. Concentrated oral liquids must be given using protein hydrolysates or amino acids to ensure

---

sepsis Presence in the blood or other tissues of pathogenic microorganisms or their toxins; conditions associated with such pathogens.

Table 22.3	Added energy cost of metabolic stress in illness and trauma, the metabolic activity factor (MAF)

MAF according to degree of stress	Examples of conditions
BEE × 1.25: minimal stress	Nutritionally sound, little stress
BEE × 1.30: moderate stress	Cancer, inflammatory bowel disease, skeletal trauma, minor surgery
BEE × 1.50: severe stress	Cancer, chemotherapy or radiation, burns, major sepsis
BEE × 1.75-2: extreme stress	Acquired immunodeficiency syndrome (AIDS), major trauma or burns

Data from Konishi CD: Metabolic support teams as nutrition educators: who supports whom? *Top Clin Nutr* 1(4):51, 1986.
MAF, Metabolic activity factor; *BEE,* basal energy expenditure.

adequate intake. Commercial formulas are usually used to supply large amounts of nourishment. Solid foods, according to individual food preferences, are added by about the second week. Tube feeding may be required by some patients in the beginning. In this case low-bulk defined formula solutions may be given through small-bore feeding tubes (see Chapter 17). In either case, continuous support and encouragement are necessary. Food should be made as attractive and appetizing as possible, supplying items particularly liked and respecting disliked foods.

2. *Parenteral feeding.* For some patients, oral intake and tube feedings may be inadequate to meet the accelerated demands or may be impossible because of associated injuries or complications. In these cases parenteral feeding through a large central vein or peripheral vein is needed to provide the essential nutritional support. Details of this often life-saving procedure are given in Chapter 17.

Stage 3: Follow-up reconstruction

Continued vigorous nutrition support is essential to maintain tissue integrity for successful skin grafting or plastic reconstructive surgery. In addition, the principles of rehabilitative care discussed in Chapter 25 apply in the case of burned patients. The patient needs not only physical rebuilding of body resources but also much personal support to rebuild the human will and spirit, since there may be disfigurement and disability. Health team members can do much to help instill the courage and confidence the person must have to face the future again. However, whatever the future demands, optimal physical stamina gained through persistent, supportive care—medical, nutritional, and nursing—helps each patient rebuild the personal resources needed to cope.

TO SUM UP

The nutritional demands of surgery begin before the patient reaches the operating table. Preoperatively the task is to correct any existing deficiencies and build nutrient reserves to meet surgical demands. Postoperatively it is to replace losses and support recovery. The additional task of encouraging eating is often required during this period.

Presurgical and postsurgical feedings are given in a variety of ways. The oral route is always preferred, but damage to the intestinal tract or a poor appetite may require other enteral or parenteral feedings. Diets are modified according to the surgical procedure performed. For the depleted surgical patient or the critically burned patient, nutritional support relies heavily on biomedical technology to facilitate enteral and parenteral feedings administered by specially trained nutrition support team members.

■ QUESTIONS FOR REVIEW

1. Describe the general impact of imbalances of the following nutritional factors during the preoperative, immediate postoperative, and later postoperative periods: protein, kcalories, vitamins, minerals, and fluids.

2. Describe the major surgical effects for which nutrition therapy must be planned following these procedures: mouth, throat, and neck surgery; gastric resection; cholecystectomy; and rectal surgery.

3. Write a 1-day meal plan for a person experiencing the postgastrectomy dumping syndrome. What general dietary guidelines are used? Why?

4. Describe the difference in care between an ileostomy and a colostomy. What are the dietary implications of each?

5. Outline the nutritional care of a burn patient from treatment for immediate shock through recovery and tissue reconstruction.

■ REFERENCES

1. Campos ACL, Meguid MM: A critical appraisal of the usefulness of perioperative nutritional support, *Am J Clin Nutr* 55:117, 1992.

2. Zuckerman J: Hip fracture, *N Engl J Med* 334(23):1519, 1996.

3. Lipkin R: Bone fracture: treatment and risks, *Sci News* 147(12):180, 1995.

4. Adama SO et al: Military RDs improve oral liquid diets, *J Am Diet Assoc* 94(1):24, 1994.

5. Sachdeva AK et al: Surgical treatment of peptic ulcer disease, *Med Clin North Am* 75(4):999, 1991.

6. Frandzel S: The incredible shrinking surgery, *Am Health* 13(3):80, 1994.

7. Stix G: Boot camp for surgeons, *Sci Am* 273(3):24, 1995.

8. Tyns FJ et al: Diet tolerance and stool frequency in patients with ileoanal reservoirs, *J Am Diet Assoc* 92(7):861, 1992.

9. Alles MS et al: Bacterial fermentation of fructooligosaccharides and resistant starch in patients with an ileal pouch–anal anastomosis, *Am J Clin Nutr* 666(June 1):1286, 1997.

10. Miedema BW et al: Absorption and motility of the bypassed human ileum, *Dis Colon Rectum* 33:829, 1990.

11. Ireton-Jones CS, Baxter CR: Nutrition for adult burn patients: a review, *Nutr Clin Pract* 6(1):3, 1990.

12. Prelack K et al: Urinary urea nitrogen is imprecise as a predictor of protein balance in burned children, *J Am Diet Assoc* 97(5):489, 1997.

13. Persinger M: Burn protocol sets goals for protein and micronutrient intake, *J Am Diet Assoc* 97(5):495, 1997.

14. Hustler DA: Nutrition monitoring of a pediatric burn patient, *Nutr Clin Pract* 6(1):11, 1991.

15. Mayes T et al: Evaluation of predicted and measured energy requirements in burned children, *J Am Diet Assoc* 96(1):24, 1996.

16. Gottschlich MM et al: Lack of effect of sleep on energy expenditure and physiologic measures in critically ill burn patients, *J Am Diet Assoc* 97(2):131, 1997.

■ FURTHER READING

Cerra FB: How nutrition intervention changes what getting sick means, *J Parenter Enter Nutr* 14(suppl 5):164, 1990.

This article provides a good review of three basic factors that influence what is observed at an ill patient's bedside when considering the effects of nutrition intervention: (1) the disease process inherent in the metabolic response to injury, (2) the presence of starvation, and (3) the presence of the nutritional intervention.

Hustler DA: Nutritional monitoring of a pediatric burn patient, *Nutr Clin Pract* 6:11, 1991.

This experienced dietitian-specialist on a burn-center team provides a case report of a young boy who sustained mostly full-thickness burns over 56% of his total body surface area. She describes in detail the challenge of initial evaluation and therapy, constant close monitoring, and appropriate responses to changing needs.

Tynes JJ et al: Diet tolerance and stool frequency in patients with ileoanal reservoirs, *J Am Diet Assoc* 92(7):861, 1992.

This brief report of a survey of patients with ileoanal reservoirs provides much helpful background information about this recently developed alternative surgical procedure to the ileostomy, with practical guidance for nutritional management and patient counseling.

Case study

The patient with a gastrectomy

Walter Reilly is a 42-year-old male admitted for a total gastrectomy 4 weeks ago. He had a history of repeated episodes of pain and bleeding, for which he had been hospitalized twice during the last 6 months.

Surgery proceeded smoothly, with an anastomosis established between the esophagus and the jejunum. Mr. Reilly received nothing orally for 48 hours postoperatively but received TPN to give nutritional support. He was then given ice chips and water, which he gradually began to tolerate.

Two days later Mr. Reilly was able to tolerate 30 to 60 ml (2 to 4 tbsp; 1 to 2 oz) of milk between sips of water. This amount increased, as did his appetite. He was graduated to servings of a single soft food (eggs, cereal, custards, potato) once or twice a day. By the end of the second week he was tolerating a full soft diet on six small feedings daily. He was cautioned to use liquids in moderation during a discharge diet session conducted 1 week later.

At a later follow-up visit with his physician, Mr. Reilly complained of general discomfort and cramping following meals. Other symptoms included a rapid heart rate, dizziness, nausea and vomiting, and breaking out into a cold sweat. He had also begun to lose weight, and appeared slightly emaciated. His physician referred him to the clinical nutritionist to explore any problem with eating habits. Mr. Reilly seemed to accept most of her recommendations. One week later he telephoned to explain that all symptoms had subsided and that he was tolerating the diet well.

Questions for Analysis

1. Do you think that the surgical procedure performed was warranted? Defend your response.
2. Explain the physiologic rationale for the refeeding program as planned.
3. What nutrient would you emphasize in this patient's diet? Why? What is its significance with surgery?
4. Why was some fluid limitation recommended?
5. Account for the symptoms that followed eating. What dietary recommendations would you make to control them?

Issues Answers

New methods for assessing nutritional status?

Traditional methods used to assess nutritional status and needs rely heavily on the use of *objective* measures such as anthropometry, clinical criteria, laboratory tests, and, in some instances, indirect calorimetry. But how does *subjective* evaluation relate? What role does it play in getting the whole picture of the patient's situation and its effect on health and illness?

Canadian researchers seeking some answers to these questions have been studying the relationships between these two basic assessment approaches. Working with hospitalized surgery patients, they demonstrated a subjective clinical assessment of nutritional needs based on a history and physical examination, which they have called a "subjective global assessment" (SGA). They have found that this subjective approach is highly correlated with assessments made using the usual objective measures. They also found that with SGA, postoperative infections could be predicted as well or better than with objective measures.

In follow-up study the investigators applied SGA to 202 patients before gastrointestinal surgery and examined the effect of individual characteristics on the SGA ratings. This study confirmed the validity of SGA as a technique of nutritional assessment. SGA ratings are based on five features of the patient history:

- Weight changes (loss) in the past 6 months and changes in the past 2 weeks

- Changes in dietary intake
- Gastrointestinal symptoms (nausea, vomiting, diarrhea, and anorexia) that have persisted over 2 weeks
- Functional capacity (ambulatory or bed-bound)
- Presence of disease and its relation to nutritional needs

Four features of the physical examination are rated as normal, mild, moderate, or severe for five parameters:

- Loss of subcutaneous fat (triceps and chest)
- Muscle wasting (quadriceps and deltoids)
- Ankle and sacral edema
- Ascites

On the basis of these features of the history and physical examination, health team members identify an SGA rank, which indicates the person's nutritional status: well nourished, moderate or suspected malnutrition, or severe malnutrition.

The researchers feel that a major advantage of SGA is its flexibility in capturing subtle patterns of change in clinical variables and relating them to the effects of disease or surgical stress.

References

Detsky AS et al: What is subjective global assessment of nutritional status? *J Parenter Enter Nutr* 11(1):8, 1987.
Detsky AS et al: Is this patient malnourished? *JAMA* 271:54, 1994.

Chapter

23

Nutrition and Acquired Immuno-deficiency Syndrome (AIDS)

In this chapter of our clinical series we focus on acquired immunodeficiency syndrome (AIDS). This modern-day plague has eluded medical science's search for a cure and left countless numbers of infected and dying young adults and children in its wake.

Here we examine the background of the AIDS epidemic and the nature of the human immunodeficiency virus-1 (HIV-1). We review the current state of medical management, especially the component of nutritional support and its relation to nutritional status and the course of the disease. As knowledge of the disease process has grown over the past decade, it has become increasingly evident that nutritional support plays a vital role in the care of HIV-infected and AIDS patients.

EVOLUTION OF HIV AND THE AIDS EPIDEMIC

In the late 1970s, physicians on the East and West coasts of the United States, centered in New York City and San Francisco, became puzzled about an uncommon medical problem appearing among their patients.[1] No known cause of immune suppression could be found. Nonetheless they were suffering and dying from complications of common infections, largely pneumonia, ordinarily handled easily by the human immune system and the usual antibiotics or other antibacterial drugs. Its **virus** source and **pandemic** effects were soon to become alarmingly evident world wide.

EVOLUTION OF HIV

Social change

Where did this new deadly virus come from and how did it gain such strength? Apparently, HIV represents not a new virus but an old one that has in recent years grown deadly in humans as it gained strength during the social upheavals of the 1960s and 1970s. The uprooting effect of this rapid social change and urbanization allowed the virus to spread rapidly through world populations and reproduce aggressively in its human host.

Parasite nature of virus

No virus can have a life of its own. All viruses by their structure and nature are **parasites**. They are mere shreds of genetic material, a small packet of genetic information encased in a protein coat. They contain only a small chromosome of nucleic acids (RNA or DNA), usually with fewer than five genes (see Chapter 24). They can only live through a host, whom they invade and infect. There they hijack the host's cell machinery to run off a multitude of copies of themselves. Their purpose is to make as many self-copies as they can. Today's viruses are those that succeeded in that task over time and are, like all plants and animals, simply descendants of earlier forms. Scientists agree that the human immunoviruses HIV-1 and HIV-2 are genetically similar to viruses found in African primates such as monkeys and apes (SIV, simian immunodeficiency virus) and were probably transmitted to humans in an earlier age.

The earliest known case of AIDS has recently been identified in an African blood sample collected in 1959 from a Bantu man living presently in the Democratic Republic of Congo, an area from which the current epidemic is believed to have spread.[2] This sample is the oldest HIV infection discovered so far, indicating that it predates the time at which the virus divided into several of the current varieties that now infect different parts of the world. Over the years HIV has mutated to form 10 different subtypes, lettered A through J. Recent reports from Africa indicate that in a stretch of sub-Saharan

countries know as the AIDS belt, nearly 25% of the urban population is infected with AIDS.[3] Although the course of the present world wide epidemic is difficult to predict, there is a growing sense of guarded optimism among the leading scientists based on the current research agenda, especially among the increasing number of young, newly trained scientists with new ideas and a changing United States culture of AIDS research that embraces more cooperative team attitudes.[4-7]

DISEASE PROGRESSION

The individual clinical course of HIV infection varies substantially. Nonetheless, three distinct stages mark the progression of the disease and are usually referred to as (1) primary HIV infection and extended asymptomatic incubation, (2) AIDS-related complex (ARC), and (3) terminal AIDS.

Primary HIV infection

After initial docking of the virus on the cell surface receptor protein CD4, initial infection takes place with the aid of the recently discovered cofactor *fusin*. The National Institutes of Health discovery team, led by Edward Berger, so named this cofactor because together with CD4, it allows cells to fuse with the HIV surface, a key step in the infection process.[8] This discovery raises the prospect of new therapies to block this binding to *fusin*, thus limiting HIV's ability to infect cells.

About 2 to 4 weeks after initial exposure and infection, a mild flu-like syndrome lasting about a week, may or may not occur. This brief response corresponds to the process of *seroconversion*, the development of antibodies to the viral infection. Subsequent HIV testing will be positive. Signs of enlarged lymph nodes may occur, and an extended asymptomatic "well" period usually continues for the next 8 to 10 years. However, this seemingly inac-

---

pandemic A widespread epidemic, distributed through a region, continent, or the world.

parasite An organism that lives on or in an organism of another species, known as the host, from whom all life cycle nourishment is obtained.

virus Minute infectious agent, characterized by lack of independent metabolism and by the ability to reproduce with genetic continuity only with living host cells. They range in decreasing size from about 200 nanometers (nm) down to only 15 nanometers (nm). (A nanometer is a linear measure equal to one-billionth of a meter; it is also called a millimicron.) Each particle (virion) consists basically of nucleic acids (genetic material) and a protein shell, which protects and contains the genetic material and any enzymes present.

tive, relatively well period can be deceiving. Recent research indicates that it is actually a crucial stage in the underlying growth of the virus.[9,10] This extended period is a critical stage of viral incubation, during which the virus appears to be inactive. In reality it is hiding in lymphoid tissues, such as lymph nodes, spleen, adenoid glands and tonsils, multiplying constantly in its parasite life cycle within its host, taking over more and more white blood cells and gaining strength.[11,12]

New research findings demonstrate the complexity and strength of this disease and the problems presented in finding a solution to stem the epidemic tide. These researchers and their colleagues underscore the crucial nature of this incubation period and the importance of earlier treatment intervention after HIV-seropositive detection, to slow this viral-strengthening hiatus while developing drugs and vaccine to combat its steady progression.

AIDS-related complex (ARC)

After the extended asymptomatic HIV-positive stage, which may last as long as 10 years, a period of associated infectious illnesses begins. This AIDS-related complex of opportunistic illnesses is so named because the HIV infection has now killed enough host protective white T-cells (mainly T-helper or CD4+ lymphocytes) to severely damage the immune system and lower the body's normal disease resistance. At this point, even the most common infections have an open opportunity to take root and grow. Common symptoms observed during this pre-AIDS period include persistent fatigue, thrush (oral *Candida albicans*), night sweats, diarrhea, fever over 100° F, unintentional weight loss of 5 kg (11 lb) or more, remarkable headache, new skin rash, new or unusual cough, sore throat or mouth, unusual bruises or skin discoloration, and shortness of breath.[13]

Final stage of AIDS

The terminal stage of HIV infection, commonly designated as AIDS, is marked by declining T-helper lymphocyte counts from the normal healthy level of about 1000 such cells in every cubic millimeter of blood ($1000/mm^3$). HIV-infected persons usually experience a decline of these cells by an average of about 40 to $80/mm^3$ every year.[13] Generally, when the falling T-helper lymphocyte counts are roughly between 500 and $200/mm^3$, diseases such as tuberculosis or Kaposi's sarcoma (the most common AIDS-associated malignancy) occur; at counts below $200/mm^3$, *Pneumocystis carinii* pneumonia and *Toxoplasma gondii* (protozoan parasites able to infect a number of body organs) appear; and at counts under $50/mm^3$, cytomegalovirus (CMV) or **lymphoma** can flourish.[14] When the virus finally kills enough white cells to overwhelm the weakened immune system resistance to the disease complications, death follows.

PUBLIC HEALTH SERVICE RESPONSIBILITIES

In any major epidemic, the Public Health Service and its related agencies have the major task of monitoring and stopping the disease spread. Thus they carry responsibilities in two major areas: (1) surveillance, including testing and counseling; and (2) community education and prevention through interrupting its spread, vaccine research, and treatment.

Surveillance

Throughout the AIDS epidemic, as knowledge of this new disease and its nature has grown, the United States Centers for Disease Control (CDC) in Atlanta has worked with state and territorial health departments and has been involved in constant world wide knowledge exchange, to conduct accurate and comprehensive AIDS surveillance in the United States.[14] Since the mid-1980s, such seroprevalence studies have provided a massive amount of information about HIV spread in various population groups and have helped CDC develop early classification guidelines for medical teams caring for HIV-infected patients. The periodic CDC revisions of surveillance criteria reflect advances in the care and understanding of disease caused by HIV infection. In accord with current knowledge and the evolution of the HIV epidemic among demographic groups, CDC has expanded the AIDS surveillance definition to include any HIV-seropositive person with a CD4+ (specific T-lymphocyte subset analysis) cell count of less than 200 cells per microliter of blood.[14]

Because of the tremendous life-changing import of a positive HIV-1 test result to the individual and his or her family and loved ones, public health testing programs have developed a coordinated pretest and posttest counseling component, especially in clinics serving high-risk areas.[15] First, a brief pretest interview assesses personal knowledge of HIV infection, provides risk-reduction education, and offers the HIV test. Then those who accept the HIV testing are given a 2-week return appointment for a longer follow-up review of test results and counseling concerning health care and personal needs.

Education and prevention

The United States Department of Health and Human Services (DHHS), through its Public Health Service and Food and Drug Administration divisions, has provided national health promotion and disease prevention objectives for the year 2000 that call for the expansion of HIV education and prevention efforts.[16] Wide community involvement in the community-based process of developing any health promotion or disease prevention program is essential for its successful outcome.[17] This need has been shown, for example, in the mobilizing of community leadership and resources to plan and implement interventions in other health problems such as heart disease or changing lifestyle habits (such as smoking) that contribute to lung disease.

The community-support need is particularly true with HIV infection. Despite its burdening social stigma, it is reaching into all communities in some form, cutting short the lives of children, adolescents, and young adults in ever increasing numbers. The Harvard Global AIDS Policy Coalition estimates that by the year 2000 between 38 million and 110 million adults and more than 10 million children will be infected world wide.[18] Such a deadly pandemic epidemic warrants mobilizing and coordinating the most realistic and effective preventive strategies possible for all ethnic and socioeconomic community groups to change sexual risk-taking behavior at all levels—local, national, and international.[19-22] New drugs are certainly lightening the horizon, but they can never be enough; *prevention* is still our best weapon for taking aim on any front.[23,24]

NATURE OF THE DISEASE PROCESS

ACTION OF HIV ON THE IMMUNE SYSTEM

HIV-1 and HIV-2 are members of a class of viruses called **retrovirus** because their unique life cycle involves a reverse transcription of RNA into DNA in the cell nucleus, which is then integrated into the host cell DNA.[2] The virus consists of an outer envelope with attached surface proteins covering the outer protective shell and an inner shell that contains the small strands of ribonucleic acid (RNA) genetic material and enzymes, including the reverse transcriptase. Of the virus's nine genes, four apparently less essential ones are poorly understood. After entering the body, the virus attaches to host cells, mostly the actively replicating T-helper (CD4+) white blood cells, major lymphocytes of the body's immune system. There it integrates itself into the host cell's DNA copying system, infecting and eventually killing the host cell. Rapidly increasing masses of virus particles erupt from the dying cells in small buds to immediately infect new cells.

METHODS OF TRANSMISSION AND GROUPS AT RISK

Throughout the world, sexual behavior is central to the epidemic spread of HIV and AIDS. An estimated 71% of HIV infection world wide is a result of heterosexual behavior and 15% is a result of homosexual behavior; only a relatively small proportion is a result of intravenous drug use with contaminated needles.[20] In the United States, in a 1995 report covering the year 1994, the Centers for Disease Control (CDC) of the Public Health Service indicated that AIDS cases by type of transmission were as follows[23]:

- 43.3% male homosexual/bisexual behavior
- 31.8% intravenous drug use with shared blood contaminated needles

- 27% women and heterosexual men
- 4.8% male homosexual/bisexual contact
- 10.3% heterosexual contact
- 1.2% perinatal transmission
- 1% blood transfusions
- 0.6% persons with hemophilia

The remaining cases were listed as "no risk reported." Of the total 80,691 reported cases, 79,674 (99%) occurred among adolescents and adults (persons 13 years or older) and 1017 occurred among children younger than 13 years. Overall, women, blacks, Hispanics, and persons in the South and Northeast accounted for higher percentages of reported cases than the previous year, and the largest decline was among homosexual/bisexual men.[23]

Vertical transmission from infected mothers to their babies during pregnancy or at birth is a growing concern. Approximately 7000 infants are born to HIV-infected women in the United States each year.[24] Questions remain about maternal transmission through breast-feeding.[25,26] The increase in pediatric cases of HIV infection brings more concern, and care of these children requires special consideration (see *Issues & Answers*, p. 506). The fastest growing subgroup of new heterosexual cases is among women, with the proportion among younger women and adolescent girls alarmingly high.[18,27]

Groups at risk

Persons at greatest risk of HIV infection are those who, if sexually active, are not consistently practicing responsible and safe sexual behavior, which consists of (1) consistent and correct condom use for protection (the regular latex male sheath, the female polyurethane condom, or a cervical cap approved for use by the Food and Drug Administration),[28-30] and (2) avoidance of sex with multiple partners and persons at risk for HIV. Others at risk are intravenous drug users who share contaminated needles. Since the public-donated blood supply for transfusions has been thoroughly cleared of HIV infection by a rigorous double-testing program, this route of infection risk by blood units for medical purposes has virtually been eliminated.

---

lymphoma General term applied to any neoplastic disorder (cancer) of the lymphoid tissue.

retrovirus Any of a family of single-strand RNA viruses having an envelope and containing a reverse coding enzyme that allows for a reversal of genetic transcription from RNA to DNA rather than the usual DNA to RNA, the newly transcribed viral DNA then being incorporated into the host cell's DNA strand for the production of new RNA retroviruses.

DIAGNOSIS OF HIV INFECTION

Testing procedures

HIV infection is diagnosed by detection of the virus or serologic response to the virus. HIV infection can be identified by detection of specific antibodies, as is done in the routine screening of blood and blood products for transfusion and in most epidemiologic studies. The recommended procedure for virus detection is a two-step process. First is *enzyme-linked immunosorbent assay (ELISA)* screening. Second, suspected positive samples from the ELISA screening are followed by *Western blot* testing for confirmation. Both of these tests are highly sensitive and specific, and both are used to confirm the results before informing the individual. Because a positive test is such a personal and life-changing event, most experienced physicians caring for HIV-infected patients repeat all positive tests again, even when they have been confirmed by Western blot, before informing the individual. Requirements for the testing procedure include pretest and posttest counseling to cover such issues as:

- **Medical significance** of the test, whether positive or negative
- **Limitations** of the test

Table

23.1   Common infectious complications of AIDS

Microorganism	Clinical manifestation
Parasites	
Pneumocystis carinii	Pneumonia
Toxoplasma gondii	Focal encephalitis, pneumonia
Cryptosporidium	Malabsorption, diarrhea
Isospora belli	Diarrhea
Microspora	Malabsorption, diarrhea
Entamoeba histolytica	Diarrhea
Giardia lamblia	Diarrhea
Acanthamoeba	Meningoencephalitis
Bacteria	
Campylobacter	Diarrhea, bacteremia
Legionella	Pneumonia
Listeria monocytogenes	Meningitis, bacteremia
Mycobacterium avium-intracellulare	Tuberculosis, diarrhea, other mycobacteria
Norcardia	Pneumonia, encephalitis
Pneumococcus	Pneumonia
Salmonella	Diarrhea, bacteremia
Shigella	Diarrhea, bacteremia
Haemophilus influenzae	Pneumonia
Streptococcus pneumoniae	Pneumonia
Staphylococcus aureus	Pneumonia
Fungi	
Aspergillus	Fungemia, pneumonia
Candida albicans	Thrush, stomatitis, esophagitis, pneumonia
Cryptococcus neoformans	Meningitis, pneumonitis
Histoplasma capsulatum	Pneumonitis, skin lesions
Coccidioides immitis	Pneumonitis
Viruses	
Cytomegalovirus	Esophagitis, pneumonitis, diarrhea
Herpes simplex virus	Ulcerative mucocutaneous lesions, stomatitis, esophagitis, pneumonia
Epstein-Barr virus	EBV-positive non-Hodgkin's lymphomas, oral hairy leukoplakia
Hepatitis B	Nausea, vomiting, fever, antigenemia
Herpes zoster	Multiple dermatomal zoster
Papillomavirus	Oral hairy leukoplakia

Modified from Gold JWM: HIV-1 infection: diagnosis and management, *Med Clin North Am* 76(1):1, 1992; Bernard EM et al: Pneumocystosis, *Med Clin North Am* 76(1):107, 1992; and Ralten DJ: Nutrition and HIV infection: a review and evaluation of the extent of knowledge of the relationship between nutrition and HIV infection, *Nutr Clin Prac* 6(3):1S, 1991.

- **Information** about HIV-1 and AIDS, how they are spread, and how to prevent their spread
- **Medical, nutritional, and psychosocial care** availability
- **Confidentiality** concept involved with documentation in the medical record; possible social and legal results of testing, personal needs and support system

Clinical symptoms and illnesses

The early clinical symptoms that may follow initial exposure to the virus add further confirmation to the HIV-seropositive testing procedures. These initial symptoms, as well as possible associated illnesses and diseases that characterize the later ARC and AIDS stages, have been generally described above in discussing the basic disease progression. Some examples of these common infectious complications of AIDS and their clinical problems are listed in Table 23.1.

BASIC ROLE OF NUTRITION IN HIV DISEASE PROCESS

Nutrition support plays a vital role throughout the HIV disease process in two basic areas. First, it is a vital component of care for the involuntary weight loss and body tissue wasting caused by the disease effects on metabolism, reflected in the severe state of protein-energy malnutrition. Second, and fundamental in all conditions associated with the body's basic immune system (see extended discussion in Chapter 24), nutrition is an intimate and integral component of care through the specific roles of key nutrients in maintaining the body's immunocompetence. Furthermore, for many of the associated diseases, individual nutritional status influences the impact of morbidity and mortality irrespective of the disease process.

MEDICAL MANAGEMENT

BASIC CURRENT GOALS

The medical management of HIV-1 infection in all its stages is constantly evolving as medical research seeks to eliminate, or at least suppress, the virus. Intensive current research is aimed at preventing the progressive immunodeficiency, stopping HIV-1 transmission to uninfected persons, and restoring depressed immune function to normal to prevent AIDS-associated complications. Thus present basic medical management objectives are to (1) delay progression of the infection and improve the patient's immune system, (2) prevent opportunistic illnesses, and (3) recognize the infection early and provide rapid treatment for any complications of immune deficiency, including infections and cancers.

INITIAL EVALUATION: AIDS TEAM

The initial medical evaluation of a newly diagnosed HIV infected patient is critical in beginning and continuing the ongoing comprehensive care by the AIDS team of professional medical, nutritional, nursing, and psychosocial health care specialists. Box 23.1 outlines an initial evaluation guide for beginning the care of a person with newly identified HIV-1 infection. These guidelines emphasize the special coordinated care by all members of the AIDS team, and the importance of personal nutritional and psychosocial support.

ANTIRETROVIRAL DRUG THERAPY

After the initial discovery and identification of HIV-1, research began in earnest to develop effective antiretroviral drugs to inhibit replication of the virus. Although the problems involved are complex and the task has been frustrating, two classes of antiretroviral drugs have been developed and are now being used: (1) reverse transcriptase inhibitors (RTIs) and (2) protease inhibitors.[31]

Reverse transcriptase inhibitors (RTIs)

One of the earliest findings in this drug research effort was that certain members of a class of compounds called

---

Box 23.1 Initial evaluation of newly diagnosed HIV-infected patients

Routine history and physical examination include:
  History of exposure to infectious complications of AIDS
  Assessment of baseline mental status
Baseline laboratory studies
  CBC, differential, platelets
  Biochemistry screening profile
  Urinalysis
  Chest x-ray examination
  Tuberculin test with anergy panel
  Serologic test for syphilis
  Toxoplasma serology
  T-lymphocyte subsets
  Hepatitis B serology (optional)
Nutritional assessment, counseling, support, and follow-up
Psychosocial and financial status assessment
Referral to and involvement in psychosocial support include:
  Social worker, nurse, psychologist or psychiatrist, patient support group, community support group, and agencies
Rehabilitation program for substance abusers
Planning for family members and children, including issues of testing and providing for their care.

Modified from Gold JWM: HIV-1 infection: diagnosis and management, *Med Clin North Am* 76(1)1, 1992.

Table 23.2 Protease inhibitor drug side effects and related food guide		
Protease inhibitor drugs	**Drug side effects**	**Related food guide**
Saquinavir	Diarrhea, nausea	Take after a high-kcalorie, high-fat meal for best absorption
Indinavir	Taste changes, nausea, vomiting, diarrhea	Best absorbed on an empty stomach or a nonfat light snack
		Increase fluids to about 24 oz/day (consider weight and age)
		Increased kcalories are needed, substitute juices
Ritonavir	Diarrhea, nausea, vomiting, appetite loss, abnormal mouth feelings (burning, prickling)	Take with high-kcalorie, high-fat foods.
	Elevated blood cholesterol and triglyceride levels	
Nelfinavir	Diarrhea, loose stools	Take with food
Nevirapine	Skin rash, mouth sores, general fatigue	Take with food on an empty stomach

Adapted from Heller LS, Shattuck, L: Nutrition support with children with HIV/AIDS, *J Am Diet Assoc* 97(5):473, 1997.

dideoxynucleosides effectively inhibited HIV-1 replication in the laboratory.[32] Subsequent clinical trials with HIV-infected patients have shown that in human cells, dideoxynucleosides act as competitive inhibitors of the virus's necessary enzyme for replicating itself, *HIV reverse transcriptase*, thus effectively preventing viral increase.[33-35] Thus drugs in this class are called *reverse transcription inhibitors (RTIs)*. Currently, five RTIs are in use:

1. *AZT* (generic name *zidovudine* [Retrovir]). AZT inhibits growth of HIV in HIV-positive patients, delaying advancing stages of ARC and HIV. It is usually given early to slow the initial viral growth.[36,37]
2. *3TC*. This RTI works synergistically with AZT to slow the development of resistance to AZT.
3. *d4T (dideoxythymidinene)*. This RTI and the two following ones form a class of RTIs called dideoxynucleosides. They have enhanced and strengthened combination therapy using several drugs in each dosage.
4. *ddc (dideoxycytidine)*
5. *ddl (dideoxyinosine)*

Protease inhibitors

Protease is the HIV enzyme that the virus depends on to assemble itself properly. This recent class of drugs helps stop HIV by inhibiting this basic enzyme essential to its development[32,33]:

1. *Saquinavir*
2. *Indinavir*
3. *Ritonavir*
4. *Nelfinavir*
5. *Nevirapine*

Some possible side effects of these drugs are shown in Table 23-2 with food uses to minimize these effects. Some of these side effects, such as nausea, may be helped by diet modifications (see Chapter 24). Micronutrient supplements, as shown in Table 23-3, are used to counteract nutrient deficiencies and malnutrition, a large risk factor in immune response and disease.

The results of AZT in patient therapy have been found to diminish over time as the virus, confronted by the drug, readily mutates into slight variations of the drug's range, making the virus slightly less efficient with each mutation.[36,37] However, this combination therapy, with two or three of the new drugs that have complementary actions being taken together, is now achieving more effective results over longer periods of time, especially in reducing reservoirs of infection hidden in lymph tissues.[38,39] But this multiple drug therapy, requiring dozens of pills daily, is expensive.[40]

Self-testing monitoring kits

The large-growing AIDS-related market has led to the development of self-testing kits used by patients and their physicians to help make treatment decisions. Most of these monitors measure levels of white blood cells with a CD4+ receptor, the receiving point used by HIV's surface protein to infect cells. These measures indicates how much damage has been done to the immune system.

CONTINUING RESEARCH AND FUTURE DEVELOPMENTS

Continuing research for a long-awaited vaccine against HIV has thus far been disappointing. Researchers are

Table 23.3 Micronutrients immune response deficiency and supplement effects		
Micronutrient	**Immune response deficiency**	**Supplement effects**
Vitamins		
Vitamin A	Impaired response; increase infections and subsequent mortality	Improves immunity; excess is toxic
Beta carotene	Impaired immunity, increased cancer risk	Enhances response, CD4+ T-cells
B vitamins	Reduced lymphoid tissue	Vitamin B_{12} enhances skin test, mitogen response; vitamin B_6 does not enhance above reactions
Vitamin C	Impaired phagocytosis	May enhance immune function
Vitamin E	T-, B-cell dysfunction	Enhances immunity, skin test response, and function
Minerals		
Copper	Impaired function of macrophages	Good repletion, but excess can be toxic
Iron	Reduced immune response	Excess can harm
Selenium	Low intake, cancer risk	Repletion contributes to survival; excess can impair immunity
Zinc	Loss of T-cell immunity	Improves with moderate supplementation; excess can harm

Modified from Cunningham-Rundles S et al: Micronutrient and cytokine interaction in congenital pediatric HIV infection, *J Nutr* 126(10S):2674S, 1996.

redoubling their efforts to find answers to basic research problems involved.[41] The search for a vaccine is nearing the stage of international trials. Sites are being selected in representative endemic areas, such as central Africa, southeast Asia, Brazil, and the United States. Although it continues to be a bumpy road with rough spots still ahead, researchers and policy makers, as well as involved drug companies, are digging in for the long haul of finding answers, perhaps based on new vaccine strategies that use gene therapy—DNA instead of protein—which has recently been proposed.[42] In the final analysis, all persons involved have learned that vaccines remain the best long-term hope for the prevention of AIDS—and they *will* come.[43]

Undoubtedly the epidemiology and treatment of HIV-1 infection will change rapidly over the next few years. Patients will live longer and have improved quality of life. Nonetheless, with longer life and treatment for known complications, new complications will probably appear, such as uncommon infections, neurologic disease, or wasting syndromes. The medical management of AIDS will continue to require highly involved health care professionals and patients, as well as community support.

demic, terminal disease, and its treatment varies according to individual status and needs—medical, nutritional, and psychosocial. Research breakthroughs will help light the course, but in every case, health care professionals and patients must remain highly involved, seeking the best possible individual care each step of the way.

There are many causes of malnutrition in HIV infection. Thus at any point, nutritional recommendations and support must be individual and integrated with other therapies. Nutritional care plans must provide a comprehensive view of the disease process through each stage, specific drug use, and the patient's wishes. All patients diagnosed as HIV infected should be considered to be at nutritional risk. Although the patient may be in an earlier, asymptomatic period, the disease process, its complications, or treatments will begin to take their toll on the person's nutritional status. The nutritional status of any HIV-infected person may be compromised in numerous ways. At all times, each patient must be viewed within the context of his or her own disease and individual lifestyle.

NUTRITIONAL MANAGEMENT

BASIC APPROACH: INDIVIDUAL STATUS AND NEEDS

Although answers will eventually come to many of our puzzling questions, HIV infection is still an elusive, epi-

dideoxynucleosides Nucleoside, basic type of chemical compound involved. A class of drugs used to treat HIV-infected persons; a nucleoside is a combination of a sugar (a pentose) with a purine or pyrimidine (two types of compounds that provide the cross-linking "ladders" of the double strands of DNA) base.

WASTING EFFECTS OF HIV INFECTION ON NUTRITIONAL STATUS

Severe malnutrition and weight loss

A fundamental effect of HIV infection is major weight loss, which eventually leads to extreme cachexia similar to that observed in cancer patients (Chapter 24). Such serious weight loss was recognized in the Centers for Disease Control classification of body weight loss over 10% of usual weight, with more than 30 days of constitutional symptoms in an HIV-positive person, as a primary diagnosis of AIDS.[44] This serious, characteristic body-wasting resulting from HIV infection also becomes a cofactor in the development of the full disease syndrome in infected persons, as the malnutrition itself suppresses cellular immune function. So striking is this chronic, relentless body wasting of AIDS that early in the AIDS epidemic outbreak in Uganda, Africa, it was given the name "slim disease."[45] Body wasting in AIDS is characterized by loss of body cell mass, primarily muscle protein. Death occurs when body weight reaches two thirds of normal weight and body cell mass reaches half of normal values. This designation implies that death may be more often a result of malnutrition, specifically negative nitrogen balance, than to the direct effects of infection or malignancy.[46] Also, the attendant diseases of the wasting process play a major role in the decreased quality of life, debilitating weakness, and fatigue seen in AIDS patients.

Causes of body wasting

The characteristic body wasting of HIV infection may be a result of any of the following processes, alone or combined:

- *Inadequate food intake.* Both clinicians and AIDS patients indicate, from their combined clinical observations and personal experience, that an important factor in the profound weight loss is severe *anorexia*. This state is probably related to both the patient's personal life-changing situation and the body's physiologic changes from the disease. Anorexia and its resulting decreased food intake, insufficient to meet body needs, clearly contributes to the body wasting.[46,47]
- *Malabsorption of nutrients.* From early reports, as well as continuing clinical experience, diarrhea and malabsorption have been common in AIDS patients. These malabsorptive symptoms have been related to both drug-diet interactions and progressive effects of HIV-infection. An "AIDS enteropathy" in the early stages of infection has been described, characterized by blunting of the intestinal villi, abnormal intestinal enzymes that cause clinical malabsorption, and HIV infection of infiltrating lymphocytes as well as enterocytes.[48] In later stages, the intestine is infected more frequently with opportunistic organisms, resulting in severe diarrhea and malabsorption.
- *Disordered metabolism.* In the final stage of weight loss in AIDS patients, changes in metabolism occur, including hypermetabolism and altered energy metabolism, usually associated with end-stage effects of the HIV infection as well as increased spread of opportunistic infections. There is progressive depletion of lean body mass as well as increased resting energy expenditure.

NUTRITION ASSESSMENT

The initial nutrition assessment must be comprehensive to provide the baseline information necessary for beginning and continuing nutritional care, including nutritional supplementation, early in the course of the disease.[49,50] Table 23.4 provides guidelines the team clinical dietitian uses for calculating daily kcalories and protein needs, assessing weight changes, and evaluating biochemical data. The calculations and evaluations are required especially for selected patients—children and adults—on special nutritional support therapies, either enteral or parenteral.[51,52]

Further, person-centered nutritional care required for all HIV-infected patients is evident in ongoing nutrition assessment (see *Practical Application* box, p. 498). Special attention is given to any taste and smell losses, which reduce appetite and food intake. These losses in appetite may be aided by increased flavor enhancement in food preparation.[52] This type of detailed initial nutrition interview includes investigation of the patient's medical history, physical and anthropometric data, biochemical indices, medications, living situation, dietary intake, general socioeconomic status, and assistance needs. All patients, at first contact with a health professional, should be referred to the AIDS team clinical dietitian for screening to evaluate the degree of any nutrition problems.[53,54] Thus together with the patient, a plan for personal ongoing nutritional care and support can be initiated.

MICRONUTRIENTS AND ANTIOXIDANT THERAPY

The role of micronutrients, that is, vitamins and minerals, in increased therapeutic amounts in the treatment of AIDS is the focus of much current research. Ongoing studies at the University of Toronto, Canada, for example, have focused on the antioxidant capacities of six basic micronutrients—vitamins A, C, E, and beta-carotene, and the trace minerals iron and zinc.[55,56] These results showed an increase in oxidative stress, resulting from metabolic overproduction of reactive oxygen intermediates, and a weakened antioxidant defense system in HIV-positive patients. Other study centers, focusing on children with AIDS, have reported similar findings.[57-60]

Table 23.4	Outline of nutritional assessment in persons with HIV infection and AIDS

I. Estimated daily kcalorie and protein requirements for adults
  A. *Kcalories (total kcal)*
      Male/female: 35-40 kcal/kg
  B. *Protein (g)*
      Male/female 2-2.5 g/kg

II. Calculated daily kcalorie and protein requirements for adults
  A. *Kcalories (total kcal) for weight maintenance*
      Male = (66.5 + (13.7 × wt [kg]) + (5 × ht [cm]) − (6.7 × age [yr]) × AP* × IF† + 500 kcal
      Female = (665.1 + (9.6 × wt [kg]) + (1.8 × ht [cm]) − (4.7 × age [yr]) × AF* x IF† + 500 kcal
      NOTE: Add 500 kcal to the equations above for weight gain.
  B. *Protein (g)*
      Male/female = Total kcal × $\dfrac{\text{g nitrogen}}{150 \text{ kcal}}$ × $\dfrac{6.25 \text{ g protein}}{\text{g nitrogen}}$

III. Nutritional assessment parameters

	Extent of malnutrition		
	Mild	**Moderate‡**	**Severe‡**
Albumin (g/dl)	2.8-3.2	2.1-2.7	<2.1
Transferrin (mg/dl)	150-200	100-150	<100
Total lymphocyte count (cells/mm3)	1200-2000	800-1200	<800
Creatinine-height index (5) (actual/ideal × 100)	60-80	40-60	<40
Ideal body weight (%)	80-90	70-80	<70
Usual body weight (%)	85-95	75-85	<75
Weight loss/unit time	<5%/mo <7.5%/3 mo <10%/6 mo	<2%/wk >5%/mo >7.5%/3 mo >10%/6 mo	>2%/wk
Skin tests (no. reactive/no. placed)	4/4 (normal)	1-2/4 (Weak)	0/4 (Anergic)
Anthropometry	Normal male	Normal female	
Triceps skinfold (mm)	12.5	16.5	
Mid-arm circumference (cm)	29.3	28.5	

Adapted from Hickey MS: Nutritional support of patients with AIDS, *Surg Clin North Am* 71(3):645, 1991.
*Activity factors (AF): Confined to bed - 1.2, ambulatory = 1.3, fever factor = 1.13/°C>37.
†Injury factor (IF): Surgery = 1.1-1.2, infection = 1.2 = 1.6, trauma = 1.1-1.8, sepsis = 1.4-1.8.
‡Nutritional therapy indicated.

NUTRITION INTERVENTION

Experienced clinical dietitians working with AIDS patients build nutrition care plans with each client or patient for appropriate nutrition intervention and guidance. Such guidance has been written into the recent position paper adopted jointly by The American Dietetic Association and The Canadian Dietetic Association.[53] Personal care planning is continually adjusted as needed according to the disease progression and personal needs. It focuses on identifying food-nutrient problems, developing a plan of action for each problem, and outlining the form of nutrition support needed. Suggested guidelines for developing such patient-centered care plans are outlined in Table 23.5. For those persons receiving nutrition support in special enteral or parenteral forms, the dietitian will work with the AIDS team physician, and other members of the hospital Nutrition Support team, to develop an appropriate formula and feeding mode, using oral or tube-fed enteral means or intravenous feeding by peripheral or central veins (see Chapter 17).

NUTRITION COUNSELING, EDUCATION, AND SUPPORTIVE STRATEGIES

Counseling principles

An adolescent client once aptly defined a counselor as "someone to talk to while I make up my mind." Client-centered counseling in the care of persons with HIV

The ABCDs of nutrition assessment in AIDS

The initial nutrition assessment visit with an HIV-infected patient is an important beginning point for the continuing nutritional care that is to follow. This encounter serves both informational and relational functions. It provides the necessary baseline information for planning practical individual nutrition support. More importantly, it establishes the essential provider-patient relationship, the human context within which this continuing nutritional care and support will be provided as needed. The basic ABCDs of nutrition assessment will provide a practical guide (see Chapter 16), with special assessment (the letters "E" and "F") added for HIV infection patients.

Anthropometry
- Age, sex, height
- Weight: current, usual, percent of usual, ideal, percent of ideal, weight loss over defined time period
- Mid-upper-arm measures: circumference, triceps skinfold thickness; calculated mid-arm muscle circumference

Biochemical indices
- Serum proteins: albumin, prealbumin, transferrin
- Liver function test (evaluate liver function)
- Blood urea nitrogen, serum electrolytes (evaluate renal function)
- Urinary urea nitrogen excretion over 24 hours (nitrogen balance)
- Creatinine height index
- Complete blood count (evaluate for anemia)
- Fasting glucose (evaluate for hyperglycemia or hypoglycemia)

Clinical observations
- General signs of nutritional status (Table 19-2)
- Drug effects

Diet evaluation
- Usual intake, current intake, restrictions, modifications (use both 24-hour recall and food diaries)
- Nutrition supplements, vitamin-mineral supplements
- Food allergies, intolerances
- Activity level (general kcalories expended per day)

- Support system (caregivers to help with nutrition care plan)

Environmental, behavioral, and psychologic assessment
- Living situation, personal support
- Food environment, types of meals, eating assistance needed

Financial assessment
- Medical insurance
- Income, financial support through caregivers
- Current medical and other expenses
- Ability to afford food, enteral supplements, added vitamins-minerals

References
Fields-Gardner C: Position of the American Dietetic Association and the Canadian Dietetic Association: nutrition intervention in the care of persons with human immunodeficiency virus infection, *J Am Diet Assoc* 94(9):1042, 1994.
Trujillo EB et al: Assessment of nutritional status, nutrient intake, and nutrition support in AIDS patients, *J Am Diet Assoc* 92(4):477, 1992.

infection must be just that. Professionals and patients must remain involved throughout the progressive course of the disease because the patient's wishes and needs are ultimately paramount in various treatments and decisions about care. The basic goal of nutrition counseling is to make the fewest possible changes in the person's lifestyle and food patterns necessary to promote optimal nutritional status while providing maximum comfort and quality of life. In this person-centered care process, several counseling principles are particularly pertinent:
- *Motivation.* Changed behavior in any area requires the motivation, desire, and ability to

achieve one's goals. Until the patient perceives food patterns and behaviors as appropriate goals, it is best to wait for a better time and begin with establishing a general supportive climate in which to continue working together. Any specific obstacle raised by the patient, such as time, physical limitations, money, or increased anxiety, can be met with related suggestions to think about. Priorities among needs should be recognized in the care plan and items should be introduced according to order of importance and immediacy of the patient's nutritional problems.

Table
23.5 Planning nutrition care for patients with AIDS

Type of problem	Possible causes	Patient care plan considerations
Food intake		
	Anorexia	Patient, caregiver roles
	Drug, food interaction	Motivation, patient decision making
	HIV, other infection	Education, counseling
	Taste alteration	Resource materials
	Food intolerances, allergies	Nutrition supplements
	Lack of access or ability to prepare food	Vitamin, mineral supplements
	Depression	Drug-food reactions
		Special enteral-parenteral nutrition support
		Monitoring, adjustments as needed
Nutrient absorption		
	HIV-related infections or cancers	Treatment of underlying disease or disorder
	Diminished gastric HCL secretion	Pancreatic enzymes supplement
	Altered mucosal absorbing surface	Drug-nutrient reactions
	Organ involvement; liver, pancreas, gallbladder, kidney	Special enteral-parenteral nutrition support, appropriate formula design
	Drug-nutrient interaction	Monitoring, adjustments as needed
Altered metabolism, excretion		
	HIV infection	Review of drug dosage, schedule
	Associated infections, diseases	Modification of diet, meal pattern
	Drug-nutrient interactions	Treatment of infection, symptoms
	Altered hormonal function	Review of diet nutrients, increase or decrease
	Organ dysfunction	Special enteral-parenteral nutrition support appropriate formula design
		Monitoring, adjustments as needed

Data from Newman CF: *Practical guidelines for improving nutritional status in HIV-related disease,* University of California, Davis, Medical School Fifth Annual Conference on Clinical Nutrition, Nutrition in the Treatment of Serious Medical Problems, Feb 28-29, 1992.

- *Rationale.* Any diet or food behavior change, with possible benefits and risks, must be clearly explained to the patient. The question "Why?" is always important to everybody.
- *Provider-patient agreement.* In the best interests of all concerned, the patient and health care provider must agree to the change. Any change should be structured around daily routines and include any caregivers as needed. The nutrition counselor should provide any needed information and encouragement throughout the process.
- *Manageable steps.* All information given and actions agreed on should proceed in manageable steps, as small as necessary, in order of complexity and difficulty. Information overload can discourage anyone. But here the particular stress load at any point can be intolerable for the patient. At such points of stress, patients are also more vulnerable to the lure of unproved HIV therapies (see *To Probe Further* box, p. 500).

Personal food management skills

The patient's living situation and general practical skills in planning, purchasing, and preparing food must be considered. Any need for information and guidance in developing skills in any aspect of procuring food, or in sources of needed help, should be provided.

Community programs

Information may be needed about any available community food programs, such as Meals-on-Wheels, for delivery of prepared meals at times when the patient is too ill to get out for food. A number of these programs in various hard-hit inner cities on the East and West coasts of the United States, for example, as well as central cities, have developed to meet these needs, and in some cases they also provide home health and nutritional care services.[61-64] Also, information may need to be provided about food assistance programs such as Food Stamps or Food Commodities (see Chapter 10), for which the lower income person may qualify.

To Probe Further

Are AIDS patients targets for nutritional hucksters?

When diseases such as acquired immunodeficiency syndrome (AIDS) lack curative therapy and have poor prognosis, many persons afflicted with such a disease are susceptible to claims of unproved, alternative therapies, that is, nutrition quackery. Some of the alternative therapies and approaches that are being touted as treatments for HIV infection include the following questionable practices.

Megadoses of nutrients

Large doses of vitamins A, C, E, B_{12}, selenium and zinc have been recommended to restore cell-mediated immunity by increasing T-cell number and activity. The value of such large doses has not been established by controlled clinical studies. In fact, the opposite is true; megadoses of these nutrients can be dangerous. Chronic intakes of vitamin A in excess of 50,000 IU/day can produce toxicity. Chronic intakes of excess zinc, as little as 25 mg/day, can cause gastrointestinal distress, nausea, and impaired immune function. Selenium is also toxic in high chronic doses, but the level at which this toxicity occurs is uncertain.

Dr. Berger's Immune Power Diet

In his book, Berger (1985) states that poor health is caused by "immune hypersensitivity" to many foods such as milk, wheat, corn, yeast, soy, sugar, and eggs. He suggests a 21-day elimination diet for foods believed to cause allergies, followed by a reintroduction phase and then a maintenance diet, to prevent food sensitivities and "revitalize" the immune system. The usefulness of this diet has not been tested or proven by scientific studies. The diet promoted in Berger's book (high in fruits and vegetables and low in fat and calcium) may produce undernutrition, and the suggestion that moldy food be consumed to test for allergy to molds may be dangerous to persons who are immunocompromised.

AL 721

This compound, developed in Israel and approved by the FDA for clinical trials, is composed of "active lipids" (AL) mixed in a ratio of 70% neutral lipid, 20% lecithin, and 10% phosphatidylethanolamine—hence the 721 designation. It has been hypothesized that 721 can reduce or inhibit HIV infection. Clinical trials found little toxicity, but no consistent trends in T cell quantitation or HIV cultures. Increases in body weight, serum total, HDL, and LDL cholesterol levels were noted. AL 721 can be made at home from soy or egg yolk lecithin or obtained already mixed, but is of unknown purity and can spoil easily if stored improperly.

Butylated Hydroxytoluene (BHT)

Claims that Butylated Hydroxytoluene (BHT) kills HIV by attacking the "coating" on the virus are unfounded and unproved. The safety of its use is also questionable.

"Maximum Immunity Diet"

Any value for megadoses of vitamin C to strengthen the immune system has not been established. Rebound scurvy has occurred on cessation of the megadoses.

Laetrile

When used in combination with a strict vegan diet and vitamin supplements, laetrile is supposed to destroy a tumor enzyme (B-glucuronidase). In addition to being proven ineffective, this low-energy diet may supply inadequate amounts of calcium, iron, niacin, vitamin B_{12}, and excessive amounts of thiamin, vitamins A and C, and zinc.

Gerson method

This program restricts all foods other than oatmeal and uncanned fresh fruits and vegetables, and advocates regular enemas, especially coffee enemas, to create an internal environment hostile to malignant cells. Efficacy has not been proven, and the diet is inadequate.

Kelley regimen

The Kelley regimen excludes meat, milk in all forms except yogurt, and peanuts from the diet to overcome supposed pancreatic enzyme deficiency. Almonds are substituted for meat, and nutritional supplements including vitamins and minerals are recommended. Deficiencies of protein and calcium and fluid and electrolyte losses are possible in addition to possible vitamin A toxicity.

Yeast-free diet

The exclusion of high-carbohydrate and yeast-containing foods is supposed to prevent opportunistic yeast infections such as candidiasis. The underlying theory behind this has been characterized as speculative, and there is a possibility that undernutrition may result.

Macrobiotic diet

A macrobiotic diet is based on oriental philosophy that it will restore balance and harmony between yin and yang forces and thereby improve health. However, it is very low in fat and high in fiber: 50% (by volume) whole-grain cereals, 20% to 30% vegetables, 10% to 15% cooked beans or seaweed; and 5% miso (fermented soy paste) or tamari broth soup. This regimen can produce protein-kcalorie malnutrition and provides inadequate intake of riboflavin, niacin, and calcium in adults, as well as pyridoxine and vitamins B_{12} and D in children (in addition to those nutrients mentioned for adults).

Although it is conceivable that there are nutrients and other dietary substances that may improve some of the symptoms associated with HIV infection, it is still too early in our understanding of the disease process to make recommendations about supplementation. Alternative therapies require further study in controlled clinical trials.

References

Dwyer JT et al: Unproven nutrition therapies for AIDS: What is the evidence? *Nutr Today* 23:25, 1988.

Raiten DJ: Nutrition and HIV infection: A review and evaluation of the extant knowledge of the relationship between nutrition and HIV infection, *Nutr Clin Prac* 6(3):S1, 1991.

Psychosocial support

Every aspect of care provided should be given within a form and context that also provides genuine psychosocial support. All health care providers working with HIV-infected patients must be particularly sensitive to the special psychologic and social issues that confront persons with AIDS. Major stress areas may include issues relating to autonomy and dependency, a sense of uncertainty and fear of the unknown, grief, change and loss, fear of symptoms, fears of abandonment, and spiritual questions that arise when someone confronts a life-threatening illness. Common emotions are hostility, denial, withdrawal, depression, anxiety, guilt, and confusion. All of these at one time or another may significantly influence treatment. Health care providers must always be aware and assess how the patient and caregivers are relating to the disease, using assistance of social workers, clinical psychologists, or psychiatrists as needed.[65,66] Stress reduction groups, including exercise training, are helpful, as they have proved to be in other life-threatening situations such as cancer and coronary heart disease.[67]

Most important, however, health care workers must examine their own values and fears regarding sexual orientation, sexual behavior, intravenous drug use, and fears of AIDS transmission. Preconceived judgments are easily picked up by patients and threaten the provider-patient relationship. Before they can be effective with patients, all health care workers must first confront their own fears and prejudices and learn to let go of such judgmental behavior.

TO SUM UP

The viral evolution and current world wide spread of human immunodeficiency virus (HIV) infection has reached epidemic proportions and is still growing. The disease progression follows three distinct stages: HIV infection, AIDS-related complex (ARC) with associated opportunistic illnesses, and full-blown AIDS with complicating diseases leading to death. This overall disease progression from initial infection to death lasts about 10 to 12 years. The Public Health Service and the CDC of the United States Department of Health and Human Services (DHHS) have responsibilities for monitoring the disease and providing leadership in research and treatment development, based on collaborative information exchange with scientists world wide.

During the initial decade of the epidemic in the 1980s, scientists learned the nature and life cycle of the new mutation of HIV and its transmission modes and population groups at risk. Development of diagnostic testing procedures has enabled population surveillance and individual detection of disease and personal care to proceed. A fundamental role of nutrition support in this personal care of HIV-infected individuals has become evident.

Medical management of HIV infection, which is without a vaccine or cure, involves supportive treatment of associated illnesses and complicating diseases. In the terminal HIV stage, the virus eventually gains sufficient strength to destroy the host's immune system white cells, and death follows. New drugs to slow the disease progression are developing.

Current ongoing research is studying the role of micronutrients in oxidation processes in the cell. Nutritional management focuses on providing personal individual nutrition support to counteract the severe body wasting and malnutrition characteristic of the disease. The process of nutritional care involves comprehensive nutrition assessment and evaluation of personal needs, planning care with each patient and caregivers, and meeting practical food needs. Throughout the care process, nutrition counseling, education, and strategic services also help provide psychosocial support to each patient.

■ QUESTIONS FOR REVIEW

1. Describe the evolutionary history of the human immunodeficiency virus (HIV-1) and its current world wide epidemic spread. How is it transmitted and why do you think it has spread so rapidly? Identify major population groups at risk.

2. Describe the nature of the AIDS virus and its action in the human body. What is a retrovirus?

3. Describe the progression of HIV infection in terms of its three basic stages of development from initial infection to death.

4. Identify some of the drugs currently used in medical management of HIV infection, and describe any associated actions, side effects, or toxicities that may relate to dietary management.

5. Outline basic parts of a comprehensive initial nutrition assessment of a patient with HIV infection and describe the reasons for each type of information and its evaluation.

6. Describe the general process of planning nutritional care on the basis of the patient assessment information and the main types of nutrition problems in HIV infection. Devise a related plan of action for each type of problem. Can you give an example of how you might follow up to see what worked or did not work and make adjustments?

■ REFERENCES

1. Piot P: AIDS: a global response (editorial), *Science* 272(5270): 1855, June 28, 1996.

2. Tuofu Z et al: An African HIV-1 sequence from 1959 and implications for the origin of the epidemic, *Nature* 391(6667):594, 1998.

3. Caldwell JC, Caldwell P: The African AIDS epidemic, *Sci Am* 274(3):62, 1996.

4. Cohen J: The changing of the guard, *Science* 272(5270):1876, 1996.

5. Holmberg SD: The estimated prevalence and incidence of HIV in 96 large US metropolitan areas, *Am J Pub Health* 86(5):642, 1996.

6. Stein Z, Susser M: AIDS—an update on global dynamics (editorial), *Am J Public Health* 97(6):901, 1997.

7. Cohen J: Failure isn't what it used to be, *Science* 279(Feb 20):1133, 1998.

8. Cohen J: Likely HIV cofactor found, *Science* 272(5262):809, 1996.

9. Pantaleo G et al: HIV infection is active and progressive in lymphoid tissue during the clinically latent stage of disease, *Nature* 362(6418):355, 1993.

10. Embretson J et al: Massive covert infection of helper T lymphocytes and macrophages by HIV during the incubation period of AIDS, *Nature* 362(6418):359, 1993.

11. Maddox J: Where the virus hides away, *Nature* 362(6418):287, 1993.

12. Hoover DR et al: The progression of untreated HIV-1 infection prior to AIDS, *Am J Public Health* 82(11):1538, 1992.

13. Mills J, Masur H: AIDS-related infections, *Sci Am* 263(2):50, 1990.

14. Gold JWM: HIV-1 infection, *Med Clin North Am* 76(1):1992.

15. Otten MW et al: Changes in sexually transmitted disease rates after HIV testing and posttest counseling, Miami, 1988 to 1989, *Am J Public Health* 83(4):529, 1993.

16. US Department of Health and Human Services, Public Health Service: *Healthy People 2000: national health promotion and disease prevention objectives,* DHHS Pub No (PHS) 91-50212, Washington, DC, 1991, US Government Printing Office.

17. Wickizer TM et al: Activating communities for health promotion: a process evaluation method, *Am J Public Health* 83(4):561, 1993.

18. Ehrhardt AA: Trends in sexual behavior and the HIV pandemic, *Am J Public Health* 82(11):1459, 1992.

19. Aggleton P et al: Risking everything? Risk behavior, behavior change, and AIDS, *Science* 265(5170):341, 1994.

20. Bayer R: Sounding board: AIDS prevention—sexual ethics and responsibility, *N Engl J Med* 334(23):1540, 1996.

21. Merson MH: My turn: how to fight AIDS, *Newsweek* 128(6):18, 1996.

22. Stevens JE: Model programs take aim at HIV rates in Indonesia, *Science* 264(5155):24, 1994.

23. Centers for Disease Control and Prevention, Public Health Service: Update: acquired immunodeficiency syndrome-United States, 1994, *MMWR* 44(4):65, 1995.

24. Centers for Disease Control and Prevention, Public Health Service: Update: AIDS among women—United States, 1994, *MMWR* 44(5):83, 1995.

25. Black RF: Transmission of HIV-1 in the breast-feeding process, *J Am Diet Assoc* 96(3):267, 1996.

26. Zimmer P, Garza C: Maternal considerations in formulating HIV-related breast feeding recommendations (editorial), *Am J Public Health* 87(6):904, 1997.

27. Cohen J: Women: absent term in the AIDS research equation, *Science* 26(5225):777, 1995.

28. Catania JA et al: Condom use in multi-ethnic neighborhoods of San Francisco: the population-based AMEN

(AIDS in multi-ethnic neighborhoods) Study, *Am J Public Health* 82:284, 1992.

29. Roper WL et al: Condoms and HIV/STD prevention: clarifying the message, *Am J Public Health* 83(4):501, 1993.

30. Gollub EL, Stein ZA: The new female condom: item 1 on a woman's AIDS prevention agenda, *Am J Public Health* 83(4):498, 1993.

31. Cohen J: The marketplace of HIV/AID$, *Science* 272(5270):1880, 1996.

32. Ho DD: Time to hit HIV, early and hard (editorial), *N Engl J Med* 333(7):450, 1995.

33. Seachrist L: AZT: attacking AIDS early and hard, *Sci News* 148(8):116, 1995.

34. Cohen J: Results of the new AIDS drugs brings cautious optimism, *Science* 271(5250):755, 1996.

35. Cohen J: Drug development: a tale of two companies, *Science* 272(5270):1882, 1996.

36. Cohen J: The media's love affair with AIDS research: hope vs. hype, *Science* 275(5298):298, 1997.

37. Cohen J: The daunting challenge of keeping HIV suppressed, *Science* 277(5322):32, 1997.

38. Cohen J: Stubborn HIV reservoirs vulnerable to new treatments, *Science* 276(5314):898, 1997.

39. Cavert W, Haase AT et al: Kinetics of response in lymphoid tissues to antiretroviral therapy of HIV-1 infection, *Science* 276(53i4):960, 1997.

40. Sternberg S: AIDS optimism high despite therapy cost, *Sci News* 150(2):21, 1996.

41. Kaiser J: AIDS vaccine trial disappointing, *Science* 272(5260):341, 1996.

42. McDonnell WM, Askari FK: Molecular medicine—DNA vaccines, *N Engl J Med* 334(1):42, 1996.

43. Bloom BR: A perspective on AIDS vaccines, *Science* 272(5270):1888, 1996.

44. Centers for Disease Control and Prevention, Center for Infectious Diseases: *Acquired immunodeficiency syndrome weekly surveillance report, Atlanta*, Sept 7, 1987, US AIDS Programs.

45. Serwadda D et al: Slim disease: a new disease in Uganda and its association with HTLV-III infection, *Lancet* 2:849, 1985.

46. Macallan DC et al: Energy expenditure and wasting in human immunodeficiency virus infection, *N Engl J Med* 333(2):83, 1995.

47. Grunfeld C: What causes wasting in AIDS, *N Engl J Med* 333(2):123, editorial, 1995.

48. Heise et al: Human immunodeficiency virus infection of enterocytes and mononuclear cells in human jejunal mucosa, *Gastroenterology* 100:1522, 1991.

49. Stack JA et al: High-energy, high-protein, oral, liquid, nutrition supplementation in patients with HIV infection: effect on weight status in relation to incidence of secondary infection, *J Am Diet Assoc* 96(4):337, 1996.

50. Chlebowski RT et al: Dietary intake and counseling, weight maintenance, and the course of HIV infection, *J Am Diet Assoc* 95(4):428, 1995.

51. Heller LS, Shattuck D: Nutrition support for children with HIV/AIDS, *J Am Diet Assoc* 97(5):473, 1997.

52. Graham CS et al: Taste and smell losses in HIV infected patients, *Physiol Behav* 58(2):287, 1995.

53. Fields-Gardner C: Position of the American Dietetic Association and the Canadian Dietetic Association: nutrition intervention in the care of persons with human immunodeficiency virus infection, *J Am Diet Assoc* 94(9):1042, 1994.

54. Young JS: HIV and medical nutrition therapy, *J Am Diet Assoc* 97(10):S161, 1997.

55. Allard JP et al: Oxidative stress and plasma antioxidant micronutrients in humans with HIV infection, *Am J Clin Nutr* 67:143, 1998.

56. Kotler D: Antioxidant therapy and HIV infection: 1998, *Am J Clin Nutr* 67:7, 1998.

57. Cunningham-Rundles S et al: Micronutrient and cytokine interaction in congenital pediatric HIV infection, *J Nutr* 126(10S):2674S, 1996.

58. Miller TL et al: Nutritional status and cardiac mass and function in children infected with the human immunodeficiency virus, *Am J Clin Nutr* 66:660, 1997.

59. Henderson RA et al: Serum and plasma markers of nutritional status in children infected with the human immunodeficiency virus, *J Am Diet Assoc* 97(12):1377.

60. Tang AM, Graham NMH: Effects of micronutrients, *Epidemiol* 143:1244, 1996.

61. Luder E et al: Assessment of nutritional, clinical, and immunologic status of HIV-infected, inner-city patients with multiple risk factors, *J Am Diet Assoc* 95(6):655, 1995.

62. Topping CM et al: A community-based, interagency approach by dietitians to provide meals, medical nutrition therapy, and education to clients with HIV/AIDS, *J Am Diet Assoc* 95(6):683, 1995.

63. Kraak VI: Home-delivered meal programs for homebound people with HIV/AIDS, *J Am Diet Assoc* 95(4):476, 1995.

64. Udine LM, Rorthkopf MM: Utilization of home health care services in HIV infection: a pilot study in Ohio, *J Am Diet Assoc* 94(1):83, 1994.

65. Antoni MH et al: Cognitive-behavior stress management intervention buffers distress responses and immunologic change following notification of HIV-1 seropositivity, *J Consult Clin Psychol* 59(6):906, 1991.

66. Jacobsberg LB, Perry S: Psychiatric disturbances, *Med Clin North Am* 76(1):99, 1992.

67. LaPerriere A et al: Aerobic exercise training in an AIDS risk group, *Int J Sports Med* 12(suppl 1):S53, 1991.

■ FURTHER READING

Bryson YL et al: Clearance of HIV infection in a perinatally infected infant, *N Engl J Med* 332(13):833, 1995.

McIntosh K, Burchett SK: Clearance of HIV-lessons from newborns, *N Engl J Med* 332(13):883, editorial, 1995.

Black RF: Transmission of HIV-1 in the breast-feeding process, *J Am Diet Assoc* 96(3):267, 1996.

These three articles provide interesting background in a case study, and its accompanying editorial, of perinatal transmission of AIDS at birth with apparent clearance afterward, in a boy now 5 years old and in kindergarten, and a discussion of the controversial question of breast-feeding by HIV mothers.

Nowak MA, McMichael AJ: How HIV defeats the immune system, *Sci Am* 273(2):58, 1995.

This excellent article by two HIV researchers, complete with many illustrations for which the *Scientific American* is famous, discusses background for understanding the virus's devastating effect and dangerous development in the body.

Timbo BB, Tollefson L: Nutrition: a cofactor in HIV disease, *J Am Diet Assoc* 94(9):1018, 1994.

This study demonstrates how poor nutritional status and infection interact and affect the body's immune system, and how nutritional status continues to affect the progression of HIV disease.

Case study

HIV infection in a young mother

Mrs. Theresa Stevens is a 25-year-old young mother, admitted to the hospital with a history of weight loss, weakness, and watery diarrhea. She is married and has a 3-year-old son. Her husband is in a rehabilitation program for intravenous drug abuse. About 1 year ago she started to notice that she was becoming easily fatigued, but attributed it to taking care of a 2-year-old child. When her appetite began to wane and her weight dropped from 150 pounds to 90 pounds she went to her physician. In addition to the fatigue and weight loss, she reported fever and night sweats. Physical examination revealed swollen lymph glands, tongue lesions of herpes simplex, and perianal ulcers. Her physician admitted her to the hospital, and further tests indicated depressed T cells, and bronchial washings showed the presence of *Pneumocystis carinii* pneumonia. She was tested for HIV infection, since *P. carinii* is uncommon in persons with healthy immune systems. Her blood test for HIV infection antibodies was positive.

While in the hospital, she developed symptoms of several infections: anorexia, fever, fatigue, nausea, vomiting, watery diarrhea, perianal ulcers, and rectal incontinence. Her temperature frequently registered 39.4° C (103° F) despite therapy with multiple antibiotics. The volume of diarrhea was measured to be 2500 ml/day, and her vomiting necessitated intravenous hydration. She also began to receive treatment for *P. carinii* pneumonia, esophageal candidiasis, oral and lingual herpes, and *Mycobacterium avium intracellulare* infection of the duodenum.

The patient did not tolerate a soft diet with nutritional supplements, continued to lose weight, and demonstrated severe anorexia, abdominal cramping, and bloating. Results of the nutritional assessment were as follows:

Height (cm) 100.1
Weight (kg) 40.9
Body weight (% ideal) 65
Body weight (% usual) 70
Triceps skinfold (% standard) 40
Midarm muscle circumference (% standard) 72
Serum albumin (g/dl) 2.2
Serum total protein (g/dl) 5.6
Serum total iron binding capacity (TIBC) (μg/dl) 192
Estimated resting energy expenditure (REE) 1750

Questions for Analysis

1. Name and describe several major clinical complications of the final stage of AIDS. How can these complicating diseases profoundly compromise a patient's nutritional status?

2. On the basis of the nutritional assessment, what is this patient's nutritional diagnosis?

3. What should be the goal of nutritional therapy based on the baseline nutritional assessment data and the patient's history?

4. By what route of feeding should nutritional support be administered?

References

Rago RR, Feurer ID: Acquired immunodeficiency syndrome (AIDS), In Blackburn GL et al, eds: *Nutritional medicine: a case management approach,* Philadelphia, 1989, WB Saunders.

Issues & Answers

Special consideration for pediatric patients with AIDS

Although limited, the available information on pediatric AIDS indicates that malnutrition, particularly undernutrition of kcalories, is a recurring problem. With adults, the disease alone impacts nutrition status, but in children, growth and development add to the impact of the disease process.

Nutritional assessments should be performed routinely in pediatric patients with AIDS so any problems can be identified and treated as they occur and nutritional deficits can be minimized. Assessments should include anthropometry, plasma protein evaluation, complete blood counts, and evaluation of appetite and intake. Eating ability should be determined and the social situation evaluated.

Providing enough kcalories to maintain linear growth and weight gain is sometimes difficult. Increasing protein intake 50% to 100% over the RDA has been recommended. However, needs are individual and should be monitored. Suggestions to provide supplemental caloric and nutrient intake are listed below:

- Use a kcalorie-dense formula (24 to 27 kcal/oz) for infants. Add glucose polymers or medium-chain triglycerides to formulas or reduce the amount of water added to powdered formulas to boost kcalories.
- Try food supplements that are high in kcalories and protein.
- Add fats such as butter, margarine, or mayonnaise to foods to boost kcalories.
- Encourage nutrient-dense snacks such as raisins and peanuts or peanut butter.
- For the older, lactose-tolerant child, add skim milk powder to whole milk to boost kcalories and proteins.
- Make adjustments in diet consistency and temperatures to overcome eating difficulties associated with disease complications and any other eating problems.

- For lactose-intolerance, which occurs frequently in children with AIDS, use lactose-free, soy-based infant formulas instead of milk.
- Add Lactaid, a commercial preparation of lactose, to milk products to permit improved digestion.
- Use low-lactose dairy foods such as yogurt and mild cheddar cheese, if tolerated.

Vitamin and mineral supplements in amounts one or two times the RDA may offset possible deficits and contribute to meeting increased requirements during hypermetabolic states. Attention should also be given to drug-nutrient interactions and other effects of drugs on nutritional status.

Proper procedures and sanitary formula preparation must be followed for infants being bottle fed. Infants should not be put to bed with a bottle of milk or juice, as they are easily contaminated. Unpasteurized milk and milk products should also be avoided, as they may be a source of *Salmonella* and other microorganisms that can cause intestinal infections.

Children should never be fed any food directly from a jar to avoid possible bacterial contamination of the remaining food from the child's mouth. Fruits and vegetables should be peeled or cooked, and meats should be well cooked. All utensils and dishes should be washed in a dishwasher or in hot sudsy water and air dried.

References

Bentler M, Stanish M: Nutrition support of the pediatric patient with AIDS, *J Am Diet Assoc* 87:488, 1987.

Berry RK: Home care of the child with AIDS, *Pediatr Nurs* 14:341, 1988.

Carrot Top Nutrition Resources: *Nutrition handbook for AIDS,* Aurora, Colo, 1988, Carrot Top Nutrition Resources.

Grossman M: Special problems in the child with AIDS. In Sande MA, Volberding PA, eds: *The medical management of AIDS,* ed 2, Philadelphia, 1990, WB Saunders.

Raiten DJ: Nutrition and HIV infection: a review and evaluation of the extant knowledge of the relationship between nutrition and HIV infection, *Nutr Clin Prac* 6(3):S1, 1991.

24

Nutrition and Cancer

Chapter Outline

The Process of Cancer Development
The Body's Defense System
Nutritional Support for Cancer Therapy
Nutritional Therapy
Nutritional Management

This chapter focuses on cancer, one of the major diseases in the Western world. We examine the nature of the cancer process and its treatments and seek to relate these processes to the nutritional factors involved.

Here we look at nutrition and cancer in two basic areas: prevention, through the environment and the body's defense system, and therapy, through nutritional support for medical treatment and rehabilitation. To understand these nutritional relationships, we must understand the nature of cancer as a growth process, the physiologic basis of cancer in the structure and function of cells, and the body's defense systems in immunity and in the healing process.

THE PROCESS OF CANCER DEVELOPMENT

MULTIPLE FORMS OF CANCER

The health toll of cancer continues to extract its price in human disease and death, despite ongoing battles around the world and the initial war declaration of the United States in its National Cancer Act of 1971. In its latest report the United States National Institutes of Health statistical cancer review program Surveillance, Epidemiology, and End Results (SEER) has indicated an overall cancer death rate rise of 6.3%.[1] Currently, about 555,000 Americans die from cancer each year. As in most developed countries of the world, 40% of Americans will develop the disease, and more than 20% will die of it.[2] The World Health Organization estimates that cancer kills about 6 million persons each year. Killing the cancer tumor is the continuing goal of all cancer researchers.[3]

The United States Department of Health and Human Services estimates that about 510,000 Americans die of cancer each year, with 30% dying of lung cancer. In its multiple forms cancer has become one of our major health problems, second only to heart disease, and accounts for about 20% of the total deaths in the United States each year.

Difficulties in the study of cancer have arisen from its varying nature and multiple forms. The word **cancer** is a general term used to designate any one of many malignant tumors, or **neoplasms** (new growths), forming in various body tissue sites. There are many different forms of cancer, varying world wide and changing with population migrations. There are multiple causes and often conflicting research results because of the large number of variables involved. We would be more correct, then, to use the plural term "cancers" in discussing this great variety of neoplasms.

To better understand cancer development we should view it as a growth process that has its physiologic basis in the structure and function of cells. Since nutrition is fundamental to all tissue growth, we need to look briefly at the cancer cell to understand the relationship of nutritional factors to cancer. This "misguided cell" and its tumor tissue represent normal cell growth that has gone wild.

THE CANCER CELL

The marvel of human life is that the normal process of cell growth and reproduction goes on almost flawlessly over and over again, guided by the cell's genes. In adult humans some 3 to 4 million cells complete the normal life-sustaining process of cell division every second, largely without mistake, guided by the genetic code. The central question in cell biology has been: How is the process and rate of cell reproduction maintained so precisely in normal cells? The question in cancer research, based on increased knowledge of normal cell physiology, then follows: How and why is this normal, precise regulation of cell reproduction and function lost in cancer cells, and why do cancer cells then remain mutant and malformed, functionally immature and imperfect, incapable of normal cell life?

The first part of the answer lies in the nature of the cell's genetic material and its regulating components. The specific genetic material in the cell's nucleus is arranged as chromosomes and genes, which hold the controlling agent, *deoxyribonucleic acid (DNA)*. Specific sites along the chromosome threads are called genes. Each gene carries specific information that controls synthesis of specific proteins and transmits genetic heritage. A single chromosome thread is made up of hundreds of genes arranged end to end, and each gene of DNA is made up of some 600 to several thousand smaller subunits called nucleotides. The nucleic acids, DNA and its companion *ribonucleic acid (RNA)*, compose the controlling system by which both the cell and thus the organism sustain life. The structure of DNA is that of a very large polynucleotide made up of many individual mononucleotides, each one of which has three parts: (1) a sugar (deoxyribose); (2) a phosphate; and (3) a specific nitrogenous base—adenine, cytosine, guanine, or thymine. It is the ladderlike pairing of these nitrogenous bases, as shown in Figure 24.1, that incorporates the "genetic code" and enables the DNA to transmit messages to guide protein structure. The DNA appears as a twisted ladder or spiral staircase in structure and is thus called a "helix," the Greek word meaning "coil."

GENE CONTROL OF CELL REPRODUCTION AND FUNCTION

The normal cell

Cells arise only by division from preexisting cells and carry the preexisting cell's genetic pattern. Normally the various cell structures and functions operate in an orderly manner under gene control, directing the cell's specific processes of protein synthesis. Gene action, however, may be switched on and off, depending on the position of a cell in the body, the stage of body development, and the external environment. Specific regulator genes control such function by producing a repressor substance as needed to regulate operator genes and structural genes. This orderly regulation of induction and repression in cell activity, however, may be lost with mutation of these regulatory genes. Control is also lost when a specific gene for some reason moves from its position to another location on the chromosome.

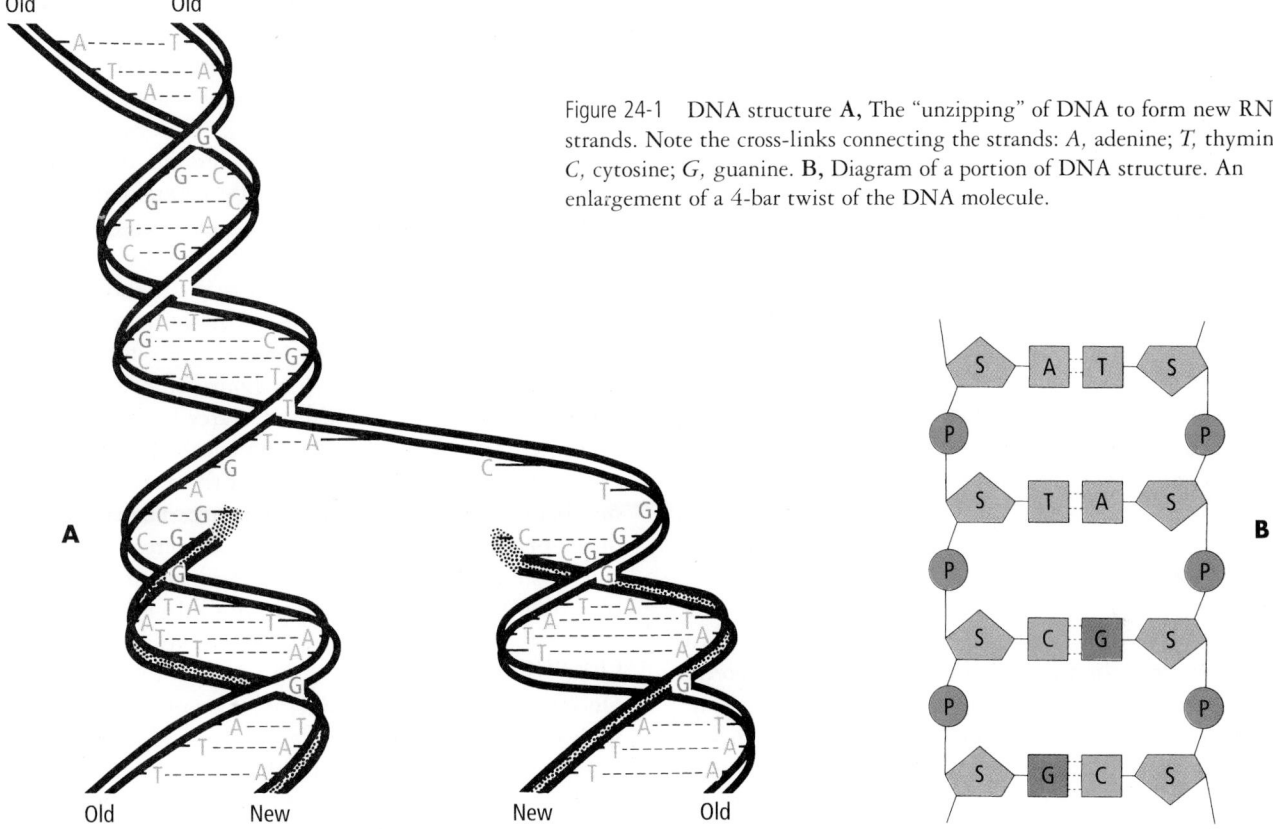

Figure 24-1 DNA structure **A,** The "unzipping" of DNA to form new RNA strands. Note the cross-links connecting the strands: *A,* adenine; *T,* thymine; *C,* cytosine; *G,* guanine. **B,** Diagram of a portion of DNA structure. An enlargement of a 4-bar twist of the DNA molecule.

The cancer cell

A cell may become malignant when one of these potentially cancer-causing genes is translocated and reinserted into a highly active part of the DNA. This has been shown to occur, for example, in patients with Burkitt's lymphoma and the blood cancer acute nonlymphocytic leukemia. Now apparently these root causes of damaged DNA and the cell's impaired ability to repair it are joined by the recently discovered cellular genes called *proto-oncogenes*, which in their developed form of **oncogenes** can cause neoplastic growth.[3] The proliferation of normal cells is regulated by a counter-balance between growth-promoting proto-oncogenes and growth-restraining tumor suppressor genes.[4,5] Search for genetic damage and the explanation of how that damage affects biochemical function in the cell are key lines of current research that hold much promise for further unfolding the mysteries of cancer.

Cancer cell source

The source of the cancer cell is now clear. It is derived from a normal cell that has lost control over cell reproduction and is thereby transformed from a normal cell into a cancer cell.

Cancer tumor types

On this basis of cell nature and differentiation, it is possible to classify cancer tumor types according to (1) type of originating tissue, with those arising from connective tissues called **sarcomas** and those from epithelial tissues called **carcinomas**; and (2) extent or degree of cell tissue change. Tumor stages are defined in relation to rate of growth, degree of autonomy, and invasiveness.

cancer A malignant cellular tumor with properties of tissue invasion and spreading to other parts of the body.

carcinoma A malignant new growth made up of epithelial cells, infiltrating the surrounding tissue and spreading to other parts of the body.

neoplasm Any new tissue growth that is abnormal, uncontrolled, and progressive.

oncogene Any of various genes that, when activated as by radiation or a virus, may cause a normal cell to become cancerous; viral genetic material carrying the potential of cancer and passed from parent to offspring.

sarcoma A tumor, usually malignant, arising from connective tissue.

Relation to the aging process

Because the incidence of cancer increases with age, a relationship exists between cancer development and the aging process in cells, tissues, and organ systems.

CAUSES OF CANCER CELL DEVELOPMENT

It is thus evident that the basic cause of cancers is the fundamental loss of control over normal cell reproduction. Researchers have discovered several interrelated causes contributing to this loss of cell control.

Mutations

Gene mutations result from loss of one or more regulatory genes in the cell nucleus. Such a mutant gene may be inherited, although some environmental agent may contribute to its expression.

Chemical carcinogens

A number of chemical carcinogens interfere with the structure or function of regulatory genes. Exposure to such agents may be by individual choice, as in cigarette smoking, which causes 30% of cancer deaths, making tobacco smoke the single most lethal carcinogen in the United States.[6] Smoking, mainly of cigarettes, is the major cause of cancer of the lungs with other primary sites in the larynx, oral cavity, and oropharynx.[6,7] Smoking also contributes to cancer of the upper respiratory tract, esophagus, bladder, and pancreas, the degree of maligancy depending on the frequency of smoking and duration of the habit, especially when started at a young age. Although the United States Food and Drug Administration has restricted the sale and distribution of cigarettes to children and teenagers, the prevalence of smoking among this vulnerable group has been increasing since 1992, with inevitable long-term mortality risks.[8-10]

Other exposure comes by general environmental substances, such as pesticide residues, water and air pollutants, food additives and contaminants, and occupational hazards. However, many of our natural environmental agents can carry more hazard, depending on the dose. The principle that "the dose makes the poison" applies to all substances, including carcinogens, natural or synthetic. Possible cancer-causing actions of such substances may be mutation, effect on regulation of gene function, or activation of a dormant virus.

Radiation

Radiation that is sufficient to damage DNA causes breakage and incorrect rejoining of chromosomes. Such radiation damage may be ionizing, such as from x-rays, radioactive materials, atomic exhausts or wastes, or it may be nonionizing, such as from sunlight. Every year an estimated 750,000 Americans develop skin cancer from overexposure to sunlight's ultraviolet radiation. This radiation mutates the recently discovered gene called *patched (PTC)* that inhibits cell growth.[11-13]

Our current pursuit of the bronzed-god look has taken a large toll: sun-related skin cancer has risen rapidly in the United States and Europe, afflicting younger and younger persons. The common forms on the head and neck are usually (1) basal cell carcinoma (about 800,000 United States cases/year), and (2) squamous cell carcinoma (about 100,000 United States cases/year).[14,15] Both of these common forms are easily cured by surgical removal. However, a far more lethal form, **malignant melanoma**, occurs in the skin cells that produce the pigment *melanin* and accounts for about 2% of all cancers. Currently, about 38,000 United States cases occur each year with approximately 7000 deaths.[14] In the United States the incidence varies with latitude, with the greater number occuring in the southern states. The rising incidence probably results from increased recreational exposure to sunlight. The currently rising incidence is probably a result of increased exposure to sunlight.

Oncogenic viruses

Oncogenic, or tumor-producing, viruses that interfere with the function of the regulatory genes have been identified. Oncogenes involved are the focus of much current research related to cell growth factors and possible new therapies for blocking tumor cell growth.[14,16] Although oncogenes were first found in viruses, their evolutionary history indicates that they are also present and functioning in normal vertebrate cells. It is their abnormal expression that can lead to cancerous growth.

A virus is little more than a packet of genetic information encased in a protein coat (see Chapter 23). It contains a small chromosome, DNA or RNA, with a relatively small number of genes, usually fewer than five and never more than several hundred. In contrast, cells of complex organisms have tens of thousands of genes. Generally, when viruses produce disease, they act as parasites, taking over the cell machinery to replicate themselves. Continuing study indicates that viruses must be thought of as the second most important risk factor for cancer development, exceeded only by tobacco use.[17]

Epidemiologic factors

Studies of cancer distribution and occurrence in relation to such factors as race, diet, region, sex, age, heredity, and occupation show variable and conflicting results. It is becoming increasingly clear, for example, that racial differences in cancer incidence between blacks and whites in the United States are great, with more cancer among blacks than whites. However, it is also clear that these differences have nothing to do with race but have much to do with poverty, which has implications for nutritional status, health care, education, and resources. The world incidence of cancer does vary a great deal from country to country, and that of specific cancer types varies from 6-fold to 300-fold. Although our cancer rates have not changed markedly over the past few decades, cancer is endemic in our population; the United States incidence rates are appreciably greater than those in many other countries.

Also, racial incidence of cancer seems to change as population groups migrate and aquire the different cancer characteristics of the new population. Although specific dietary factors have been hard to pinpoint in the cause of cancer, world wide epidemiologic studies do show significant correlation of mortality from breast cancer, for example, with the consumption of fat in the diet. Overall epidemiologic evidence from case-control studies provides a basis for a primary prevention approach for reducing cancer risks (see Issues and Answers).[17,18]

STRESS FACTORS

The idea that emotions may play a part in malignancy is not new. Galen, a second century Greek physician, wrote of such relationships, as have many different kinds of "healers" since that time. However, these relationships are difficult to measure. Even with great technologic and scientific advances, Western medicine holds fast to its basic tenet that a thing must be measurable under controlled conditions to be said to exist.

Nonetheless, increasing observations are being made of relationships between cancer and less measurable factors of stress. Clinicians and researchers have reported that psychic trauma, especially the loss of a central relationship, does seem to carry with it a strong cancer correlation. The cause of a possible relationship between such trauma and cancer may lie in two physiologic areas: (1) damage to the thymus gland and the immune system, and (2) neuroendocrine effects mediated through the hypothalamus, pituitary, and adrenal cortex. This automatic "cascade of physiologic events" triggered by stress may well provide the neurologic currency that converts anxiety to malignancy. Such a stressful state may also make a person more vulnerable to other factors present, influencing the integrity of the immune system, food behaviors, and the nutritional status. Once cancer occurs, however, today's cancer patients have many options for easing their distress and improving the quality of their lives through supportive relations and current positive medical approaches to pain management.[19,20]

THE BODY'S DEFENSE SYSTEM

COMPONENTS OF THE IMMUNE SYSTEM

The human body's defense system is remarkably efficient and complex. Several components of special type cells protect not only against external invaders such as bacteria and viruses but also against internal "aliens" such as malignant tumor cells. These malignant cells from developing tumors in the body can spread invading cells into other body tissues and form secondary tumors, or **metastases**, that become life-threating.[21]

Two major populations of cells provide the immune system's primary line of defense for detecting and destroying malignant cells that arise daily in the body. These cells mediate specific **cellular immunity** and **humoral immunity**, as well as providing supportive backup biologic systems. These two populations of lymphoid cells, or *lymphocytes*, a type of white blood cell, develop early in life from a common stem cell in fetal liver and bone marrow (Figure 24.2). They then differentiate and populate the peripheral lymphoid organs during the latter stages of gestation. One type is called *T cells*, traced from the thymus-derived cells. The other *B cells*, are preprocessed by the liver and bone marrow.

T cells

After precursor cells migrate to the thymus, the T cell population is differentiated in this small gland, which lies posterior to the sternum and anterior to the great vessels partly covering the trachea. The majority of the circulating small lymphocytes in blood, lymph, and certain areas of the lymph nodes and spleen are T cells. These cells recognize invading antigens by means of specific specialized receptors on their surfaces. When T-cells meet an *antigen*—a foreign intruder, a "non-self," or alien substance such as abnormal cancer cells—they proliferate and initiate specific cellular immune responses: (1) they activate the *phagocytes*, special cells that have intracellular killing and degrading mechanisms for destroying invaders; and (2) they cause an inflammatory response through chemical mediators released by the antigen-stimulated T cells. Scientists have now discovered that some T lymphocytes can do even more, not only proliferating in response to an antigen but also attacking it. These special T cells are called "helper cell–independent cytotoxic T lymphocytes," abbreviated more graphically to the name *HIT cells*.

B cells

The B cell population matures first in the bone marrow and then, following migration, in the solid peripheral lymphoid tissues of the body—the lymph nodes, spleen, and gut. These cells are responsible for synthesis and secretion of specialized protein known as *antibodies*. When the B cells contact an antigen, they increase and initiate specific humoral immune responses: (1) they pro-

---

malignant melanoma A tumor tending to become progressively worse, composed of melanin (the dark pigment of the skin and other body tissues), usually arising from the skin and aggravated by excessive sun exposure.

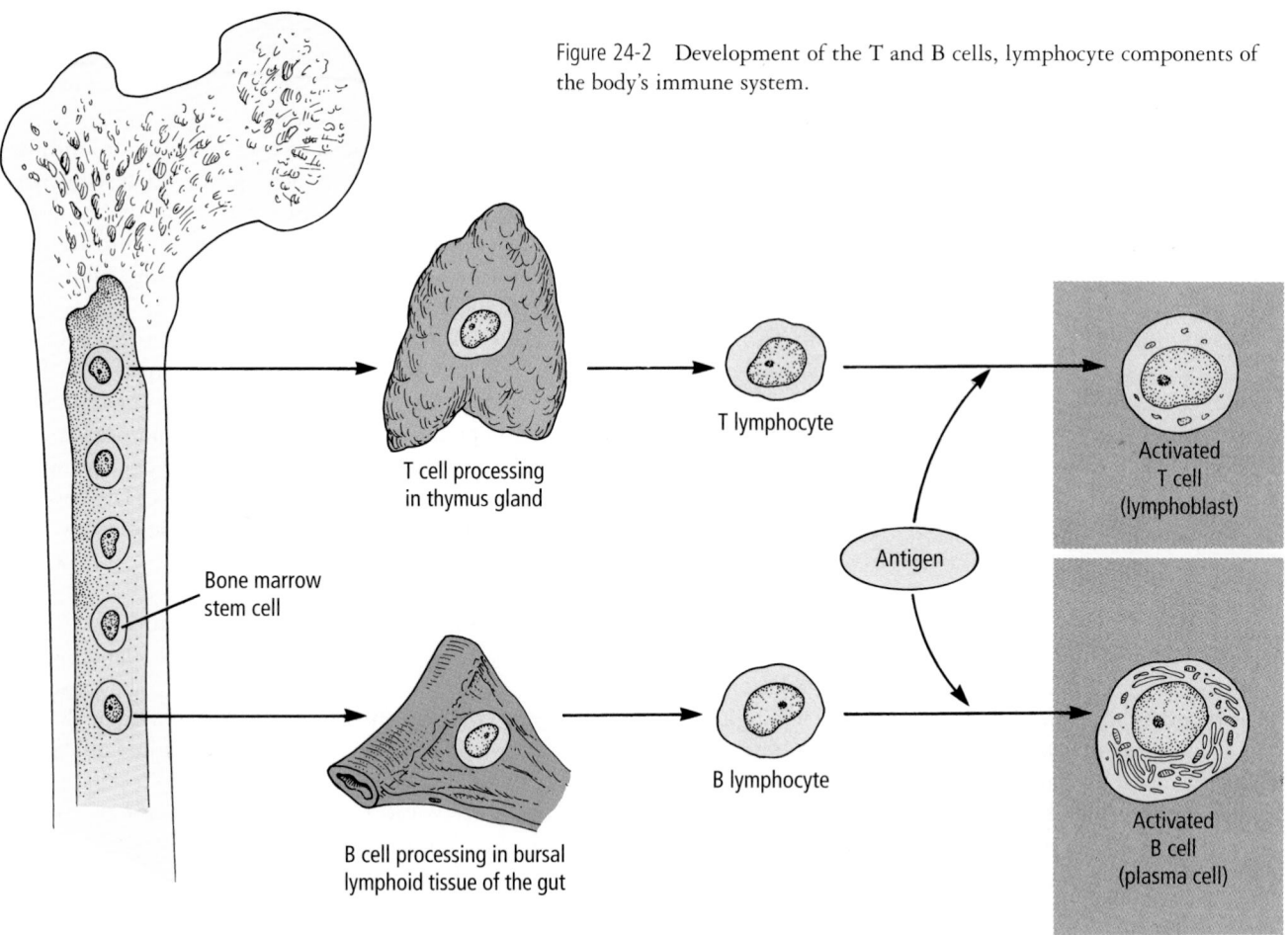

Figure 24-2   Development of the T and B cells, lymphocyte components of the body's immune system.

duce specific antibodies or *immunoglobulins* in the blood; and (2) they produce a particular antibody secretion, immunoglobulin A, in the bowel and upper respiratory mucosa. This combination of antigen and antibody then activates the *complement system*, which attracts phagocytes and initiates the inflammatory response for healing.

RELATION TO NUTRITION

Immune system

Integrity of the body's immune system components requires nutritional support. Severely malnourished persons show changes in the structure and function of the immune system with atrophy of the liver, bowel wall, bone marrow, spleen, and lymphoid tissue.[22,23] Clearly, sound nutrition maintains normal immunity and combats sustained attacks in malignancy. Recent studies in *nutritional immunology* have shown that wise and early use of vigorous nutrition support for cancer patients provides recovery of normal nutritional status, including immunocompetence, thereby improving their response to therapy and prognosis.[22] States of malnutrition, especially alcohol-induced, create a high risk of nutritional immunosupression.[23,24]

The healing process

Tissue integrity, essential for the healing process, is maintained through protein synthesis. Such strength of tissue is a front line of the body's defense system. This process of healing requires optimal nutritional intake to support (1) cell function and structure of all its parts involving DNA, RNA, amino acids, and proteins, and (2) the integrity of all the immune system components.

NUTRITIONAL SUPPORT FOR CANCER THERAPY

Current cancer therapy takes three major forms: *surgery, radiation,* and *chemotherapy.* Nutritional support for any form of cancer therapy enhances its potentional success.

SURGERY

Operable tumors

Early diagnosis of operable tumors has led to successful surgical treatment of a large number of cancer patients. The success of any surgery depends in large measure on the sound nutritional status of the patient (see Chapter 22). But this is especially true of cancer patients because their general condition may be weakened. Prevention of problems through early detection and surgical treatment has significantly increased cancer cure rates. Surgical treatment may also be used with other forms of therapy for removal of single metastases or for prevention and alleviation of symptoms. Optimal nutritional status preoperatively and maximal nutritional support postoperatively are fundamenmtal to the healing process.

Nutrition relationships

Nutrition has both general and specific relationships: (1) support of the general healing process and overall body metabolism, and (2) specific modifications of nutrient factors, texture, or feeding method according to the surgical site and organ function involved.

RADIATION

After the discovery of **radiation** in the 19th century, scientists soon found that it could damage body tissue. Continued study of its use and control revealed that normal tissue could largely withstand an amount of radiation that would damage and destroy cancer tissue. The subsequent role of radiation in cancer treatment has developed around controlled use with two types of tumor: (1) those responsive to radiation therapy, or radiotherapy, within a dose level tolerable to health of normal tissue, and (2) those that can be targeted without damage to overlying vital organ tissue.

Forms

Radiation used in cancer therapy is produced from three main sources: (1) *x-rays*, the oldest form of cancer treatment, which are electromagnetic waves similar to heat and light rays, with varying penetration according to the speed at which the electrons strike the target, as well as modern clinical linear accelarators that can be rotated easily around the patient to irradiate the tumor from different directions; (2) *radioisotopes*, such as cobalt 60, and (3) *atomic particles*, such as neutrons, protons, and electrons, derived from radioactive materials.

Effects

Radiotherapy may be used alone or in conjunction with other therapies both for curative and **palliative** care for some 50% of all cancer patients at some time during the course of their disease. Radiation effects will influence nutritional status and therapy a great deal, depending on the site and intensity of treatment:

1. *Head and neck* radiation will affect the oral mucosa and salivary secretions, as well as the esophagus, influencing taste sensations and sensitivity to food temperature and texture.

2. *Abdomen* radiation may produce denuded bowel mucosa, loss of villi and absorbing surface area, vascular changes from intimal thickening, thrombosis, ulcer formation, or inflammation. Obstruction, fistula formation, or strictures may further contribute to general malabsorption, compounded by curtailment of food intake caused by anorexia and nausea.

CHEMOTHERAPY

Drug development

Although chemotherapy has been recognized as a valid cancer therapy over the past few decades, the most effective agents currently in use have largely been developed only within the past few years. Intensive research has resulted in the development of a large number of effective *antineoplastic drugs*. Their therapeutic use is based on two general principles related to rate and mode of action.

Rate of action

The so-called cell or log (logarithm)–kill hypothesis of the action of chemotherapeutic agents on tumors indicates that a single dose can only be as much as 99.9% effective in killing the tumor cells. Thus if as large a tumor as is compatible with life can be treated with a drug tolerable at a toxicity level that is 99.9% effective, the tumor is gradually reduced with successive doses that cause "fractional killing" with each dose. This process finally brings the tumor within the capability of the body's own immune system to take over and make the final kill and cure. The smaller the tumor, either because of early detection or initial treatment by surgery or radiation, the greater the possible effectiveness of the chemotherapeutic agents. Also, two other principles of dosage rate for greater effectiveness are important: (1) aggressive use of maximal tolerable dosages in repeated series, and (2) use of several drugs together for a *synergistic* effect. Many malignacies such as leukemias, lymphomas, and testicular cancer are now successfully treated by such combination therapy.[25] However, most common cancers such as breast, lung, colorectal, and prostate are not yet curable by chemotherapy alone and require an overall program also involving surgery and radiation.

Mode of action

Chemotherapeutic agents are effective because they disrupt the normal processes in the cell responsible for cell growth and reproduction. Some agents interfere with

---

palliative Care affording relief but not cure; useful for comfort when cure is still unknown or obscure.

radiation A highly controlled treatment for cancer, using radioactive substances in limited, controlled exposure to kill cancerous cells.

DNA synthesis. Others disrupt DNA structure and RNA replication. Others prevent cell division by mitosis, cause hormonal imbalances, or make unavailable the specific amino acids necessary for protein synthesis. It is this diversity in mode of action that provides a basis for grouping drugs into certain classes of chemotherapeutic agents: (1) alkaloids, (2) alkylating agents, (3) antibiotics, (4) antimetabolites, (5) enzymes, and (6) hormones. They are usually used in combined therapy or as adjuvant therapy in conjunction with surgery or radiation.

Toxic effects

Chemotherapeutic agents have the same effects on rapidly reproducing normal cells as they do on the rapidly reproducing cancer cells. Interference with normal function is most apparent in normal cells of the bone marrow, the gastrointestinal tract, and the hair follicles, accounting for a number of the toxic side effects and problems in nutritional management:

1. *Bone marrow effects* include interference with production of red blood cells (anemia), white cells (infections), and platelets (bleeding).
2. *Gastrointestinal effects* include nausea and vomiting, **stomatitis**, anorexia, ulcers, and diarrhea.
3. *Hair follicle effects* include alopecia (baldness) and general hair loss.

Modes of drug use

Chemotherapy may be used alone or in conjunction with other treatments such as surgery or radiotherapy to increase the cure rate.

Chemotherapy research

Researchers are working to find substances, either in food or drugs, that can prevent or halt cancer development. Their goal is to develop drugs or modify foods as a preventive strategy for people at high risk for cancer.[26] Food itself has been found to be a source of some promising chemopreventive compounds from plants. These chemical compounds produced by plants or in persons eating the plants are now termed *phytochemicals* (see discussion in Chapter 7). For example, members of this group of compounds include alpha- and beta-carotene found in carrots; beta-cryptoxanthin found in oranges, peaches, and tangerines; and lutein found in vegetables such as corn, green beans, spinach and other greens. There are many of these phytochemicals, found in a wide variety of vegetables and fruits, that provide specific health benefits. Another group called disease preventive agents is being studied. This group is the dithiolthiones found in cruciferous vegetables such as broccoli, cauliflower, and cabbage are potential preventive agents; a synthetic form called Oltipraz has inhibited tumor growth in animal tests and is under further study.[26]

NUTRITIONAL THERAPY

THERAPEUTIC PROBLEMS AND GOALS

Numerous problems present needs for nutritional therapy and care of patients with cancer. In general, nutritional therapy deals with two types of problems: (1) those related to the disease process itself, and (2) those related to medical treatment of the disease. Thus the basic objectives of nutritional therapy in cancer are to (1) meet the increased metabolic demands of the disease and prevent catabolism as much as possible, and (2) alleviate symptoms resulting from the disease and its treatment through adaptations of food and the feeding process.

PROBLEMS RELATED TO THE DISEASE PROCESS

Feeding problems forming the basic challenge to nutritional therapy are caused by general systemic effects of the neoplastic disease process and by specific responses related to the type of cancer.

General systemic reactions

The disease process causes three basic systemic effects: (1) *anorexia*, (2) *hypermetabolic state*, and (3) *negative nitrogen balance*, which are often accompanied by a continuing weight loss. These effects may vary widely with individual patients, according to type and stage of the disease, from mild, scarcely discernible responses to the extreme forms of debilitating cachexia seen in advanced disease, and estimated to cause more than 50% of the cancer deaths.[27,28] This extreme weight loss and weakness is caused by abnormalities in glucose metabolism, in which cancer patients cannot produce glucose efficiently from carbohydrates and instead "feed" off their own tissue protein and convert it to glucose.[27,29] The "new-old" drug, hydrazine sulfate, seems to correct this metabolic error, allowing patients to conserve more energy and show modest improvements in survival, but no remissions have been documented.[30]

Anorexia is frequently accompanied by depression or discomfort during normal eating. This contributes further to a limited nutrient intake at the very time the disease process causes an increased metabolic rate and nutrient demand. Often this imbalance of decreased intake and increased demand creates a negative nitrogen balance, an indication of body-tissue wasting. Sometimes a true tissue loss of protein is masked by outward nitrogen equilibrium as the growing tumor retains nitrogen at the expense of the host, further compounding the problem.

Specific responses related to type of cancer

Interrelated functional and metabolic problems stem from specific types of cancer and their effects on the body. All of these factors contribute to nutritional depletion. In addition to the primary nutritional deficiencies induced by the disease process itself, secondary difficulties in ingestion and use of nutrients relate to specific tumors that cause obstructions or lesions in the gastrointestinal tract or adjacent tissue. These conditions that curtail intake or absorption of adequate nutrients include: (1) malabsorption, (2) bypass problems and subsequent diarrhea, (3) fluid-electrolyte imbalances, (4) hormonal imbalances, and (5) anemia. Additional contributory factors may be increased hemolysis, bleeding of ulcerated lesions, or the presence of gastrointestinal fistulas.

PROBLEMS RELATED TO CANCER TREATMENT

Medical treatments for cancer entail physiologic stress. These results include toxic tissue effects, often with damage to cell DNA structure and changes in normal body function. Thus the benefit achieved is not without attendant problems. Nutritional support seeks to alleviate these problems.

Problems related to surgery

Beyond the regular nutritional needs surrounding any surgical procedure and its healing process, gastrointestinal surgery poses special problems for normal eating and digesting and absorbing of food nutrients. Head and neck surgery, or resections in the oropharyngeal area, are sometimes necessitated by cancer. In such cases food intake is greatly affected. A creative variety of food forms and semiliquid textures as well as modes of feeding must be devised. Often the mechanical problems of food ingestion make long-term tube feeding necessary (see Chapter 17).

Gastrectomy may cause numerous postgastrectomy "dumping" problems requiring frequent, small, low-carbohydrate feedings (see Chapter 22). Vagotomy contributes to gastric stasis. Various intestinal resections or tumor excisions may cause steatorrhea because of general malabsorption, fistulas, or stenosis. Pancreatectomy causes loss of digestive enzymes, induced insulin-dependent diabetes mellitus, and general weight loss.

Problems related to radiation

Radiation to the oropharyngeal area often produces a loss of taste sensation, with increasing anorexia and nausea. Other means of tempting appetite through food appearance and aroma, as well as texture, must be developed. Abdominal radiation may cause intestinal damage, with tissue edema and congestion, decreased peristalsis, or endarteritis in small blood vessels. In the intestinal wall there may be fibrosis, stenosis, necrosis, or ulceration. General malabsorption or fistulas may develop, as well as hemorrhage, obstruction, and diarrhea, all contributing to nutritional problems. The liver is somewhat more resistant to damage from radiation in adults, but children are more vulnerable.

Chemotherapy

The major nutritional problems during chemotherapy relate to (1) the gastrointestinal symptoms caused by the effect of the toxic drugs on the rapidly developing mucosal cells; (2) the anemia associated with bone marrow effects; and (3) the general systemic toxicity effect on appetite. Stomatitis, nausea, diarrhea, and malabsorption contribute to many food intolerances. Antiemetic drugs such as prochlorperazine (Compazine) may be used (Table 24.1). Such drugs act on the vomiting center in the brain to prevent the nausea response. Prolonged vomiting seriously affects fluid and electrolyte balance, especially in elderly patients, and needs to be controlled. In breast cancer patients, relief from nausea has been achieved with use of the antiemetic drug megestrol acetate (Megase), a synthetic female sex hormone similar to the natural hormone progesterone. Increased appetites and food intakes were accompanied by weight gains in true body mass rather than fluid retention.[31] Two new drugs that act as serotonin blockers, granisetron hydrochloride (Kytril) and ondansetron hydrochloride (Zofran), administered in combination therapy with dexamethasone, an adrenal cortical steroid, have been added to the list of drugs that help control episodic nausea and vomiting.[32]

In some cases of chronic long-term drug therapy, special nutritional management restricting conditioned, or learned, food aversions to odors and colors has been effective. For example, patients receiving periodic treatments of the drug cisplatin (Platinol), who had a special diet of three meals a day of plain colorless, odorless foods, including items such as cottage cheese, applesauce, vanilla ice cream, and other predetermined foods, experienced little nausea and increased food intake.[33] The potential for developing conditioned food aversions while on long-term chemotherapy is diminished by use of food having little or no odor or color because the drug-related *dysgeusis* (perverted sense of taste) and *dysosmia* (impaired sense of smell) are correlated with visual olfactory stimulation factors.[33,34]

Certain chemotherapeutic drugs also have special effects. For example, monoaminoxidase (MAO) inhibitors may be used for pretreatment relief of mental and emotional depression or for palliative therapy. These antidepressant drugs cause well-known pressor effects when used with tyramine-rich foods (Table 24.2). Thus these foods should be avoided when using such drugs (see Chapter 16).

---

stomatitis Inflammation of the oral mucosa, especially the buccal tissue lining the inside of the cheeks, but also may involve the tongue, palate, floor of mouth, and the gums.

Table

24.1 Medications used to control nausea and vomiting in patients receiving chemotherapy

Antiemetic drug/action	Cancer chemotherapeutic drug counteracted	Dosage used	Side effects	Comments
Phenothiazines Action: blocks CTZ* stimulation by dopamine Examples Compazine (prochlorperazine) Torecan (thiethylperazine) Phenergan (promethazine)	Moderate emetic-potential drugs	5-10 mg, orally or parenterally before chemotherapy; every 4-6 hr after, for 24-48 hr	Sedation Orthostatic hypertension	Less effective when given on "as needed" basis
Droperidol (Inapsine) Action: sedative and antiemetic	Cisplatin	0.5 mg intravenously 1 hr before chemotherapy; every 4 hr after chemotherapy	Somnolence	Some patients given up to 1.5 mg intravenously developed a tolerance for the drug
Corticosteroids Dexamethasone (Hexadrol, Decadron) Methylprednisone (Solu-Medrol)	Cyclophosphmide Doxorubicin Nitrogen mustard Mitomycin Methyl-CCNU†	10 mg intramuscular before chemotherapy 250 mg intravenously every 6 hr for 4 doses beginning 2 hr after chemotherapy	Perianal stinging if given too rapidly Swelling Facial rash Weakness, lethargy	Moderate to high relief in 70% of the patients Effects of methylprednisolone considered disappointing
Tetrahydrocannabinol (THC, marijuana)	Variety of agents studied Methotrexate 5-FU‡ Methyl-CCNU Cyclophosphamide Doxorubicin Nitrosoureas Mechorethamine	10 mg/m²	Somnolence Visual hallucinations	Patients (usually older) not used to THC refused to continue it because of CNS effects§ Response associated with extent of THC-induced "high" Most effective with flourouracil, cyclophosphamide, methotrexate, doxorubicin "High" by giving a phenothiazine
Metoclopramide (Reglan)	Cisplatin	Single 20-mg dose, given orally halfway through a 6-hr infusion of cisplatin (100 mg/m²); higher doses might be possible intravenously (1-3 mg/kg/dose)	Sedation	Works well for patients who do not respond to other antiemetic drugs

Data modified from studies reported by Huber SL, Ballentine R: *Nutr Support Serv* 2(10):30, 1982.

*CTZ, chemoreceptor zone, vomiting center in brain.

†Methyl-CCNU, methyl-1-(chloroethyl)-3-cyclohexyl-1-nitrosourea.

‡5-FU, 5-flurouracil.

§CNS, central nervous system.

Table 24.2	Tyramine-restricted diet

General directions

- Designed for patients on monoamine oxidase inhibitors, drugs that have been reported to cause hypertensive crises when used with tyramine-rich foods. These include foods in which aging, protein breakdown, and putrefaction are used to increase flavor. Studies indicate that as little as 5 to 6 mg of tyramine may produce a response, and 25 mg is a dangerous dose.
- Food sources of other pressor amines such as histamine, dihydroxyphenylalanine, and hydroxytyramine are also avoided.
- Avoid all foods listed. Limited amounts of foods with a lower amount of tyramine, such as yeast bread, may be included in a specific diet.
- Avoid over-the-counter drugs such as decongestants, cold remedies, and antihistamines.

Foods to avoid	Representative Tyramine Values in μg/g or ml	Additional foods to avoid
Cheeses		Other aged cheeses
New York State cheddar	1416	Blue
Gruyère	516	Boursalt
Stilton	466	Brick
Emmentaler	225	Cheddars (other)
Brie	180	Gouda
Camembert	86	Mozzarella
Processed American	50	Parmesan
Wines		Provolone
Chianti	25.4	Romano
Sherry	3.6	Roquefort
Riesling	0.6	Yeast and products made with yeast
Sauternes	0.4	Homemade bread
Beer, ale (varies with brand)		Yeast extracts such as soup cubes, canned meats, and marmite
Highest	4.4	Italian broad beans with pod (fava beans)
Average	2.3	Meat
Least	1.8	Aged game
		Liver
		Canned meats with yeast extracts
		Fish (salted dried)
		Herring, cod, capelin
		Pickled herring
		Other
		Chocolate
		Cream (especially sour cream)
		Salad dressings
		Soy sauce
		Vanilla
		Yogurt

PRINCIPLES OF NUTRITIONAL THERAPY FOR CANCER

Two important principles of nutritional therapy, vital in any sound nutrition practice but especially essential in care of patients with cancer, provide the basis for planning nutritional care of each patient: (1) personal nutritional assessment, and (2) vigorous nutrition therapy to maintain good nutritional status and support medical treatment.

Nutrition assessment

It is far more difficult to replenish a nutritionally depleted patient than to maintain a good nutritional status from the outset of the disease process. Therefore a primary goal in nutritional therapy is to prevent a depleted state. Initial assessment for baseline data and regular monitoring thereafter during treatment are necessary. A detailed personal history is essential to determine individual needs, desires, and tolerances. To be valid, the interview should be conducted as a conversation, using verbal and nonverbal probes and pauses rather than a cross fire of separate questions and answers (see Chapter 15).

Nutritional therapy and plan of care

Based on careful individual nutritional assessment, the team clinical dietitian prepares a plan for optimal nutritional therapy to meet needs. This nutritional therapy outline is then incorporated into the nursing care plan as the clinical dietitian works with the nursing staff to carry it out. Primary care provided by the dietitian and the nurse on a regular basis is a necessary part of the oncology team practice. This early, vigorous care often makes the difference in the success rate of medical therapy. Thus working closely with the oncology nurse and physician, the clinical dietitian assesses personal needs, determines nutritional requirements, plans and manages nutritional care, monitors progress and responses to therapy, and makes adjustments in care according to status and tolerances.

NUTRITIONAL NEEDS

Each of the nutrient factors related to tissue protein synthesis and energy metabolism requires careful attention. The increased needs for energy, protein, vitamins and minerals, and fluid are based on demands made by the disease and its treatment. Individual needs and food tolerances vary, but general guidelines are the same.

Energy

Great energy demands are placed on the cancer patient. These demands result from the hypermetabolic state of the disease process and the tissue-healing requirements. Of this total dietary kcalorie value, sufficient carbohydrate to spare protein for vital tissue synthesis is essential. For the adult patient with good nutritional status, about 2000 kcal/day will provide for maintenance needs. A more malnourished patient may require 3000 to 4000 kcalories, depending on the degree of malnutrition and body trauma. Carbohydrate should supply the majority of the energy intake, with fat restricted to 30% or less of the total kcalories.

Dietary fat

Numerous studies have related excessive dietary fat to cancer metastasis and effectiveness of cancer therapy.[35-37] The practical feasibility of dietary intervention programs to reduce fat intake has been demonstrated by recent studies of the National Cancer Institute, a large multi-centered pilot study, and the Women's Health Trial.[38,39] In these studies women with breast cancer and women at high risk of breast cancer were able to reduce their fat intake from a baseline of 40% of total kcalories to 22% while increasing their intakes of all the vitamins and minerals. These results indicate that a nutritionally sound low-fat diet can be successfully implemented in highly motivated, free-living groups of individuals.

Protein

Tissue protein synthesis, a necessary component of healing and rehabilitation, requires essential amino acids and nitrogen. Efficient protein use, which depends on an optimum protein/kcalorie ratio, promotes tissue building, prevents tissue wastage (catabolism), and helps make up tissue deficits. An adult patient with good nutritional status will need about 80 to 100 g/day of protein to meet maintenance needs and assure anabolism. A malnourished patient will need more to replenish tissue and restore positive nitrogen balance.

Vitamins and minerals

Key vitamins and minerals control protein and energy metabolism through their roles in cell enzyme systems. They also play a necessary part in structural development and tissue integrity. The B-complex vitamins in general serve as necessary coenzyme agents in energy and protein metabolism, Vitamins A and C are necessary for the development and integrity of body tissues. Vitamin A also has a significant role in protective immunity and cell differentiation; vitamin C has significant antioxidant, enzymatic, and immune biologic functions related to cancer.[40,41] Increased dietary consumption of vegetables and fruits is a primary means of obtaining these vitamins.[42] Recent study of nutritional molecular carcinogens suggest also that the expression of certain oncogenes may be reduced by vitamins A, E, and D.[43] Vitamin D hormone ensures proper calcium and phosphorus metabolism in bone and blood serum. Vitamin E protects the integrity of cell wall materials and hence tissue integrity. Many minerals function in structural and enzymatic roles in vital metabolic and tissue-building processes. Thus an optimal intake of vitamins and minerals, at least to the recommended dietary allowances (RDA) levels but frequently augmented with supplements according to individual patient nutritional status, is indicated.

Fluids

Adequate fluid intake is important for two reasons: (1) to replace gastrointestinal losses or losses caused by infection and fever, and (2) to help the kidneys dispose of the metabolic breakdown products from the destroyed cancer cells as well as from the toxic drugs used in treatment. For example, some toxic drugs such as cyclophosphamide (Cytoxan) require as much as 2 to 3 L of forced fluids daily to prevent hemorrhagic cystitis.

NUTRITIONAL MANAGEMENT

The specific feeding method used depends on the individual patient's condition. However, the classic dictum of nutritional management should prevail: *"If the gut works, use it."* Details of available enteral and parenteral modes of nutritional support are provided in Chapter 17. If at all possible, an oral diet with supplementation is the most desired form of feeding, of course. A carefully designed personal plan of care based on nutrition assessment data and including adjustments in texture, temperature, food choices, and tolerances, as well as family food patterns, can often meet needs (see *Practical Application* box, p. 520). Often the hospitalized patient's diet can be supplemented with familiar foods from home as the clinical nutritionist plans with the family. Personal food tolerances will vary according to the current treatment and nature of the disease. A number of adjustments in food texture, temperature, amount, timing, taste, appearance, and form can be made to help alleviate symptoms stemming from common problems in successive parts of the gastrointestinal tract.[44]

Difficulties in eating may be caused by loss of appetite, problems in the mouth, or swallowing problems.

Loss of appetite

Anorexia is a major problem and curtails food intake when it is needed most. It is a general systemic effect of the cancer disease process itself, often further induced by the cancer treatment and progressively enhanced by personal anxiety, depression, and stress of the illness. Such a vicious cycle, if not countered by much effort, can lead to more malnutrition and the well-recognized starvation "cancer cachexia," a syndrome of emaciation, debilitation, and malnutrition.[45-46]

A vigorous program of eating, *not dependent on appetite for stimulus,* must be planned and maintained with the patient and family. It is helpful sometimes to develop protein and caloric goals, discussing the role of nutrients and key foods in combatting the disease and providing support for therapy. With such support both patient and family are better able to build a positive mental attitude toward the diet as an integral part of the treatment, and are thus more able to accept responsibility for this aspect of therapy. Often this positive attitude of the vital role patients play in their own treatment is a means of gaining some sense of control of their own lives, a sense frequently lost in the bewildering world of cancer and its therapy.

The overall goal is to provide food with as much nutrient density as possible so that "every bite will count." If appetite is better in the morning, a good breakfast should be emphasized. Food texture may be varied as tolerated, with appeal to sensory perceptions of color, aroma, and taste. A series of small meals with a wide variety of foods is better tolerated than regular larger meals. Getting some exercise before meals and maintaining surroundings that reduce stress may also help in the eating process.

Mouth problems

Eating difficulties may stem from sore mouth, stomatitis, or taste changes. Sore mouth often results from chemotherapy or from radiation to the head and neck area. It is increased by any state of malnutrition or from infections such as **candidiasis** (thrush), with numerous ulcerations of the oral and throat mucosa. Frequent small meals and snacks, soft in texture, bland in nature, and cool or cold in temperature, are often better tolerated. There may also be alterations in the tongue's taste buds, causing taste distortion ("taste blindness") and inability to distinguish the basic tastes of salt, sweet, sour, or bitter, with consequent food aversions. Since the aversion is often toward basic protein foods, a high-protein, high-energy liquid drink supplement may be needed. *Dental problems* may also contribute to mouth difficulties and should be corrected. *Salivary secretions* are also affected by cancer treatment, so foods with a high liquid content should be used. Solid foods may be swallowed more easily with use of sauces, gravies, broth, yogurt, or salad dressings. A food processor or blender can render foods in semisolid or liquid forms and make them easier to swallow. If the swallowing problem is especially severe because of tumor growth or therapy, guides for a special swallowing training program, including progressive food textures, exercises, and positions, can be followed.

Gastrointestinal problems

Eating difficulties may include nausea and vomiting, general indigestion, bloating, or specific surgery responses such as the postgastrectomy "dumping" syndrome (see Chapter 22). Nausea is often enhanced by foods that are hot, sweet, fatty, or spicy, so these can be avoided according to individual tolerance. Other lower gastrointestinal problems may include general diarrhea, constipation, flatuence, or specific lactose intolerance or surgery responses, such as occur with intestinal resections and various ostomies. Helpful guidance for patients with colostomies, ileostomies, or ileoanal reservoirs is necessary (see Chapter 22). The effect of chemotherapy or radiation treatment on the mucosal cells secreting lactase contributes to lactose intolerance. In such cases a nutrient supplement formula with a nonmilk soy protein base may be needed.[47]

A number of commercial nutrient supplement products are available. A comparative review of these products will provide the basis for developing a formulary in the hospital setting for a limited number of such products (see Chapter 17). A food processor or blender can be used at home to produce creative solid and liquid food combinations from regular foods for interval liquid supplementation.

Involving cancer patients in their personal nutritional care plan is necessary for its personal success.[48]

---

candidiasis Infection with the fungus of the genus *Candida,* generally caused by *C. albicans,* so named for the whitish appearance of its small lesions; usually a superficial infection in moist areas of the skin or inner mucous membranes.

Promoting oral intake in cancer patients

Encouraging and maintaining adequate oral intake for cancer patients is one of the most difficult aspects of cancer treatment. It is time consuming and often frustrating, but may be one of the most rewarding experiences in patient care. By identifying feeding problems, initiating appropriate interventions, and providing individual education, adequate oral nutrition is promoted. The dietitian is the key figure for coordinating the nutritional program, but its success requires the full support and cooperation of the entire health care team, especially the nurse.

The patient interview is one of the most important parts of the nutritional assessment. Information that helps identify adequacy of current nutritional intake and potential nutritional problems is obtained during the interview. The following list of questions may assist in gathering accurate information about the patient's ability to obtain oral nutrition:

- How would you describe your appetite?
- Has it changed recently?
- Are you eating differently than you have most of your life?
- Do you usually eat three meals each day? Has this changed recently?

- Are you nauseated or experiencing vomiting? Is this food-related or medication-related? How long have you been experiencing this? How often do you vomit or feel nauseated?
- Do you have a bowel movement every day? Has this changed?
- Do you have diarrhea? If so, do you think this may be food-related?
- Do food smells or cooking odors bother you?
- Do you have difficulty chewing?
- Do your dentures (if any) fit? Do you wear them?
- Do you have difficulty swallowing?
- Is your mouth dry? Does your saliva seem to be different? Is it thicker or decreased in amounts?
- Do you find it easier to drink liquids than to eat solid foods?
- What were you able to eat yesterday? (Obtain a brief 24-hour dietary recall.)
- Are you unable to eat certain foods right now?
- Do some foods taste different to you? Can you give an example?

- Have you ever taken any high-kcalorie, high-protein supplements? When? What kind? How often? Were you able to tolerate them?
- Do you take a multivitamin supplement?
- Do you have any food allergies or intolerances? Are these new, or have you always experienced these intolerances?
- Do you prepare your own meals? If so, do you ever feel too tired to prepare something to eat?

The success of the interview depends on the dietitian's professional competence, interviewing skills, and bedside manner. If the dietitian establishes a feeling of comfort and trust with the patient, the opportunity to accomplish successful dietary interventions is great.

References

Bloch AS: Nutrition and cancer: the paradox, *Diet Curr* 23(2):1996.

Marian M: Cancer cachexia: prevalence, mechanisms, and interventions, *Support Line* 20(2):3, 1998.

Nahikian-Nelms ML: Encouraging oral intake. In Bloch AS, ed: *Nutrition management of the cancer patient*, Rockville, Md, 1990, Aspen.

They need to feel some sense of personal control. By starting with small amounts, the patient and the nutrition team can then set goals for the quantities that need to be ingested. Individual patients may need to schedule their supplements as medications, which commits the entire health care team to the nutritional care plan. This team involvement helps the patient to understand the importance of adequate nutrition.[49]

FEEDING IN TERMINAL ILLNESS

Although many advances have been made in the detection and treatment of cancer, mortality rates for some cancers have not declined and in some cancers have actually increased.[2] We feel these results in our work with cancer patients. We see the progressive weight loss and malnutrition that occurs, caused by the primary tumor and its spread, that leads to profound nutritional depletion and is a major cause of morbidity and mortality.[49] For some patients a time comes when the spread of the disease overcomes the body's capacity to combat it. When the patient is no longer able to eat, enteral tube-feeding or parenteral feeding may be used. Ultimately, however, ethical questions about continued feeding efforts are faced in many cases (see *To Probe Further* box, p. 522). Answers lie with the patient, as long as possible, and with the family. But sensitive and supportive counseling is needed from the cancer team members, especially the clinical dietitian responsible for the nutrition support therapy and the nurse responsible for administering the continued feeding and for personal care. These skilled and sensitive professionals, along with the physician, the patient, and the family, face these decisions together.[50]

NUTRITION AND CANCER: THE FINAL ANALYSIS

What, then, are our overall final conclusions? As Bloch, an experienced oncology nutrition specialist, has well reminded us, we see that nutrition has a dual role in relation to cancer—both prevention and therapy.[32]

Preventive role

Nutrition and health professionals have a major wellness role in maintaining health and preventing illness, especially in relation to cancer. This role is embodied in the American Cancer Society's new dietary guidelines[51]:

1. Choose most of the foods you eat from plant sources; eat a variety of fruits, vegetables, and grains.
2. Limit your intake of high-fat foods, particularly from animal sources.
3. Be physically active, achieve and maintain a healthy weight.
4. Limit consumption of alcoholic beverages, if you drink at all.

These guidelines are similar to the overall 1995 Dietary Guidelines for Americans (see Chapter 1). They are displayed in the Food Guide Pyramid and emphasized in national and state "5 a Day for Better Health" programs to encourage Americans to eat five or more servings of fruits and vegatables every day.[52] This emphasis stems from certain compounds found in plants, thus called phytochemicals ("plant chemicals"), which ongoing research indicates have promising effects in the chemoprevention of cancer.[26] As indicated, these compounds include food nutrients—vitamins A (and its analogues), C, and E—as well as nonnutritive substances such as indoles, isothiocyanates, dithiolthiones, and organosulfur (see p. 514).[26] A recent position paper of the American Dietetic Association indicates that the Association will continue to work with the government and the food industry to ensure that the public has accurate scientific information in this emerging field.[53]

Therapeutic role

For the cancer patient the clinical dietitian must shift into a therapeutic role, in which the patient is central in diet planning during disease stages and therapy effects. Nutrition therapy must now focus constantly on proactive assessment with early and continuing preventive measures to intervene wisely before malnutrition occurs. For example, anticipate possible gastrointestinal needs or psychosocial situations that relate to appetite, eating various foods, or drug effects. Provide information concerning mouth care, symptoms exerienced, or drug actions and effects. A recent study of elderly advanced cancer patients has indicated that with adequate medical management of pain and distressing symptoms, 92% of them could eat well until the day they died. Throughout the study the aim was to create an optimal individual adaptation to meals and snacks based on food preferences and dislikes, subjective intolerance of certain foods, and difficulties in chewing and swallowing.[54] Always there is a special need for building nutritional quality on personal food desires with constant support and encouragement.

TO SUM UP

Cancer is a term applied to abnormal, malignant growths in various body tissue sites. The cancerous cell is derived from a normal cell that loses control over cell reproduction. Cancer cell development occurs via mutation, carcinogens, radiation, and oncogenic viruses. It is also influenced by many epidemiologic factors such as diet, alcohol, and smoking, as well as physical and psychologic stress factors. Cell development is mediated by the body's immune system, primarily its T cells, a type of white cell found in blood, lymph, and certain parts of the lymph nodes and spleen, and B cells, which manufacture and secrete antibodies.

Cancer therapy consists primarily of surgery, radiation, and chemotherapy. Supportive nutritional therapy for the cancer patient should be highly individualized and depends on the response of each body system to the disease and to the treatment itself. It is based on a thorough nutritional assessment and provided by a number of routes—oral, tube feeding, peripheral vein, TPN. The oral route is preferred if at all possible. Nutrient requirements and feeding mode must be designed for specific physical and psychologic needs of individual patients.

QUESTIONS FOR REVIEW

1. What is cancer? Identify and describe several major causes of cancer cell formation.
2. How does your body attempt to defend itself against cancer? What nutritional factors may diminish this ability?

To Probe Further

When does feeding become an ethical issue?

Plato believed that the moral person and the physician both should abide by the Hippocratic principle of medicine, "Above all, do no harm." In recent times others have returned to Plato's use of this medical model of ethics. Current writers assert that an ethic of care rests on the "premise of nonviolence—that no one should be hurt."

Technology such as enteral and parenteral nutrition may sometimes support a caring intent and compassionate spirit, while at other times such modern technology becomes a value in and of itself with its own standard of efficiency. Enteral and parenteral feeding techniques may be used to maintain indefinitely patients who are unable to take food orally.

Concerned ethical thinkers use the following moral principles for decisions in regard to life-sustaining treatment that encompasses enteral or parenteral nutrition: benefit to patient; respect for patient autonomy or self-determination; maintenance of moral integrity of health professionals; and justice in distributing scarce medical resources among eligible patients. They offer helpful views to guide clinicians in coming to a reasoned and defensible resolution of moral conflict.

Alternatives to artificial nutrition

All options of nutritional support should be explored, not simply considering "Give food or fluids" versus "Do not give food or fluids." Dietitians are particularly useful in identifying alternative feeding strategies. The full range of therapeutic options should be carefully explored instead of assuming that the question is "Let the patient die" versus "Keep the patient alive."

Patient prognosis for recovery of functions

A widely held ethically defensible view is that aggressive means of life prolongation becomes less morally desirable in proportion to the inability of the patient to regain what he or she considers to be useful function. The persistent vegetative state and permanent loss of consciousness are examples of extreme cases where recovery of function is not possible. Accurately determining the prognosis for recovery is essential.

Total management plans and goals of therapy

The patient's prognosis and nature of the illness might determine whether the goal of medical care is to attempt cure, to manage a chronic illness that cannot be cured so as to maintain maximal patient func-

tion, or to allow a terminally ill patient to die with maximal comfort and symptom control. Nutritional treatment may make sense within one plan of care but no sense at all in another.

Wishes of the patient or patient surrogate

It is legally and ethically acceptable that in almost all cases the voluntary choice of an informed patient should override all other concerns. When the patient cannot choose, a surrogate or other substitute decision maker who is familiar with the patient's values and wishes may be consulted.

Ability of the patient to choose

It is important to assess the patient's ability to make the particular medical care choice that is relevant to the matter at hand. In some circumstances, expert psychiatric or psychologic evaluation is needed to determine this.

Benefits and burdens of artificial treatment

The medical team often tends to overestimate the benefits and underestimate the burdens of the treatments they use routinely. When the means of administering nutrition become invasive and painful, then the burdens may become substantial. Restraining the patient or repeated blood draws to monitor the effects of total parenteral nutrition may be deemed burdens unacceptable to the patient. Patients may feel that being kept alive by artificial means is an indignity itself and that life is no longer useful or meaningful to them. Spiritual and emotional burdens should be assessed equally with physical burdens in making accurate assessments of the moral obligations to patients.

Modern medical technology has produced circumstances that caregivers and patients alike have never faced before. Decisions regarding nutrition and hydration in terminally ill patients are becoming more frequent. Ethical and moral questions do not always have black or white solutions; they are often grey. The ethics task for dietitians may be to achieve balance between what works and who cares.

References

Brody H, Noel MB: Dietitians' role in decisions to withhold nutrition and hydration, *J Am Diet Assoc* 91(5):580, 1991.

Dalton S: What are the sources and standards of ethical judgment in dietetics? *J Am Diet Assoc* 91(5):545, 1991.

Edelstein S, Anderson S: Bioethics and dietetics: education and attitudes, *J Am Diet Assoc* 91(5):546, 1991.

Wall MG et al: Feeding the terminally ill: dietitians attitudes and beliefs, *J Am Diet Assoc* 91(5):549, 1991.

3. List and describe the rationale and mode of action of the types of therapies used to treat cancer.
4. Differentiate those factors challenging cancer recovery that are associated with the disease versus the type of therapy used.
5. Outline the general procedure for the nutritional management of a cancer patient.

REFERENCES

1. National Institutes of Health, National Cancer Institute: *SEER statistics review, 1973-1992,* NIH Pub No 96-2789, 1995.
2. Rennie J, Rusting R: Making headway against cancer, *Sci Am* 275(3(:56, 1996.
3. Cavenee WK, White RL: The genetic basis of cancer, *Sci Am* 27(3):72, 1995.
4. Weinberg RA: Tumor suppressor genes, *Sci Am* 275(3):62, 1996.
5. Weinberg RA: Tumor suppressor genes, *Science* 254:1138, 1991.
6. Trichopoulos D et al: What causes cancer? *Sci Am* 275(3):80, 1996.
7. Brennan JA et al: Association between cigarette smoking and mutation of the p53 gene in squamous-cell carcinoma of the head and neck, *N Engl J Med* 332(11):712, 1995.
8. Kessler DA et al: The Food and Drug Administration's regulation of tobacco products, *N Engl J Med* 335:988, 1996.
9. US Department of Health and Human Services, Public Health Services, Centers for Disease Control, National Center for Chronic Disease Prevention and Health Promotion, Office on Smoking and Health: Projected smoking-related deaths among youth—United States, *MMWR* 45(44):971, 1996.
10. Thun MJ: Excess mortality among cigarette smokers: changes in a 20-year interval, *Am J Public Health* 85(9):1223, 1995.
11. Pennisi E: Gene linked to commonest cancer, *Science* 272(5268):1583, 1996.
12. Johnson RL et al: Human homolog of *patched*, a candidate gene for the basal cell nervus syndrome, *Science* 272(5268):1668, 1886.
13. Travis J: Gene for the most common cancer found, *Sci News* 149(24):1996.
14. Leffell DJ, Brash DE: Sunlight and skin cancer, *Sci Am* 275(1):52, 1996.
15 Perera FP: Uncovering new clues to cancer risk, *Sci Am* 274(5):54, 1996.
16. Hausen H: Viruses in human cancer, *Science* 254(5035):1167, 1991.
17. Henderson BE et al: Toward the primary prevention of cancer, *Science* 254:1131, 1991.
18. Willett WC et al: Strategies for minimizing cancer risk, *Sci Am* 275(3):88, 1996.
19. Holland JC: Cancer's psychological challenges, *Sci Am* 275(3):158, 1996.
20. Foley KM: Controlling the pain of cancer, *Sci Am* 275(3):164, 1996.
21. Liotta LA: Cancer invasion and metatasis, *Sci Am* 266(2):54, 1992.
22. Beisel WP: History of nutritional immunology: introduction and overview, *J Nutr* 122:591, 1992.
23. Chandra RK: Protein-energy malnutrition and immunological responses, *J Nutr* 122:597, 1992.
24. Watzl B, Watson RR: Role of alcohol abuse in nutrition immunosuppression, *J Nutr* 122:733, 1992.
25. Hellman S, Vokes EE: Advancing current treatments for cancer, *Sci Am* 275(3):118, 1996.
26. Greenwald P: Chemoprevention of cancer, *Sci Am* 275(3):96, 1996.
27. Tayek JA, Chlebowski RT: Metabolic response to chemotherapy in colon cancer patients, *J Parenter Enter Nutr* 16(suppl 6):65, 1992.
28. Shaw JHF et al: Leucine kinetics in patients with benign disease, non-weight-losing cancer and cancer cachexia: studies at the whole body level and the response to nutritional support, *Surgery* 109:37, 1991.
29. Tayck JA: A review of cancer cachexia and abnormal glucose metabolism in humans with cancer, *J Am Coll Nutr* 11:445, 1992.
30. Aulas J-J: Alternative cancer treatments, *Sci Am* 275(3):162, 1996.
31. Tchekmedyian NS et al: Nutrition in advanced cancer: anorexia as an outcome variable and target of therapy, *J Parenter Enter Nutr* 16(suppl 6):88, 1992.
32. Bloch AS: Nutrition and cancer: the paradox, *Diet Curr* 23(2):1, 1996.
33. Menashian L et al: Improved food intake and reduced nausea and vomiting in patients given a restricted diet while receiving cisplatin chemotherapy, *J Am Diet Assoc* 92(1):58, 1992.
34. Darbinian J, Coulston A: Impact of chemotherapy on the nutritional status of the cancer patient. In Bloch AS, ed: *Nutrition management of the cancer patient,* Rockville, Md, 1990, Aspen.
35. Djuric Z et al: Effects of a low-fat diet on levels of oxidative damage to DNA in human peripheral nucleated blood cells, *J Natl Cancer Inst* 83(11):766, 1991.
36. Erikson KL, Hubbard NE: Dietary fat and tumor metastasis, *Nutr Rev* 48(1):6, 1990.
37. Burns CP, Spector AA: Effects of lipids on cancer therapy, *Nutr Rev* 48(6):233, 1990.
38. Buzzard IM et al: Diet intervention methods to reduce fat intake: nutrient and food group composition of self-selected low-fat diets, *J Am Diet Assoc* 90(1):42, 1990.
39. Gorbach SL et al: Changes in food patterns during a low-fat dietary intervention in women, *J Am Diet Assoc* 90(6):802, 1990.
40. Ross C: Vitamin A and protective immunity, *Nutr Today* 27(4):18, 1992.
41. Henson DE et al: Ascorbic acid: biologic functions and relation to cancer, *J Natl Cancer Inst* 83(8):547, 1991.

42. Negri E et al: Vegetable and fruit consumption and cancer risk, *Int J Cancer* 48:350, 1991.

43. Prasad KN, Edwards-Prasad J: Expressions of some molecular cancer risk factors and their modification by vitamins, *J Am Coll Nutr* 9(1):28, 1990.

44. Shils ME: Nutrition and diet in cancer management. In Shils ME, Olson JA, Shike M, eds: *Modern nutrition in health and disease,* ed 8, vol 2, Philadelphia, 1994, Lea & Febiger.

45. Ottery FD: Cancer cachexia: prevention, early diagnosis, and management, *Cancer Pract* 2:123, 1994.

46. Marian M: Cancer cachexia: prevalence, mechanisms, and interventions, *Support Line* 20(April):3, 1998.

47. Messina M, Messina V: Increasing use of soyfoods and their potential role in cancer prevention, *J Am Diet Assoc* 91(7):836, 1991.

48. Nahikian-Nelms ML: Encouraging oral intake. In Bloch AS, ed: *Nutrition management of the cancer patient*, Rockville, Md, 1990, Aspen.

49. Daly JM: Nutritional support in the cancer patient, *J Parenter Enter Nutr* 14(suppl 5):244S, 1990.

50. Brody H, Noel MB: Dietitians' role in decisions to withhold nutrition and hydration, *J Am Diet Assoc* 91(5):580, 1991.

51. American Cancer Society: Guidelines on diet, nutrition, and health, *Nation's Health* 26(9):23, 1996.

52. Foerster SB et al: California's "5-a-day—for better health" campaign: an innovative population-based effort to effect large-scale dietary change, *Am J Prev Med* 11:124, 1995.

53. Bloch AS, Thomson CA: Position of the American Dietetic Association: phytochemicals and functional foods, *J Am Diet Assoc* 95(4):493, 1995.

54. Fuez A, Rapin C-H: An observational study of the role of pain control and food adaption of elderly patients with terminal cancer, *J Am Diet Assoc* 94(7):767, 1994.

▬ FURTHER READING

Bloch AS, ed: *Nutrition management of the cancer patient,* Rockville, Md, 1990, Aspen.

This helpful reference by an experienced oncology dietitian and her contributors provides a comprehensive background for a better understanding of the complexities of caring for cancer patients.

Bloch AS, Thomson CA: Position of the American Dietetic Association: Phytochemicals and functional foods, *J Am Diet Association* 95(4):493,1995.

Steinmetz, KA, Potter JD: Vegetables, fruit, and cancer prevention: a review, *J Am Diet Assoc* 96(10):1027, 1996.

These two statements, one an American Dietetic Association position paper and the other a review of the role of certain foods in cancer prevention, provide important information for counseling.

Kalman D, Villani LJ: Nutritional aspects of cancer-related fatigue, *J Am Diet Assoc* 97(6):650, 1997.

This article describes the fatigue associated with cancer and its treatment and ways in which all cancer team members may contribute to using nutrition management to minimize these side effects and broaden the patient's nutritional limits and food choices.

Case study

Patient with cancer

Catherine Schofield is a 35-year-old mother of three young children. She was admitted to Green Hills Hospital 3 weeks ago with multiple enterocutaneous fistulas. She weighed 52 kg (116 lb) on admission and is 165 cm (5 ft 6 in) tall. Mrs. Schofield had undergone a hysterectomy 4 months before admission, following a recurrence of cervical cancer. During the chemotherapy that followed for 7 months, she had regular bouts with nausea and anorexia. Surgery was performed again. Her fistulas continued to drain for 2 weeks postoperatively, during which she tolerated clear liquids only. An intravenous drip of 10% glucose and 45% normal saline was ordered to supplement fluids and kcalories. This week she developed peritonitis and has had a fever of 39° C (102° F) for the past 24 hours. Her weight has dropped to 41 kg (90 lb); drainage from the fistulas has become odorous. The patient was placed in isolation today and was advised by her physician that he intended to start her on TPN and take some more tests to determine her progress.

Questions for analysis

1. What types of nutritional assessment procedures would be used by the TPN team for planning Mrs. Schofield's nutritional therapy? Explain the purpose of each.
2. Calculate Mrs. Schofield's energy and protein needs, and account for increased needs.
3. Why did Mrs. Schofield develop nausea and anorexia during chemotherapy?

    What are the implications of this for recovery? Outline a plan for evaluating and controlling nausea and vomiting in patients undergoing chemotherapy.
4. What personal concerns would you expect Mrs. Schofield to have? What resources would you use to help her obtain the personal and physical support she probably needs?

Issues & Answers

Toward the prevention of cancer

Studies of geographic, socioeconomic, chronologic, and immigration patterns of cancer distribution indicate that the vast majority of cases of cancer are primarily caused by environmental factors. The logical conclusion is that reduction of these causative factors may reduce or eliminate most forms of cancer.

The American Cancer Society suggests that two thirds of all cases of cancer in the United States are caused by only two factors: inhaled smoke and ingested food.

Tobacco, alone or in combination with alcohol, remains the most important cause of cancer, accounting for about one of every three cancer deaths in the United States. Cigarettes are the most important cause of tobacco-related cancer, but other forms of tobacco (chewing tobacco and snuff) are also established carcinogens. The cancer risk of ex-smokers remains elevated with lifetime nonsmokers. However, quitting smoking, even late in life after heavy long-term abuse, greatly reduces cancer risk when compared with the risk of continued smoking. Despite the rhetoric of tobacco companies, even regular smokers of low-tar cigarettes still have a much higher cancer risk than nonsmokers.

Alcohol, in addition to its synergistic effects with tobacco, increases risk of cancers of the oral cavity, pharynx, liver, and esophagus. Alcohol use has also been consistently linked to colorectal cancer and female breast cancer. Liquor, wine, and beer seem to be equal in effect on cancer risk.

Major incriminating dietary factors that appear now to be carcinogenic are the food changes that contrast current Western diets with those of our paleolithic hunter-gatherer ancestors. We have reduced the amount of energy we obtain from starchy foods by one half to two thirds. We have decreased our intake of dietary fiber by 75%. We have more than doubled the proportion of energy we derive from fat and changed from mostly unsaturated fats to saturated fats. We have increased our salt intake fivefold. And sugar now accounts for one fifth of our total energy intake. The diet of our ancestors was energy dilute, whereas our modern diet is energy dense.

Many studies link what we eat and don't eat to the development of cancer. Direct relationships between preserved or salty foods and nasopharynx and stomach cancer have been consistently observed in case-control and correlational studies. Generous use of fresh fruits and vegetables has consistently been found to decrease the risk of stomach cancer. Epidemiologic studies suggest a relation between high–animal fat, low-fiber intakes and colorectal cancer. The basis for this relationship lies in the decreased transit time through the colon associated with high-fiber diets, and the increased water content in the intestinal lumen that dilutes other nutrients such as animal fat.

Considerable, although not yet conclusive, evidence exists that ascorbic acid has a protective effect against cancer of the esophagus, larynx, and oral cavity. Nutrients such as vitamin A, beta-carotene, vitamin E, and ascorbic acid are thought to lower cancer risk in patients with elevated risk for cancers of the lung, esophagus, colon, and skin. Clinical and laboratory studies support findings that adequate intakes of vitamin D and calcium are associated with reduced incidence of colorectal cancer. These studies did not necessarily utilize supplemental amounts of these nutrients in addition to the RDAs but were based more on low levels of intake of these nutrients, which would parallel the low levels of fresh fruit and vegetable intakes that are prevalent in our society.

The majority of the causes of cancer—such as tobacco, alcohol, animal fat, obesity, and ultraviolet light—are associated with lifestyle, that is, personal choices and not environmental causes. This fact reinforces the basic truth that the best cure is prevention. Lifestyle changes, including regular exercise, are the best prevention.

References

Garland CF et al: Can colon cancer incidence and death rates be reduced with calcium and vitamin D? *Am J Clin Nutr* 54:193S, 1991.

Henderson BE et al: Toward the primary prevention of cancer, *Science* 254:1131, 1991.

Kalman DS, Villani LJ: Exercise and the cancer patient, *On-Line,*6(1):1, American Dietetic Association.

Leffell DJ, Brash DE: Sunlight and skin cancer, *Sci Am* 275(1):52, 1996.

Trichopoulos D et al: What causes cancer? *Sci Am* 275(3):80, 1996.

Willett WC et al: Strategies for minimizing cancer risk, *Sci Am* 275(3):88, 1996.

Wynder EL: Primary prevention of cancer: planning and policy considerations, *J Natl Cancer Inst* 83(7):475, 1991.

Nutritional Support in Disabling Disease and Rehabilitation

This chapter completes our clinical nutrition series. In addition to the primary care clinical problems we have reviewed in the preceding chapters of this section, we conclude with a focus on long-term disabling disease requiring rehabilitative care. Such situations often involve profound trauma and devastating effects that call for tremendous coping resources.

In this final chapter, we examine the supportive role of nutrition in the rehabilitative process. We look at musculoskeletal disease, neuromuscular disease, and progressive neurologic disorders. In each case we see that personalized nutritional care plays a vital role in the healing and restoring process. Such care demands special knowledge and skills and much personal strength.

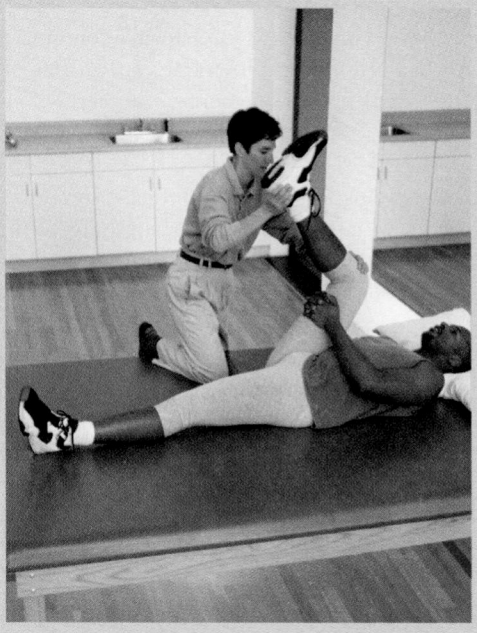

NUTRITIONAL SUPPORT AND REHABILITATIVE CARE

GOALS OF SUPPORTIVE CARE

Positive goals guide care for those with disabling disease or injury. Successful support is rooted in a positive philosophy based on the optimal potential of each person affected. This approach requires a specialized team working with the patient and family to meet individual needs. It is built on clearly defined *preventive* and *restorative* personal care objectives. To the greatest degree possible within each situation, two goals are fundamental in planning care: (1) to prevent further **disability**, and (2) to restore potential function. Health workers and their clients have developed many creative techniques of care to meet these twin goals. Both of these key principles apply to nutritional support. Together with the other specialized therapists on the rehabilitation team, the registered dietitian functions as the nutrition specialist and carries numerous nutritional care responsibilities[1]:

- *Nutritional assessment*—initial comprehensive evaluation and continuing reassessment at appropriate intervals
- *Nutritional therapy*—to meet fundamental nutrient and energy requirements, as well as any specialized requirements
- *Eating or feeding assessment*—needs for self-help eating devices of food marketing and preparation
- *Coordination of community services*—referrals and communication to meet individual needs, home health care, rehabilitation, public health, vocational agencies, financial assistance, or other services
- *Nutritional education and counseling*—with the individual client, the family, and other caregivers

TEAM APPROACH METHOD

How can these goals be met? How can the health care system draw on its various resources and levels of care to meet these tremendous needs? In some devastating cases, obstacles may seem almost insurmountable. In others, when the underlying disease may lack a cure, the prognosis is poor. Nonetheless, these support goals remain valid. Often the patient's initial reaction is one of defeat and resignation or withdrawal. Certainly the patient and family cannot carry the overwhelming burden alone or accomplish the necessary care alone. Such a complex and complicated process requires a strong *team approach*. Rehabilitation team specialists include the physician (physiatrist), clinical nutritionist, nurse, occupational therapist, physical therapist, psychologist, and social worker. These sensitive and skilled specialists lend their particular expertise, bringing their unique training, insights, and resources to identify specific personal needs.

At all times, however, these health care specialists remember that the most important member of the team is the patient. They always work *with*, not for, the patient and family to help develop solutions. Goal setting is always personal. These three partners—the professional specialists, the client, and the family—form a greater health team. It is always a shared, supportive undertaking, whatever the individual limitations or outcome (see *To Probe Further* box, p. 529).

SOCIOECONOMIC AND PSYCHOLOGIC FACTORS

Social attitudes

The general attitudes of society toward disabled persons varies between extremes of overprotection and avoidance. These social attitudes result mainly from years of negative conditioning and are not easily changed. Some people are repelled by deformities or severe illness, perhaps because they sense their own vulnerability and mortality. Others completely ignore them. Neither extreme is helpful. But at the same time, overprotection robs persons of their selfhood and smothers the *will* to fight against surrounding odds and develop self-acceptance. However, disabled persons do have varying special needs, and social avoidance of these needs creates additional problems in everyday living. There are doorways not made for wheelchairs, unmanageable stairs and curbings, lack of access to public transportation, and many more daily barriers.

Economic problems

Care for disabling injury or severe illness is a long and costly process. A major area of exploration for the health care team is one of financial resources and assistance needed. Also, continuing long-term economic problems may revolve around employment capabilities or earning capacities, or the means for providing care.

Living situation

Disabled persons face many practical problems of everyday living. Whether a person needs long-term hospital care or can maintain independent living, perhaps with an attendant, depends on a number of physical and situational factors (see *Issues & Answers*, p. 549). If with help the person can maintain a home, then the necessary special equipment for maximal self-care enables the person to do more things for themselves and helps preserve their sense of self-accomplishment.[2]

Psychologic barriers

Positive resolution of many practical and emotional problems requires tremendous psychologic adjustment. Each person struggles with self-image and physical body

To Probe Further

Invisible disability

Persons with obvious disabling conditions receive cues from others that help them adapt to their disabilities. Anyone with a disability undergoes some revision of self-concept, a disruption in familiar role patterns, and a period of adjustment to the limitations. This adjustment usually involves going through the stages of the classic medical model of the "sick role": (1) exemption from normal responsibility, (2) wanting to get well, and (3) cooperation with health professionals.

However, the person with an invisible disability, such as kidney failure, some types of cancer, cardiovascular disease, or diabetes, often does not receive these supportive cues and feedback in the difficult task of adjustment, and is often denied obtaining employment. These conditions are not apparent or easily observed by casual acquaintances. Often this reinforces the human desire to deny the actual limitations and creates more damage through poor self-care. The person with an invisible disability is tempted to avoid the adjustment process and ignore the condition's limitations. Yet these persons need rehabilitative support and training as much as those with more obvious disabilities.

These psychologic aspects of invisible disability carry implications for all members of the health team. Because the loss is not tangible, the patient or client often lacks the support for living a normal life in the home or workplace, especially support for the initial grieving and adjustment needed for living with a chronic condition, which hinders adjustment. Health professionals must be aware of the psychodynamics of the adaptive process, anticipate needs, offer guidance, and assist the client in mourning outwardly. Then the healing process can begin.

References
Cross EW: Implementing the Americans with Disabilities Act, *J Am Diet Assoc* 93(3):273, 1993.

Falvo DR, Allen H, Maki DR: Psychosocial aspects of invisible disability, *Rehabil Lit* 43:2, 1982

---

trauma. It is no wonder that they often withdraw in defeat and exhaustion. Personality changes occur during rehabilitation processes that test both inner strength and physical stamina. Depending on personal resources and strengths, the person may or may not be able to function. Much of the health team's keen insight and concern are directed toward supporting each person's efforts to meet individual needs. That many disabled persons do reach self-care goals in some measure is evident in the remarkable achievements some of them attain, despite or perhaps because of their difficulties.

SPECIAL NEEDS OF OLDER DISABLED PERSONS

America is aging. Population projections indicate that by the year 2000, 13% of the population will be over 65 years; by 2030, 22% will be over 65 years old. Over the next decade the most rapid population increase will be among those over 85 years of age.[3] And with older age comes an increased number of disabled elderly persons. The United States Rehabilitation Services Administration, using a baseline of one disabled American in 10, estimates that the odds of being disabled increase to 1 in 3 after the age of 65 years. Increased services, including rehabilitation services, are needed. But rehabilitation needs of older persons differ from those of younger people. Three life-changing events of aging determine these needs: retirement, chronic illnesses, and general physical decline.

Vocational rehabilitation

Without adequate planning, many older persons experience stressful disorientation with retirement. They have had a lifetime occupation of active involvement in a familiar working environment and now that sense of stability and identity is no longer there. Supportive activities focus on vocational planning and effective use of leisure time. At this point, many persons have not been accustomed to viewing leisure activities in a positive manner and need help in making this adjustment. In

---

disability A mental or physical impairment that prevents an individual from performing one or more gainful activities; not synonymous with *handicap,* which implies serious disadvantage.

addition, vocational programs can help persons find gainful employment after they retire from work. They can also help retired healthy Americans find ways of contributing their wisdom and skills to others now working in the same field. In turn, such activity can enhance the health and social assets of the older person.

Residual disabilities from illnesses

In the age period of 60 to 75 years (the young-old), rehabilitation must focus on problems of chronic diseases of aging—heart disease, hypertension, stroke, or cancer. Chronic illnesses may also be related to damaging health behaviors such as alcoholism, smoking, excessive eating of foods high in fat and salt, and a sedentary life. Survival after a heart attack or stroke, which now occurs more frequently with modern medical care, may leave an older person with chronic disabilities. With more than 3 million stroke survivors currently incapacitated, it is the leading cause of disability in the United States.[4] A number of new drugs are being developed to treat strokes, and in one drug's clinical trials (Cerestat [Cambridge Neuroscience]) a number of subjects with moderately severe strokes recovered completely.[5] In any case, early efforts at rehabilitation help prevent disability, avoid complications, and restore reasonable function.

Physical decline in aging

In persons between 75 to 85 years of age and older (the old-old), disability increases sharply. Much of this increase comes from falls and resulting fractures, chronic brain failure, disorders in locomotion, impaired senses of perception, and increased problems with drug reactions and interactions. Older persons may have several different diseases and take a number of different drugs or receive a variety of medical treatments. In this age group, minor disabilities often result in major handicaps. Mental and physical dependency may require supportive care in the home or long-term care facility. Common health problems in both the young-old and old-old groups involve nutritional care as well. These problems include arthritis, cardiorespiratory and cardiovascular insufficiency, depression, sensory deprivation, infections, skin and foot disorders, and nutritional deficiencies from poor dentition and fad diets.

In general, however, disease and disability do not affect only the young-old and old-old, nor are all of these groups disabled. Many of the disabled are young people, and many older adults continue to be fit and healthy. But the increasing age of the general population inevitably brings with it an increasing number of older adults with chronic disease and various disabilities of aging. Even minor disabilities may cause major **handicaps** in everyday living, and minor injuries may bring major debilitating results. In any case, the twin goals of rehabilitation care continue to be prevention of further disability and restoration of the maximal function available.

PRINCIPLES OF SUPPORTIVE NUTRITIONAL CARE

PREVENTION OF MALNUTRITION

Kilocalories

The rehabilitative process of physical therapy involves hard work. The patient tires easily, and the energy intake must be sufficient to meet the energy output demands. Excess kcalories must be avoided to prevent obesity, but sufficient energy for tissue metabolism is essential.

Protein

General protein needs are based on maintaining strength of tissue structure and function. Tissue and organ integrity protect against catabolism, infections, negative nitrogen balance, and **decubitus ulcers**.[6] Dietary protein in optimal quantity and quality ensures the necessary supply of all essential amino acids required for tissue synthesis. In addition to these general needs, severe trauma such as that involved in spinal cord injury brings special needs to meet the catabolic response.

Carbohydrate

General energy needs are great. They are met by optimal dietary carbohydrate as the body's major fuel source (see Chapters 3 and 14). Severe trauma requires maximal carbohydrate, especially in the early stages following injury. More breakdown of tissue protein and fat occurs to provide needed energy, but this only adds to the negative nitrogen balance. Thus sufficient carbohydrate foods are important to provide the needed energy and spare protein for its essential tissue rebuilding function.

Fat

At any point in rehabilitation care the diet must supply linoleic acid, the essential fatty acid, and a moderate amount of fat for the body's general metabolic activities and tissue integrity. The general dietary recommendation that fat supply about 30% of the total kcalories is sufficient. Some fat for food palatability also aids appetite, which tends to be poor in the course of long-term illness.

Vitamins and minerals

Optimal intake of vitamins and minerals for metabolic activity and maintenance of tissue reserves is needed. The normal RDA standards for age and sex are adequate in most cases. However, a deficiency state such as anemia indicates need for supplementation. In some rehabilitation centers multivitamin preparations are given routinely to ensure adequate amounts.

RESTORATION OF EATING ABILITY

Normal development of the eating process

In the normal growth and development of a child, the feeding and eating process develops through an overlapping and interdependent series of physical and psychologic stages. The usual activities of eating—swallowing, chewing, hand and utensil use—gradually develop with motor ability. The learning comes with much practice and patience. In a sense, the injured person must "start over" and relearn these basic skills.

Thus with an understanding of these normal patterns, the disabled person works with the professional team of occupational and physical therapists, nutritionists, and nurses to find adaptive procedures to restore basic eating ability. For each client, four aspects of the eating process will require individual attention: (1) the nature and degree of motor control; (2) eating position; (3) use of adapted utensils; and (4) support of individual needs. For example, blind persons will need a description of the food served, its placement on the plate (named generally in a clockwise direction to help them remember), and a follow-up training course in preparing food with a number of assistive tools and techniques.

Nutritional base

The personal food plan must fulfill basic nutritional needs, in increased amounts to meet additional metabolic demands. In addition, appetite and motivation must be supported to accomplish the task. Sensory stimuli such as variety in food texture, color, and flavor can enhance appetite and help motivate the learning of new adapted modes of eating. Also, "comfort foods" or familiar ethnic dishes and well-liked foods can encourage the client with the sometimes frustrating and difficult process of relearning how to eat.

Independence in daily living

With each disabled person the goal is to achieve as much independence in daily living as possible (see *Issues & Answers,* p. 549). Maximal use is made of individual neuromotor resources and emotional reserves. These personal resources are aided by self-help devices as needed. A large number of these creative devices are available.

A number of representative disabling conditions can illustrate various areas of need for supportive nutritional care. Here we briefly review examples of such conditions in three types of problems: (1) musculoskeletal disease, (2) neuromuscular disease, and (3) progressive neurologic disorders.

MUSCULOSKELETAL DISEASE

RHEUMATOID ARTHRITIS

Clinical characteristics

The general term arthritis comes from the Greek word *arthron,* meaning "joint." Its underlying chronic, systemic, inflammatory disease process usually occurs in the young adult years. It is a severe type of *autoimmune* disorder in which the body's immune system acts against its own tissues. It mainly attacks the joints of the hands, arms, and feet, causing them to become extremely painful, stiff, and deformed. The precise triggering antigen is still unknown. However, a number of possible primary causes (a virus or several viruses) that stimulate the immune response in the genetically susceptible host are under study.[7] The joint damage involves tissue changes in the **synosheaths**. Progressive joint deformity and destruction usually progress rapidly.

This disability dramatically affects activities of daily living, especially the fundamental necessity of obtaining and eating food. There is hand and wrist involvement, including destruction of wrist ligaments and tendons, with weakened finger and hand grip strength, and limited finger movement (Figure 25.1). All of these changes limit ability to self-feed, shop for food, or prepare it. Also, elbow and shoulder involvement hinder bringing food to the mouth. Further tissue damage of the *temporomandibular joint (TMJ)* of the jaws limits normal opening and closing of the mouth and alters chewing ability. Other nonjoint problems—such as anemia of chronic disease, decrease in salivary secretions, dysphagia, and bone disease—further complicate nutrition problems, leading to overall malnutrition. In its juvenile form in children and adolescents, this resulting malnutrition can cause serious growth retardation.

Medical management

Medical treatment may involve a number of drugs for control of the inflammatory process. Aspirin, as well as other nonsteroidal antiinflammatory drugs (NSAIDs), is still a mainstay of medical therapy, with the use of enteric-coated preparations to avoid gastric irritation (see Chapter 18). Other drugs used to control the inflammatory process include gold salts, D-penicillamine, steroids, and immunosuppressive agents.[7] Weekly low-dose therapy with the anticancer drug methotrexate, which acts as an antimetabolite to folic acid in DNA synthesis, is sometimes used but may cause the complicating viral

decubitus ulcer Pressure sores in long-term bed-bound or immobile patients at points of bony protuberances, where prolonged pressure of body weight in one position cuts off adequate blood circulation to that area, causing tissue death and ulceration.

handicap A mental or physical defect that may or may not be congenital, which prevents the individual from participating in normal life activities; implies disadvantage.

synosheath Protective pliable connective tissue surrounding the bony collagen mesh and fluid that come together in the synovial area between major bone heads in joints, which allows normal padded and lubricated joint movement and motion.

Ulna

Figure 25.1 **A,** Arthritic hand showing ulnar drift. **B,** Self-help device for stirring food during preparation and for eating assistance.

condition **herpes zoster**.[8] Sometimes combination drug therapy is used as with cyclosporine and methotrexate.[9] When irreversible destruction of cartilage occurs in advanced stages of the disease, reconstructive joint surgery along with physical therapy and occupational therapy gives the best results.[7]

 Nutritional management

In all settings, planning nutritional support must begin with early assessment of individual patient status and needs, especially to detect any degree of malnutrition.[10] An initial history must thus assess potential drug-nutrition-food interactions and their nutritional effects (see Chapters 15,16). Also, the history should include any of the numerous unproved regimens for arthritis that the patient may be using.[10] In addition, attention may be given to dietary modifications under study that have shown therapeutic promise. Results indicate that supplementation with the omega-3 fatty acids (see Chapter 4) suppresses synthesis of **cytokines** with potent inflammatory activities.[11]

Special functional assessment of eating ability is also needed. Classic guidelines for this assessment and training have been provided.[12] Such guidelines should include any swallowing problem from lack of salivary secretions and dysphagia (see *Practical Application* box, p. 533). Standard nutritional assessment is essential (see Chapter 15). On the basis of these data, nutritional needs can be determined and monitored.

1. *Energy.* Energy needs, especially for children, vary widely and must be determined on an individual basis. In general, needs will involve basal energy expenditure plus added kcalories for increased metabolic activity factors (MAFs), such as stress of disease activity, sepsis, fever, skeletal injury, or surgery (see Chapter 22). If the client is receiving physical therapy, an additional physical activity factor is used. Total kcalories are increased as needed to achieve desirable weight gain during growth, or decreased if indicated for obese adults. Follow-up monitoring determines any needed adjustments in energy estimates.

References
Price ME, Dilorio C: Swallowing: a practice guide, *Am J Nurs* 90(7):42, 1990.

practical application

Tilt and swallow

The swallowing reflex is frequently diminished or absent in disabled persons. The reflex may be enhanced, however, by the use of an ice collar or by brushing the neck with a small brush, such as a paint brush, just before eating. The liquid or semisolid food should be placed behind the front teeth, and the patient should slowly tilt the head back and swallow. This routine may be learned as the helper uses the repeated statement, "Tilt and swallow...tilt and swallow..."

2. *Protein.* Protein needs vary with protein status, surgical therapy, proteinuria, and nitrogen balance. A well-nourished adult patient needs about 0.5 to 1 g of protein/kg/day during quiet disease periods. An increase to 1.5 to 2g/kg/day is needed during active inflammatory disease periods. The RDA standards for age and sex can guide protein needs for children to meet basic growth needs. States of malnutrition will require more.
3. *Vitamins and minerals.* Standard recommendations for vitamins and minerals are used. Specific supplementation may be used if needed, such as supplying calcium and vitamin D if bone disease is involved.
4. *Special enteral and parenteral feeding.* Tube feeding may be used either to supplement oral intake or to supply total nutrition support (see Chapter 17). Parenteral nutrition support is seldom used, except for preoperative and postoperative needs or when bowel rest is indicated.

The course of rheumatoid arthritis is unpredictable. The disease is usually progressive and some degree of permanent disability results. But many persons after years of disease are capable of self-care with rehabilitation training and are fully employable. Continuing optimal nutritional support is important maintenance therapy.

Osteoarthritis

This milder form of arthritis in older adults is more appropriately called *degenerative joint disease* because there is minimal inflammation involved. Osteoarthritis affects approximately 44% of persons over the age of 40 years in the United States. It is chronic and may progress, limiting movement of affected joints, mainly the hands, knees, and hips. Marked disability is uncommon, but osteoarthritis may become a chronic disabling disease in the elderly.[10] There is no cure for the disease process,

which ultimately destroys cartilage between rubbing heads of bones in involved joints. However, damaged joints can be replaced by **arthroplasty**, surgical removal of the degenerated joint and replacement of a joint made with metal or plastic components. Hip replacements have been performed since the early 1960s, and the technique is now being refined and applied to other joints. In general, appropriate pain-controlling medication and nutritional support for general health promotion help relieve symptoms. Depending on the degree of hand joint involvement, self-feeding devices may assist eating.

OSTEOPOROSIS

The metabolic bone disorder *osteoporosis* is the most common skeletal disorder in the United States, affecting about 24 million individuals. Approximately one third of the postmenopausal women of the United States have osteoporosis and suffer from some 1.3 million associated fractures each year.[13] Over age 70 years, osteoporosis affects men and women after a slow, steady rate of bone loss and increasing fracture potential develop over many decades. When the porous bone

arthroplasty Plastic surgery of nonfunctioning body joints to form movable joints with replacement metal or plastic materials.

cytokines Substances, produced in tissues, that can cause inflammatory changes in tissue cells (such as tumor necrosis factor and interleukin-1).

herpes zoster An acute self-limiting viral inflammatory disease of posterior nerve roots causing skin eruptions in a lateral pattern across the back of the torso served by these nerves, accompanied by neuralgic pain; caused by the virus of chickenpox and commonly called *shingles.*

mass finally falls below a fracture threshold, fractures occur spontaneously or with little trauma.[14] These fractures in the elderly are a major cause of disabling illness and death. Bones of the vertebrae and the hip are most vulnerable, but hip fractures are more serious. The annual cost of treating patients with osteoporosis ranges from $7 to $12 billion.[15]

Medical treatment of postmenopausal osteoporosis in women is most effectively managed with estrogen replacement therapy. The slow, steadily developing form of osteoporosis in men and women responds more readily to nutritional therapy with a sound diet including a calcium intake of 1200 to 1500 mg/day (see Chapters 8 and 13), increased physical activity, and weight control. Newer medical treatments under investigation include the cyclic use of bisphosphonate (etidronate), a structural analog of the naturally occurring pyrophosphate, a component of the hydroxyapatite crystals forming bone.[15,16] The best approach, of course, is prevention. This is achieved by ensuring that adolescents and young adults have sufficient dietary calcium for building bone mass, which peaks by the age of 30 years, stimulated by physical activity. Then a continuing sound diet and physical activity help to sustain this normal bone mass.

NEUROMUSCULAR DISEASE

GROWING PROBLEM OF NEUROLOGIC INJURIES

In the United States traumatic injury is the leading cause of death in the first four decades of life.[17,18] It is also the third leading cause of death for all ages. In 1 year some 150,000 persons are killed by automobile and industrial accidents, gunshot wounds and homicides, and sports injuries.[17,19] Increasingly, the strain on urban medical care centers comes into focus as special investigation reports in our local city newspapers remind us in bold front page Sunday headlines—"Trauma Care in Crisis."[20] Further realization of the problem of traumatic injury comes from the fact that more Americans die of highway trauma each year than have died of acquired immune deficiency syndrome (AIDS) since that disease was first identified in 1981, and in both conditions the majority of the victims are young males between 16 and 30 years of age.[17]

BRAIN AND SPINAL CORD INJURY

With current advances in emergency medicine, the number of persons surviving traumatic brain and spinal cord injury has increased dramatically. Here we review nutritional care of the injured patient in the acute care setting and follow-up nutritional management in rehabilitation.

TRAUMATIC BRAIN INJURY

Postinjury metabolic alterations

The brain is the control center of body functions and activities. Thus brain injury brings an immediate cascade of systemic metabolic responses that affect the entire body as the body resources are mobilized to protect itself. The systemic inflammatory response is activated, and a sustained state of *hypermetabolism* develops. Ultimately, if the process continues unchecked, a sequence of organ failure follows. Any complication prolongs the hypermetabolic phase, and the increasing protein *catabolism* causes depletion of lean body mass.[21,22] Increased energy expenditure and urinary nitrogen excretion mark this increased metabolic demand in response to trauma.

 ### Initial nutrition management

The immediate goals of the trauma team are control of the injury, maintenance of oxygen transport, and metabolic support.[21] Nutritional support as soon as possible is vital to meet the hypermetabolic drain on the body tissue resources for increased energy and protein demands.[22,23] Regular monitoring of energy needs is essential, often more than once a day. Most trauma centers now use indirect calorimetry at the bedside with a mobile calorimeter unit (see Chapter 6).

Early nutrition support may be delivered by either enteral or parenteral route (Chapter 17). Successful use has been reported of enteral feedings as early as 2 to 3 days after injury, achieving full caloric intake of 3020 kcal/day by day 7 (Vital HN-Ross: 10% fat, 16% hydrolyzed protein, 74% carbohydrate, continuous infusion).[23] Parenteral nutrition is an alternate option because it can be started within the first 24 hours after injury and may be immediately adjusted to the nutritional requirements of each patient according to daily metabolic profile and urinary nitrogen analysis.[24-26] Some trauma centers prefer a combination of early total parenteral nutrition (TPN) through a central vein catheter (Chapter 17) within 24 hours, starting enteral nutrition as soon as it can be tolerated, gradually tapering the TPN and discontinuing it when the enteral feeding is considered adequate.[21]

 ### Rehabilitation nutrition

Nutritional rehabilitation of the person with traumatic brain injury presents a complex of individual problems that require skilled and sensitive nutrition management. To develop individual nutritional care plans, the rehabilitation dietitian works closely with other team members, especially the nurse, occupational therapist, speech pathologist, cognitive rehabilitation therapist, and physical therapist.[26] Together they assess the degree of *dysphagia*, difficulty with chewing and swallowing, level of language deficits and communication, and ability to perform basic daily living skills, including food preparation and eating. Short- and long-range goals, as well as strategies to reach these goals, are developed along with many practical suggestions for adapting food forms and textures to meet eating problems.[27]

SPINAL CORD INJURY

After-injury management

The cervical region of the spine at the neck is the most mobile portion and hence the most common site of spinal cord injuries.[28] Each year catastrophic spinal cord injury in the United States affects some 10,000 trauma survivors between ages 16 and 30 years. Over 200,000 quadriplegic and paraplegic patients now require lifetime care at an estimated annual cost of approximately $600,000.[29,30] Because of advanced medical care the number of survivors, and consequent costs, is increasing each year.[31] Most of these spinal cord injuries are a result of automobile accidents (48%); other factors include falls (21%), sports injuries (14%), and physical assaults (15%).[28] Injury and loss of neurologic function in the upper cervical area of the spinal cord results in *quadriplegia*, paralysis from the neck down. Injuries and loss of neurologic function in the lower thoracic, lumbar, and sacral areas of the spine result in *paraplegia*, paralysis of the lower portion of the body. This spinal cord damage disrupts the nerve transmission of impulses from the brain to peripheral nerves and muscles so that muscle function below the level of injury is lost. Immobilization brings complicating illnesses. Protein-energy malnutrition is common. About half of the hospitalized patients and two thirds of the patients admitted to a rehabilitation unit have clinical signs of malnutrition.[32,33]

 ### Nutrition management

Enteral feeding tubes placed beyond the pylorus usually make it possible to start nutrition support within 3 to 5 days. The patients are usually well-nourished at the time of the sudden injury. Thus the goal of starting the feeding process as early as possible is to counteract the initial acute phase of spinal shock, and to prevent the onset of a malnutrition decline and secondary illnesses. There is wide variation in metabolic rates and energy needs, but they tend to be lower than those of other trauma patients as a result of decreased metabolic activity of denervated muscle.[32] The higher the injury to the spinal column, the greater the denervated muscle mass and the lower the measure of energy expenditure. Daily guidelines for energy needs are 23 kcal/kg for quadriplegics and 28 kcal/kg for paraplegics.[32]

 ### Rehabilitation nutrition

When the acute phase passes and the patient is stabilized, usually within 2 to 3 months after injury, the extended rehabilitation training phase begins. This complex process of many parts is designed to restore the client to the best functional capacity possible to promote independent living.[33] The goal is to prevent and treat any complications associated with spinal cord injury. Combined therapies are used from the team of rehabilitation specialists: physiatrist, registered dietitian, registered nurse, physical therapist, occupational therapist, speech therapist, psychologist, social worker, and vocational counselor. Nutritional management involves individual assessment and care of (1) basic energy-nutrient needs and feeding capacities, and (2) complications associated with the spinal cord injury.

Basic nutritional needs

Energy needs are based on sufficient kcalories to maintain an ideal body weight somewhat below that for a comparative person given in standard weight-height tables for healthy populations (see inside back book cover). For example, general weight goals for paraplegics have been recommended at 10 to 15 lb below standard body weight, and for quadriplegics, 15 to 20 lb below standard weight.[31] Excess weight gain is common in spinal cord injury clients as a result of the decreased metabolic rate that persists from the preceding acute after-injury phase and the continued relative immobilization.[29] Obesity contributes to medical problems, as well as adding physical problems in the frequent turning necessary in bed to prevent bed sores and the transfers between bed to wheelchair. Adequate protein intake is essential for maintaining muscle mass and tissue integrity to prevent negative nitrogen balance, ulcer formation, or infection. Palatable high-protein supplements between meals may be needed to maintain an adequate intake. The client may be at risk for vitamin or mineral deficiencies if appetite and food intake are poor as a result of depression or fatigue. A standard multiple vitamin-mineral preparation is frequently recommended.

Associated complications

Several nutrition-related complications in rehabilitation for spinal cord injury patients require special attention:

- *Pressure sores.* Decubitus ulcers are caused by immobilization, loss of pressure sensation around bony prominences, decreased blood circulation, skin breakdown, and ulcer formation that is open to infection and difficult to heal. They occur in 60% of quadriplegic patients and 52% of paraplegics. Nutritional factors involved include anemia, which reduces oxygen supply to tissues, excessive weight loss, which reduces padding of bony prominences, and low levels of plasma proteins such as albumin, which lead to edema and loss of skin elasticity. The protein deficiency requires an increased protein intake. More severe ulcers require more intense nutritional intervention, with protein needs of 1.5 to 2 g/kg. Other nutrients important to the healing process include supplements of vitamin C and zinc.

- *Hypercalciuria.* Immobility leads to an imbalance in calcium metabolism with a loss of bone calcium and its increased excretion in the urine. In the long term this loss of bone calcium leads to osteoporosis, which has been found to be present and progressive in 88% of the patients with spinal cord injury, affecting the denervated musculoskeletal tissue below the level of injury.[32] A balance of calcium–vitamin D therapy, and a prudent control of excessive protein intake, which causes increased calcium withdrawal, are indicated. Bone fractures result in about 7% of these patients.

- *Kidney stones.* The hypercalciuria also contributes to formation of kidney stones. The neurogenic effects following spinal cord injury cause loss of normal bladder control, resulting in problems of urinary reflux, retention, incontinence, infection, and stone formation.[33] Regular catheterization is necessary to prevent accumulation of bacteria and solutes such as calcium and other particles that can easily form stones. A high fluid intake of 2 to 3 L/day must be a part of the overall nutrition care plan to dilute the urine and reduce the solute concentration.

- *Neurogenic bowel.* Gastrointestinal complications from loss of normal neuromuscular controls include decreased peristalsis and loss of bowel control. A regularly scheduled program for emptying the bowel is necessary. About 12 hours before the scheduled time, 4 ounces (120 ml) of prune juice with a little lemon juice is taken. Then twenty to thirty minutes before the scheduled evacuation time, one or two glycerine suppositories are placed well above the anal sphincter, at least 21/2 inches (6.5 cm) into the rectum, against the rectal mucosa. The patient is then placed on the toilet or bedside commode and provided with adequate support. This daily schedule and recording of results continues with no interruption by enemas. The patient is taught manual evacuation for continuing care at home. A vital part of this care is a high-fiber diet to provide added bulk and ample fluid intake to prevent impaction.

- *Depression.* During the initial days of shock and survival, the full impact of the disability is not realized. When transfer to the rehabilitation unit occurs and the full extent of the disability is realized, a period of depression is a normal part of the personal grieving and healing process. Its severity and duration depends in large measure on the patient's personal strengths and resources. But it also requires the sensitive yet realistic support of family and the rehabilitation team for the serious and demanding work of rehabilitation to be successful. The nutritionist must help ensure that adequate energy, protein, and fluid intake is maintained. Nutritional status is repleted with appetizing foods, especially when the patient's human spirit is low. Even subtle improvements in muscle mass and function from the nutritional care can be a source of strength to mind and body.

CEREBROVASCULAR ACCIDENT (CVA)—STROKE

Brain injury resulting from a stroke also causes varying degrees of nerve damage and body paralysis (Chapter 19). Cerebrovascular disease from underlying atherosclerosis ranks third as a cause of death and second as a cause of disability in the United States.[34] In recent years the incidence of strokes has declined, largely as a result of the improvement in control of hypertension and increased public education concerning hypertension. Nutrition management is detailed in Chapter 19. Rehabilitation care follows the same general goals and methods discussed in this chapter (see the *Case Study,* p. 548).

DEVELOPMENTAL DISABILITIES

During the developmental period of childhood, neuromuscular conditions such as cerebral palsy, epilepsy, spina bifida, and Down syndrome cause eating problems that can contribute to poor growth and delayed development.

Cerebral palsy

Cerebral palsy is a general term for nonprogressive disorders of muscle control of movements and posture. It has many causes and results from brain damage that occurs largely before or at birth, probably as result of *hypoxia,* poor oxygen supply to the brain.[35,36] Most affected children fall into one of two groups: (1) *spastic*—muscles of one or more limbs permanently contracted, making normal movements very difficult or impossible; and (2) *athetoid*—involuntary writhing movements. These continuous involuntary movements increase energy needs, with research reports indicating increased resting metabolic rates that are approximately 15% higher (about 1700 kcal/day) than those of control subjects.[35-39] Because the immune system is often compromised in persons with developmental disabilities, they are at high risk for problems related to food safety. Thus all caretakers involved should have food safety training.[38,39]

Mental retardation, with an IQ below 70, occurs in about 75% of persons with cerebral palsy, mostly in the spastic group. Important exceptions occur, mostly among athetoids. Some of these individuals are highly intelligent. Some features of the condition during childhood change as the child grows older, often for the better with patience and skillful treatment.

Early nutritional management focuses mainly on feeding problems. When the infant or young child cannot obtain sufficient nourishment as a result of oral motor dysfunction, or when satisfactory oral feeding is interrupted for a prolonged period because of illness or surgery, enteral nutrition support by nasoenteric or gastrostomy tube feeding (Chapter 17) may be necessary. In such cases, transition to oral feeding is usually difficult. In any case, oral feeding poses numerous problems, both functional and behavioral. Feeding problems of oral motor dysfunction (e.g., difficulties in sucking, swallowing, or chewing), gross motor/self-feeding impairment, lack of appetite, and food aversions, as well as alternate feeding practices of prolonged assisted feeding and use of pureed foods, significantly reduce energy and nutrient intake. In persons with severe physical and developmental difficulties, malnutrition and growth failure are common.[35,40,41]

Early and ongoing nutrition assessment, intervention, and counseling are essential components of rehabilitation team care. In cases where accurate height measures to assess growth are difficult because of joint contractures, spasticity, or inability to stand, reasonably accurate stature can be calculated from knee height measures (see Chapter 17), using the standard equations given in Table 25.1.[42,43] Growth retardation seen in children persists with age. Studies have shown that at age 2 years they are 2% shorter than their peers and at 8 years of age they are more than 10% shorter.[42,43] As adults, persons with spastic cerebral palsy need about 500 extra kcal/day to cover the added energy need for *athetosis*, the continuous involuntary writhing motions of the disease.[40] Many still have feeding problems, but exercise helps promote better nutrition.[44]

Epilepsy

World wide, about 50 million people have epilepsy. It occurs mainly in childhood and plateaus from ages 15 to 65 years and then rises again among the elderly.[45] Epilepsy, literally "seizures," is a neuromuscular disorder in which abnormal electrical activity in the brain causes recurring transient seizures. Normally, the brain regulates all human activities, thoughts, perceptions, and emotions through the regular orderly electrical excitation of its nerve cells. But in an epileptic state during a seizure, an unregulated, chaotic electrical discharge occurs. Seizures often appear spontaneously, or in some cases they may be set off by some stimulus such as a flashing light. This brain dysfunction may develop for no obvious reason or there may be an inherited predisposition. In other cases it may result from a wide variety of diseasees or injuries such as birth trauma, a metabolic

Table 25.1	Equations for estimating stature from knee height*
Age/sex group	**Equation**
White males	
6-18 years	stature = (knee height × 2.22) + 40.54
19-59 years	stature = (knee height × 1.88) + 71.85
White females	
6-18 years	stature = (knee height × 2.15) + 43.21
19-59 years	stature = (knee height × 1.86) −(age × 0.05) ± 70.25

Adapted from Estimating stature from knee height. In *Direction for the Ross Knee Height Caliper,* Columbus, Ohio, Ross Laboratories, 1990.
*Equations are based on normal, healthy individuals. Stature and knee height are measured in centimeters.

imbalance in the body, head injury, brain infection (meningitis, encephalitis), stroke, brain tumor, drug intoxication, or alcohol or drug withdrawal states. Epilepsy occurs in about 1 person in 200; the number of epileptics in the United States is about 1 million. Usually the disorder starts in childhood or adolescence. About a third of these persons will outgrow the condition and do not need medication. Another third find their seizures well controlled by drug treatment and require less medication over time. The remaining third find that their condition remains the same or becomes more resistant to drug therapy. Anticonvulsant drugs are the first line of treatment for epilepsy and in most cases do lessen seizure frequency. In cases of the Lennox-Gastaut syndrome, a severe form of epilepsy that usually begins in early childhood and is difficult to treat, the new antiepileptic drug lamotrigine (Lamictal, Glaxo Wellcome) has proved to be an effective and well-tolerated treatment for associated seizures.[46]

Nutritional management of epilepsy functions in several areas of care. First, it helps to ensure an appropriate diet for normal growth during childhood and adolescence and for health maintenance in adulthood. Second, it seeks to ameliorate side effects of the anticonvulsant drugs used. Some of the most commonly used ones and their relation to food and nutrients are shown in Table 25.2. Third, if a *ketogenic* diet is used, the clinical nutritionist is responsible for its calculations and education of staff, patient, and family in its use. This special high-fat diet was developed to control epilepsy before current anticonvulsant drugs became widely available in the 1940s. It is still successfully

Table 25.2 Anticonvulsant drugs used to control basic types of epilepsy and their nutrition-related side effects		
Most commonly used drug	**Drug trade name**	**Nutrition-based side effects**
Grand mal (tonic/clonic) seizures		
Phenytoin (adults)	Dilantin	Nausea, vomiting, and constipation; reduced taste sensation; vitamins D and K catabolism; reduced serum calcium, vitamins B_6 and B_{12}, folate, and serum magnesium levels; overgrowth of gums
Phenobarbitol	Luminal	Increased appetite or anorexia, nausea, vomiting, vitamins D and K catabolism, reduced bone density
Primidone	Mysoline	Gastrointestinal upset, weight loss
Carbamazepine	Tegretol	Nausea, vomiting, diarrhea, abdominal pain, xerostomia (dry mouth), glossitis (sore tongue), stomatitis (sore mouth), increased blood urea nitrogen
Petit mal (absence seizures)		
Ethosuximide	Zarontin	Gastrointestinal upset, nausea, vomiting, anorexia, weight loss
Valproic acid	Depakane, Depakote	Nausea, vomiting, indigestion, diarrhea, abdominal pain, constipation, anorexia and weight loss, or increased appetite and weight gain
Clonazepam	Klonopin	Hyperactivity, short attention span, impulsive behavior, weight gain
Partial seizures		
Phenytoin (adults)	Dilantin	Nausea, vomiting, and constipation; reduced taste sensation; vitamins D and K catabolism; reduced levels of serium calcium, vitamins B_6 and B_{12}, folate, and serum magnesium; overgrowth of gums
Phenobarbitol	Luminal	Increased appetite or anorexia, nausea, vomiting, vitamins D and K catabolism, reduced bone density
Carbamazepine	Tegretol	Nausea, vomiting, diarrhea, abdominal pain, xerostomia (dry mouth), glossitis (sore tongue), stomatitis (sore mouth), increased blood urea nitrogen

used for those children with intractable myoclonic epilepsy that resists drug therapy. [47,48] Details of the strict calculations required to achieve the necessary high-fat to low-carbohydrate ratios are outlined in The American Dietetic Association's *Manual of Dietetics*.[49]

Spina bifida

Spina bifida is a congenital defect in the formation of the spine that contributes to serious developmental disabilities in the United States.[50] It develops during early embryonic life when the neural tube, which forms the spinal cord, does not close completely, leaving part of one or more vertebrae of the of the spinal cord exposed at birth.[51] The vertebral canal usually closes within 4 weeks of conception. Thus this congenital defect can often be diagnosed early in the pregnancy by *ultrasound scanning* or by high levels of **alpha-fetoprotein** in the amniotic fluid or maternal blood, so that appropriate genetic counseling can be provided for the parents. Recent discovery of the cell enzyme error involved indicates that folic acid and vitamin B_{12} supplementation at the time of conception through the first few months of pregnancy reduces a woman's risk that the baby will develop this devastating neural tube defect.[52,53] The defect can occur anywhere along the spine but is more common in the lower back. As Atensio's group study of children with myelomeningocele indicates, the neurologic damage that occurs depends on the severity and level of the lesion on the spine.[54] The incidence is about one case per 1000 babies born, but it increases with either very young or old maternal age. A mother who has had one affected child is 10 times more likely than the average rate of having another affected child.

There are three main forms of spina bifida:

- *Spina bifida occulta.* This is the least serious and most common form. The name indicates an "unseen cleft in the spine." It often goes unnoticed in otherwise healthy children save for a small dimple over the area of the underlying abnormality.
- *Myelomeningocele.* Also known as myelocele, this is the most severe form, and the child is usually severely disabled. Here the spinal cord ("myelo") and its enveloping membranes ("meninges") protrude from the spine in a sac ("cele").
- *Meningocele.* This form is less severe because the nerve tissue of the spinal cord is usually intact. Outer skin covers the bulging sac, and therefore there are usually no functional problems. Ideally, necessary surgical repairs are performed in the first few days of life.

Nutrition management of spina bifida children focuses on growth pattern and individual degree of problems with growth retardation and short stature, low muscle mass and weakness, deformities or paralysis of lower extremities, and reduced ability to control bladder and bowels. Normal growth charts have been revised for use with nutrition assessment of these children.[51] Nutrition care plans give attention to the main problems of short stature and poor growth, increased weight, and constipation. Obesity is a particular problem because of several factors: (1) low basal metabolic rate related to lowered amount of lean body mass; (2) little physical activity related to the disabled condition and dependency on a wheelchair; and (3) use of food and overfeeding by parents or other caregivers to reward or show love or to counteract what is seen as frailty or weakness caused by the disability. All of these factors become part of ongoing nutrition counseling.

Down syndrome

A chromosomal abnormality accounts for the mental retardation and characteristic appearance of children with Down syndrome, a condition first described in the previous century by the English physician John L.H. Down (1828-1896). Its cause remained a mystery until 1959, when modern researchers discovered that persons with Down syndrome had one too many chromosomes in each of their cells-47 instead of the normal 46. Then because the extra chromosome is usually number 21, they gave it the alternate name of *trisomy 21*. The two parent chromosomes numbered 21 fail to go into separate daughter cells during the first stage of sperm or egg cell formation, and some eggs or sperm are thus formed with an extra number 21 chromosome. If one of these takes part in fertilization, the resulting baby will have the extra chromosome and Down syndrome. This event is more likely if the mother is over 35 years of age, indicating that defective egg formation, rather than sperm formation, is usually the cause.

Down syndrome occurs in about one in 650 babies born. The rate rises steeply with increased maternal age to about one in 40 among mothers over 40 years. The degree of mental retardation varies, with an IQ anywhere between 30 to 80, but all are capable of limited learning. These children are usually affectionate, cheerful, friendly, and get along well with family and friends. They thrive to their full potential in a loving family.

Nutritional needs focus on delayed feeding skills; inappropriate, excessive, or inadequate intakes of food energy and nutrients; and poor eating habits. Studies indicate frequent obesity, possibly resulting from excessive fat, low physical activity, or both.[55,56] Diets need to be individualized because these children tend to gain excess weight if they are given the intakes recommended for most children. Plans for increasing physical activity are important.

PROGRESSIVE NEUROLOGIC DISORDERS

Progressive neurologic disorders, especially through the middle and older years of adulthood, have disabling effects on the personal lives of many individuals. Examples reviewed here illustrate some of these effects and nutrition approaches to providing support.

PARKINSON'S DISEASE

Parkinson's disease is a long-known neurologic disease, first described by the English physician James Parkinson (1755-1824) nearly two centuries ago, when in 1817 he described its characteristic symptoms in "An Essay on the

---

alpha-fetoprotein A fetal antigen in amniotic fluid that provides an early pregnancy test for fetal malformations such as neural tube defect.

spina bifida A congenital defect in the fetal closing of the neural tube to form a portion of the lower spine, leaving the spine unclosed and the spinal cord open in various degrees of exposure and damage.

Shaking Palsy."[57] Its underlying origin remains unknown, but current researchers speculate that the triggering cause may be related to some environmental factor such as a toxin.[58,59] Genetic factors are not the cause, but in some families genetic factors may predispose persons to the disease. It is a common disorder reported in every race and region of the world, usually with onset of motor symptoms after the age of 40 years, rising in incidence with advancing age. In the United States, about one person in 200, mostly elderly, is affected by the disease, with some 50,000 new cases a year.[60] Men are more likely to be affected than women.

The disorder affects the *basal ganglia* of the brain, a cluster of nerve cells at the central base of the brain. Signals from the brain's motor cortex pass, via the brainstem *reticular formation* and the spinal cord, to the muscles, which contract. Other signals pass through the basal ganglia, which provides a *damping effect* to help smooth and control the signal flow to reticular formation and the spinal cord, thus preventing uncoordinated muscle contraction responses. This damping effect is produced by the balancing action of two neurotransmitters: (1) *dopamine*, which is made in the basal ganglia and is necessary for the damping effect, stimulates the signal flow, and (2) *acetylcholine*, a widespread neurotransmitter in the body, inhibits it. In Parkinson's disease, degeneration of key parts of the basal ganglia causes a lack of dopamine within this part of the brain, thus preventing the basal ganglia from modifying nerve pathways that control muscle function.[61] The muscles become overly tense, causing joint rigidity and a general body stiffness, a fine constant tremor even at rest, and slow movements.

Medical management

Although there is no cure for Parkinson's disease, drug management has helped to minimize symptoms for many patients. A dramatic change in treatment came in the 1960s with the advent of the drug levodopa, which the body can transform into the needed dopamine. Dopamine itself cannot be used, since it does not cross the blood-brain barrier as does levadopa.[61] New methods of drug delivery to achieve a slow steady release, and means of slowing down the progression of Parkinson's disease are the major goals of present research.[62] Current surgical research is investigating transplants of dopamine-secreting adrenal medulla tissue and the brain grafting of fetal dopamine neurons.[63,64] The new discovery of a mutant form of the Parkinson's disease gene in several generations of a large Italian family with Greek origins has now provided scientists, including geneticist Mihael Polymeropoulos' discovery group at the United States National Institutes of Health, with a major clue to the disease origins in the much larger number of patients with nonhereditary Parkinson's.[65,66]

 Nutritional management

Nutritional care focuses on nutrition-related drug effects, eating problems, and malnutrition. Common side effects of levodopa include severe nausea that affects food intake and, when the patient also takes anticholinergics, causes dryness of secretions. Excessive intake of vitamin B_6 should be avoided because it interacts with levodopa and reduces the drug's beneficial effect. Hand tremors make obtaining and preparing food, as well as eating movements of carrying food from bowl or plate to the mouth, difficult. Thus, for example, soups should be avoided and more textured foods used. As the disease progresses, there may be problems with chewing, swallowing, or aspiration of small food items such as peas or nuts, as well as discomfort from constipation, flatulence, or delayed gastric emptying. Small frequent meals of increased carbohydrate and decreased fat, chewing thoroughly and eating slowly with special utensils as needed, with appropriate energy intake to maintain optimal weight and adequate fiber and fluid to prevent constipation, will be helpful.

Paré's recent group study indicates that a special diet of daytime protein restriction to about 10 g has provided a helpful adjunct therapy for patients experiencing unpredictable motor-response fluctuations from the drug levodopa.[67] Protein foods such as meat and dairy products, to a day's total RDA intake (0.8 g/kg/day), are reserved for use in the evening meal and later snack. These beneficial effects of steady symptom control appear to result from a decrease during the day in the plasma concentration of dietary protein–derived large neutral amino acids that compete with levodopa for transport into the brain. Unintentional weight loss and body composition changes are common in Parkinson's disease patients. They are at greater nutritional risk than a matched population and should have continuing nutritional assessment and guidance.[68]

HUNTINGTON'S CHOREA

First described in a landmark 1872 paper by American physician George Huntington (1850-1916), Huntington's **chorea** is an uncommon genetic disease in which degeneration of the basal ganglia of the brain results in *chorea*—rapid, jerky, involuntary movements, and *dementia*—progressive mental impairment. Currently, after a decade-long search, a large group of scientists from six institutions have finally discovered the defective gene that causes the disease, opening the way to future therapies and possibly to an eventual cure.[69,70] Symptoms do not usually appear until about age 35 to 50 years; cases of symptomatic effects beginning in childhood are rare. This genetic disease is inherited in an autosomal dominant pattern with each child having a 50% chance of the condition developing. The highest concentration of persons world wide with Huntington's chorea in one family has been found and its gene linkage studied by Wesler's group in the little town of San Luis on the shores of Lake Maracaibo high in the Andes mountains of Venezuela.[71] In the United States, the disease develops in about 5 persons out of 100,000. Generally, the symptoms do not appear until middle adulthood, so affected persons may have children before knowing that they have the disease. Continuing study has identified gene mutation that causes an abnormal protein product the scientists have called *huntingtin*.[72]

Medical management

As a result of recent advances in genetics, a test is now available for young adults whose parents have Huntington's chorea to learn, with 95% accuracy, if they carry the gene and thus have the disorder. This test can then help them decide whether or not to have children themselves. There is no known cure, so medical management helps to lessen the characteristic chorea, which affects face, arms, and trunk with random grimaces, twitches, and general clumsiness. The drug chlorpromazine (Thorazine), the most widely used antipsychotic drug for its tranquilizing effect (it suppresses brain centers that control abnormal emotions and behaviors), has been found useful. The mental impairment causes behavior changes, difficulty making decisions, apathy, irritability, and memory loss.

Nutritional management

The excessive muscular activity requires adequate energy and nutrient intake to prevent malnutrition and excess weight loss. As the disease progresses, patients become cachectic and even with an adequate food intake show a progressively catabolic state. Nutritional counseling involves help in planning energy-nutrient dense diets to combat malnutrition, and assistance with dysphagia or feeding problems and the drug side effect of constipation. Persons with advanced disease accompanied by dysphagia, marasmus, and depression may be fed an enteral support formula through a percutaneous endoscopic gastrostomy (PEG) tube (see Chapter 17).[73]

GUILLAIN-BARRÉ SYNDROME

This acute postinfectious polyneuritis was first described by two 20th-century French neurologists, Georges Guillain (1876-1961) and Jean Alexander Barré (1880-1965). It is a rare form of damage to the peripheral nerves in which the myelin sheaths covering nerve axons, and sometimes the axons themselves, deteriorate, causing loss of nerve conduction and partial or complete paralysis.[74] Nerve inflammation occurs particularly where their roots leave the spine, impairing both movement and sensation. Muscular weakness in the legs, often accompanied by numbness and tingling, progresses upward to trunk and arms, as well as face and head. A low-grade fever persists, and there may be urinary tract infection, respiratory failure requiring a ventilator, and personality changes. This acute syndrome is an autoimmune reaction, often following a viral infection and sometimes an immunization. Recent study has indicated that infection with *Campylobacter jejuni* often precedes the Guillain-Barré syndrome and is associated with axonal degeneration, slow recovery, and sometimes severe residual disability.[75] In general, the United States incidence is about 15 cases per million population per year.

Medical management

Hospitalization for close monitoring of acute condition is essential, especially if a breathing difficulty occurs. In severe cases, *plasmapheresis*, in which blood plasma is withdrawn from the patient, treated to remove antibodies, and replaced, may be done. Most people recover completely without specific treatment other than general supportive care, but some are left with permanent weakness in affected areas.

Nutritional management

During early acute phases, enteral or parenteral nutrition support may be necessary, with attention to increased energy and protein needs in the formula solutions (see Chapter 17). Also, if respiratory distress occurs requiring ventilator assistance, increased use of fat for needed energy fuel rather than increased carbohydrate, such as the need for patients with chronic obstructive pulmonary disease (COPD), would be indicated (see Chapter 19). Food consistency and texture may need to be adjusted in early oral feedings to accommodate any chewing and swallowing problems from weak facial and throat muscles. Continuing attention to energy and nutrient needs during convalescence is required to restore lost body weight and muscle mass.

AMYOTROPHIC LATERAL SCLEROSIS (ALS)

Amyotrophic lateral sclerosis (ALS), also known as Lou Gehrig disease for the famous United States baseball player who developed ALS at the height of his successful Major League career, is the most common of the motor neuron diseases, affecting approximately one person in 10,000.[76] In these rare neuron disorders, nerves that control muscular activity degenerate within the brain and

---

amyotrophic lateral sclerosis   A progressive neuromuscular disease characterized by the degeneration of the neurons of the spinal cord and the motor cells of the brainstem, causing a deficit of upper and lower motor neurons; death usually occurs in 2 to 3 years.

chorea   A wide variety of ceaseless involuntary movements that are rapid, complex, and jerky, yet appear to be well coordinated; characteristic movements of Huntington's disease.

spinal cord. Researchers have recently reported the discovery of the gene causing a hereditary form of the disease.[77,78] The gene controls the synthesis of an enzyme that helps cells get rid of highly toxic and destructive superoxide free radicals, which are produced by a variety of oxidative cell reactions.[79,80] If the enzyme were abnormal because of the defective ALS gene, free cell radicals might well build up, causing the death of the motor neurons affected in ALS. As it is now, this relentless nerve degeneration of ALS progresses to involve the muscles of respiration and swallowing, usually killing its victims in about 3 years.[78-80] This giant step of identifying the responsible defective gene will lead to more knowledge of how the progressive destructive course of ALS may be slowed, controlled, or prevented.

 ## Nutritional management

Nutrition care planning and counseling will focus on increased energy intake and adjusted nutrient needs as the disease progresses.[81] Weakness of hands and arms, as well as problems with chewing, swallowing, delayed or absent response of gag reflex and risk of aspiration will require eating assistance and modification of food textures. Frequent small meals are better tolerated. In advanced stages, enteral and parenteral nutrition support can supply needed energy and nutrients in a variety of individualized formulas (see Chapter 17).

MULTIPLE SCLEROSIS

Multiple sclerosis (MS) is a progressive disease of the central nervous system in which scattered patches of insulating myelin, the fatty covering of nerve fibers in the brain and spinal cord that protects the neurons and facilitates the passage of neuromuscular impulses, are destroyed. In these denuded patches, the myelin is replaced by nonfunctional plaques of scar tissue so that the nerve fiber can no longer conduct normal electrical impulses. The severity of the condition varies markedly among the persons it affects. The precise cause of multiple sclerosis is unknown, but it is an autoimmune disease in which the body's defense system begins to treat the myelin tissue in the central nervous system as a foreign substance and gradually sets out to destroy it, with subsequent scarring left in its wake.

Ongoing studies at the Weizmann Institute of Science in Israel have been developing and testing a new approach. They are investigating triggering events for this mutiny in the immune system involving T cells and the protein antigens produced, and the possibilities of using these autoimmune components as treatment strategies in a similar manner to that of vaccines.[82] After successful trials with multiple sclerosis patients at 11 centers in the United States, the new drug produced by Teva Pharmaceutical Industries in Israel is now marketed under the trade name Copaxone.[83]

An as yet unknown genetic factor is probably involved, since relatives of affected persons are eight times more likely than others to develop the disease. Environment seems to play a role. Multiple sclerosis is five times more common in temperate zones, such as the United States and Europe, than in the tropics.[84] Perhaps it is induced by a virus picked up in the first 15 years of life in these temperate climates. Approximately two thirds of the persons affected experience the beginning symptoms between ages 20 to 40 years, more women than men are affected at a 2:1 ratio, and it is most commonly found in white populations. In the relatively high-risk temperate areas the incidence of multiple sclerosis is about 1 in every 1000 people.

Depending on how extensive the tissue involvement and which parts of the brain and spinal cord are affected, the effects of multiple sclerosis vary widely from mild periodic feelings of tingling, numbness, constriction, or stiffness in any part of the body to more severe disabling disease. The role of dietary factors remains uncertain, but considerable investigation has implicated a high-fat diet as an agent.[84]

Medical management

Physicians have lacked specific means of treatment while the search for a cure goes on. Corticosteroid drugs have been used to alleviate symptoms of an acute attack. Currently, however, three new, more specifically effective drugs are being used. The first one to be approved by the United States Food and Drug Administration is beta-interferon (Betaseron), followed by Avonex. The newest one is copolymer 1 (Copaxone), developed in Israel and approved by the FDA for use in the United States.[85] These drugs reduce the frequency and severity of attacks. Adjunct physical therapy helps maintain muscle strength and the ability to remain mobile and independent.

 ## Nutritional management

General nutritional care responds to basic nutrition needs for adequate energy and nutrient intake to maintain or restore optimal nutritional status and assist with symptomatic gastrointestinal problems with eating and elimination, as discussed with other neuromuscular diseases above.[81] If steroid therapy is used, dietary sodium is reduced. Low-fat foods are wise in any case, in possible relation to disease control,[84] and to healthy weight management.[85] Nasoenteric or gastrostomy tube feeding may be needed in advanced disease to provide enteral nutrition support.

MYASTHENIA GRAVIS

The neuromuscular disease **myasthenia gravis** occurs in about 1 out of every 20,000 persons, causing the affected person to become paralyzed as a result of the inability of the neuromuscular junctions to transmit nerve fiber signals to the muscles.[86] It is an autoimmune disorder, in which, for unknown reasons, the body's immune system attacks and gradually destroys the receptors in muscles that are responsible for picking up nerve impulses. As a result, the affected muscles respond only weakly or not at all to nerve impulses. Only about 2 to 5 new cases of this rare disease per 100,000 people are diagnosed annually. It affects more women than men in a ratio of 3:2. Although it can occur at any age, it usually occurs between ages 20 to 30 years in women and 50 to 70 years in men. Facial muscles are usually involved first, causing drooped eyelids, double vision, and sometimes a lack of facial animation with an absent stare appearance. Weak muscles of the face, throat, larynx, and neck cause difficulties in speaking and eating. As muscles in the arms and legs become involved, problems with other daily living activities such as food procurement and preparation, as well as dressing, combing the hair, and climbing stairs, also develop. In severe cases, respiratory muscles in the chest weaken and cause breathing difficulty.

Medical management

Treatment may involve a thymectomy, that is, removal of the thymus gland, a small gland in the upper chest thought to be partly responsible for the abnormal antibody activity, especially if a small tumor is found there. Temporary relief may be obtained by regular plasmapheresis, exchanges of the patient's antibody-containing blood for antibody-free blood. These antibodies produced by the disease attack the receptors on the muscle cells that bind the acetylcholine neurotransmitter necessary for muscle contraction, thus effectively reducing stimulation of muscle cells and weakening muscle action. Drugs used to treat myasthenia gravis, such as neostigmine (Prostigmin) or pyridostigmine (Mestinon, Regonol), increase the amount of the neurotransmitter acetylcholine at the nerve ending by blocking the action of the enzyme that normally breaks it down.[86,87] The blocking action of these drugs increases levels of the acetylcholine transmitter by allowing more of it to accumulate in the synaptic cleft between nerve and muscle-fiber endings, thus permitting the remaining receptors to function more efficiently.

 ## Nutritional management

Nutritional care has three main goals: (1) to maintain optimal energy-nutrient intake for muscle strength and good nutritional status; (2) to solve any associated eating problems by adjusting meal patterns to a major meal at breakfast when the patient is more rested and frequent small meals through the day, and by modifying food texture and supplementing with enteral feedings as needed; and (3) to help counteract drug side effects of nausea and vomiting. The drugs described should be taken with liquid or food to lessen stomach irritation.

ALZHEIMER'S DISEASE

Alzheimer's disease was named for the German neurologist Alois Alzheimer (1864-1915), who in 1907 first described the characteristic neurofibrillary tangles found in the postmortem brain of a 51-year-old demented woman named Auguste who died in 1906.[88-90] The disease is a form of progressive dementia in which nerve cells degenerate in the brain and the brain substance shrinks. The hallmark of the disease is the development of abnormal intracellular filaments in tangles of neurofibrils and extracellular deposits of amyloid-forming protein in senile plaques (**amyloid** plaques) and cerebral blood vessels, as first reported by Alzheimer. The density of these plaques has become the basis for the postmortem diagnosis of Alzheimer's disease; there is no absolute diagnostic test for the disease during life. Alzheimer's disease accounts for 60% to 80% of dementia cases over the age of 65 years, and afflicts 5% to 11% of the population over the age of 65 years and about half of the population over the age of 85 years.[91]

In addition to its human cost to patient and family, Alzheimer's disease levies a tremendous social and financial burden. Currently, more than 4 million Americans have been diagnosed, many of whom require institutional care at a cost that exceeds $50 billion a year and is expected to increase to $80 billion in the next few years.[91] Based on these trends, the Alzheimer's Association estimates that there may be 14 million cases by the middle of the next century, carrying the related soaring costs.[92] With the rapidly increasing elderly population of persons over 85 years, the health care problem of Alzheimer's disease is assuming enormous proportions.

Research into causes and treatment has greatly expanded in recent years. Current reports describe the discovery of genes for early onset familial Alzheimer's disease and the more common late-onset form.[93,94] However, the direct cause remains unknown and there is still no means of stopping the progressive years of mental and personal decline until death. This declining progression of Alzheimer's disease has been divided into

---

amyloid   A glycoprotein substance having a relation to starchlike structure but more a protein compound; an abnormal complex material forming characteristic brain deposits of fibrillary tangles always found in postmortem examinations of patients with Alzheimer's disease, the only means of definitive diagnosis; found in various body tissues that, when advanced, form lesions that destroy functional cells and injure the organ.

myasthenia gravis   A progressive neuromuscular disease caused by faulty nerve conduction resulting from the presence of antibodies to acetylcholine receptors at the neuromuscular junction.

three broad stages: (1) Stage one, the early period of increasing forgetfulness and anxious depression; (2) Stage two, a middle period of severe memory loss for recent events, disorientation, and personality changes; and (3) Stage three, the final period of severe confusion, psychosis, memory loss, personal neglect, bed-bound, feeding problems, full-time nursing care, and finally death from an infection such as pneumonia.[95]

Medical management

There is no treatment for the disease itself, except for suitable day-to-day nursing and social care for both the patient and the family. Keeping the patient well nourished, occupied, and exercised helps to lessen anxiety and personal distress, especially in the earlier stages when the person is sufficiently aware of his or her condition. Some use of tranquilizing medication often helps improve difficult behavior and enables the patient to sleep. Research

into drug therapy continues. Family counseling and respite care are essential.

 ## Nutritional management

Nutritional care in each stage of Alzheimer's disease becomes increasingly difficult and challenging. Adequate nutrition throughout the course of the disease is essential to improve physical well-being, help maximize the patient's functioning, and improve the quality of life. Nutrition-related changes occur at each progressive stage of the illness, as shown in Table 25.3, and illustrate the major goals of maintaining adequate nutrition and preventing malnutrition, and devising practical ways of dealing with feeding problems.[95,96] Because these patients have lower body weight and require higher energy intakes than normal elderly persons, they often require high-caloric supplement beverages to help supply added nourishment. In general, they have more risk factors and major indicators of poor nutritional status than the overall elderly population.[97] Four major factors help promote optimal intake in long-term care:

- Using skillful individual feeding techniques
- Selecting appropriate food consistency
- Providing adequate time in which to feed
- Focusing on the midday meal when peak cognitive abilities occur

Table 25.3	Progression of Alzheimer's disease	
	General Symptoms	**Nutrition-related effects**
Stage 1 (early)	Loss of memory	Difficulty in shopping, cooking
	Decrease in social and vocational skills	Forgetting to eat
	Careless work, housekeeping, finances	Changes in taste and smell
	Easily lost	Unusual food choices
	Personality changes	Degeneration of appetite regulation
	Recognition of faces	
	Well-oriented to time	
Stage 2 (middle)	Inability to recall names	Increased energy requirement from agitation
	Disorientation to times	Holding food in mouth
	Delusions	Forgetting to swallow
	Depression	Losing ability to use utensils
	Agitation	Use spoon only
	Language problems	Eating with hands
Stage 3 (final)	Complete disorientation	No recognition of food
	Forgetting own name	Refusal to eat or open mouth for feeding
	Not recognizing family	Need for nasogastric feeding
	Loss of verbal skills	
	Loss of basic self-care skills	
	Urinary and fecal incontinence	
	Bed-bound	

Data from Gray GE: Nutrition and dementia, *J Am Diet Assoc* 89(12):1795, 1989.

TO SUM UP

Individuals facing disabling illness and injury confront a myriad of interacting challenges, including social attitudes and financial, physical, and psychologic barriers. The team approach, involving family and friends in addition to health professionals, becomes an essential basis of care.

The basic principles of nutrition care involve the *prevention* of malnutrition and *restoration* of eating ability. To avoid malnutrition, the nutritionist must assess individual nutritional needs to meet basal energy expenditure (BEE) needs, added metabolic activity factors (MAF) resulting from any underlying disease process, as well as requirements to meet physical therapy and other activities. There must be sufficient nutrient intake to meet a variety of needs: protein and fat (linoleic acid) to promote tissue and organ integrity; carbohydrate to counteract impaired postinjury metabolism; and optimal intake of vitamins and minerals, which sometimes requires the use of supplements to guard against deficiencies. To restore eating ability, the occupational therapist and nurse play significant roles in promoting adequate swallowing, chewing, and hand and utensil usage skills. To meet the individual's nutritional needs, the nutritionist must assess eating skills, estimate eating desire (sensory stimuli, "comfort foods") and help the client develop new ways of eating with various self-help devices.

Disabling conditions that require special nutrition support and modifications to treat underlying disease effects include: (1) *musculoskeletal disease*, such as various forms of arthritis; (2) *neuromuscular disease*, caused by a sudden brain or spinal cord injury or a stroke, or by developmental disabilities resulting from cerebral palsy, epilepsy, or spina bifida; and (3) *progressive neurologic disorders*, such as Parkinson's and Huntington's diseases, ALS, multiple sclerosis, or dementia as seen in Alzheimer's disease.

■ QUESTIONS FOR REVIEW

1. What are the two major goals of rehabilitative therapy for disabling conditions? How do the basic principles of nutritional care help meet these goals?

2. Describe the functions of major nutrients in preventing or retarding the catabolic process that often occurs in long-term disabling illness or injury.

3. Select six of the different disease processes or injuries discussed that result in eating disabilities. Describe the nature of the disease or injury and relate it to disability involved. Outline the medical and nutritional therapy used in each case, giving the rationale for the nutritional management.

■ REFERENCES

1. Gines DJ: Introduction to nutrition and rehabilitation. In Gines DJ, ed: *Nutrition management in rehabilitation,* Rockville, Md, 1990, Aspen.

2. Verbrugge LM et al: The great efficacy of personal and equipment assistance in reducing disability, *Am J Public Health* 87(3):384, 1997.

3. National Institutes of Health, Institute of Medicine: *The second fifty years: promoting health and preventing disability,* Washington, DC, 1991, National Academy Press.

4. Doyle R: Stroke mortality in men ages 35 to 74, *Sci Am* 274(3):26, 1996.

5. Barinaga M: Finding new drugs to treat stroke, *Science* 272(5263):664, 1996.

6. Breslow RA et al: Malnutrition in tube-fed nursing home patients with pressure sores, *J Parenter Enter Nutr* 15(6):663, 1991.

7. Harris ED: Rheumatoid arthritis: pathophysiology and implications for therapy, *N Engl J Med* 322(18):1277, 1990.

8. Antonelli MAS et al: Herpes zoster in patients with rheumatoid arthritis treated with weekly, low-dose methotrexate, *Am J Med* 90:295, 1991.

9. Tugwell P et al: Combination therapy with cyclosporine and methotrexate in severe rheumatoid arthritis, *N Engl J Med* 333(3): 137, 1995.

10. Wolman PG: Arthritis. In Gines DJ, ed: *Nutrition management in rehabilitation,* Rockville, Md, 1990, Aspen.

11. Kremer JM et al: Dietary fish oil and olive oil supplementation in patients with rheumatoid arthritis: clinical and immunologic effects, *Arthritis Rheum* 33(6):810, 1990.

12. Price ME, Dilorio C: Swallowing: a practice guide, *Am J Nurs* 90(7):42, 1990.

13. Raloff J: Hip fracture risks go beyond bone loss, *Sci News* 150(4):54, 1996.

14. Cummings SR et al: Risk factors for hip fracture in women, *N Engl J Med* 332(12):767, 1995.

15. Tolstoi LG, Levin RM: Osteoporosis—the treatment controversy, *Nutr Today* 27(4):6, 1992.

16. Chesnut CH: Osteoporosis and its treatment, *N Engl J Med* 326:406, 1992.

17. US Department of Health and Human Services, Public Health Service: *Healthy people 2000: national health promotion and disease prevention objectives,* Pub No 91-50212, Washington, DC, 1990, US Government Printing Office.

18. Kearns P: Nutrition in neurological injury, *Nutr Clin Prac* 6(6):211, 1991.

19. National Center for Health Statistics: *Health, United States, 1989 and prevention profile,* Pub No 90-1232, Hyattsville, Md, 1990, US Department of Health and Human Services.

20. Hubert C: Trauma care crisis, *Sacramento Bee* 273:1, 1993.

21. Konvolinka CW, Morell VO: Nutrition in head trauma, *Nutr Clin Prac* 6(6):223, 1991.

22. Ott L, Young B: Nutrition in the neurologically injured patient, *Nutr Clin Prac* 6(6):223, 1991.

23. Varella L: Barbiturate therapy and nutrition support in head-injured patients, *Nutr Clin Prac* 6(6):239, 1991.

24. Kirby DF et al: Early enteral nutrition after brain injury by percutaneous endoscopic gastrojejunostomy, *J Parenter Enter Nutr* 15(3):298, 1991.

25. Weakes E, Elia M: Observations on the patterns of 24-hour energy expenditure change in body composition and gastric emptying in head-injuries patients receiving nasogastric tube feeding, *J Parenter Enter Nutr* 20(1):31, 1996.

26. Annis K et al: Nutritional support of the severe head-injured patient, *Nutr Clin Prac* 6(6):245, 1991.

27. Yankelson S: Traumatic brain injury. In Gines DJ, ed: *Nutrition management in rehabilitation,* Rockville, Md, 1990, Aspen.

28. Chiles BW, Cooper PR: Acute spinal injury, *N Engl J Med* 334(8):514, 1996.

29. Rice DP, MacKenzie EJ: *Cost of injury in the United States: a report to Congress, 1989,* San Francisco, 1989, Institute on Health and Aging, University of California, and Injury Prevention Center, Johns Hopkins University.

30. Rice DR, Max W: Annotation: The high cost of injuries in the United States, *Am J Public Health* 86(1):14, 1996.

31. Young W: Spinal cord regeneration, *Science* 273(July 26):451, 1996.

32. Doolittle ND: Advances in the neurosciences and implications for nursing care, *J Neurosci Nurs* 23(4):207, 1991.

33. Rouch W: Are pushy axons a key to spinal cord repair? *Science* 276(5321):1917, 1997.

34. Johnson RK et al: *Athetosis* increases resting metabolic rate in adults with cerebral palsy, *J Am Diet Assoc* 96(2):145, 1996.

35. Johnson RK et al: Total energy expenditure in adults with cerebral palsy as assessed by doubly labeled water, *J Am Diet Assoc* 97(9):966, 1997.

36. Walter A et al: Food safety training needs exist for staff and consumers in a variety of community-based homes for people with developmental disabilities, *J Am Diet Assoc* 97(6):611, 1997.

37. Hogan SE, Evers SE: A multinational rehabilitation program for persons with severe physical and developmental disabilities, *J Am Diet Assoc* 97(2):162, 1997.

38. Lucas BL, Blyler E: Position of the American Dietetic Association: Nutrition in comprehensive program planning for persons with developmental disabilities, *J Am Diet Assoc* 97(2):189, 1997.

39. Stallings VA et al: Body composition in children with spastic quadriplegic cerebral palsy, *J Pediatr* 126:1883, 1995.

40. Ross Laboratories: Estimating stature from the knee height. In Ross Laboratories: *Directions for the Ross knee height caliper,* Columbus, Ohio, 1992, Ross.

41. Johnson RK, Ferrara MS: Estimating stature from knee height for persons with cerebral palsy: an evaluation of estimating equations, *J Am Diet Assoc* 91(10):1283, 1991.

42. Krick J et al: Pattern of growth in children with cerebral palsy, *J Am Diet Assoc* 96(7):680, 1996.

43. Tolia V et al: Gastrointestinal tolerance of a pediatric fiber formula in developmentally disabled children, *J Am Coll Nutr* 16(3):224, 1997.

44. Ferrang TM et al: Dietary and anthropomorphic assessment of adults with cerebral palsy, *J Am Diet Assoc* 92(9):1083, 1992.

45. Brodie MJ, Dichter MA: Antiepileptic drugs, *N Engl J Med* 334(2):168, 1996.

46. Motte J et al: Lamotrigine for generalized seizures associated with the Lennox-Gastaut syndrome, *N Engl J Med* 337(25):1807, 1997.

47. Gasch AT: Use of the traditional ketogenic diet for treatment of intractable epilepsy, *J Am Diet Assoc* 90(10):1433, 1990.

48. Edelstein SF, Chisholm M: Management of intractable childhood seizures using the non-MCT oil ketogenic diet in 20 patients, *J Am Diet Assoc* 96(11):1181, 1996.

49. Sutton M et al: Pediatric diets. In Chicago Dietetic Association and the South Suburban Dietetic Association: *Manual of clinical dietetics,* ed 4, 1992, American Dietetic Association.

50. Lary JM, Edmonds LD: Prevalence of spina bifida at birth—United States, 1983-1990: a comparison of two surveillance systems, *MMWR* 45(SS-2): 15, 1996.

51. Dustrude A, Prince A: Provision of optimal nutrition care in myelomeningocele, *Top Clin Nutr* 5(2):34, 1990.

52. Raloff J: Enzyme error behind neural tube defects, *Sci News* 147(4):53, 1995.

53. Rush D: Periconceptional folate and neural tube defect, *Am J Clin Nutr* 59(suppl 2S):511S, 1994.

54. Atencio PL et al: Effect of level of lesion and quality of ambulation on growth chart measurements in children with myelomeningocele, *J Am Diet Assoc* 92(7):858, 1992.

55. Unonu JN, Johnson AA: Feeding patterns, food energy, nutrient intakes, and anthropometric measurements of selected black preschool children with Down syndrome, *J Am Diet Assoc* 92(7):856, 1992.

56. Luke A et al: Nutrient intake and obesity in prepubescent children with Down syndrome, *J Am Diet Assoc* 96(12):1262, 1996.

57. Youdim MBH, Riederer P: Understanding Parkinson's Disease, *Sci Am* 276(1):52, 1997.

58. Rajput AH: Frequency and cause of Parkinson's disease, *Can J Neurol Sci* 19:103, 1992.

59. Branddmann O et al: Association of the slow acetylator genotype for N-acetyltransferase 2, *Lancet* 350(Oct 18): 1136, 1997.

60. Goldberg J: Fetal attraction, *Discover* 16(7):86, 1995.

61. Guyton AC: *Textbook of medical physiology,* ed 9, Philadelphia, 1996, WB Saunders.

62. Tsui JKC: Future treatment of Parkinson's disease, *Can J Neurol Sci* 19:160, 1992.

63. Lindvall O et al: Grafts of fetal dopamine neurons survive and improve motor function in Parkinson's disease, *Science* 247:574, 1990.

64. Fackelmann K: Fetal cells thrive in a Parkinsonian brain, *Sci News* 147(17):262, 1995.

65. Vogel G: Gene discovery offers tentative clues to Parkinson's, *Science* 276(5321:1973, 1997.

66. Polymeropoulos MH et al: Mutation in the α-synuclein gene identified in families with Parkinson's disease, *Science* 276(5321):2045, 1997.

67. Paré S et al: Effect of daytime protein restriction on nutrient intakes of free-living Parkinson's disease patients, *Am J Clin Nutr* 55:701, 1992.

68. Beyer PI et al: Weight change and body composition in patients with Parkinson's disease, *JAMA* 95(9):979, 1995.

69. Revkin A: Hunting down Huntington's, *Discover* 14(12):98, 1993.

70. Wexler NS et al: Huntington's disease in Venezuela and gene kinkage, *Cytogenet Cell Genet* 37:605, 1984.

71. Barinaga M: An intriguing new lead on Huntington's disease, *Science* 271(5253):1233, 1996.

72. Burcin R et al: Nutritional therapy in Huntington's disease: a case report, *Support Line* 17(6):6, 1995.

73. Honavar M et al: A clinicopathological study of the Guillain-Barré syndrome, *Brain* 114(3):1245, 1991.

74. Rees JH et al: *Campylobacter jejuni* infection and Guillain-Barré syndrome, *N Engl J Med* 333(21):1374, 1995.

75. Hughes RAC, Swan AV: Double-blind trial of intravenous methylprednisolone in Guillian-Barré syndrome, *Lancet* 341(Mar 16):586, 1993.

76. McNamara JO, Fridovich I: Did radicals strike Lou Gehrig? *Nature* 362(6415):20, 1993.

77. Rosen DR et al : Mutations in Cu/Zn superoxide dismutase gene are associated with familial amyotrophic lateral sclerosis, *Nature* 362(6415):59, 1993.

78. Marx J: Gene linked to Lou Gehrig's disease, *Science* 259(5100):1393, 1993.

79. Pennisi E: Free-radical scavenger gene tied to ALS, *Sci News* 143(10):148, 1993.

80. Wiedau-Pazas M et al: Altered reactivity of superoxide dismutase in familial amyotrophic lateral sclerosis, *Science* 271(5247):515, 1996.

81. Miller CA: Nutritional needs and care in amyotrophic lateral sclerosis, *Top Clin Nutr* 4(1):15, 1989.

82. Hoffman M: On the trail of the errant T cells of multiple sclerosis, *Science* 254(5031):521, 1991.

83. Staff: New multiple sclerosis drug clears hurdle, *Sci News* 150(13):199, 1996.

84. Lowis GW: The social epidemiology of multiple sclerosis, *Sci Total Environ* 90:163, 1990.

85. Wozniak-Wowk SC: Nutrition intervention in the management of multiple sclerosis, *Nutr Today* 28(6):12, 1993.

86. Guyton AC, Hall JE: *Textbook of medical physiology,* ed 9, Philadelphia, 1996, WB Saunders.

87. Dobkin BH: Vital signs—standing tall, *Discover* 15(9):58, 1994.

88. Alzheimer A: *Uber eine eigenartige Erkrankung der Hirnrinde, Allgemeine Zeitschrift fur Psychiatrie* 64:146, 1907. (English translation, *Arch Neurol* 21:109, 1969.)

89. Campion EW: When a mind dies (editorial), *N Engl J Med* 334(12):791, 1996.

90. O'Brien C: Auguste D. and Alzheimer's disease, *Science* 273(5271):28, 1996.

91. Yankner BA, Mesulam M: μ-Amyloid and the pathogenesis of Alzheimer's disease, *N Engl J Med* 325(26):1849, 1991.

92. Marx J: Searching for drugs that combat Alzheimer's, *Science* 273(5271):29, 1996.

93. Barinaga M: New Alzheimer's gene found, *Science* 2685(219):1845, 1996.

94. Reiman EM et al: Preclinical evidence of Alzheimer's disease in persons homozygous for the e4 allele for apolipoprotein E, *N Engl J Med* 334(12):752, 1996.

95. Gray GE: Nutrition and dementia, *J Am Diet Assoc* 89(12):1795, 1989.

96. Renvall NJ et al: Nutritional care of ambulatory residents in special care units for Alzheimer's patients, *J Nutr Elderly* 12(4):5, 1993.

97. Zabler LP et al: Nutritional care of ambulatory residents in special care units for Alzheimer's patients, *J Nutr Elderly* 12(4):5, 1993.

■ FURTHER READING

Hogan SE, Evers SE: A nutritional rehabilitation program for persons with severe physical and developmental disabilities, *J Am Diet Assoc* 97(2):162, 1997.

These nutritionists describe their process of designing and implementing a nutritional rehabilitation program for all residents of a long-term care facility for persons with severe disabilities and an auxiliary group home in southwestern Ontario, Canada. The authors provide an excellent example of the challenging needs of these patients and the team approach needed for their care.

Johnson RK et al: Athetosis increases resting metabolic rate in adults with cerebral palsy, *J Am Diet Assoc* 96(2):145, 1996.

Krick J et al: Pattern of growth in children with cerebral palsy, *J Am Diet Assoc* 96(7):680, 1996.

These two articles provide helpful background information about cerebral palsy, the most common cause of physical disability in children and adults. Based on studies of these growth patterns in children, Krick's group developed special charts for parents and health care professionals to use in evaluating and monitoring nutritional status. Johnson's group studied the influence of athetosis, the continuous involuntary writhing movements of cerebral palsy in adults, and its influence on increased energy requirements.

Youdim MBH, Riederer P: Understanding Parkinson's disease, *Sci Am* 276(1):52, 1997.

In this interesting and informative article, with its numerous illustrations, these two scientists studying Parkinson's disease and developing treatment substances describe their fascinating work in seeking its cause. They indicate their progress with the terse observation that the "smoking gun" may still be missing, but the highly reactive free radicals in the cell are certainly central suspects.

Case study

Patient with a cerebrovascular accident

James Braddock is a tall (182 cm, or 6 ft 1 in), 57-year-old black man who, until 6 weeks ago, was residing at a rehabilitation center to recover from the results of a cerebrovascular accident (CVA, stroke) that occurred 6 months ago. At that time he was brought to the local hospital emergency room, accompanied by his wife, who found him unconscious on the bathroom floor after hearing a fall. He had flaccid paralysis on the right side. Pinprick response on the left side was normal, but it was questionable on the right.

Within an hour Mr. Braddock began to regain consciousness but appeared to be confused, disoriented, and apprehensive. An examination conducted by his personal physician revealed a weight of 155 kg (345 lb), which was usual for the patient, pulse rate of 140, and a blood pressure of 190/100. The physician's impression was cerebral hemorrhage in the left-middle cerebral artery prefrontal area with massive extension, paralysis on the right side, and aphasia.

Laboratory tests were ordered, including blood urea nitrogen, fasting blood glucose, and serum cholesterol, hemoglobin, hematocrit, sodium, potassium, and chloride levels and carbon dioxide-combining power. The physician also ordered an intravenous infusion composed of 500 ml of 2.5% dextrose in 0.5% saline every 8 hours. The diet order was clear liquids by mouth as tolerated. Later the laboratory reported these results: blood urea nitrogen, 16 mg/dl; blood glucose, 140 mg/dl; cholesterol, 290 mg/dl; hemoglobin, 14 gm/100ml; hematocrit, 40 ml/100 ml; carbon dioxide, 60 vol/dl; sodium, 135 mEq/l; potassium, 4.2 mEq/l; and chloride, 98 mEq/l.

The diet was changed to full liquid the following day, and the intravenous infusion was discontinued. Mr. Braddock was advanced to a soft diet 4 days later. Nurses' notes indicated he was being fed by the staff. Two weeks later he was able tolerate a full diet. The occupational therapist, together with the clinical nutritionist and the nurse, developed eating aids that would help him learn to feed himself.

After 4 weeks Mr. Braddock was transferred to the rehabilitation center for follow-up therapy. At that time a vigorous physical and speech therapy program began. Self-feeding skills helped him gain more independence, and a diet plan of 1500 kcalories with cholesterol limited to 300 mg and sodium restricted to 1000 mg was designed to promote weight loss and help control his hypertension and vascular disease.

Response to therapy was good. In 6 months Mr. Braddock was able to walk with a cane and had regained much of his ability to speak. He was released to home care, following careful instructions regarding his home-care needs. Follow-up home visit reports indicate that Mr. Braddock has been losing weight gradually, has stopped smoking, and is practicing prescribed exercises daily. He is now inquiring about future job possibilities.

Questions for analysis

1. What underlying conditions may have been responsible for the CVA? What factors indicate this possible association?
2. What was the purpose of each laboratory test ordered? Which values were elevated? Which values were inadequate?
3. What members of the rehabilitative support team are identified? Was any member underused? How could this role have been expanded?
4. Outline the instructions you would give Mrs. Braddock to help her plan nutritional care for her husband at home.

Issues Answers

Independent living versus the kindness of strangers

If Tennessee Williams' famous line, "I have always relied on the kindness of strangers," in his play *A Streetcar Named Desire* for his lead character, Blanche, conjures up images of a blithe Southern belle, you're right—but think again. In today's reality, you may well think of a once-independent career woman now confined to her wheelchair, much of her financial resources gone to pay for lengthy and highly specialized care. Before 1978 she would have relied heavily on the "kindness of strangers" to meet most of her basic needs, including transportation to keep medical appointments and to purchase food and help in meal preparation and personal care.

In 1978 the Rehabilitation Act of 1973 was amended to allocate federal funds to establish independent living centers for disabled persons. The number of Americans who cannot perform even simple activities of daily living because of a major illness, disabling injury, or chronic health condition rose dramatically by 83.2% in the decade between 1966 and 1976, and has been gradually rising during the 1980s. In 1980 about 15% of the free living population was disabled. This rise is caused primarily by new technologies that have virtually wiped out the infectious diseases that used to kill the disabled, as well as those that together with nutrition have extended the general life span. The causes of disability have changed also, with rheumatoid arthritis and diabetes replacing heart disease and other causes.

Disabled persons have traditionally been barred from many activities because of limited mobility. Jobs, education, and recreational facilities have often been denied to them because of inadequate physical access or facilities and even fear and prejudice. Promotion of access, as well as independent living and access to employment, has been a strong civil rights issue in many parts of the United States with many positive results.

The passage of legislation establishing independent living centers across the United States enabled disabled persons to meet their basic needs. It also promoted political awareness among local communities. This legislation has opened the door to disabled persons who can and want to be self-reliant individuals capable of enriching their lives and contributing to their communities. Economic realities have meant that federal authorities have been reluctant to issue costly new regulations regarding the needs of disabled persons, although employment access is now guaranteed under the Americans With Disabilities Act of 1990. But the recent record is mixed, since cutbacks have occurred in programs providing income support via the Social Security Administration. Public support for these programs is also lessening, since the proportion of the public being served is relatively small and their needs are highly specialized.

Will the disabled person once again find it necessary to rely on "the kindness of strangers"? How will the loss of contributed income from working disabled persons affect the economy? Will the kind strangers be capable of filling the gap?

References

Cross EW: Implementing the Americans with Disabilities Act, *J Am Diet Assoc* 93(3):273, 1993.

DeJong G, Lifchez R: Physical disability and public policy, *Sci Am* 248(6):40, 1983.

Appendix A

Food Composition Table

The following Food Composition Table was developed by Positive Input Corp. and includes all of the foods listed in *Mosby's NutriTrac Nutrition Analysis CD-ROM,* which accompanies every copy of this text. Please note, however, that you will be able to find some nutrient information in *Mosby's NutriTrac Nutrition Analysis CD-ROM* that is not listed here in the Food Composition Table.

USDA ID Code	Food Name	Weight in Grams*	Quantity of Units	Unit of Measure	Protein (gm)	Fat (gm)	Carbohydrates (gm)	Kcalories	Caffeine (gm)	Fiber (gm)	Cholesterol (mg)	Saturated Fat (gm)
3117	Babyfood, Applesauce	28.35	3	Ounce	0	0	2.92	10.49	0	0.48	0	0
3280	Babyfood, Bananas w/ Tapioca	28.35	3	Ounce	0.11	0.06	5.05	18.99	0	0.45	0	0
3681	Babyfood, Barley, Ppd w/ Whole Milk	28.35	3	Ounce	1.3	0.94	4.62	31.47	0	0	0	0
3003	Babyfood, Beef	28.35	3	Ounce	4.11	1.39	0	30.05	0	0	0	0.73
3049	Babyfood, Beef and Rice	28.35	3	Ounce	1.42	0.82	2.49	23.25	0	0	0	0
3043	Babyfood, Beef Lasagna	28.35	3	Ounce	1.19	0.6	2.84	21.83	0	0	0	0
3287	Babyfood, Beef Noodle	28.35	3	Ounce	0.71	0.54	2.1	16.16	0	0.31	0	0
3052	Babyfood, Beef Stew	28.35	3	Ounce	1.45	0.34	1.56	14.46	0	0.31	3.55	0.16
3098	Babyfood, Beets	28.35	3	Ounce	0.37	0.03	2.18	9.64	0	0.54	0	0
3100	Babyfood, Carrots	28.35	3	Ounce	0.23	0.06	2.04	9.07	0	0.48	0	0
3013	Babyfood, Chicken	28.35	3	Ounce	4.17	2.72	0	42.24	0	0	0	0.7
3069	Babyfood, Chicken Noodle	28.35	3	Ounce	0.54	0.4	2.13	14.46	0	0.31	0	0
3070	Babyfood, Chicken Soup	28.35	3	Ounce	0.45	0.48	2.04	14.18	0	0.31	0	0
3014	Babyfood, Chicken Sticks	10	3	Stick	1.46	1.44	0.14	18.8	0	0.02	0	0
3214	Babyfood, Cookies, Arrowroot	28.35	3	Ounce	2.15	4.05	20.19	125.31	0	0.06	0.3	0.94
3120	Babyfood, Corn, Creamed	28.35	3	Ounce	0.4	0.11	4.62	18.43	0	0.6	0	0
3028	Babyfood, Cottage Cheese w/ Fruit	28.35	3	Ounce	0.85	0.2	4.51	22.11	0	0	0	0
3018	Babyfood, Egg Yolks	28.35	3	Ounce	2.84	4.9	0.28	57.55	0	0	208.37	1.47
3201	Babyfood, Egg Yolks and Bacon	28.35	3	Ounce	0.71	1.42	1.76	22.4	0	0.26	0	0
3236	Babyfood, Fruit Dessert	28.35	3	Ounce	0.09	0	4.88	17.86	0	0.17	0	0
3092	Babyfood, Green Beans	28.35	3	Ounce	0.34	0.03	1.62	7.09	0	0.54	0	0
3009	Babyfood, Ham	28.35	3	Ounce	4.28	1.9	0	35.44	0	0	0	0.64
3166	Babyfood, Juice, Apple	247.791	0.75	Cup	0	0.25	28.99	116.46	0	0.25	0	0
3179	Babyfood, Juice, Mixed Fruit	247.791	0.75	Cup	0.25	0.25	28.74	116.46	0	0.25	0	0
3172	Babyfood, Juice, Orange	247.791	0.75	Cup	1.49	0.74	25.27	109.03	0	0.25	0	0
3090	Babyfood, Macaroni and Cheese	28.35	3	Ounce	0.74	0.57	2.32	17.29	0	0.09	0	0
3045	Babyfood, Macaroni and Tomato and Beef	28.35	3	Ounce	0.71	0.31	2.66	16.73	0	0.31	0	0
3021	Babyfood, Meat Sticks	10	3	Stick	1.34	1.46	0.11	18.4	0	0.02	0	0.58
3279	Babyfood, Mixed Vegetable	28.35	3	Ounce	0.28	0	2.24	9.36	0	0	0	0
3076	Babyfood, Noodles and Chicken	28.35	3	Ounce	0.48	0.62	2.58	18.14	0	0.31	0	0
3228	Babyfood, Peach Cobbler	28.35	3	Ounce	0.09	0	5.19	18.99	0	0.2	0	0
3230	Babyfood, Peach Melba	28.35	3	Ounce	0.09	0	4.65	17.01	0	0	0	0
3131	Babyfood, Peaches w/ Sugar	28.35	3	Ounce	0.14	0.06	5.36	20.13	0	0.43	0	0
3133	Babyfood, Pears	28.35	3	Ounce	0.09	0.03	3.29	12.19	0	1.02	0	0
3124	Babyfood, Peas, Buttered	28.35	3	Ounce	0.99	0.37	3.2	17.01	0	0	0	0

The easiest way to look for a food is to use the "Search For" feature in *Mosby's NutriTrac Nutrition Analysis CD-ROM*. However, if you do not have access to a computer or your computer time is limited, you can easily look for a food using this Food Composition Table. The foods in the table are arranged alphabetically, within in groups.

The code number before each food corresponds to the food data bank in *Mosby's Nutrition Analysis CD-ROM*. When you input your Nutri-intake into the CD-ROM program, you may use these code numbers. Alternatively, you may to enter your dietary intake into *Mosby's NutriTrac Analysis CD-ROM* by typing a food's name or name and using the "Search For" option.

Column heading key: *gm* = grams; *mg* = milligrams; *mcg* = micrograms; *re* = retinol equivalent
*Please note that the "Weight in Grams" column provides the weight in grams of the serving or of one unit of measure. (For example, if a serving is 3 ounces, the "Weight in Grams" column may incidate the weight of 1 ounce.)

Monounsaturated Fat (gm)	Polyunsaturated Fat (gm)	Vitamin D (mg)	Vitamin K (mg)	Vitamin E (mg)	Vitamin A (re)	Vitamin C (mg)	Thiamin (mg)	Riboflavin (mg)	Niacin (mg)	Vitamin B6 (mg)	Folate (mg)	Vitamin B12 (mcg)	Calcium (mg)	Iron (mg)	Magnesium (mg)	Phosphorus (mg)	Potassium (mg)	Sodium (mg)	Zinc (mg)
0	0	0	0	0.17	0.28	10.72	0	0.01	0.02	0.01	0.48	0	1.42	0.06	0.85	1.7	21.83	0.57	0.01
0	0	0	0	0.17	1.13	7.29	0	0.01	0.06	0.04	1.81	0	2.27	0.09	3.4	2.55	30.62	2.55	0.02
0	0	0	0	0	0	0	0.14	0.16	1.7	0.03	2.52	0.09	65.21	3.5	8.51	42.53	54.43	13.89	0.24
0.52	0.05	0	0	0.11	8.79	0.54	0	0.05	0.93	0.03	1.62	0.42	2.27	0.47	2.55	20.41	53.87	18.71	0.57
0	0	0	0	0	22.4	1.11	0	0.02	0.38	0.04	1.7	0.14	3.12	0.2	2.27	9.92	34.02	101.21	0.26
0	0	0	0	0	44.23	0.54	0.02	0.03	0.38	0.02	1.7	0.14	5.1	0.25	3.12	11.34	34.59	128.71	0.2
0	0	0	0	0.11	24.95	0.4	0.01	0.01	0.16	0.01	1.56	0.03	2.27	0.12	1.98	8.51	13.04	4.82	0.11
0.12	0.03	0	0	0.07	65.49	0.85	0	0.02	0.37	0.02	1.7	0.14	2.55	0.2	3.12	12.47	40.26	97.81	0.25
0	0	0	0	0.15	0.85	0.68	0	0.01	0.04	0.01	8.73	0	3.97	0.09	3.97	3.97	51.6	23.53	0.03
0	0	0	0	0.15	334.81	1.56	0.01	0.01	0.14	0.02	4.9	0	6.52	0.11	3.12	5.67	57.27	13.89	0.05
1.23	0.66	0	0	0.11	15.88	0.43	0	0.05	0.97	0.05	3.15	0.11	15.59	0.28	3.12	25.52	34.59	14.46	0.29
0	0	0	0	0.07	30.33	0.34	0.01	0.01	0.15	0.01	1.5	0.04	4.82	0.11	2.55	6.8	9.92	4.82	0.08
0	0	0	0	0.07	62.65	0.28	0	0.01	0.08	0.01	1.47	0.03	10.49	0.08	1.42	6.8	18.71	4.54	0.06
0	0	0	0	0.04	95.4	0.17	0	0.02	0.2	0.01	1.11	0.04	7.3	0.16	1.4	12.1	10.6	47.9	0.1
2.55	0.24	0	0	0.13	0	1.56	0.14	0.12	1.63	0.01	2.84	0.02	9.07	0.85	6.24	32.89	44.23	104.9	0.15
0	0	0	0	0.15	2.27	0.62	0	0.01	0.14	0.01	3.6	0.01	5.1	0.08	2.27	9.36	22.96	14.74	0.07
0	0	0	0	0.17	0.57	6.75	0	0.01	0.01	0	1.45	0.02	8.79	0.04	1.13	11.06	11.91	14.46	0.05
1.96	0.64	0	0	0.22	106.6	0.4	0.02	0.08	0.01	0.05	26.11	0.44	21.55	0.78	1.98	81.36	21.83	11.06	0.54
0	0	0	0	0.08	7.94	0.26	0.01	0.02	0.08	0.01	1.16	0.03	7.94	0.13	1.42	14.18	9.92	13.61	0.08
0	0	0	0	0.07	6.8	0.85	0.01	0	0.04	0.01	0.99	0	2.55	0.06	1.42	2.27	26.93	3.69	0.01
0	0	0	0	0.15	12.19	2.38	0.01	0.03	0.09	0.01	9.27	0	18.43	0.31	6.24	5.39	36.29	0.57	0.05
0.9	0.26	0	0	0.11	2.84	0.6	0.04	0.05	0.81	0.06	0.6	0.03	1.42	0.29	3.12	25.23	59.54	18.99	0.48
0	0	0	0	1.49	4.96	143.47	0.02	0.04	0.21	0.07	0.25	0	9.91	1.41	7.43	12.39	225.49	7.43	0.07
0	0	0	0	0.5	9.91	157.59	0.06	0.03	0.3	0.11	16.6	0	19.82	0.84	12.39	12.39	250.27	9.91	0.07
0	0	0	0	1.49	14.87	154.87	0.11	0.07	0.59	0.13	65.42	0	29.73	0.42	22.3	27.26	455.93	2.48	0.14
0	0	0	0	0.07	0.85	0.37	0.02	0.02	0.15	0	0.43	0.01	14.46	0.09	1.98	16.73	12.47	21.55	0.09
0	0	0	0	0.07	30.9	0.43	0.01	0.02	0.21	0.01	1.84	0.07	3.97	0.1	1.98	12.47	20.41	4.82	0.1
0.65	0.16	0	0	0.04	2.1	0.24	0.01	0.02	0.15	0.01	0.89	0.03	3.4	0.14	1.1	10.3	11.4	54.7	0.19
0	0	0	0	0	69.17	0.94	0	0.01	0.12	0.02	1.9	0	4.82	0.09	2.84	6.24	31.75	2.55	0.07
0	0	0	0	0.07	36.86	0.23	0.01	0.01	0.19	0.01	0.96	0.03	7.37	0.14	3.12	9.36	16.73	7.37	0.09
0	0	0	0	0.07	3.97	5.81	0	0	0.07	0	0.31	0	1.13	0.03	0.57	1.7	15.88	2.55	0.01
0	0	0	0	0	5.67	7.37	0	0.01	0.08	0	0.54	0	3.12	0.09	0.57	1.42	26.37	2.55	0.08
0	0	0	0	0.17	5.1	5.36	0	0.01	0.18	0.01	1.11	0	1.42	0.08	1.42	3.12	43.94	1.42	0.02
0	0	0	0	0.17	0.85	6.24	0	0.01	0.05	0	1.08	0	2.27	0.07	2.55	3.4	32.6	0.57	0.02
0	0	0	0	0	11.62	3.6	0.02	0.02	0.39	0	10.26	0	12.76	0.29	0	0	33.17	1.42	0

USDA ID Code		Weight in Grams*	Quantity of Units	Unit of Measure	Protein (gm)	Fat (gm)	Carbohydrates (gm)	Kcalories	Caffeine (gm)	Fiber (gm)	Cholesterol (mg)	Saturated Fat (gm)
	food, Plums w/ Tapioca	28.35	3	Ounce	0.03	0	5.78	20.98	0	0.34	0	0
	yfood, Rice, Ppd w/ Whole Milk	28.35	3	Ounce	1.11	1.02	4.73	32.6	0	0	0	0
	byfood, Rice, w/ Mixed Fruit	28.35	3	Ounce	0.28	0.06	5.3	23.81	0	0.28	0	0
	abyfood, Spaghetti and Tomato and Meat	28.35	3	Ounce	0.71	0.37	2.86	17.86	0	0.31	0	0
	Babyfood, Spinach, Creamed	28.35	3	Ounce	0.85	0.4	1.81	11.91	0	0.51	0	0
	Babyfood, Split Pea and Ham	28.35	3	Ounce	0.94	0.37	3.2	20.13	0	0.31	0	0
	Babyfood, Squash	28.35	3	Ounce	0.23	0.06	1.59	6.8	0	0.6	0	0
	Babyfood, Sweetpotatoes	28.35	3	Ounce	0.31	0.03	3.94	17.01	0	0.43	0	0
	Babyfood, Teething Biscuits	11	3	Biscuit	1.18	0.46	8.4	43.12	0	0.15	0	0
	Babyfood, Tropical Fruit	28.35	3	Ounce	0.06	0	4.65	17.01	0	0	0	0
6	Babyfood, Turkey	28.35	3	Ounce	4.37	2.01	0	36.57	0	0	0	0.65
83	Babyfood, Turkey and Rice	28.35	3	Ounce	0.51	0.4	2.04	13.89	0	0.31	0	0.12
017	Babyfood, Turkey Sticks	10	3	Stick	1.37	1.42	0.14	18.2	0	0.05	0	0
19186	Apple Crisp	282	1	Cup	5.08	10.15	91.09	459.66	0	0	0	2.03
18001	Bagels, Blueberry	71	1	3¹/2 In.	7.98	1.14	42.9	205.77	0	1.66	0	0.16
18005	Bagels, Cinnamon-raisin	71	1	3¹/2 In.	6.96	1.21	39.19	194.54	0	0	0	0.19
18006	Bagels, Cinnamon-raisin, Toasted	66	1	3¹/2 In.	7	1.19	39.14	194.04	0	0	0	0.19
18003	Bagels, Egg	71	1	3¹/2 In.	7.53	1.49	37.63	197.38	0	0	17.04	0.3
18004	Bagels, Egg, Toasted	66	1	3¹/2 In.	7.52	1.45	37.62	197.34	0	0	17.16	0.3
18007	Bagels, Oat Bran	71	1	3¹/2 In.	7.6	0.85	37.84	181.05	0	0	0	0.14
18008	Bagels, Oat Bran, Toasted	66	1	3¹/2 In.	7.59	0.86	37.82	180.84	0	0	0	0.14
18001	Bagels, Plain	71	1	3¹/2 In.	7.46	1.14	37.91	195.25	0	1.49	0	0.16
18409	Bagels, Plain, Toasted	66	1	3¹/2 In.	7.46	1.12	37.95	194.7	0	0	0	0.16
18009	Biscuits, Plain or Buttermilk	35	1	Each	2.17	5.78	16.98	127.4	0	0	0.35	0.87
18086	Cake, Angelfood	28.35	1	Slice	1.67	0.23	16.39	73.14	0	0.43	0	0.03
18090	Cake, Boston Cream Pie	92	1	Slice	2.21	7.82	39.47	231.84	0	1.2	34.04	2.33
18094	Cake, Carrot, w/ Cream Cheese Frosting	111	1	Slice	5.11	29.3	52.39	483.96	0	0	59.94	5.43
18096	Cake, Chocolate w/ Chocolate Frosting	64	1	Slice	2.62	10.5	34.94	234.88	0	1.79	29.44	2.97
18110	Cake, Fruitcake	43	1	Piece	1.25	3.91	26.49	139.32	0	1.51	2.15	0.48
18113	Cake, German Chocolate, w/ Frosting	111	1	Slice	3.89	20.65	55.17	404.04	0	0	53.28	5.26
18115	Cake, Gingerbread	67	1	Slice	2.68	6.83	33.97	207.03	0	2.14	23.45	1.74
18119	Cake, Pineapple Upside-down	115	1	Slice	4.03	13.92	58.08	366.85	0	0	25.3	3.35
18120	Cake, Pound	28.35	1	Slice	1.56	5.64	13.83	110	0	0	62.65	3.15
18133	Cake, Sponge	38	1	Slice	2.05	1.03	23.22	109.82	0	0	38.76	0.3
18102	Cake, White, w/ Coconut Frosting	112	1	Slice	4.93	11.54	70.78	398.72	0	0	1.12	4.36
18139	Cake, White, w/o Frosting	74	1	Slice	4	9.18	42.33	264.18	0	0	1.48	2.42
18140	Cake, Yellow, w/ Chocolate Frosting	64	1	Slice	2.43	11.14	35.46	242.56	0	1.15	35.2	3.02
18141	Cake, Yellow, w/ Vanilla Frosting	64	1	Slice	2.24	9.28	37.63	238.72	0	0	35.84	1.52
18147	Cheesecake, Commercially Prepared	85	1	Slice	4.68	19.13	21.68	272.85	0	1.79	46.75	9.79
18149	Cheesecake, Homemade	85	1	Slice	0.5	22.1	21.42	303.45	0	0	102.85	12.21
18148	Cheesecake, No-bake Type	80	1	Slice	4.4	10.16	28.4	219.2	0	1.52	33.6	5.64
18382	Cheesecake, Plain, w/ Cherry Topping	90	1	Slice	4.5	16.65	23.85	258.3	0	0	76.5	9.11
18444	Cherry Pie, Fast Food	128	1	Pie	3.84	20.61	54.53	404.48	0	0	0	3.09
18104	Coffeecake	63	1	Slice	4.28	14.68	29.42	263.34	0	2.08	20.16	3.63
18103	Coffeecake, Cheese	76	1	Slice	5.32	11.55	33.67	257.64	0	0.91	25.84	3.8
18106	Coffeecake, Fruit	50	1	Slice	2.6	5.1	25.75	155.5	0	1.25	11	1.22
18238	Cream Puffs, Shell, w/ Custard Filling	130	1	Each	8.71	20.15	29.77	335.4	0	0	174.2	4.78
18240	Croissant, Apple	57	1	Medium	4.22	4.96	21.15	144.78	0	1.43	28.5	2.53
18239	Croissant, Butter	57	1	Medium	4.67	11.97	26.11	231.42	0	1.6	42.75	6.68
18241	Croissant, Cheese	57	1	Medium	5.24	11.91	26.79	235.98	0	2.17	36.48	5.49
	Croissant, Chocolate	56	1	Medium	5.21	14.07	25.15	234.61	0	2.2	38	8.07
18245	Danish Pastry, Cheese	71	1	Each	5.68	15.55	26.41	265.54	0	0	31.95	4.94
18244	Danish Pastry, Cinnamon	65	1	Each	4.55	14.56	28.99	261.95	0	0.78	19.5	3.73
18246	Danish Pastry, Fruit,	71	1	Each	3.83	13.14	33.94	263.41	0	1.35	14.91	3.35
18433	Danish Pastry, Lemon	71	1	Each	3.83	13.14	33.94	263.41	0	0	0	3.35

Monounsaturated Fat (gm)	Polyunsaturated Fat (gm)	Vitamin D (mg)	Vitamin K (mg)	Vitamin E (mg)	Vitamin A (re)	Vitamin C (mg)	Thiamin (mg)	Riboflavin (mg)	Niacin (mg)	Vitamin B6 (mg)	Folate (mg)	Vitamin B12 (mcg)	Calcium (mg)	Iron (mg)	Magnesium (mg)	Phosphorus (mg)	Potassium (mg)	Sodium (mg)	Zinc (mg)
0	0	0	0	0.17	2.55	0.23	0	0.01	0.06	0.01	0.26	0	1.7	0.06	1.13	1.7	23.53	13	0.02
0	0	0	0	0	0	0	0.13	0.14	1.48	0.03	2.32	0.09	67.76	3.46	12.76	49.61	53.87	13	0.18
0	0	0	0	0.09	0.57	5.73	0.07	0.17	0.77	0.07	0.77	0.01	5.67	1.34	1.42	6.52	9.36	3.1	0.05
0	0	0	0	0.07	37.71	0.62	0.02	0.02	0.31	0.02	2.01	0	5.1	0.16	2.27	10.49	30.62	5.6	0.12
0	0	0	0	0.15	104.33	1.02	0.01	0.02	0.07	0.02	19.5	0.02	32.04	0.4	17.86	13.89	62.65	15.59	0.1
0	0	0	0	0.07	22.68	0.54	0.01	0.01	0.14	0.01	3.69	0.01	6.52	0.14	0	13.89	38.56	3.97	18
0	0	0	0	0.15	56.98	2.21	0	0.02	0.11	0.02	4.37	0	6.8	0.1	3.4	4.54	52.45	0.28	2
0	0	0	0	0.15	188.24	2.72	0.01	0.01	0.11	0.03	2.92	0	4.54	0.11	3.4	6.8	68.89	6.24	
0	0	0	0	0.05	1.32	1	0.03	0.06	0.48	0.01	2.2	0.01	28.93	0.39	3.85	18.04	35.53	39.82	
0	0	0	0	0	0.57	5.33	0	0.01	0.02	0.01	0.94	0	2.84	0.07	1.42	2.27	16.44	1.98	
0.75	0.5	0	0	0.11	48.48	0.68	0	0.07	0.99	0.05	3.43	0.3	7.94	0.38	3.4	26.93	51.03	20.41	0.
0.16	0.09	0	0	0.07	41.96	0.34	0	0.01	0.08	0.01	0.88	0.03	6.52	0.08	2.27	4.82	9.64	4.25	0.0
0	0	0	0	0.04	6.8	0.15	0	0.02	0.18	0.01	1.13	0.1	7.2	0.12	1.6	10.3	9.1	48.3	0.18
4.31	2.99	0	0	0	87.42	6.49	0.24	0.2	2.19	0.12	14.1	0	78.96	2.12	19.74	70.5	273.54	513.24	0.45
0.09	0.49	0	0	0	12.88	19.77	0.38	0.22	3.24	0.04	15.62	0	52.54	2.53	20.59	68.16	99.5	379.14	0.62
0.12	0.48	0	0	0	5.68	0.5	0.27	0.2	2.19	0.04	14.91	0	13.49	2.7	14.91	54.67	107.92	228.62	0.53
0.12	0.48	0	0	0	4.62	0.4	0.22	0.18	1.97	0.04	10.56	0	13.2	2.7	15.18	54.78	107.58	228.36	0.53
0.3	0.46	0	0	0	23.43	0.43	0.38	0.17	2.44	0.06	15.62	0.11	9.23	2.83	17.75	59.64	48.28	358.55	0.55
0.3	0.46	0	0	0	21.12	0.33	0.3	0.15	2.2	0.06	11.22	0.11	9.24	2.82	17.82	59.4	48.18	358.38	0.55
0.18	0.35	0	0	0	0	0.14	0.24	0.24	2.1	0.14	32.66	0	8.52	2.19	40.47	117.15	144.84	359.97	1.48
0.18	0.35	0	0	0	0	0.07	0.19	0.22	1.89	0.13	23.1	0	8.58	2.18	40.92	116.82	144.54	359.7	1.48
0.09	0.49	0	0	0	0	0	0.38	0.22	3.24	0.04	15.62	0	52.54	2.53	20.59	68.16	71.71	379.14	0.62
0.09	0.49	0	0	0	0	0	0.31	0.2	2.91	0.03	11.22	0	12.54	2.52	20.46	67.98	71.94	378.84	0.62
2.42	2.17	0	0	0	0.35	0	0.15	0.1	1.17	0.02	2.45	0.05	17.15	1.16	5.95	150.5	78.4	368.2	0.17
0.02	0.1	0	0	0	0	0	0.03	0.14	0.25	0.01	0.85	0	39.69	0.15	3.4	65.77	26.37	212.34	0.02
4.08	0.93	0	0	0	21.16	0.09	0.38	0.25	0.18	0.02	7.36	0.15	21.16	0.35	5.52	45.08	35.88	132.48	0.15
7.24	15.1	0	0	0	426.24	1.22	0.15	0.17	1.13	0.08	13.32	0.11	27.75	1.39	19.98	78.81	124.32	273.06	0.54
5.76	1.22	0	0	0	17.92	0.06	0.02	0.09	0.37	0	5.12	0.08	27.52	1.41	21.76	78.08	128	213.76	0.44
1.79	1.39	0	0	0	8.17	0.17	0.02	0.04	0.34	0.02	1.29	0.03	14.19	0.89	6.88	22.36	65.79	116.1	0.12
8.71	5.46	0	0	0	23.31	0	0.11	0.14	1.1	0.02	4.44	0.1	53.28	1.22	18.87	173.16	150.96	368.52	0.49
3.75	0.9	0	0	0	10.72	0.07	0.13	0.12	1.05	0.03	6.7	0.05	46.23	2.22	10.72	112.56	161.47	306.86	0.27
5.97	3.77	0	0	0	74.75	1.38	0.18	0.18	1.37	0.04	8.05	0.09	138	1.7	14.95	94.3	128.8	366.85	0.36
1.58	0.31	0	0	0	44.23	0.03	0.04	0.06	0.37	0.01	3.12	0.05	9.92	0.39	3.12	38.84	33.74	112.83	0.13
0.36	0.17	0	0	0	17.48	0	0.09	0.1	0.73	0.02	4.94	0.09	26.6	1.03	4.18	52.06	37.62	92.72	0.19
4.14	2.42	0	0	0	12.32	0.11	0.14	0.21	1.19	0.03	5.6	0.07	100.8	1.3	13.44	78.4	110.88	318.08	0.37
3.93	2.33	0	0	0	11.84	0.15	0.14	0.18	1.13	0.02	5.18	0.06	96.2	1.12	8.88	68.82	70.3	241.98	0.24
6.19	1.34	0	0	0	17.28	0.06	0.08	0.1	0.8	0.02	5.12	0.08	23.68	1.33	19.2	103.04	113.92	215.68	0.4
3.91	3.28	0	0	0	12.16	0.13	0.06	0.04	0.32	0.02	5.76	0.13	39.68	0.68	3.84	91.52	33.92	220.16	0.16
6.58	1.17	0	0	0	136.85	0.51	0.02	0.16	0.17	0.04	12.75	0.14	43.35	0.54	9.35	79.05	76.5	175.95	0.43
6.87	1.75	0	0	0	272.85	0.34	0.03	0.18	0.34	0.04	10.2	0.21	49.3	1.06	6.8	81.6	86.7	240.55	0.47
3.12	0.52	0	0	0	79.2	0.4	0.1	0.21	0.39	0.04	14.4	0.25	137.6	0.38	15.2	187.2	168.8	304	0.37
5.21	1.38	0	0	0	216.9	0.63	0.03	0.14	0.32	0.04	9	0.15	38.7	1.11	6.3	63.9	83.7	182.7	0.36
9.53	6.92	0	0	0	21.76	1.66	0.18	0.14	1.82	0.04	3.84	0.1	28.16	1.56	12.8	55.04	83.2	478.72	0.29
8.31	1.8	0	0	0	18.27	0.19	0.13	0.14	1.06	0.02	20.16	0.07	34.02	1.2	13.86	68.04	77.49	221.13	0.51
5.71	1.25	0	0	0	53.96	0.08	0.08	0.1	0.52	0.04	44.08	0.11	44.84	0.49	11.4	75.24	219.64	257.64	0.45
2.86	0.71	0	0	0	10	0.4	0.02	0.1	1.29	0.02	9.5	0.03	22.5	1.22	8.5	59	45	192.5	0.33
8.49	5.4	0	0	0	258.7	0.39	0.16	0.36	1.09	0.08	19.5	0.47	85.8	1.52	15.6	141.7	149.5	443.3	0.78
1.35	0.42	0	0	0	41.61	0.23	0.13	0.09	0.91	0.02	7.41	0.13	17.1	0.63	7.41	33.06	51.3	156.18	0.59
3.25	0.74	0	0	0	78.09	0.11	0.22	0.14	1.25	0.03	15.96	0.17	21.09	1.16	9.12	59.85	67.26	424.08	0.43
3.74	1.55	0	0	0	89.49	0.11	0.3	0.19	1.23	0.04	18.81	0.18	30.21	1.23	13.68	87re	75.24	316.35	0.54
3.31	0.89	0	0	0	76.41	0.11	0.22	0.15	1.22	0.02	16.11	0.16	23.89	1.18	10.89	63.2	69.69	376.34	0.43
7.84	1.73	0	0	0	44.02	0.07	0.13	0.18	1.42	0.03	17.75	0.17	24.85	1.14	10.65	76.68	69.58	319.5	0.56
8.1	1.86	0	0	0	7.15	0.13	0.2	0.17	1.86	0.03	21.45	0.11	46.15	1.27	12.35	69.55	81.25	241.15	0.47
7.32	1.7	0	0	0	11.36	2.77	0.19	0.16	1.41	0	11.36	0.06	32.66	1.26	10.65	63.19	58.93	251.34	0.38
7.32	1.7	0	0	0	37.63	2.77	0.05	0.07	0.55	0	11.36	0	32.66	0.53	10.65	63.19	58.93	251.34	0.38

USDA ID Code	Food Name	Weight in Grams*	Quantity of Units	Unit of Measure	Protein (gm)	Fat (gm)	Carbohydrates (gm)	Kcalories	Caffeine (gm)	Fiber (gm)	Cholesterol (mg)	Saturated Fat (gm)
18247	...h Pastry, Nut	65	1	Each	4.62	16.38	29.71	279.5	0	1.5	29.9	3.54
18435	...sh Pastry, Raspberry	71	1	Each	3.83	13.14	33.94	263.41	0	0	0	3.35
18251	...oughnuts, Chocolate, Sugared or Glazed	42	1	Each	1.89	8.36	24.11	175.14	0	0.92	23.94	2.25
18253	...oughnuts, French Crullers, Glazed	41	1	Each	1.27	7.5	24.4	168.92	0	0	4.51	1.92
1825...	...oughnuts, Glazed	60	1	Each	3.84	13.68	26.58	241.8	0	1.26	3.6	3.49
182...	Doughnuts, Plain	47	1	Each	2.35	10.76	23.36	197.87	0	0.8	17.39	1.76
18...	Doughnuts, Plain, Chocolate-coated or Frosted	43	1	Each	2.15	13.33	20.64	203.82	0	0.86	24.94	3.59
1...	Doughnuts, Plain, Sugared or Glazed	45	1	Each	2.34	10.31	22.86	191.7	0	0	14.4	2.4
	Doughnuts, w/ Creme Filling	85	1	Each	5.44	20.83	25.5	306.85	0	0	20.4	5.74
	Doughnuts, w/ Jelly Filling	85	1	Each	5.02	15.9	33.15	289	0	0	22.1	4.05
...2	Doughnuts, Whole Wheat, Sugared or Glazed	45	1	Each	2.84	8.69	19.17	162	0	0	9	1.39
...57	Eclairs, Custard-filled w/ Chocolate Glaze	62	1	Each	3.97	9.73	15	162.44	0	0	78.74	2.55
...319	Fruit Pie, Fried	128	1	Pie	3.84	20.61	54.53	404.48	0	3.33	0	3.09
...320	Lemon Meringue Pie	113	1	Slice	1.7	9.83	53.34	302.84	0	1.36	50.85	1.75
...8445	Lemon Pie, Fried	128	1	Pie	3.84	20.61	54.53	404.48	0	0	0	3.09
	Muffins, Banana Nut	95	1	Each	6	12	53	340	0	2	35	0.9
18274	Muffins, Blueberry	65	1	Large	3.58	4.23	31.2	180.05	0	2.34	19.5	0.81
18279	Muffins, Corn	65	1	Large	3.84	5.46	33.09	198.25	0	0	33.15	0.98
18283	Muffins, Oat Bran	65	1	Large	4.55	4.81	31.4	175.5	0	4.88	0	0.58
18273	Muffins, Plain	65	1	Large	4.49	7.41	26.91	192.4	0	1.76	25.35	1.4
18287	Muffins, Wheat Bran	65	1	Large	4.62	7.93	27.24	183.95	0	0	21.45	1.47
18302	Pie, Apple	155	1	Slice	3.72	19.38	57.51	410.75	0	0	0	4.73
18304	Pie, Banana Cream	148	1	Slice	6.51	20.13	48.69	398.12	0	0	75.48	5.56
18305	Pie, Blueberry	125	1	Slice	2.25	12.5	43.63	290	0	0	0	2.35
18307	Pie, Butterscotch Pudding	127	1	Slice	5.97	18.16	42.29	354.33	0	0	77.47	5.09
18308	Pie, Cherry	125	1	Slice	2.5	13.75	49.75	325	0	1	0	2.6
18310	Pie, Chocolate Crème	113	1	Slice	2.94	21.92	37.97	343.52	0	2.26	5.65	5.96
18312	Pie, Chocolate Mousse	95	1	Slice	3.33	14.63	28.12	247	0	0	20.9	7.79
18313	Pie, Coconut Crème	64	1	Slice	1.34	10.62	23.81	190.72	0	0	0	4.81
18316	Pie, Coconut Custard	104	1	Slice	6.14	13.73	31.41	270.4	0	1.87	36.4	6
18317	Pie, Egg Custard	105	1	Slice	5.78	12.18	21.84	220.5	0	1.26	34.65	2.92
18322	Pie, Mince Meat	165	1	Slice	4.29	17.82	79.2	476.85	0	0	0	4.43
18324	Pie, Pecan	113	1	Slice	4.52	20.91	64.64	452	0	3.96	36.16	4.25
18326	Pie, Pumpkin	109	1	Slice	4.25	10.36	29.76	228.9	0	2.94	21.8	2.2
18328	Pie, Vanilla Crème	126	1	Slice	6.05	18.14	41.08	350.28	0	0	78.12	5.08
18354	Strudel, Apple	71	1	Each	2.34	7.95	29.18	194.54	0	1.56	19.88	2.08
18359	Sweet Rolls w/ Raisins and Nuts	57	1	Each	3.76	7.3	29.58	196.08	0	0	13.11	1.35
18355	Sweet Rolls, Cheese	66	1	Each	4.69	12.08	28.84	237.6	0	0	36.96	3.81
18356	Sweet Rolls, Cinnamon w/ Raisins	60	1	Each	3.72	9.84	30.54	223.2	0	0.78	39.6	2.53
14114	Beef Broth and Tomato Juice, Cnd	243.998	0.75	Cup	1.46	0.24	20.74	90.28	0	0	0	0.08
	Beer - Dark	29.5	12	Fl Oz	0.089	0	1.099	12.177	0	0.059	0	0
	Beer - Killians	29.5	12	Fl Oz	0.089	0	1.099	12.177	0	0.059	0	0
14006	Beer, Light	29.5	12	Fl Oz	0.059	0	0.383	8.26	0	0	0	0
14003	Beer, Regular	29.5	12	Fl Oz	0.089	0	1.099	12.177	0	0.059	0	0
14008	Bloody Mary	29.7	1	Fl Oz	0.15	0.03	0.98	23.17	0	0	0	0
14413	Bourbon and Soda	29	1	Fl Oz	0	0	0	26.1	0	0	0	0
14187	Clam and Tomato Juice, Cnd	241.396	0.75	Cup	1.45	0.24	26.31	111.04	0	0	0	0.02
14121	Club Soda	355.2	12	Fl Oz	0	0	0	0	0	0	0	0
14209	Coffee, Brewed	29.6	6	Fl Oz	0.03	0	0.12	0.59	17.1	0	0	0
62685	Coffee, Brewed, Decaf.	29.6	6	Fl Oz	0.03	0	0.12	0.59	0.18	0	0	0
14418	Coffee, Instant, Cappuccino Flavor	29.3	6	Fl Oz	0.06	0.32	1.64	9.38	12.16	0	0	0.28
14219	Coffee, Instant, Decaffeinated	29.858	6	Fl Oz	0.03	0	0.12	0.6	0.3	0	0	0
14420	Coffee, Instant, Mocha Flavor	29.3	6	Fl Oz	0.09	0.29	1.32	7.91	6.83	0	0	0.25
14215	Coffee, Instant, Regular	29.858	6	Fl Oz	0.03	0	0.12	0.6	9.5	0	0	0
14400	Cola	369	12	Fl Oz	0.1	0.1	38.5	151	7.6	0	0	0

Monounsaturated Fat (gm)	Polyunsaturated Fat (gm)	Vitamin D (mg)	Vitamin K (mg)	Vitamin E (mg)	Vitamin A (re)	Vitamin C (mg)	Thiamin (mg)	Riboflavin (mg)	Niacin (mg)	Vitamin B6 (mg)	Folate (mg)	Vitamin B12 (mcg)	Calcium (mg)	Iron (mg)	Magnesium (mg)	Phosphorus (mg)	Potassium (mg)	Sodium (mg)	Zinc (mg)
8.19	3.74	0	0	0	9.1	1.11	0.14	0.16	1.5	0.06	17.55	0.11	61.1	1.17	20.8	71.5	61.75	235.95	0.57
7.32	1.7	0	0	0	42.6	2.77	0.05	0.07	0.55	0	11.36	0	32.66	0.53	10.65	63.19	58.93	251.34	0.38
4.61	1.03	0	0	0	10.92	0.04	0.02	0.03	0.2	0.02	7.14	0.07	89.46	0.95	14.28	68.04	49.56	142.8	0.24
4.28	0.94	0	0	0	0	0.04	0.07	0.09	0.63	0.01	3.28	0.03	10.66	0.63	4.92	50.43	31.98	141.45	0.11
7.74	1.72	0	0	0	0	0	0.22	0.13	1.71	0.03	13.2	0.05	25.8	1.22	13.2	55.8	64.8	205.2	0.46
4.53	3.83	0	0	0	7.99	0.09	0.1	0.11	0.87	0.03	3.76	0.11	20.68	0.92	9.4	126.43	59.69	256.62	0.26
7.39	1.61	0	0	0	13.33	0.04	0.05	0.05	0.56	0.02	7.31	0.16	15.05	1.06	17.2	86.86	49.02	184.47	0.26
5.38	1.17	0	0	0	1.35	0.05	0.1	0.09	0.68	0.01	5.4	0.09	27	0.48	7.65	52.65	45.9	180.9	0.2
11.46	2.53	0	0	0	6.8	0	0.29	0.13	1.91	0.02	11.9	0.08	21.25	1.56	17	64.6	68	262.65	0.68
8.98	1.99	0	0	0	6.8	1.02	0.27	0.12	1.82	0.02	14.45	0.05	21.25	1.5	17	72.25	67.15	249.05	0.64
3.6	3.11	0	0	0	8.55	0.09	0.1	0.11	0.83	0.03	6.75	0.1	22.05	0.5	9.9	46.8	66.6	159.75	0.31
4.02	2.45	0	0	0	118.42	0.19	0.07	0.16	0.5	0.04	8.68	0.21	39.06	0.73	9.3	66.34	72.54	208.94	0.38
9.53	6.92	0	0	0	3.84	1.66	0.18	0.14	1.82	0.04	3.84	0.1	28.16	1.56	12.8	55.04	83.2	478.72	0.29
4.1	3.27	0	0	0	58.76	3.62	0.07	0.24	0.73	0.03	9.04	0.17	63.28	0.69	16.95	118.65	100.57	164.98	0.55
9.53	6.92	0	0	0	3.84	0	0.18	0.14	1.82	0.04	3.84	0.1	28.16	1.56	12.8	55.04	83.2	478.72	0.29
1.5	2.4	0	0	0	21	0.033	0.18	0.12	0.035	0.01	13.2	0	44	1.01	16.1	108.2	371	210	0.2
1.59	1.32	0	0	0	0	0.72	0.09	0.08	0.72	0.01	10.4	0.38	37.05	1.05	10.4	128.05	79.95	290.55	0.32
2.17	1.84	0	0	0	23.4	0.07	0.18	0.21	1.32	0.05	22.1	0.12	48.1	1.83	24.05	184.6	44.85	338.65	0.47
0.92	2.96	0	0	0	0	0.33	0.17	0.06	0.27	0.1	11.7	0	40.95	2.73	102.05	244.4	329.55	255.45	1.2
1.79	3.72	0	0	0	26	0.2	0.18	0.2	1.5	0.03	8.45	0.1	130	1.55	11.05	99.45	78.65	303.55	0.36
1.91	4.09	0	0	0	162.5	5.07	0.22	0.29	2.62	0.21	33.8	0.09	121.55	2.72	50.7	185.25	206.7	382.2	1.79
8.36	5.17	0	0	0	18.6	2.64	0.23	0.17	1.91	0.05	6.2	0	10.85	1.74	10.85	43.4	122.45	327.05	0.29
8.46	4.87	0	0	0	103.6	2.37	0.21	0.31	1.56	0.2	16.28	0.37	111	1.54	23.68	136.16	244.2	355.2	0.71
6.69	2.43	0	0	0	42.5	3.38	0.01	0.04	0.38	0.05	5	0	10	0.38	6.25	26.25	62.5	406.25	0.2
7.64	4.35	0	0	0	106.68	0.64	0.18	0.27	1.26	0.07	13.97	0.38	128.27	1.64	21.59	134.62	220.98	335.28	0.69
7.49	2.5	0	0	0	0	0.88	0.03	0.04	0.25	0.01	10	0	15	0.6	10	36.25	101.25	307.5	0.23
12.34	2.59	0	0	0	0	0.34	0.04	0.12	0.77	0.02	7.91	0.05	40.68	1.21	23.73	76.84	143.51	153.68	0.26
4.83	0.77	0	0	0	95.95	0.48	0.05	0.14	0.57	0.03	2.85	0.2	73.15	1.03	30.4	219.45	270.75	437	0.57
4.33	0.94	0	0	0	12.8	0	0.03	0.05	0.13	0.04	3.2	0	18.56	0.51	12.8	54.4	41.6	163.2	0.41
5.79	1.24	0	0	0	28.08	0.31	0.09	0.15	0.42	0.01	4.16	0.09	84.24	0.83	18.72	126.88	182	348.4	0.71
6.05	2.02	0	0	0	52.5	0.32	0.04	0.22	0.31	0.05	21	0.45	84	0.61	11.55	117.6	111.3	252	0.55
7.68	4.69	0	0	0	3.3	9.74	0.25	0.17	1.96	0.11	8.25	0	36.3	2.46	23.1	69.3	334.95	419.1	0.36
12.14	3.35	0	0	0	53.11	1.24	0.1	0.14	0.28	0.02	6.78	0.09	19.21	1.18	20.34	87.01	83.62	479.12	0.64
5.46	1.75	0	0	0	523.2	1.64	0.06	0.17	0.2	0.06	16.35	0.43	65.4	0.86	16.35	77.39	167.86	307.38	0.49
7.61	4.33	0	0	0	107.1	0.63	0.18	0.27	1.24	0.06	13.86	0.38	113.4	1.29	16.38	131.04	158.76	327.6	0.67
4.38	1.01	0	0	0	6.39	1.21	0.03	0.02	0.23	0.03	4.26	0.11	10.65	0.3	6.39	23.43	68.87	190.99	0.13
2.66	2.85	0	0	0	60.42	0.34	0.16	0.16	1.33	0.05	17.67	0.06	36.48	1.46	15.96	62.7	123.12	185.25	0.38
6.13	1.36	0	0	0	40.92	0.13	0.1	0.09	0.55	0.04	20.46	0.11	77.88	0.5	12.54	64.68	87.12	235.62	0.42
5.46	1.27	0	0	0	38.4	1.2	0.19	0.16	1.43	0.06	14.4	0.07	43.2	0.96	10.2	45.6	66.6	229.8	0.35
0.07	0.05	0	0	0	31.72	2.2	0	0.07	0.4	0.06	10.49	0.12	26.84	1.42	7.32	31.72	234.24	319.64	0.05
0	0	0	0	0	0	0	0.002	0.008	0.135	0.015	1.782	0.006	1.485	0.009	1.782	3.564	7.425	1.485	0.006
0	0	0	0	0	0	0	0.002	0.008	0.135	0.015	1.782	0.006	1.485	0.009	1.782	3.564	7.425	1.485	0.006
0	0	0	0	0	0	0	0.003	0.009	0.116	0.015	1.209	0.003	1.475	0.012	1.475	3.54	5.31	0.885	0.009
0	0	0	0	0	0	0	0.002	0.008	0.135	0.015	1.782	0.006	1.485	0.009	1.782	3.564	7.425	1.485	0.006
0	0.01	0	0	0	10.1	4.1	0.01	0.01	0.13	0.02	3.95	0	2.08	0.11	2.38	4.16	43.36	66.53	0.03
0	0	0	0	0	0	0	0	0	0.01	0	0	0	0.87	0.01	0.29	0.58	0.58	4.06	0.02
0.02	0.05	0	0	0	53.11	9.9	0.1	0.07	0.46	0.2	38.38	73.87	28.97	1.45	53.11	188.29	217.26	965.58	2.61
0	0	0	0	0	0	0	0	0	0	0	0	0	1.48	0	0.3	0	0.59	6.22	0.03
0	0	0	0	0	0	0	0	0	0.07	0	0.03	0	0.59	0.01	1.48	0.3	15.98	0.59	0.01
0	0	0	0	0	0	0	0	0	0.07	0	0.03	0	0.59	0.01	1.48	0.3	15.98	0.59	0.01
0.02	0.01	0	0	0	0	0	0	0	0.05	0	0	0	1.17	0.02	1.47	4.1	18.17	15.82	0.01
0	0	0	0	0	0	0	0	0	0.08	0	0	0	0.9	0.01	1.19	0.9	10.45	0.9	0.01
0.02	0.01	0	0	0	0	0	0	0	0.04	0	0	0	1.17	0.04	1.47	4.4	18.46	5.57	0.02
0	0	0	0	0	0	0	0	0	0.08	0	0	0	0.9	0.01	1.19	0.9	10.75	0.9	0.01
0	0	0	0	0	0	0	0	0	0	0	0	0	0	0.13	3	46	4	14	0.05

USDA ID Code	Food Name	Weight in Grams*	Quantity of Units	Unit of Measure	Protein (gm)	Fat (gm)	Carbohydrates (gm)	Kcalories	Caffeine (gm)	Fiber (gm)	Cholesterol (mg)	Saturated Fat (gm)
62530	Cola, Diet	369	12	Fl Oz	0.2	0	0.3	2	7.6	0	0	0
14238	Cranberry-apple Juice Drink, Bottled	244.593	0.75	Cup	0.24	0	41.83	163.88	0	0.24	0	0
14240	Cranberry-apricot Juice Drink, Bottled	244.593	0.75	Cup	0.49	0	39.62	156.54	0	0.24	0	0
14241	Cranberry-grape Juice Drink, Bottled	244.593	0.75	Cup	0.49	0.24	34.24	136.97	0	0.24	0	0.08
14130	Cream Soda	371	12	Fl Oz	0	0	49.3	191	0	0	0	0
14034	Creme De Menthe, 72 Proof	33.6	1	Fl Oz	0	0.1	13.98	124.66	0	0	0	0
62635	Crystal Lite	29.575	8	Fl Oz	0	0	0	0.63	0	0	0	0
14010	Daiquiri	30.2	1	Fl Oz	0.03	0.03	2.05	56.17	0	0	0	0
14009	Daiquiri, Bottled	30.5	1	Fl Oz	0	0	4.79	38.13	0	0	0	0
14153	Dr. Pepper	360	12	Fl Oz	0	0.4	38.2	151	41	0	0	0.02
14267	Fruit Punch Drink, Cnd	247.791	0.75	Cup	0	0	29.49	116.46	0	0.25	0	0
	Gatorade Thirst Quencher	244	8	Fl Oz	0	0	14	50	0	0	0	0
	Gatorlode High Carb, Loading Recovery Drink	354	11.6	Fl Oz	0	0	71	280	0	0	0	0
	Gatorpro Sports Nutrition Sup.	336	11	Fl Oz	17	6	59	360	0	0	0	0.5
14011	Gin and Tonic	30	1	Fl Oz	0	0	2.1	22.8	0	0	0	0
14136	Ginger Ale	366	12	Fl Oz	0.1	0	31.9	124	0	0	0	0
62532	Ginger Ale, Diet	366	12	Fl Oz	0	0	0	0	0	0	0	0
14277	Grape Drink, Cnd	250.189	0.75	Cup	0	0	28.77	112.58	0	0	0	0.01
14282	Grape Juice Drink, Cnd	250.189	0.75	Cup	0.25	0	32.27	125.09	0	0.25	0	0
14142	Grape Soda	372	12	Fl Oz	0	0	41.7	161	0	0	0	0
62547	Iced Tea, Bottled, All Flavors	236.6	1	Cup	0	0	28.59	118.3	44	0	0	0
62548	Iced Tea, Bottled, All Flavors, Diet	236.6	1	Cup	0	0	0.99	0	54	0	0	0
62643	Kool-Aid	236	8	Fl Oz	0	0	25.1	98	0	0	0	0
14297	Lemonade Flavor Drink	266	1	Cup	0	0	28.73	111.72	0	0	0	0.05
14543	Lemonade, Pink	247.791	1	Cup	0.25	0	26.02	99.12	0	0	0	0.01
14290	Lemonade, Low Calorie	243.698	1	Cup	0	0	1.22	4.87	0	0	0	0
14293	Lemonade, White	247.791	1	Cup	0.25	0	26.02	99.12	0	0	0	0.01
14145	Lemon-lime Soda	355	12	Fl Oz	0	0	38.4	149	0	0	0	0
62529	Lemon-lime Soda, Diet	355	12	Fl Oz	0	0	0	0	0	0	0	0
14415	Liqueur, Coffee w/ Cream, 34 Proof	31.1	1	Fl Oz	0.87	4.88	6.5	101.7	0	0	4.67	3.01
14414	Liqueur, Coffee, 53 Proof	34.8	1	Fl Oz	0.03	0.1	16.29	116.93	0	0	0	0.04
14534	Liqueur, Coffee, 63 Proof	34.8	1	Fl Oz	0.03	0.1	11.21	107.18	0	0	0	0.04
14533	Liquor, Distilled, All 100 Proof	27.8	1	Fl Oz	0	0	0	82.01	0	0	0	0
14037	Liquor, Distilled, All 80 Proof	27.8	1	Fl Oz	0	0	0	64.22	0	0	0	0
14550	Liquor, Distilled, All 86 Proof	27.8	1	Fl Oz	0	0	0.03	69.5	0	0	0	0
14551	Liquor, Distilled, All 90 Proof	27.8	1	Fl Oz	0	0	0	73.11	0	0	0	0
14532	Liquor, Distilled, All 94 Proof	27.8	1	Fl Oz	0	0	0	76.45	0	0	0	0
14012	Manhattan	28.5	6	Fl Oz	0.03	0	0.91	63.84	0	0	0	0
62645	Margarita	29.575	6	Fl Oz	0	0	4.5	28.75	0	0	0	0
14014	Martini	28.2	6	Fl Oz	0	0	0.08	62.89	0	0	0	0
1110	Milk Shakes, Thick Chocolate	345.436	1.5	Cup	10.54	9.33	73.06	409.71	0	1.04	36.27	5.81
1111	Milk Shakes, Thick Vanilla	345.436	1.5	Cup	13.33	10.47	61.31	386.23	0	0	40.76	6.51
62659	Mountain Dew	360	12	Fl Oz	0	0	44.4	179	54	0	0	0
14327	Orange and Apricot Juice Drink, Cnd	249.389	0.75	Cup	0.75	0.25	31.67	127.19	0	0.25	0	0.02
14323	Orange Drink, Cnd	247.791	0.75	Cup	0	0	31.96	126.37	0	0.25	0	0
14017	Pina Colada	31.4	6	Fl Oz	0.13	0.6	8.89	77.26	0	0	0	0.27
14334	Pineapple and Grapefruit Juice Drink, Cnd	250.189	0.75	Cup	0.5	0.25	29.02	117.59	0	0.25	0	0.02
14341	Pineapple and Orange Juice Drink, Cnd	250.189	0.75	Cup	3.25	0	29.52	125.09	0	0.25	0	0
14157	Root Beer	355	12	Fl Oz	0.1	0	39.2	152	0	0	0	0
62531	Root Beer, Diet	355	12	Fl Oz	0	0	0.355	0	0	0	0	0
14018	Screwdriver	30.4	6	Fl Oz	0.15	0	2.61	24.93	0	0	0	0
14346	Shake, Chocolate	226.4	1.5	Cup	7.7	8.38	46.41	287.53	0	0	29.43	5.24
14428	Shake, Strawberry	226.4	1.5	Cup	7.7	6.34	42.79	255.83	0	0	24.9	3.93
14347	Shake, Vanilla	226.4	1.5	Cup	7.92	6.79	40.53	251.3	0	0	24.9	4.21
14351	Strawberry Flavor Beverage	266	1	Cup	7.98	8.25	32.72	234.08	0	0	31.92	5.08

Monounsaturated Fat (gm)	Polyunsaturated Fat (gm)	Vitamin D (mg)	Vitamin K (mg)	Vitamin E (mg)	Vitamin A (re)	Vitamin C (mg)	Thiamin (mg)	Riboflavin (mg)	Niacin (mg)	Vitamin B6 (mg)	Folate (mg)	Vitamin B12 (mcg)	Calcium (mg)	Iron (mg)	Magnesium (mg)	Phosphorus (mg)	Potassium (mg)	Sodium (mg)	Zinc (mg)
0	0	0	0	0	0	0	0	0	0	0	0	0	0	0.11	4	30	0	21	0.28
0	0	0	0	0	0	78.27	0.01	0.05	0.15	0.05	0.49	0	17.12	0.15	4.89	7.34	66.04	4.89	0.1
0	0	0	0	0	112.51	0	0.01	0.02	0.29	0.05	1.47	0	22.01	0.37	7.34	12.23	149.2	4.89	0.1
0	0	0	0	0	0	78.27	0.02	0.04	0.29	0.07	1.71	0	19.57	0.02	7.34	9.78	58.7	7.34	0.1
0	0	0	0	0	0	0	0	0	0	0	0	0	19	0.19	3	0	4	43	0.24
0.01	0.06	0	0	0	0	0	0	0	0	0	0	0	0	0.02	0	0	0	1.68	0.01
0	0	0	0	0	0	0.75	0	0	0	0	0	0	0	0	0	0	0	0	0
0	0	0	0	0	0	0.48	0	0	0.01	0	0.6	0	0.91	0.05	0.6	1.81	6.34	1.51	0.02
0	0	0	0	0	0	0.4	0	0	0	0	0.24	0	0	0	0.31	0.61	3.36	12.2	0.01
0	0	0	0	0	0	0	0	0	0	0	0	0	0.92	0.01	0	3.38	0.31	3.07	0.01
0	0.01	0	0	0	2.48	73.35	0.05	0.06	0.05	0	3.22	0	19.82	0.52	4.96	2.48	61.95	54.51	0.3
0	0	0	0	0	0	0	0	0	0	0	0	0	0	0	0	0	30	110	0
0	0	0	0	0	0	18	0.11	0.39	4.5	0.45	0	0	0	0	0	0	0	0	0
0	0	2	0	3.5	160	50	1.1	0.5	6	0.64	63	0.8	280	3	70	400	1310	300	3.6
0	0	0	0	0	0	0.12	0	0	0	0	0.15	0	0.6	0.01	0.3	0.3	1.5	1.2	0.02
0	0	0	0	0	0	0	0	0	0	0	0	0	12	0.66	3	1	5	25	0.18
0	0	0	0	0	0	0	0	0	0	0	0	0	0	0	0	0	0	2.5	0
0	0.01	0	0	0	0	85.31	0.01	0.01	0.07	0.02	0.75	0	7.51	0.43	5	2.5	12.51	15.01	0.28
0	0	0	0	0	0	40.03	0.03	0.03	0.25	0.05	2	0	7.51	0.25	10.01	10.01	87.57	2.5	0.08
0	0	0	0	0	0	0	0	0	0	0	0	0	12	0.31	4	0	3	57	0.26
0	0	0	0	0	0	0	0	0	0	0	0	0	0	0	0	0	0	9.86	0
0	0	0	0	0	0	0	0	0	0	0	0	0	0	0	0	0	0	0	0
0	0	0	0	0	0	6	0	0	0	0	0	0	15	0	0	8	1	8	0
0.01	0.01	0	0	0	0	34.05	0	0	0	0	0	0	29.26	0.05	2.66	2.66	2.66	18.62	0.08
0	0.03	0	0.07	0	0	9.66	0.01	0.05	0.04	0.01	5.45	0	7.43	0.4	4.96	4.96	37.17	7.43	0.1
0	0	0	0	0	0	6.09	0	0	0	0	0.24	0	5.12	0.1	2.44	24.37	0	7.31	0.07
0	0.03	0	0	0	4.96	9.66	0.01	0.05	0.04	0.01	5.45	0	7.43	0.4	4.96	4.96	37.17	7.43	0.1
0	0	0	0	0	0	0	0	0	0.1	0	0	0	9	0.25	2	1	4	41	0.18
0	0	0	0	0	0	0	0	0	0	0	0	0	0	0	0	0	0	2.5	0
1.39	0.21	0	0	0	13.37	0	0	0.02	0.02	0.01	0	0.04	4.98	0.04	0.62	15.55	9.95	28.61	0.05
0.01	0.04	0	0	0	0	0	0	0	0.05	0	0	0	0.35	0.02	1.04	2.09	10.44	2.78	0.01
0.01	0.04	0	0	0	0	0	0	0	0.05	0	0	0	0.35	0.02	1.04	2.09	10.44	2.78	0.01
0	0	0	0	0	0	0	0	0	0	0	0	0	0	0.01	0	1.11	0.56	0.28	0.01
0	0	0	0	0	0	0	0	0	0	0	0	0	0	0.01	0	1.11	0.56	0.28	0.01
0	0	0	0	0	0	0	0	0	0	0	0	0	0	0.01	0	1.11	0.56	0.28	0.01
0	0	0	0	0	0	0	0	0	0	0	0	0	0	0.01	0	1.11	0.56	0.28	0.01
0	0	0	0	0	0	0	0	0	0.03	0	0.03	0	0.57	0.03	0.57	2	7.41	0.86	0.01
0	0	0	0	0	0	0	0	0	0	0	0	0	0	0	0	0	0	11.88	0
0	0	0	0	0	0	0	0	0	0	0	0.06	0	0.56	0.03	0.56	0.85	5.08	0.85	0.01
2.69	0.35	0	0	0.35	72.54	0	0.16	0.77	0.43	0.09	16.93	1.09	455.98	200	55.27	435.25	773.78	383.43	1.66
3.02	0.39	0	0	0.35	96.72	0	0.1	0.67	0.5	0.15	22.8	1.8	504.68	300	40.62	397.94	631.11	329.55	1.35
0	0	0	0	0	0	0	0	0	0	0	0	0	0	0	0	0	10	31	0
0.08	0.05	0	0	0	144.65	49.88	0.05	0.02	0.5	0.07	14.46	0	12.47	0.25	9.98	19.95	199.51	4.99	0.12
0	0.01	0	0	0	4.96	84.5	0.01	0.01	0.08	0.02	5.45	0	14.87	0.69	4.96	2.48	44.6	39.65	0.22
0.05	0.11	0	0	0	0	1.48	0.01	0	0.04	0.01	3.2	0	2.51	0.07	2.51	2.2	22.29	1.88	0.04
0.03	0.07	0	0	0	10.01	115.09	0.08	0.04	0.67	0.11	26.27	0	17.51	0.78	15.01	15.01	152.61	35.03	0.15
0	0	0	0	0	132.6	56.29	0.08	0.05	0.52	0.12	27.27	0	12.51	0.68	15.01	10.01	115.09	7.51	0.15
0	0	0	0	0	0	0	0	0	0	0	0	0	19	0.18	4	2	3	49	0.26
0	0	0	0	0	0	0	0	0	0	0	0	0	0	0	0	0	0	2.5	0
0	0	0	0	0	1.82	9.48	0.02	0	0.05	0.01	10.67	0	2.13	0.02	2.43	4.26	46.51	0.3	0.01
2.43	0.32	0.91	0	0	52.07	0.91	0.13	0.55	0.36	0.11	7.92	0.77	255.83	0.7	38.49	230.93	452.8	219.61	0.93
0	0	0.45	0	0	65.66	1.81	0.1	0.44	0.4	0.1	6.79	0.7	255.83	0.25	29.43	226.4	412.05	187.91	0.82
1.95	0.25	0.45	0	0	72.45	1.81	0.1	0.41	0.42	0.12	7.47	0.82	276.21	0.2	27.17	230.93	393.94	185.65	0.82
2.36	0.3	0	0	0	74.48	2.39	0.09	0.42	0.22	0.1	12.24	0.88	292.6	0.21	31.92	228.76	369.74	127.68	0.93

USDA ID Code	Food Name	Weight in Grams*	Quantity of Units	Unit of Measure	Protein (gm)	Fat (gm)	Carbohydrates (gm)	Kcalories	Caffeine (gm)	Fiber (gm)	Cholesterol (mg)	Saturated Fat (gm)
	Swiss Miss Hot Choc Mix - No Sugar	20	1	Packet	3	1.5	13	70	4	0	0	0
	Swiss Miss Hot Choc Mix - No Sugar, Fat Free	15	1	Packet	4	0	9	50	4	0	0	0
14355	Tea, Brewed	236	8	Fl Oz	0	0	0.09	0.3	48	0	0	0
14381	Tea, Herb, Brewed	236	8	Fl Oz	0	0	0.06	0.3	0	0	0	0
14371	Tea, Instant, Sweetened	236	8	Fl Oz	0.03	0	2.75	11.01	29	0	0	0
14367	Tea, Instant, Unsweetened	236	8	Fl Oz	0	0	0.06	0.3	36	0	0	0
14020	Tequila Sunrise	31.2	6	Fl Oz	0.09	0.03	2.68	34.32	0	0	0	0
14382	Thirst Quencher Drink, Bottled	236	8	Fl Oz	0	0.1	15.2	60	0	0	0	0
14023	Tom Collins	29.6	1	Fl Oz	0	0	0.38	16.28	0	0	0	0
14155	Tonic Water	29.6	12	Fl Oz	0	0	2.68	10.37	0	0	0	0
14269	Tropical Fruit Juice, Blend	246.99	0.75	Cup	0	0	28.9	113.62	0	0	0	0
	Vodka, 80 Proof	42	1.5	Fl Oz	0	0	0	97.02	0	0	0	0
	Water, Bottled, Perrier	192	6.5	Fl Oz	0	0	0	0	0	0	0	0
	Water, Municipal	240	8	Fl Oz	0	0	0	0	0	0	0	0
14032	Whiskey Sour	29.9	1	Fl Oz	0.06	0.03	1.67	40.66	0	0	0	0.01
14536	Wine, Dessert, Dry, 3.5 Oz Glass	103	1	Glass	0.206	0	12.154	157.59	0	0	0	0
14057	Wine, Dessert, Sweet, 3.5 Oz Glass	103	1	Glass	0.206	0	12.154	157.59	0	0	0	0
14084	Wine, Table, All, 3.5 Oz Glass	103	1	Glass	0.206	0	1.442	72.1	0	0	0	0
14096	Wine, Table, Red, 3.5 Oz Glass	103	1	Glass	0.206	0	1.751	74.16	0	0	0	0
14104	Wine, Table, Rose, 3.5 Oz Glass	103	1	Glass	0.206	0	1.442	73.13	0	0	0	0
14106	Wine, Table, White, 3.5 Oz Glass	103	1	Glass	0.103	0	0.824	70.04	0	0	0	0
8053	Cereals, 100% Bran	66	1	Cup	8.25	3.3	48.11	177.54	0	19.54	0	0.59
8054	Cereals, 100% Natural Cereal, Plain	104	1	Cup	12.17	22.36	65.21	488.8	0	8.84	0.66	15.05
8055	Cereals, 100% Natural Cereal, w/ apple and cinn.	104	1	Cup	10.71	19.55	69.78	477.36	0	6.86	0	15.46
	Cereals, 100% Natural Cereal, w/ oats and honey	48	0.5	Cup	5.054	7.896	32.947	213.12	0	3.6	0.48	3.466
8056	Cereals, 100% Natural Cereal, w/ raisins and dates	110	1	Cup	11.22	20.35	72.38	496.1	0	7.26	0	13.68
8028	Cereals, 40% Bran Flakes, Kellogg's	39	1	Cup	4.91	0.74	30.54	127.14	0	5.5	0	0
8029	Cereals, 40% Bran Flakes, Post	47	1	Cup	5.31	0.75	37.27	152.28	0	9.17	0	0
8153	Cereals, 40% Bran Flakes, Ralston Purina	49	1	Cup	5.64	0.69	39.1	158.76	0	6.91	0	0
8001	Cereals, All-bran	30	0.5	Cup	3.861	1.02	22.01	81.3	0	9.72	0	0.21
	Cereals, Almond Crunch	55	1	Cup	4.35	0.83	46.915	198	0	4.62	0	0.165
	Cereals, Alpha-Bits	34	1	Cup	2.584	0.782	29.444	133.28	0	1.462	0	0.128
62668	Cereals, Apple Cinnamon Cheerios	30	0.75	Cup	1.86	1.632	25.05	117.9	0	1.59	0	0.3
	Cereals, Apple Jacks	30	1	Cup	1.44	0.39	26.84	115.5	0	0.57	0	0.09
	Cereals, Apple Raisin Crisp	55	1	Cup	3.465	0.495	46.695	184.8	0	4.4	0	0.11
	Cereals, Basic 4	55	1	Cup	4.18	2.838	41.97	200.75	0	3.355	0	0.424
	Cereals, Berry Berry Kix	30	0.75	Cup	1.308	1.161	26.13	120	0	0.18	0	0.195
	Cereals, Blueberry Squares	55	0.75	Cup	4.18	0.99	43.78	181.5	0	4.84	0	0.22
8006	Cereals, Bran Chex	49	1	Cup	5.05	1.37	39.05	156.31	0	7.94	0	0.198
	Cereals, Bran Flakes, Kellogg's	29	0.75	Cup	3.016	0.638	23.159	94.83	0	4.611	0	0.116
	Cereals, Bran Flakes, Post	47	1	Cup	5.311	0.752	37.27	152.28	0	9.165	0	0.117
8008	Cereals, C.W. Post, Plain	97	1	Cup	7.95	12.804	72.653	420.98	0	7.18	0.18	1.668
8009	Cereals, C.W. Post, w/ Raisins	103	1	Cup	8.86	14.73	73.95	445.99	0	13.6	0.2	10.97
8010	Cereals, Cap'n Crunch	27	0.75	Cup	1.35	0.37	23.04	107.19	0	0.864	0	0.37
8011	Cereals, Cap'n Crunch's Crunchberries	35	1	Cup	1.82	2.94	28.53	145.95	0	0.67	0.07	1.93
8012	Cereals, Cap'n Crunch's Peanut Butter	35	1	Cup	2.52	4.52	26.5	153.65	0	0.46	0	1.9
8013	Cereals, Cheerios	30	1	Cup	3.144	1.77	22.86	109.5	0	2.64	0	0.351
	Cereals, Cinnamon Life	50	1	Cup	4.355	1.735	40.4	189.5	0	2.95	0	0.325
	Cereals, Cinnamon Mini Buns	30	0.75	Cup	1.47	0.63	26.61	115.2	0	0.66	0	0.15
	Cereals, Cinnamon Oatmeal Squares	60	1	Cup	7.566	2.568	47.154	231.6	0	4.56	0	0.504
	Cereals, Cinnamon Toast Crunch	30	0.75	Cup	1.68	3.042	23.838	124.2	0	1.5	0	0.501
8014	Cereals, Cocoa Krispies	31	0.75	Cup	1.55	0.806	27.249	120.28	0	0.403	0	0.589
	Cereals, Cocoa Puffs	30	1	Cup	1.14	0.903	26.715	118.8	0	0.18	0	0.204
8017	Cereals, Cookie-crisp, Choc Chip and Van.	30	1	Cup	1.53	1.08	26.25	120	0	0.42	0	0
8018	Cereals, Corn Bran	36	1	Cup	2.45	1.26	30.35	124.56	0	6.84	0	0

Monounsaturated Fat (gm)	Polyunsaturated Fat (gm)	Vitamin D (mg)	Vitamin K (mg)	Vitamin E (mg)	Vitamin A (re)	Vitamin C (mg)	Thiamin (mg)	Riboflavin (mg)	Niacin (mg)	Vitamin B6 (mg)	Folate (mg)	Vitamin B12 (mcg)	Calcium (mg)	Iron (mg)	Magnesium (mg)	Phosphorus (mg)	Potassium (mg)	Sodium (mg)	Zinc (mg)
0	0	0	0	0	0	0	0	0	0	0	0	0	80	0.4	0	0	0	220	0
0	0	0	0	0	0	0	0	0	0	0	0	0	80	0.2	0	0	0	180	0
0	0	0	0.01	0	0	0	0	0	0	0	1.54	0	0	0.01	0.89	0.3	10.95	0.89	0.01
0	0	0	0	0	0	0	0	0	0	0	0.18	0	0.59	0.02	0.3	0	2.66	0.3	0.01
0	0	0	0	0	0	0	0	0.01	0.01	0	1.2	0	0.65	0.01	0.65	0.32	6.15	0.97	0.01
0	0	0	0	0	0	0	0	0	0.01	0	0.09	0	0.59	0.01	0.59	0.3	5.92	0.89	0.01
0.01	0.01	0	0	0	3.12	6.02	0.01	0	0.06	0.02	3.31	0	1.87	0.09	2.18	3.12	32.45	1.25	0.02
0	0	0	0	0	0	0	0	0	0	0	0	0	0	0.12	1	22	26	96	0.05
0	0	0	0	0	0	0.5	0	0	0	0	0.21	0	1.18	0	0.3	0.3	2.37	5.03	0.02
0	0	0	0	0	0	0	0	0	0	0	0	0	0.31	0	0	0	0	1.22	0.03
0	0	0	0	0	2.47	108.43	0.02	0.03	0.05	0.01	2.22	0	9.88	0.22	4.94	2.47	32.11	9.88	0.1
0	0	0	0	0	0	0	0	0	0	0	0	0	0	0	0	2.1	0.42	0.42	0
0	0	0	0	0	0	0	0	0	0	0	0	0	26.88	0	0	0	0	1.92	0
0	0	0	0	0	0	0	0	0	0	0	0	0	0	0	0	0	0	0	0
0	0.01	0	0	0	0.3	3.77	0.06	0	0.04	0.01	1.55	0	1.79	0.02	1.2	2.09	15.85	3.29	0.01
0	0	0	0	0	0	0	0.02	0.02	0.219	0	0.412	0	8.24	0.247	9.27	9.27	94.76	9.27	0.072
0	0	0	0	0	0	0	0.02	0.02	0.219	0	0.412	0	8.24	0.247	9.27	9.27	94.76	9.27	0.072
0	0	0	0	0	0	0	0.004	0.016	0.079	0.025	1.133	0.01	8.24	0.442	10.3	14.42	91.67	8.24	0.072
0	0	0	0	0	0	0	0.005	0.029	0.083	0.035	2.06	0.01	8.24	0.443	13.39	14.42	115.36	5.15	0.093
0	0	0	0	0	0	0	0.004	0.016	0.076	0.025	1.133	0.01	8.24	0.391	10.3	15.45	101.97	5.15	0.062
0	0	0	0	0	0	0	0.004	0.005	0.069	0.014	0.206	0	9.27	0.33	10.3	14.42	82.4	5.15	0.072
0.57	1.87	0	0	1.53	0	62.7	1.58	1.78	20.92	2.11	46.86	6.27	46.2	8.12	312.18	801.24	652.08	457.38	5.74
4.27	2.01	0	0	0.73	0	0	0.31	0.56	2.37	0.19	31.2	0.13	180.96	3.07	124.8	382.72	513.76	44.72	2.35
1.83	1.33	0	0	0.73	6.24	1.04	0.33	0.57	1.87	0.11	16.64	0.3	157.04	2.89	71.76	350.48	513.76	52	2
3.475	1.042	0	0	0.548	0.48	0.144	0.168	0.077	0.85	0.086	12	0.053	46.08	1.435	50.4	148.8	210.72	12.96	1.152
3.72	1.71	0	0	0.77	6.6	0	0.31	0.65	2.09	0.17	45.1	0.15	159.5	3.12	124.3	347.6	537.9	47.3	2.11
0	0	1.37	0	0.45	516.36	0	0.51	0.58	6.86	0.7	137.67	2.07	19.11	24.76	70.98	191.88	247.65	302.64	5.15
0	0	0	0	0.54	622.28	0	0.61	0.7	8.27	0.85	165.91	2.49	20.68	7.47	101.52	296.1	250.51	430.99	2.49
0	0	0	0	0.56	648.76	25.97	0.64	0.73	8.62	0.88	172.97	2.6	22.54	7.79	117.6	272.93	286.16	456.19	2.04
0.18	0.66	2.98	0	0.55	225.3	15	0.39	0.42	5.01	0.51	105.9	1.5	105.9	4.5	128.7	294	300.3	275.4	3.75
0.22	0.44	0	0	3	47.3	0	0.523	0.594	7	0.69	99	2.101	26.4	5.99	48.95	129.8	170.5	284.35	1.43
0.26	0.291	0	0	0.02	450.16	0	0.442	0.51	5.984	0.612	120.02	1.802	9.86	3.23	20.06	61.54	65.96	215.9	1.802
0.642	0.21	0	0	0.296	225.3	15	0.375	0.426	5.001	0.501	99.9	0	35.4	4.5	20.1	65.1	60	150.3	3.75
0.12	0.18	0	0	0.049	225.3	15	0.39	0.42	5.01	0.51	105.9	0	3.3	4.5	8.7	30	31.8	134.4	3.75
0.165	0.22	0	0	0.457	233.75	0	0.385	0.44	5.17	0.495	110	1.54	14.85	1.87	9.9	85.8	85.25	373.45	1.54
0.99	1.1	0	0	0.676	375.1	14.96	0.37	0.424	4.999	0.501	99.55	0	309.65	4.499	40.15	231.55	161.7	322.85	3.751
0.462	0.06	0	0	0.171	225.3	15	0.375	0.426	5	0.501	99.9	0	66	4.5	5.7	37.2	23.7	184.5	3.75
0.22	0.55	0	0	0.849	0	0	0.385	0.44	5.115	0.495	110	1.54	19.25	16.5	51.15	161.7	183.15	20.35	1.54
0.254	0.671	0	0	0.56	10.78	25.97	0.64	0.26	8.62	0.88	172.97	2.6	29.4	13.99	69.09	172.97	216.09	345.45	6.48
0.116	0.406	0	0	5.365	362.79	14.993	0.377	0.435	5	0.493	102.37	1.45	13.92	8.12	60.03	149.93	175.16	226.2	3.75
0.107	0.369	0	0	0.541	622.28	0	0.611	0.705	8.272	0.846	165.91	2.491	20.68	13.442	101.52	296.1	250.51	430.99	2.491
5.995	4.656	0	0	0.679	1284.28	0	1.261	1.455	17.072	1.75	342.41	5.14	46.56	15.42	66.93	224.07	197.88	166.84	1.64
1.67	1.38	0	0	0.72	1363.72	0	1.34	1.55	18.13	1.85	363.59	5.46	50.47	16.38	74.16	231.75	260.59	160.68	1.64
0.273	0.189	0	0	0.134	3.51	0	0.375	0.424	5	0.499	100.17	0	5.4	4.504	9.45	28.62	34.56	208.44	3.753
0.39	0.47	0	0	0.09	4.55	0	0.6	0.67	8.13	0.93	127.75	2.5	10.85	9.04	13.65	46.55	49	243.6	3.56
1.37	1.01	0	0	0.09	5.6	0	0.6	0.7	8.97	1.04	243.6	2.3	7	9.11	18.55	48.65	56.7	267.75	3.79
0.642	0.216	0.8	0	0.206	357.3	15	0.375	0.426	5	0.501	99.9	0	55.2	8.1	32.7	114	88.5	284.1	3.75
0.57	0.77	0	0	0.225	1.5	0.1	0.625	0.71	8.38	0.835	167.5	0	134.5	74.54	41.5	181	113	220	6.285
0.18	0.3	0	0	0.053	225.3	15	0.39	0.42	5.01	0.51	90	0	3.9	4.5	11.1	24	36.6	207.6	3.75
0.864	1.074	0	0	2.219	165	6.6	0.408	0.462	5.484	0.546	109.8	0	41.4	14.55	70.2	181.8	250.2	266.4	4.11
0.93	0.528	0	0	0.279	225.3	15	0.375	0.426	5.001	0.501	99.9	0	42.3	4.5	13.5	74.4	44.1	210.3	3.75
0.093	0.124	0	0	0.143	225.06	15.004	0.372	0.434	4.991	0.496	93	0	4.03	1.798	11.47	29.45	60.14	210.18	1.488
0.348	0.045	0	0	0.137	0	15	0.375	0.426	5.001	0.501	99.9	0	33	4.5	6.6	42.6	52.2	180.6	3.75
0	0	0	0	0.08	397.2	15.9	0.39	0.45	5.28	0.54	3.3	1.59	5.7	4.77	8.4	24	29.4	206.7	0.29
0	0	0	0	0.84	7.56	0	0.37	0.7	10.86	0.86	232.2	1.39	41.4	12.24	18.36	51.84	70.2	309.6	4

USDA ID Code	Food Name	Weight in Grams*	Quantity of Units	Unit of Measure	Protein (gm)	Fat (gm)	Carbohydrates (gm)	Kcalories	Caffeine (gm)	Fiber (gm)	Cholesterol (mg)
8019	Cereals, Corn Chex	29	1	Cup	2059	0.116	25.433	113.68	0	0.522	0	0.016
8020	Cereals, Corn Flakes, Kellogg's	28	1	Cup	1.84	0.199	24.217	102.2	0	0.784	0	0.056
8022	Cereals, Corn Flakes, Low Sodium	25	1	Cup	1.93	0.08	22.2	99.75	0	0.28	0	0
8021	Cereals, Corn Flakes, Ralston Purina	25	1	Cup	1.95	0.1	21.65	97.5	0	0.48	0	0
	Cereals, Corn Pops	31	1	Cup	1.147	0.18	28.427	118.11	0	0.434	0	0.062
8023	Cereals, Cracklin' Oat Bran	55	0.75	Cup	4.615	6.969	40.095	224.95	0	6.545	0	2.919
8168	Cereals, Cream Of Rice, Ckd	244	1	Cup	2.2	0.24	28.06	126.88	0	0	0	0
8171	Cereals, Cream Of Wheat, Instant	241	1	Cup	4.34	0.48	31.57	154.24	0	0	0	0
8170	Cereals, Cream Of Wheat, Quick	239	1	Cup	3.59	0.48	26.77	129.06	0	0	0	0
8169	Cereals, Cream Of Wheat, Regular	251	1	Cup	3.76	0.5	27.61	133.03	0	0	0	0
8024	Cereals, Crisp Rice, Low Sodium	26	1	Cup	1.43	0.08	23.66	104.52	0	0	0	0
62634	Cereals, Crispex	29	1	Cup	2.146	0.29	24.998	108.46	0	0.638	0	0.087
8025	Cereals, Crispy Rice	28	1	Cup	1.79	0.11	24.81	110.88	0	0.34	0	0
8026	Cereals, Crispy Wheats 'n Raisins	55	1	Cup	4.466	0.759	44.33	191.4	0	3.41	0	0.154
	Cereals, Fiber One	30	0.5	Cup	2.778	0.843	24.006	61.5	0	14.25	0	0.132
8027	Cereals, Fortified Oat Flakes	48	1	Cup	8.98	0.72	34.75	177.12	0	1.44	0	0
	Cereals, Frosted Flakes	31	0.75	Cup	1.212	0.155	28.21	117.18	0	0.496	0	0.062
62637	Cereals, Frosted Mini-Wheats	55	1	Cup	5.17	0.88	45.375	186.45	0	5.885	0	0.165
8030	Cereals, Fruit Loops	30	1	Cup	1.47	0.87	26.46	117.3	0	0.57	0	0.39
	Cereals, Fruity Pebbles	32	1	Cup	1.28	1.664	27.552	129.6	0	0.416	0	1.373
8035	Cereals, Golden Grahams	30	0.75	Cup	1.596	1.08	25.689	115.5	0	0.93	0	0.177
8036	Cereals, Graham Crackos	30	1	Cup	2.25	0.18	25.92	108.3	0	1.83	0	0
8037	Cereals, Granola, Homemade	122	1	Cup	17.934	30.012	64.66	569.74	0	12.81	0	5.795
8038	Cereals, Grape-nuts	109	1	Cup	12.753	0.436	89.38	389.13	0	10.9	0	0.059
8039	Cereals, Grape-nuts Flakes	39	1	Cup	3.939	0.36	26.55	116.2	0	3.21	0	0
62639	Cereals, Great Grains	79.46	1	Cup	1.131	9	56.97	329.84	0	6	0	1.5
8040	Cereals, Heartland Natural Cereal, Plain	115	1	Cup	11.615	17.71	78.545	499.1	0	7.015	0	4.52
8041	Cereals, Heartland Natural Cereal, w/ coconut	105	1	Cup	10.92	17.12	71.3	463.05	0	7.46	0	0
8042	Cereals, Heartland Natural Cereal, w/ raisins	110	1	Cup	10.67	15.62	75.9	467.5	0	6.05	0	3.985
8043	Cereals, Honey and Nut Corn Flakes	37.867	1	Cup	2.42	2.08	31.13	150.71	0	0.45	0	0
	Cereals, Honey Graham Oh!	27	0.75	Cup	1.35	1.909	22.745	111.78	0	0.702	0	0.55
8045	Cereals, Honey Nut Cheerios	30	1	Cup	2.778	1.239	24.261	114.9	0	1.56	0	0.228
8044	Cereals, Honeybran	35	1	Cup	3.08	0.735	28.63	119.35	0	3.885	0	0.255
8046	Cereals, Honeycomb	22	1	Cup	1.28	0.4	19.6	86.02	0	0.62	0	0
62641	Cereals, Just Right	55	1	Cup	4.235	1.485	46.035	204.05	0	2.805	0	0.11
	Cereals, Just Right, Fruit & Nut	55	1	Cup	4.125	1.595	44.275	192.5	0	2.75	0	0.275
8048	Cereals, Kix	30	1.33	Cup	1.965	0.621	25.914	114.3	0	0.81	0	0.171
8049	Cereals, Life	44	1	Cup	8.1	0.84	31.5	162.36	0	2.64	0	0
	Cereals, Low Fat Granola, w/ raisins	55	0.67	Cup	4.51	2.75	43.67	201.85	0	3.3	0	0.935
	Cereals, Low Fat Granola, w/o raisins	55	0.5	Cup	4.62	3.245	44.165	213.4	0	3.245	0	0.495
62642	Cereals, Low-Fat Granola, Kellogg's	82.459	1	Cup	7.5	4.5	64.47	314.84	0	4.5	0	1.5
8050	Cereals, Lucky Charms	30	1	Cup	2.154	1.083	25.17	116.1	0	1.2	0	0.219
8178	Cereals, Malt-o-meal, Plain and Choc	240	1	Cup	3.6	0.24	25.92	122.4	0	0	0	0
8179	Cereals, Maypo, Ckd w/ water, w/ salt	240	1	Cup	5.76	2.4	31.92	170.4	0	0	0	0
8119	Cereals, Maypo, Ckd w/ water, w/o salt	240	1	Cup	5.76	2.4	31.92	170.4	0	5.76	0	0
	Cereals, Mueslix, Apple & Almond Crunch	55	0.75	Cup	5.39	4.95	40.865	210.65	0	4.675	0	1.045
	Cereals, Multigrain Cheerios	30	1	Cup	2.556	1.089	24.45	111.9	0	1.92	0	0.249
8052	Cereals, Nature Valley Granola	113	1	Cup	11.53	19.66	75.48	502.85	0	5.99	0	13.03
	Cereals, Nut & Honey Crunch	55	1.25	Cup	4.015	2.475	45.98	222.75	0	0.88	0	0.495
8149	Cereals, Nutri-grain, Barley	41	1	Cup	4.47	0.33	33.95	152.52	0	2.38	0	0
8150	Cereals, Nutri-grain, Corn	42	1	Cup	3.36	0.97	35.45	160.02	0	2.6	0	0
8151	Cereals, Nutri-grain, Rye	40	1	Cup	3.48	0.28	33.88	143.6	0	2.56	0	0
8152	Cereals, Nutri-grain, Wheat	30	0.75	Cup	3.03	0.99	24	100.5	0	3.78	0	0.06
	Cereals, Oat Bran Cereal	57	1.25	Cup	8.539	2.947	41.393	212.61	0	5.985	0	0.542
	Cereals, Oat Flakes	48	1	Cup	7.872	0.96	36.096	180.48	0	1.44	0	0.163

Monounsaturated Fat (gm)	Polyunsaturated Fat (gm)	Vitamin D (mg)	Vitamin K (mg)	Vitamin E (mg)	Vitamin A (re)	Vitamin C (mg)	Thiamin (mg)	Riboflavin (mg)	Niacin (mg)	Vitamin B6 (mg)	Folate (mg)	Vitamin B12 (mcg)	Calcium (mg)	Iron (mg)	Magnesium (mg)	Phosphorus (mg)	Potassium (mg)	Sodium (mg)	Zinc (mg)
0.029	0.05	0	0	0.072	14.5	51.37	0.377	0.07	5.104	0.522	102.37	1.537	3.19	8.282	4.06	11.31	23.49	316.97	0.101
0.028	0.112	0.8	0	0.035	210.28	14	0.364	0.392	4.676	0.476	98.84	0	1.12	8.68	3.36	10.92	25.48	297.92	0.168
0	0	0	0	0.03	9.5	0	0	0.05	0.11	0.02	1.75	0	10.75	0.56	3.25	12.25	18.25	2.5	0.07
0	0	0	0	0.06	9.5	0	0.13	0.03	1.05	0.02	1.75	0	1.75	0.63	2.75	9.75	22	239	0.06
0.062	0.031	0	0	0.033	232.81	15.5	0.403	0.434	5.177	0.527	109.43	0	2.48	1.86	2.48	6.51	22.63	123.07	1.55
3.249	0.754	2.1	0	0.364	253	16.83	0.421	0.477	5.612	0.561	152.9	0	24.75	2.035	76.45	186.45	254.65	195.25	1.65
0	0	0	0	0	0	0	0	0	0.98	0.07	7.32	0	7.32	0.49	7.32	41.48	48.8	422.12	0.39
0	0	0	0	0	0	0	0.24	0	1.69	0.03	9.64	0	60.25	12.05	14.46	43.38	48.2	363.91	0.41
0	0	0	0	0	0	0	0.24	0	1.43	0.03	9.56	0	50.19	10.28	11.95	100.38	45.41	463.66	0.33
0	0	0	0	0	0	0	0.25	0	1.51	0.04	10.04	0	50.2	10.29	10.04	42.67	42.67	336.34	0.33
0	0	0	0	0	0	0	0	0.05	0.36	0.04	2.86	0	17.42	0.8	10.14	27.04	20.28	2.6	0.39
0.058	0.116	0.5	0	0.119	225.33	14.993	0.377	0.435	4.988	0.493	87	0	3.48	1.798	6.96	26.68	35.09	240.12	1.508
0	0	0	0	0.03	0	1.12	0.11	0.03	1.99	0.04	3.08	0.08	5.04	0.7	11.76	30.52	26.6	205.52	0.46
0.121	0.156	0	0	0.574	375.1	0	0.374	0.424	4.999	0.501	99.55	0	69.3	4.499	42.35	140.25	229.9	284.9	1.083
0.138	0.06	0	0	0.332	0	9	0.375	0.426	5.001	0.501	99.9	0	58.5	4.5	68.1	168.3	216.9	142.5	1.239
0	0	0	0	0.34	635.52	0	0.62	0.72	8.45	0.86	169.44	2.54	68.16	13.73	57.6	176.16	343.2	429.12	1.5
0.031	0.093	0	0	0.04	232.81	15.5	0.403	0.434	5.177	0.527	109.43	0	0.62	4.65	2.79	8.06	20.46	202.12	0.155
0.11	0.605	0	0	0.496	0	0	0.385	0.44	5.005	0.495	102.3	1.485	19.8	61.225	55.55	159.5	183.15	1.65	1.485
0.21	0.27	0.99	0	0.11	211.2	14.07	0.39	0.42	5.01	0.51	90	0	3.3	4.23	8.7	20.7	31.5	140.7	3.75
0.102	0.075	0	0	0.032	423.68	0	0.416	0.48	5.632	0.576	112.96	1.696	3.84	2.016	9.28	18.88	24.32	177.6	1.696
0.279	0.159	1.37	0	0.226	225.3	15	0.375	0.426	5.001	0.501	99.9	0	14.4	4.5	9.3	36	52.8	274.5	3.75
0	0	0	0	0.02	397.2	15.9	0.39	0.45	5.28	0.54	105.9	0	13.8	1.89	24.9	65.7	108.3	195.9	1.59
9.601	12.895	0	0	15.708	4.88	1.708	0.903	0.342	2.501	0.39	104.92	0	98.82	5.124	217.16	563.64	656.36	29.28	4.953
0.057	0.194	3.98	0	0.273	1443.16	0	1.417	1.635	19.184	1.962	384.77	5.777	10.355	31.174	73.03	273.59	364.06	757.55	2.398
0	0	0	0	0.08	429.73	0	0.42	0.49	5.71	0.58	114.57	1.72	12.98	9.28	35.7	96.72	112.95	183.06	0.65
0	0	0.75	0	0	374.81	0	0.56	0.64	7.12	0.75	74.96	0.75	35.98	2.25	52.47	179.91	179.91	224.89	1.8
4.799	7.089	0	0	0.805	6.9	1.15	0.356	0.161	1.61	0.194	64.4	0	74.75	4.336	147.2	416.3	385.25	293.25	3.036
0	0	0	0	0.74	0	1.05	0.35	0.15	1.79	0.16	56.7	0	66.15	5.39	137.55	380.1	384.3	213.15	2.74
4.228	6.241	0	0	0.77	6.6	1.1	0.319	0.143	1.54	0.198	44	0	66	4.015	140.8	376.2	414.7	225.5	2.83
0	0	0	0	0.09	501.35	20.07	0.49	0.57	6.66	0.68	133.67	0	4.54	2.39	7.57	17.42	47.71	300.66	0.14
1.064	0.276	0	0	0.109	301.32	12.042	0.375	0.472	5.017	0.499	100.44	0	12.42	4.514	12.69	41.85	45.09	177.93	3.761
0.48	0.189	1.16	0	0.312	225.3	15	0.375	0.426	5.001	0.501	99.9	0	20.4	4.5	29.4	102.9	85.2	258.9	3.75
0.08	0.262	0	0	0.812	463.4	18.55	0.455	0.525	6.16	0.63	23.45	1.855	16.1	5.565	45.85	131.95	150.5	202.3	0.903
0	0	0.77	0	0.09	291.28	0	0.29	0.33	3.87	0.4	77.66	1.17	3.74	2.09	7.48	21.78	70.4	123.86	1.17
0.275	1.045	0	0	2.238	375.65	0	0.385	0.44	5.005	0.495	102.3	1.485	14.3	16.225	34.1	106.15	121	337.7	0.88
0.77	0.55	0	0	2.997	344.3	0	0.33	0.385	4.565	0.44	110	1.375	0	14.85	33	108.9	155.65	265.65	1.045
0.147	0.036	0.66	0	0.018	375.3	15	0.375	0.426	5.001	0.501	99.9	0	43.5	8.1	9.3	42	41.1	263.1	3.75
0	0	0	0	0.31	0	0	0.95	1	11.63	0.08	36.96	0	154	11.62	14.08	237.6	196.68	229.24	1.45
0.66	1.155	0	0	5.533	206.25	0	0.33	0.385	4.565	0.44	110	1.375	24.2	1.925	45.65	127.05	155.65	123.75	3.465
0.66	2.09	0	0	5.533	253	0	0.44	0.495	5.61	0.55	110	1.705	22.55	2.035	46.75	134.75	137.5	134.75	4.235
0	0	0.75	0	0	224.89	0	0.56	0.64	7.12	0.75	74.96	0.75	35.98	1.5	52.47	179.91	254.87	202.4	5.62
0.393	0.15	1.12	0	0.128	225.3	15	0.375	0.426	5.001	0.501	99.9	0	32.4	4.5	19.5	75.6	54	203.1	3.75
0	0	0	0	0	0	0	0.48	0.24	5.76	0.02	4.8	0	4.8	9.6	4.8	24	31.2	324	0.17
0	0	0	0	0	703.2	28.8	0.72	0.72	9.36	0.96	9.6	2.88	124.8	8.4	50.4	247.2	211.2	259.2	1.49
0	0	0	0	1.68	703.2	28.8	0.72	0.72	9.36	0.96	9.6	2.88	124.8	8.4	50.4	247.2	211.2	9.6	1.49
2.585	1.045	0	0	5.775	233.75	0	0.385	0.44	5.17	0.495	110	1.265	33.55	4.675	62.7	175.45	209	270.05	3.135
0.297	0.15	0	0	0.191	225.3	15	0.375	0.426	5	0.501	99.9	0	57	8.1	29.7	114.3	97.2	254.1	3.75
2.93	2.75	0	0	3.39	0	0	0.4	0.19	0.82	0.09	84.75	0	71.19	3.77	115.26	353.69	388.72	232.78	2.19
1.155	0.825	0	0	0.138	225.5	15.015	0.385	0.44	5.005	0.495	110	0	5.5	4.51	4.95	36.3	59.95	370.15	0.385
0	0	0	0	10.82	542.84	21.73	0.53	0.62	7.22	0.74	144.73	2.17	11.07	1.45	32.39	126.28	107.83	277.16	5.41
0	0	0	0	11.09	556.08	22.26	0.55	0.63	7.39	0.76	148.26	2.23	1.26	0.89	26.88	120.54	97.86	276.36	5.54
0	0	0	0	10.56	529.6	21.2	0.52	0.6	7.04	0.72	141.2	2.12	8.4	1.13	30.4	104	71.6	272	5.28
0.24	0.69	0	0	5.4	0	15	0.39	0.42	5.01	0.51	90	1.5	9.6	0.99	24.3	108.3	109.5	220.8	3.75
0.963	1.214	0	0	2.096	155.61	6.213	0.388	0.439	5.187	0.519	103.74	0	30.21	15.96	99.18	306.09	257.07	205.2	3.887
0.276	0.36	0	0	0.336	635.52	0	0.624	0.72	8.448	0.864	169.44	2.544	68.16	13.728	57.6	176.16	228	220.32	2.544

USDA ID Code	Food Name	Weight in Grams*	Quantity of Units	Unit of Measure	Protein (gm)	Fat (gm)	Carbohydrates (gm)	Kcalories	Caffeine (gm)	Fiber (gm)	Cholesterol (mg)	Saturated Fat (gm)
	Cereals, Oatmeal Raisin Crisp	55	1	Cup	4.351	2.447	43.703	204.05	0	3.52	0	0.385
	Cereals, Oatmeal Squares	56	1	Cup	7.274	2.587	43.316	216.16	0	4.256	0	0.476
8123	Cereals, Oats, Instant, Plain	177	1	Pkt.	4.43	1.77	18.05	104.43	0	3.01	0	0
8125	Cereals, Oats, Instant, w/ apples and cinn	149	1	Pkt.	3.87	1.64	26.37	135.59	0	0	0	0
8127	Cereals, Oats, Instant, w/ bran & rsns	195	1	Pkt.	4.88	1.95	30.42	157.95	0	0	0	0
8129	Cereals, Oats, Instant, w/ cinn and spice	161	1	Pkt.	4.83	1.93	35.1	177.1	0	2.58	0	0
8131	Cereals, Oats, Instant, w/ mapl & brn sug flav	155	1	Pkt.	4.65	1.86	31.93	162.75	0	0	0	0
8133	Cereals, Oats, Instant, w/ raisins and spice	158	1	Pkt	4.27	1.74	31.92	161.16	0	2.21	0	0
8180	Cereals, Oats, Reg and Quick and Instant	234	1	Cup	6.08	2.34	25.27	145.08	0	0	0	0.44
8058	Cereals, Product 19	30	1	Cup	2.295	0.39	25.089	109.8	0	1.23	0	0.03
	Cereals, Puffed Rice	14	1	Cup	0.98	0.126	12.288	53.62	0	0.196	0	0.045
	Cereals, Puffed Wheat	15	1.25	Cup	2.439	0.323	11.459	54.9	0	1.14	0	0.016
8059	Cereals, Quisp	30	1	Cup	1.5	2.16	24.99	124.2	0	0.54	0	1.48
8060	Cereals, Raisin Bran, Kellogg's	61	1	Cup	5.49	1.427	46.72	196.42	0	7.808	0	0.143
8061	Cereals, Raisin Bran, Post	56	1	Cup	5.208	1.064	42.336	171.92	0	7.896	0	0.176
8062	Cereals, Raisin Bran, Ralston Purina	56	1	Cup	4.368	0.28	46.48	178.08	0	7.504	0	0.046
	Cereals, Raisin Bran, Total, General Mills	55	1	Cup	3.998	1.006	42.752	178.2	0	5.005	0	0.231
	Cereals, Raisin Nut Bran	55	1	Cup	5.164	4.4	41.454	209	0	5.06	0	0.715
	Cereals, Raisin Squares	55	0.75	Cup	4.4	1.54	42.9	187	0	5.17	0	0.165
8063	Cereals, Raisins, Rice and Rye	46	1	Cup	2.62	0.14	39.28	154.56	0	2.62	0	0
	Cereals, Reese's Peanut Butter Puffs	30	0.75	Cup	2.571	3.195	22.98	129.3	0	0.39	0	0.636
8064	Cereals, Rice Chex	33	1	Cup	1.749	0.132	29.436	130.35	0	0.594	0	0.036
8065	Cereals, Rice Krispies	33	1.25	Cup	2.079	0.363	28.545	124.41	0	0.363	0	0.132
8156	Cereals, Rice, Puffed	14	1	Cup	0.88	0.07	12.57	56.28	0	0	0	0
	Cereals, Shredded Wheat, Large	23.6	1	Biscuit	2.572	0.389	19.187	84.96	0	2.313	0	0.065
	Cereals, Shredded Wheat, Small	30	1	Cup	3.3	0.495	24.12	107.1	0	2.94	0	0.083
	Cereals, S'mores Grahams	30	0.75	Cup	1.677	1.2	25.59	117	0	0.84	0	0.177
8067	Cereals, Special K	31	1	Cup	6.355	0.279	22.444	114.7	0	0.961	0	0
8068	Cereals, Sugar Corn Pops	28.4	1	Cup	1.42	0.09	25.7	108.49	0	0.23	0	0
8069	Cereals, Sugar Frosted Flakes	38	1	Cup	2.014	0.532	34.238	148.58	0	0.836	0	0.305
	Cereals, Sun Country Granola w/ almonds	57	0.5	Cup	6.709	10.271	38.304	266.19	0	2.964	0	1.265
	Cereals, Sun Country Granola, w/ raisins & dates	31	0.5	Cup	3.019	4.225	22.382	135.16	0	1.86	0	0.642
	Cereals, Super Sugar Crisp	33	1	Cup	2.145	0.297	29.766	123.42	0	0.495	0	0.052
8074	Cereals, Tasteeos	24	1	Cup	3.07	0.67	18.984	94.32	0	2.544	0	0.23
8075	Cereals, Team	42	1	Cup	2.69	0.76	36.04	164.22	0	0.55	0	0
	Cereals, Toasted Brown Sugar Squares	55	1.25	Cup	5.225	1.045	44.99	189.2	0	5.115	0	0.181
	Cereals, Toasted Oatmeal Cereal, Honey Nut	49	1	Cup	4.89	2.71	38.955	190.61	0	3.332	0.49	0.519
	Cereals, Toasted Oats Granola	55	0.75	Cup	5.803	9.691	36.234	238.05	0	3.52	0	1.271
	Cereals, Toasties	23	1	Cup	1.836	0.046	19.734	89.01	0	0.782	0	0.006
8077	Cereals, Total	30	0.75	Cup	2.988	0.696	23.88	105.3	0	2.64	0	0.18
	Cereals, Triples	30	1	Cup	2.379	1.011	24.984	116.1	0	0.84	0	0.291
8078	Cereals, Trix	30	1	Cup	0.954	1.707	26.04	122.4	0	0.72	0	0.407
	Cereals, Waffelos	30	1	Cup	1.68	1.26	25.89	121.5	0	0	0	0
8082	Cereals, Wheat Chex	46	1	Cup	4.55	1.15	37.81	168.82	0	4.09	0	0.198
	Cereals, Wheat Germ, Toasted	28.35	1	Oz.	8.25	3.033	14.062	108.297	0	3.657	0	0.519
8080	Cereals, Wheat 'n Raisin Chex	54	1	Cup	5.08	0.43	42.98	185.22	0	3.56	0	0
8143	Cereals, Wheatena, Ckd w/ water	243	1	Cup	4.86	1.22	28.67	136.08	0	6.56	0	0
8182	Cereals, Wheatena, Ckd w/ water, w/ Salt	243	1	Cup	4.86	1.22	28.67	136.08	0	0	0	0
8089	Cereals, Wheaties	30	1	Cup	3.24	0.927	23.79	110.1	0	2.1	0	0.198
8183	Cereals, Whole Wheat Hot Natural Cereal	242	1	Cup	4.84	0.97	33.15	150.04	0	0	0	0
18268	French Toast, Frozen, Ready-to-heat	59	1	Slice	4.37	3.6	18.94	125.67	0	1.65	48.38	1.15
18269	French Toast, Made w/ Lowfat (2%) Milk	65	1	Slice	5.01	7.02	16.25	148.85	0	0	75.4	1.77
18381	French Toast, Made w/ Whole Milk	65	1	Slice	5.01	7.35	16.19	150.8	0	0	76.05	1.95
3189	Oatmeal, Dry	38.368	0.33	Cup	4.6	1.9	18.4	109	0	2.53	0	0
3689	Oatmeal, Prepared	359.999	0.75	Cup	4.5	1.8	18.9	108	0	1.6	0	0.3

Monounsaturated Fat (gm)	Polyunsaturated Fat (gm)	Vitamin D (mg)	Vitamin K (mg)	Vitamin E (mg)	Vitamin A (re)	Vitamin C (mg)	Thiamin (mg)	Riboflavin (mg)	Niacin (mg)	Vitamin B6 (mg)	Folate (mg)	Vitamin B12 (mcg)	Calcium (mg)	Iron (mg)	Magnesium (mg)	Phosphorus (mg)	Potassium (mg)	Sodium (mg)	Zinc (mg)
1.155	0.363	0	0	1.355	225.5	0	0.374	0.424	5.005	0.501	100.1	0	37.95	4.499	44.55	117.15	211.75	223.85	3.751
0.806	1.047	0	0	2.278	169.12	6.776	0.42	0.476	5.628	0.56	112.56	0	35.84	15.68	70	185.92	227.92	263.2	4.222
0	0	0	0	0.21	453.12	0	0.53	0.28	5.47	0.74	150.45	0	162.84	6.3	42.48	132.75	99.12	284.97	0.87
0	0	0	0	0	435.08	0	0.48	0.28	5.14	0.7	137.08	0	157.94	6.06	34.27	117.71	107.28	222.01	0.7
0	0	0	0	0	479.7	0	0.57	0.64	8.13	0.76	156	0	173.55	7.62	56.55	206.7	235.95	247.65	1.35
0	0	0	0	0.35	473.34	0	0.56	0.34	5.65	0.77	152.95	0	172.27	6.63	51.52	144.9	104.65	280.14	0.97
0	0	0	0	0	451.05	0	0.53	0.33	5.35	0.74	145.7	0	161.2	6.36	41.85	142.6	102.3	279	0.87
0	0	0	0	0.16	440.82	0	0.51	0.36	5.48	0.75	150.1	0	165.9	6.59	36.34	132.72	150.1	225.94	0.71
0.84	0.96	0	0	0	0	0	0.26	0.05	0.3	0.05	9.36	0	18.72	1.59	56.16	177.84	131.04	374.4	1.15
0.15	0.21	1.16	0	22.2	225.3	60	1.5	1.71	20.01	2.01	423.6	6	2.7	18	12.3	39.9	51.9	282	15
0.025	0.048	0	0	0.014	0	0	0.057	0.007	0.875	0	1.4	0	1.26	0.407	4.2	16.52	16.24	0.7	0.154
0.046	0.16	0	0	0.101	0.15	0	0.06	0.041	1.791	0.02	5.1	0.063	3.6	0.702	19.95	49.65	54.6	0.75	0.461
0.26	0.31	0	0	0.08	4.8	0	0.54	0.76	5.8	0.91	8.1	2.58	9.3	6.32	12.3	24.9	44.7	240.9	0.18
0.119	0.428	1.23	0	0.556	250.1	0	0.427	0.488	5.551	0.549	113.46	1.647	40.62	5.002	89.06	214.11	349.53	390.4	4.148
0.146	0.503	2.16	0	1.299	741.44	0	0.728	0.84	9.856	1.008	197.68	2.968	26.32	8.904	95.2	234.64	344.96	365.12	2.968
0.038	0.132	0	0	1.299	556.08	1.68	0.56	0.616	7.392	0.728	148.4	2.24	26.88	27.328	84.56	247.52	287.28	486.08	1.674
0.17	0.17	0	0	29.975	375.1	0	1.502	1.7	20.02	2.002	399.85	6.353	238.15	18.001	44.55	258.5	287.1	239.8	14.999
1.925	0.456	0	0	2.032	0	0	0.374	0.424	4.999	0.501	99.55	0	73.7	4.499	53.9	162.8	218.35	245.85	1.105
0.11	0.495	0	0	0.291	0	0	0.385	0.44	5.17	0.495	110	1.54	18.7	16.83	47.85	159.5	259.6	3.3	1.54
0	0	0	0	0.25	467.82	0.46	0.46	0.55	6.26	0.64	124.66	1.89	10.12	5.61	19.78	49.68	143.52	349.6	4.69
1.431	0.6	0	0	0.565	225.3	15	0.375	0.426	5.001	0.501	99.9	0	21	4.5	15.9	43.2	61.5	177.3	3.75
0.041	0.035	0	0	0.043	1.98	17.49	0.429	0.01	5.808	0.594	116.49	1.749	4.62	9.438	8.25	32.34	38.28	275.88	0.455
0.099	0.165	0.99	0	0.041	247.83	16.5	0.429	0.462	5.511	0.561	116.49	0	3.3	1.98	15.84	43.56	42.24	353.76	0.597
0	0	0	0	0	0	0	0.36	0.25	4.94	0.01	2.66	0	0.84	4.44	3.5	13.72	15.82	0.42	0.14
0.062	0.207	0	0	0.125	0	0	0.066	0.066	1.079	0.06	11.8	0	9.676	0.743	40.12	85.668	77.172	0.472	0.592
0.079	0.263	0	0	0.159	0	0	0.078	0.084	1.575	0.076	15	0	11.4	1.266	39.6	105.9	108.3	3	0.99
0.393	0.15	0	0	0.218	225.3	15	0.375	0.426	5.001	0.501	99.9	0	14.4	4.5	10.8	40.5	48	212.4	3.75
0	0.217	0.75	0	0.077	225.06	14.88	0.527	0.589	7.006	0.713	93	0	4.65	8.401	17.67	50.84	54.56	249.86	3.751
0	0	0.99	0	0.07	376.01	15.05	0.37	0.43	5	0.51	100.25	0	1.14	1.79	1.99	28.12	17.32	103.66	1.51
0.072	0.098	1.23	0	0.095	503.12	20.14	0.494	0.57	6.688	0.684	2.66	2.014	4.18	0.95	2.66	9.5	23.94	246.62	0.817
3.329	1.813	0	0	1.194	0	0.057	0.177	0.103	0.542	0.068	19.38	0.04	49.02	2.479	51.87	167.58	221.16	18.81	1.14
1.423	0.803	0	0	0.483	0	0.124	0.087	0.065	0.257	0.04	9.61	0.062	23.87	1.29	26.04	91.76	132.68	7.75	0.496
0.06	0.116	0	0	0.122	436.92	0	0.429	0.495	5.808	0.594	116.49	1.749	6.93	2.079	19.8	43.89	47.85	50.82	1.749
0.173	0.184	0	0	0.168	317.76	12.72	0.312	0.36	4.22	0.43	87.72	1.272	11.04	6.864	26.16	95.76	71.04	182.88	0.686
0	0	0	0	0.1	556.08	22.26	0.55	0.63	7.39	0.76	6.72	2.23	6.3	2.57	18.48	65.1	70.98	259.56	0.58
0.154	0.429	0	0	2.997	51.15	0	0.55	0.605	7.15	0.715	110	2.145	18.7	6.435	59.4	194.15	213.95	1.65	1.54
1.151	0.75	0	0	2.012	150.43	5.978	0.372	0.421	4.998	0.5	99.96	0.015	26.95	4.498	53.41	166.11	184.73	165.62	3.92
6.49	1.87	0	0	3.878	0	0	0.17	0.06	0.611	0.076	8.25	0	41.25	1.716	52.25	160.05	182.6	189.1	1.105
0.011	0.02	0	0	0.058	304.52	0	0.299	0.345	4.048	0.414	81.91	1.219	0.92	0.605	3.45	10.12	26.68	241.04	0.067
0.135	0.081	1.16	0	23.492	375.3	60	1.5	1.701	20.1	2.001	399.9	7.671	258.3	18	32.1	210.9	96.9	198.6	15
0.27	0.03	0	0	0.141	375.3	15	0.375	0.426	5.001	0.501	99.9	0	41.1	8.1	6.9	35.4	30.6	191.4	3.75
0.903	0.291	0.98	0	0.598	225.3	15	0.376	0.426	5.001	0.501	99.9	0	32.1	4.5	3.6	26.1	17.7	196.8	3.75
0	0	0	0	0	397.2	15.9	0.39	0.45	5.28	0.54	3.3	1.59	8.4	4.77	6.3	244.5	26.4	124.8	0.243
0.143	0.479	0	0	0.17	0	24.38	0.598	0.166	8.096	0.828	126.38	2.438	17.94	13.138	58.42	181.7	173.42	308.2	1.233
0.425	1.877			5.143	0	1.701	0.473	0.232	1.585	0.277	99.792	0	12.758	2.577	90.72	324.891	268.475	1.134	4.726
0	0	0	0	0.31	0	1.62	0.54	0.59	7.13	0.7	143.1	2.16	24.3	7.72	52.92	163.08	226.8	305.64	1.19
0	0	0	0	0.9	0	0	0.02	0.05	1.34	0.05	17.01	0	9.72	1.36	48.6	145.8	187.11	4.86	1.68
0	0	0	0	0	0	0	0.02	0.05	1.34	0.05	17.01	0	9.72	1.36	48.6	145.8	187.11	578.34	1.68
0.222	0.15	1.02	0	0.369	225.3	15	0.375	0.426	5.001	0.501	99.9	0	54.6	8.1	31.8	95.4	104.1	222.3	0.708
0	0	0	0	0	0	0	0.17	0.12	2.15	0.18	26.62	0	16.94	1.5	53.24	166.98	171.82	563.86	1.16
1.23	0.7	0	0	0	31.86	0.3	0.16	0.22	1.61	0.29	14.16	0.99	63.13	1.3	10.03	82.01	79.06	292.05	0.45
2.94	1.69	0	0	0	85.8	0.2	0.13	0.21	1.06	0.05	14.95	0.2	65	1.09	11.05	76.05	87.1	311.35	0.44
3.03	1.7	0	0	0	80.6	0.2	0.13	0.21	1.06	0.05	14.95	0.2	64.35	1.09	11.05	76.05	86.45	310.7	0.44
0	0	0	0	0.15	0	1.23	0.19	0.03	0.2	0.06	29	0	14	1.08	40	128	105	1	1
0	0.7	0	0	0	0	0	0.19	0.04	0.2	0.04	7	0	15	1.19	42	133	99	1	0.86

USDA ID Code	Food Name	Weight in Grams*	Quantity of Units	Unit of Measure	Protein (gm)	Fat (gm)	Carbohydrates (gm)	Kcalories	Caffeine (gm)	Fiber (gm)	Cholesterol (mg)	Saturated Fat (gm)
18288	Pancakes Plain, Frozen	9	1	4 In.	0.47	0.3	3.92	20.61	0	0	0.81	0.07
18294	Pancakes, Blueberry	9.5	1	4 In.	0.58	0.87	2.76	21.09	0	0	5.32	0.19
18390	Pancakes, Buttermilk	9.5	1	4 In.	0.65	0.88	2.73	21.57	0	0	5.51	0.17
18298	Pancakes, Dietary	22	1	3 In.	1.12	0.18	9.28	43.78	0	0	0	0.03
18293	Pancakes, Plain	9.5	1	4 In.	0.61	0.92	2.69	21.57	0	0	5.61	0.2
18300	Pancakes, Whole-wheat	44	1	4 In.	3.74	2.86	12.94	91.52	0	0	26.84	0.77
18392	Waffles, Buttermilk	75	1	Each	6.23	10.2	24.75	216.75	0	0	50.25	1.88
18367	Waffles, Homemade, Plain	75	1	Each	5.93	10.58	24.68	218.25	0	0	51.75	2.15
18403	Waffles, Plain, Frozen, Toasted	33	1	Each	2.05	2.71	13.43	87.12	0	0	7.92	0.47
62670	Cheddar Cheese, Non-Fat	28.35	1.5	Ounce	8.1	0	2.03	45.56	0	0	4.05	0
1150	Cheese Spread, Past. Processed, American	28.35	2	Ounce	4.65	6.02	2.47	82.35	0	0	15.65	3.78
62671	Cheese Stick, Mozzarella	28	1	Each	8	5	0	80	0	0	15	3
1147	Cheese, American, Pasteurized Processed	28.35	2	Ounce	6.28	8.86	0.45	106.44	0	0	26.76	5.58
1004	Cheese, Blue	28.35	1.5	Ounce	6.07	8.15	0.66	100.09	0	0	21.32	5.29
1005	Cheese, Brick	28.35	1.5	Ounce	6.59	8.41	0.79	105.16	0	0	26.76	5.32
1006	Cheese, Brie	28.35	1.5	Ounce	5.88	7.85	0.13	94.59	0	0	28.35	4.94
1008	Cheese, Caraway	28.35	1.5	Ounce	7.14	8.28	0.87	106.6	0	0	26.37	5.27
1009	Cheese, Cheddar	28.35	1.5	Ounce	7.06	9.4	0.36	114.13	0	0	29.74	5.98
62577	Cheese, Cheddar, Reduced Fat	28.35	1.5	Ounce	8	5	1	80	0	0	15	3
1011	Cheese, Colby	28.35	1.5	Ounce	6.74	9.1	0.73	111.6	0	0	26.9	5.73
1012	Cheese, Cottage, Creamed	28.35	1.5	Ounce	3.54	1.28	0.76	29.3	0	0	4.22	0.81
1013	Cheese, Cottage, Creamed, w/ Fruit	28.35	1.5	Ounce	2.81	0.96	3.77	35.05	0	0	3.18	0.61
62690	Cheese, Cottage, Fat Free	226	0.5	Cup	26	0	0	140	0	0	20	0
1016	Cheese, Cottage, Lowfat, 1% Fat	28.35	1.5	Ounce	3.51	0.29	0.77	20.52	0	0	1.25	0.18
1015	Cheese, Cottage, Lowfat, 2% Fat	28.35	1.5	Ounce	3.9	0.55	1.03	25.43	0	0	2.38	0.35
1014	Cheese, Cottage, Uncreamed, Dry	28.35	1.5	Ounce	4.9	0.12	0.52	23.98	0	0	1.9	0.08
1017	Cheese, Cream	28.35	1.5	Ounce	2.14	9.89	0.75	98.95	0	0	31.1	6.23
62554	Cheese, Cream, Fat Free	17.508	2	Tbsp.	2.5	0	1	17.51	0	0	2.5	0
62553	Cheese, Cream, Light	16.014	2	Tbsp.	1.5	2.5	1	35.03	0	0	7.51	1.75
	Cheese, Cream, w/Strawberry	30	1	Ounce	4	0	2	35	0	0	3	0
1018	Cheese, Edam	28.35	1.5	Ounce	7.08	7.88	0.41	101.1	0	0	25.29	4.98
62579	Cheese, Fat Free Slices, White	21.263	1	Slice	5	0	2	30	0	0	0	0
62578	Cheese, Fat Free Slices, Yellow	21.263	1	Slice	5	0	2	30	0	0	0	0
1019	Cheese, Feta	28.35	1.5	Ounce	4.03	6.03	1.16	74.72	0	0	25.23	4.24
1020	Cheese, Fontina	28.35	1.5	Ounce	7.26	8.83	0.44	110.29	0	0	32.89	5.44
1156	Cheese, Goat, Hard Type	28.35	1.5	Ounce	8.65	10.09	0.62	128.14	0	0	29.77	6.98
1157	Cheese, Goat, Semisoft Type	28.35	1.5	Ounce	6.12	8.46	0.72	103.19	0	0	22.4	5.85
1159	Cheese, Goat, Soft Type	28.35	1.5	Ounce	5.25	5.98	0.25	75.98	0	0	13.04	4.13
1022	Cheese, Gouda	28.35	1.5	Ounce	7.07	7.78	0.63	101.01	0	0	32.32	4.99
1023	Cheese, Gruyere	28.35	1.5	Ounce	8.45	9.17	0.1	117.07	0	0	31.19	5.36
1024	Cheese, Limburger	28.35	1.5	Ounce	5.68	7.73	0.14	92.71	0	0	25.52	4.75
1025	Cheese, Monterey	28.35	1.5	Ounce	6.94	8.58	0.19	105.84	0	0	25.23	5.41
62576	Cheese, Monterey, Reduced Fat	28.35	1.5	Ounce	8	5	1	80	0	0	15	3
1028	Cheese, Mozzarella, Part Skim Milk	28.35	1.5	Ounce	6.88	4.51	0.79	72.08	0	0	16.39	2.87
1029	Cheese, Mozzarella, Part Skim Milk, Low Moisture	28.35	1.5	Ounce	7.79	4.85	0.89	79.36	0	0	15.31	3.08
1161	Cheese, Mozzarella, Substitute	28.35	1.5	Ounce	3.25	3.46	6.71	70.31	0	0	0	1.05
1026	Cheese, Mozzarella, Whole Milk	28.35	1.5	Ounce	5.51	6.12	0.63	79.77	0	0	22.23	3.73
1027	Cheese, Mozzarella, Whole Milk, Low Moisture	28.35	1.5	Ounce	6.12	6.99	0.7	90.26	0	0	25.34	4.41
1030	Cheese, Muenster	28.35	1.5	Ounce	6.64	8.52	0.32	104.43	0	0	27.1	5.42
1032	Cheese, Parmesan, Grated	5	1	Tbsp.	2.08	1.5	0.19	22.79	0	0	3.94	0.95
62608	Cheese, Parmesan, Grated, Fat Free	5.002	1	Tbsp.	0.67	0	0.67	5	0	0	1.67	0
1033	Cheese, Parmesan, Piece	28.35	1.5	Ounce	10.14	7.32	0.91	111.18	0	0	19.19	4.65
1146	Cheese, Parmesan, Shredded	28.35	1.5	Ounce	10.73	7.75	0.97	117.65	0	0	20.41	4.92
1025	Cheese, Pepper	28.35	1.5	Ounce	7.12	8.13	0.21	107.98	0	0	27.81	5.39
1035	Cheese, Provolone	28.35	1.5	Ounce	7.25	7.55	0.61	99.65	0	0	19.53	4.84

Monounsaturated Fat (gm)	Polyunsaturated Fat (gm)	Vitamin D (mg)	Vitamin K (mg)	Vitamin E (mg)	Vitamin A (re)	Vitamin C (mg)	Thiamin (mg)	Riboflavin (mg)	Niacin (mg)	Vitamin B6 (mg)	Folate (mg)	Vitamin B12 (mcg)	Calcium (mg)	Iron (mg)	Magnesium (mg)	Phosphorus (mg)	Potassium (mg)	Sodium (mg)	Zinc (mg)
0.11	0.09	0	0	0	2.61	0.04	0.03	0.04	0.36	0	1.26	0.01	5.58	0.31	1.26	33.48	6.57	45.81	0.06
0.22	0.4	0	0	0	4.85	0.21	0.02	0.03	0.14	0	1.14	0.02	19.57	0.16	1.52	14.35	13.11	39.14	0.05
0.22	0.43	0	0	0	2.85	0.04	0.02	0.03	0.15	0	1.24	0.02	14.92	0.16	1.43	13.21	13.78	49.59	0.06
0.03	0.08	0	0	0	2.2	0	0.04	0.02	0.37	0	1.1	0	12.76	0.39	5.94	74.8	84.92	57.64	0.15
0.24	0.42	0	0	0	5.13	0.03	0.02	0.03	0.15	0	1.14	0.02	20.81	0.17	1.52	15.11	12.54	41.71	0.05
0.77	1.06	0	0	0	28.16	0.22	0.09	0.23	1.02	0.05	9.24	0.13	110	1.37	20.24	164.12	122.76	251.68	0.46
2.52	5.09	0	0	0	26.25	0.38	0.2	0.27	1.55	0.04	11.25	0.16	136.5	1.63	13.5	123.75	128.25	450.75	0.56
2.64	5.09	0	0	0	48.75	0.3	0.2	0.26	1.55	0.04	11.25	0.19	191.25	1.73	14.25	142.5	119.25	383.25	0.51
1.06	0.92	0	0	0	120.12	0	0.13	0.16	1.46	0.3	11.55	0.83	76.56	1.48	7.26	138.6	42.24	259.71	0.19
0	0	0	0	0	60.75	0	0	0	0	0	0	0	243	0	0	0	0	283.5	0
1.76	0.18	0	0	0	53.58	0	0.01	0.12	0.04	0.03	1.98	0.11	159.3	0.09	8.09	248.06	68.58	460.69	0.73
0	0	0	0	0	40	0	0	0	0	0	0	0	240	0	0	0	0	170	0
2.54	0.28	0	0	0	82.22	0	0.01	0.1	0.02	0.02	2.21	0.2	174.49	0.11	6.31	125.87	45.93	184.28	0.85
2.21	0.23	0	0	0.18	64.64	0	0.01	0.11	0.29	0.05	10.32	0.35	149.57	0.09	6.5	109.83	72.66	395.57	0.75
2.44	0.22	0	0	0.14	85.62	0	0	0.1	0.03	0.02	5.76	0.36	190.99	0.12	6.89	127.86	38.5	158.65	0.74
2.27	0.23	0	0	0.19	51.6	0	0.02	0.15	0.11	0.07	18.43	0.47	52.16	0.14	5.67	53.3	43.09	178.43	0.67
2.35	0.24	0	0	0	81.93	0	0.01	0.13	0.05	0.02	5.16	0.08	190.88	0.18	6.27	138.92	26.37	195.62	0.83
2.66	0.27	0.09	0	0.1	85.9	0	0.01	0.11	0.02	0.02	5.16	0.23	204.49	0.19	7.88	145.18	27.9	175.91	0.88
0	0	0	0	0	60	0	0	0	0	0	0	0	240	0	0	0	23	180	0
2.63	0.27	0	0	0.1	77.96	0	0	0.11	0.03	0.02	5.16	0.23	194.08	0.22	7.32	129.42	35.86	171.29	0.87
0.36	0.04	0	0	0.03	13.61	0	0.01	0.05	0.04	0.02	3.46	0.18	17.01	0.04	1.49	37.37	23.9	114.76	0.1
0.27	0.03	0	0	0.03	10.21	0	0	0.04	0.03	0.02	2.75	0.14	13.49	0.03	1.18	29.63	18.97	114.76	0.08
0	0	0	0	0	0	0	0	0	0	0	0	0	240	0	0	0	0	840	0
0.08	0.01	0	0	0.03	3.12	0	0.01	0.05	0.04	0.02	3.52	0.18	17.27	0.04	1.51	37.93	24.24	115.1	0.11
0.16	0.02	0	0	0.02	5.67	0	0.01	0.05	0.04	0.02	3.71	0.2	19.42	0.05	1.7	42.67	27.27	115.1	0.12
0.03	0	0	0	0.03	2.27	0	0.01	0.04	0.04	0.02	4.2	0.23	8.99	0.07	1.12	29.48	9.19	3.63	0.13
2.79	0.36	0	0	0.27	123.89	0	0	0.06	0.03	0.01	3.74	0.12	22.65	0.34	1.83	29.6	33.85	83.77	0.15
0	0	0	0	0	50.02	0	0	0	0	0	0	0	60.03	0	0	0	0	90.04	0
0	0	0	0	0	40.03	0	0	0	0	0	0	0	24.02	0	0	0	0	75.06	0
0	0	0	0	0	10	0	0	0	0	0	0	0	24	0	0	0	0	200	0
2.3	0.19	0.26	0	0.21	71.73	0	0.01	0.11	0.02	0.02	4.59	0.44	207.24	0.12	8.44	151.84	53.21	273.58	1.06
0	0	0	0	0	40	0	0	0	0	0	0	0	120	0	0	0	18	310	0
0	0	0	0	0	40	0	0	0	0	0	0	0	120	0	0	0	18	310	0
1.31	0.17	0	0	0.01	36.29	0	0.04	0.24	0.28	0.12	9.07	0.48	139.62	0.18	5.45	95.6	17.52	316.41	0.82
2.46	0.47	0	0	0.1	82.22	0	0.01	0.06	0.04	0.02	1.7	0.48	155.93	0.07	3.97	98.18	18	226.8	0.99
2.3	0.24	0	0	0	442.26	0	0.04	0.34	0.68	0.02	1.13	0.03	253.73	0.53	15.31	206.67	13.61	98.09	0.45
1.93	0.2	0	0	0	467.78	0	0.02	0.19	0.33	0.02	0.57	0.06	84.48	0.46	8.22	106.31	44.79	146	0.19
1.36	0.14	0	0	0	385.56	0	0.02	0.11	0.12	0.07	3.4	0.05	39.69	0.54	4.54	72.58	7.37	104.33	0.26
2.2	0.19	0	0	0.1	49.33	0	0.01	0.09	0.02	0.02	5.93	0.44	198.39	0.07	8.22	154.88	34.16	232.27	1.11
2.85	0.49	0	0	0.1	85.33	0	0.02	0.08	0.03	0.02	2.95	0.45	286.62	0.05	10.18	171.6	22.96	95.26	1.11
2.44	0.14	0	0	0.18	89.59	0	0.02	0.14	0.04	0.02	16.3	0.29	140.81	0.04	5.95	111.42	36.29	226.8	0.6
2.48	0.25	0	0	0.1	71.73	0	0	0.11	0.03	0.02	5.16	0.23	211.6	0.2	7.66	125.87	22.88	152.04	0.85
0	0	0	0	0	60	0	0	0	0	0	0	0	240	0	0	0	18	180	0
1.28	0.13	0	0	0.12	50.18	0	0.01	0.09	0.03	0.02	2.49	0.23	183.06	0.06	6.58	131.26	23.73	132.11	0.78
1.37	0.14	0	0	0.13	54.15	0	0.01	0.1	0.03	0.02	2.81	0.26	207.32	0.07	7.45	148.58	26.89	149.6	0.89
1.77	0.49	0	0	0	123.89	0.03	0.01	0.13	0.09	0.01	3.12	0.23	172.94	0.11	11.62	165.28	128.99	194.2	0.54
1.86	0.22	0	0	0.1	68.32	0	0	0.07	0.02	0.02	1.98	0.19	146.57	0.05	5.27	105.09	19.02	105.77	0.63
1.99	0.22	0	0	0.19	77.68	0	0	0.08	0.03	0.02	2.21	0.21	162.98	0.06	5.86	116.89	21.15	117.65	0.7
2.47	0.19	0	0	0.13	89.59	0	0	0.09	0.03	0.02	3.43	0.42	203.35	0.12	7.75	132.59	38.1	177.95	0.8
0.44	0.03	0	0	0.04	8.65	0	0	0.02	0.02	0.01	0.4	0.07	68.79	0.05	2.54	40.36	5.36	93.08	0.16
0	0	0	0	0	0	0	0	0	0	0	0	0	16.01	0	0	0	10	15.01	0
2.13	0.16	0.2	0	0.23	42.24	0	0.01	0.09	0.08	0.03	1.96	0.34	335.52	0.23	12.39	196.86	26.14	454.03	0.78
2.48	0.19	0	0	0	49.05	0	0.01	0.1	0.08	0.03	2.27	0.4	355.23	0.25	14.4	208.37	27.5	480.82	0.9
2.46	0.24	0	0	0.1	79.89	0	0	0.12	0.03	0.02	6.13	0.22	212.76	0.2	6.23	122.77	25.76	172.77	0.81
2.1	0.22	0	0	0.1	74.84	0	0.01	0.09	0.04	0.02	2.95	0.41	214.3	0.15	7.82	140.64	39.21	248.2	0.92

USDA ID Code	Food Name	Weight in Grams*	Quantity of Units	Unit of Measure	Protein (gm)	Fat (gm)	Carbohydrates (gm)	Kcalories	Caffeine (gm)	Fiber (gm)	Cholesterol (mg)	Saturated Fat (gm)
1037	Cheese, Ricotta, Part Skim Milk	28.35	1.5	Ounce	3.23	2.24	1.46	39.14	0	0	8.73	1.4
1036	Cheese, Ricotta, Whole Milk	28.35	1.5	Ounce	3.19	3.68	0.86	49.31	0	0	14.35	2.35
1038	Cheese, Romano	28.35	1.5	Ounce	9.02	7.64	1.03	109.61	0	0	29.48	4.85
1039	Cheese, Roquefort	28.35	1.5	Ounce	6.11	8.69	0.57	104.62	0	0	25.52	5.46
1040	Cheese, Swiss, Domestic	28.35	1.5	Ounce	8.06	7.78	0.96	106.53	0	0	26	5.04
1044	Cheese, Swiss, Pasteurized Processed	28.35	2	Ounce	7.01	7.09	0.6	94.56	0	0	24.04	4.55
1067	Cream Substitute, Nondairy, Liquid	15	1	Tbsp.	0.15	1.5	1.71	20.35	0	0	0	0.29
1069	Cream Substitute, Nondairy, Powdered	2	1	Tsp.	0.1	0.71	1.1	10.93	0	0	0	0.65
1049	Cream, Half and Half, Cream and Milk	15	1	Tbsp.	0.44	1.72	0.64	19.55	0	0	5.53	1.07
1053	Cream, Heavy Whipping	15	1	Tbsp.	0.31	5.55	0.42	51.72	0	0	20.56	3.45
1052	Cream, Light Whipping	15	1	Tbsp.	0.33	4.64	0.44	43.86	0	0	16.65	2.9
1050	Cream, Light, Coffee or Table	15	1	Tbsp.	0.4	2.9	0.55	29.31	0	0	9.91	1.8
1051	Cream, Medium, 25% Fat	15	1	Tbsp.	0.37	3.75	0.52	36.56	0	0	13.12	2.33
1054	Cream, Whipped, Pressurized	3	1	Tbsp.	0.1	0.67	0.37	7.72	0	0	2.28	0.41
1073	Dessert Topping, Nondairy	4	1	Tbsp.	0.05	1.01	0.92	12.73	0	0	0	0.87
1142	Egg Substitute, Frozen	240	1	Cup	27.1	26.66	7.68	383.57	0	0	4.8	4.63
1143	Egg Substitute, Liquid	251	1	Cup	30.12	8.31	1.61	210.98	0	0	2.51	1.65
1124	Egg, White Only, w/o Yolk	33.4	2	Large	3.51	0	0.34	16.7	0	0	0	0
1057	Eggnog	254	1	Cup	9.68	19	34.39	341.9	0	0	149.1	11.29
62680	Eggnog, Reduced-Fat	246	1	Cup	12	8	48	320	0	0	90	5
1128	Eggs, Chicken, Whole, Ckd, Fried	46	1	Large	6.23	6.9	0.63	91.54	0	0	211.14	1.92
1129	Eggs, Chicken, Whole, Ckd, Hard-boiled	50	1	Large	6.29	5.31	0.56	77.5	0	0	212	1.63
1130	Eggs, Chicken, Whole, Ckd, Omelet	59	1	Large	6.09	6.75	0.61	89.68	0	0	206.5	1.88
1131	Eggs, Chicken, Whole, Ckd, Poached	50	1	Large	6.22	4.99	0.61	74.5	0	0	211.5	1.54
1132	Eggs, Chicken, Whole, Ckd, Scrambled	220	0.5	Cup	24.4	26.86	4.84	365.2	0	0	774.4	8.09
1123	Eggs, Chicken, Whole, Fresh, and Frozen	50	1	Large	6.25	5.01	0.61	74.5	0	0	212.5	1.55
1075	Milk Substitutes, Fluid w/ hydr Vegetable Oils	244	1	Cup	4.27	8.32	15.03	149.95	0	0	0.49	1.87
1076	Milk Substitutes, Fluid, w/ lauric Acid Oil	244	1	Cup	4.27	8.32	15.03	149.95	0	0	0.49	7.41
1088	Milk, Buttermilk	245	1	Cup	8.11	2.16	11.74	98.99	0	0	8.57	1.34
1104	Milk, Chocolate Drink, Lowfat, 1% Fat	250	1	Cup	8.1	2.5	26.1	157.57	0	0	7.25	1.54
1103	Milk, Chocolate Drink, Lowfat, 2% Fat	250	1	Cup	8.02	5	26	178.84	0	3.75	17	3.1
1102	Milk, Chocolate Drink, Whole	250	1	Cup	7.92	8.47	25.85	208.37	0	3.75	30.5	5.26
1105	Milk, Chocolate Homemade Hot Cocoa	250	1	Cup	9.1	9.05	25.77	218.15	0	3.75	33.25	5.61
1095	Milk, Cnd, Condensed, Sweetened	305.342	0.25	Cup	24	26.4	165.6	976	0	0	26	4.2
1153	Milk, Cnd, Evaporated	251.787	0.25	Cup	17.15	19.04	25.28	338.37	0	0	74.03	11.56
1097	Milk, Cnd, Evaporated, Skim	254.984	1	Cup	19.25	0.51	28.94	198.69	0	0	9.18	0.31
1082	Milk, Light, 1% Fat	244	1	Cup	8.03	2.59	11.66	102.15	0	0	9.76	1.61
1099	Milk, Malted, Beverage	265	1	Cup	10.34	9.81	27.3	235.85	0	0	37.1	5.95
1101	Milk, Malted, Chocolate Flavor, Beverage	265	1	Cup	9.01	9.01	29.95	227.9	7.95	0	34.45	5.53
1085	Milk, Non-Fat	245	1	Cup	8.35	0.44	11.88	85.53	0	0	4.41	0.29
1079	Milk, Reduced, 2% Fat	244	1	Cup	8.13	4.68	11.71	121.2	0	0	18.3	2.92
1077	Milk, Whole, 3.3% Fat	244	1	Cup	8.03	8.15	11.37	149.92	0	0	33.18	5.07
1078	Milk, Whole, 3.7% Fat	244	1	Cup	8	8.93	11.35	156.58	0	0	34.89	5.56
1056	Sour Cream	12	1	Tbsp.	0.38	2.52	0.51	25.71	0	0	5.33	1.57
62556	Sour Cream, Fat Free	16.014	1	Tbsp.	0.5	0	2.5	12.51	0	0	2.5	0
1074	Sour Cream, Imitation, Nondairy, Cultured	14.35	1	Tbsp.	0.34	2.8	0.95	29.91	0	0	0	2.55
62555	Sour Cream, Light	16.014	1	Tbsp.	0.92	1.14	0.92	16.01	0	0	4.58	0.69
62660	Sour Cream, Non-Fat	16	2	Tbsp.	0.5	0	2.5	12.5	0	0	2.5	0
	Yogurt, Dannon, 99% Fat Free	227	8	Ounce	9	3	45	240	0	0	15	1.5
	Yogurt, Dannon, Light	227	8	Ounce	9	0	45	240	0	0	15	1.5
	Yogurt, Dannon, Non Fat, No Sugar w/ Granola	227	8	Ounce	9	0	26	140	0	0	5	0
62657	Yogurt, Frozen	148	0.5	Cup	6	12	48	320	0	0	20	4
62552	Yogurt, Frozen, Fat Free	133.916	0.5	Cup	7.99	0	43.97	199.87	0	0	0	0
62658	Yogurt, Frozen, Low-Fat	148	0.5	Cup	6	6	48	280	0	0	20	4
62604	Yogurt, Fruit, Fat Free	247.957	1	Cup	10.21	0	48.13	233.37	0	0	7.29	0

Monounsaturated Fat (gm)	Polyunsaturated Fat (gm)	Vitamin D (mg)	Vitamin K (mg)	Vitamin E (mg)	Vitamin A (re)	Vitamin C (mg)	Thiamin (mg)	Riboflavin (mg)	Niacin (mg)	Vitamin B6 (mg)	Folate (mg)	Vitamin B12 (mcg)	Calcium (mg)	Iron (mg)	Magnesium (mg)	Phosphorus (mg)	Potassium (mg)	Sodium (mg)	Zinc (mg)
0.66	0.07	0	0	0.06	32.04	0	0.01	0.05	0.02	0.01	3.71	0.08	77.11	0.12	4.19	51.77	35.44	35.35	0.38
1.03	0.11	0	0	0.1	37.99	0	0	0.06	0.03	0.01	3.46	0.1	58.68	0.11	3.2	44.82	29.65	23.84	0.33
2.22	0.17	0	0	0.21	39.97	0	0.01	0.1	0.02	0.02	1.93	0.32	301.59	0.22	11.6	215.46	24.47	340.2	0.73
2.4	0.37	0	0	0	84.77	0	0.01	0.17	0.21	0.04	13.89	0.18	187.62	0.16	8.37	111.16	25.71	512.85	0.59
2.06	0.28	0.31	0	0.14	71.73	0	0.01	0.1	0.03	0.02	1.81	0.48	272.42	0.05	10.18	171.4	31.38	73.71	1.11
2	0.18	0	0	0.19	64.92	0	0	0.08	0.01	0.01	1.67	0.35	218.83	0.17	8.26	215.89	61.09	388.48	1.02
1.13	0	0	0	0.24	1.35	0	0	0	0	0	0	0	1.4	0	0.05	9.63	28.58	11.88	0
0.02	0	0	0	0.01	0.4	0	0	0	0	0	0	0	0.45	0.02	0.08	8.44	16.24	3.62	0.01
0.5	0.06	0	0	0.02	16.05	0.13	0.01	0.02	0.01	0.01	0.37	0.05	15.73	0.01	1.53	14.28	19.44	6.1	0.08
1.6	0.21	0.19	0	0.09	63.15	0.09	0	0.02	0.01	0	0.55	0.03	9.69	0	1.05	9.36	11.31	5.64	0.03
1.36	0.13	0	0	0.09	44.25	0.09	0	0.02	0.01	0	0.55	0.03	10.41	0	1.08	9.16	14.52	5.14	0.04
0.84	0.11	0	0	0.02	27.3	0.11	0	0.02	0.01	0	0.34	0.03	14.43	0.01	1.3	11.98	18.25	5.94	0.04
1.08	0.14	0	0	0.09	34.8	0.11	0	0.02	0.01	0	0.34	0.03	13.53	0.01	1.26	10.59	17.17	5.55	0.04
0.19	0.02	0	0	0.02	6.21	0	0	0	0	0	0.08	0.01	3.03	0	0.32	2.68	4.42	3.9	0.01
0.06	0.02	0	0	0.01	3.44	0	0	0	0	0	0	0	0.25	0	0.07	0.31	0.73	1.01	0
5.84	14.98	0	0	5.07	324	1.13	0.29	0.93	0.34	0.32	39.36	0.81	174.72	4.75	35.9	172.08	511.92	478.56	2.35
2.25	4.02	0	0	1.22	542.16	0	0.28	0.75	0.28	0.01	37.4	0.75	133.03	5.27	21.89	303.71	828.3	444.27	3.26
0	0	0	0.01	0	0	0	0	0.15	0.03	0	1	0.07	2	0.01	3.67	4.34	47.76	54.78	0
5.67	0.86	0	0	0.58	203.2	3.81	0.09	0.48	0.27	0.13	2.29	1.14	330.2	0.51	46.99	277.88	419.61	138.18	1.17
0	0	0	0	0	160	2.4	0	0	0	0	0	0	480	0.4	0	0	0	280	0
2.75	1.28	0	0	1.57	114.08	0	0.03	0.24	0.04	0.07	17.48	0.42	25.3	0.72	5.06	89.24	60.72	162.38	0.55
2.04	0.71	0	0	0.98	84	0	0.03	0.26	0.03	0.06	22	0.56	25	0.6	5	86	63	62	0.53
2.69	1.26	0	0	1.54	110.33	0	0.03	0.24	0.03	0.06	17.11	0.41	24.78	0.7	5.31	87.32	59.59	159.3	0.54
1.9	0.68	0	0	0.45	95	0	0.02	0.22	0.03	0.06	17.5	0.4	24.5	0.72	5	88.5	60	140	0.55
10.49	4.73	0	0	1.85	429	0.44	0.11	0.96	0.17	0.26	66	1.69	156.2	2.64	26.4	374	303.6	616	2.2
1.9	0.68	0.65	25	1.03	95.5	0	0.03	0.25	0.04	0.07	23.5	0.5	24.5	0.72	5	89	60.5	63	0.55
4.88	1.19	0	0	2.57	0	0	0.03	0.21	0	0	0	0	79.3	250	15.57	181.05	278.89	191.05	2.88
0.43	0.02	0	0	0	0	0	0.03	0.21	0	0	0	0	79.3	250	15.57	181.05	278.89	191.05	2.88
0.62	0.08	0	0	0.15	19.6	2.4	0.08	0.38	0.14	0.08	12.25	0.54	285.18	285	26.83	218.54	370.68	257	1.03
0.75	0.09	2.5	0	0	147.5	2.32	0.09	0.41	0.32	0.1	12	0.85	286.75	285	33.32	256.5	425.5	151.75	1.03
1.47	0.18	2.5	0	0.13	142.5	2.3	0.09	0.41	0.31	0.1	12	0.85	284	285	33	254.25	422	150.5	1.03
2.47	0.31	2.5	0	0.23	72.5	2.27	0.09	0.4	0.31	0.1	11.75	0.83	280.25	280	32.57	251.25	417.25	149	1.03
2.65	0.33	0	0	0.26	85	2.4	0.1	0.43	0.36	0.11	12.25	0.87	298.25	315	55.5	270	479.75	122.75	1.23
0	0.2	0	0	0.65	62	2	0.06	0.32	0.2	0.04	8	0.34	216	108	20	194	284	98	0.98
5.88	0.62	0	0	0	135.97	4.73	0.12	0.8	0.49	0.13	19.89	0.41	656.66	0.48	60.91	509.87	763.17	266.39	1.94
0.16	0.02	5.1	0	0.01	298.33	0.06	0.11	0.79	0.44	0.14	21.93	0.61	738.18	0.74	68.85	496.96	845.27	293.23	2.29
0.75	0.1	2.44	0	0.1	143.96	2.37	0.1	0.41	0.21	0.1	12.44	0.9	300.12	0.12	33.72	234.73	380.88	123.22	0.95
2.78	0.56	0	0	0	95.4	2.92	0.2	0.59	1.31	0.19	21.73	1.03	355.1	0.27	53	302.1	530	222.6	1.14
2.57	0.38	0	0	0	79.5	2.65	0.13	0.44	0.63	0.14	16.43	0.93	304.75	0.61	47.7	265	498.2	172.25	1.09
0.12	0.02	2.45	9.8	0.1	149.45	2.4	0.09	0.34	0.22	0.1	12.74	0.93	302.33	0.1	27.83	247.2	405.72	126.17	0.98
1.35	0.17	2.44	0	0.17	139.08	2.32	0.1	0.4	0.21	0.1	12.44	0.89	296.7	0.12	33.35	232.04	376.74	121.76	0.95
2.35	0.3	2.44	9.76	0.24	75.64	2.29	0.09	0.4	0.2	0.1	12.2	0.87	291.34	0.12	32.79	227.9	369.66	119.56	0.93
2.58	0.33	0	0	0	82.96	3.59	0.09	0.39	0.2	0.1	12.2	0.87	290.36	0.12	32.7	227.16	368.44	119.07	0.93
0.73	0.09	0	0	0.07	23.4	0.1	0	0.02	0.01	0	1.3	0.04	13.97	0.01	1.35	10.19	17.28	6.4	0.03
0	0	0	0	0	30.03	0	0	0	0	0	0	0	36.03	0	0	0	0	17.51	0
0.08	0.01	0	0	0.02	0	0	0	0	0	0	0	0	0.36	0.06	0.92	6.39	23.03	14.64	0.17
0	0	0	0	0	18.3	0	0	0	0	0	0	0	21.96	0	0	0	27.45	9.15	0
0	0	0	0	0	30	0	0	0	0	0	0	0	36	0	0	0	0	17.5	0
0	0	0	0	0	0	12	0	0	0	0	0	0	280	0	0	0	0	140	0
0	0	0	0	0	0	12	0	0	0	0	0	0	280	0	0	0	0	130	0
0	0	0	0	0	0	2.4	0	0	0	0	0	0	280	0.4	0	0	0	125	0
0	0	0	0	0	40	0	0	0	0	0	0	0	192	0	0	0	0	100	0
0	0	0	0	0	39.97	0	0	0	0	0	0	0	191.88	0	0	0	0	139.91	0
0	0	0	0	0	40	0	0	0	0	0	0	0	192	0	0	0	0	100	0
0	0	0	0	0	0	0	0	0	0	0	0	0	437.57	0	0	0	422.99	153.15	0

USDA ID Code	Food Name	Weight in Grams*	Quantity of Units	Unit of Measure	Protein (gm)	Fat (gm)	Carbohydrates (gm)	Kcalories	Caffeine (gm)	Fiber (gm)	Cholesterol (mg)	Saturated Fat (gm)
62627	Yogurt, Fruit, Fat Free, Light	247.957	1	Cup	10	0	19	109.98	0	0	5	0
1121	Yogurt, Fruit, Lowfat, 10 Gm Protein Per 8 Oz	227	1	Cup	9.92	2.45	43.24	231.26	0	0	9.53	1.58
1122	Yogurt, Fruit, Lowfat, 11 Gm Protein Per 8 Oz	227	1	Cup	11.03	3.2	42.22	238.64	0	0	12.48	2.06
1120	Yogurt, Fruit, Lowfat, 9 Gm Protein Per 8 Oz	227	1	Cup	9.03	2.61	42.31	225.27	0	0	10.21	1.68
62603	Yogurt, Plain, Fat Free	247.957	1	Cup	13	0	17	119.98	0	0	5	0
1117	Yogurt, Plain, Lowfat, 12 Gm Protein Per 8 Oz	227	1	Cup	11.92	3.52	15.98	143.66	0	0	13.85	2.27
1118	Yogurt, Plain, Skim Milk, 13 Gm Protein Per 8 Oz	227	1	Cup	13.01	0.41	17.43	126.6	0	0	4.09	0.26
1116	Yogurt, Plain, Whole Milk, 8 Gm Protein Per 8 Oz	227	1	Cup	7.88	7.38	10.58	139.42	0	0	28.83	4.76
1119	Yogurt, Vanilla, Lowfat, 11 Gm Protein Per 8 Oz	227	1	Cup	11.19	2.84	31.33	193.96	0	0	11.12	1.83
4136	Butter, w/ Salt	5	1	Pat	0.05	4.06	0.01	35.85	0	0	10.95	2.53
1145	Butter, w/o Salt	5	1	Pat	0.04	4.06	0	35.84	0	0	10.95	2.52
1002	Butter, Whipped	11.011	1	Tbsp.	0.09	8.93	0.01	78.93	0	0	24.1	5.56
4002	Lard	205	0.25	Cup	0	51.2	0	460	0	0	48	20
4067	Margarine, Hard, Corn&sybn	4.7	1	Tsp.	0.04	3.78	0.04	33.78	0	0	0	0.71
4071	Margarine, Hard, Corn(hydr)	4.7	1	Tsp.	0.04	3.78	0.04	33.78	0	0	0	0.62
4128	Margarine, Imitation (appx 40% Fat)	4.805	1	Tsp.	0.02	1.86	0.02	16.59	0	0	0	0.37
4132	Margarine, Regular, w/ Salt Added	4.7	1	Tsp.	0.04	3.78	0.04	33.78	0	0	0	0.74
4131	Margarine, Regular, w/o Added Salt	4.7	1	Tsp.	0.02	3.77	0.02	33.56	0	0	0	0.71
4130	Margarine, Soft, w/ Salt Added	4.701	1	Tsp.	0.04	3.78	0.02	33.68	0	0	0	0.65
4129	Margarine, Soft, w/o Added Salt	4.701	1	Tsp.	0.04	3.78	0.04	33.68	0	0	0	0.65
4018	Mayonnaise	14.7	1	Tbsp.	0.13	4.91	3.51	57.29	0	0	3.82	0.72
62610	Mayonnaise, Fat Free	15.007	1	Tbsp.	0	0	3	10	0	0	0	0
62609	Mayonnaise, Light	15.007	1	Tbsp.	0	2	1	25.01	0	0	5	0
4053	Oil, Olive	13.511	1	Tbsp.	0	13.51	0	119.44	0	0	0	1.82
4042	Oil, Peanut	13.511	1	Tbsp.	0	13.51	0	119.44	0	0	0	2.28
4058	Oil, Sesame	13.637	1	Tbsp.	0	13.64	0	120.55	0	0	0	1.94
4044	Oil, Soybean	13.637	1	Tbsp.	0	13.64	0	120.55	0	0	0	1.96
4034	Oil, Soybean, (hydr)	13.637	1	Tbsp.	0	13.64	0	120.55	0	0	0	2.03
4543	Oil, Soybean, (hydr)&cttnsd	13.637	1	Tbsp.	0	13.64	0	120.55	0	0	0	2.45
4518	Oil, Vegetable Corn	13.637	1	Tbsp.	0	13.64	0	120.55	0	0	0	1.73
4582	Oil, Vegetable, Canola	13.637	1	Tbsp.	0	13.64	0	120.55	0	0	0	0.97
4501	Oil, Vegetable, Cocoa Butter	13.637	1	Tbsp.	0	13.64	0	120.55	0	0	0	8.14
4502	Oil, Vegetable, Cottonseed	13.637	1	Tbsp.	0	13.64	0	120.55	0	0	0	3.53
4055	Oil, Vegetable, Palm	13.637	1	Tbsp.	0	13.64	0	120.55	0	0	0	6.72
4513	Oil, Vegetable, Palm Kernel	13.637	1	Tbsp.	0	13.64	0	117.55	0	0	0	11.11
4510	Oil, Vegetable, Safflower, Linoleic	13.637	1	Tbsp.	0	13.64	0	120.55	0	0	0	1.24
4511	Oil, Vegetable, Safflower, Oleic	13.637	1	Tbsp.	0	13.64	0	120.55	0	0	0	0.83
4584	Oil, Vegetable, Sunflower	13.637	1	Tbsp.	0	13.64	0	120.55	0	0	0	1.33
62541	Salad Dressing, Blue Cheese	16.014	2	Tbsp.	0.5	3.5	2.5	45.04	0	0	5	2
62542	Salad Dressing, Blue Cheese, Fat Free	17.508	2	Tbsp.	0.25	0	6	25.01	0	0	0	0
	Salad Dressing, Ceasar	17.12	2	Tbsp.	0.17	17.12	1.31	155	0	0	1.11	3.22
	Salad Dressing, Creamy Italian	29.4	2	Tbsp.	0.03	16.12	2.33	147.43	0	0	1.22	2.43
4120	Salad Dressing, French	15.638	2	Tbsp.	0.09	6.41	2.74	67.2	0	0	9.07	1.49
62545	Salad Dressing, French, Fat Free	17.508	2	Tbsp.	0	0	6	25.01	0	0	0	0
4020	Salad Dressing, French, Lo Fat	16.264	2	Tbsp.	0.03	0.94	3.53	21.83	0	0.05	0.98	0.13
	Salad Dressing, Honey Mustard	31.2	2	Tbsp.	0.05	6.33	14.22	102.11	0	0.23	0	1.33
4114	Salad Dressing, Italian	14.7	2	Tbsp.	0.1	7.1	1.5	68.69	0	0	0	1.03
62543	Salad Dressing, Italian, Fat Free	15.51	2	Tbsp.	0	0	1	5	0	0	0	0
4021	Salad Dressing, Italian, Lo Cal	15.013	2	Tbsp.	0.02	1.47	0.74	15.82	0	0.02	0.9	0.2
	Salad Dressing, Peppercorn	26.8	2	Tbsp.	0.02	16.22	1.1	151.22	0	0	13.11	3.11
	Salad Dressing, Poppy Seed	29.4	2	Tbsp.	0.02	12.31	6.41	130.44	0	0	0	2.33
62539	Salad Dressing, Ranch	14.519	2	Tbsp.	0	9.01	1	85.11	0	0	2.5	1.5
62540	Salad Dressing, Ranch, Fat Free	17.508	2	Tbsp.	0	0	5.5	25.01	0	0	0	0
	Salad Dressing, Raspberry Vinegrette	14.7	2	Tbsp.	0.1	7.1	1.5	68.69	0	0	0	1.03
4015	Salad Dressing, Russian	15.325	2	Tbsp.	0.25	7.79	1.59	75.71	0	0	2.76	1.12

Monounsaturated Fat (gm)	Polyunsaturated Fat (gm)	Vitamin D (mg)	Vitamin K (mg)	Vitamin E (mg)	Vitamin A (re)	Vitamin C (mg)	Thiamin (mg)	Riboflavin (mg)	Niacin (mg)	Vitamin B6 (mg)	Folate (mcg)	Vitamin B12 (mcg)	Calcium (mg)	Iron (mg)	Magnesium (mg)	Phosphorus (mg)	Potassium (mg)	Sodium (mg)	Zinc (mg)
0	0	0	0	0	0	15	0	0	0	0	0	0	419.93	0.2	0	0	509.91	159.97	0
0.67	0.07	0	0	0.07	24.97	1.5	0.08	0.4	0.22	0.09	21.11	1.06	344.81	0.16	33.07	271.04	441.51	132.57	1.68
0.88	0.09	0	0	0	34.05	1.68	0.09	0.45	0.24	0.1	23.61	1.18	383.4	0.16	36.77	301.23	491	147.32	1.86
0.72	0.07	0	0	0.07	27.24	1.36	0.08	0.37	0.2	0.08	19.29	0.97	313.94	0.14	30.12	246.75	402.02	120.76	1.52
0	0	0	0	0	0	3.6	0	0.25	0	0	0	0	479.92	0	0	0.21	599.9	169.97	0
0.97	0.1	0	0	0.1	36.32	1.82	0.1	0.49	0.26	0.11	25.42	1.28	414.5	0.18	39.61	325.74	530.73	159.35	2.02
0.11	0.01	0	0	0.01	4.54	1.97	0.11	0.53	0.28	0.12	27.69	1.39	451.96	0.2	43.36	355.25	578.62	173.65	2.2
2.03	0.21	0	0	0.2	68.1	1.2	0.07	0.32	0.17	0.07	16.8	0.84	273.99	0.11	26.29	215.42	350.94	105.33	1.34
0.78	0.08	0	0	0.08	29.51	1.7	0.1	0.46	0.24	0.1	23.83	1.2	388.85	0.16	37.3	305.54	497.81	149.37	1.88
1.17	0.15	0	0	0.08	37.7	0	0	0	0	0	0.15	0.01	1.2	0.01	0.1	1.15	1.3	41.3	0
1.17	0.15	0	0	0.08	37.7	0	0	0	0	0	0.14	0.01	1.18	0.01	0.11	1.14	1.3	0.55	0
2.58	0.33	0	0	0.17	83.02	0	0	0	0	0	0.31	0.01	2.59	0.02	0.24	2.51	2.86	91.01	0.01
92.46	5.6	0	0	2.46	0	0	0	0	0	0	0	0	0.14	0	0.04	0	0.04	0.02	0.23
1.73	1.18	0	0	0.52	46.67	0.01	0	0	0	0	0.06	0	1.41	0	0.12	1.08	1.99	44.34	0
2.15	0.85	0	0	0.55	46.67	0.01	0	0	0	0	0.06	0	1.41	0	0.12	1.08	1.99	44.34	0
0.75	0.66	0	0	0.11	47.71	0	0	0	0	0	0.03	0	0.86	0	0.07	0.66	1.22	46.1	0
1.68	1.19	0	0	0.6	46.67	0.01	0	0	0	0	0.06	0	1.41	0	0.12	1.08	1.99	44.34	0
1.72	1.18	0	0	0.6	46.67	0	0	0	0	0	0.03	0	0.82	0	0.07	0.63	1.16	0.1	0
1.34	1.63	0	0	0.56	46.68	0.01	0	0	0	0	0.05	0	1.25	0	0.11	0.95	1.77	50.71	0
1.75	1.21	0	0	0.41	46.68	0.01	0	0	0	0	0.05	0	1.25	0	0.11	0.95	1.77	1.29	0
1.32	2.65	0	0	0.59	12.35	0	0	0	0	0	0.92	0.03	2.06	0.03	0.29	3.82	1.32	104.48	0.03
0	0	0	0	0	0	0	0	0	0	0	0	0	0	0	0	0	10	105.05	0
0	0	0	0	0	0	0	0	0	0	0	0	0	0	0	0	0	5	130.06	0
9.96	1.13	0	7.84	1.62	0	0	0	0	0	0	0	0	0.02	0.05	0	0.16	0	0.01	0.01
6.24	4.32	0	0.27	1.75	0	0	0	0	0	0	0	0	0.01	0	0.01	0	0	0.01	0
5.41	5.69	0	1.64	0.56	0	0	0	0	0	0	0	0	0	0	0	0	0	0	0
3.18	7.9	0	0	0.85	0	0	0	0	0	0	0	0	0.01	0	0	0.03	0	0	0
5.86	5.13	0	0	2.21	0	0	0	0	0	0	0	0	0	0	0	0	0	0	0
4.02	6.56	0	0	0.63	0	0	0	0	0	0	0	0	0	0	0	0	0	0	0
3.3	8	0	0.68	2.88	0	0	0	0	0	0	0	0	0	0	0	0	0	0	0
8.03	4.04	0	113.18	0	0	0	0	0	0	0	0	0	0	0	0	0	0	0	0
4.49	0.41	0	0	0.25	0	0	0	0	0	0	0	0	0	0	0	0	0	0	0
2.43	7.08	0	0	5.22	0	0	0	0	0	0	0	0	0	0	0	0	0	0	0
5.05	1.27	0	1.09	2.97	0	0	0	0	0	0	0	0	0	0	0	0	0.02	0	0
1.55	0.22	0	0	0.52	0	0	0	0	0	0	0	0	0	0	0	0	0	0	0
1.65	10.16	0	0.95	4.69	0	0	0	0	0	0	0	0	0	0	0	0	0	0	0
10.27	1.94	0	0	4.65	0	0	0	0	0	0	0	0	0	0	0	0	0	0	0
11.4	0.52	0	0	0	0	0	0	0	0	0	0	0	0	0	0	0	0	0	0
0	0	0	0	0	0	0	0	0	0	0	0	0	12.01	0	0	0	0	235.2	0
0	0	0	0	0.2	0	0	0	0	0	0	0	0	0	0	0	0	0	170.08	0
2.22	5.89	0	0	0.77	0.44	0	0	0	0	0	0	0	12.01	0	0	0	0	317.33	0
1.77	4.13	0	0	0.43	9.77	0	0	0	0	0	0	0	0.74	0.05	0	0	0	2.33	0
1.25	3.39	0	0	1.32	3.13	15	0	0	0	0	0.66	0.02	1.72	0.06	0	2.19	12.35	214.24	0.01
0	0	0	0	0	50.02	0	0	0	0	0	0	0	0	0	0	0	0	150.07	0
0.23	0.55	0	0	0.24	0	0	0	0	0	0	0	0	1.79	0.07	0	2.28	12.85	128	0.03
1.64	3.22	0	0	0.98	0	0.3	0	0	0	0	0	0	10.11	0.11	0	0	0	74.33	0
1.65	4.12	0	0	1.52	3.53	0	0	0	0	0	0.72	0.02	1.47	0.03	0.09	0.73	2.2	115.69	0.02
0	0	0	0	0	0	0	0	0	0	0	0	0	0	0	0	0	0	145.1	0
0.3	0.9	0	0	0.23	0	0	0	0	0	0	0	0	0.3	0.03	0	0.75	2.25	118.15	0.02
1.77	4.11	0	0	0	0	0.3	0	0	0	0	0	0	0.22	0.02	0	0	0	285.32	0
1.33	2.88	0	0	0	0	0.3	0	0	0	0	0	0	0.22	0.02	0	0	0	127.11	0
0	0	0	0	0	0	0	0	0	0	0	0	0	0	0	0	0	0	135.18	0
0	0	0	0	0.3	0	0	0	0	0	0	0	0	0	0	0	0	0	155.07	0
1.65	4.12	0	0	1.52	3.53	0	0	0	0	0	0.72	0.02	1.47	0.03	0.09	0.73	2.2	115.69	0.02
1.81	4.51	0	0	1.56	31.72	0.92	0.01	0.01	0.09	0	1.59	0.05	2.91	0.09	0.23	5.67	24.06	133.02	0.07

USDA ID Code	Food Name	Weight in Grams*	Quantity of Units	Unit of Measure	Protein (gm)	Fat (gm)	Carbohydrates (gm)	Kcalories	Caffeine (gm)	Fiber (gm)	Cholesterol (mg)	Saturated Fat (gm)
4022	Salad Dressing, Russian, Low Cal	16.264	2	Tbsp.	0.08	0.65	4.49	23	0	0.05	0.98	0.1
4016	Salad Dressing, Sesame Seed	15.325	2	Tbsp.	0.48	6.93	1.32	67.91	0	0	0	0.95
4017	Salad Dressing, Thousand Island	15.638	2	Tbsp.	0.14	5.58	2.38	59	0	0.31	4.07	0.94
62544	Salad Dressing, Thousand Island, Fat Free	17.508	2	Tbsp.	0	0	5.5	22.51	0	0	0	0
4023	Salad Dressing, Thousand Island, Lo Cal	15.325	2	Tbsp.	0.12	1.64	2.48	24.31	0	0.18	2.3	0.25
4135	Salad Dressing, Vinegar and Oil	15.638	2	Tbsp.	0	7.83	0.39	70.18	0	0	0	1.42
11001	Alfalfa Seeds, Sprouted, Fresh	33	0.5	Cup	1.32	0.23	1.25	9.57	0	0.83	0	0.02
9007	Apples, Cnd, Sweetened	204	0.5	Cup	0.37	1	34.07	136.68	0	3.47	0	0.16
9009	Apples, Dehydrated, Sulfured	60	0.25	Cup	0.79	0.35	56.12	207.6	0	7.44	0	0.06
9003	Apples, Fresh, w/ Skin	138	1	Medium	0.26	0.5	21.05	81.42	0	3.73	0	0.08
9004	Apples, Fresh, w/o Skin	128	1	Medium	0.19	0.4	19	72.96	0	2.43	0	0.07
9028	Apricots, Cnd, Heavy Syrup Pack	258	1	Cup	1.32	0.23	55.34	214.14	0	0	0	0.02
9024	Apricots, Cnd, Juice Pack	248	1	Cup	1.56	0.1	30.6	119.04	0	3.22	0	0.01
9026	Apricots, Cnd, Light Syrup Pack	253	1	Cup	1.34	0.13	41.72	159.39	0	3.29	0	0.01
9022	Apricots, Cnd, Water Pack	243	0.5	Cup	1.73	0.39	15.53	65.61	0	3.16	0	0.03
9030	Apricots, Dehydrated, Sulfured	119	0.5	Cup	5.83	0.74	98.64	380.8	0	0	0	0.05
9032	Apricots, Dried, Sulfured	130	0.5	Cup	4.75	0.6	80.28	309.4	0	11.7	0	0.04
9021	Apricots, Fresh	35.333	3	Medium	1.5	0.4	11.8	51	0	1.4	0	0.01
9035	Apricots, Frozen, Sweetened	242	1	Cup	1.69	0.24	60.74	237.16	0	4.11	0	0.02
	Artichoke, Boiled, Hearts w/ Salt	84	0.5	Cup	2.923	0.134	9.391	42	0	4.536	0	0.031
	Artichoke, Boiled, Hearts w/o Salt	84	0.5	Cup	2.923	0.134	9.391	42	0	4.536	0	0.031
11705	Asparagus, Ckd	180	0.5	Cup	4.66	0.56	7.92	45	0	0	0	0.13
11015	Asparagus, Cnd	242	0.5	Cup	5.18	1.57	6	45.98	0	3.87	0	0.36
11011	Asparagus, Fresh	134	0.5	Cup	3.06	0.27	6.08	30.82	0	2.81	0	0.06
11019	Asparagus, Frz, Ckd	200	0.5	Cup	5.31	0.84	9.74	56	0	0	0	0.19
9037	Avocados, Fresh	201	1	Medium	3.98	30.79	14.85	323.61	0	11.86	0	4.9
11028	Bamboo Shoots, Cnd	131	0.5	Cup	2.25	0.52	4.22	24.89	0	3.93	0	0.12
11026	Bamboo Shoots, Fresh	151	0.5	Cup	3.93	0.45	7.85	40.77	0	3.32	0	0.1
	Banana, Dehydrated, Chips	100	1	Cup	3.89	1.81	88.28	346	0	7.5	0	0.698
9040	Bananas, Fresh	114	1	Medium	1.17	0.55	26.71	104.88	0	2.74	0	0.21
11924	Bean Sprouts	133.333	0.5	Cup	17.47	9.47	12.53	166.67	0	0	0	0
11056	Beans, Green, Cnd	136	0.5	Cup	1.56	0.14	6.12	27.2	0	2.58	0	0.03
11052	Beans, Green, Fresh	110	0.5	Cup	2	0.13	7.85	34.1	0	3.74	0	0.03
11061	Beans, Green, Fzn	135	0.5	Cup	1.84	0.19	8.26	35.1	0	4.46	0	0.04
11040	Beans, Lima, Fzn	180	1	Cup	11.97	0.54	35.01	189	0	0	0	0.12
11932	Beans, Yellow, Cnd	136	0.5	Cup	1.56	0.14	6.12	27.2	0	1.77	0	0.03
11722	Beans, Yellow, Fresh	110	0.5	Cup	2	0.13	7.85	34.1	0	1.98	0	0.03
11081	Beets, Ckd	170	1.5	Cup	2.86	0.31	16.93	74.8	0	2.89	0	0.05
9052	Blueberries, Cnd, Heavy Syrup	256	1	Cup	1.66	0.84	56.47	225.28	0	3.84	0	0
9050	Blueberries, Fresh	145	1	Cup	0.97	0.55	20.49	81.2	0	3.92	0	0
9055	Blueberries, Frozen, Sweetened	230	1	Cup	0.92	0.3	50.49	186.3	0	4.83	0	0
9054	Blueberries, Frozen, Unsweetened	155	1	Cup	0.65	0.99	18.86	79.05	0	4.19	0	0
11091	Broccoli, Ckd	156	0.5	Cup	4.65	0.55	7.89	43.68	0	4.52	0	0.08
11740	Broccoli, Flower Clusters, Fresh	88	1	Cup	2.62	0.31	4.61	24.64	0	0	0	0.05
11093	Broccoli, Frz, Chopped, Ckd	184	1	Cup	5.7	0.22	9.84	51.52	0	5.52	0	0.03
11099	Brussels Sprouts, Ckd	156	1	Cup	3.98	0.8	13.53	60.84	0	6.71	0	0.16
	Cabbage, Chinese (pak-choi)	70	1	Cup	1.05	0.14	1.56	9.1	0	0.7	0	0.018
11110	Cabbage, Ckd	150	0.5	Cup	1.53	0.65	6.69	33	0	4.2	0	0.08
11749	Cabbage, Fresh	70	1	Cup	0.85	0.13	3.76	16.8	0	0	0	0.02
11960	Carrots, Baby, Fresh	10	3	Medium	0.7	0.1	7.3	31	0	1.1	0	0.1
11125	Carrots, Ckd	156	1	Cup	1.7	0.28	16.35	70.2	0	5.15	0	0.05
11128	Carrots, Cnd, Reg Pk	146	1	Cup	0.93	0.28	8.09	33.58	0	2.19	0	0.05
11124	Carrots, Fresh	60	1	Medium	0.62	0.11	6.08	25.8	0	1.8	0	0.02
11131	Carrots, Frz, Ckd	146	0.5	Cup	1.74	0.16	12.05	52.56	0	5.11	0	0.03
11136	Cauliflower, Ckd, Boiled	124	0.5	Cup	2.28	0.56	5.1	28.52	0	3.35	0	0.09

Monounsaturated Fat (gm)	Polyunsaturated Fat (gm)	Vitamin D (mg)	Vitamin K (mg)	Vitamin E (mg)	Vitamin A (re)	Vitamin C (mg)	Thiamin (mg)	Riboflavin (mg)	Niacin (mg)	Vitamin B6 (mg)	Folate (mg)	Vitamin B12 (mcg)	Calcium (mg)	Iron (mg)	Magnesium (mg)	Phosphorus (mg)	Potassium (mg)	Sodium (mg)	Zinc (mg)
0.15	0.37	0	0	0.12	2.6	0.98	0	0	0	0	0.57	0.02	3.09	0.1	0.07	6.02	25.53	141.17	0.02
1.82	3.85	0	0	0.77	31.72	0	0	0	0	0	0	0	2.91	0.09	0	5.67	24.06	153.25	0.02
1.3	3.1	0	0	0.18	15.01	0	0	0	0	0	0.98	0.03	1.72	0.09	0.31	2.66	17.67	109.47	0.02
0	0	0	0	0	0	0	0	0	0	0	0	0	0	0	0	0	0	150.07	0
0.37	0.95	0	0	1.16	14.71	0	0	0	0	0	0.86	0.03	1.69	0.09	0.11	2.61	17.32	153.25	0.02
2.31	3.77	0	0	1.38	0	0	0	0	0	0	0	0	0	0	0	0	1.17	0.08	0
0.02	0.13	0	0	0.01	5.28	2.71	0.03	0.04	0.16	0.01	11.88	0	10.56	0.32	8.91	23.1	26.07	1.98	0.3
0.04	0.29	0	0	0.1	10.2	0.82	0.02	0.02	0.15	0.09	0.61	0	8.16	0.47	4.08	10.2	138.72	6.12	0.06
0.01	0.1	0	0	2.15	4.8	1.32	0.03	0.08	0.41	0.17	0.6	0	11.4	1.2	13.2	33	384	74.4	0.17
0.02	0.14	0	5.52	0.81	6.9	7.87	0.02	0.02	0.11	0.07	3.86	0	9.66	0.25	6.9	9.66	158.7	0	0.06
0.02	0.12	0	0.59	0.35	5.12	5.12	0.02	0.01	0.12	0.06	0.51	0	5.12	0.09	3.84	8.96	144.64	0	0.05
0.1	0.04	0	0	0	319.92	7.22	0.05	0.06	1.07	0.14	4.39	0	23.22	1.11	20.64	33.54	345.72	28.38	0.26
0.04	0.02	0	0	2.21	419.12	12.15	0.04	0.05	0.85	0.13	4.22	0	29.76	0.74	24.8	49.6	409.2	9.92	0.27
0.05	0.03	0	0	2.25	333.96	6.83	0.04	0.05	0.77	0.14	4.3	0	27.83	0.99	20.24	32.89	349.14	10.12	0.28
0.17	0.08	0	0	2.16	313.47	8.26	0.05	0.06	0.96	0.13	4.13	0	19.44	0.78	17.01	31.59	466.56	7.29	0.27
0.32	0.14	0	0	0	1507.73	11.31	0.05	0.18	4.26	0.62	5.24	0	72.59	7.51	74.97	186.83	2201.5	15.47	1.19
0.26	0.12	0	0	0	941.2	3.12	0.01	0.2	3.9	0.2	13.39	0	58.5	6.11	61.1	152.1	1791.4	13	0.96
0.06	0.1277	0	0	0.31	277	11	0.03	0.04	0.6	0.06	9	0	15	0.58	8	21	313	1	0.28
0.11	0.05	0	0	2.15	406.56	21.78	0.05	0.1	1.94	0.15	4.11	0	24.2	2.18	21.78	45.98	554.18	9.68	0.24
0.004	0.057	0	0	0.16	15.12	8.4	0.055	0.055	0.841	0.093	42.84	0	37.8	1.084	50.4	72.24	297.36	278.04	0.412
0.004	0.057	0	0	0.16	15.12	8.4	0.055	0.055	0.841	0.093	42.84	0	37.8	1.084	50.4	72.24	297.36	79.8	0.412
0.02	0.25	0	0	0	149.4	48.78	0.18	0.22	1.89	0.25	176.58	0	43.2	1.19	34.2	109.8	558	432	0.86
0.05	0.69	0	0	0	128.26	44.53	0.15	0.24	2.31	0.27	231.35	0	38.72	4.43	24.2	104.06	416.24	943.8	0.97
0.01	0.12	0	52.26	2.68	77.72	17.69	0.19	0.17	1.57	0.18	171.52	0	28.14	1.17	24.12	75.04	365.82	2.68	0.62
0.03	0.37	0	0	0	164	48.8	0.13	0.21	2.08	0.04	269.4	0	46	1.28	26	110	436	8	1.12
19.31	3.93	0	0	2.69	122.61	15.88	0.22	0.25	3.86	0.56	124.42	0	22.11	2.05	78.39	82.41	1203.99	20.1	0.84
0.01	0.23	0	0	0.5	1.31	1.44	0.03	0.03	0.18	0.18	4.19	0	10.48	0.42	5.24	32.75	104.8	9.17	0.85
0.01	0.2	0	0	1.51	3.02	6.04	0.23	0.11	0.91	0.36	10.72	0	19.63	0.76	4.53	89.09	804.83	6.04	1.66
0.153	0.337	0	0	0	31	7	0.18	0.24	2.8	0.44	14	0	22	1.15	108	74	1491	3	0.61
0.05	0.1	0	0.57	0.31	9.12	10.37	0.05	0.11	0.62	0.66	21.77	0	6.84	0.35	33.06	22.8	451.44	1.14	0.18
0	0	0	0	0	2.67	16	0.56	0.25	1.47	0.22	169.87	0	109.33	0.53	128	288	756	333.33	2.8
0.01	0.07	0	0	0.19	47.6	6.53	0.02	0.08	0.27	0.05	43.25	0	35.36	1.22	17.68	25.84	148.24	341.36	0.39
0.01	0.06	0	30.8	0.45	73.7	17.93	0.09	0.12	0.83	0.08	40.15	0	40.7	1.14	27.5	41.8	229.9	6.6	0.26
0.01	0.09	0	0	0.19	71.55	11.07	0.06	0.1	0.56	0.08	11.07	0	60.75	1.11	28.35	32.4	151.2	17.55	0.84
0.03	0.26	0	0	0	30.6	10.44	0.13	0.1	1.39	0.21	27.9	0	50.4	3.53	100.8	201.6	739.8	52.2	0.99
0.01	0.07	0	0	0.39	14.96	6.53	0.02	0.08	0.27	0.05	43.25	0	35.36	1.22	17.68	25.84	148.24	341.36	0.39
0.01	0.06	0	0	0.09	12.1	17.93	0.09	0.12	0.83	0.08	40.15	0	40.7	1.14	27.5	41.8	229.9	6.6	0.26
0.06	0.11	0	0	0.51	6.8	6.12	0.05	0.07	0.56	0.11	136	0	27.2	1.34	39.1	64.6	518.5	130.9	0.6
0	0	0	1.28	2.56	15.36	2.82	0.09	0.14	0.29	0.09	4.1	0	12.8	0.84	10.24	25.6	102.4	7.68	0.18
0	0	0	0	1.45	14.5	18.85	0.07	0.07	0.52	0.05	9.28	0	8.7	0.25	7.25	14.5	129.05	8.7	0.16
0	0	0	0	1.63	9.2	2.3	0.05	0.12	0.58	0.14	15.41	0	13.8	0.9	4.6	16.1	138	2.3	0.14
0	0	0	0	1.55	12.4	3.88	0.05	0.06	0.81	0.09	10.39	0	12.4	0.28	7.75	17.05	83.7	1.55	0.11
0.04	0.26	0	0	0.75	216.84	116.38	0.09	0.18	0.9	0.22	78	0	71.76	1.31	37.44	92.04	455.52	40.56	0.59
0.02	0.15	0	0	0	264	82.02	0.06	0.1	0.56	0.14	62.48	0	42.24	0.77	22	58.08	286	23.76	0.35
0.01	0.1	0	0	0.88	347.76	73.78	0.1	0.15	0.84	0.24	103.78	0	93.84	1.12	36.8	101.2	331.2	44.16	0.55
0.06	0.41	0	0	1.33	112.32	96.72	0.17	0.12	0.95	0.28	93.6	0	56.16	1.87	31.2	87.36	494.52	32.76	0.51
0.011	0.067	0	0	0.084	210	31.5	0.028	0.049	0.35	0.136	45.99	0	73.5	0.56	13.3	25.9	176.4	45.5	0.133
0.05	0.29	0	0	0.16	19.5	30.15	0.09	0.08	0.42	0.17	30	0	46.5	0.26	12	22.5	145.5	12	0.14
0.01	0.06	0	0	0	9.1	35.7	0.04	0.02	0.21	0.07	39.69	0	32.9	0.39	10.5	16.1	172.2	12.6	0.13
0	0.03	0	0	0	2025	7	0.07	0.04	0.7	0.11	10	0	19	0.36	11	32	233	25	0.14
0.01	0.14	0	0	0.66	3829.8	3.59	0.05	0.09	0.79	0.38	21.68	0	48.36	0.97	20.28	46.8	354.12	102.96	0.47
0.01	0.13	0	0	0	2010.42	3.94	0.03	0.04	0.81	0.16	13.43	0	36.5	0.93	11.68	35.04	261.34	351.86	0.38
0	0.05	0	7.8	0.28	1687.8	5.58	0.06	0.04	0.56	0.09	8.4	0	16.2	0.3	9	26.4	193.8	21	0.12
0.01	0.08	0	0	0.61	2584.2	4.09	0.04	0.05	0.64	0.19	15.77	0	40.88	0.69	14.6	37.96	230.68	86.14	0.35
0.04	0.27	0	0	0.05	2.48	54.93	0.05	0.06	0.51	0.21	54.56	0	19.84	0.41	11.16	39.68	176.08	18.6	0.22

USDA ID Code	Food Name	Weight in Grams*	Quantity of Units	Unit of Measure	Protein (gm)	Fat (gm)	Carbohydrates (gm)	Kcalories	Caffeine (gm)	Fiber (gm)	Cholesterol (mg)	Saturated Fat (gm)
11135	Cauliflower, Fresh	100	0.5	Cup	1.98	0.21	5.2	25	0	2.5	0	0.03
11138	Cauliflower, Frz, Ckd	180	0.5	Cup	2.9	0.4	6.75	34.2	0	3.96	0	0.06
11144	Celery, Ckd	150	0.5	Cup	1.25	0.24	6.02	27	0	2.4	0	0.06
11143	Celery, Fresh	120	0.5	Cup	0.9	0.17	4.38	19.2	0	2.04	0	0.04
9066	Cherries, Sour, Red, Cnd, Heavy Syrup Pack	256	1	Cup	1.87	0.26	59.57	232.96	0	2.05	0	0.05
9065	Cherries, Sour, Red, Cnd, Light Syrup Pack	252	1	Cup	1.86	0.25	48.64	189	0	0	0	0.06
9064	Cherries, Sour, Red, Cnd, Water Pack	244	1	Cup	1.88	0.24	21.81	87.84	0	1.95	0	0.06
9067	Cherries, Sour, Red, Cnd, X-heavy Syrup Pack	261	1	Cup	1.85	0.23	76.29	297.54	0	0	0	0.05
9063	Cherries, Sour, Red, Fresh	103	0.5	Cup	1.03	0.31	12.55	51.5	0	1.24	0	0.07
9074	Cherries, Sweet, Cnd, Heavy Syrup Pack	257	1	Cup	1.54	0.39	54.66	213.31	0	1.8	0	0.09
9072	Cherries, Sweet, Cnd, Juice Pack	250	1	Cup	2.27	0.05	34.52	135	0	1.75	0	0.01
9073	Cherries, Sweet, Cnd, Light Syrup Pack	252	1	Cup	1.54	0.38	43.57	168.84	0	1.76	0	0.09
9071	Cherries, Sweet, Cnd, Water Pack	248	1	Cup	1.91	0.32	29.16	114.08	0	1.74	0	0.07
9075	Cherries, Sweet, Cnd, X-heavy Syrup Pack	261	1	Cup	1.54	0.39	68.46	266.22	0	0	0	0.09
9070	Cherries, Sweet, Fresh	145	0.5	Cup	1.74	1.39	24	104.4	0	3.34	0	0.31
9076	Cherries, Sweet, Frozen, Sweetened	259	1	Cup	2.98	0.34	57.91	230.51	0	2.59	0	0.08
	Chives, Raw	1	1	Tsp.	0.033	0.007	0.043	0.3	0	0.025	0	0.001
11159	Coleslaw	127.892	0.5	Cup	1.65	3.34	15.87	88.25	0	0	10.23	0.49
11162	Collards, Ckd	128	0.5	Cup	1.73	0.24	7.85	34.56	0	2.56	0	0
11161	Collards, Fresh	36	1	Cup	0.57	0.08	2.56	11.16	0	1.33	0	0
11164	Collards, Frz, Chopped, Ckd	170	1	Cup	5.05	0.7	12.09	61.2	0	0	0	0
20092	Corn, Ckd	140	0.5	Cup	3.68	1.02	39.07	176.4	0	6.72	0	0.14
11901	Corn, Sweet, White, Ckd	164	1	Cup	5.44	2.1	41.18	177.12	0	9.35	0	0.32
11905	Corn, Sweet, White, Cnd	164	1	Cup	4.3	1.64	30.49	132.84	0	2.3	0	0.25
11906	Corn, Sweet, White, Cnd, Cream Style	256	1	Cup	4.45	1.08	46.41	184.32	0	3.07	0	0.17
11900	Corn, Sweet, White, Fresh	154	1	Cup	4.96	1.82	29.29	132.44	0	4.93	0	0.28
11168	Corn, Sweet, Yellow, Ckd	164	1	Cup	5.44	2.1	41.18	177.12	0	4.59	0	0.32
11172	Corn, Sweet, Yellow, Cnd, Brine Pk	164	1	Cup	4.3	1.64	30.49	132.84	0	3.28	0	0.25
11174	Corn, Sweet, Yellow, Cnd, Cream Style	256	1	Cup	4.45	1.08	46.41	184.32	0	3.07	0	0.17
11167	Corn, Sweet, Yellow, Fresh	154	1	Cup	4.96	1.82	29.29	132.44	0	4.16	0	0.28
9077	Crabapples, Fresh	110	1	Cup	0.44	0.33	21.95	83.6	0	0	0	0.05
9078	Cranberries, Fresh	95	1	Cup	0.37	0.19	12.05	46.55	0	3.99	0	0
9081	Cranberry Sauce, Cnd, Sweetened	277	1	Cup	0.55	0.42	107.75	418.27	0	2.77	0	0
9082	Cranberry-orange Relish, Cnd	275	1	Cup	0.82	0.27	127.05	489.5	0	0	0	0
11205	Cucumber, Fresh	104	0.5	Cup	0.72	0.14	2.87	13.52	0	0.83	0	0.04
9087	Dates, Domestic, Natural and Dry	178	1	Cup	3.51	0.8	130.85	489.5	0	13.35	0	0
11210	Eggplant, Ckd	96	0.5	Cup	0.8	0.22	6.37	26.88	0	2.4	0	0.04
11209	Eggplant, Fresh	82	0.5	Cup	0.84	0.15	4.98	21.32	0	2.05	0	0.03
	Endive, Raw	25	0.5	Cup	0.313	0.05	0.837	4.25	0	0.775	0	0.012
9100	Fruit Hvy Syrup	255	1	Cup	0.99	0.18	48.22	186.15	0	2.81	0	0.03
9097	Fruit Juice Pack	248	1	Cup	1.14	0.02	29.41	114.08	0	2.73	0	0
9099	Fruit Lt Syrup	252	1	Cup	1.01	0.18	37.62	143.64	0	2.77	0	0.03
9105	Fruit Salad, Hvy Syrup	255	1	Cup	0.87	0.18	48.73	186.15	0	2.81	0	0.03
9103	Fruit Salad, Juice Pack	249	1	Cup	1.27	0.07	32.49	124.5	0	0	0	0.01
9104	Fruit Salad, Lt Syrup	252	1	Cup	0.86	0.18	38.15	146.16	0	0	0	0.02
9102	Fruit Salad, Water Pack	245	1	Cup	0.86	0.17	19.28	73.5	0	0	0	0.02
9096	Fruit Water Pack	245	1	Cup	1.03	0.12	20.85	78.4	0	2.69	0	0.01
9188	Fruit, Mixed, Dried	150.004	0.5	Cup	3.69	0.74	96.09	364.51	0	0	0	0.06
9189	Fruit, Mixed, Frzn, Swtnd, Thawd	250	1	Cup	3.55	0.45	60.57	245	0	4.75	0	0.06
9187	Fruit, Mixed, Hvy Syrup	255	1	Cup	0.94	0.26	47.84	183.6	0	0	0	0.04
	Garlic, Raw	3	1	Clove	0.191	0.015	0.992	4.47	0	0.063	0	0.003
9112	Grapefruit, Fresh, Pink&red	146	0.5	Medium	0.8	0.15	11.21	43.8	0	0	0	0.02
9116	Grapefruit, Fresh, White	136	0.5	Medium	0.94	0.14	11.44	44.88	0	1.5	0	0.02
9120	Grapefruit, Sections, Cnd, Juice Pack	249	1	Cup	1.74	0.22	22.93	92.13	0	1	0	0.03
9121	Grapefruit, Sections, Cnd, Light Syrup Pack	254	1	Cup	1.42	0.25	39.22	152.4	0	1.02	0	0.04

Monounsaturated Fat (gm)	Polyunsaturated Fat (gm)	Vitamin D (mg)	Vitamin K (mg)	Vitamin E (mg)	Vitamin A (re)	Vitamin C (mg)	Thiamin (mg)	Riboflavin (mg)	Niacin (mg)	Vitamin B6 (mg)	Folate (mg)	Vitamin B12 (mcg)	Calcium (mg)	Iron (mg)	Magnesium (mg)	Phosphorus (mg)	Potassium (mg)	Sodium (mg)	Zinc (mg)
0.01	0.1	0	191	0.04	2	46.4	0.06	0.06	0.53	0.22	57	0	22	0.44	15	44	303	30	0.28
0.03	0.19	0	0	0.07	3.6	56.34	0.07	0.1	0.56	0.16	73.8	0	30.6	0.74	16.2	43.2	250.2	32.4	0.23
0.05	0.11	0	0	0.54	19.5	9.15	0.06	0.07	0.48	0.13	33	0	63	0.63	18	37.5	426	136.5	0.21
0.03	0.08	0	0	0.43	15.6	8.4	0.06	0.05	0.39	0.1	33.6	0	48	0.48	13.2	30	344.4	104.4	0.16
0.07	0.07	0	0	0.33	181.76	5.12	0.04	0.1	0.43	0.11	19.46	0	25.6	3.33	15.36	25.6	238.08	17.92	0.15
0.07	0.07	0	0	0	183.96	5.04	0.04	0.1	0.43	0.11	19.4	0	25.2	3.33	15.12	25.2	239.4	17.64	0.18
0.07	0.07	0	0	0.32	183	5.12	0.04	0.1	0.43	0.11	19.52	0	26.84	3.34	14.64	24.4	239.12	17.08	0.17
0.07	0.07	0	0	0	182.7	4.96	0.04	0.1	0.43	0.11	19.31	0	26.1	3.29	13.05	23.49	237.51	18.27	0.16
0.08	0.09	0	0	0.13	131.84	10.3	0.03	0.04	0.41	0.05	7.73	0	16.48	0.33	9.27	15.45	178.19	3.09	0.1
0.11	0.12	0	0	0.15	38.55	9.25	0.05	0.1	1.02	0.08	10.79	0	23.13	0.9	23.13	46.26	372.65	7.71	0.26
0.01	0.01	0	0	0.25	32.5	6.25	0.04	0.06	1.02	0.07	10.5	0	35	1.45	30	55	327.5	7.5	0.25
0.11	0.12	0	0	0.33	40.32	9.32	0.05	0.1	1.02	0.08	10.58	0	22.68	0.91	22.68	45.36	372.96	7.56	0.25
0.08	0.09	0	0	0.32	39.68	5.46	0.05	0.1	1.02	0.07	10.42	0	27.28	0.89	22.32	37.2	324.88	2.48	0.2
0.1	0.12	0	0	0	39.15	9.4	0.05	0.1	1.01	0.08	10.96	0	23.49	0.91	20.88	44.37	370.62	7.83	0.26
0.38	0.42	0	0	0.19	30.45	10.15	0.07	0.09	0.58	0.05	6.09	0	21.75	0.57	15.95	27.55	324.8	0	0.09
0.09	0.1	0	0	0.34	49.21	2.59	0.07	0.12	0.46	0.09	10.88	0	31.08	0.91	25.9	41.44	515.41	2.59	0.1
0.001	0.003	0	0	0.002	4.35	0.581	0.001	0.001	0.006	0.001	1.05	0	0.92	0.016	0.42	0.58	2.96	0.03	0.006
0.91	1.73	0	0	0	104.87	41.82	0.08	0.08	0.35	0.16	33.89	0	57.55	0.75	12.79	40.93	231.48	29.42	0.26
0	0	0	0	1.13	349.44	15.49	0.03	0.07	0.37	0.07	7.68	0	29.44	0.2	8.96	10.24	167.68	20.48	0.14
0	0	0	0	0.81	119.88	8.39	0.01	0.02	0.13	0.02	4.32	0	10.44	0.07	3.24	3.6	60.84	7.2	0.05
0	0	0	0	0	1016.6	44.88	0.08	0.2	1.08	0.19	129.37	0	357	1.9	51	45.9	426.7	85	0.46
0.27	0.46	0	0	0.46	8.4	0	0.07	0.03	0.78	0.08	8.4	0	1.4	0.35	50.4	106.4	43.4	0	0.88
0.61	0.99	0	0	0.15	0	10.17	0.35	0.12	2.65	0.1	76.1	0	3.28	1	52.48	168.92	408.36	27.88	0.79
0.48	0.77	0	0	0.15	0	13.94	0.05	0.13	1.96	0.08	79.7	0	8.2	1.41	32.8	106.6	319.8	529.72	0.64
0.31	0.51	0	0	0.23	0	11.78	0.06	0.14	2.46	0.16	114.69	0	7.68	0.97	43.52	130.56	343.04	729.6	1.36
0.53	0.86	0	0	0.42	0	10.47	0.31	0.09	2.62	0.08	70.53	0	3.08	0.8	56.98	137.06	415.8	23.1	0.69
0.61	0.99	0	0	0.15	36.08	10.17	0.35	0.12	2.65	0.1	76.1	0	3.28	1	52.48	168.92	408.36	27.88	0.79
0.48	0.77	0	0	0.25	26.24	13.94	0.05	0.13	1.96	0.08	79.7	0	8.2	1.41	32.8	106.6	319.8	529.72	0.64
0.31	0.51	0	0	0.23	25.6	11.78	0.06	0.14	2.46	0.16	114.69	0	7.68	0.97	43.52	130.56	343.04	729.6	1.36
0.53	0.86	0	10.78	0.14	43.12	10.47	0.31	0.09	2.62	0.08	70.53	0	3.08	0.8	56.98	137.06	415.8	23.1	0.69
0.01	0.1	0	0	0	4.4	8.8	0.03	0.02	0.11	0	0	0	19.8	0.4	7.7	16.5	213.4	1.1	0
0	0	0	0	0.1	4.75	12.83	0.03	0.02	0.1	0.06	1.62	0	6.65	0.19	4.75	8.55	67.45	0.95	0.12
0	0	0	3.88	0.28	5.54	5.54	0.04	0.06	0.28	0.04	0	0	11.08	0.61	8.31	16.62	72.02	80.33	0.14
0	0	0	0	0	19.25	49.5	0.08	0.05	0.27	0	0	0	30.25	0.55	11	22	104.5	88	0
0	0.06	0	5.2	0.08	21.84	5.51	0.02	0.02	0.23	0.04	13.52	0	14.56	0.27	11.44	20.8	149.76	2.08	0.21
0	0	0	0	0.18	8.9	0	0.16	0.18	3.92	0.34	22.43	0	56.96	2.05	62.3	71.2	1160.56	5.34	0.52
0.02	0.09	0	0	0.03	5.76	1.25	0.07	0.02	0.58	0.08	13.82	0	5.76	0.34	12.48	21.12	238.08	2.88	0.14
0.01	0.06	0	0	0.02	6.56	1.39	0.04	0.03	0.49	0.07	15.58	0	5.74	0.22	11.48	18.04	177.94	2.46	0.11
0.001	0.022	0	0	0.11	51.25	1.625	0.02	0.019	0.1	0.005	35.5	0	13	0.207	3.75	7	78.5	5.5	0.197
0.03	0.08	0	0	0.74	51	4.85	0.05	0.05	0.95	0.13	6.63	0	15.3	0.74	12.75	28.05	224.4	15.3	0.2
0.01	0.01	0	0	0.5	76.88	6.7	0.03	0.04	1	0.13	6.2	0	19.84	0.52	17.36	34.72	235.6	9.92	0.22
0.04	0.08	0	0	0.73	52.92	4.79	0.05	0.05	0.96	0.13	6.8	0	15.12	0.73	12.6	27.72	224.28	15.12	0.23
0.04	0.08	0	0	1.17	127.5	6.12	0.04	0.05	0.88	0.08	6.38	0	15.3	0.71	12.75	22.95	204	15.3	0.18
0.01	0.03	0	0	0	149.4	8.22	0.03	0.03	0.89	0.07	6.47	0	27.39	0.62	19.92	34.86	288.84	12.45	0.35
0.03	0.07	0	0	0	108.5	6.3	0.04	0.05	0.92	0.08	6.55	0	17.64	0.73	12.6	22.68	206.64	15.12	0.18
0.03	0.07	0	0	0	107.8	4.65	0.04	0.05	0.92	0.08	6.37	0	17.15	0.73	12.25	22.05	191.1	7.35	0.2
0.02	0.05	0	0	0.71	61.25	5.14	0.04	0.03	0.89	0.13	6.61	0	12.25	0.61	17.15	26.95	230.3	9.8	0.22
0.35	0.17	0	0	0	366.01	5.7	0.07	0.24	2.89	0.24	5.85	0	57	4.07	58.5	115.5	1194.04	27	0.75
0.08	0.19	0	0	1.13	80	187.5	0.04	0.09	0.99	0.06	19	0	17.5	0.7	15	30	327.5	7.5	0.12
0.05	0.11	0	0	0	48.45	175.95	0.04	0.1	1.53	0.09	7.65	0	2.55	0.92	12.75	25.5	214.2	10.2	0.18
0	0.007	0	0	0	0	0.936	0.006	0.003	0.021	0.037	0.093	0	5.43	0.051	0.75	4.59	12.03	0.51	0.035
0.02	0.04	0	0	0	37.96	55.63	0.05	0.03	0.28	0.06	17.81	0	16.06	0.18	11.68	13.14	188.34	0	0.1
0.02	0.03	0	0	0.34	1.36	45.29	0.05	0.03	0.37	0.06	13.6	0	16.32	0.08	12.24	10.88	201.28	0	0.1
0.03	0.05	0	0	0.62	0	84.41	0.07	0.04	0.62	0.05	21.91	0	37.35	0.52	27.39	29.88	420.81	17.43	0.2
0.03	0.06	0	0	0.64	0	54.1	0.1	0.05	0.62	0.05	21.59	0	35.56	1.02	25.4	25.4	327.66	5.08	0.2

USDA ID Code	Food Name	Weight in Grams*	Quantity of Units	Unit of Measure	Protein (gm)	Fat (gm)	Carbohydrates (gm)	Kcalories	Caffeine (gm)	Fiber (gm)	Cholesterol (mg)	Saturated Fat (gm)
9119	Grapefruit, Sections, Cnd, Water Pack	244	1	Cup	1.42	0.24	22.33	87.84	0	0.98	0	0.03
9131	Grapes, Fresh	92	1	Cup	0.58	0.32	15.78	57.96	0	1.1	0	0.1
9400	Juice, Apple, Unsweetened	247.791	0.75	Cup	0.15	0.27	28.94	116.46	0	0	0	0.05
11655	Juice, Carrot, Cnd.	246	0.75	Cup	2.34	0.37	22.85	98.4	0	1.97	0	0.07
9080	Juice, Cranberry, Bottled	252.586	0.75	Cup	0	0.25	36.37	143.97	0	0	0	0
9135	Juice, Grape, Cnd. Or Bottle, Unsweetened	252.586	0.75	Cup	1.41	0.2	37.79	154.08	0	0.25	0	0.06
9124	Juice, Grapefruit, Cnd. Sweetened	249.389	0.75	Cup	1.45	0.22	27.76	114.72	0	0.25	0	0.03
9123	Juice, Grapefruit, Cnd. Unsweetened	246.991	0.75	Cup	1.28	0.25	22.13	93.86	0	0.25	0	0.03
9404	Juice, Grapefruit, Pink, Fresh	247	0.75	Cup	1.24	0.25	22.72	96.33	0	0	0	0.03
9128	Juice, Grapefruit, White, Fresh	247	0.75	Cup	1.24	0.25	22.72	96.33	0	0.25	0	0.03
62534	Juice, Guava	239.912	0.75	Cup	0	0	21.63	87.86	0	0	0	0
62535	Juice, Mango	239.912	0.75	Cup	0	0	21.63	87.86	0	0	0	0
9206	Juice, Orange, Fresh	248	0.75	Cup	1.74	0.5	25.79	111.6	0	0.5	0	0.06
9215	Juice, Orange, From Concentrate	248.59	0.75	Cup	1.69	0.15	26.8	111.87	0	0.5	0	0.02
62558	Juice, Orange, w/ Added Calcium	248.59	0.75	Cup	1.69	0.15	26.8	111.87	0	0.5	0	0.02
9232	Juice, Passion-fruit, Purple, Fresh	246.991	1	Cup	0.96	0.12	33.59	125.97	0	0.49	0	0
9233	Juice, Passion-fruit, Yellow, Fresh	246.991	1	Cup	1.65	0.44	35.69	148.19	0	0.49	0	0
9273	Juice, Pineapple, Cnd.	250.189	1	Cup	0.8	0.2	34.48	140.11	0	0.25	0	0.01
9294	Juice, Prune, Cnd	255.784	1	Cup	1.56	0.08	44.63	181.61	0	2.56	0	0.01
9223	Juice, Tangerine, Cnd. Sweetened	248.59	1	Cup	1.24	0.5	29.83	124.29	0	0.5	0	0.03
9221	Juice, Tangerine, Fresh	246.991	1	Cup	1.23	0.49	24.95	106.21	0	0.49	0	0.06
11886	Juice, Tomato, Cnd w/o Salt	244	1	Cup	1.85	0.15	10.32	41.48	0	1.95	0	0.02
11540	Juice, Tomato, Cnd.w/ Added Salt	244	1	Cup	1.85	0.15	10.32	41.48	0	0.98	0	0.02
62644	Juice, V-8, Low Salt	243	8	Fl Oz	1.6	0	8.2	40	0	0.25	0	0
11578	Juice, Vegetable, Cnd.	242	1	Cup	1.52	0.22	11.01	45.98	0	1.94	0	0.03
9148	Kiwifruit, Fresh	76	1	Medium	0.75	0.33	11.31	46.36	0	2.58	0	0
11247	Leeks, Ckd	104	0.5	Cup	0.84	0.21	7.92	32.24	0	0	0	0.03
11246	Leeks, Fresh	104	0.5	Cup	1.56	0.31	14.72	63.44	0	1.87	0	0.04
9150	Lemons, Fresh, w/o Peel	58	1	Medium	0.64	0.17	5.41	16.82	0	1.62	0	0.02
11250	Lettuce, Butterhead, Fresh	56	1	Cup	0.72	0.12	1.3	7.28	0	0.56	0	0.02
11252	Lettuce, Iceberg, Fresh	56	1	Cup	0.57	0.11	1.17	7.28	0	0.78	0	0.01
11253	Lettuce, Looseleaf, Fresh	56	1	Cup	0.73	0.17	1.96	10.08	0	1.06	0	0.02
11251	Lettuce, Romaine, Fresh	56	1	Cup	0.91	0.11	1.33	8.96	0	1.34	0	0.01
	Lime, Raw	67	1	Medium	0.469	0.134	7.062	20.1	0	1.876	0	0.015
9176	Mangos, Fresh	165	0.5	Cup	0.84	0.45	28.05	107.25	0	2.97	0	0.11
9185	Melon Balls, Frozen, Unthawed	173	1	Cup	1.45	0.43	13.74	57.09	0	1.21	0	0
9181	Melons, Cantaloupe, Fresh	80	1	Wedge	0.7	0.22	6.69	28	0	0.64	0	0
9183	Melons, Casaba, Fresh	164	1	Wedge	1.48	0.16	10.17	42.64	0	1.31	0	0
9184	Melons, Honeydew, Fresh	129	1	Wedge	0.59	0.13	11.84	45.15	0	0.77	0	0
11261	Mushrooms, Ckd	156	0.5	Cup	3.39	0.73	8.02	42.12	0	3.43	0	0.1
11264	Mushrooms, Cnd, Drained Solids	156	0.5	Cup	2.92	0.45	7.74	37.44	0	3.74	0	0.06
11950	Mushrooms, Enoki, Fresh	3	1	Medium	0.07	0.01	0.21	1.02	0	0	0	0
11260	Mushrooms, Fresh	70	0.5	Cup	1.46	0.29	3.26	17.5	0	0.84	0	0.04
11269	Mushrooms, Shiitake, Ckd	145	0.5	Cup	2.26	0.32	20.71	79.75	0	3.05	0	0.08
11268	Mushrooms, Shiitake, Dried	3.6	1	Medium	0.34	0.04	2.71	10.66	0	0.41	0	0.01
9403	Nectar, Apricot, Cnd, w/ Added Vit C	250.988	0.75	Cup	0.93	0.23	36.12	140.55	0	0	0	0.02
9036	Nectar, Apricot, Cnd, w/o Vit C	250.988	0.75	Cup	0.93	0.23	36.12	140.55	0	1.51	0	0.02
9229	Nectar, Papaya, Cnd.	249.389	1	Cup	0.42	0.37	36.19	142.15	0	1.5	0	0.12
9251	Nectar, Peach, Cnd, w/o Added Vit. C	248.59	1	Cup	0.67	0.05	34.6	134.24	0	1.49	0	0
	Nectarine, Raw	136	1	Medium	1.278	0.626	16.021	66.64	0	2.176	0	0.069
11279	Okra, Ckd	160	1	Cup	2.99	0.27	11.54	51.2	0	4	0	0.07
11278	Okra, Fresh	100	0.5	Cup	2	0.1	7.63	38	0	2.6	0	0.03
11281	Okra, Frz, Ckd	184	1	Cup	3.83	0.55	15.03	68.08	0	5.15	0	0.15
11280	Okra, Frz, Unprepared	142.514	0.5	Cup	2.41	0.36	9.46	42.75	0	3.14	0	0.09
62648	Olives, Green	3	5	Each	0	0.5	0	5	0	0	0	0

Monounsaturated Fat (gm)	Polyunsaturated Fat (gm)	Vitamin D (mg)	Vitamin K (mg)	Vitamin E (mg)	Vitamin A (re)	Vitamin C (mg)	Thiamin (mg)	Riboflavin (mg)	Niacin (mg)	Vitamin B6 (mg)	Folate (mcg)	Vitamin B12 (mcg)	Calcium (mg)	Iron (mg)	Magnesium (mg)	Phosphorus (mg)	Potassium (mg)	Sodium (mg)	Zinc (mg)
0.03	0.06	0	0	0.61	0	53.19	0.1	0.05	0.61	0.05	21.47	0	36.6	1	24.4	24.4	322.08	4.88	0.22
0.01	0.09	0	0	0.31	9.2	3.68	0.08	0.05	0.28	0.1	3.59	0	12.88	0.27	4.6	9.2	175.72	1.84	0.04
0.01	0.08	0	0	0.02	0	103.08	0.05	0.04	0	0.07	0.25	0	17.35	0.92	7.43	17.35	294.87	7.43	0.07
0.02	0.17	0	0	0.02	6334.5	20.91	0.23	0.14	0.95	0.53	9.35	0	59.04	1.13	34.44	103.32	718.32	71.34	0.44
0	0	0	0	0	0	89.42	0.02	0.02	0.09	0.05	0.51	0	7.58	0.38	5.05	5.05	45.47	5.05	0.18
0.01	0.06	0	0	0	2.53	0.25	0.07	0.09	0.66	0.16	6.57	0	22.73	0.61	25.26	27.78	333.41	7.58	0.13
0.03	0.05	0	0	0.12	0	67.09	0.1	0.06	0.8	0.05	25.94	0	19.95	0.9	24.94	27.43	404.01	4.99	0.15
0.03	0.06	0	0	0.12	2.47	72.12	0.1	0.05	0.57	0.05	25.69	0	17.29	0.49	24.7	27.17	377.9	2.47	0.22
0.03	0.06	0	0	0	108.68	93.86	0.1	0.05	0.49	0.11	25.19	0	22.23	0.49	29.64	37.05	400.14	2.47	0.12
0.03	0.06	0	0.05	0.12	2.47	93.86	0.1	0.05	0.49	0.11	25.19	0	22.23	0.49	29.64	37.05	400.14	2.47	0.12
0	0	0	0	0	0	40.55	0	0	0	0	0	0	0	0	0	0	0	23.65	0
0	0	0	0	0	0	40.55	0	0	0	0	0	0	0	0	0	0	0	23.65	0
0.09	0.1	0	0.1	0.22	49.6	124	0.22	0.07	0.99	0.1	75.14	0	27.28	0.5	27.28	42.16	496	2.48	0.12
0.02	0.03	0	0	0.47	19.89	96.7	0.2	0.04	0.5	0.11	108.88	0	22.37	0.25	24.86	39.77	472.32	2.49	0.12
0.02	0.03	0	0	0	19.89	96.7	0.2	0.04	0.5	0.11	108.88	0	298.31	0.25	24.86	39.77	472.32	2.49	0.12
0	0	0	0	0.12	177.83	73.6	0	0.32	3.61	0	0	0	9.88	0.59	41.99	32.11	686.64	14.82	0
0	0	0	0	0.12	595.25	44.95	0	0.25	5.53	0	0	0	9.88	0.89	41.99	61.75	686.64	14.82	0
0.02	0.07	0	0	0.05	0	26.77	0.14	0.06	0.64	0.24	57.79	0	42.53	0.65	32.52	20.02	335.25	2.5	0.28
0.05	0.02	0	0	0.03	0	10.49	0.04	0.18	2.01	0.56	1.02	0	30.69	3.02	35.81	63.95	705.96	10.23	0.54
0.04	0.06	0	0	0.22	104.41	54.69	0.15	0.05	0.25	0.08	11.44	0	44.75	0.5	19.89	34.8	442.49	2.49	0.07
0.09	0.1	0	0	0.22	103.74	76.57	0.15	0.05	0.25	0.1	11.36	0	44.46	0.49	19.76	34.58	439.64	2.47	0.07
0.02	0.06	0	0	2.22	136.64	44.65	0.11	0.08	1.64	0.27	48.56	0	21.96	1.42	26.84	46.36	536.8	24.4	0.34
0.02	0.06	0	0	2.22	136.64	44.65	0.11	0.08	1.64	0.27	48.56	0	21.96	1.42	26.84	46.36	536.8	880.84	0.34
0	0	0	0	0	62.5	39	0.04	0.05	0	0	0	0	31	1.2	0	0	439	41	0
0.03	0.09	0	0	0.77	283.14	67.03	0.1	0.07	1.76	0.34	51.06	0	26.62	1.02	26.62	41.14	467.06	883.3	0.48
0	0	0	0	0.85	13.68	74.48	0.02	0.04	0.38	0	0	0	19.76	0.31	22.8	30.4	252.32	3.8	0
0	0.12	0	0	0	5.2	4.37	0.03	0.02	0.21	0.12	25.27	0	31.2	1.14	14.56	17.68	90.48	10.4	0.06
0	0.17	0	0	0.96	10.4	12.48	0.06	0.03	0.42	0.24	66.66	0	61.36	2.18	29.12	36.4	187.2	20.8	0.12
0.01	0.05	0	0	0.14	1.74	30.74	0.02	0.01	0.06	0.05	6.15	0	15.08	0.35	4.64	9.28	80.04	1.16	0.03
0	0.07	0	0	0.25	54.32	4.48	0.03	0.03	0.17	0.03	41.05	0	17.92	0.17	7.28	12.88	143.92	2.8	0.1
0	0.06	0	63.28	0.06	18.48	2.18	0.03	0.02	0.1	0.02	31.36	0	10.64	0.28	5.04	11.2	88.48	5.04	0.12
0.01	0.09	0	0	0.25	106.4	10.08	0.03	0.04	0.22	0.03	27.89	0	38.08	0.78	6.16	14	147.84	5.04	0.16
0	0.06	0	0	0.25	145.6	13.44	0.06	0.06	0.28	0.03	75.99	0	20.16	0.62	3.36	25.2	162.4	4.48	0.14
0.013	0.037	0	0	0.161	0.67	19.49	0.02	0.013	0.134	0.029	5.49	0	22.11	0.402	4.02	12.06	68.34	1.34	0.074
0.17	0.08	0	0	1.85	641.85	45.71	0.1	0.09	0.96	0.22	0	0	16.5	0.21	14.85	18.15	257.4	3.3	0.07
0	0	0	0	0.26	306.21	10.73	0.29	0.04	1.11	0.18	44.46	0	17.3	0.5	24.22	20.76	484.4	53.63	0.29
0	0	0	0	0.12	257.6	33.76	0.03	0.02	0.46	0.09	13.6	0	8.8	0.17	8.8	13.6	247.2	7.2	0.13
0	0	0	0	0.25	4.92	26.24	0.1	0.03	0.66	0	0	0	8.2	0.66	13.12	11.48	344.4	19.68	0
0	0	0	0	0.19	5.16	31.99	0.1	0.02	0.77	0.08	0	0	7.74	0.09	9.03	12.9	349.59	12.9	0
0.01	0.29	0	0	0.19	0	6.24	0.11	0.47	6.96	0.15	28.39	0	9.36	2.71	18.72	135.72	555.36	3.12	1.36
0.01	0.18	0	0	0.19	0	0	0.13	0.03	2.49	0.1	19.19	0	17.16	1.23	23.4	102.96	201.24	663	1.12
0	0	0	0	0	0.03	0.36	0	0	0.11	0	0.9	0	0.03	0.03	0.48	3.39	11.43	0.09	0.02
0	0.12	1.33	5.6	0.08	0	2.45	0.07	0.31	2.88	0.07	14.77	0	3.5	0.87	7	72.8	259	2.8	0.51
0.1	0.04	0	0	0.17	0	0.44	0.05	0.25	2.18	0.23	30.31	0	4.35	0.64	20.3	42.05	169.65	5.8	1.93
0.01	0.01	1.49	0	0	0	0.13	0.01	0.05	0.51	0.03	5.88	0	0.4	0.06	4.75	10.58	55.22	0.47	0.28
0.1	0.04	0	0	0	331.3	136.54	0.02	0.04	0.65	0.06	3.26	0	17.57	0.95	12.55	22.59	286.13	7.53	0.23
0.1	0.04	0	0	0.2	331.3	1.51	0.02	0.04	0.65	0.06	3.26	0	17.57	0.95	12.55	22.59	286.13	7.53	0.23
0.1	0.09	0	0	0.05	27.43	7.48	0.01	0.01	0.37	0.02	5.24	0	24.94	0.85	7.48	0	77.31	12.47	0.37
0.02	0.03	0	0	0.02	64.63	13.18	0.01	0.03	0.72	0.02	3.48	0	12.43	0.47	9.94	14.92	99.44	17.4	0.2
0.237	0.313	0	0	1.21	100.64	7.34	0.023	0.056	1.346	0.034	5.032	0	6.8	0.099	10.88	21.76	288.32	0	0.122
0.04	0.07	0	0	1.1	92.8	26.08	0.21	0.09	1.39	0.3	73.12	0	100.8	0.72	91.2	89.6	515.2	8	0.88
0.02	0.03	0	0	0.69	66	21.1	0.2	0.06	1	0.22	87.8	0	81	0.8	57	63	303	8	0.6
0.09	0.15	0	0	1.27	93.84	22.45	0.18	0.23	1.44	0.09	267.9	0	176.64	1.23	93.84	84.64	430.56	5.52	1.14
0.06	0.09	0	0	0.98	65.56	17.67	0.13	0.15	1.01	0.06	210.35	0	115.44	0.81	61.28	59.86	300.7	4.28	0.76
0	0	0	0	0	0	0	0	0	0	0	0	0	0	0	0	0	0	13	0

USDA ID Code	Food Name	Weight in Grams*	Quantity of Units	Unit of Measure	Protein (gm)	Fat (gm)	Carbohydrates (gm)	Kcalories	Caffeine (gm)	Fiber (gm)	Cholesterol (mg)	Saturated Fat (gm)
9194	Olives, Ripe, Canned (jumbo-super colossal)	8.3	1	Jumbo	0.08	0.57	0.47	6.72	0	0	0	0.08
9193	Olives, Ripe, Canned (small-extra large)	3.2	1	Small	0.03	0.34	0.2	3.68	0	0	0	0.05
11283	Onions, Ckd	239.797	2	Cup	3.26	0.46	24.34	105.51	0	3.36	0	0.07
11285	Onions, Cnd, Sol&liq	224	0.5	Cup	1.9	0.2	8.98	42.56	0	2.91	0	0.04
11282	Onions, Fresh	159.865	1	Cup	1.85	0.26	13.8	60.75	0	2.88	0	0.04
9200	Oranges, Fresh	131	1	Medium	1.23	0.16	15.39	61.57	0	3.14	0	0.02
9226	Papayas, Fresh	304	1	Medium	1.85	0.43	29.82	118.56	0	5.47	0	0.13
11808	Parsnips, Ckd, w/ Salt	156	0.5	Cup	2.06	0.47	30.47	126.36	0	0	0	0.08
11299	Parsnips, Ckd, w/o Salt	156	0.5	Cup	2.06	0.47	30.47	126.36	0	6.24	0	0.08
11298	Parsnips, Fresh	133	0.5	Cup	1.6	0.4	23.93	99.75	0	6.52	0	0.07
9241	Peaches, Cnd, Heavy Syrup Pack	256	1	Cup	1.15	0.26	51.05	189.44	0	2.56	0	0.03
9238	Peaches, Cnd, Juice Pack	248	1	Cup	1.56	0.07	28.69	109.12	0	2.48	0	0.01
9240	Peaches, Cnd, Light Syrup Pack	251	1	Cup	1.13	0.08	36.52	135.54	0	2.51	0	0.01
9237	Peaches, Cnd, Water Pack	244	1	Cup	1.07	0.15	14.91	58.56	0	2.44	0	0.01
9242	Peaches, Cnd, X-heavy Syrup Pack	262	1	Cup	1.23	0.08	68.28	251.52	0	0	0	0.01
9239	Peaches, Cnd, X-light Syrup	247	1	Cup	0.99	0.25	27.42	103.74	0	0	0	0.03
9244	Peaches, Dehydrated, Sulfured	116	0.25	Cup	5.67	1.19	96.49	377	0	0	0	0.13
9246	Peaches, Dried, Sulfured	160	0.25	Cup	5.78	1.22	98.13	382.4	0	13.12	0	0.13
9236	Peaches, Fresh	87	1	Medium	0.61	0.08	9.66	37.41	0	1.74	0	0.01
9250	Peaches, Frozen, Sliced, Sweetened	250	1	Cup	1.57	0.32	59.95	235	0	3.5	0	0.03
9340	Pears, Asian, Fresh	122	1	Medium	0.61	0.28	12.99	51.24	0	4.39	0	0.01
9257	Pears, Cnd, Heavy Syrup Pack	255	1	Cup	0.51	0.33	48.88	188.7	0	5.1	0	0.02
9254	Pears, Cnd, Juice Pack	248	1	Cup	0.84	0.17	32.09	124	0	4.96	0	0.01
9256	Pears, Cnd, Light Syrup Pack	251	1	Cup	0.48	0.08	38.08	143.07	0	5.02	0	0.01
9253	Pears, Cnd, Water Pack	244	1	Cup	0.46	0.07	19.06	70.76	0	4.88	0	0
9258	Pears, Cnd, X-heavy Syrup Pack	261	1	Cup	0.5	0.34	65.9	253.17	0	0	0	0.02
9255	Pears, Cnd, X-light Syrup Pack	247	1	Cup	0.74	0.25	30.13	116.09	0	0	0	0.01
9252	Pears, Fresh	166	1	Medium	0.65	0.66	25.08	97.94	0	3.98	0	0.04
11318	Peas and Carrots, Cnd	151.897	0.5	Cup	3.3	0.41	12.88	57.72	0	5.01	0	0.07
11323	Peas and Carrots, Frz, Ckd	160	0.5	Cup	4.94	0.67	16.19	76.8	0	5.76	0	0.12
11324	Peas and Onions, Cnd	120	0.5	Cup	3.94	0.46	10.28	61.2	0	0	0	0.08
11327	Peas and Onions, Frz, Ckd	180	0.5	Cup	4.57	0.36	15.53	81	0	5.4	0	0.06
11300	Peas, Edible-podded, Fresh	145	0.5	Cup	4.06	0.29	10.96	60.9	0	3.77	0	0.06
11305	Peas, Green, Ckd	160	0.5	Cup	8.58	0.35	25.02	134.4	0	8.8	0	0.06
11308	Peas, Green, Cnd	170	0.5	Cup	7.51	0.6	21.39	117.3	0	6.97	0	0.11
11310	Peas, Green, Cnd, Seasoned	170	0.5	Cup	5.25	0.46	15.73	85	0	0	0	0.08
11304	Peas, Green, Fresh	145	0.5	Cup	7.86	0.58	20.97	117.45	0	7.4	0	0.1
11313	Peas, Green, Frz, Ckd	160	0.5	Cup	8.24	0.43	22.82	124.8	0	8.8	0	0.08
11329	Peppers, Hot Chili, Green, Cnd	73	1	Each	0.66	0.07	4.45	18.25	0	1.39	0	0.01
11670	Peppers, Hot Chili, Green, Fresh	45	1	Each	0.9	0.09	4.26	18	0	0.68	0	0.01
11820	Peppers, Hot Chili, Red, Cnd	73	1	Each	0.66	0.07	4.45	18.25	0	0.95	0	0.01
11819	Peppers, Hot Chili, Red, Fresh	45	1	Each	0.9	0.09	4.26	18	0	0.68	0	0.01
11632	Peppers, Jalapeno, Cnd	136	0.25	Cup	1.09	0.82	6.66	32.64	0	0	0	0.08
11333	Peppers, Sweet, Green, Fresh	74	1	Medium	0.66	0.14	4.76	19.98	0	1.33	0	0.02
11821	Peppers, Sweet, Red, Fresh	74	1	Medium	0.66	0.14	4.76	19.98	0	1.7	0	0.02
11951	Peppers, Sweet, Yellow, Fresh	74	1	Medium	0.74	0.16	4.68	19.98	0	0	0	0
	Persimmon, Japanese, Raw	168	1	Medium	0.974	0.319	31.23	117.6	0	6.048	0	0.034
11941	Pickle, Cucumber ,Sour	7	1	Slice	0.02	0.01	0.16	0.77	0	0.08	0	0
11937	Pickle, Cucumber, Dill	6	1	Slice	0.04	0.01	0.25	1.08	0	0.07	0	0
11947	Pickle, Cucumber, Dill, Low Sodium	6	1	Slice	0.04	0.01	0.25	1.08	0	0	0	0
11946	Pickle, Cucumber, Sour, Low Sodium	7	1	Slice	0.02	0.01	0.16	0.77	0	0.08	0	0
11940	Pickle, Cucumber, Sweet	6	1	Slice	0.02	0.02	1.91	7.02	0	0.07	0	0
11948	Pickle, Cucumber, Sweet, Low Sodium	6	1	Slice	0.02	0.02	1.91	7.02	0	0.09	0	0
9270	Pineapple, Cnd, Heavy Syrup Pack	255	1	Cup	0.89	0.28	51.51	198.9	0	1.79	0	0.02
9268	Pineapple, Cnd, Juice Pack	250	1	Cup	1.05	0.2	39.25	150	0	1.75	0	0.01

Monounsaturated Fat (gm)	Polyunsaturated Fat (gm)	Vitamin D (mg)	Vitamin K (mg)	Vitamin E (mg)	Vitamin A (re)	Vitamin C (mg)	Thiamin (mg)	Riboflavin (mg)	Niacin (mg)	Vitamin B6 (mg)	Folate (mcg)	Vitamin B12 (mcg)	Calcium (mg)	Iron (mg)	Magnesium (mg)	Phosphorus (mg)	Potassium (mg)	Sodium (mg)	Zinc (mg)
0.42	0.05	0	0	0	2.91	0.12	0	0	0	0	0	0	7.8	0.28	0.33	0.25	0.75	74.53	0.02
0.25	0.03	0	0	0	1.28	0.03	0	0	0	0	0	0	2.82	0.11	0.13	0.1	0.26	27.9	0.01
0.06	0.18	0	0	0.31	0	12.47	0.1	0.06	0.4	0.31	35.97	0	52.76	0.58	26.38	83.93	398.06	7.19	0.5
0.03	0.08	0	0	0.43	0	9.63	0.07	0.01	0.14	0.31	21.73	0	100.8	0.29	13.44	62.72	248.64	831.04	0.65
0.04	0.1	0	0.83	0.21	0	10.23	0.07	0.03	0.24	0.19	30.37	0	31.97	0.35	15.99	52.76	250.99	4.8	0.3
0.03	0.03	0	1.77	0.31	27.51	69.69	0.11	0.05	0.37	0.08	39.69	0	52.4	0.13	13.1	18.34	237.11	0	0.09
0.12	0.09	0	0	3.4	85.12	187.87	0.08	0.1	1.03	0.06	115.52	0	72.96	0.3	30.4	15.2	781.28	9.12	0.21
0.17	0.07	0	0	0	0	20.28	0.13	0.08	1.13	0.15	90.79	0	57.72	0.9	45.24	107.64	572.52	383.76	0.41
0.17	0.07	0	0	1.56	0	20.28	0.13	0.08	1.13	0.15	90.79	0	57.72	0.9	45.24	107.64	572.52	15.6	0.41
0.15	0.06	0	0	1.33	0	22.61	0.12	0.07	0.93	0.12	88.84	0	47.88	0.78	38.57	94.43	498.75	13.3	0.78
0.09	0.12	0	0	2.28	84.48	7.17	0.03	0.06	1.57	0.05	8.19	0	7.68	0.69	12.8	28.16	235.52	15.36	0.23
0.03	0.04	0	7.44	3.72	94.24	8.93	0.02	0.04	1.44	0.05	8.43	0	14.88	0.67	17.36	42.16	317.44	9.92	0.27
0.03	0.04	0	0	2.23	87.85	6.02	0.02	0.06	1.49	0.05	8.28	0	7.53	0.9	12.55	27.61	243.47	12.55	0.23
0.05	0.07	0	0	2.17	129.32	7.08	0.02	0.05	1.27	0.05	8.3	0	4.88	0.78	12.2	24.4	241.56	7.32	0.22
0.03	0.04	0	0	0	34.06	3.14	0.03	0.06	1.36	0.05	8.12	0	7.86	0.76	13.1	28.82	217.46	20.96	0.24
0.09	0.12	0	0	0	66.69	7.41	0.05	0.05	1.98	0.05	8.15	0	12.35	0.74	12.35	27.17	182.78	12.35	0.22
0.44	0.58	0	0	0	164.72	12.3	0.05	0.13	5.6	0.18	7.66	0	44.08	6.39	66.12	187.92	1567.16	11.6	0.9
0.44	0.59	0	0	0	345.6	7.68	0	0.34	7	0.11	0.48	0	44.8	6.5	67.2	190.4	1593.6	11.2	0.91
0.03	0.04	0	0	0.61	46.98	5.74	0.01	0.04	0.86	0.02	2.96	0	4.35	0.1	6.09	10.44	171.39	0	0.12
0.12	0.16	0	0	2.22	70	235.5	0.03	0.09	1.63	0.04	8	0	7.5	0.92	12.5	27.5	325	15	0.12
0.06	0.07	0	0	0.61	0	4.64	0.01	0.01	0.27	0.03	9.76	0	4.88	0	9.76	13.42	147.62	0	0.02
0.07	0.08	0	0	1.28	0	2.81	0.03	0.06	0.62	0.04	3.06	0	12.75	0.56	10.2	17.85	165.75	12.75	0.2
0.03	0.04	0	1.14	1.24	2.48	3.97	0.03	0.03	0.5	0.03	2.98	0	22.32	0.72	17.36	29.76	238.08	9.92	0.22
0.02	0.02	0	0	1.26	0	1.76	0.03	0.04	0.39	0.04	3.01	0	12.55	0.7	10.04	17.57	165.66	12.55	0.2
0.01	0.02	0	0	1.22	0	2.44	0.02	0.02	0.13	0.03	2.93	0	9.76	0.51	9.76	17.08	129.32	4.88	0.22
0.07	0.08	0	0	0	0	2.87	0.03	0.06	0.62	0.04	3.13	0	13.05	0.57	10.44	18.27	167.04	13.05	0.21
0.05	0.06	0	0	0	0	4.94	0.02	0.05	0.99	0.03	2.96	0	17.29	0.49	12.35	17.29	111.15	4.94	0.17
0.14	0.16	0	0	0.83	3.32	6.64	0.03	0.07	0.17	0.03	12.12	0	18.26	0.42	9.96	18.26	207.5	0	0.2
0.03	0.2	0	0	0.64	876.45	10.03	0.11	0.08	0.88	0.13	27.8	0	34.94	1.14	21.27	69.87	151.9	394.93	0.88
0.06	0.32	0	0	0.51	1241.6	12.96	0.36	0.1	1.85	0.14	41.6	0	36.8	1.5	25.6	78.4	252.8	108.8	0.72
0.04	0.21	0	0	0	19.2	3.6	0.12	0.08	1.54	0.23	31.92	0	20.4	1.04	19.2	61.2	115.2	530.4	0.7
0.03	0.17	0	0	0.27	63	12.42	0.27	0.12	1.88	0.16	35.82	0	25.2	1.69	23.4	61.2	210.6	66.6	0.52
0.03	0.13	0	0	0.57	20.3	87	0.22	0.12	0.87	0.23	60.47	0	62.35	3.02	34.8	76.85	290	5.8	0.39
0.03	0.16	0	0	0.62	96	22.72	0.41	0.24	3.23	0.35	101.28	0	43.2	2.46	62.4	187.2	433.6	4.8	1.9
0.05	0.28	0	0	0.65	130.9	16.32	0.21	0.13	1.24	0.11	75.31	0	34	1.62	28.9	113.9	294.1	372.3	1.21
0.04	0.22	0	0	0	73.1	19.55	0.16	0.12	1.17	0.17	48.62	0	25.5	2.04	25.5	91.8	207.4	431.8	1.11
0.05	0.27	0	0	0.57	92.8	58	0.39	0.19	3.03	0.25	94.25	0	36.25	2.13	47.85	156.6	353.8	7.25	1.8
0.04	0.21	0	0	0.27	107.2	15.84	0.45	0.16	2.37	0.18	93.76	0	38.4	2.51	46.4	144	268.8	139.2	1.5
0	0.04	0	0	0.5	44.53	49.64	0.01	0.04	0.58	0.11	7.3	0	5.11	0.37	10.22	12.41	136.51	856.29	0.12
0	0.05	0	0	0.31	34.65	109.13	0.04	0.04	0.43	0.13	10.53	0	8.1	0.54	11.25	20.7	153	3.15	0.14
0	0.04	0	0	0.34	867.97	49.64	0.01	0.04	0.58	0.11	7.3	0	5.11	0.37	10.22	12.41	136.51	856.29	0.12
0	0.05	0	0	0.31	483.75	109.13	0.04	0.04	0.43	0.13	10.53	0	8.1	0.54	11.25	20.7	153	3.15	0.14
0.05	0.44	0	0	0	231.2	17.68	0.04	0.07	0.68	0.28	18.36	0	35.36	3.81	16.32	23.12	184.96	1989.68	0.26
0.01	0.08	0	0	0.51	46.62	66.08	0.05	0.02	0.38	0.18	16.28	0	6.66	0.34	7.4	14.06	130.98	1.48	0.09
0.01	0.08	0	0	0.51	421.8	140.6	0.05	0.02	0.38	0.18	16.28	0	6.66	0.34	7.4	14.06	130.98	1.48	0.09
0	0	0	0	0	17.76	135.79	0.02	0.02	0.66	0.12	19.24	0	8.14	0.34	8.88	17.76	156.88	1.48	0.13
0.062	0.072	0	0	0.991	364.56	12.6	0.05	0.034	0.168	0.168	12.6	0	13.44	0.252	15.12	28.56	270.48	1.68	0.185
0	0.01	0	0	0.01	1.05	0.07	0	0	0	0	0.05	0	0	0.03	0.28	0.98	1.61	84.56	0
0	0	0	0	0.01	1.98	0.11	0	0	0	0	0.06	0	0.54	0.03	0.66	1.26	6.96	76.92	0.01
0	0	0	0	0.01	1.98	0.11	0	0	0	0	0.06	0	0.54	0.03	0.66	1.26	6.96	1.08	0.01
0	0.01	0	0	0	1.05	0.07	0	0	0	0	0	0	0	0.03	0.28	0.98	1.61	1.26	0
0	0.01	0	0	0.01	0.78	0.07	0	0	0.01	0	0.06	0	0.24	0.04	0.24	0.72	1.92	56.34	0
0	0.01	0	0	0.01	0.78	0.07	0	0	0.01	0	0.06	0	0.24	0.04	0.24	0.72	1.92	1.08	0
0.03	0.1	0	0	0.26	2.55	18.87	0.23	0.06	0.73	0.19	11.73	0	35.7	0.97	40.8	17.85	265.2	2.55	0.31
0.02	0.07	0	0	0.25	10	23.75	0.24	0.05	0.71	0.18	12	0	35	0.7	35	15	305	2.5	0.25

USDA ID Code	Food Name	Weight in Grams*	Quantity of Units	Unit of Measure	Protein (gm)	Fat (gm)	Carbohydrates (gm)	Kcalories	Caffeine (gm)	Fiber (gm)	Cholesterol (mg)	Saturated Fat (gm)
9269	Pineapple, Cnd, Light Syrup Pack	252	1	Cup	0.91	0.3	33.89	131.04	0	1.76	0	0.02
9267	Pineapple, Cnd, Water Pack	246	1	Cup	1.06	0.22	20.42	78.72	0	1.72	0	0.01
9271	Pineapple, Cnd, X-heavy Syrup Pack	260	1	Cup	0.88	0.29	55.9	215.8	0	0	0	0.02
9266	Pineapple, Fresh	84	1	Slice	0.33	0.36	10.41	41.16	0	1.01	0	0.03
	Plantain, Raw	179	1	Medium	2.327	0.662	57.08	218.38	0	4.117	0	0.256
9284	Plums, Cnd, Purple, Heavy Syrup Pack	258	1	Cup	0.93	0.26	59.96	229.62	0	2.58	0	0.02
9282	Plums, Cnd, Purple, Juice Pack	252	1	Cup	1.29	0.05	38.18	146.16	0	2.52	0	0.01
9283	Plums, Cnd, Purple, Light Syrup Pack	252	1	Cup	0.93	0.25	41.03	158.76	0	2.52	0	0.02
9281	Plums, Cnd, Purple, Water Pack	249	1	Cup	0.97	0.02	27.46	102.09	0	2.49	0	0
9285	Plums, Cnd, Purple, X-heavy Syrup Pack	261	1	Cup	0.94	0.26	68.67	263.61	0	0	0	0.02
9279	Plums, Fresh	66	1	Medium	0.52	0.41	8.59	36.3	0	0.99	0	0.03
11672	Potato Pancakes, Home-prepared	28.35	1	Ounce	1.75	4.32	8.12	77.11	0	0.57	27.22	0.86
11399	Potato Puffs, Frz, Prepared	7	1	Each	0.23	0.75	2.13	15.54	0	0.22	0	0.36
11414	Potato Salad	250	0.5	Cup	6.7	20.5	27.92	357.5	0	0	170	3.57
11843	Potatoes, Au Gratin, Home-prepared	245	1	Cup	12.4	18.6	27.61	323.4	0	0	36.75	8.65
11363	Potatoes, Baked w/o Skin	202	1	Medium	3.96	0.2	43.55	187.86	0	3.03	0	0.05
11364	Potatoes, Baked, Skin only	58	1	Each	2.49	0.06	26.72	114.84	0	2.32	0	0.02
11674	Potatoes, Baked, w/ Skin	202	1	Medium	4.65	0.2	50.96	220.18	0	4.85	0	0.05
11365	Potatoes, Boiled, Ckd In Skin w/o Skin	202	1	Medium	3.78	0.2	40.66	175.74	0	3.64	0	0.05
11367	Potatoes, Boiled, Ckd w/o Skin	202	1	Medium	3.45	0.2	40.42	173.72	0	3.64	0	0.05
11366	Potatoes, Boiled, Skin only	34	1	Each	0.97	0.03	5.85	26.52	0	0	0	0.01
11376	Potatoes, Cnd, Drained Solids	180	0.5	Cup	2.54	0.38	24.5	108	0	0	0	0.1
11374	Potatoes, Cnd, Solids and Liquids	300	0.5	Cup	4.08	0.45	25.98	120	0	4.8	0	0.12
11370	Potatoes, Hashed Brown	156	0.5	Cup	3.78	21.7	11.58	238.68	0	3.12	0	8.48
11657	Potatoes, Mashed, Home-prepared	210	1	Cup	4.07	1.24	36.86	161.7	0	4.2	4.2	0.7
11930	Potatoes, Mashed, Prepared From Flakes	210	1	Cup	3.99	11.76	31.54	237.3	0	0	8.4	3.07
11368	Potatoes, Microwaved w/o Skin	156	0.5	Cup	3.28	0.16	36.32	156	0	0	0	0.04
11369	Potatoes, Microwaved, Skin only	58	1	Each	2.55	0.06	17.19	76.56	0	0	0	0.02
11675	Potatoes, Microwaved, w/ Skin	202	1	Medium	4.93	0.2	48.74	212.1	0	0	0	0.05
11671	Potatoes, O'brien, Home-prepared	194	1	Cup	4.56	2.48	30.01	157.14	0	0	7.76	1.55
11844	Potatoes, Scalloped	245	0.5	Cup	7.03	9.02	26.41	210.7	0	0	14.7	3.37
9289	Prunes, Dehydrated	132	0.5	Cup	4.88	0.96	117.57	447.48	0	0	0	0.08
9293	Prunes, Dried, Stewed, w/ Added Sugar	238	0.5	Cup	2.59	0.52	78.25	295.12	0	9.04	0	0.04
9292	Prunes, Dried, Stewed, w/o Added Sugar	212	0.5	Cup	2.48	0.49	59.53	226.84	0	13.99	0	0.04
9291	Prunes, Dried, Uncooked	161	0.5	Cup	4.2	0.84	101	384.79	0	11.43	0	0.07
11423	Pumpkin, Ckd	245	1	Cup	1.76	0.17	11.98	49	0	0	0	0.09
11424	Pumpkin, Cnd, w/o Salt	245	1	Cup	2.69	0.69	19.8	83.3	0	6.86	0	0.36
11429	Radishes, Fresh	116	0.5	Cup	0.7	0.63	4.16	19.72	0	1.86	0	0.03
11431	Radishes, Oriental, Ckd	147	0.5	Cup	0.98	0.35	5.04	24.99	0	2.35	0	0.11
11432	Radishes, Oriental, Dried	116	1	Cup	9.16	0.84	73.51	314.36	0	0	0	0.25
11430	Radishes, Oriental, Fresh	88	0.5	Cup	0.53	0.09	3.62	15.84	0	1.41	0	0.03
11637	Radishes, White Icicle, Fresh	100	0.5	Cup	1.1	0.1	2.63	14	0	0	0	0.03
9297	Raisins, Golden Seedless	145	0.66	Cup	3.4	0.5	79.5	302	0	5.8	0	0.22
9299	Raisins, Seeded	145	0.66	Cup	2.5	0.5	78.5	296	0	9.86	0	0.26
9298	Raisins, Seedless	145	0.66	Cup	3.2	0.5	79.1	300	0	5.8	0	0.22
9304	Raspberries, Cnd, Red, Heavy Syrup Pack	256	1	Cup	2.12	0.31	59.8	232.96	0	8.45	0	0.01
9302	Raspberries, Fresh	123	1	Cup	1.12	0.68	14.23	60.27	0	8.36	0	0.02
9306	Raspberries, Frozen, Red, Sweetened	250	1	Cup	1.75	0.4	65.4	257.5	0	11	0	0.01
62546	Salsa	16.517	2	Tbsp.	0	0	2.5	10.01	0	0	0	0
11439	Sauerkraut, Cnd, Sol&liq	236	0.5	Cup	2.15	0.33	10.1	44.84	0	5.9	0	0.08
11640	Shallots, Freeze-dried	14.388	1	Cup	1.77	0.07	11.61	50.07	0	0	0	0.01
11677	Shallots, Fresh	159.865	1	Cup	4	0.16	26.86	115.1	0	0	0	0.03
11458	Spinach, Ckd	180	0.5	Cup	5.35	0.47	6.75	41.4	0	4.32	0	0.08
11461	Spinach, Cnd, Drained Solids	214	0.5	Cup	6.01	1.07	7.28	49.22	0	0	0	0.17
11459	Spinach, Cnd, Reg Pk, Sol&liq	234	0.5	Cup	4.94	0.87	6.83	44.46	0	5.15	0	0.14

Monounsaturated Fat (gm)	Polyunsaturated Fat (gm)	Vitamin D (mg)	Vitamin K (mg)	Vitamin E (mg)	Vitamin A (re)	Vitamin C (mg)	Thiamin (mg)	Riboflavin (mg)	Niacin (mg)	Vitamin B6 (mg)	Folate (mg)	Vitamin B12 (mcg)	Calcium (mg)	Iron (mg)	Magnesium (mg)	Phosphorus (mg)	Potassium (mg)	Sodium (mg)	Zinc (mg)
0.03	0.1	0	0	0.25	2.52	18.9	0.23	0.06	0.74	0.19	11.84	0	35.28	0.98	40.32	17.64	264.6	2.52	0.3
0.03	0.08	0	0	0.25	4.92	18.94	0.23	0.06	0.73	0.18	11.81	0	36.9	0.98	44.28	9.84	312.42	2.46	0.3
0.03	0.1	0	0	0	2.6	18.98	0.23	0.07	0.73	0.19	11.96	0	36.4	0.99	39	18.2	265.2	2.6	0.29
0.04	0.12	0	0	0.08	1.68	12.94	0.08	0.03	0.35	0.07	8.9	0	5.88	0.31	11.76	5.88	94.92	0.84	0.07
0.057	0.124	0	0	0.483	202.27	32.936	0.093	0.097	1.228	0.535	39.38	0	5.37	1.074	66.23	60.86	893.21	7.16	0.251
0.17	0.06	0	0	1.81	67.08	1.03	0.04	0.1	0.75	0.07	6.45	0	23.22	2.17	12.9	33.54	234.78	49.02	0.18
0.04	0.01	0	0	1.76	254.52	7.06	0.06	0.15	1.19	0.07	6.55	0	25.2	0.86	20.16	37.8	388.08	2.52	0.28
0.17	0.06	0	0	1.76	65.52	1.01	0.04	0.1	0.75	0.07	6.55	0	22.68	2.17	12.6	32.76	234.36	50.4	0.2
0.01	0	0	0	1.74	226.59	6.72	0.05	0.1	0.92	0.07	6.47	0	17.43	0.4	12.45	32.37	313.74	2.49	0.2
0.17	0.05	0	0	0	65.25	1.04	0.04	0.1	0.74	0.07	6.53	0	23.49	2.14	13.05	31.32	232.29	49.59	0.18
0.27	0.09	0	0	0.4	21.12	6.27	0.03	0.06	0.33	0.05	1.45	0	2.64	0.07	4.62	6.6	113.52	0	0.07
1.32	1.85	0	0	0.04	3.97	6.24	0.04	0.05	0.61	0.11	6.8	0.05	6.8	0.44	9.36	31.47	222.83	144.02	0.24
0.3	0.06	0	0	0	0.14	0.48	0.01	0.01	0.15	0.02	1.16	0	2.1	0.11	1.33	3.36	26.6	52.22	0.02
6.2	9.34	0	0	0	82.5	25	0.19	0.15	2.22	0.35	16.75	0	47.5	1.62	37.5	130	635	1322.5	0.77
6.34	2.64	0	0	0	93.1	24.25	0.16	0.28	2.43	0.43	19.84	0	291.55	1.57	49	276.85	970.2	1060.85	1.69
0	0.09	0	0.44	0.08	0	25.86	0.21	0.04	2.82	0.61	18.38	0	10.1	0.71	50.5	101	789.82	10.1	0.59
0	0.02	0	0	0.02	0	7.83	0.07	0.06	1.78	0.36	12.53	0	19.72	4.08	24.94	58.58	332.34	12.18	0.28
0	0.09	0	1.07	0.1	0	26.06	0.22	0.07	3.32	0.7	22.22	0	20.2	2.75	54.54	115.14	844.36	16.16	0.65
0	0.09	0	0	0.1	0	26.26	0.21	0.04	2.91	0.6	20.2	0	10.1	0.63	44.44	88.88	765.58	8.08	0.61
0	0.09	0	0	0.1	0	14.95	0.2	0.04	2.65	0.54	17.98	0	16.16	0.63	40.4	80.8	662.56	10.1	0.55
0	0.01	0	0	0	0	1.77	0.01	0.01	0.42	0.08	3.3	0	15.3	2.06	10.2	18.36	138.38	4.76	0.15
0.01	0.16	0	0	0	0	9.18	0.12	0.02	1.65	0.34	11.16	0	9	2.27	25.2	50.4	412.2	468	0.5
0.01	0.19	0	0	0.12	0	37.2	0.1	0.06	2.67	0.41	13.5	0	90	2.91	42	66	729	903	1.17
9.69	2.5	0	0	0.3	0	8.89	0.12	0.03	3.12	0.43	12.01	0	12.48	1.26	31.2	65.52	500.76	37.44	0.47
0.31	0.12	0	0	0.11	39.9	14.07	0.18	0.08	2.35	0.49	17.22	0	54.6	0.57	37.8	100.8	627.9	636.3	0.61
4.84	3.26	0	0	0	44.1	20.37	0.23	0.11	1.41	0.02	15.54	0	102.9	0.46	37.8	117.6	489.3	697.2	0.38
0	0.07	0	0	0	0	23.56	0.2	0.04	2.54	0.5	19.34	0	7.8	0.64	39	170.04	641.16	10.92	0.51
0	0.02	0	0	0	0	8.87	0.04	0.04	1.29	0.29	9.63	0	26.68	3.45	21.46	47.56	377	9.28	0.3
0	0.09	0	0	0	0	30.5	0.24	0.06	3.46	0.69	24.24	0	22.22	2.5	54.54	212.1	902.94	16.16	0.73
0.67	0.11	0	0	0	110.58	32.4	0.15	0.11	1.96	0.41	16.1	0	69.84	0.91	34.92	97	516.04	420.98	0.58
3.31	1.83	0	0	0	46.55	25.97	0.17	0.23	2.58	0.44	21.31	0	139.65	1.4	46.55	154.35	926.1	820.75	0.98
0.64	0.21	0	0	0	232.32	0	0.16	0.22	3.95	0.98	2.51	0	95.04	4.65	84.48	147.84	1396.56	6.6	0.99
0.34	0.11	0	0	0	69.02	6.43	0.05	0.22	1.61	0.48	0.24	0	49.98	2.48	45.22	78.54	742.56	4.76	0.52
0.32	0.11	0	0	0	65.72	6.15	0.05	0.21	1.53	0.46	0.21	0	48.76	2.35	42.4	74.2	708.08	4.24	0.51
0.55	0.18	0	0	2.33	320.39	5.31	0.13	0.26	3.16	0.43	5.96	0	82.11	3.99	72.45	127.19	1199.45	6.44	0.85
0.02	0.01	0	0	0	264.6	11.51	0.08	0.19	1.01	0.11	20.82	0	36.75	1.4	22.05	73.5	563.5	2.45	0.56
0.09	0.04	0	36.75	2.6	5404.7	10.29	0.06	0.13	0.9	0.14	30.13	0	63.7	3.41	56.35	85.75	504.7	12.25	0.42
0.02	0.05	0	0	0	1.16	26.45	0.01	0.05	0.35	0.08	31.32	0	24.36	0.34	10.44	20.88	269.12	27.84	0.35
0.06	0.16	0	0	0	0	22.2	0	0.03	0.22	0.06	25.58	0	24.99	0.22	13.23	35.28	418.95	19.11	0.19
0.14	0.38	0	0	0	0	0	0.31	0.79	3.94	0.72	341.85	0	729.64	7.81	197.2	236.64	4053.04	322.48	2.47
0.01	0.04	0	0	0	0	19.36	0.02	0.02	0.18	0.04	24.82	0	23.76	0.35	14.08	20.24	199.76	18.48	0.13
0.02	0.05	0	0	0	0	29	0.03	0.02	0.3	0.08	14	0	27	0.8	9	28	280	16	0.13
0.03	0.2	0	0	1.02	4	3	0.1	0.19	1.1	0.32	3	0	53	1.79	35	115	746	12	0.32
0.03	0.23	0	0	1.02	0	5	0.16	0.18	1.1	0.19	3	0	28	2.59	30	79	825	28	0.18
0.03	0.2	0	0	1.02	1.45	3	0.16	0.09	0.8	0.36	4.79	0	49	2.08	33	97	751	12	0.27
0.03	0.17	0	0	1.15	7.68	22.27	0.05	0.08	1.13	0.11	26.88	0	28.16	1.08	30.72	23.04	240.64	7.68	0.41
0.07	0.38	0	0	0.55	15.99	30.75	0.04	0.11	1.11	0.07	31.98	0	27.06	0.7	22.14	14.76	186.96	0	0.57
0.04	0.22	0	0	1.13	15	41.25	0.05	0.11	0.57	0.08	65	0	37.5	1.62	32.5	42.5	285	2.5	0.45
0	0	0	0	0	40.04	1.8	0	0	0	0	0	0	0	0	0	0	0	120.12	0
0.03	0.14	0	0	0.24	4.72	34.69	0.05	0.05	0.34	0.31	55.93	0	70.8	3.47	30.68	47.2	401.2	1559.96	0.45
0.01	0.03	0	0	0	807.16	5.61	0.04	0.01	0.14	0.24	16.72	0	26.33	0.86	14.96	42.59	237.4	8.49	0.28
0.02	0.06	0	0	0	1995.11	12.79	0.1	0.03	0.32	0.55	54.67	0	59.15	1.92	33.57	95.92	533.95	19.18	0.64
0.01	0.19	0	0	1.72	1474.2	17.64	0.17	0.42	0.88	0.44	262.44	0	244.8	6.43	156.6	100.8	838.8	126	1.37
0.03	0.45	0	0	0	1878.92	30.6	0.03	0.3	0.83	0.21	209.29	0	271.78	4.92	162.64	94.16	740.44	57.78	0.98
0.02	0.36	0	0	2.23	1504.62	31.59	0.04	0.25	0.63	0.19	135.72	0	194.22	3.7	131.04	74.88	538.2	746.46	0.98

USDA ID Code	Food Name	Weight in Grams*	Quantity of Units	Unit of Measure	Protein (gm)	Fat (gm)	Carbohydrates (gm)	Kcalories	Caffeine (gm)	Fiber (gm)	Cholesterol (mg)	Saturated Fat (gm)
11457	Spinach, Fresh	56	1	Cup	1.6	0.2	1.96	12.32	0	1.51	0	0.03
11464	Spinach, Frz, Ckd	190	1	Cup	5.97	0.4	10.15	53.2	0	5.7	0	0.06
11463	Spinach, Frz, Unprepared	156	0.5	Cup	4.56	0.48	6.24	37.44	0	4.68	0	0.08
11483	Squash, Acorn, Ckd. w/o Salt	205	1	Cup	2.3	0.29	29.89	114.8	0	0	0	0.06
11486	Squash, Butternut, Ckd. w/o Salt	205	1	Cup	1.85	0.18	21.5	82	0	0	0	0.04
11493	Squash, Spaghetti, Ckd. w/o Salt	155	0.5	Cup	1.02	0.4	10.01	44.95	0	2.17	0	0.1
11642	Squash, Summer, Ckd	180	0.5	Cup	1.64	0.56	7.76	36	0	2.52	0	0.12
11641	Squash, Summer, Fresh	130	0.5	Cup	1.53	0.27	5.66	26	0	2.47	0	0.06
11644	Squash, Winter, Baked	205	0.5	Cup	1.82	1.29	17.94	79.95	0	5.74	0	0.27
11643	Squash, Winter, Fresh	116	0.5	Cup	1.68	0.27	10.21	42.92	0	1.74	0	0.05
11953	Squash, Zucchini, Baby, Fresh	11	1	Medium	0.3	0.04	0.34	2.31	0	0	0	0.01
9316	Strawberries, Fresh	149	1	Cup	0.91	0.55	10.46	44.7	0	3.43	0	0.03
9320	Strawberries, Frozen, Sweetened	255	1	Cup	1.35	0.33	66.1	244.8	0	4.85	0	0.02
9318	Strawberries, Frozen, Unsweetened	149	1	Cup	0.64	0.16	13.6	52.15	0	3.13	0	0.01
11508	Sweetpotatoes, Baked In Skin	200	1	Cup	3.44	0.22	48.54	206	0	6	0	0.05
11510	Sweetpotatoes, Boiled, w/o Skin	328	1	Cup	5.41	0.98	79.64	344.4	0	8.2	0	0.21
11659	Sweetpotatoes, Candied	226.795	1	Cup	1.97	7.37	63.19	310.71	0	0	18.14	3.06
11514	Sweetpotatoes, Mashed	255	1	Cup	5.05	0.51	59.16	257.55	0	0	0	0.11
11647	Sweetpotatoes, Syrup Pack, Drained Solids	196	1	Cup	2.51	0.63	49.71	211.68	0	0	0	0.14
9219	Tangerines, Cnd, Juice Pack	249	1	Cup	1.54	0.07	23.83	92.13	0	1.74	0	0.01
9220	Tangerines, Cnd, Light Syrup Pack	252	1	Cup	1.13	0.25	40.8	153.72	0	1.76	0	0.03
9218	Tangerines, Fresh	84	1	Medium	0.53	0.16	9.4	36.96	0	1.93	0	0.02
62654	Tator Tots	2.835	10	Each	0.3	0.5	2	14	0	0.3	0	0.1
11954	Tomatillos, Fresh	34	1	Medium	0.33	0.35	1.98	10.88	0	0.65	0	0
11883	Tomatoes, Cherry	10	1	Each	0.09	0.03	0.46	2.1	0	0	0	
11530	Tomatoes, Ckd, Boiled	240	1	Cup	2.57	0.98	13.99	64.8	0	2.4	0	0.14
11660	Tomatoes, Ckd, Stewed	101	1	Cup	1.98	2.71	13.18	79.79	0	1.72	0	0.53
11533	Tomatoes, Cnd, Stewed	255	1	Cup	2.37	0.36	16.47	66.3	0	0	0	0.05
11537	Tomatoes, Cnd, w/ Green Chilies	241	1	Cup	1.66	0.19	8.72	36.15	0	0	0	0.03
11535	Tomatoes, Cnd, Wedges In Tomato Juice	261	1	Cup	2.06	0.42	16.47	67.86	0	0	0	0.06
11531	Tomatoes, Cnd, Whole, Reg Pk	240	1	Cup	2.23	0.58	10.3	48	0	2.4	0	0.08
11529	Tomatoes, Fresh	123	1	Medium	1.05	0.41	5.71	25.83	0	1.35	0	0.06
11527	Tomatoes, Green, Fresh	123	1	Medium	1.48	0.25	6.27	29.52	0	1.85	0	0.03
11955	Tomatoes, Sun-dried	54	0.25	Cup	7.62	1.6	30.11	139.32	0	6.64	0	0.23
11956	Tomatoes, Sun-dried, Packed In Oil	110	0.25	Cup	5.57	15.49	25.66	234.3	0	0	0	2.08
11565	Turnips, Ckd	156	0.5	Cup	1.11	0.12	7.64	28.08	0	3.12	0	0.01
11564	Turnips, Fresh	130	0.5	Cup	1.17	0.13	8.1	35.1	0	2.34	0	0.01
11581	Vegetables, Mixed, Cnd	163	0.5	Cup	4.22	0.41	15.09	76.61	0	0	0	0.08
11584	Vegetables, Mixed, Frz	182	0.5	Cup	5.21	0.27	23.82	107.38	0	9.83	0	0.06
62687	Veggie Burger	90	1	Each	18	4	8	140	0	5	0	1.5
	Watercress, Raw	2.5	1	Sprig	0.058	0.003	0.032	0.275	0	0.038	0	0.001
9326	Watermelon	160	1	Cup	0.99	0.69	11.49	51.2	0	0.8	0	0
11602	Yam, Baked	136	1	Cup	2.03	0.19	37.54	157.76	0	5.3	0	0.04
20004	Barley, Cooked	193	1	Cup	3.6	0.7	44.3	157	0	31.83	0	0.1
18080	Bread Sticks, Plain	10	1	Stick	1.2	0.95	6.84	41.2	0	0	0	0.14
18083	Bread Stuffing, Plain	232	1	Cup	8.82	16.7	51.5	389.76	0	0	0	3.39
18020	Bread, Banana	60	1	Slice	2.58	7.08	33.06	202.8	0	0	25.8	1.83
18024	Bread, Cornbread	65	1	Piece	4.36	4.62	28.28	172.9	0	0	26	1.01
18025	Bread, Cracked-wheat	25	1	Slice	2.18	0.98	12.38	65	0	1.33	0	0.23
18026	Bread, Cracked-wheat, Toasted	23	1	Slice	2.19	0.97	12.37	65.09	0	0	0	0.23
18344	Bread, Dinner Roll, Egg	35	1	Each	3.33	2.24	18.2	107.45	0	1.33	17.5	0.56
18349	Bread, Dinner Roll, French	38	1	Each	3.27	1.63	19.08	105.26	0	0	0	0.36
18345	Bread, Dinner Roll, Oat Bran	33	1	Each	3.14	1.52	13.27	77.88	0	1.35	0	0.2
18342	Bread, Dinner Roll, Plain	35	1	Each	2.94	2.56	17.64	105	0	1.05	0.35	0.61
18346	Bread, Dinner Roll, Rye	35	1	Each	3.61	1.19	18.59	100.1	0	0	0	0.21

Monounsaturated Fat (gm)	Polyunsaturated Fat (gm)	Vitamin D (mg)	Vitamin K (mg)	Vitamin E (mg)	Vitamin A (re)	Vitamin C (mg)	Thiamin (mg)	Riboflavin (mg)	Niacin (mg)	Vitamin B6 (mg)	Folate (mcg)	Vitamin B12 (mcg)	Calcium (mg)	Iron (mg)	Magnesium (mg)	Phosphorus (mg)	Potassium (mg)	Sodium (mg)	Zinc (mg)
0.01	0.08	0	148.96	1.06	376.32	15.74	0.04	0.11	0.41	0.11	108.86	0	55.44	1.52	44.24	27.44	312.48	44.24	0.3
0.01	0.16	0	0	1.81	1478.2	23.37	0.11	0.32	0.8	0.28	204.25	0	277.4	2.89	131.1	91.2	566.2	163.4	1.33
0.01	0.2	0	215.28	1.49	1210.56	37.91	0.13	0.24	0.68	0.22	186.58	0	173.16	3.2	90.48	63.96	503.88	115.44	0.69
0.02	0.12	0	0	0	88.15	22.14	0.34	0.03	1.81	0.4	38.34	0	90.2	1.91	88.15	92.25	895.85	8.2	0.35
0.01	0.08	0	0	0	1435	30.96	0.15	0.03	1.99	0.25	39.36	0	84.05	1.23	59.45	55.35	582.2	8.2	0.27
0.03	0.2	0	0	0.19	17.05	5.43	0.06	0.03	1.26	0.15	12.4	0	32.55	0.53	17.05	21.7	181.35	27.9	0.31
0.04	0.24	0	0	0.22	52.2	9.9	0.08	0.07	0.92	0.12	36.18	0	48.6	0.65	43.2	70.2	345.6	1.8	0.7
0.02	0.12	0	0	0.16	26	19.24	0.08	0.05	0.72	0.14	33.28	0	26	0.6	29.9	45.5	253.5	2.6	0.34
0.1	0.54	0	0	0.25	729.8	19.68	0.17	0.05	1.44	0.15	57.4	0	28.7	0.68	16.4	41	895.85	2.05	0.53
0.02	0.11	0	0	0.14	470.96	14.27	0.11	0.03	0.93	0.1	25.17	0	35.96	0.67	24.36	37.12	406	4.64	0.15
0	0.02	0	0	0	5.39	3.75	0	0	0.08	0.02	2.2	0	2.31	0.09	3.63	10.23	50.49	0.33	0.09
0.08	0.28	0	20.86	0.21	4.47	84.48	0.03	0.1	0.34	0.09	26.37	0	20.86	0.57	14.9	28.31	247.34	1.49	0.19
0.05	0.16	0	0	0.36	5.1	105.57	0.04	0.13	1.02	0.08	38	0	28.05	1.5	17.85	33.15	249.9	7.65	0.15
0.02	0.08	0	0	0.4	5.96	61.39	0.03	0.06	0.69	0.04	25.03	0	23.84	1.12	16.39	19.37	220.52	2.98	0.19
0.01	0.1	0	0	9.14	4364	49.2	0.15	0.25	1.21	0.48	45.2	0	56	0.9	40	110	696	20	0.58
0.04	0.43	0	0	14.99	5592.4	56.09	0.17	0.46	2.1	0.8	36.41	0	68.88	1.84	32.8	88.56	603.52	42.64	0.89
1.42	0.33	0	0	0	950.27	15.2	0.04	0.1	0.89	0.09	25.85	0	58.97	2.56	24.95	58.97	428.64	158.76	0.34
0.02	0.23	0	0	0	3858.15	13.26	0.07	0.23	2.44	0.6	27.29	0	76.5	3.39	61.2	132.6	535.5	191.25	0.54
0.02	0.28	0	0	0	1403.36	21.17	0.05	0.07	0.67	0.12	15.48	0	33.32	1.86	23.52	49	378.28	76.44	0.31
0.01	0.01	0	0	1.25	211.65	85.16	0.2	0.07	1.11	0.1	11.45	0	27.39	0.67	27.39	24.9	331.17	12.45	1.27
0.05	0.05	0	0	0.86	211.68	49.9	0.13	0.11	1.12	0.11	11.59	0	17.64	0.93	20.16	25.2	196.56	15.12	0.6
0.03	0.03	0	0	0.2	77.28	25.87	0.09	0.02	0.13	0.06	17.14	0	11.76	0.08	10.08	8.4	131.88	0.84	0.2
0	0	0	0	0	0	0	0	0	0	0	0	0	0	0	0	0	24	24	0
0	0	0	0	0.13	3.74	3.98	0.01	0.01	0.63	0.02	2.38	0	2.38	0.21	6.8	13.26	91.12	0.34	0.07
0.01	0.01	0	0	0.03	6.2	2.6	0.01	0	0.06	0.01	1.5	0	0.5	0.05	1.1	2.4	22.2	0.9	0.01
0.15	0.41	0	0	0.91	177.6	54.72	0.17	0.14	1.8	0.23	31.2	0	14.4	1.34	33.6	74.4	669.6	26.4	0.26
1.06	0.89	0	0	1.28	67.67	18.38	0.11	0.08	1.12	0.09	11.11	0	26.26	1.07	15.15	38.38	249.47	459.55	0.18
0.05	0.15	0	0	0	140.25	33.92	0.12	0.09	1.82	0.04	13.77	0	84.15	1.86	30.6	51	609.45	647.7	0.43
0.03	0.07	0	0	0	93.99	14.94	0.08	0.05	1.54	0.25	21.93	0	48.2	0.63	26.51	33.74	257.87	966.41	0.31
0.06	0.17	0	0	0	151.38	38.63	0.15	0.07	1.76	0.31	26.36	0	67.86	1.2	28.71	60.03	655.11	566.37	0.42
0.09	0.24	0	0	0.77	144	36.24	0.11	0.07	1.76	0.22	18.72	0	62.4	1.46	28.8	45.6	530.4	391.2	0.38
0.06	0.17	0	28.29	0.47	76.26	23.49	0.07	0.06	0.77	0.1	18.45	0	6.15	0.55	13.53	29.52	273.06	11.07	0.11
0.04	0.1	0	57.81	0.47	78.72	28.78	0.07	0.05	0.62	0.1	10.82	0	15.99	0.63	12.3	34.44	250.92	15.99	0.09
0.26	0.6	0	0	0.01	46.98	21.17	0.29	0.26	4.89	0.18	36.72	0	59.4	4.91	104.76	192.24	1850.58	1131.3	1.07
9.53	2.27	0	0	0	141.9	111.98	0.21	0.42	3.99	0.35	25.3	0	51.7	2.94	89.1	152.9	1721.5	292.6	0.86
0.01	0.07	0	0	0.05	0	18.1	0.04	0.04	0.47	0.1	14.35	0	34.32	0.34	12.48	29.64	210.6	78	0.31
0.01	0.07	0	0	0.04	0	27.3	0.05	0.04	0.52	0.12	18.85	0	39	0.39	14.3	35.1	248.3	87.1	0.35
0.03	0.19	0	0	0	1898.95	8.15	0.07	0.08	0.94	0.13	38.47	0	44.01	1.71	26.08	68.46	474.33	242.87	0.67
0.02	0.13	0	0	0.66	778.96	5.82	0.13	0.22	1.55	0.13	34.58	0	45.5	1.49	40.04	92.82	307.58	63.7	0.89
0	0.5	0	0	0	0	0	0.25	0	4	0	0	0	96	1.5	0	0	0	380	7.5
0	0.001	0	0	0.025	11.75	1.075	0.002	0.003	0.005	0.003	0.23	0	3	0.005	0.525	1.5	8.25	1.025	0.003
0	0	0	0	0.24	59.2	15.36	0.13	0.03	0.32	0.23	3.52	0	12.8	0.27	17.6	14.4	185.6	3.2	0.11
0.01	0.08	0	6.22	0	16.46		0.13	0.04	0.75	0.31	21.76	0	19.04	0.71	24.48	66.64	911.2	10.88	0.27
0.1	0.3	0	0	1.05	3.68	0	1.19	0.52	3.2	0.18	26	0	17	2.09	35	85	145	5	1.29
0.37	0.36	0	0	0	0	0	0.06	0.06	0.53	0.01	3	0	2.2	0.43	3.2	12.1	12.4	65.7	0.09
7.4	4.89	0	0	0	160.08	3.94	0.39	0.33	3.69	0.12	39.44	0	148.48	3.8	34.8	113.68	303.92	1069.52	0.74
3.02	1.77	0	0	0	14.4	1.02	0.1	0.12	0.87	0.09	6.6	0.05	10.8	0.84	8.4	33.6	78.6	118.8	0.22
1.19	2.08	0	0	0	35.1	0.2	0.19	0.19	1.47	0.07	12.35	0.1	161.85	1.63	16.25	109.85	95.55	427.7	0.39
0.48	0.17	0	0	0	0	0	0.09	0.06	0.92	0.08	9.75	0.01	10.75	0.7	13	38.25	44.25	134.5	0.31
0.48	0.17	0	0	0	0	0	0.07	0.05	0.83	0.07	6.9	0.01	10.81	0.7	13.11	38.18	44.16	134.55	0.31
1.06	0.37	0	0	0	7.7	0	0.18	0.18	1.15	0.03	18.55	0.08	20.65	1.23	8.75	34.65	36.75	190.75	0.32
0.75	0.32	0	0	0	0	0	0.2	0.11	1.65	0.02	12.54	0	34.58	1.03	7.6	31.92	43.32	231.42	0.29
0.49	0.52	0	0	0	0.33	0	0.15	0.1	1.63	0.01	10.23	0	28.05	1.37	9.9	33.99	35.97	136.29	0.28
1.3	0.43	0	0	0	0	0.04	0.17	0.11	1.41	0.02	10.5	0.01	41.65	1.1	8.05	40.6	46.55	182.35	0.27
0.43	0.25	0	0	0	0	0	0.13	0.09	1.37	0.03	7.7	0	10.5	0.95	18.9	55.65	63	312.2	0.35

USDA ID Code	Food Name	Weight in Grams*	Quantity of Units	Unit of Measure	Protein (gm)	Fat (gm)	Carbohydrates (gm)	Kcalories	Caffeine (gm)	Fiber (gm)	Cholesterol (mg)	Saturated Fat (gm)
18347	Bread, Dinner Roll, Wheat	33	1	Each	2.84	2.08	15.18	90.09	0	0	0	0.5
18348	Bread, Dinner Roll, Whole-wheat	33	1	Each	2.87	1.55	16.86	87.78	0	0	0	0.28
18027	Bread, Egg	40	1	Slice	3.8	2.4	19.12	114.8	0	0	20.4	0.59
18028	Bread, Egg, Toasted	37	1	Slice	3.89	2.44	19.46	116.55	0	0	20.72	0.6
18029	Bread, French or Vienna	25	1	Slice	2.2	0.75	12.98	68.5	0	0.7	0	0.16
18030	Bread, French or Vienna, Toasted	23	1	Slice	2.21	0.76	12.97	68.54	0	0	0	0.16
18033	Bread, Italian	30	1	Slice	2.64	1.05	15	81.3	0	0.93	0	0.26
18034	Bread, Italian, Toasted	27	1	Slice	2.62	1.05	14.85	80.46	0	0	0	0.25
18049	Bread, Lo Cal, Oat Bran	23	1	Slice	1.84	0.74	9.5	46.23	0	0	0	0.1
18050	Bread, Lo Cal, Oat Bran, Toasted	19	1	Slice	1.81	0.72	9.35	45.41	0	0	0	0.1
18051	Bread, Lo Cal, Oatmeal	23	1	Slice	1.75	0.81	9.96	48.3	0	0	0	0.14
18052	Bread, Lo Cal, Oatmeal, Toasted	19	1	Slice	1.71	0.8	9.79	47.69	0	0	0	0.14
18053	Bread, Lo Cal, Rye	23	1	Slice	2.09	0.67	9.32	46.69	0	0	0	0.08
18054	Bread, Lo Cal, Rye, Toasted	19	1	Slice	2.05	0.65	9.16	45.79	0	0	0.19	0.08
18055	Bread, Lo Cal, Wheat	23	1	Slice	2.09	0.53	10.03	45.54	0	2.6	0	0.08
18056	Bread, Lo Cal, Wheat, Toasted	19	1	Slice	2.05	0.51	9.86	44.84	0	0	0	0.08
18057	Bread, Lo Cal, White	23	1	Slice	2	0.58	10.19	47.61	0	2.14	0	0.13
18058	Bread, Lo Cal, White, Toasted	19	1	Slice	1.96	0.57	10.01	46.93	0	0	0	0.12
18035	Bread, Mixed-grain	26	1	Slice	2.6	0.99	12.06	65	0	1.85	0	0.21
18036	Bread, Mixed-grain, Toasted	24	1	Slice	2.62	0.98	12.1	65.28	0	0	0	0.21
18037	Bread, Oat Bran	30	1	Slice	3.12	1.32	11.94	70.8	0	1.35	0	0.21
18038	Bread, Oat Bran, Toasted	27	1	Slice	3.08	1.3	11.8	69.93	0	0	0	0.21
18039	Bread, Oatmeal	27	1	Slice	2.27	1.19	13.1	72.63	0	1.05	0	0.19
18040	Bread, Oatmeal, Toasted	25	1	Slice	2.3	1.2	13.18	73	0	0	0	0.19
18041	Bread, Pita, White, Enriched	60	1	Pita	5.46	0.72	33.42	165	0	0.96	0	0.1
18042	Bread, Pita, Whole-wheat	64	1	Pita	6.27	1.66	35.2	170.24	0	4.8	0	0.26
18044	Bread, Pumpernickel	32	1	Slice	2.78	0.99	15.2	80	0	1.89	0	0.14
18045	Bread, Pumpernickel, Toasted	29	1	Slice	2.76	0.99	15.14	79.75	0	0	0	0.14
18046	Bread, Pumpkin	60	1	Slice	2.4	7.68	30.72	198.6	0	0	26.4	1.23
18047	Bread, Raisin	26	1	Slice	2.05	1.14	13.6	71.24	0	1.12	0	0.28
18048	Bread, Raisin, Toasted	24	1	Slice	2.06	1.15	13.66	71.28	0	0	0	0.28
18059	Bread, Rice Bran	27	1	Slice	2.4	1.24	11.75	65.61	0	0	0	0.19
18384	Bread, Rice Bran, Toasted	25	1	Slice	2.43	1.25	11.83	66	0	0	0	0.19
18353	Bread, Rolls, Hard (includes Kaiser)	57	1	Each	5.64	2.45	30.04	167.01	0	0	0	0.35
18060	Bread, Rye	32	1	Slice	2.72	1.06	15.46	82.88	0	1.98	0	0.2
18061	Bread, Rye, Toasted	29	1	Slice	2.73	1.04	15.4	82.36	0	0	0	0.2
18064	Bread, Wheat (includes Wheat Berry)	25	1	Slice	2.28	1.03	11.8	65	0	1.08	0	0.22
18066	Bread, Wheat Bran	36	1	Slice	3.17	1.22	17.21	89.28	0	3.06	0	0.28
18067	Bread, Wheat Bran, Toasted	33	1	Slice	3.2	1.22	17.33	90.09	0	0	0	0.28
18065	Bread, Wheat, Toasted	23	1	Slice	2.28	1.01	11.8	64.86	0	0	0	0.22
18069	Bread, White	25	1	Slice	2.05	0.9	12.38	66.75	0	0.58	0.25	0.2
18070	Bread, White, Toasted	23	1	Slice	2.07	0.92	12.51	67.39	0	0	0.23	0.21
18075	Bread, Whole Wheat	25	1	Slice	2.43	1.05	11.53	61.5	0	1.73	0	0.23
18078	Bread, Whole Wheat, Toasted	25	1	Slice	2.3	1.48	14.1	76.25	0	0	0	0.22
18351	Buns, Hamburger or Hot Dog, Mixed-grain	43	1	Each	4.13	2.58	19.18	113.09	0	1.85	0	0.61
18350	Buns, Hamburger or Hot Dog, Plain	43	1	Each	3.66	2.19	21.63	122.98	0	0	0	0.51
	Cornstarch	128	1	Cup	0.333	0.064	116.826	487.68	0	1.152	0	0.012
	Couscous, Cooked	157	1	Cup	5.95	0.251	36.455	175.84	0	2.198	0	0.046
18214	Crackers, Cheese, Regular	1	1	Each	0.1	0.25	0.58	5.03	0	0.02	0.13	0.09
18215	Crackers, Cheese, w/ Peanut Butter Filling	7	1	Each	0.88	1.62	3.99	33.74	0	0.08	0.35	0.36
62592	Crackers, Cinn. Graham Snacks, Fat Free-SnackWell	0.67	20	Each	0.04	0	0.58	2.46	0	0.02	0	0
62606	Crackers, Cracked Pepper, Fat Free-SnackWell	2.14	7	Each	0.29	0	1.85	8.56	0	0.07	0	0
18216	Crackers, Crispbread, Rye	10	1	Each	0.79	0.13	8.22	36.6	0	1.62	0	0.01
18173	Crackers, Graham, Plain or Honey	7	1	Each	0.48	0.71	5.38	29.61	0	0.19	0	0.18
18218	Crackers, Matzo, Egg	28.35	1	Each	3.49	0.6	22.28	110.85	0	0	24.95	0.16

Monounsaturated Fat (gm)	Polyunsaturated Fat (gm)	Vitamin D (mg)	Vitamin K (mg)	Vitamin E (mg)	Vitamin A (re)	Vitamin C (mg)	Thiamin (mg)	Riboflavin (mg)	Niacin (mg)	Vitamin B6 (mg)	Folate (mg)	Vitamin B12 (mcg)	Calcium (mg)	Iron (mg)	Magnesium (mg)	Phosphorus (mg)	Potassium (mg)	Sodium (mg)	Zinc (mg)
1.07	0.35	0	0	0	0	0	0.14	0.09	1.34	0.03	4.95	0	58.08	1.17	13.86	38.94	43.89	112.2	0.34
0.4	0.71	0	0	0	0	0	0.08	0.05	1.21	0.06	9.9	0	34.98	0.8	28.05	73.92	89.76	157.74	0.66
1.09	0.42	0	0	0	9.2	0	0.18	0.17	1.94	0.03	28	0.04	37.2	1.22	7.6	42.4	46	196.8	0.32
1.11	0.43	0	0	0	8.51	0	0.14	0.16	1.77	0.02	19.98	0.04	37.74	1.24	7.77	43.29	46.62	199.8	0.32
0.3	0.17	0	0	0	0	0	0.13	0.08	1.19	0.01	7.75	0	18.75	0.63	6.75	26.25	28.25	152.25	0.22
0.3	0.17	0	0	0	0	0	0.1	0.07	1.07	0.01	5.52	0	18.63	0.63	6.9	26.22	28.06	152.03	0.22
0.24	0.42	0	0	0	0	0	0.14	0.09	1.31	0.01	9	0	23.4	0.88	8.1	30.9	33	175.2	0.26
0.24	0.41	0	0	0	0	0	0.11	0.08	1.17	0.01	6.21	0	22.95	0.87	8.1	30.78	32.67	173.34	0.26
0.16	0.38	0	0	0	0	0	0.08	0.05	0.87	0.02	7.82	0	13.11	0.72	10.58	27.83	23.46	80.73	0.23
0.15	0.38	0	0	0	0	0	0.06	0.04	0.77	0.02	5.32	0	12.92	0.71	10.45	27.36	23.18	79.42	0.23
0.19	0.31	0	0	0	0.23	0.05	0.08	0.06	0.7	0.01	7.82	0	26.45	0.53	6.67	27.37	35.19	89.24	0.22
0.19	0.31	0	0	0	0.19	0.04	0.06	0.06	0.62	0.01	5.32	0.03	26.03	0.52	6.46	26.98	34.58	87.78	0.21
0.15	0.17	0	0	0	0	0.02	0.08	0.06	0.58	0.01	5.29	0.02	17.48	0.71	3.91	19.32	22.54	93.15	0.18
0.15	0.17	0	0	0	0	0.02	0.07	0.05	0.51	0.01	3.61	0.02	17.29	0.7	3.99	18.81	22.23	91.77	0.17
0.06	0.22	0	0	0	0	0.02	0.1	0.07	0.89	0.03	6.44	0.01	18.4	0.68	6.44	0	28.52	117.53	0.19
0.06	0.22	0	0	0	0	0.02	0.08	0.06	0.79	0.03	4.37	0.01	18.24	0.67	6.46	20.71	27.93	115.52	0.19
0.25	0.13	0	0	0	0	0.09	0.09	0.07	0.84	0.01	7.82	0.06	21.62	0.73	5.98	30.82	17.48	104.19	0.31
0.24	0.13	0	0	0	0.19	0.08	0.07	0.06	0.74	0.01	5.51	0.06	21.28	0.72	5.89	30.21	17.29	102.41	0.3
0.4	0.24	0	0	0	0	0.08	0.11	0.09	1.13	0.09	12.48	0.02	23.66	0.9	13.78	45.76	53.04	126.62	0.33
0.4	0.24	0	0	0	0	0.07	0.08	0.08	1.02	0.08	8.88	0.02	23.76	0.9	13.92	45.84	53.28	127.2	0.33
0.48	0.51	0	0	0	0	0	0.15	0.1	1.45	0.01	7.5	0	19.5	0.94	9.3	31.8	33.6	122.1	0.29
0.47	0.5	0	0	0	0	0	0.12	0.09	1.29	0.01	5.13	0	19.17	0.93	9.18	31.32	33.21	120.96	0.28
0.43	0.46	0	0	0	0.54	0.11	0.11	0.06	0.85	0.02	7.29	0	17.82	0.73	9.99	34.02	38.34	161.73	0.28
0.43	0.46	0	0	0	0.5	0.08	0.09	0.06	0.77	0.02	5.25	0.01	18	0.74	10.25	34.25	38.5	162.75	0.28
0.06	0.32	0	0	0	0	0	0.36	0.2	2.78	0.02	14.4	0	51.6	1.57	15.6	58.2	72	321.6	0.5
0.22	0.68	0	0	0	0	0	0.22	0.05	1.82	0.15	22.4	0	9.6	1.85	44.16	115.2	108.8	340.48	0.97
0.3	0.4	0	0	0	0	0	0.1	0.1	0.99	0.04	10.88	0	21.76	0.92	17.28	56.96	66.56	214.72	0.47
0.3	0.39	0	0	0	0	0	0.08	0.09	0.89	0.04	7.54	0	21.46	0.91	17.4	56.55	66.12	214.02	0.47
1.85	4.11	0	0	0	334.2	0.6	0.09	0.1	0.79	0.02	6.6	0.05	10.8	0.99	7.8	31.8	55.2	187.8	0.2
0.6	0.18	0	0	0	0	0.13	0.09	0.1	0.9	0.02	8.84	0	17.16	0.75	6.76	28.34	59.02	101.4	0.19
0.6	0.18	0	0	0	0	0.1	0.07	0.09	0.81	0.02	6.24	0	17.28	0.76	6.72	28.32	59.04	101.76	0.19
0.45	0.48	0	0	0	0	0	0.18	0.08	1.84	0.06	8.1	0	18.63	0.97	18.9	43.2	52.65	118.8	0.34
0.45	0.48	0	0	0	0	0	0.14	0.07	1.67	0.05	5.75	0	18.75	0.98	19	43.5	53	119.5	0.35
0.65	0.98	0	0	0	0	0	0.27	0.19	2.42	0.03	8.55	0	54.15	1.87	15.39	57	61.56	310.08	0.54
0.42	0.26	0	0	0	0	0	0.14	0.11	1.22	0.02	16.32	0	23.36	0.91	12.8	40	53.12	211.2	0.36
0.42	0.25	0	0	0	0	0.06	0.11	0.1	1.09	0.02	11.31	0	23.2	0.9	12.47	40.02	53.07	210.25	0.36
0.43	0.23	0	0	0	0	0	0.1	0.07	1.03	0.02	10.25	0	26.25	0.83	11.5	37.5	50.25	132.5	0.26
0.58	0.23	0	0	0	0	0	0.14	0.1	1.58	0.06	9	0	26.64	1.11	29.16	66.6	81.72	174.96	0.49
0.59	0.24	0	0	0	0	0	0.12	0.09	1.44	0.06	6.6	0	26.73	1.11	29.37	67.32	82.17	176.22	0.49
0.43	0.23	0	0	0	0	0	0.08	0.06	0.93	0.02	7.13	0	26.22	0.83	11.5	37.49	50.14	132.48	0.26
0.4	0.19	0	0	0	0	0	0.12	0.09	0.99	0.02	8.5	0	27	0.76	6	23.5	29.75	134.5	0.16
0.41	0.19	0	0	0	0	0	0.1	0.08	0.9	0.01	5.98	0	27.37	0.77	5.98	23.69	30.13	136.16	0.16
0.42	0.25	0	0	0	0	0	0.09	0.05	0.96	0.04	12.5	0	18	0.83	21.5	57.25	63	131.75	0.49
0.32	0.81	0	0	0	0	0	0.07	0.06	0.99	0.05	9	0	9	0.85	22.25	51.25	86.25	95.25	0.41
1.28	0.49	0	0	0	0	0	0.2	0.13	1.92	0.04	12.04	0	40.85	1.7	20.64	52.03	64.5	196.94	0.46
1.07	0.39	0	0	0	0	0	0.21	0.13	1.69	0.02	11.61	0.01	59.77	1.36	8.6	37.84	60.63	240.8	0.27
0.02	0.032	0	0	0	0	0	0	0	0	0	0	0	2.56	0.602	3.84	16.64	3.84	11.52	0.077
0.035	0.1	0	0	0.02	0	0	0.099	0.042	1.543	0.08	23.55	0	12.56	0.597	12.56	34.54	91.06	7.85	0.408
0.09	0.05	0	0	0	0.3	0	0.01	0	0.05	0.01	0.25	0	1.51	0.05	0.36	2.18	1.45	9.95	0.01
0.85	0.31	0	0	0	0	0	0.03	0.02	0.46	0.1	1.75	0	5.53	0.2	4.06	22.68	17.15	69.44	0.08
0	0	0	0	0	0	0	0	0	0	0	0	0	0	0.01	0	0	0	2.01	0
0	0	0	0	0	0	0	0	0	0	0	0	0	3.42	0.06	0	0	0	21.4	0
0.02	0.06	0	0	0	0	0	0.02	0.01	0.1	0.02	2.2	0	3.1	0.24	7.8	26.9	31.9	26.4	0.24
0.35	0.11	0	0	0	0	0	0.02	0.02	0.29	0	1.19	0	1.68	0.26	2.1	7.28	9.45	42.35	0.06
0.17	0.13	0	0	0	3.69	0	0.18	0.18	1.44	0.02	8.22	0.14	11.34	0.77	6.52	45.08	42.53	5.95	0.21

USDA ID Code	Food Name	Weight in Grams*	Quantity of Units	Unit of Measure	Protein (gm)	Fat (gm)	Carbohydrates (gm)	Kcalories	Caffeine (gm)	Fiber (gm)	Cholesterol (mg)	Saturated Fat (gm)
18400	Crackers, Matzo, Egg and Onion	28.35	1	Each	2.84	1.11	21.86	110.85	0	1.42	15.03	0.27
18217	Crackers, Matzo, Plain	28.35	1	Each	2.84	0.4	23.73	111.98	0	0.85	0	0.06
18219	Crackers, Matzo, Whole-wheat	28.35	1	Each	3.71	0.43	22.37	99.51	0	3.29	0	0.07
18220	Crackers, Melba Toast, Plain	5	1	Each	0.61	0.16	3.83	19.5	0	0.33	0	0.02
18424	Crackers, Melba Toast, Plain, w/o Salt	5	1	Each	0.61	0.16	3.83	19.5	0	0	0	0.02
18221	Crackers, Melba Toast, Rye	5	1	Each	0.58	0.17	3.87	19.45	0	0.4	0	0.02
18222	Crackers, Melba Toast, Wheat	5	1	Each	0.65	0.12	3.82	18.7	0	0.37	0	0.02
18229	Crackers, Ritz	3	1	Each	0.22	0.76	1.83	15.06	0	0.06	0	0.15
18427	Crackers, Ritz, Low Sodium	3	1	Each	0.22	0.76	1.83	15.06	0	0	0	0.15
18225	Crackers, Rye, w/ Cheese Filling	7	1	Each	0.64	1.56	4.26	33.67	0	0	0.63	0.4
18226	Crackers, Rye, Wafers, Plain	25	1	Each	2.4	0.23	20.1	83.5	0	0	0	0.03
18227	Crackers, Rye, Wafers, Seasoned	22	1	Each	1.98	2.02	16.24	83.82	0	0	0	0.34
18228	Crackers, Saltines	3	1	Each	0.28	0.35	2.15	13.02	0	0.08	0	0.06
62688	Crackers, Saltines, Fat Free	3	1	Each	0.4	0	2.4	12	0	0	0	0
18425	Crackers, Saltines, Low Salt	3	1	Each	0.28	0.35	2.15	13.02	0	0	0	0.06
18230	Crackers, Snack-type, w/ Cheese Filling	7	1	Each	0.65	1.48	4.32	33.39	0	0	0.14	0.4
18231	Crackers, Snack-type, w/ Peanut Butter Filling	7	1	Each	0.78	1.67	4.11	34.16	0	0	0	0.36
62590	Crackers, Wheat, Fat Free - SnackWell	3	5	Each	0.4	0	2.4	12	0	0.2	0	0
18428	Crackers, Wheat, Low Salt	2	1	Each	0.17	0.41	1.3	9.46	0	0	0	0.07
18232	Crackers, Wheat, Regular	2	1	Each	0.17	0.41	1.3	9.46	0	0.11	0	0.07
18233	Crackers, Wheat, w/ Cheese Filling	7	1	Each	0.69	1.75	4.07	34.79	0	0	0.49	0.46
18234	Crackers, Wheat, w/ Peanut Butter Filling	7	1	Each	0.95	1.87	3.77	34.65	0	0	0	0.4
18235	Crackers, Whole-wheat	4	1	Each	0.35	0.69	2.74	17.72	0	0.42	0	0.12
18429	Crackers, Whole-wheat, Low Salt	4	1	Each	0.35	0.69	2.74	17.72	0	0	0	0.12
18260	English Muffins, Mixed-grain (includes Granola)	66	1	Each	6.01	1.19	30.56	155.1	0	0	0	0.15
18261	English Muffins, Mixed-grain, Toasted	61	1	Each	6.04	1.16	30.68	155.55	0	0	0	0.15
18258	English Muffins, Plain	57	1	Each	4.39	1.03	26.22	133.95	0	0	0	0.15
18259	English Muffins, Plain, Toasted	52	1	Each	4.37	1.04	26	132.6	0	0	0	0.15
18262	English Muffins, Raisin-cinnamon	57	1	Each	4.28	1.54	27.76	138.51	0	0	0	0.22
18263	English Muffins, Raisin-cinnamon, Toasted	52	1	Each	4.26	1.51	27.56	137.28	0	0	0	0.22
18264	English Muffins, Wheat	57	1	Each	4.96	1.14	25.54	127.11	0	0	0	0.16
18265	English Muffins, Wheat, Toasted	52	1	Each	4.89	1.09	25.32	126.36	0	0	0	0.16
18266	English Muffins, Whole-wheat	66	1	Each	5.81	1.39	26.66	133.98	0	4.16	0	0.22
18267	English Muffins, Whole-wheat, Toasted	61	1	Each	5.86	1.4	26.9	134.81	0	0	0	0.22
20081	Flour, White	125	1	Cup	12.91	1.23	95.39	455	0	4.13	0	0.19
20080	Flour, Whole Grain	120	1	Cup	16.44	2.24	87.08	406.8	0	14.64	0	0.39
20030	Grits	160	0.5	Cup	2.37	1.41	22.82	115.2	0	4	0	0.2
20330	Hominy, Cnd, Yellow	160	0.5	Cup	2.37	1.41	22.82	115.2	0	0	0	0.2
18270	Hush Puppies	22	1	Each	1.69	2.97	10.12	74.14	0	0.62	9.9	0.46
20100	Macaroni, Ckd, Enriched	140	1	Cup	6.68	0.94	39.68	197.4	0	1.82	0	0.13
20400	Macaroni, Ckd, Unenriched	140	1	Cup	6.68	0.94	39.68	197.4	0	1.82	0	0.13
20106	Macaroni, Vegetable, Ckd, Enriched	134	1	Cup	6.07	0.15	35.66	171.52	0	5.76	0	0.02
20108	Macaroni, Whole-wheat, Ckd	140	1	Cup	7.46	0.76	37.16	173.6	0	6.16	0	0.14
20113	Noodles, Chinese, Chow Mein	45	0.5	Cup	3.77	13.84	25.89	237.15	0	1.76	0	1.97
20310	Noodles, Egg, Ckd, Enriched	160	1	Cup	7.6	2.35	39.74	212.8	0	0	52.8	0.5
20510	Noodles, Egg, Ckd, Unenriched	160	1	Cup	7.6	2.35	39.74	212.8	0	0	52.8	0.5
20112	Noodles, Egg, Spinach, Ckd, Enriched	160	1	Cup	8.06	2.51	38.8	211.2	0	3.68	52.8	0.58
20115	Noodles, Japanese, Soba, Ckd	114	0.5	Cup	5.77	0.11	24.44	112.86	0	0	0	0.02
62647	Noodles, Ramen	86	1	Each	10	16	52	380	0	2	0	8
20321	Pasta, Ckd, Enriched, w/ Added Salt	140	1	Cup	6.68	0.94	39.68	197.4	0	0	0	0.13
20121	Pasta, Ckd, Enriched, w/o Added Salt	140	1	Cup	6.68	0.94	39.68	197.4	0	2.38	0	0.13
20094	Pasta, Fresh-refrigerated, Plain, Ckd	146	1	Cup	7.52	1.53	36.4	191.26	0	0	48.18	0.22
20096	Pasta, Fresh-refrigerated, Spinach, Ckd	146	1	Cup	7.39	1.37	36.56	189.8	0	0	48.18	0.32
20097	Pasta, Homemade, Made w/ Egg, Ckd	147.2	1	Cup	7.77	2.56	34.65	191.36	0	0	60.35	0.6
20098	Pasta, Homemade, Made w/o Egg, Ckd	147.2	1	Cup	6.43	1.44	36.98	182.53	0	0	0	0.21

Monounsaturated Fat (gm)	Polyunsaturated Fat (gm)	Vitamin D (mg)	Vitamin K (mg)	Vitamin E (mg)	Vitamin A (re)	Vitamin C (mg)	Thiamin (mg)	Riboflavin (mg)	Niacin (mg)	Vitamin B6 (mg)	Folate (mg)	Vitamin B12 (mcg)	Calcium (mg)	Iron (mg)	Magnesium (mg)	Phosphorus (mg)	Potassium (mg)	Sodium (mg)	Zinc (mg)
0.28	0.28	0	0	0	5.1	0.06	0.16	0.12	1.39	0.03	2.84	0.06	10.21	1.24	8.51	25.23	23.53	80.8	0.21
0.04	0.17	0	0	0	0	0	0.11	0.08	1.1	0.03	3.97	0	3.69	0.9	7.09	25.23	31.75	0.57	0.19
0.05	0.19	0	0	0	0	0	0.1	0.08	1.53	0.05	9.92	0	6.52	1.32	37.99	86.47	89.59	0.57	0.74
0.04	0.06	0	0	0	0	0	0.02	0.01	0.21	0	1.3	0	4.65	0.19	2.95	9.8	10.1	41.45	0.1
0.04	0.06	0	0	0	0	0	0.02	0.01	0.21	0	1.3	0	4.65	0.19	2.95	9.8	10.1	0.95	0.1
0.05	0.07	0	0	0	0	0.01	0.02	0.01	0.24	0	1.1	0	3.9	0.18	1.95	9.15	9.65	44.95	0.07
0.03	0.05	0	0	0	0	0	0.02	0.01	0.25	0.01	1.2	0	2.15	0.23	2.8	8.25	7.4	41.85	0.08
0.32	0.25	0	0	0	0	0	0.01	0.01	0.12	0	0.42	0	3.6	0.11	0.81	6.84	3.99	25.41	0.02
0.32	0.25	0	0	0	0	0	0.01	0.01	0.12	0	0.42	0	3.6	0.11	0.81	6.84	10.65	11.19	0.02
0.84	0.2	0	0	0	0.14	0.01	0.04	0.03	0.25	0.01	1.12	0	15.54	0.17	2.59	23.73	23.94	73.08	0.05
0.04	0.1	0	0	0	0.5	0.03	0.11	0.07	0.4	0.07	11.25	0	10	1.49	30.25	83.5	123.75	198.5	0.7
1.05	0.37	0	0	0	0	0.02	0.07	0.05	0.54	0.04	11.44	0	9.68	0.67	23.32	67.54	99.88	195.14	0.56
0.19	0.06	0	0	0	0	0	0.02	0.01	0.16	0	0.93	0	3.57	0.16	0.81	3.15	3.84	39.06	0.02
0	0	0	0	0	0	0	0	0	0	0	0	0	0	0.12	0	0	25.6	36	0
0.19	0.06	0	0	0	0	0	0.02	0.01	0.16	0	0.93	0	3.57	0.16	0.81	3.15	21.72	19.08	0.02
0.8	0.19	0	0	0	0.49	0	0.03	0.05	0.26	0	0.98	0	17.99	0.17	2.52	28.42	30.03	98.07	0.04
0.88	0.32	0	0	0	0	0	0.03	0.02	0.41	0.01	2.38	0	6.79	0.21	3.71	16.87	15.61	65.94	0.07
0	0	0	0	0	0	0	0	0	0	0	0	0	4.8	0.08	0	0	9	34	0
0.23	0.06	0	0	0	0	0	0.01	0.01	0.1	0	0.36	0	0.98	0.09	1.24	4.4	4.06	5.66	0.03
0.23	0.06	0	0	0	0	0	0.01	0.01	0.1	0	0.36	0	0.98	0.09	1.24	4.4	3.66	15.9	0.03
0.95	0.23	0	0	0	0.63	0.11	0.03	0.03	0.22	0.02	1.33	0.01	14.28	0.18	3.78	26.74	21.42	63.91	0.06
0.98	0.36	0	0	0	0	0	0.03	0.02	0.41	0.01	2.59	0	11.9	0.19	2.66	24.29	20.79	56.49	0.06
0.38	0.11	0	0	0	0	0	0.01	0	0.18	0.01	1.12	0	2	0.12	3.96	11.8	11.88	26.36	0.09
0.38	0.11	0	0	0	0	0	0.01	0	0.18	0.01	1.12	0	2	0.12	3.96	11.8	11.88	9.88	0.09
0.55	0.37	0	0	0	0.66	0	0.28	0.21	2.36	0.06	23.1	0	129.36	1.99	29.04	98.34	102.96	274.56	0.64
0.55	0.37	0	0	0	0.61	0	0.23	0.19	2.14	0.06	16.47	0	129.93	2.01	29.28	98.82	103.09	276.33	0.64
0.17	0.51	0	0	0	0	0.06	0.25	0.16	2.21	0.02	21.09	0.02	99.18	1.43	11.97	75.81	74.67	264.48	0.4
0.17	0.5	0	0	0	0	0.05	0.2	0.14	1.98	0.02	15.08	0.02	98.28	1.41	11.44	75.4	74.36	262.08	0.4
0.29	0.78	0	0	0	0	0.17	0.22	0.17	2.03	0.04	18.24	0	83.79	1.38	8.55	43.89	118.56	254.79	0.57
0.29	0.78	0	0	0	0	0.16	0.17	0.15	1.81	0.04	13	0	82.68	1.37	8.84	43.68	117.52	252.72	0.57
0.16	0.48	0	0	0	0	0	0.25	0.17	1.91	0.05	22.23	0	101.46	1.64	22.23	65.55	106.02	217.74	0.64
0.16	0.47	0	0	0	0	0	0.2	0.15	1.71	0.05	15.6	0	100.36	1.62	21.84	64.48	105.04	215.8	0.63
0.34	0.55	0	0	0	0	0	0.2	0.09	2.25	0.11	32.34	0	174.9	1.62	46.86	186.12	138.6	420.42	1.06
0.34	0.55	0	0	0	0	0	0.16	0.08	2.03	0.1	22.57	0	175.68	1.62	46.97	187.27	139.08	422.12	1.06
0.11	0.52	0	0.63	0.46	0	0	0.98	0.62	7.38	0.06	32.5	0	18.75	5.8	27.5	135	133.75	2.5	0.88
0.28	0.93	0	1.32	1.48	0	0	0.54	0.26	7.64	0.41	52.8	0	40.8	4.66	165.6	415.2	486	6	3.52
0.37	0.64	0	0	0	0	0	0	0.01	0.05	0.01	1.6	0	16	0.99	25.6	56	14.4	336	1.68
0.37	0.64	0	0	0	17.6	0	0	0.01	0.05	0.01	1.6	0	16	0.99	25.6	56	14.4	336	1.68
0.72	1.59	0	0	0	9.46	0.04	0.08	0.07	0.61	0.02	4.4	0.04	61.16	0.67	5.28	41.58	31.68	146.96	0.15
0.11	0.38	0	0	0.04	0	0	0.29	0.14	2.34	0.05	9.8	0	9.8	1.96	25.2	75.6	43.4	1.4	0.74
0.11	0.38	0	0	0.04	0	0	0.03	0.03	0.56	0.05	9.8	0	9.8	0.7	25.2	75.6	43.4	1.4	0.74
0.02	0.06	0	0	0.05	6.7	0	0.15	0.08	1.44	0.03	8.04	0	14.74	0.66	25.46	67	41.54	8.04	0.59
0.11	0.3	0	0	0.14	0	0	0.15	0.06	0.99	0.11	7	0	21	1.48	42	124.6	61.6	4.2	1.13
3.46	7.8	0	0	0.07	4.05	0	0.26	0.19	2.68	0.05	9.9	0	9	2.13	23.4	72.45	54	197.55	0.63
0.69	0.65	0	0	0	9.6	0	0.3	0.13	2.38	0.06	11.2	0.14	19.2	2.54	30.4	110.4	44.8	264	0.99
0.69	0.65	0	0	0	9.6	0	0.05	0.03	0.64	0.06	11.2	0.14	19.2	0.96	30.4	110.4	44.8	264	0.99
0.79	0.56	0	0	0.08	22.4	0	0.39	0.2	2.36	0.18	33.6	0.22	30.4	1.74	38.4	91.2	59.2	19.2	1.01
0.03	0.04	0	0	0	0	0	0.11	0.03	0.58	0.05	7.98	0	4.56	0.55	10.26	28.5	39.9	68.4	0.14
0	0	0	0	0	0	0	0	0	0	0	0	0	0	1.6	0	0	0	1560	0
0.11	0.38	0	0	0	0	0	0.29	0.14	2.34	0.05	9.8	0	9.8	1.96	25.2	75.6	43.4	140	0.74
0.11	0.38	0	0	0.08	0	0	0.29	0.14	2.34	0.05	9.8	0	9.8	1.96	25.2	75.6	43.4	1.4	0.74
0.18	0.63	0	0	0	8.76	0	0.31	0.22	1.45	0.05	10.22	0.2	8.76	1.66	26.28	91.98	35.04	8.76	0.82
0.43	0.31	0	0	0	20.44	0	0.26	0.2	1.48	0.16	26.28	0.2	26.28	1.62	35.04	83.22	54.02	8.76	0.92
0.75	0.77	0	0	0	25.02	0	0.25	0.26	1.85	0.05	27.97	0.15	14.72	1.71	20.61	76.54	30.91	122.18	0.65
0.28	0.75	0	0	0	0	0	0.27	0.22	1.98	0.04	25.02	0	8.83	1.66	20.61	58.88	27.97	108.93	0.54

USDA ID Code	Food Name	Weight in Grams*	Quantity of Units	Unit of Measure	Protein (gm)	Fat (gm)	Carbohydrates (gm)	Kcalories	Caffeine (gm)	Fiber (gm)	Cholesterol (mg)	Saturated Fat (gm)
20127	Pasta, Spinach, Ckd	140	1	Cup	6.41	0.88	36.61	182	0	0	0	0.13
20125	Pasta, Whole-wheat, Ckd	140	1	Cup	7.46	0.76	37.16	173.6	0	6.3	0	0.14
62557	Red Beans and Rice	28.35	2	Ounce	3.98	0.5	19.89	94.5	0	3.48	0	0
20037	Rice, Brown, Long-grain, Ckd	195	1	Cup	5.03	1.76	44.77	216.45	0	3.51	0	0.35
20041	Rice, Brown, Medium-grain, Ckd	195	1	Cup	4.52	1.62	45.84	218.4	0	0	0	0.32
20045	Rice, White, Long-grain, Ckd	158	1	Cup	4.25	0.44	44.51	205.4	0	0.63	0	0.12
20049	Rice, White, Long-grain, Instant, Enriched	165	1	Cup	3.4	0.26	35.1	161.7	0	0.99	0	0.07
20051	Rice, White, Medium-grain, Ckd	186	1	Cup	4.43	0.39	53.18	241.8	0	0.56	0	0.11
20053	Rice, White, Short-grain, Ckd	186	1	Cup	4.39	0.35	53.44	241.8	0	0	0	0.09
20057	Rice, White, w/ Pasta, Ckd	202	1	Cup	5.13	5.7	43.29	246.44	0	7.88	2.02	1.09
62653	Tabouli	28.35	1	Ounce	1	2	2	30	0	1	0	0
18360	Taco Shells, Baked	13	1	Medium	0.94	2.94	8.11	60.84	0	1.05	0	0.44
18448	Taco Shells, Baked, w/o Added Salt	13	1	Medium	0.94	2.94	8.11	60.84	0	0	0	0.44
18363	Tortillas, Corn	25	1	Medium	1.43	0.63	11.65	55.5	0	1.3	0	0.08
18449	Tortillas, Corn, w/o Added Salt	25	1	Medium	1.43	0.63	11.65	55.5	0	0	0	0.08
18364	Tortillas, Flour	35	1	Medium	3.05	2.49	19.46	113.75	0	1.09	0	0.39
18450	Tortillas, Flour, w/o Added Salt	35	1	Medium	3.05	2.49	19.46	113.75	0	0	0	0.39
20089	Wild Rice, Ckd	164	1	Cup	6.54	0.56	35	165.64	0	2.95	0	0.08
62663	Wild Rice, Unkle Ben's	56	1	Cup	6	0.5	41	190	0	1	0	0
10124	Bacon	6	1	Slice	1.83	2.95	0.04	34.56	0	0	5.1	1.05
10131	Bacon, Canadian-style Bacon, Grilled	21	1	Slice	5.09	1.77	0.28	38.85	0	0	12.18	0.6
62528	Bacon, Turkey	14	1	Slice	3	2	0	25	0	0	10	0.5
7001	Barbecue Loaf, Lunch Meat	23	1	Slice	3.64	2.05	1.47	39.79	0	0	8.51	0.73
16006	Beans, Baked, Cnd, Vegetarian	254	0.5	Cup	6.1	13	54.1	382	0	13.9	13	4.9
16007	Beans, Baked, Cnd, w/ Beef	266	0.5	Cup	16.97	9.18	44.98	321.86	0	0	58.52	4.46
16008	Beans, Baked, Cnd, w/ Franks	257	0.5	Cup	17.35	16.88	39.55	364.94	0	17.73	15.42	6.04
16009	Beans, Baked, Cnd, w/ Pork	253	0.5	Cup	13.13	3.92	50.55	268.18	0	13.92	17.71	1.52
16005	Beans, Baked, Home Prepared	253	0.5	Cup	6.1	13	54.1	382	0	13.92	13	4.9
16315	Beans, Black, Ckd	256	0.5	Cup	15.2	1.2	45	214	0	0	0	0.12
16058	Beans, Garbanzo, Cnd.	240	0.5	Cup	11.9	2.7	54.3	286	0	10.6	0	0.3
16029	Beans, Kidney, Cnd	256	0.5	Cup	13.3	0.8	38.1	107	0	0	0	0.1
16073	Beans, Lima, Cnd	241	0.5	Cup	11.9	0.4	35.9	190	0	11.6	0	0.1
16039	Beans, Navy, Cnd	262	0.5	Cup	19.7	1.1	53.6	296	0	13.4	0	0.3
16044	Beans, Pinto, Cnd	240	0.5	Cup	11.7	1.9	36.6	206	0	11	0	0.4
16103	Beans, Refried, Cnd	253	0.5	Cup	13.9	3.2	39.3	238	0	13.4	0	1.2
62632	Beans, Refried,Lowfat, Cnd.	268	0.5	Cup	16	0	42	240	0	14	0	0
13347	Beef, Corned, Brisket, Ckd	28.35	3	Ounce	5.15	5.38	0.13	71.16	0	0	27.78	1.8
13353	Beef, Cured, Lunch Meat, Jellied	28.35	3	Ounce	5.39	0.94	0	31.47	0	0	9.64	0.4
13355	Beef, Cured, Pastrami	28.35	3	Ounce	4.89	8.27	0.86	98.94	0	0	26.37	2.95
13357	Beef, Cured, Sausage, Smoked	28.35	3	Ounce	4	7.63	0.69	88.45	0	0	18.99	3.24
13358	Beef, Cured, Smoked, Chopped Beef	28.35	3	Ounce	5.72	1.25	0.53	34.87	0	0	13.04	0.51
13360	Beef, Cured, Thin-sliced Beef	28.35	3	Ounce	7.97	1.09	1.62	50.18	0	0	11.62	0.47
	Beef, Filet, Tnderloin, Broiled	85	3	Ounce	23.55	9.75	0	188.7	0	0	70.55	3.681
13298	Beef, Ground, Extra Lean, Broiled	28.35	3	Ounce	7.2	4.63	0	72.58	0	0	23.81	1.82
13300	Beef, Ground, Extra Lean, Pan-fried	28.35	3	Ounce	7.08	4.66	0	72.29	0	0	22.96	1.83
13305	Beef, Ground, Lean, Broiled	28.35	3	Ounce	7.01	5.23	0	77.11	0	0	24.66	2.06
13307	Beef, Ground, Lean, Pan-fried	28.35	3	Ounce	6.87	5.4	0	77.96	0	0	23.81	2.12
13312	Beef, Ground, Regular, Broiled	28.35	3	Ounce	6.82	5.87	0	81.93	0	0	25.52	2.3
13314	Beef, Ground, Regular, Pan-fried	28.35	3	Ounce	6.78	6.4	0	86.75	0	0	25.23	2.51
13326	Beef, Liver, Ckd, Braised	28.35	3	Ounce	6.91	1.39	0.97	45.64	0	0	110.28	0.54
13327	Beef, Liver, Ckd, Pan-fried	28.35	3	Ounce	7.58	2.27	2.23	61.52	0	0	136.65	0.76
7042	Beef, Loaved, Lunch Meat	28.35	1	Slice	4.08	7.43	0.82	87.32	0	0	18.14	3.17
13504	Beef, Steaks and Roasts, Ckd, 1/2 in. Fat	28.35	3	Ounce	7.07	7.62	0	98.94	0	0	25.8	3.15
13361	Beef, Steaks and Roasts, Ckd, Fat Trimmed	28.35	3	Ounce	7.75	4.92	0	77.4	0	0	24.66	1.94
13004	Beef, Steaks and Roasts, Ckd., 1/4 in. Fat	28.35	3	Ounce	7.35	6.11	0	86.47	0	0	24.95	2.42

Monounsaturated Fat (gm)	Polyunsaturated Fat (gm)	Vitamin D (mg)	Vitamin K (mg)	Vitamin E (mg)	Vitamin A (re)	Vitamin C (mg)	Thiamin (mg)	Riboflavin (mg)	Niacin (mg)	Vitamin B6 (mg)	Folate (mcg)	Vitamin B12 (mcg)	Calcium (mg)	Iron (mg)	Magnesium (mg)	Phosphorus (mg)	Potassium (mg)	Sodium (mg)	Zinc (mg)
0.1	0.36	0	0	0	21	0	0.14	0.14	2.14	0.13	16.8	0	42	1.46	86.8	151.2	81.2	19.6	1.51
0.11	0.3	0	0	0.07	0	0	0.15	0.06	0.99	0.11	7	0	21	1.48	42	124.6	61.6	4.2	1.13
0	0	0	0	0	49.74	2.98	0.11	0	1.42	0	0	0	23.87	0.75	0	0	0	392.92	0
0.64	0.63	0	0	1.4	0	0	0.19	0.05	2.98	0.28	7.8	0	19.5	0.82	83.85	161.85	83.85	9.75	1.23
0.59	0.58	0	0	0	0	0	0.2	0.02	2.59	0.29	7.8	0	19.5	1.03	85.8	150.15	154.05	1.95	1.21
0.14	0.12	0	0	0.08	0	0	0.26	0.02	2.33	0.15	4.74	0	15.8	1.9	18.96	67.94	55.3	1.58	0.77
0.08	0.07	0	0	0.08	0	0	0.12	0.08	1.45	0.02	6.6	0	13.2	1.04	8.25	23.1	6.6	4.95	0.4
0.12	0.1	0	0	0	0	0	0.31	0.03	3.41	0.09	3.72	0	5.58	2.77	24.18	68.82	53.94	0	0.78
0.11	0.09	0	0	0	0	0	0.31	0.03	2.78	0.11	3.72	0	1.86	2.72	14.88	61.38	48.36	0	0.74
2.26	1.91	0	0	0	0	0.4	0.25	0.16	3.6	0.2	14.14	0.12	16.16	1.9	24.24	74.74	84.84	1147.36	0.57
0	0	0	0	0	100	12	0	0	0	0	0	0	0	0.4	0	0	0	75	0
1.23	1.12	0	0	0	4.55	0	0.03	0.01	0.18	0.05	0.78	0	20.8	0.33	13.65	32.24	23.27	47.71	0.18
1.23	1.12	0	0	0	0	0	0.03	0.01	0.18	0	0.78	0	20.8	0.33	13.65	32.24	23.27	1.95	0.18
0.16	0.28	0	0	0	6	0	0.03	0.02	0.37	0.05	3.75	0	43.75	0.35	16.25	78.5	38.5	40.25	0.24
0.16	0.28	0	0	0	0	0	0.03	0.02	0.37	0.05	3.75	0	43.75	0.35	16.25	78.5	38.5	2.75	0.24
1.01	0.98	0	0	0	0	0	0.19	0.1	1.25	0.02	4.2	0	43.75	1.16	9.1	43.4	45.85	167.3	0.25
1.01	0.98	0	0	0	0	0	0.19	0.1	1.25	0.02	4.2	0	13.65	1.16	9.1	43.4	45.85	167.3	0.25
0.08	0.35	0	0	0	0	0	0.09	0.14	2.11	0.22	42.64	0	4.92	0.98	52.48	134.48	165.64	4.92	2.2
0	0	0	0	0	2.4	0	0	0	0	0	0	0	24	1	0	0	0	620	0
1.42	0.35	0	0	0.03	2.01		0.04	0.02	0.44	0.02	0.3	0.11	0.72	0.1	1.44	20.16	29.16	95.76	0.2
0.85	0.17	0	0	0.05	0	4.54	0.17	0.04	1.45	0.09	0.84	0.16	2.1	0.17	4.41	62.16	81.9	324.66	0.36
0	0	0	0	0	0	0	0	0	0	0	0	0	0	0	0	0	0	170	0
0.95	0.19	0.21	0	0	1.61	4.37	0.08	0.06	0.52	0.06	2.07	0.39	12.65	0.27	3.91	30.36	75.67	306.82	0.57
5.4	1.9	0	0	0.32	0	5.06	0.13	0.1	1.13	0.16	91.84	0	134.09	4.3	86.02	273.24	781.77	1047.42	3.69
3.68	0.55	0	0	0	55.86	4.79	0.14	0.12	2.5	0.24	115.44	0	119.7	4.26	66.5	215.46	851.2	1263.5	3.19
7.27	2.15	0	0	1.21	38.55	5.91	0.15	0.14	2.32	0.12	77.1	0	123.36	4.45	71.96	267.28	603.95	1105.1	4.81
1.7	0.5	0	0	1.37	45.54	5.06	0.13	0.1	1.13	0.16	91.84	0	134.09	4.3	86.02	273.24	781.77	1047.42	3.69
5.4	1.9	0	0	0.32	0	3	0.34	0.12	0.23	0.23	122	0	154	5.03	109	276	906	1068	1.85
0.04	0.2	0	0	0	0.86	0	0.21	0.05	0.435	0.06	128	0	46	1.8	120	240	610	408	0.97
0.6	1.2	0	0	0	5	9	0.07	0.08	0.3	1.14	160	0	77	3.24	70	216	413	718	2.54
0.1	0.4	0	0	0	0	3	0.28	0.18	1.3	0.18	126	0	69	3.15	79	134.4	658	888	1.41
0	0.2	0	0	1.74	0	0	0.13	0.08	0.6	0.22	121	0	51	4.36	94	178	530	810	1.57
0.1	0.5	0	0	1	0	2	0.37	0.14	1.3	0.27	163	0	123	4.85	123	351	755	1174	2.02
0.4	0.7	0	0	0	0	2	0.24	0.15	0.7	0.18	144	0	103	3.5	65	221	583	706	1.66
1.4	0.4	0	0	0	0	15	0.07	0.04	0.8	0.36	28	0	89	4.2	83	218	676	756	2.96
0	0	0	0	0	0	0	0	0	0	0	0	0	0	2	0	0	0	960	0
2.61	0.19	0	0	0.05	0	4.54	0.01	0.05	0.86	0.07	1.7	0.46	2.27	0.53	3.4	35.44	41.11	321.49	1.3
0.41	0.05	0	0	0	0	4.88	0.04	0.08	1.37	0.07	1.98	1.46	2.84	0.98	5.1	39.41	113.97	374.79	1.01
4.1	0.28	0	0	0.07	0	0.85	0.03	0.05	1.44	0.05	1.98	0.5	2.55	0.54	5.1	42.53	64.64	347.85	1.21
3.68	0.3	0	0	0	0	3.4	0.01	0.04	0.9	0.03	1.13	0.53	1.98	0.5	3.69	29.77	49.9	320.64	0.79
0.52	0.07	0	0	0.03	0	5.87	0.02	0.05	1.3	0.1	2.27	0.49	2.27	0.81	5.95	51.31	106.88	356.64	1.11
0.48	0.06	0	0	0.04	0	4.05	0.02	0.05	1.49	0.1	3.12	0.73	3.12	0.77	5.39	47.63	121.62	407.96	1.13
3.808	0.442	0	0	0	0	0	0.085	0.264	2.898	0.246	7.65	2.303	5.95	3.13	22.95	203.15	332.35	51.85	4.07
2.03	0.17	0	0	0.05	0	0	0.02	0.08	1.41	0.08	2.55	0.62	1.98	0.67	5.95	45.64	88.74	19.85	1.55
2.04	0.17	0	0	0.05	0	0	0.02	0.07	1.34	0.08	2.55	0.57	1.98	0.67	5.95	45.36	88.45	19.85	1.54
2.29	0.2	0	0	0.06	0	0	0.01	0.06	1.46	0.07	2.55	0.67	3.12	0.6	5.95	44.79	85.33	21.83	1.52
2.36	0.2	0	0	0.06	0	0	0.01	0.06	1.36	0.08	2.55	0.64	2.84	0.62	5.67	45.08	84.77	21.83	1.47
2.57	0.22	0	0	0.07	0	0	0.01	0.05	1.64	0.08	2.55	0.83	3.12	0.69	5.67	48.2	82.78	23.53	1.47
2.8	0.24	0	0	0.07	0	0	0.01	0.06	1.65	0.07	2.55	0.77	3.12	0.69	5.67	48.48	85.05	23.81	1.44
0.18	0.3	0	0	0	3005.67	6.52	0.06	1.16	3.04	0.26	61.52	20.13	1.98	1.92	5.67	114.53	66.62	19.85	1.72
0.46	0.48	0	0	0.18	3041.67	6.52	0.06	1.17	4.09	0.41	62.37	31.7	3.12	1.78	6.52	130.69	103.19	30.05	1.55
3.47	0.25	0	0	0.06	0	3.69	0.03	0.06	1.04	0.05	1.42	1.1	3.12	0.66	3.97	33.74	58.97	376.77	0.72
3.41	0.29	0	0	0	0	0	0.02	0.06	0.98	0.09	1.98	0.68	2.84	0.74	5.95	54.72	81.36	16.73	1.56
2.1	0.18	0	0	0.05	0	0	0.02	0.06	1.04	0.09	1.98	0.71	2.55	0.77	6.52	59.82	91.57	17.58	1.72
2.61	0.22	0	0	0.06	0	0	0.02	0.06	1.03	0.09	1.98	0.69	2.84	0.74	6.24	57.55	88.74	17.58	1.66

USDA ID Code	Food Name	Weight in Grams*	Quantity of Units	Unit of Measure	Protein (gm)	Fat (gm)	Carbohydrates (gm)	Kcalories	Caffeine (gm)	Fiber (gm)	Cholesterol (mg)	Saturated Fat (gm)
7043	Beef, Thin Sliced	4.2	1	Slice	1.18	0.16	0.24	7.43	0	0	1.72	0.07
10126	Bologna	23	1	Slice	3.52	4.57	0.17	56.81	0	0	13.57	1.58
7007	Bologna, Beef	28.35	1	Slice	3.46	8.08	0.23	88.45	0	0	16.44	3.42
62601	Buffalo (Chicken) Wings	22.75	4	Each	4.5	3	0.5	47.5	0	0	25	0.75
5280	Chicken Roll, Light Meat	28.35	3	Ounce	5.54	2.09	0.69	45.08	0	0	14.18	0.57
5283	Chicken Salad Sandwich Spread	28.35	3	Ounce	3.3	3.83	2.1	56.7	0	0	8.51	0.98
5281	Chicken Spread, Cnd	28.35	3	Ounce	4.37	3.32	1.53	54.43	0	0	14.74	0.96
5054	Chicken, Back, Meat Only, Ckd, Fried	28.35	3	Ounce	8.5	4.34	1.61	81.65	0	0	26.37	1.17
5055	Chicken, Back, Meat Only, Ckd, Roasted	28.35	3	Ounce	7.99	3.73	0	67.76	0	0	25.52	1.02
5056	Chicken, Back, Meat Only, Ckd, Stewed	28.35	3	Ounce	7.18	3.17	0	59.25	0	0	24.1	0.86
5049	Chicken, Back, Meat&skin, Ckd, Fried, Batter	28.35	3	Ounce	6.23	6.21	2.91	93.84	0	0	24.95	1.65
5050	Chicken, Back, Meat&skin, Ckd, Fried, Flr	28.35	3	Ounce	7.88	5.88	1.84	93.84	0	0	25.23	1.59
5051	Chicken, Back, Meat&skin, Ckd, Roasted	28.35	3	Ounce	7.36	5.94	0	85.05	0	0	24.95	1.65
5052	Chicken, Back, Meat&skin, Ckd, Stewed	28.35	3	Ounce	6.29	5.14	0	73.14	0	0	22.11	1.42
5063	Chicken, Breast, Meat Only, Ckd, Fried	28.35	3	Ounce	9.48	1.34	0.14	53.01	0	0	25.8	0.37
5064	Chicken, Breast, Meat Only, Ckd, Roasted	28.35	3	Ounce	8.79	1.01	0	46.78	0	0	24.1	0.29
5065	Chicken, Breast, Meat Only, Ckd, Stewed	28.35	3	Ounce	8.22	0.86	0	42.81	0	0	21.83	0.24
5058	Chicken, Breast, Meat&skin, Ckd, Fried, Batter	28.35	3	Ounce	7.04	3.74	2.55	73.71	0	0.09	24.1	1
5059	Chicken, Breast, Meat&skin, Ckd, Fried, Flr	28.35	3	Ounce	9.03	2.51	0.46	62.94	0	0	25.23	0.69
5060	Chicken, Breast, Meat&skin, Ckd, Roasted	28.35	3	Ounce	8.45	2.21	0	55.85	0	0	23.81	0.62
5061	Chicken, Breast, Meat&skin, Ckd, Stewed	28.35	3	Ounce	7.77	2.1	0	52.16	0	0	21.26	0.59
5277	Chicken, Cnd.	28.35	3	Ounce	6.17	2.25	0	46.78	0	0	17.58	0.62
5044	Chicken, Dark Meat, Meat Only, Ckd, Fried	28.35	3	Ounce	8.22	3.29	0.73	67.76	0	0	27.22	0.88
5045	Chicken, Dark Meat, Meat Only, Ckd, Roasted	28.35	3	Ounce	7.76	2.76	0	58.12	0	0	26.37	0.75
5046	Chicken, Dark Meat, Meat Only, Ckd, Stewed	28.35	3	Ounce	7.36	2.55	0	54.43	0	0	24.95	0.69
5035	Chicken, Dark Meat, Meat&skin, Ckd, Fried, Batter	28.35	3	Ounce	6.19	5.28	2.66	84.48	0	0	25.23	1.4
5036	Chicken, Dark Meat, Meat&skin, Ckd, Fried, Flr	28.35	3	Ounce	7.72	4.79	1.16	80.8	0	0	26.08	1.3
5037	Chicken, Dark Meat, Meat&skin, Ckd, Roasted	28.35	3	Ounce	7.36	4.47	0	71.73	0	0	25.8	1.24
5038	Chicken, Dark Meat, Meat&skin, Ckd, Stewed	28.35	3	Ounce	6.66	4.16	0	66.06	0	0	23.25	1.15
5072	Chicken, Drumstick, Meat Only, Ckd, Fried	28.35	3	Ounce	8.11	2.29	0	55.28	0	0	26.65	0.6
5073	Chicken, Drumstick, Meat Only, Ckd, Roasted	28.35	3	Ounce	8.02	1.6	0	48.76	0	0	26.37	0.42
5074	Chicken, Drumstick, Meat Only, Ckd, Stewed	28.35	3	Ounce	7.8	1.62	0	47.91	0	0	24.95	0.43
5067	Chicken, Drumstick, Meat&skin, Ckd, Fried, Batter	28.35	3	Ounce	6.22	4.47	2.35	75.98	0	0	24.38	1.17
5068	Chicken, Drumstick, Meat&skin, Ckd, Fried, Flr	28.35	3	Ounce	7.64	3.89	0.46	69.46	0	0	25.52	1.04
5069	Chicken, Drumstick, Meat&skin, Ckd, Roasted	28.35	3	Ounce	7.66	3.16	0	61.24	0	0	25.8	0.86
5070	Chicken, Drumstick, Meat&skin, Ckd, Stewed	28.35	3	Ounce	7.18	3.02	0	57.83	0	0	23.53	0.82
5021	Chicken, Giblets, Ckd, Fried	28.35	3	Ounce	9.23	3.82	1.23	78.53	0	0	126.44	1.08
5022	Chicken, Giblets, Ckd, Simmered	28.35	3	Ounce	7.33	1.35	0.27	44.51	0	0	111.42	0.42
5026	Chicken, Heart, Ckd, Simmered	28.35	3	Ounce	7.49	2.25	0.03	52.45	0	0	68.61	0.64
5081	Chicken, Leg, Meat Only, Ckd, Fried	28.35	3	Ounce	8.05	2.64	0.18	58.97	0	0	28.07	0.71
5082	Chicken, Leg, Meat Only, Ckd, Roasted	28.35	3	Ounce	7.66	2.39	0	54.15	0	0	26.65	0.65
5083	Chicken, Leg, Meat Only, Ckd, Stewed	28.35	3	Ounce	7.44	2.29	0	52.45	0	0	25.23	0.62
5076	Chicken, Leg, Meat&skin, Ckd, Fried, Batter	28.35	3	Ounce	6.17	4.58	2.47	77.4	0	0	25.52	1.21
5077	Chicken, Leg, Meat&skin, Ckd, Fried, Flour	28.35	3	Ounce	7.61	4.09	0.71	72.01	0	0	26.65	1.11
5078	Chicken, Leg, Meat&skin, Ckd, Roasted	28.35	3	Ounce	7.36	3.82	0	65.77	0	0	26.08	1.05
5079	Chicken, Leg, Meat&skin, Ckd, Stewed	28.35	3	Ounce	6.85	3.66	0	62.37	0	0	23.81	1.01
5028	Chicken, Liver, Ckd, Simmered	28.35	3	Ounce	6.91	1.55	0.25	44.51	0	0	178.89	0.52
5012	Chicken, Meat Only, Ckd, Fried	28.35	3	Ounce	8.67	2.59	0.48	62.09	0	0.03	26.65	0.7
5013	Chicken, Meat Only, Roasted	28.35	3	Ounce	8.2	2.1	0	53.87	0	0	25.23	0.58
5014	Chicken, Meat Only, Stewed	28.35	3	Ounce	7.74	1.9	0	50.18	0	0	23.53	0.52
5097	Chicken, Thigh, Meat Only, Ckd, Fried	28.35	3	Ounce	7.99	2.92	0.33	61.8	0	0	28.92	0.79
5098	Chicken, Thigh, Meat Only, Ckd, Roasted	28.35	3	Ounce	7.35	3.08	0	59.25	0	0	26.93	0.86
5099	Chicken, Thigh, Meat Only, Ckd, Stewed	28.35	3	Ounce	7.09	2.78	0	55.28	0	0	25.52	0.77
5092	Chicken, Thigh, Meat&skin, Ckd, Fried, Batter	28.35	3	Ounce	6.13	4.69	2.57	78.53	0	0	26.37	1.25
5093	Chicken, Thigh, Meat&skin, Ckd, Fried, Flr	28.35	3	Ounce	7.58	4.25	0.9	74.28	0	0	27.5	1.16

Monounsaturated Fat (gm)	Polyunsaturated Fat (gm)	Vitamin D (mg)	Vitamin K (mg)	Vitamin E (mg)	Vitamin A (re)	Vitamin C (mg)	Thiamin (mg)	Riboflavin (mg)	Niacin (mg)	Vitamin B6 (mg)	Folate (mg)	Vitamin B12 (mcg)	Calcium (mg)	Iron (mg)	Magnesium (mg)	Phosphorus (mg)	Potassium (mg)	Sodium (mg)	Zinc (mg)
0.07	0.01	0	0	0.01	0	0.6	0	0.01	0.22	0.01	0.46	0.11	0.46	0.11	0.8	7.06	18.02	60.44	0.17
2.25	0.49	0	0	0.06	0	8.12	0.12	0.04	0.9	0.06	1.15	0.21	2.53	0.18	3.22	31.97	64.63	272.32	0.47
3.91	0.31	0.2	0	0.05	0	5.95	0.01	0.03	0.68	0.04	1.42	0.4	3.4	0.47	3.4	24.95	44.51	278.11	0.61
0	0	0	0	0	15	0.3	0	0	0	0	0	0	6	0.1	0	0	0	225	0
0.84	0.45	0	0	0.08	6.8	0	0.02	0.04	1.5	0.06	0.57	0.04	12.19	0.27	5.39	44.51	64.64	165.56	0.2
0.92	1.76	0	0	0	11.91	0.34	0.01	0.02	0.47	0.03	1.42	0.11	2.84	0.17	2.84	9.36	51.88	106.88	0.29
1.38	0.71	0	0	0	7.09	0	0	0.03	0.78	0.04	0.85	0.04	35.44	0.66	3.4	25.23	30.05	109.43	0.33
1.62	1.03	0	0	0	8.22	0	0.03	0.07	2.18	0.1	2.55	0.09	7.37	0.47	7.09	49.9	71.16	28.07	0.79
1.37	0.86	0	0	0.08	7.94	0	0.02	0.06	2	0.1	1.98	0.09	6.8	0.39	6.24	46.78	67.19	27.22	0.75
1.14	0.74	0	0	0.08	7.65	0	0.01	0.05	1.29	0.06	1.98	0.06	5.95	0.36	4.82	36.86	44.79	18.99	0.67
2.53	1.47	0	0	0	10.21	0	0.03	0.06	1.65	0.07	2.55	0.07	7.37	0.42	5.39	38.84	51.03	89.87	0.56
2.32	1.36	0	0	0	10.49	0	0.03	0.07	2.07	0.09	2.27	0.08	6.8	0.46	6.52	47.06	64.07	25.52	0.7
2.35	1.31	0	0	0.08	28.07	0	0.02	0.06	1.9	0.08	1.7	0.08	5.95	0.4	5.67	43.66	59.54	24.66	0.64
2.02	1.13	0	0	0.08	24.95	0	0.01	0.04	1.23	0.04	1.42	0.05	5.1	0.35	4.54	34.02	41.11	18.14	0.55
0.49	0.3	0	0	0.12	1.98	0	0.02	0.04	4.19	0.18	1.13	0.1	4.54	0.32	8.79	69.74	78.25	22.4	0.31
0.35	0.22	0	0	0.08	1.7	0	0.02	0.03	3.89	0.17	1.13	0.1	4.25	0.29	8.22	64.64	72.58	20.98	0.28
0.29	0.19	0	0	0.08	1.7	0	0.01	0.03	2.4	0.09	0.85	0.07	3.69	0.25	6.8	46.78	53.01	17.86	0.27
1.55	0.87	0	0	0.3	5.67	0	0.03	0.04	2.98	0.12	1.7	0.09	5.67	0.35	6.8	52.45	56.98	77.96	0.27
0.99	0.56	0	0	0	4.25	0	0.02	0.04	3.9	0.16	1.13	0.1	4.54	0.34	8.51	66.06	73.43	21.55	0.31
0.86	0.47	0	0	0.08	7.65	0	0.02	0.03	3.6	0.16	1.13	0.09	3.97	0.3	7.65	60.67	69.46	20.13	0.29
0.82	0.45	0	0	0.08	6.8	0	0.01	0.03	2.21	0.08	0.85	0.06	3.69	0.26	6.24	44.23	50.46	17.58	0.27
0.89	0.5	0	0	0.06	9.64	0.57	0	0.04	1.79	0.1	1.13	0.08	3.97	0.45	3.4	31.47	39.12	142.6	0.4
1.22	0.79	0	0	0	6.8	0	0.03	0.07	2	0.1	2.55	0.09	5.1	0.42	7.09	53.01	71.73	27.5	0.82
1.01	0.64	0	0	0.08	6.24	0	0.02	0.06	1.86	0.1	2.27	0.09	4.25	0.38	6.52	50.75	68.04	26.37	0.79
0.92	0.59	0	0	0.08	5.95	0	0.02	0.06	1.34	0.06	1.98	0.06	3.97	0.39	5.67	40.54	51.31	20.98	0.75
2.15	1.26	0	0	0	8.79	0	0.03	0.06	1.59	0.07	2.55	0.08	5.95	0.41	5.67	41.11	52.45	83.63	0.59
1.89	1.11	0	0	0	8.79	0	0.03	0.07	1.94	0.09	2.27	0.09	4.82	0.43	6.8	49.9	65.21	25.23	0.74
1.75	0.99	0	0	0	16.44	0	0.02	0.06	1.8	0.09	1.98	0.08	4.25	0.39	6.24	47.63	62.37	24.66	0.71
1.63	0.92	0	0	0	15.31	0	0.01	0.05	1.28	0.05	1.7	0.06	3.97	0.37	5.1	37.71	47.06	19.85	0.64
0.83	0.56	0	0	0	5.1	0	0.02	0.07	1.74	0.11	2.55	0.1	3.4	0.37	6.8	52.73	70.59	27.22	0.91
0.53	0.39	0	0	0.08	5.1	0	0.02	0.07	1.72	0.11	2.55	0.1	3.4	0.37	6.8	52.16	69.74	26.93	0.9
0.55	0.39	0	0	0.08	4.82	0	0.02	0.06	1.22	0.07	2.27	0.07	3.12	0.39	5.95	42.53	56.42	22.68	0.86
1.82	1.07	0	0	0	7.37	0	0.03	0.06	1.44	0.08	2.55	0.08	4.82	0.38	5.67	41.67	52.73	76.26	0.66
1.54	0.92	0	0	0	7.09	0	0.02	0.06	1.71	0.1	2.27	0.09	3.4	0.38	6.52	49.9	64.92	25.23	0.82
1.2	0.71	0	0	0.08	8.51	0	0.02	0.06	1.7	0.1	2.27	0.09	3.4	0.38	6.52	49.61	64.92	25.52	0.81
1.15	0.67	0	0	0.08	7.65	0	0.01	0.05	1.19	0.05	1.98	0.06	3.12	0.38	5.67	39.97	52.16	21.55	0.75
1.25	0.96	0	0	0	1014.65	2.47	0.03	0.43	3.11	0.17	107.45	3.77	5.1	2.93	7.09	81.08	93.56	32.04	1.78
0.34	0.31	0	0	0.37	631.92	2.27	0.02	0.27	1.16	0.1	106.6	2.87	3.4	1.83	5.67	64.92	44.79	16.44	1.3
0.57	0.65	0	0	0	2.55	0.51	0.02	0.21	0.79	0.09	22.68	2.07	5.39	2.56	5.67	56.42	37.42	13.61	2.07
0.97	0.63	0	0	0	5.67	0	0.02	0.07	1.9	0.11	2.55	0.1	3.69	0.4	7.09	54.72	72.01	27.22	0.84
0.86	0.56	0	0	0.08	5.39	0	0.02	0.07	1.79	0.1	2.27	0.09	3.4	0.37	6.8	51.88	68.61	25.8	0.81
0.83	0.53	0	0	0.08	5.1	0	0.02	0.06	1.36	0.06	2.27	0.07	3.12	0.4	5.95	42.24	53.87	22.11	0.79
1.87	1.09	0	0	0	7.65	0	0.03	0.06	1.54	0.08	2.55	0.08	5.1	0.4	5.67	43.09	53.58	79.1	0.62
1.61	0.94	0	0	0	7.94	0	0.02	0.07	1.86	0.1	2.27	0.09	3.69	0.41	6.8	51.6	66.06	24.95	0.76
1.49	0.85	0	0	0.08	11.06	0	0.02	0.06	1.76	0.09	1.98	0.09	3.4	0.38	6.52	49.33	63.79	24.66	0.74
1.43	0.81	0	0	0.08	10.21	0	0.02	0.05	1.3	0.05	1.7	0.06	3.12	0.38	5.67	39.41	49.9	20.7	0.69
0.38	0.26	0	0	0.41	1392.84	4.48	0.04	0.5	1.26	0.16	218.3	5.5	3.97	2.4	5.95	88.45	39.69	14.46	1.23
0.95	0.61	0	0	0.13	5.1	0	0.02	0.06	2.74	0.14	1.98	0.1	4.82	0.38	7.65	58.12	72.86	25.8	0.64
0.75	0.48	0	0	0.08	4.54	0	0.02	0.05	2.6	0.13	1.7	0.09	4.25	0.34	7.09	55.28	68.89	24.38	0.6
0.68	0.44	0	0	0.08	4.25	0	0.01	0.05	1.73	0.07	1.7	0.06	3.97	0.33	5.95	42.53	51.03	19.85	0.56
1.08	0.69	0	0	0	5.95	0	0.02	0.07	2.02	0.11	2.55	0.09	3.69	0.41	7.37	56.42	73.43	26.93	0.79
1.18	0.7	0	0	0.08	5.67	0	0.02	0.07	1.85	0.1	2.27	0.09	3.4	0.37	6.8	51.88	67.47	24.95	0.73
1.05	0.64	0	0	0.08	5.39	0	0.02	0.06	1.47	0.06	1.98	0.06	3.12	0.4	5.95	42.24	51.88	21.26	0.73
1.9	1.11	0	0	0	8.22	0	0.03	0.06	1.62	0.07	2.55	0.08	5.1	0.41	5.95	43.94	54.43	81.65	0.58
1.66	0.97	0	0	0	8.22	0	0.03	0.07	1.97	0.09	2.27	0.09	3.97	0.42	7.09	53.01	67.19	24.95	0.71

USDA ID Code	Food Name	Weight in Grams*	Quantity of Units	Unit of Measure	Protein (gm)	Fat (gm)	Carbohydrates (gm)	Kcalories	Caffeine (gm)	Fiber (gm)	Cholesterol (mg)	Saturated Fat (gm)
5094	Chicken, Thigh, Meat&skin, Ckd, Roasted	28.35	3	Ounce	7.1	4.39	0	70.02	0	0	26.37	1.23
5095	Chicken, Thigh, Meat&skin, Ckd, Stewed	28.35	3	Ounce	6.59	4.18	0	65.77	0	0	23.81	1.17
5106	Chicken, Wing, Meat Only, Ckd, Fried	28.35	3	Ounce	8.55	2.59	0	59.82	0	0	23.81	0.71
5107	Chicken, Wing, Meat Only, Ckd, Roasted	28.35	3	Ounce	8.64	2.3	0	57.55	0	0	24.1	0.64
5108	Chicken, Wing, Meat Only, Ckd, Stewed	28.35	3	Ounce	7.71	2.04	0	51.31	0	0	20.98	0.57
5101	Chicken, Wing, Meat&skin, Ckd, Fried, Batter	28.35	3	Ounce	5.63	6.18	3.1	91.85	0	0	22.4	1.65
5102	Chicken, Wing, Meat&skin, Ckd, Fried, Flr	28.35	3	Ounce	7.4	6.28	0.68	91	0	0	22.96	1.72
5103	Chicken, Wing, Meat&skin, Ckd, Roasted	28.35	3	Ounce	7.61	5.52	0	82.22	0	0	23.81	1.55
5104	Chicken, Wing, Meat&skin, Ckd, Stewed	28.35	3	Ounce	6.46	4.77	0	70.59	0	0	19.85	1.34
16059	Chili w/ Beans, Cnd	255	0.5	Cup	14.56	14	30.37	285.6	0	11.22	43.35	6
7020	Corned Beef Loaf, Jellied	28.35	1	Slice	6.49	1.73	0	43.38	0	0	13.32	0.74
	Cornish Game Hen	110	0.5	Bird	25.63	4.257	0	147.4	0	0	116.6	1.089
5142	Duck, Domesticated, Meat Only, Roasted	28.35	3	Ounce	6.66	3.18	0	56.98	0	0	25.23	1.18
5140	Duck, Domesticated, Meat&skin, Roasted	28.35	3	Ounce	5.38	8.04	0	95.54	0	0	23.81	2.74
7021	Dutch Brand Loaf, Lunch Meat	28.35	1	Slice	3.8	5.05	1.58	68.04	0	0	13.32	1.8
7032	Ham and Cheese Loaf(or Roll), Lunch Meat	28.35	1	Slice	4.71	5.73	0.41	73.43	0	0	16.16	2.13
7033	Ham and Cheese Spread, Lunch Meat	15	1	Tbsp.	2.43	2.78	0.34	36.75	0	0	9.15	1.29
7031	Ham Salad Spread	15	1	Tbsp.	1.3	2.33	1.6	32.4	0	0	5.55	0.76
7029	Ham, Approx 11% Fat, Sliced	28.35	1	Slice	4.98	3	0.88	51.6	0	0	16.16	0.96
7027	Ham, Chopped, Not Cnd	28.35	3	Ounce	4.85	4.89	0	64.92	0	0	14.46	1.62
7026	Ham, Chopped, Spiced, Cnd	28.35	3	Ounce	4.55	5.34	0.08	67.76	0	0	13.89	1.78
7028	Ham, Extra Lean, Appx 5% Fat	28.35	1	Slice	5.49	1.41	0.27	37.14	0	0	13.32	0.46
7030	Ham, Minced	28.35	3	Ounce	4.62	5.86	0.52	74.56	0	0	19.85	2.04
62626	Hamburger Patty, Meatless	90	1	Each	18	4	8	140	0	5	0	1.5
7035	Honey Loaf, Lunch Meat	28.35	1	Slice	4.47	1.27	1.51	36.29	0	0	9.64	0.41
7022	Hot Dog, Beef	57	1	Each	6.84	16.25	1.03	179.55	0	0	34.77	6.87
7024	Hot Dog, Chicken	45	1	Each	5.82	8.77	3.06	115.65	0	0	45.45	2.49
62605	Hot Dog, Fat Free	50	1	Each	7	0	2	40	0	0	15	0
7025	Hot Dog, Turkey	45	1	Each	6.43	7.97	0.67	101.7	0	0	48.15	2.65
16137	Hummus, Fresh	246	0.5	Cup	12.1	20.8	49.6	421	0	12.5	0	3.1
17225	Lamb, Ground, Ckd, Broiled	28.35	3	Ounce	7.02	5.57	0	80.23	0	0	27.5	2.3
17016	Lamb, Leg, Shank, Meat and Fat, Ckd, Rstd	28.35	3	Ounce	7.49	3.53	0	63.79	0	0	25.52	1.44
17018	Lamb, Leg, Shank, Meat Only, Ckd, Rstd	28.35	3	Ounce	7.99	1.89	0	51.03	0	0	24.66	0.67
17020	Lamb, Leg, Sirloin, Meat and Fat, Ckd, Rstd	28.35	3	Ounce	6.98	5.86	0	82.78	0	0	27.5	2.48
17022	Lamb, Leg, Sirloin, Meat Only, Ckd, Rstd	28.35	3	Ounce	8.04	2.6	0	57.83	0	0	26.08	0.93
17012	Lamb, Leg, Whole, Meat and Fat, Ckd, Rstd	28.35	3	Ounce	7.24	4.67	0	73.14	0	0	26.37	1.95
17014	Lamb, Leg, Whole, Meat Only, Ckd, Rstd	28.35	3	Ounce	8.02	2.19	0	54.15	0	0	25.23	0.78
17024	Lamb, Loin, Meat and Fat, Ckd, Broiled	28.35	3	Ounce	7.14	6.54	0	89.59	0	0	28.35	2.79
17025	Lamb, Loin, Meat and Fat, Ckd, Roasted	28.35	3	Ounce	6.39	6.69	0	87.6	0	0	26.93	2.9
17027	Lamb, Loin, Meat Only, Ckd, Broiled	28.35	3	Ounce	8.5	2.76	0	61.24	0	0	26.93	0.98
17028	Lamb, Loin, Meat Only, Ckd, Roasted	28.35	3	Ounce	7.54	2.77	0	57.27	0	0	24.66	1.05
17002	Lamb, Meat and Fat, Ckd	28.35	3	Ounce	6.95	5.94	0	83.35	0	0	27.5	2.5
17004	Lamb, Meat Only, Ckd	28.35	3	Ounce	8	2.7	0	58.4	0	0	26.08	0.96
17030	Lamb, Rib, Meat and Fat, Ckd, Broiled	28.35	3	Ounce	6.27	8.39	0	102.34	0	0	28.07	3.6
17031	Lamb, Rib, Meat and Fat, Ckd, Roasted	28.35	3	Ounce	5.99	8.45	0	101.78	0	0	27.5	3.62
17033	Lamb, Rib, Meat Only, Ckd, Broiled	28.35	3	Ounce	7.86	3.67	0	66.62	0	0	25.8	1.32
17034	Lamb, Rib, Meat Only, Ckd, Roasted	28.35	3	Ounce	7.42	3.77	0	65.77	0	0	24.95	1.35
10161	Olive Loaf, Lunch Meat	28.35	1	Slice	3.36	4.68	2.6	66.62	0	0	10.77	1.66
7051	Olive Loaf, Pork, Lunch Meat	28.35	1	Slice	3.35	4.68	2.61	66.62	0	0	10.77	1.66
10162	Pickle and Pimento Loaf, Lunch Meat	28.35	1	Slice	3.26	5.98	1.67	74.28	0	0	10.49	2.23
7058	Pickle and Pimiento Loaf, Pork, Lunch Meat	28.35	1	Slice	3.26	5.98	1.67	74.28	0	0	10.49	2.22
7062	Picnic Loaf, Lunch Meat	28.35	1	Slice	4.23	4.72	1.35	65.77	0	0	10.77	1.72
10193	Pork, Backribs	28.35	3	Ounce	6.88	8.39	0	104.9	0	0	33.45	3.12
10127	Pork, Braunschweiger	28.35	3	Ounce	3.83	9.1	0.89	101.78	0	0	44.23	3.09
7045	Pork, Cnd, Lunch Meat	21	1	Slice	2.63	6.36	0.44	70.14	0	0	13.02	2.27

Monounsaturated Fat (gm)	Polyunsaturated Fat (gm)	Vitamin D (mg)	Vitamin K (mg)	Vitamin E (mg)	Vitamin A (re)	Vitamin C (mg)	Thiamin (mg)	Riboflavin (mg)	Niacin (mg)	Vitamin B6 (mg)	Folate (mg)	Vitamin B12 (mcg)	Calcium (mg)	Iron (mg)	Magnesium (mg)	Phosphorus (mg)	Potassium (mg)	Sodium (mg)	Zinc (mg)
1.74	0.97	0	0	0.08	13.61	0	0.02	0.06	1.8	0.09	1.98	0.08	3.4	0.38	6.24	49.33	62.94	23.81	0.67
1.66	0.92	0	0	0.08	12.47	0	0.02	0.05	1.39	0.05	1.7	0.05	3.12	0.39	5.39	39.41	48.2	20.13	0.64
0.87	0.59	0	0	0	5.1	0	0.01	0.04	2.05	0.17	1.13	0.1	4.25	0.32	5.95	46.49	58.97	25.8	0.6
0.74	0.5	0	0	0.08	5.1	0	0.01	0.04	2.07	0.17	1.13	0.1	4.54	0.33	5.95	47.06	59.54	26.08	0.61
0.65	0.45	0	0	0.08	4.54	0	0.01	0.03	1.47	0.09	0.85	0.06	3.69	0.32	5.1	37.99	43.38	20.7	0.57
2.54	1.44	0	0	0	9.64	0	0.03	0.04	1.49	0.09	1.7	0.07	5.67	0.37	4.54	34.3	39.12	90.72	0.39
2.52	1.4	0	0	0	10.77	0	0.02	0.04	1.9	0.12	0.85	0.08	4.25	0.35	5.39	42.53	50.18	21.83	0.5
2.17	1.17	0	0	0.08	13.32	0	0.01	0.04	1.88	0.12	0.85	0.08	4.25	0.36	5.39	42.81	52.16	23.25	0.52
1.87	1.01	0	0	0.08	11.34	0	0.01	0.03	1.31	0.06	0.85	0.05	3.4	0.32	4.54	34.3	39.41	18.99	0.46
5.95	0.92	0	0	1.87	86.7	4.34	0.12	0.27	0.91	0.34	57.89	0	119.85	8.75	114.75	392.7	930.75	1331.1	5.1
0.76	0.09	0	0	0.05	0	2.27	0	0.03	0.5	0.03	2.27	0.36	3.12	0.58	3.12	20.7	28.63	270.18	1.16
1.364	1.034	0	0	0.291	22	0.66	0.083	0.25	6.9	0.394	2.2	0.33	14.3	0.847	20.9	163.9	275	69.3	1.683
1.05	0.41	0	0	0.2	6.52	0	0.07	0.13	1.45	0.07	2.84	0.11	3.4	0.77	5.67	57.55	71.44	18.43	0.74
3.66	1.03	0	0	0.2	17.86	0	0.05	0.08	1.37	0.05	1.7	0.09	3.12	0.77	4.54	44.23	57.83	16.73	0.53
2.36	0.54	0.28	0	0.06	0	5.1	0.09	0.08	0.68	0.07	0.57	0.37	23.81	0.35	5.95	45.93	106.6	354.38	0.49
2.63	0.62	0.31	0	0.08	6.52	7.09	0.17	0.05	0.98	0.07	0.85	0.23	16.44	0.26	4.54	71.73	83.35	380.74	0.57
1.06	0.21	0	0	0	13.65	1.05	0.05	0.03	0.32	0.02	0.45	0.11	32.55	0.11	2.7	74.25	24.3	179.55	0.34
1.08	0.4	0	0	0.26	0	0.9	0.07	0.02	0.31	0.02	0.15	0.11	1.2	0.09	1.5	18	22.5	136.8	0.16
1.4	0.34	0	0	0.08	0	7.94	0.24	0.07	1.49	0.1	0.85	0.24	1.98	0.28	5.39	70.02	94.12	373.37	0.61
2.32	0.6	0	0	0	0	5.67	0.18	0.06	1.1	0.1	0.28	0.26	1.98	0.24	4.54	43.94	90.44	388.68	0.55
2.6	0.58	0	0	0.07	0	0.57	0.15	0.05	0.91	0.09	0.28	0.2	1.98	0.27	3.69	39.41	80.51	386.98	0.52
0.67	0.14	0	0	0.08	0	7.37	0.26	0.06	1.37	0.13	1.13	0.21	1.98	0.22	4.82	61.8	99.23	405.12	0.55
2.71	0.7	0	0	0	0	8.51	0.2	0.05	1.18	0.07	0.28	0.27	2.84	0.22	4.54	44.51	88.17	352.96	0.54
0	0.5	0	0	0	0	0	0.25	0	4	0	0	0	96	1.5	0	0	0	380	7.5
0.57	0.13	0.26	0	0.06	0	5.95	0.14	0.07	0.89	0.09	2.27	0.31	4.82	0.38	4.82	40.54	97.24	374.22	0.69
7.76	0.79	0.51	0	0.11	0	13.68	0.03	0.06	1.38	0.07	2.28	0.88	11.4	0.82	1.71	49.59	94.62	584.82	1.24
3.82	1.82	0	0	0.1	17.1	0	0.03	0.05	1.39	0.14	1.8	0.11	42.75	0.9	4.5	48.15	37.8	616.5	0.47
0	0	0	0	0	0	0	0	0	0	0	0	0	0	0.2	0	0	0	460	0
2.51	2.25	0	0	0.28	0	0	0.02	0.08	1.86	0.1	3.6	0.13	47.7	0.83	6.3	60.3	80.55	641.7	1.4
8.7	7.8	0	0	2.4	5	19	0.23	0.13	1	0.98	146	0	123	3.86	71	276	428	600	2.71
2.36	0.4	0	0	0.07	0	0	0.03	0.07	1.9	0.04	5.39	0.74	6.24	0.51	6.8	56.98	96.11	22.96	1.32
1.5	0.25	0	0	0.05	0	0	0.03	0.08	1.86	0.05	6.24	0.76	2.84	0.56	7.09	56.13	92.42	18.43	1.32
0.83	0.12	0	0	0.05	0	0	0.03	0.08	1.81	0.05	6.8	0.77	2.27	0.58	7.37	58.97	96.96	18.71	1.42
2.47	0.42	0	0	0.04	0	0	0.03	0.08	1.88	0.04	4.82	0.72	3.12	0.57	6.24	51.88	85.33	19.28	1.17
1.14	0.17	0	0	0.05	0	0	0.03	0.09	1.78	0.05	5.95	0.73	2.27	0.62	7.09	57.55	94.41	20.13	1.37
1.97	0.33	0	0	0.04	0	0	0.03	0.08	1.87	0.04	5.67	0.73	3.12	0.56	6.8	54.15	88.74	18.71	1.25
0.96	0.14	0	0	0.05	0	0	0.03	0.08	1.8	0.05	6.52	0.75	2.27	0.6	7.37	58.4	95.82	19.28	1.4
2.75	0.48	0	0	0.04	0	0	0.03	0.07	2.01	0.04	5.1	0.7	5.67	0.51	6.8	55.57	92.7	21.83	0.99
2.74	0.53	0	0	0.03	0	0	0.03	0.07	2.01	0.03	5.39	0.63	5.1	0.6	6.52	51.03	69.74	18.14	0.97
1.21	0.18	0	0	0.05	0	0	0.03	0.08	1.94	0.05	6.8	0.71	5.39	0.57	7.94	64.07	106.6	23.81	1.17
1.12	0.24	0	0	0.05	0	0	0.03	0.08	1.94	0.05	7.09	0.61	4.82	0.69	7.65	58.4	75.69	18.71	1.15
2.5	0.43	0	0	0	0	0	0.03	0.07	1.89	0.04	5.1	0.72	4.82	0.53	6.52	53.3	87.89	20.41	1.26
1.18	0.18	0	0	0.05	0	0	0.03	0.08	1.79	0.05	6.52	0.74	4.25	0.58	7.37	59.54	97.52	21.55	1.49
3.44	0.67	0	0	0.03	0	0	0.03	0.06	1.98	0.03	3.97	0.72	5.39	0.53	6.52	50.46	76.55	21.55	1.13
3.55	0.62	0	0	0.03	0	0	0.03	0.06	1.91	0.03	4.25	0.63	6.24	0.45	5.67	47.06	76.83	20.7	0.99
1.48	0.33	0	0	0.05	0	0	0.03	0.07	1.86	0.04	5.95	0.75	4.54	0.63	8.22	60.39	88.74	24.1	1.49
1.65	0.25	0	0	0.04	0	0	0.03	0.07	1.75	0.04	6.24	0.61	5.95	0.5	6.52	55.28	89.3	22.96	1.27
2.23	0.55	0	0	0	5.67	2.49	0.08	0.07	0.52	0.07	0.57	0.36	30.9	0.15	5.39	36	84.2	420.71	0.39
2.23	0.55	0.31	0	0.07	0	2.55	0.08	0.07	0.52	0.07	0.57	0.36	30.9	0.15	5.39	36	84.2	420.71	0.39
2.72	0.73	0	0	0	1.98	3.83	0.08	0.07	0.58	0.05	1.42	0.33	26.93	0.29	5.1	39.69	96.39	393.78	0.4
2.72	0.73	0.31	0	0.07	8505	3.97	0.08	0.07	0.58	0.05	1.42	0.33	26.93	0.29	5.1	39.69	96.39	393.78	0.4
2.18	0.54	0.34	0	0	0	5.1	0.11	0.07	0.65	0.09	0.57	0.43	13.32	0.29	4.25	35.44	75.69	329.99	0.62
3.82	0.66	0	0	0	0.85	0.09	0.12	0.06	1.01	0.09	0.85	0.18	12.76	0.39	5.95	55.28	89.3	28.63	0.96
4.23	1.06	0	0	0	1196.37	2.72	0.07	0.43	2.37	0.09	12.47	5.7	2.55	2.65	3.12	47.63	56.42	324.04	0.8
3	0.75	0	0	0	0	0.21	0.08	0.04	0.66	0.04	1.26	0.19	1.26	0.15	2.1	17.22	45.15	270.69	0.31

USDA ID Code	Food Name	Weight in Grams*	Quantity of Units	Unit of Measure	Protein (gm)	Fat (gm)	Carbohydrates (gm)	Kcalories	Caffeine (gm)	Fiber (gm)	Cholesterol (mg)	Saturated Fat (gm)
10220	Pork, Ground, Ckd	28.35	3	Ounce	7.28	5.89	0	84.2	0	0	26.65	2.19
10154	Pork, Ham and Cheese Loaf or Roll	28.35	3	Ounce	4.71	5.73	0.41	73.43	0	0	16.16	2.13
10147	Pork, Ham Patties, Grilled	28.35	3	Ounce	3.77	8.75	0.48	96.96	0	0	20.41	3.14
10148	Pork, Ham Salad Spread	28.35	3	Ounce	2.46	4.4	3.02	61.24	0	0	10.49	1.43
10143	Pork, Ham, Chopped, Cnd	28.35	3	Ounce	4.55	5.34	0.08	67.76	0	0	13.89	1.78
10138	Pork, Ham, Cnd, Extra Lean (appx 4% Fat), Roasted	28.35	3	Ounce	6	1.38	0.15	38.56	0	0	8.51	0.45
10185	Pork, Ham, Cnd, Extra Lean and Reg, Roasted	28.35	3	Ounce	5.94	2.39	0.14	47.34	0	0	11.62	0.8
10184	Pork, Ham, Cnd, Extra Lean and Reg, Unheated	28.35	3	Ounce	5.09	2.11	0	40.82	0	0	10.77	0.69
10140	Pork, Ham, Cnd, Regular (approx 13% Fat), Roasted	28.35	3	Ounce	5.82	4.31	0.12	64.07	0	0	17.58	1.43
10134	Pork, Ham, Extra Lean (5% Fat), Roasted	28.35	3	Ounce	5.93	1.57	0.43	41.11	0	0	15.03	0.51
10133	Pork, Ham, Extra Lean (5% Fat), Unheated	28.35	3	Ounce	5.49	1.41	0.27	37.14	0	0	13.32	0.46
10183	Pork, Ham, Extra Lean and Reg, Roasted	28.35	3	Ounce	6.23	2.17	0.14	46.78	0	0	16.16	0.74
10182	Pork, Ham, Extra Lean and Reg, Unheated	28.35	3	Ounce	5.18	2.38	0.65	45.93	0	0	15.03	0.77
10151	Pork, Ham, Meat and Fat, Roasted	28.35	3	Ounce	6.12	4.75	0	68.89	0	0	17.58	1.7
10153	Pork, Ham, Meat Only, Roasted	28.35	3	Ounce	7.1	1.56	0	44.51	0	0	15.59	0.52
10136	Pork, Ham, Regular (11% Fat), Roasted	28.35	3	Ounce	6.41	2.56	0	50.46	0	0	16.73	0.88
10135	Pork, Ham, Regular (11% Fat), Unheated	28.35	3	Ounce	4.98	3	0.88	51.6	0	0	16.16	0.96
10172	Pork, Smoked Link Sausage, Grilled	28.35	3	Ounce	6.29	9	0.6	110.28	0	0	19.28	3.21
10089	Pork, Spareribs, Meat and Fat, Ckd, Braised	28.35	3	Ounce	8.24	8.59	0	112.55	0	0	34.3	3.15
10221	Pork, Tenderloin, Meat and Fat, Ckd, Broiled	28.35	3	Ounce	8.47	2.3	0	56.98	0	0	26.65	0.83
10223	Pork, Tenderloin, Meat Only, Ckd, Broiled	28.35	3	Ounce	8.62	1.79	0	53.01	0	0	26.65	0.64
7003	Sausage, Beerwurst, Pork	23	1	Slice	3.28	4.32	0.47	54.74	0	0	13.57	1.44
7006	Sausage, Bockwurst	65	1	Link	8.66	17.92	0.31	199.55	0	0	38.35	6.58
7013	Sausage, Bratwurst	85	1	Link	11.97	21.99	1.76	255.85	0	0	51	7.92
7089	Sausage, Italian, Ckd	83	1	Link	16.62	21.33	1.25	268.09	0	0	64.74	7.53
7037	Sausage, Kielbasa, Kolbassy	85	1	Link	11.27	23.08	1.82	263.5	0	0	56.95	8.42
7038	Sausage, Knockwurst	68	1	Link	8.08	18.88	1.2	209.44	0	0	39.44	6.94
7075	Sausage, Link, Pork and Beef	68	1	Link	9.11	20.62	0.97	228.48	0	0	48.28	7.22
7057	Sausage, Pepperoni	5.5	1	Slice	1.15	2.42	0.16	27.34	0	0	4.35	0.89
7059	Sausage, Polish-style	84	1	Each	12	24.3	1.5	276	0	0	60	8.7
7064	Sausage, Pork, Links or Bulk, Ckd	13	1	Link	2.55	4.05	0.13	47.97	0	0	10.79	1.41
7072	Sausage, Salami, Beef and Pork, Dry	10	1	Slice	2.29	3.44	0.26	41.8	0	0	7.9	1.22
7068	Sausage, Salami, Beef, Ckd	23	1	Slice	3.46	4.76	0.65	60.26	0	0	14.95	2.07
7074	Sausage, Smoked Link, Pork	68	1	Link	15.1	21.56	1.43	264.52	0	0	46.24	7.7
62661	Sausage, Turkey	28.35	3	Ounce	4	2.5	1.5	45	0	0	15	1.25
5297	Turkey Bologna	21	1	Slice	2.88	3.19	0.2	41.79	0	0	20.79	1.06
7079	Turkey Breast Meat	21	1	Slice	4.73	0.33	0	23.1	0	0	8.61	0.1
5292	Turkey Burger, Breaded, Battered, Fried	28.35	3	Ounce	3.97	5.1	4.45	80.23	0	0.14	17.58	1.33
5287	Turkey Lunch Meat	28.35	1	Slice	5.37	1.44	0.1	36.29	0	0	15.88	0.48
5289	Turkey Pastrami	28.35	1	Slice	5.21	1.76	0.47	39.97	0	0	15.31	0.51
5296	Turkey Roast, Roasted	28.35	3	Ounce	6.04	1.64	0.87	43.94	0	0	15.03	0.54
5291	Turkey Roll, Light and Dark Meat	28.35	3	Ounce	5.14	1.98	0.6	42.24	0	0	15.59	0.58
5290	Turkey Roll, Light Meat	28.35	3	Ounce	5.3	2.05	0.15	41.67	0	0	12.19	0.57
5299	Turkey Salami	28.35	1	Slice	4.64	3.91	0.16	55.57	0	0	23.25	1.14
5300	Turkey Sticks, Breaded, Battered, Fried	28.35	3	Ounce	4.03	4.79	4.82	79.1	0	0	18.14	1.24
5294	Turkey Thigh, Prebasted, Meat&skin, Ckd, Roasted	28.35	3	Ounce	5.33	2.42	0	44.51	0	0	17.58	0.75
5190	Turkey, Back, Meat&skin, Ckd, Roasted	28.35	3	Ounce	7.54	4.08	0	68.89	0	0	25.8	1.19
5192	Turkey, Breast, Meat&skin, Ckd, Roasted	28.35	3	Ounce	8.14	2.1	0	53.58	0	0	20.98	0.6
5164	Turkey, Ckd, Roasted, Meat&skin&giblets&neck	28.35	3	Ounce	7.93	2.68	0.02	58.12	0	0	26.93	0.79
5188	Turkey, Dark Meat, Ckd, Roasted	28.35	3	Ounce	8.1	2.05	0	53.01	0	0	24.1	0.69
5184	Turkey, Dark Meat, Meat&skin, Ckd, Roasted	28.35	3	Ounce	7.79	3.27	0	62.65	0	0	25.23	0.99
5172	Turkey, Giblets, Ckd, Simmered, Some Giblet Fat	28.35	3	Ounce	7.53	1.44	0.59	47.34	0	0	118.5	0.44
5306	Turkey, Ground, Ckd	28.35	3	Ounce	7.76	3.73	0	66.62	0	0	28.92	0.96
5194	Turkey, Leg, Meat&skin, Ckd, Roasted	28.35	3	Ounce	7.9	2.78	0	58.97	0	0	24.1	0.87
5186	Turkey, Light Meat, Ckd, Roasted	28.35	3	Ounce	8.48	0.91	0	44.51	0	0	19.56	0.29

Monounsaturated Fat (gm)	Polyunsaturated Fat (gm)	Vitamin D (mg)	Vitamin K (mg)	Vitamin E (mg)	Vitamin A (re)	Vitamin C (mg)	Thiamin (mg)	Riboflavin (mg)	Niacin (mg)	Vitamin B6 (mg)	Folate (mg)	Vitamin B12 (mcg)	Calcium (mg)	Iron (mg)	Magnesium (mg)	Phosphorus (mg)	Potassium (mg)	Sodium (mg)	Zinc (mg)
2.62	0.53	0	0	0	0.57	0.2	0.2	0.06	1.19	0.11	1.7	0.15	6.24	0.37	6.8	64.07	102.63	20.7	0.91
2.63	0.62	0	0	0	6.52	7.12	0.17	0.05	0.98	0.07	0.85	0.23	16.44	0.26	4.54	71.73	83.35	380.74	0.57
4.16	0.94	0	0	0.07	0	0	0.1	0.05	0.92	0.05	0.85	0.2	2.55	0.46	2.84	28.63	69.17	301.36	0.54
2.04	0.77	0	0	0	0	1.7	0.12	0.03	0.59	0.04	0.28	0.22	2.27	0.17	2.84	34.02	42.53	258.55	0.31
2.6	0.58	0	0	0	0	0.51	0.15	0.05	0.91	0.09	0.28	0.2	1.98	0.27	3.69	39.41	80.51	386.98	0.52
0.71	0.12	0	0	0.07	0	7.8	0.29	0.07	1.39	0.13	1.42	0.2	1.7	0.26	5.95	59.25	98.66	321.77	0.63
1.15	0.26	0	0	0.07	0	6.49	0.27	0.07	1.43	0.11	1.42	0.24	1.98	0.3	5.67	62.65	99.51	302.78	0.66
1.01	0.22	0	0	0.07	0	7.14	0.25	0.07	1.3	0.13	1.7	0.23	1.7	0.26	4.54	58.68	94.69	361.75	0.52
2	0.5	0	0	0	0	3.97	0.23	0.07	1.5	0.09	1.42	0.3	2.27	0.39	4.82	68.89	101.21	266.77	0.71
0.74	0.15	0	0	0.07	0	5.95	0.21	0.06	1.14	0.11	0.85	0.18	2.27	0.42	3.97	55.57	81.36	341.05	0.82
0.67	0.14	0	0	0.07	0	7.46	0.26	0.06	1.37	0.13	1.13	0.21	1.98	0.22	4.82	61.8	99.23	405.12	0.55
1.06	0.3	0	0	0.07	0	6.24	0.21	0.08	1.51	0.1	0.85	0.19	2.27	0.4	5.39	70.31	102.63	392.65	0.75
1.12	0.26	0	0	0.07	0	7.71	0.25	0.07	1.44	0.11	0.85	0.23	1.98	0.26	5.1	66.91	84.2	362.31	0.58
2.23	0.51	0	0	0.07	0	0	0.17	0.06	1.26	0.11	0.85	0.18	1.98	0.25	5.39	60.67	81.08	336.51	0.66
0.72	0.18	0	0	0.07	0	0	0.19	0.07	1.42	0.13	1.13	0.2	1.98	0.27	6.24	64.35	89.59	376.2	0.73
1.26	0.4	0	0	0.07	0	6.44	0.21	0.09	1.74	0.09	0.85	0.2	2.27	0.38	6.24	79.66	115.95	425.25	0.7
1.4	0.34	0	0	0.07	0	7.85	0.24	0.07	1.49	0.1	0.85	0.24	1.98	0.28	5.39	70.02	94.12	373.37	0.61
4.15	1.07	0	0	0.09	0	0.51	0.2	0.07	1.28	0.1	1.42	0.46	8.51	0.33	5.39	45.93	95.26	425.25	0.8
3.82	0.77	0	0	0.07	0.85	0	0.12	0.11	1.55	0.1	1.13	0.31	13.32	0.52	6.8	73.99	90.72	26.37	1.3
0.95	0.21	0	0	0	0.57	0.28	0.27	0.11	1.43	0.15	1.7	0.28	1.42	0.39	9.92	82.22	125.87	18.14	0.82
0.73	0.16	0	0	0	0.57	0.28	0.28	0.11	1.46	0.15	1.7	0.28	1.42	0.41	10.21	83.63	127.86	18.43	0.84
2.07	0.54	0.21	0	0.06	0	6.67	0.13	0.04	0.75	0.08	0.69	0.2	1.84	0.17	2.99	23.69	58.19	285.2	0.4
8.45	1.94	0	0	0.09	3.9	0	0.27	0.11	2.68	0.15	3.9	0.53	10.4	0.42	11.7	94.9	175.5	718.25	1.01
10.36	2.33	0	0	0.21	0	0.85	0.43	0.16	2.72	0.18	1.7	0.81	37.4	1.1	12.75	126.65	180.2	473.45	1.96
9.92	2.73	0	0	0.21	0	1.66	0.52	0.19	3.46	0.27	4.15	1.08	19.92	1.25	14.94	141.1	252.32	765.26	1.98
11	2.62	0	0	0.19	0	17.85	0.19	0.18	2.45	0.15	4.25	1.37	37.4	1.23	13.6	125.8	230.35	914.6	1.72
8.71	1.99	0	0	0.39	0	18.36	0.23	0.1	1.86	0.12	1.36	0.8	7.48	0.62	7.48	66.64	135.32	686.8	1.13
9.65	2.22	0	0	0.15	0	12.92	0.18	0.12	2.19	0.12	1.36	1.03	6.8	0.99	8.16	72.76	128.52	642.6	1.43
1.16	0.24	0	0	0.01	0	0	0.02	0.01	0.27	0.01	0.22	0.14	0.55	0.08	0.88	6.55	19.09	112.2	0.14
11.4	2.7	0	0	0	0	0	0.42	0.12	3	0.15	3	0.84	9	1.23	12	117	201	744	1.65
1.81	0.5	0	0	0.02	0	0.26	0.1	0.03	0.59	0.04	0.26	0.22	4.16	0.16	2.21	23.92	46.93	168.22	0.33
1.71	0.32	0	0	0.03	0	2.6	0.06	0.03	0.49	0.05	0.2	0.19	0.8	0.15	1.7	14.2	37.8	186	0.32
2.17	0.24	0.28	0	0.04	0	3.98	0.02	0.04	0.74	0.04	0.46	0.7	2.07	0.5	3.22	25.99	51.52	270.48	0.5
9.96	2.56	0	0	0.17	0	1.36	0.48	0.17	3.08	0.24	3.4	1.11	20.4	0.79	12.92	110.16	228.48	1020	1.92
0	0	0	0	0	10	6	0	0	0	0	0	0	12	1.75	0	0	0	300	0
1.01	0.9	0	0	0	0	0	0.01	0.03	0.74	0.05	1.47	0.06	17.64	0.32	2.94	27.51	41.79	184.38	0.37
0.09	0.06	0	0	0	0	0	0.01	0.02	1.75	0.08	0.84	0.42	1.47	0.08	4.2	48.09	58.38	300.51	0.24
2.12	1.34	0	0	0.68	3.12	0	0.03	0.05	0.65	0.06	2.27	0.06	3.97	0.62	4.25	76.55	77.96	226.8	0.41
0.33	0.43	0	0	0.18	0	0	0.01	0.07	1	0.07	1.7	0.07	2.84	0.78	4.54	54.15	92.14	282.37	0.83
0.58	0.45	0	0	0.06	0	0	0.02	0.07	1	0.08	1.42	0.07	2.55	0.47	3.97	56.7	73.71	296.26	0.61
0.34	0.47	0	0	0.11	0	0	0.01	0.05	1.78	0.08	1.42	0.43	1.42	0.46	6.24	69.17	84.48	192.78	0.72
0.65	0.5	0	0	0.1	0	0	0.03	0.08	1.36	0.08	1.42	0.07	9.07	0.38	5.1	47.63	76.55	166.13	0.57
0.71	0.49	0	0	0	0	0	0.03	0.06	1.98	0.09	1.13	0.07	11.34	0.36	4.54	51.88	71.16	138.63	0.44
1.29	1	0	0	0	0	0	0.02	0.05	1	0.07	1.13	0.06	5.67	0.46	4.25	30.05	69.17	284.63	0.51
1.96	1.24	0	0	0	3.4	0	0.03	0.05	0.6	0.06	2.55	0.07	3.97	0.62	4.25	66.34	73.71	237.57	0.41
0.72	0.67	0	0	0	0	0	0.02	0.07	0.68	0.07	1.7	0.07	2.27	0.43	4.82	48.48	68.32	123.89	1.17
1.42	1.05	0	0	0.17	0	0	0.02	0.06	0.98	0.09	2.27	0.1	9.36	0.62	6.24	53.58	73.71	20.7	1.11
0.69	0.51	0	0	0	0	0	0.02	0.04	1.8	0.14	1.7	0.1	5.95	0.4	7.65	59.54	81.65	17.86	0.58
0.86	0.69	0	0	0	19.28	0.03	0.02	0.06	1.4	0.11	5.67	0.36	7.37	0.57	6.8	56.7	77.11	18.99	0.89
0.46	0.61	0	0	0.18	0	0	0.02	0.07	1.03	0.1	2.55	0.1	9.07	0.66	6.8	57.83	82.22	22.4	1.26
1.03	0.88	0	0	0.17	0	0	0.02	0.07	1	0.09	2.55	0.1	9.36	0.64	6.52	55.57	77.68	21.55	1.18
0.33	0.33	0	0	0.41	508.88	0.48	0.01	0.26	1.28	0.09	97.81	6.81	3.69	1.9	4.82	57.83	56.7	16.73	1.04
1.39	0.92	0	0	0.1	0	0	0.02	0.05	1.37	0.11	1.98	0.09	7.09	0.55	6.8	55.57	76.55	30.33	0.81
0.81	0.77	0	0	0.18	0	0	0.02	0.07	1.01	0.09	2.55	0.1	9.07	0.65	6.52	56.42	79.38	21.83	1.21
0.16	0.24	0	0	0.03	0	0	0.02	0.04	1.94	0.15	1.7	0.1	5.39	0.38	7.94	62.09	86.47	18.14	0.58

USDA ID Code	Food Name	Weight in Grams*	Quantity of Units	Unit of Measure	Protein (gm)	Fat (gm)	Carbohydrates (gm)	Kcalories	Caffeine (gm)	Fiber (gm)	Cholesterol (mg)	Saturated Fat (gm)
5182	Turkey, Light Meat, Meat&skin, Ckd, Roasted	28.35	3	Ounce	8.1	2.36	0	55.85	0	0	21.55	0.66
5168	Turkey, Meat Only, Ckd, Roasted	28.35	3	Ounce	8.31	1.41	0	48.2	0	0	21.55	0.46
5166	Turkey, Meat&skin, Ckd, Roasted	28.35	3	Ounce	7.97	2.76	0	58.97	0	0	23.25	0.81
5288	Turkey, Thin Sliced	28.35	3	Ounce	6.38	0.45	0	31.19	0	0	11.62	0.14
5196	Turkey, Wing, Meat&skin, Ckd, Roasted	28.35	3	Ounce	7.76	3.52	0	64.92	0	0	22.96	0.96
17089	Veal, Meat and Fat, Ckd	28.35	3	Ounce	8.53	3.23	0	65.49	0	0	32.32	1.21
17091	Veal, Meat Only, Ckd	28.35	3	Ounce	9.04	1.87	0	55.57	0	0	33.45	0.52
17165	Venison, Ckd, Roasted	28.35	3	Ounce	8.56	0.9	0	44.79	0	0	31.75	0.35
	Almond Butter, w/ salt	16	1	Tbsp.	2.43	9.456	3.395	101.28	0	0.592	0	0.896
	Almond Butter, w/o salt	16	1	Tbsp.	2.43	9.456	3.395	101.28	0	0.592	0	0.896
12067	Almonds, Toasted, Unblanched	141.96	0.5	Cup	28.93	72.07	32.52	836.14	0	15.9	0	6.83
12078	Brazilnuts, Dried, Unblanched	224	1	Ounce	4.1	18.8	3.6	186	0	1.5	0	4.6
12585	Cashews, Dry Roasted	112	0.5	Cup	17.2	52.4	37.2	652	0	3.6	0	10.4
12586	Cashews, Oil Roasted	112	0.5	Cup	17.2	52.4	37.2	652	0	3.6	0	10.4
12131	Macadamias, Dried	112	0.5	Cup	9.6	83.6	15.6	769	0	10.4	0	13.6
12633	Macadamias, Oil Roasted	112	0.5	Cup	9.6	83.6	15.6	769	0	10.4	0	13.6
12635	Mixed w/ Peanuts, Dry Roasted	112	0.5	Cup	20	64	24	680	0	12.33	0	8
12637	Mixed w/ Peanuts, Oil Roasted	112	0.5	Cup	19.2	64	24.4	700	0	11.2	0	10
12638	Mixed w/o Peanuts, Oil Roasted	112	0.5	Cup	19.2	64	24.4	700	0	11.2	0	10
16097	Peanut Butter, Chunk Style, w/ Salt	16.139	2	Tbsp.	3.88	8.06	3.48	95.06	0	1.07	0	1.55
16397	Peanut Butter, Chunk Style, w/o Salt	16.139	2	Tbsp.	3.88	8.06	3.48	95.06	0	1.07	0	1.55
62689	Peanut Butter, Reduced Fat	18	2	Tbsp.	4	6	7.5	95	0	1	0	1.25
16098	Peanut Butter, Smooth Style, w/ Salt	16.139	2	Tbsp.	3.97	8.07	3.34	94.9	0	0.95	0	1.55
16398	Peanut Butter, Smooth Style, w/o Salt	16.139	2	Tbsp.	3.97	8.07	3.34	94.9	0	0	0	1.55
12681	Peanut Kernels, Oil Roasted	112	0.5	Cup	37.94	70.99	27.26	836.64	0	12.67	0	9.85
16088	Peanuts, All Types, Ckd, Boiled, w/ Salt	112	0.5	Cup	6.8	7	6.8	102	0	2.8	0	1.92
16090	Peanuts, All Types, Dry-roasted, w/ Salt	112	0.5	Cup	34.57	72.5	31.4	854.1	0	11.68	0	10.06
16390	Peanuts, All Types, Dry-roasted, w/o Salt	112	0.5	Cup	34.57	72.5	31.4	854.1	0	11.68	0	10.06
16087	Peanuts, All Types, Fresh	112	0.5	Cup	37.67	71.89	23.56	827.82	0	12.41	0	9.98
16089	Peanuts, All Types, Oil-roasted, w/ Salt	112	0.5	Cup	37.94	70.99	27.26	836.64	0	13.25	0	9.85
16389	Peanuts, All Types, Oil-roasted, w/o Salt	112	0.5	Cup	37.94	70.99	27.26	836.64	0	13.25	0	9.85
16091	Peanuts, Spanish, Fresh	112	0.5	Cup	38.18	72.42	23.1	832.2	0	13.87	0	11.16
16092	Peanuts, Spanish, Oil-roasted, w/ Salt	112	0.5	Cup	41.17	72.09	25.65	851.13	0	0	0	11.11
16392	Peanuts, Spanish, Oil-roasted, w/o Salt	112	0.5	Cup	41.17	72.09	25.65	851.13	0	0	0	11.11
16093	Peanuts, Valencia, Fresh	112	0.5	Cup	36.63	69.47	30.53	832.2	0	0	0	10.7
16094	Peanuts, Valencia, Oil-roasted, w/ Salt	112	0.5	Cup	38.94	73.79	23.47	848.16	0	0	0	11.37
16394	Peanuts, Valencia, Oil-roasted, w/o Salt	112	0.5	Cup	38.94	73.79	23.47	848.16	0	0	0	11.37
16095	Peanuts, Virginia, Fresh	112	0.5	Cup	36.78	71.18	24.15	821.98	0	0	0	9.29
16096	Peanuts, Virginia, Oil-roasted, w/ Salt	112	0.5	Cup	36.99	69.53	28.4	826.54	0	0	0	9.07
16396	Peanuts, Virginia, Oil-roasted, w/o Salt	112	0.5	Cup	36.99	69.53	28.4	826.54	0	0	0	9.07
12142	Pecans, Dried	112	0.5	Cup	8.37	73.05	19.7	720.36	0	8.21	0	5.85
12147	Pine Nuts	10	1	Tbsp.	2.4	5.07	1.42	51.5	0	0.45	0	0.78
12151	Pistachios, Dried	112	0.5	Cup	26.34	61.94	31.76	738.56	0	13.82	0	7.84
12652	Pistachios, Dry Roasted	112	0.5	Cup	19.11	67.61	35.24	775.68	0	13.82	0	8.56
16107	Sausage, Meatless	25	1	Link	4.63	4.54	2.46	64	0	0.7	0	0.73
	Seeds, Sesame, Toasted, w/o salt	28.35	1	Ounce	4.808	13.608	7.382	160.745	0	4.791	0	1.906
	Seeds, Sesame, Toasted, w/salt	28.35	1	Ounce	4.808	13.608	7.382	160.745	0	4.791	0	1.906
12036	Seeds, Sunflower, Dried	112	0.5	Cup	32.8	71.38	27.01	820.8	0	15.12	0	7.48
12537	Seeds, Sunflower, Dry Roasted, w/ Salt added	112	0.5	Cup	24.74	63.74	30.81	744.96	0	8.7	0	6.68
12037	Seeds, Sunflower, Dry Roasted, w/o Salt	112	0.5	Cup	24.74	63.74	30.81	744.96	0	11.52	0	6.68
12538	Seeds, Sunflower, Oil Roasted, w/ Salt added	112	0.5	Cup	28.84	77.56	19.89	830.25	0	9.18	0	8.13
12038	Seeds, Sunflower, Oil Roasted, w/o Salt	112	0.5	Cup	28.84	77.56	19.89	830.25	0	9.18	0	8.13
12539	Seeds, Sunflower, Toasted, w/ Salt added	112	0.5	Cup	23.06	76.11	27.59	829.46	0	0	0	7.98
12039	Seeds, Sunflower, Toasted, w/o Salt	112	0.5	Cup	23.06	76.11	27.59	829.46	0	0	0	7.98
	Sesame Butter, Tahini, Toasted	15	1	Tbsp.	2.55	8.064	3.179	89.25	0	1.395	0	1.129

Monounsaturated Fat (gm)	Polyunsaturated Fat (gm)	Vitamin D (mg)	Vitamin K (mg)	Vitamin E (mg)	Vitamin A (re)	Vitamin C (mg)	Thiamin (mg)	Riboflavin (mg)	Niacin (mg)	Vitamin B6 (mg)	Folate (mg)	Vitamin B12 (mcg)	Calcium (mg)	Iron (mg)	Magnesium (mg)	Phosphorus (mg)	Potassium (mg)	Sodium (mg)	Zinc (mg)
0.81	0.57	0	0	0.04	0	0	0.02	0.04	1.78	0.13	1.7	0.1	5.95	0.4	7.37	58.97	80.8	17.86	0.58
0.29	0.41	0	0	0.09	0	0	0.02	0.05	1.54	0.13	1.98	0.1	7.09	0.5	7.37	60.39	84.48	19.85	0.88
0.9	0.7	0	0	0.1	0	0	0.02	0.05	1.44	0.12	1.98	0.1	7.37	0.51	7.09	57.55	79.38	19.28	0.84
0.13	0.08	0	0	0.03	0	0	0.01	0.03	2.36	0.1	1.13	0.57	1.98	0.11	5.67	64.92	78.81	405.69	0.32
1.32	0.83	0	0	0.05	0	0	0.01	0.04	1.63	0.12	1.7	0.1	6.8	0.41	7.09	55.85	75.41	17.29	0.6
1.25	0.23	0	0	0.11	0	0	0.02	0.09	2.26	0.09	4.25	0.45	6.24	0.33	7.37	67.76	92.14	24.66	1.35
0.67	0.17	0	0	0.12	0	0	0.02	0.1	2.39	0.09	4.54	0.47	6.8	0.33	7.94	70.88	95.82	25.23	1.45
0.25	0.18	0	0	0	0	0	0.05	0.17	1.9	0	0	0	1.98	1.27	6.8	64.07	94.97	15.31	0.78
6.14	1.984	0	0	3.242	0	0.112	0.021	0.098	0.46	0.012	10.432	0	43.2	0.592	48.48	83.68	121.28	72	0.488
6.14	1.984	0	0	3.248	0	0.112	0.021	0.098	0.46	0.012	10.432	0	43.2	0.592	48.48	83.68	121.28	1.76	0.488
46.8	15.12	0	0	22.71	0	0.99	0.19	0.85	4.02	0.11	91	0	401.75	6.98	432.98	780.78	1097.35	15.62	6.98
6.5	6.8	0	0	3.5	0	0	0.28	0.03	0.5	0.07	1	0	50	0.96	64	170	170	1	1.3
30.8	8.8	0	0	0.78	0	0	0.24	0.24	1.6	0.28	80	0	52	6.8	296	556	640	20	6.36
30.8	8.8	0	0	0.78	0	0	0.24	0.23	1.6	0.28	80	0	52	6.8	296	556	640	20	6.36
66	1.6	0	0	0.5	0	0	0.4	0.12	2.4	0.24	16	0	80	2.72	132	156	416	4	1.92
66	1.77	0	0	0.55	0	0	0.4	0.15	2.71	0.27	16	0	80	2.41	156.78	156	440.86	8	1.47
36	16	0	0	8.22	1.37	0.55	0.27	0.27	6.44	0.41	69.05	0	95.9	5.07	308.25	595.95	680	440	5.21
36	15.2	0	0	8.52	20	0	0.71	0.24	5.6	0.14	96	0	124	3.64	268	528	660	12	5.76
36	15.2	0	0	8.64	20	0	0.73	0.24	5.6	0.14	96	0	124	3.7	268	528	660	12	5.76
3.8	2.32	0	0	1.61	0	0	0.02	0.02	2.21	0.07	14.85	0	6.62	0.31	25.66	51.16	120.56	78.43	0.45
3.8	2.32	0	0	1.61	0	0	0.02	0.02	2.21	0.07	14.85	0	6.62	0.31	25.66	51.16	120.56	2.74	0.45
0	0	0	0	0	0	0	0	0	2.38	0.06	6	0	0	0.2	26.25	0	360.5	125	0.45
3.81	2.32	0	0.02	1.61	0	0	0.02	0.02	2.11	0.06	12.62	0	5.49	0.27	25.34	52.13	116.36	77.14	0.41
3.81	2.32	0	0	0	0	0	0.02	0.02	2.11	0.06	12.62	0	5.49	0.27	25.34	52.13	116.36	2.74	0.41
35.23	22.44	0	0	10.67	0	0	0.36	0.16	20.56	0.37	181.01	0	126.72	2.64	266.4	744.48	982.08	623.52	9.55
3.5	2.2	0	0	2	0	0	0.8	0.02	1.7	0.05	24	0	18	0.32	33	63	58	240	0.59
35.97	22.91	0	0	10.82	0	0	0.64	0.14	19.75	0.37	212.14	0	78.84	3.3	256.96	522.68	960.68	1186.98	4.83
35.97	22.91	0	0	11.39	0	0	0.64	0.14	19.75	0.37	212.14	0	78.84	3.3	256.96	522.68	960.68	8.76	4.83
35.67	22.72	0	0	13.33	0	0	0.93	0.2	17.62	0.51	350.11	0	134.32	6.69	245.28	548.96	1029.3	26.28	4.77
35.23	22.44	0	0	10.67	0	0	0.36	0.16	20.56	0.37	181.01	0	126.72	2.64	266.4	744.48	982.08	623.52	9.55
35.23	22.44	0	0	10.67	0	0	0.36	0.16	20.56	0.37	181.01	0	126.72	2.64	266.4	744.48	982.08	8.64	9.55
32.6	25.12	0	0	0	0	0	0.99	0.2	23.25	0.51	350.4	0	154.76	5.71	274.48	566.48	1086.24	32.12	3.1
32.45	25	0	0	0	0	0	0.47	0.12	21.95	0.38	185.07	0	147	3.35	246.96	568.89	1140.72	636.51	2.94
32.45	25	0	0	0	0	0	0.47	0.12	21.95	0.38	185.07	0	147	3.35	246.96	568.89	1140.72	8.82	2.94
31.26	24.09	0	0	0	0	0	0.93	0.44	18.8	0.5	358.43	0	90.52	3.05	268.64	490.56	484.72	1.46	4.88
33.21	25.59	0	0	0	0	0	0.13	0.22	20.65	0.35	180.72	0	77.76	2.38	230.4	459.36	881.28	1111.68	4.44
33.21	25.59	0	0	0	0	0	0.13	0.22	20.65	0.35	180.72	0	77.76	2.38	230.4	459.36	881.28	8.64	4.44
36.92	21.47	0	0	0	0	0	0.95	0.19	18.07	0.51	348.5	0	129.94	3.72	249.66	554.8	1007.4	14.6	6.47
36.07	20.98	0	0	0	0	0	0.39	0.16	21.02	0.36	179.32	0	122.98	2.39	268.84	723.58	932.36	619.19	9.47
36.07	20.98	0	0	0	0	0	0.39	0.16	21.02	0.36	179.32	0	122.98	2.39	268.84	723.58	932.36	8.58	9.47
45.53	18.09	0	0	3.35	14.04	2.16	0.92	0.14	0.96	0.2	42.34	0	38.88	2.3	138.24	314.28	423.36	1.08	5.91
1.91	2.13	0	0	0.35	0.3	0.19	0.08	0.02	0.36	0.01	5.73	0	2.6	0.92	23.3	50.8	59.9	0.4	0.43
41.82	9.36	0	0	6.67	29.44	9.22	1.05	0.22	1.38	0.32	74.24	0	172.8	8.68	202.24	643.84	1399.04	7.68	1.72
45.64	10.22	0	0	8.26	30.72	9.34	0.54	0.31	1.8	0.33	75.65	0	89.6	4.06	166.4	609.28	1241.6	998.4	1.74
1.12	2.32	0	0	0.53	16	0	0.59	0.1	2.8	0.21	6.5	0	15.75	0.93	9	56.25	57.75	222	0.37
5.139	5.965	0	0	0.644	1.985	0	0.342	0.132	1.542	0.041	27.159	0	37.139	2.206	98.091	219.429	115.101	11.057	2.9
5.139	5.965	0	0	0.644	1.985	0	0.342	0.132	1.542	0.041	27.159	0	37.139	2.206	98.091	219.429	115.101	166.698	2.9
13.63	47.14	0	0	72.39	7.2	2.02	3.3	0.36	6.48	1.11	327.46	0	167.04	9.75	509.76	1015.2	992.16	4.32	7.29
12.17	42.09	0	0	64.35	0	1.79	0.14	0.31	9.01	1.03	303.87	0	89.6	4.86	165.12	1478.4	1088	998.4	6.77
12.17	42.09	0	0	64.35	0	1.79	0.14	0.31	9.01	1.03	303.87	0	89.6	4.86	165.12	1478.4	1088	3.84	6.77
14.8	51.21	0	0	54	6.75	1.89	0.43	0.38	5.58	1.07	315.9	0	75.6	9.05	171.45	1537.65	652.05	814.05	7.03
14.8	51.21	0	0	67.86	6.75	1.89	0.43	0.38	5.58	1.07	315.9	0	75.6	9.05	171.45	1537.65	652.05	4.05	7.03
14.53	50.26	0	0	0	0	1.88	0.44	0.38	5.63	1.08	318.65	0	76.38	9.13	172.86	1551.72	657.94	821.42	7.1
14.53	50.26	0	0	0	0	1.88	0.44	0.38	5.63	1.08	318.65	0	76.38	9.13	172.86	1551.72	657.94	4.02	7.1
3.045	3.535	0	0	0.341	1.05	0	0.183	0.071	0.817	0.022	14.655	0	63.9	1.342	14.25	109.8	62.1	17.25	0.693

USDA ID Code	Food Name	Weight in Grams*	Quantity of Units	Unit of Measure	Protein (gm)	Fat (gm)	Carbohydrates (gm)	Kcalories	Caffeine (gm)	Fiber (gm)	Cholesterol (mg)	Saturated Fat (gm)
16109	Soybeans, Boiled	172	0.5	Cup	28.62	15.43	17.06	297.56	0	10.32	0	2.23
16111	Soybeans, Dry Roasted	172	0.5	Cup	68.08	37.19	56.28	774	0	13.93	0	5.38
16126	Tofu, Fresh, Firm	28.35	1	Ounce	4.47	2.47	1.21	41.11	0	0.65	0	0.36
16127	Tofu, Fresh, Regular	28.35	1	Ounce	2.29	1.36	0.53	21.55	0	0.34	0	0.2
16129	Tofu, Fried	28.35	1	Ounce	4.87	5.72	2.98	76.83	0	1.11	0	0.83
16429	Tofu, Fried, Prepared w/ Calcium Sulfate	28.35	1	Ounce	4.87	5.72	2.98	76.83	0	0	0	0.83
16130	Tofu, Okara	28.35	1	Ounce	0.91	0.49	3.56	21.83	0	0	0	0.05
16132	Tofu, Salted and Fermented (fuyu)	28.35	1	Ounce	2.31	2.27	1.46	32.89	0	0	0	0.33
12154	Walnuts, Black, Dried	125	0.5	Cup	30.44	70.73	15.13	758.75	0	6.25	0	4.54
12155	Walnuts, English, Dried	120	0.5	Cup	17.15	74.24	22.01	770.4	0	5.76	0	6.7
	Vitamin Supplement, Centrum	1	1	Each	0	0	0	0	0	0	0	0
	Vitamin Supplement, One-A-Day	1	1	Each	0	0	0	0	0	0	0	0
	Vitamin Supplement, StressTab	1	1	Each	0	0	0	0	0	0	0	0
55188	Angel Hair Pasta, Lean Cuisine-Stouffer's	283.493	1	Each	10	5	38	240	0	0	10	1
55189	Baked Cheese Ravioli, Lean Cuisine-Stouffer's	240.969	1	Each	13	8	30	240	0	0	55	3
41297	Baked Cheese Ravioli-Healthy Choice	255.144	1	Each	14	2	44	250	0	0	20	1
55190	Baked Potato w/ Sour Cream, Lean Cuisine-Stouffer's	294.124	1	Each	9	5	38	230	0	0	15	2
41240	Banana Nut Muffin-Healthy Choice	70.873	1	Each	3	6	32	180	0	0	0	0
41276	Bean and Ham Soup-Healthy Choice	212.62	1	Each	12	4	35	220	0	0	5	1
41335	Beef and Bean Burritos (medium)-Healthy Choice	148.834	1	Each	12	7	42	270	0	0	15	3
41334	Beef and Bean Burritos (mild)-Healthy Choice	148.834	1	Each	11	5	45	250	0	0	10	1
55191	Beef and Bean Enchiladas, Lean Cuisine-Stouffer's	262.231	1	Each	15	6	32	240	0	0	45	3
41270	Beef and Potato Soup-Healthy Choice	212.62	1	Each	9	1	17	110	0	0	20	0
55192	Beef Cannelloni w/ Sauce, Lean Cuisine-Stouffer's	272.862	1	Each	14	3	28	200	0	0	25	1
62692	Beef Chow Mein	247	1	Cup	10	1.5	15	110	0	4	10	1
41249	Beef Enchilada-Healthy Choice	379.172	1	Each	15	5	66	370	0	0	30	2
55149	Beef Pie-Stouffer's	283.493	1	Each	18	27	37	460	0	0	0	0
57806	Beef Pot Pie-Swanson	198.445	1	Pie	12	19	36	370	0	0	0	0
43405	Beef Ravioli, Micro Cup-Hormel	212.62	1	Each	9	11	34	270	0	0	20	4
41251	Beef Sirloin Tips-Healthy Choice	318.93	1	Each	22	7	29	270	0	0	65	3
43413	Beef Stew, Micro Cup-Hormel	212.62	1	Each	13	15	11	230	0	0	45	5
55158	Beef Stroganoff w/ Parsley Noodles-Stouffer's	276.406	1	Each	24	20	28	390	0	0	0	0
41286	Boneless Beef Ribs w/ Barbecue Sauce-Healthy Choice	311.843	1	Each	28	6	40	330	0	0	70	2
41348	Breaded Fish-Healthy Choice	9.745	1	Stick	1	0.5	1.75	15	0	0	2.5	0
43400	Breast of Chicken w/ Spanish Rice, Top Shelf-Hormel	283.493	1	Each	27	15	38	400	0	0	75	7
41252	Breast of Turkey-Healthy Choice	297.668	1	Each	21	5	39	290	0	0	45	2
62616	Broccoli and Cheese Baked Potato-Weight Watchers	283.5	1	Each	12	7	34	230	0	6	10	2
55177	Canadian Style Bacon, French Bread Pizzas-Stouffer's	163.008	1	Each	18	15	40	370	0	0	0	0
55832	Cheddar Cheese Sauce-Stouffer's	283.92	1	Cup	26.04	60.09	22.03	731.1	0	0	130.2	0
55764	Cheddar Cheese Soup-Stouffer's	283.92	1	Cup	21.03	31.05	18.03	440.66	0	0	70.11	0
55772	Cheddar Cheese, Heat'n Serve Soup -Stouffer's	307.58	1	Cup	21.7	35.8	21.7	488.23	0	0	97.65	0
55196	Cheese Cannelloni, Lean Cuisine-Stouffer's	258.688	1	Each	23	8	27	270	0	0	25	4
55108	Cheese Enchiladas-Stouffer's	276.406	1	Each	23	29	33	490	0	0	0	0
41331	Cheese French Bread Pizza-Healthy Choice	159.465	1	Each	19	4	46	290	0	0	15	2
41300	Cheese Manicotti-Healthy Choice	262.231	1	Each	15	3	34	220	0	0	30	2
55796	Cheese Manicotti-Stouffer's	28.35	1	Ounce	1.6	1.3	2.6	29	0	0	4	0
55822	Cheese Ravioli-Stouffer's	28.35	1	Ounce	2.8	1.9	6.4	54	0	0	14	0
55808	Cheese Stuffed Shells-Stouffer's	28.35	1	Ounce	1.5	0.9	3.4	28	0	0	3	0
55819	Cheese Tortellini w/ Egg Pasta-Stouffer's	145.29	1	Each	11.29	8.47	22.22	211.64	0	0	63.49	0
55821	Cheese Tortellini w/ Spinach Pasta-Stouffer's	28.35	1	Ounce	3	2.4	5.7	56	0	0	19	0
55109	Chicken a la King w/ Rice-Stouffer's	269.319	1	Each	18	5	38	270	0	0	0	0
43397	Chicken a la King, Top Shelf-Hormel	283.493	1	Each	18	10	49	360	0	0	37	4
57799	Chicken a la King-Swanson	250	1	Each	16.8	20.16	15.12	319.15	0	0	0	0
55197	Chicken a la Orange, Lean Cuisine-Stouffer's	226.795	1	Each	27	4	33	280	0	0	55	1
41301	Chicken a la Orange-Healthy Choice	255.144	1	Each	20	2	36	240	0	0	45	2

Monounsaturated Fat (gm)	Polyunsaturated Fat (gm)	Vitamin D (mg)	Vitamin K (mg)	Vitamin E (mg)	Vitamin A (re)	Vitamin C (mg)	Thiamin (mg)	Riboflavin (mg)	Niacin (mg)	Vitamin B6 (mg)	Folate (mg)	Vitamin B12 (mcg)	Calcium (mg)	Iron (mg)	Magnesium (mg)	Phosphorus (mg)	Potassium (mg)	Sodium (mg)	Zinc (mg)
3.41	8.71	0	0	3.35	1.72	2.92	0.27	0.49	0.69	0.4	92.54	0	175.44	8.84	147.92	421.4	885.8	1.72	1.98
8.21	21	0	0	3.35	3.44	7.91	0.73	1.3	1.82	0.39	351.91	0	464.4	6.79	392.16	1116.28	2346.08	3.44	8.2
0.55	1.4	0	0	0	4.82	0.06	0.04	0.03	0.11	0.03	8.31	0	58.12	2.97	26.65	53.87	67.19	3.97	0.45
0.3	0.77	0	0	0	2.55	0.03	0.02	0.01	0.06	0.01	4.25	0	29.77	1.52	29.2	27.5	34.3	1.98	0.23
1.26	3.23	0	0	0.01	0	0	0.05	0.01	0.03	0.03	7.6	0	105.46	1.38	17.01	81.36	41.39	4.54	0.56
1.26	3.23	0	0	0	0	0	0.05	0.01	0.03	0.03	7.6	0	272.44	1.38	26.93	81.36	41.39	4.54	0.56
0.08	0.21	0	0	0	0	0	0.01	0.01	0.03	0.03	7.48	0	22.68	0.37	7.37	17.01	60.39	2.55	0.16
0.5	1.28	0	0	0	4.82	0.06	0.04	0.03	0.11	0.03	8.25	0	13.04	0.56	14.74	20.7	21.26	814.5	0.44
15.91	46.87	0	0	3.28	37.5	4	0.27	0.14	0.86	0.69	81.88	0	72.5	3.84	252.5	580	655	1.25	4.28
17.01	46.95	0	0	3.14	14.4	3.84	0.46	0.18	1.25	0.67	79.2	0	112.8	2.93	202.8	380.4	602.4	12	3.28
0	0	5	0	10	1000	60	1.5	1.7	20	2	400	6	162	18	100	109	40	0	15
0	0	5	0	10	1000	60	1.5	1.7	20	2	400	6	0	0	0	0	0	0	0
0	0	0	0	10	0	500	10	0	100	5	400	12	0	18	0	0	0	0	0
0	1	0	0	0	250	6	0.3	0.34	2.85	0	0	0	80	1.5	0	0	500	410	0
0	0	0	0	0	60	36	0.06	0.26	1.14	0	0	0	160	0.8	0	0	380	590	0
0	0	0	0	0	500	4.8	0.3	0.26	1.9	0	0	0	200	1.5	0	240	590	420	0
0	0	0	0	0	350	30	0.23	0.26	1.14	0	0	0	160	0.6	0	0	900	570	0
0	3	0	0	0	0	0	0.15	0.14	0.76	0	0	0	80	1	0	160	250	80	0
0	1	0	0	0	60	2.4	0.23	0.17	1.14	0	0	0	48	1	0	220	630	480	0
0	3	0	0	0	20	3.6	0.38	0.17	1.9	0	0	0	48	1.5	0	180	270	520	0
0	2	0	0	0	20	1.2	0.38	0.17	2.85	0	0	0	32	2	0	130	330	450	0
0	1	0	0	0	80	6	0.23	0.26	1.9	0	0	0	80	1	0	0	470	480	0
0	0	0	0	0	0	2.4	0.03	0	0.38	0	0	0	0	0.2	0	0	100	550	0
0	0	0	0	0	350	6	0.12	0.17	2.85	0	0	0	120	1.5	0	0	800	490	0
0	0	0	0	0	40	12	0	0	0	0	0	0	24	0.4	0	0	0	760	0
0	2	0	0	0	250	24	0.3	0.26	1.9	0	0	0	120	1	0	260	600	450	0
0	0	0	0	0	700	2.4	0.3	0.43	3.8	0	0	0	32	1.5	0	0	300	1130	0
0	0	0	0	0	250	0	0.23	0.17	2.85	0	0	0	16	1.5	0	0	0	730	0
5	1	0	0	0.5	100	11.4	0.15	0.27	2.47	0	0	0	48	0.9	28	0	359	920	1.05
0	2	0	0	0	700	42	0.15	0.17	2.85	0	0	0	16	1	0	190	520	360	0
4	0	0	0	0.28	320	2.4	0.05	0.1	2.28	0	0	0	16	0.9	21	0	487	1140	2.4
0	0	0	0	0	40	1.2	0.12	0.34	2.85	0	0	0	48	1.5	0	0	300	1090	0
0	2	0	0	0	60	4.8	0.23	0.26	2.85	0	0	0	48	1	0	220	670	530	0
0	0.13	0	0	0	0	0	0.01	0.02	0.1	0	0	0	0	0.1	0	0	20	31.25	0
4	3	0	0	0.07	100	3.6	0.09	0.26	7.6	0	0	0	80	0.4	35	0	584	810	1.65
0	0	0	0	0	40	48	0.45	0.26	5.7	0	0	0	32	1	0	270	540	420	0
0	0	0	0	0	200	9	0	0	0	0	0	0	300	0.8	0	0	830	510	0
0	0	0	0	0	80	6	0.6	0.43	3.8	0	0	0	160	1	0	0	300	1070	0
0	0	0	0	0	0	0	0.01	0	0	0	0	0	6.33	0.1	0	0	340.51	1392.09	0
0	0	0	0	0	0	0	0.01	0.19	0	0	0	0	4.97	0	0	0	510.77	681.02	0
0	0	0	0	0	0	0	0.02	0.21	0	0	0	0	4.95	0.11	0	0	553.33	770.32	0
0	0	0	0	0	60	21	0.12	0.26	1.52	0	0	0	240	0.4	0	0	400	590	0
0	0	0	0	0	150	6	0.09	0.34	1.52	0	0	0	480	0.8	0	0	400	550	0
0	1	0	0	0	20	0	0.45	0.26	2.85	0	0	0	240	2	0	240	310	390	0
0	0	0	0	0	250	6	0.3	0.26	1.9	0	0	0	120	1.5	0	210	590	310	0
0	0	0	0	0	0	2.4	0	0	0.04	0	0	0	296.01	0.02	0	0	45	108	0
0	0	0	0	0	0	0	0	0	0.02	0	0	0	336.01	0.01	0	0	16	52	0
0	0	0	0	0	0	0.6	0	0	0.06	0	0	0	248.01	0.02	0	0	53	59	0
0	0	0	0	0	0	0	0	0	0.2	0	0	0	1.52	0.07	0	0	70.55	271.61	0
0	0	0	0	0	0	0	0	0	0.06	0	0	0	0	0.02	0	0	26	79	0
0	0	0	0	0	20	1.2	0.09	0.17	2.85	0	0	0	160	0.8	0	32	260	800	0
4	2	0	0	0.17	250	1.2	0.12	0.17	8.55	0	0	0	48	0.2	28	0	476	890	1.2
0	0	0	0	0	0	0	0.05	0.23	3.19	0	0	0	53.75	0.34	0	0	0	1159.01	0
0	0	0	0	0	80	12	0.23	0.17	9.5	0	0	0	32	0.4	0	0	490	290	0
0	0	0	0	0	150	27	0.15	0.1	5.7	0	0	0	16	0.8	0	230	430	220	0

USDA ID Code	Food Name	Weight in Grams*	Quantity of Units	Unit of Measure	Protein (gm)	Fat (gm)	Carbohydrates (gm)	Kcalories	Caffeine (gm)	Fiber (gm)	Cholesterol (mg)	Saturated Fat (gm)
55792	Chicken and Dumplings-Stouffer's	220	1	Each	14.74	16.3	24.06	302.65	0	0	69.84	0
57801	Chicken and Dumplings-Swanson	200	1	Each	10.35	10.35	17.87	206.94	0	0	0	0
41253	Chicken and Pasta Divan-Healthy Choice	340.192	1	Each	25	4	41	300	0	0	50	2
55794	Chicken and Veg. Oriental-Stouffer's	220	1	Each	11.64	9.31	13.97	186.25	0	0	31.04	0
55198	Chicken and Veg. w/ Vermicelli, Lean Cuisine-Stouffer's	333.105	1	Each	18	5	30	240	0	0	30	1
41302	Chicken and Vegetables-Healthy Choice	326.017	1	Each	20	1	31	210	0	0	35	0
55199	Chicken Cacciatore, Lean Cuisine-Stouffer's	308.299	1	Each	22	7	31	280	0	0	45	2
43398	Chicken Cacciatore, Top Shelf-Hormel	283.493	1	Each	21	3	25	210	0	0	50	0
55200	Chicken Chow Mein w/ Rice, Lean Cuisine-Stouffer's	255.144	1	Each	14	5	34	240	0	0	30	1
55110	Chicken Chow Mein w/ Rice-Stouffer's	304.755	1	Each	13	5	39	250	0	0	0	0
41303	Chicken Chow Mein-Healthy Choice	240.969	1	Each	18	3	31	220	0	0	45	1
62611	Chicken Chow Mein-Weight Watchers	255.15	1	Each	12	2	34	200	0	3	25	0.5
55807	Chicken Classica -Stouffer's	28.35	1	Ounce	1.8	0.7	2.3	22	0	0	5	0
41336	Chicken Con Queso Burritos (mild)-Healthy Choice	148.834	1	Each	15	8	40	280	0	0	20	2
41254	Chicken Dijon-Healthy Choice	311.843	1	Each	21	3	40	250	0	0	40	1
55111	Chicken Divan-Stouffer's	226.795	1	Each	24	10	11	220	0	0	0	0
62618	Chicken Enchiladas Suiza-Weight Watchers	255.15	1	Each	15	8	28	250	0	4	25	3
55201	Chicken Enchiladas, Lean Cuisine-Stouffer's	279.95	1	Each	17	9	34	290	0	0	55	3
41304	Chicken Enchiladas-Healthy Choice	269.319	1	Each	14	9	44	310	0	0	35	3
55112	Chicken Enchiladas-Stouffer's	283.493	1	Each	21	31	31	490	0	0	0	0
41305	Chicken Fajitas-Healthy Choice	198.445	1	Each	17	3	25	200	0	0	35	1
55203	Chicken Fettucini, Lean Cuisine-Stouffer's	255.144	1	Each	23	6	33	280	0	0	35	3
41306	Chicken Fettucini-Healthy Choice	240.969	1	Each	19	7	39	240	0	0	45	2
62620	Chicken Fettucini-Weight Watchers	233.89	1	Each	22	9	25	280	0	2	40	3
55763	Chicken Gumbo Soup-Stouffer's	283.92	1	Cup	7.01	5.01	9.01	110.17	0	0	20.03	0
55202	Chicken in BBQ Sauce, Lean Cuisine-Stouffer's	248.057	1	Each	20	6	32	260	0	0	50	1
55204	Chicken Italiano, Lean Cuisine-Stouffer's	255.144	1	Each	22	6	33	270	0	0	40	1
55789	Chicken Italienne-Stouffer's	28.35	1	Ounce	2.2	0.9	1.2	22	0	0	7	0
55755	Chicken Noodle Soup-Stouffer's	283.92	1	Cup	7.01	7.01	10.02	130.2	0	0	20.03	0
55768	Chicken Noodle, Heat'n Serve Soup-Stouffer's	283.92	1	Cup	13.02	17.03	28.04	320.48	0	0	60.09	0
55205	Chicken Oriental, Lean Cuisine-Stouffer's	255.144	1	Each	22	7	31	280	0	0	35	2
41256	Chicken Oriental-Healthy Choice	318.93	1	Each	19	1	32	200	0	0	35	0
41257	Chicken Parmigiana-Healthy Choice	326.017	1	Each	22	4	45	280	0	0	45	2
41271	Chicken Pasta Soup-Healthy Choice	212.62	1	Each	7	2	13	100	0	0	15	0
55113	Chicken Pie-Stouffer's	283.493	1	Each	16	27	32	440	0	0	0	0
57807	Chicken Pot Pie-Swanson	198.445	1	Each	11	22	35	380	0	0	0	0
55790	Chicken Primavera-Stouffer's	28.35	1	Ounce	1.6	0.6	1.2	17	0	0	5	0
41295	Chicken Stir Fry w/ Broccoli-Healthy Choice	340.192	1	Each	21	6	35	280	0	0	55	3
55206	Chicken Tenderloins, Lean Cuisine-Stouffer's	269.319	1	Each	29	5	19	240	0	0	60	2
55820	Chicken Tortellini w/ Egg Pasta-Stouffer's	28.35	1	Ounce	3.1	1.5	6.2	51	0	0	20	0
41248	Chicken w/ Barbecue Sauce-Healthy Choice	361.454	1	Each	24	6	65	410	0	0	55	2
41277	Chicken w/ Rice Soup-Healthy Choice	212.62	1	Each	5	1	14	90	0	0	10	0
41272	Chili Beef Soup-Healthy Choice	212.62	1	Each	11	1	22	150	0	0	15	0
55114	Chili Con Carne w/ Beans-Stouffer's	248.057	1	Each	20	10	28	280	0	0	0	0
43411	Chili Mac, Micro Cup-Hormel	212.62	1	Each	10	9	18	192	0	0	22	4
43408	Chili no Beans, Micro Cup-Hormel	209.076	1	Each	18	17	15	290	0	0	60	8
55767	Chili w/ Beans Soup-Stouffer's	283.92	1	Cup	14.02	9.01	25.04	240.36	0	0	30.04	0
43409	Chili w/ Beans, Micro Cup-Hormel	209.076	1	Each	15	11	23	250	0	0	49	4
43369	Chili w/ Beans-Hormel	253.162	1	Cup	17.86	17.86	32.15	357.2	0	0	65.49	5.95
43368	Chili w/o Beans-Hormel	253.162	1	Cup	19.05	32.15	16.67	428.64	0	0	71.44	13.1
62691	Chili, Fat Free	240	0.5	Cup	14	0	30	160	0	14	0	0
43370	Chunky Chili w/ Beans-Hormel	253.162	1	Cup	17.86	16.67	29.77	345.3	0	0	59.53	0
55799	Confetti Rice-Stouffer's	28.35	1	Ounce	0.5	0.3	4.8	24	0	0	1	0
55824	Corn Pudding-Stouffer's	28.35	1	Ounce	1.2	1.7	4.5	38	0	0	15	0
55168	Corn Souffle-Stouffer's	170.096	1	Each	7	11	27	240	0	0	0	0

Monounsaturated Fat (gm)	Polyunsaturated Fat (gm)	Vitamin D (mg)	Vitamin K (mg)	Vitamin E (mg)	Vitamin A (re)	Vitamin C (mg)	Thiamin (mg)	Riboflavin (mg)	Niacin (mg)	Vitamin B6 (mg)	Folate (mg)	Vitamin B12 (mcg)	Calcium (mg)	Iron (mg)	Magnesium (mg)	Phosphorus (mg)	Potassium (mg)	Sodium (mg)	Zinc (mg)
0	0	0	0	0	0	0	0	0.01	0.44	0	0	0	1.06	0.16	0	0	248.33	659.63	0
0	0	0	0	0	75.25	0	0.03	0.1	1.79	0	0	0	15.05	0.38	0	0	0	921.83	0
0	1	0	0	0	800	72	0.38	0.26	4.75	0	0	0	120	1	0	270	500	520	0
0	0	0	0	0	0	4.66	0	0	0.59	0	0	0	372.49	0.08	0	0	349.21	1078.68	0
0	1	0	0	0	150	6	0.3	0.26	5.7	0	0	0	64	1	0	0	500	500	0
0	0	0	0	0	150	9	0.3	0.17	3.8	0	0	0	32	1.5	0	190	390	490	0
0	1	0	0	0	100	9	0.23	0.17	5.7	0	0	0	32	0.8	0	0	560	570	0
0	0	0	0	0.46	100	2.4	0.15	0.26	6.65	0	0	0	80	1	0	0	0	810	0
0	1	0	0	0	60	6	0.15	0.17	4.75	0	0	0	32	0.6	0	0	350	530	0
0	0	0	0	0	80	12	0.03	0.17	1.9	0	0	0	16	0.4	0	0	340	720	0
0	1	0	0	0	80	3.6	0.15	0.14	3.8	0	0	0	16	0.8	0	290	290	440	0
0	0	0	0	0	300	36	0	0	0	0	0	0	48	0.4	0	0	360	570	0
0	0	0	0	0	0	1.2	0	0	0.1	0	0	0	112	0.01	0	0	50	83	0
0	3	0	0	0	20	6	0.45	0.34	2.85	0	0	0	80	1.5	0	170	260	500	0
0	0	0	0	0	100	9	0.23	0.14	9.5	0	0	0	16	1	0	300	350	470	0
0	0	0	0	0	60	3.6	0.45	0.17	3.8	0	0	0	200	2	0	32	490	610	0
0	0	0	0	0	40	1.2	0	0	0	0	0	0	360	0.8	0	0	470	570	0
0	2	0	0	0	250	6	0.23	0.34	2.85	0	0	0	120	1.5	0	0	450	500	0
0	1	0	0	0	80	21	0.15	0.17	4.75	0	0	0	80	0.8	0	160	380	480	0
0	0	0	0	0	60	2.4	0.09	0.34	2.85	0	0	0	240	0.6	0	0	420	860	0
0	1	0	0	0	150	9	0.23	0.17	3.8	0	0	0	64	1.5	0	210	360	310	0
0	0	0	0	0	0	0	0.3	0.43	5.7	0	0	0	120	0.8	0	0	420	500	0
0	2	0	0	0	0	0	0.23	0.17	2.85	0	0	0	64	1	0	210	190	370	0
0	0	0	0	0	40	0	0	0	0	0	0	0	240	1	0	0	730	590	0
0	0	0	0	0	0	0	0	0	0.19	0	0	0	160.24	0.1	0	0	180.27	1422.13	0
0	2	0	0	0	250	18	0.15	0.17	5.7	0	0	0	48	0.8	0	0	650	500	0
0	2	0	0	0	100	24	0.3	0.26	5.7	0	0	0	80	0.8	0	0	600	590	0
0	0	0	0	0	0	1.2	0	0	0.1	0	0	0	48	0.01	0	0	57	128	0
0	0	0	0	0	0	0	0	0	0.19	0	0	0	80.12	0.1	0	0	140.21	1281.92	0
0	0	0	0	0	0	6.01	0	0	0.57	0	0	0	240.36	0.2	0	0	310.46	1792.69	0
0	2	0	0	0	40	6	0.23	0.17	6.65	0	0	0	32	1	0	0	470	480	0
0	0	0	0	0	250	36	0.15	0.14	7.6	0	0	0	32	0.8	0	200	400	440	0
0	0	0	0	0	900	12	0.15	0.17	9.5	0	0	0	80	1	0	260	500	370	0
0	0	0	0	0	60	0	0.03	0	0.38	0	0	0	0	0	0	0	70	560	0
0	0	0	0	0	500	1.2	0.3	0.43	4.75	0	0	0	80	1	0	0	320	750	0
0	0	0	0	0	400	0	0.23	0.17	2.85	0	0	0	16	1	0	0	0	760	0
0	0	0	0	0	0	1.2	0	0	0.06	0	0	0	48	0.01	0	0	40	119	0
0	0	0	0	0	20	0	0.23	0.34	2.85	0	0	0	48	1.5	0	260	630	500	0
0	1	0	0	0	200	4.8	0.23	0.34	7.6	0	0	0	120	0.4	0	0	750	490	0
0	0	0	0	0	0	0	0	0	0.13	0	0	0	72	0.03	0	0	31	57	0
0	2	0	0	0	100	12	0.12	0.14	8.55	0	0	0	48	1.5	0	250	670	550	0
0	0	0	0	0	80	6	0.03	0.07	1.9	0	0	0	16	0.2	0	70	140	510	0
0	0	0	0	0	20	6	0.09	0.03	0.38	0	0	0	16	0.6	0	0	290	560	0
0	0	0	0	0	200	15	0.15	0.26	2.85	0	0	0	64	2	0	0	700	910	0
4	0	0	0	0.17	210	0	0.08	0.17	2.09	0	0	0	0	1.5	35	0	443	977	2.1
8	1	0	0	0.01	400	0	0.08	0.24	2.47	0	0	0	48	1.6	35	0	507	830	3.9
0	0	0	0	0	0	0	0	0	0.57	0	0	0	0	0.3	0	0	711.07	991.49	0
4	0	0	0	18.9	190	0	0.14	0.15	1.71	0	0	0	48	1.9	45.5	0	677	977	2.7
7.14	1.19	0	0	0.01	250.04	0	0.11	0.2	2.04	0	0	0	57.15	1.91	58.34	0	913.25	1226.4	2.5
15.48	1.19	0	0	0.6	785.85	0	0.11	0.26	2.94	0	0	0	47.63	1.67	41.67	0	591.77	1023.98	3.21
0	0	0	0	0	2000	24	0	0	0	0	0	0	48	2	0	0	0	320	0
0	0	0	0	0	0	0	0	0	0	0	0	0	0	0	0	0	0	928.73	0
0	0	0	0	0	0	0	0	0	0.04	0	0	0	24	0	0	0	14	136	0
0	0	0	0	0	0	0.6	0	0	0.06	0	0	0	88	0.02	0	0	51	125	0
0	0	0	0	0	60	0	0.15	0.26	1.14	0	0	0	48	0.4	0	0	200	760	0

USDA ID Code	Food Name	Weight in Grams*	Quantity of Units	Unit of Measure	Protein (gm)	Fat (gm)	Carbohydrates (gm)	Kcalories	Caffeine (gm)	Fiber (gm)	Cholesterol (mg)	Saturated Fat (gm)
43366	Corned Beef Hash-Hormel	253.162	1	Cup	26.79	26.79	17.86	419.71	0	0	80.37	8.93
41278	Country Vegetable Soup-Healthy Choice	212.62	1	Each	3	1	23	120	0	0	0	0
55762	Cream of Broccoli Soup-Stouffer's	283.92	1	Cup	12.02	21.03	16.02	300.45	0	0	60.09	0
55765	Cream of Potato Soup-Stouffer's	283.92	1	Cup	11.02	13.02	34.05	300.45	0	0	30.04	0
55788	Creamed Chicken-Stouffer's	28.35	1	Ounce	2.8	3.5	1.2	48	0	0	14	0
55777	Creamed Chipped Beef-Stouffer's	28.35	1	Ounce	2.1	3.3	1.6	45	0	0	13	0
55169	Creamed Spinach-Stouffer's	127.572	1	Each	4	16	8	190	0	0	0	0
55756	Creamy Chicken Soup-Stouffer's	283.92	1	Cup	17.03	8.01	25.04	240.36	0	0	20.03	0
43375	Dinty Moore Beef Stew-Hormel	253.162	1	Cup	12.28	14.51	17.86	245.58	0	0	33.49	6.7
43376	Dinty Moore Chicken Stew-Hormel	253.162	1	Cup	13.1	21.43	17.86	309.58	0	0	95.25	4.76
43377	Dinty Moore Meatball Stew-Hormel	253.162	1	Cup	12.28	17.86	15.63	267.9	0	0	33.49	7.81
43378	Dinty Moore Vegetable Stew-Hormel	253.162	1	Cup	5.58	6.7	22.33	173.02	0	0	15.63	2.23
62636	Egg Roll	85	1	Each	7	5	21	160	0	2	10	1
41242	English Muffin Sandwich-Healthy Choice	120.484	1	Each	16	3	30	200	0	0	20	1
55170	Escalloped Apples-Stouffer's	170.096	1	Each	0	4	41	200	0	0	0	0
55117	Escalloped Chicken and Noodles-Stouffer's	283.493	1	Each	21	24	30	420	0	0	0	0
21002	Fast Food-Biscuit w/ Egg	136	1	Each	11.12	20.2	24.17	315.52	0	0	232.56	6.18
21003	Fast Food-Biscuit w/ Egg and Bacon	150	1	Each	17	31.1	28.59	457.5	0	0	352.5	9.93
21004	Fast Food-Biscuit w/ Egg and Ham	192	1	Each	20.43	27.03	30.32	441.6	0	0	299.52	8.37
21005	Fast Food-Biscuit w/ Egg and Sausage	180	1	Each	19.15	38.7	41.15	581.4	0	0	302.4	14.98
21007	Fast Food-Biscuit w/ Egg, Cheese, and Bacon	144	1	Each	16.26	31.39	33.42	476.64	0	0	260.64	11.4
21008	Fast Food-Biscuit w/ Ham	113	1	Each	13.39	18.42	43.79	386.46	0	0	24.86	11.41
21009	Fast Food-Biscuit w/ Sausage	124	1	Each	12.11	31.78	40.04	484.84	0	1.36	34.72	14.22
21010	Fast Food-Biscuit w/ Steak	141	1	Each	13.1	25.99	44.39	455.43	0	0	25.38	6.93
21001	Fast Food-Biscuit, Plain	74	1	Each	4.31	13.35	34.43	276.02	0	0	5.18	8.74
21027	Fast Food-Brownie	60	1	Each	2.74	10.1	38.97	243	0	0	9.6	3.13
21060	Fast Food-Burrito w/ Beans	108.5	1	Each	7.03	6.75	35.72	223.51	0	0	2.17	3.44
21061	Fast Food-Burrito w/ Beans and Cheese	93	1	Each	7.53	5.85	27.48	188.79	0	0	13.95	3.42
21062	Fast Food-Burrito w/ Beans and Chili Peppers	102	1	Each	8.19	7.33	29.04	206.04	0	0	16.32	3.8
21063	Fast Food-Burrito w/ Beans and Meat	115.5	1	Each	11.24	8.91	33.01	254.1	0	0	24.26	4.16
21064	Fast Food-Burrito w/ Beans, Cheese, and Beef	101.5	1	Each	7.29	6.65	19.84	165.45	0	0	61.92	3.57
21065	Fast Food-Burrito w/ Beans, Cheese, and Chili Peppers	167	1	Each	16.55	11.42	42.33	328.99	0	0	78.49	5.56
21066	Fast Food-Burrito w/ Beef	110	1	Each	13.3	10.41	29.26	261.8	0	0	31.9	5.23
21067	Fast Food-Burrito w/ Beef and Chili Peppers	100.5	1	Each	10.75	8.27	24.72	213.06	0	0	27.14	4
21068	Fast Food-Burrito w/ Beef, Cheese, and Chili Peppers	152	1	Each	20.46	12.39	31.86	316.16	0	0	85.12	5.2
21069	Fast Food-Burrito w/ Fruit (Apple or Cherry)	74	1	Each	2.5	9.52	34.98	230.88	0	0	3.7	4.57
21100	Fast Food-Cheeseburger, Large, Double Patty	258	1	Each	37.98	43.65	39.65	704.34	0	0	141.9	17.67
21098	Fast Food-Cheeseburger, Large, Single Patty	219	1	Each	28.19	32.94	38.39	562.83	0	0	87.6	15.04
21097	Fast Food-Cheeseburger, Large, Single Patty w/ Bcn&cond	195	1	Each	32	36.76	37.13	608.4	0	0	111.15	16.24
21096	Fast Food-Cheeseburger, Large, Single Patty, Plain	185	1	Each	30.14	32.99	47.42	608.65	0	0	96.2	14.84
21095	Fast Food-Cheeseburger, Regular, Double Patty	228	1	Each	29.73	35.27	53.12	649.8	0	0	93.48	12.77
21091	Fast Food-Cheeseburger, Regular, Single Patty	154	1	Each	17.83	19.79	28.14	358.82	0	0	52.36	9.19
21089	Fast Food-Cheeseburger, Regular, Single Patty, Plain	102	1	Each	14.77	15.15	31.75	319.26	0	0	49.98	6.47
21101	Fast Food-Cheeseburger, Triple Patty, Plain	304	1	Each	56.06	50.95	26.69	796.48	0	0	161.12	21.71
21103	Fast Food-Chicken Fillet Sandwich w/ Cheese	228	1	Each	29.41	38.76	41.59	631.56	0	0	77.52	12.45
21102	Fast Food-Chicken Fillet Sandwich, Plain	182	1	Each	24.12	29.45	38.69	515.06	0	0	60.06	8.53
21037	Fast Food-Chicken Nuggets, Plain	17	1	Each	2.82	2.95	2.58	48.28	0	0.07	10.2	0.92
21038	Fast Food-Chicken Nuggets, w/ Barb. Sauce	17	1	Each	2.24	2.35	3.27	43.18	0	0	7.99	0.73
21039	Fast Food-Chicken Nuggets, w/ Honey	17	1	Each	2.48	2.59	3.97	48.62	0	0	9.01	0.81
21040	Fast Food-Chicken Nuggets, w/ Must. Sauce	17	1	Each	2.28	2.48	2.73	42.16	0	0	7.99	0.75
21041	Fast Food-Chicken Nuggets, w/ Sweet and Sour	17	1	Each	2.22	2.35	3.79	45.22	0	0	7.99	0.72
21042	Fast Food-Chili Con Carne	252.999	1	Cup	24.62	8.27	21.93	255.53	0	0	134.09	3.43
21070	Fast Food-Chimichanga, w/ Beef	174	1	Each	19.61	19.68	42.8	424.56	0	0	8.7	8.51
21071	Fast Food-Chimichanga, w/ Beef and Cheese	183	1	Each	20.06	23.44	39.33	442.86	0	0	51.24	11.18
21030	Fast Food-Chocolate Chip Cookies	55	1	Box	2.89	12.14	36.22	232.65	0	0	11.55	5.34

Monounsaturated Fat (gm)	Polyunsaturated Fat (gm)	Vitamin D (mg)	Vitamin K (mg)	Vitamin E (mg)	Vitamin A (re)	Vitamin C (mg)	Thiamin (mg)	Riboflavin (mg)	Niacin (mg)	Vitamin B6 (mg)	Folate (mg)	Vitamin B12 (mcg)	Calcium (mg)	Iron (mg)	Magnesium (mg)	Phosphorus (mg)	Potassium (mg)	Sodium (mg)	Zinc (mg)
17.86	0	0	0	0.43	0	0	0	0.15	3.39	0	0	0	71.44	1.79	31.26	0	625.11	991.24	4.02
0	0	0	0	0	200	6	0.06	0.07	1.52	0	0	0	32	0.4	0	100	380	540	0
0	0	0	0	0	0	0	0	0.01	0	0	0	0	2.48	0	0	0	430.64	791.19	0
0	0	0	0	0	0	0	0	0.01	0.19	0	0	0	2.08	0.1	0	0	791.19	1422.13	0
0	0	0	0	0	0	0	0	0	0.1	0	0	0	352	0.01	0	0	37	119	0
0	0	0	0	0	0	0	0	0	0.21	0	0	0	184	0.02	0	0	57	176	0
0	0	0	0	0	400	6	0.03	0.17	0	0	0	0	80	0.4	0	0	400	400	0
0	0	0	0	0	0	0	0.02	0.01	0.19	0	0	0	2.48	0	0	0	510.77	1281.92	0
5.58	1.12	0	0	0	814.87	2.68	0.03	0.13	2.55	0	0	0	26.79	1	23.44	0	588.27	971.15	2.85
7.14	8.33	0	0	0	476.27	2.14	0.05	0.28	3.62	0	0	0	38.1	0.71	25	0	609.63	1012.08	1.25
7.81	1.12	0	0	2.59	279.06	1.34	0.07	0.15	3.18	0	0	0	26.79	1.23	27.35	0	586.04	1093.93	2.68
1.12	2.23	0	0	0.6	714.41	2.01	0.08	0.09	1.7	0	0	0	35.72	0.67	31.26	0	509.01	948.82	0.84
0	0	0	0	0	100	1.2	0	0	0	0	0	0	24	0.2	0	0	0	350	0
0	1	0	0	0	60	3.6	0.45	0.43	2.85	0	0	0	120	2	0	220	200	510	0
0	0	0	0	0	0	30	0.03	0	0	0	0	0	0	0	0	0	90	15	0
0	0	0	0	0	20	0	0.15	0.34	3.8	0	0	0	80	0.8	0	0	300	840	0
8.19	4.22	0	0	0	178.16	0	0.34	0.34	0.71	0.08	29.92	0.75	153.68	3.13	20.4	184.96	160.48	654.16	1.1
13.28	5.7	0	0	0	52.5	2.7	0.14	0.23	2.4	0.14	30	1.04	189	3.74	24	238.5	250.5	999	1.64
11.32	5.18	0	0	0	240	0	0.67	0.6	2	0.27	32.64	1.19	220.8	4.55	30.72	316.8	318.72	1382.4	2.23
16.4	4.45	0	0	0	163.8	0	0.5	0.45	3.6	0.2	39.6	1.37	154.8	3.96	25.2	489.6	320.4	1141.2	2.16
14.23	3.49	0	0	0	165.6	1.58	0.3	0.43	2.3	0.1	37.44	1.05	164.16	2.55	20.16	184.96	230.4	1260	1.54
4.83	1.04	0	0	0	33.9	0.11	0.51	0.32	3.48	0.14	7.91	0.03	160.46	2.72	22.6	553.7	196.62	1432.84	1.65
12.82	3.03	0	0	3.08	13.64	0.12	0.4	0.29	3.27	0.11	8.68	0.51	127.72	2.58	19.84	446.4	198.4	1071.36	1.55
11.08	6.42	0	0	0	15.51	0.14	0.35	0.39	4.16	0.16	11.28	0.94	115.62	4.3	26.79	204.45	234.06	795.24	2.66
3.41	0.52	0	0	0	24.42	0	0.27	0.18	1.62	0.03	5.92	0.1	89.54	1.63	8.88	260.48	86.58	583.86	0.29
3.83	2.64	0	0	0	2.4	3.18	0.07	0.13	0.58	0.02	4.2	0.16	25.2	1.29	16.2	87.6	83.4	153	0.55
2.37	0.6	0	0	0	16.28	0.98	0.31	0.3	2.03	0.15	58.59	0.54	56.42	2.26	43.4	48.83	326.59	492.59	0.76
1.24	0.89	0	0	0	119.04	0.84	0.11	0.35	1.79	0.12	40.92	0.45	106.95	1.13	39.99	90.21	248.31	583.11	0.82
2.68	0.48	0	0	0	10.2	0.61	0.22	0.36	2.19	0.14	59.16	0.58	49.98	2.27	35.7	57.12	289.68	522.24	1.7
3.51	0.61	0	0	0	32.34	0.92	0.27	0.42	2.7	0.18	36.96	0.87	53.13	2.45	41.58	70.46	328.02	667.59	1.92
2.23	0.51	0	0	0	75.11	2.54	0.15	0.36	1.93	0.11	30.45	0.55	64.96	1.87	25.38	70.04	205.03	495.32	1.18
4.2	0.63	0	0	0	190.38	3.34	0.27	0.6	3.82	0.2	71.81	0.99	143.62	3.82	48.43	141.95	402.47	1023.71	3.02
3.7	0.43	0	0	0	14.3	0.55	0.12	0.46	3.22	0.15	19.8	0.98	41.8	3.05	40.7	86.9	369.6	745.8	2.37
3.04	0.49	0	0	0	23.12	0.8	0.2	0.4	2.54	0.15	18.09	0.64	43.22	2.22	30.15	70.35	249.24	557.78	2.16
4.97	1.11	0	0	0	56.24	1.82	0.3	0.62	4.16	0.18	28.88	1.03	110.96	3.91	34.96	158.08	332.88	1045.76	3.95
3.42	1.06	0	0	0	37	0.74	0.17	0.18	1.86	0.07	3.7	0.51	15.54	1.07	7.4	14.8	104.34	211.64	0.4
17.35	4.7	0	0	0	54.18	1.03	0.36	0.49	7.25	0.41	49.02	3.41	239.94	5.91	51.6	394.74	595.98	1148.1	6.68
12.61	2.03	0	0	1.18	129.21	7.88	0.39	0.46	7.38	0.28	28.47	2.56	205.86	4.66	43.8	310.98	444.57	1108.14	4.6
14.49	2.71	0	0	0	79.95	2.15	0.31	0.41	6.63	0.31	33.15	2.34	161.85	4.74	44.85	399.75	331.5	1043.25	6.83
12.74	2.44	0.56	0	0	148	0	0.48	0.57	11.17	0.28	38.85	2.53	90.65	5.46	38.85	421.8	643.8	1589.15	5.55
12.64	6.37	0	0	1.98	84.36	2.74	0.57	0.43	8.34	0.27	34.2	2.07	168.72	4.72	36.48	348.84	389.88	921.12	4.13
7.17	1.47	0	0	0	70.84	2.31	0.32	0.23	6.38	0.15	21.56	1.23	181.72	2.65	26.18	215.6	229.46	976.36	2.62
5.77	1.54	0.31	0	0	36.72	0	0.4	0.4	3.7	0.09	26.52	0.97	140.76	2.44	21.42	195.84	164.22	499.8	2.37
21.52	3.15	0	0	0	85.12	2.74	0.61	0.64	11.46	0.61	51.68	5.9	282.72	8.3	60.8	541.12	820.8	1212.96	10.88
13.65	9.95	0	0	0	127.68	2.96	0.41	0.46	9.07	0.41	45.6	0.46	257.64	3.63	43.32	405.84	332.88	1238.04	2.9
10.41	8.38	0	0	0	30.94	8.92	0.33	0.24	6.81	0.2	29.12	0.38	60.06	4.68	34.58	232.96	353.08	957.32	1.87
1.45	0.37	0	0	0.33	5.1	0.07	0.02	0.02	1.14	0.05	1.87	0.05	2.72	0.21	3.4	34	41.82	90.44	0.18
1.15	0.31	0	0	0	6.12	0.1	0.01	0.02	0.92	0.04	3.57	0.04	2.72	0.19	3.23	28.05	41.65	108.46	0.15
1.27	0.33	0	0	0	4.42	0.07	0.01	0.02	1.01	0.05	1.7	0.04	2.55	0.2	2.89	29.92	37.74	79.39	0.16
1.18	0.38	0	0	0	4.25	0.05	0.02	0.02	0.91	0.04	1.53	0.04	3.23	0.19	3.4	28.56	36.55	103.36	0.15
1.13	0.29	0	0	0	9.52	0.1	0.01	0.03	0.9	0.04	1.53	0.05	2.72	0.19	3.06	27.54	36.21	88.57	0.14
3.41	0.53	0	0	0	166.98	1.52	0.13	1.14	2.48	0.33	30.36	1.14	68.31	5.19	45.54	197.34	690.69	1006.94	3.57
8.06	1.14	0	0	0	15.66	4.7	0.49	0.64	5.78	0.28	31.32	1.51	62.64	4.54	62.64	123.54	586.38	910.02	4.96
9.43	0.73	0	0	0	126.27	2.75	0.38	0.86	4.67	0.22	32.94	1.3	237.9	3.84	60.39	186.66	203.13	957.09	3.37
5.05	1.03	0	0	0.37	14.85	0.55	0.09	0.19	1.39	0.03	15.95	0.1	19.8	1.47	16.5	52.25	81.95	188.1	0.34

USDA ID Code	Food Name	Weight in Grams*	Quantity of Units	Unit of Measure	Protein (gm)	Fat (gm)	Carbohydrates (gm)	Kcalories	Caffeine (gm)	Fiber (gm)	Cholesterol (mg)	Saturated Fat (gm)
21043	Fast Food-Clams, Breaded and Fried	28.35	3	Ounce	3.16	6.51	9.57	111.13	0	0	21.55	1.63
21128	Fast Food-Corn On The Cob w/ Butter	146	1	Each	4.47	3.43	31.94	154.76	0	0	5.84	1.64
21045	Fast Food-Crab, Soft-shell, Fried	125	1	Each	10.99	17.86	31.2	333.75	0	0	45	4.4
21011	Fast Food-Croissant w/ Egg and Cheese	127	1	Each	12.79	24.7	24.31	368.3	0	0	215.9	14.07
21012	Fast Food-Croissant w/ Egg, Cheese, and Bacon	129	1	Each	16.23	28.35	23.65	412.8	0	0	215.43	15.43
21013	Fast Food-Croissant w/ Egg, Cheese, and Ham	152	1	Each	18.92	33.58	24.2	474.24	0	0	212.8	17.48
21014	Fast Food-Croissant w/ Egg, Cheese, and Sausage	160	1	Each	20.3	38.16	24.72	523.2	0	0	216	18.23
21015	Fast Food-Danish Pastry, Cheese	91	1	Each	5.83	24.62	28.69	353.08	0	0	20.02	5.12
21016	Fast Food-Danish Pastry, Cinnamon	88	1	Each	4.8	16.72	46.85	349.36	0	0	27.28	3.48
21017	Fast Food-Danish Pastry, Fruit	94	1	Each	4.76	15.93	45.06	334.64	0	0	18.8	3.32
21104	Fast Food-Egg and Cheese Sandwich	146	1	Each	15.61	19.42	25.93	340.18	0	0	290.54	6.63
21018	Fast Food-Egg, Scrambled	47	2	Eggs	13.2	14.7	2.5	175	0	0	346	2.89
21074	Fast Food-Enchilada w/ Cheese	163	1	Each	9.63	18.84	28.54	319.48	0	0	44.01	10.59
21075	Fast Food-Enchilada w/ Cheese and Beef	192	1	Each	11.92	17.64	30.47	322.56	0	0	40.32	9.05
21076	Fast Food-Enchirito w/ Cheese, Beef, and Beans	193	1	Each	17.89	16.08	33.79	343.54	0	0	50.18	7.95
21019	Fast Food-Eng. Muffin w/ Butter	63	1	Each	4.87	5.76	30.36	189	0	0	12.6	2.43
21020	Fast Food-Eng. Muffin w/ Cheese and Sausage	115	1	Each	15.34	24.27	29.16	393.3	0	0	58.65	9.85
21021	Fast Food-Eng. Muffin w/ Egg, Cheese, and Can. Bacon	146	1	Each	19.81	19.75	31.45	382.52	0	0	233.6	9.05
21022	Fast Food-Eng. Muffin w/ Egg, Cheese, and Sausage	165	1	Each	21.66	30.86	30.97	486.75	0	0	273.9	12.42
21047	Fast Food-Fish Fillet, Battered and Fried	91	1	Each	13.34	11.18	15.44	211.12	0	0	30.94	2.57
21105	Fast Food-Fish Sandwich w/ Tartar Sauce	158	1	Each	16.94	22.77	41.02	431.34	0	0	55.3	5.23
21106	Fast Food-Fish Sandwich w/ Tartar Sauce and Cheese	183	1	Each	20.61	28.6	47.63	523.38	0	0	67.71	8.14
21023	Fast Food-French Toast w/ Butter	67.5	1	Slice	5.17	9.38	18.02	178.2	0	0	58.05	0
21031	Fast Food-Fried Pie, Fruit (Apple, Cherry, or Lemon)	85	1	Each	2.41	14.37	33.05	266.05	0	0	12.75	6.51
21077	Fast Food-Frijoles w/ Cheese	28.35	3	Ounce	1.93	1.32	4.87	38.27	0	0	6.24	0.69
21116	Fast Food-Ham and Cheese Sandwich	146	1	Each	20.69	15.48	33.35	351.86	0	0	58.4	6.44
21117	Fast Food-Ham, Egg, and Cheese Sandwich	143	1	Each	19.25	16.3	30.95	347.49	0	0	245.96	7.4
21114	Fast Food-Hamburger, Double Patty w/ Cond and Veg	226	1	Each	34.28	26.56	40.27	540.14	0	0	122.04	10.52
21111	Fast Food-Hamburger, Double Patty w/ Condiments	215	1	Each	31.82	32.47	38.74	576.2	0	0	103.2	12
21110	Fast Food-Hamburger, Double Patty, Plain	176	1	Each	29.92	27.9	42.93	543.84	0	0	98.56	10.38
21113	Fast Food-Hamburger, Large, Single Patty w/ Cond&veg	218	1	Each	25.83	27.36	40	512.3	0	0	87.2	10.42
21112	Fast Food-Hamburger, Large, Single Patty, Plain	137	1	Each	22.62	22.92	31.73	426.07	0	0	71.24	8.38
21108	Fast Food-Hamburger, Single Patty w/ Condiments	107	1	Each	13.6	10.23	32.68	274.99	0	0	42.8	3.51
21107	Fast Food-Hamburger, Single Patty, Plain	90	1	Each	12.32	11.82	30.51	274.5	0	0	35.1	4.14
21115	Fast Food-Hamburger, Triple Patty w/ Condiments	259	1	Each	49.99	41.47	28.59	691.53	0	0	142.45	15.92
21119	Fast Food-Hot Dog w/ Chili	114	1	Each	13.51	13.44	31.29	296.4	0	0	51.3	4.85
21120	Fast Food-Hot Dog w/ Corn Flour Coating (corndog)	175	1	Each	16.8	18.9	55.79	460.25	0	0	78.75	5.16
21118	Fast Food-Hot Dog, Plain	98	1	Each	10.39	14.54	18.03	242.06	0	0	44.1	5.11
21028	Fast Food-Ice Milk, Vanilla, Soft-serve w/ Cone	103	1	Each	3.89	6.12	24.11	163.77	0	0	27.81	3.53
21078	Fast Food-Nachos w/ Cheese	28.35	3	Ounce	2.28	4.75	9.11	86.75	0	0	4.54	1.95
21079	Fast Food-Nachos w/ Cheese and Jalapeno Peppers	28.35	3	Ounce	2.34	4.75	8.35	84.48	0	0	11.62	1.95
21080	Fast Food-Nachos w/ Cheese, Beans, Ground Beef	28.35	3	Ounce	2.2	3.41	6.21	63.22	0	0	2.27	1.39
21081	Fast Food-Nachos w/ Cinnamon and Sugar	28.35	3	Ounce	1.87	9.36	16.49	153.94	0	0	10.21	4.74
21130	Fast Food-Onion Rings, Breaded and Fried	10	1	Each	0.45	1.87	3.77	33.2	0	0	1.7	0.84
21048	Fast Food-Oysters, Battered or Breaded, and Fried	28.35	3	Ounce	2.56	3.66	8.13	75.13	0	0	22.11	0.93
21025	Fast Food-Pancakes w/ Butter and Syrup	74	1	Each	2.63	4.46	28.99	165.76	0	0	18.5	1.87
21049	Fast Food-Pizza w/ Cheese	63	1	Slice	7.68	3.21	20.5	140.49	0	0	9.45	1.54
21050	Fast Food-Pizza w/ Cheese, Sausage, and Vegetables	79	1	Slice	13.01	5.36	21.29	184.07	0	0	20.54	1.53
21051	Fast Food-Pizza w/ Pepperoni	71	1	Slice	10.12	6.96	19.87	181.05	0	0	14.2	2.24
21131	Fast Food-Potato, Baked w/ Cheese Sauce	296	1	Each	14.62	28.74	46.5	473.6	0	0	17.76	10.56
21132	Fast Food-Potato, Baked w/ Cheese Sauce and Bacon	299	1	Each	18.42	25.89	44.43	451.49	0	0	29.9	10.13
21133	Fast Food-Potato, Baked w/ Cheese Sauce and Broccoli	339	1	Each	13.66	21.42	46.58	403.41	0	0	20.34	8.51
21134	Fast Food-Potato, Baked w/ Cheese Sauce and Chili	395	1	Each	23.23	21.84	55.85	481.9	0	0	31.6	13.04
21135	Fast Food-Potato, Baked w/ Sour Cream and Chives	302	1	Each	6.67	22.32	50.01	392.6	0	0	24.16	10.01
21136	Fast Food-Potato, French Fried In Beef Tallow	115	1	Large	4.59	18.5	44.36	358.8	0	0	20.7	8.52

Monounsaturated Fat (gm)	Polyunsaturated Fat (gm)	Vitamin D (mg)	Vitamin K (mg)	Vitamin E (mg)	Vitamin A (re)	Vitamin C (mg)	Thiamin (mg)	Riboflavin (mg)	Niacin (mg)	Vitamin B6 (mg)	Folate (mg)	Vitamin B12 (mcg)	Calcium (mg)	Iron (mg)	Magnesium (mg)	Phosphorus (mg)	Potassium (mg)	Sodium (mg)	Zinc (mg)
2.82	1.67	0	0	0	9.07	0	0.05	0.07	0.71	0.01	2.27	0.27	5.1	0.75	7.65	58.68	65.49	205.54	0.4
1	0.61	0	0	0	96.36	6.86	0.25	0.1	2.18	0.32	43.8	0	4.38	0.88	40.88	108.04	359.16	29.2	0.91
7.69	4.88	0	0	0	3.75	0.75	0.1	0.08	1.75	0.15	20	4.48	55	1.81	25	131.25	162.5	1117.5	1.06
7.54	1.37	0	0	0	255.27	0.13	0.19	0.38	1.51	0.1	36.83	0.77	243.84	2.2	21.59	347.98	173.99	551.18	1.75
9.18	1.76	0	0	0	119.97	2.19	0.35	0.34	2.19	0.12	34.83	0.86	150.93	2.19	23.22	276.06	201.24	888.81	1.9
11.39	2.36	0	0	0	117.04	11.4	0.52	0.3	3.19	0.23	36.48	1	144.4	2.13	25.84	335.92	272.08	1080.72	2.17
14.25	3.01	0	0	0	108.8	0.16	0.99	0.32	4	0.11	38.4	0.9	144	3.04	24	289.6	283.2	1115.2	2.14
15.6	2.42	0	0	0	42.77	2.64	0.26	0.21	2.55	0.05	14.56	0.23	70.07	1.85	15.47	80.08	116.48	319.41	0.63
10.59	1.65	0	0	0	5.28	2.55	0.26	0.19	2.2	0.05	14.08	0.22	36.96	1.8	14.08	73.92	95.92	326.48	0.48
10.1	1.57	0	0	0	24.44	1.6	0.29	0.21	1.8	0.06	15.04	0.24	21.62	1.4	14.1	68.62	109.98	332.76	0.48
8.27	2.58	0	0	0	181.04	1.46	0.26	0.57	2.07	0.13	36.5	1.14	224.84	2.98	21.9	302.22	188.34	804.46	1.65
2.77	0.93	0.8	0	0.45	125.96	1	0.08	0.6	0.3	0.19	63	0.95	60	2.59	13	230	154	226	1.64
6.31	0.82	0	0	0	185.82	0.98	0.08	0.42	1.91	0.39	34.23	0.75	324.37	1.32	50.53	133.66	239.61	784.03	2.51
6.15	1.39	0	0	0	142.08	1.34	0.1	0.4	2.52	0.27	192	1.02	228.48	3.07	82.56	167.04	574.08	1319.04	2.69
6.52	0.33	0	0	0	133.17	4.63	0.17	0.69	2.99	0.21	252.83	1.62	218.09	2.39	71.41	223.88	559.7	1250.64	2.76
1.53	1.35	0	0	0.13	33.39	0.76	0.25	0.32	2.61	0.04	17.01	0.02	102.69	1.59	13.23	85.05	69.3	386.19	0.42
10.08	2.69	0	0	0	86.25	1.27	0.7	0.25	4.14	0.15	18.4	0.68	167.9	2.25	24.15	186.3	215.05	1036.15	1.68
6.76	2.06	1.17	0	0.6	157.68	1.31	0.48	0.53	3.93	0.16	43.8	0.8	207.32	3.29	33.58	319.74	213.16	784.02	1.81
12.75	3.32	0	0	0	171.6	1.49	0.84	0.5	4.46	0.2	54.45	1.37	196.35	3.47	29.7	287.1	293.7	1135.2	2.36
2.35	5.71	0	0	0	10.92	0	0.1	0.1	1.91	0.09	50.96	1.01	16.38	1.92	21.84	155.61	291.2	484.12	0.4
7.69	8.25	0	0	0.87	30.02	2.84	0.33	0.22	3.4	0.11	44.24	1.07	83.74	2.61	33.18	211.72	339.7	614.62	1
8.92	9.43	0.92	0	1.83	96.99	2.75	0.46	0.42	4.23	0.11	31.11	1.08	184.83	3.5	36.6	311.1	353.19	938.79	1.17
0	0	0	0	0	72.9	0.07	0.29	0.25	1.96	0.03	14.85	0.18	36.45	0.95	8.1	72.9	88.43	256.5	0.3
5.83	1.16	0	0	0.37	33.15	1.11	0.1	0.08	0.98	0.03	4.25	0.08	12.75	0.88	7.65	37.4	51	324.7	0.17
0.44	0.12	0	0	0	11.91	0.26	0.02	0.06	0.25	0.03	18.99	0.12	32.04	0.38	14.46	29.77	102.63	149.69	0.29
6.74	1.38	0	0	0.29	75.92	2.77	0.31	0.48	2.69	0.2	71.54	0.54	129.94	3.24	16.06	151.84	290.54	770.88	1.37
5.74	1.69	0	0	0	148.72	2.72	0.43	0.56	4.2	0.16	42.9	1.23	211.64	3.1	25.74	346.06	210.21	1005.29	1.99
10.33	2.8	0	0	0	11.3	1.13	0.36	0.38	7.57	0.54	27.12	4.07	101.7	5.85	49.72	314.14	569.52	791	5.67
14.13	2.76	0	0	0	4.3	1.08	0.34	0.41	6.73	0.37	45.15	3.33	92.45	5.55	45.15	283.8	526.75	741.75	5.81
12.11	2.34	0.7	0	1.32	0	0	0.33	0.37	8.25	0.32	36.96	2.92	86.24	4.56	36.96	234.08	362.56	554.4	5.72
11.42	2.2	0	0	0	32.7	2.62	0.41	0.37	7.28	0.33	37.06	2.38	95.92	4.93	43.6	233.26	479.6	824.04	4.88
9.88	2.14	0.55	0	0	0	0	0.29	0.29	6.25	0.23	31.51	2.06	73.98	3.58	27.4	175.36	267.15	474.02	4.11
3.72	1.77	0	0	0.43	12.84	2.57	0.26	0.32	4.7	0.13	17.12	0.83	51.36	2.46	22.47	110.21	215.07	563.89	2.05
5.46	0.92	0.27	0	0.5	0	0	0.33	0.27	3.72	0.06	25.2	0.89	63	2.4	18.9	102.6	144.9	387	2
18.23	2.74	0	0	0	15.54	1.3	0.31	0.54	10.96	0.62	31.08	4.92	64.75	8.31	54.39	393.68	784.77	712.25	10.75
6.59	1.19	0	0	0	5.7	2.74	0.22	0.4	3.74	0.05	50.16	0.3	19.38	3.28	10.26	191.52	166.44	479.94	0.78
9.11	3.5	0	0	0	36.75	0	0.28	0.7	4.17	0.09	59.5	0.44	101.5	6.18	17.5	166.25	262.5	973	1.31
6.85	1.71	0	0	0	0	0.1	0.24	0.27	3.65	0.05	29.4	0.51	23.52	2.31	12.74	97.02	143.08	670.32	1.98
1.82	0.36	0.21	0	0.38	51.5	1.13	0.05	0.26	0.31	0.06	5.15	0.21	153.47	0.15	15.45	139.05	168.92	91.67	0.57
2.01	0.56	0	0	0	22.96	0.31	0.05	0.09	0.39	0.05	2.55	0.21	68.32	0.32	13.89	69.17	43.09	204.69	0.45
2	0.56	0	0	0	65.49	0.14	0.02	0.07	0.39	0.05	2.55	0.14	86.18	0.34	15.03	54.72	40.82	241.26	0.4
1.22	0.63	0	0	0	52.16	0.54	0.03	0.08	0.37	0.05	4.25	0.11	42.81	0.31	10.77	43.09	50.18	200.15	0.41
3.08	1.07	0	0	0	2.84	2.07	0.05	0.12	1.02	0.05	1.98	0.45	22.11	0.75	5.1	8.51	20.41	114.25	0.15
0.8	0.08	0	0	0.04	0.1	0.07	0.01	0.01	0.11	0.01	1.4	0.02	2.8	0.1	1.9	10.4	15.6	51.8	0.04
1.41	0.95	0	0	0	22.11	0.85	0.06	0.07	0.9	0.01	2.55	0.21	5.67	0.91	4.82	39.97	37.14	138.06	3.19
1.68	0.62	0	0	0.44	22.2	1.11	0.13	0.18	1.08	0.04	11.1	0.07	40.7	0.84	15.54	151.7	79.92	352.24	0.33
0.99	0.49	0	0	0	73.71	1.26	0.18	0.16	2.48	0.04	58.59	0.33	116.55	0.58	15.75	112.77	109.62	335.79	0.81
2.54	0.91	0	0	0	101.12	1.58	0.21	0.17	1.96	0.09	26.86	0.36	101.12	1.53	18.17	131.14	178.54	382.36	1.11
3.14	1.17	0	0	0	54.67	1.63	0.13	0.23	3.05	0.06	52.54	0.18	64.61	0.94	8.52	75.26	152.65	266.96	0.52
10.7	6.04	0	0	0	227.92	26.05	0.24	0.21	3.34	0.71	26.64	0.18	310.8	3.02	65.12	319.68	1166.24	381.84	1.89
9.71	4.75	0	0	0	173.42	28.7	0.27	0.24	3.98	0.75	29.9	0.33	307.97	3.14	68.77	346.84	1178.06	971.75	2.15
7.68	4.18	0	0	0	277.98	48.48	0.27	0.27	3.59	0.78	61.02	0.34	335.61	3.32	77.97	345.78	1440.75	484.77	2.03
6.84	0.9	0	0	0	173.8	31.6	0.28	0.36	4.19	0.95	51.35	0.24	410.8	6.12	110.6	497.7	1572.1	699.15	3.79
7.87	3.32	0	0	0	277.84	33.82	0.27	0.18	3.71	0.79	33.22	0.21	105.7	3.11	69.46	184.22	1383.16	181.2	0.91
8.03	0.93	0	0	0.02	3.45	6.1	0.16	0.05	2.6	0.3	37.95	0.14	18.4	1.55	37.95	152.95	818.8	187.45	0.6

USDA ID Code	Food Name	Weight in Grams*	Quantity of Units	Unit of Measure	Protein (gm)	Fat (gm)	Carbohydrates (gm)	Kcalories	Caffeine (gm)	Fiber (gm)	Cholesterol (mg)	Saturated Fat (gm)
21137	Fast Food-Potato, French Fried In Beef Tallow and Veg Oil	115	1	Large	4.59	18.5	44.36	357.65	0	0	16.1	7.63
21138	Fast Food-Potato, French Fried In Vegetable Oil	115	1	Large	4.59	18.5	44.36	355.35	0	0	0	5.74
21139	Fast Food-Potato, Mashed	240.024	0.5	Cup	5.54	2.9	38.69	199.22	0	0	4.8	1.15
21026	Fast Food-Potatoes, Hashed Brown	144	0.5	Cup	3.89	18.43	32.3	302.4	0	0	18.72	8.65
21122	Fast Food-Roast Beef Sandwich w/ Cheese	176	1	Each	32.23	18	45.37	473.44	0	0	77.44	9.03
21121	Fast Food-Roast Beef Sandwich, Plain	139	1	Each	21.5	13.76	33.44	346.11	0	0	51.43	3.61
21052	Fast Food-Salad, w/o Dressing	138.667	0.5	Cup	1.73	0.1	4.47	22.19	0	0	0	0.01
21053	Fast Food-Salad, w/o Dressing, w/ Cheese and Egg	144.666	0.5	Cup	5.84	3.86	3.17	67.99	0	0	65.1	1.98
21054	Fast Food-Salad, w/o Dressing, w/ Chicken	145.333	0.5	Cup	11.63	1.45	2.49	69.76	0	0	47.96	0.39
21055	Fast Food-Salad, w/o Dressing, w/ Pasta and Seafood	277.998	0.5	Cup	10.95	13.9	21.32	252.98	0	0	33.36	1.71
21056	Fast Food-Salad, w/o Dressing, w/ Shrimp	157.333	0.5	Cup	9.68	1.65	4.41	70.8	0	0	119.57	0.43
21058	Fast Food-Scallops, Breaded and Fried	24	1	Each	2.63	3.23	6.42	64.32	0	0	18	0.81
21059	Fast Food-Shrimp, Breaded and Fried	28.35	1	Ounce	3.26	4.3	6.91	78.53	0	0	34.59	0.93
21123	Fast Food-Steak Sandwich	140	1	Each	20.82	9.66	35.66	315	0	0	50.4	2.62
21124	Fast Food-Submarine Sandwich w/ Coldcuts	228	1	Each	21.84	18.63	51.05	456	0	0	36.48	6.81
21125	Fast Food-Submarine Sandwich w/ Roast Beef	216	1	Each	28.64	12.96	44.3	410.4	0	0	73.44	7.09
21126	Fast Food-Submarine Sandwich w/ Tuna Salad	256	1	Each	29.7	27.98	55.37	583.68	0	0	48.64	5.33
21032	Fast Food-Sundae, Caramel	155	1	Each	7.3	9.27	49.31	303.8	0	0	24.8	4.51
21033	Fast Food-Sundae, Hot Fudge	158	1	Each	5.64	8.63	47.67	284.4	0	0	20.54	5.02
21034	Fast Food-Sundae, Strawberry	153	1	Each	6.26	7.85	44.65	267.75	0	0	21.42	3.74
21082	Fast Food-Taco	263	1	Large	31.77	31.61	41.11	568.08	0	0	86.79	17.48
21083	Fast Food-Taco Salad	132	0.5	Cup	8.82	9.85	15.72	186.12	0	0	29.04	4.55
21084	Fast Food-Taco Salad w/ Chili Con Carne	174	0.5	Cup	11.61	8.75	17.71	193.14	0	0	3.48	4
21088	Fast Food-Tostada w/ Guacamole	28.35	1	Ounce	1.36	2.53	3.48	39.12	0	0	4.25	1.07
21085	Fast Food-Tostada, w/ Beans and Cheese	144	1	Each	9.6	9.86	26.52	223.2	0	0	30.24	5.37
21086	Fast Food-Tostada, w/ Beans, Beef, and Cheese	225	1	Each	16.09	16.94	29.66	333	0	0	74.25	11.48
21087	Fast Food-Tostada, w/ Beef and Cheese	163	1	Each	18.99	16.35	22.77	314.59	0	0	40.75	10.39
62621	Fettucini Alfredo with Broccoli-Weight Watchers	240.975	1	Each	15	6	24	220	0	6	15	2.5
55208	Fettucini Alfredo, Lean Cuisine-Stouffer's	255.144	1	Each	14	7	41	280	0	0	15	3
55171	Fettucini Alfredo-Stouffer's	141.746	1	Each	8	14	22	245	0	0	0	0
55209	Fettucini Primavera, Lean Cuisine-Stouffer's	283.493	1	Each	14	8	32	260	0	0	45	3
55831	Fettucini Sauce (Alfredo Style)-Stouffer's	283.92	1	Cup	14.02	67.1	11.02	701.05	0	0	180.27	0
41288	Fettucini w/ Turkey and Vegetables-Healthy Choice	354.367	1	Each	29	6	45	350	0	0	60	3
62612	Fiesta Chicken-Weight Watchers	240.975	1	Each	12	2	38	220	0	5	25	0.5
55773	Fiesta Mexicali Heat'n Serve Soup -Stouffer's	283.92	1	Cup	3	3	18.03	110.17	0	0	10.02	0
55210	Filet of Fish Divan, Lean Cuisine-Stouffer's	294.124	1	Each	27	5	13	210	0	0	65	2
55211	Filet of Fish Florentine, Lean Cuisine-Stouffer's	272.862	1	Each	26	7	13	220	0	0	65	3
55178	French Bread Pizza, Cheese-Stouffer's	145.29	1	Each	16	14	40	350	0	0	0	0
41332	French Bread Pizza, Deluxe-Healthy Choice	180.727	1	Each	23	7	41	330	0	0	35	3
55181	French Bread Pizza, Deluxe-Stouffer's	173.639	1	Each	21	19	40	420	0	0	0	0
55180	French Bread Pizza, Double Cheese-Stouffer's	166.552	1	Each	22	18	43	420	0	0	0	0
55182	French Bread Pizza, Hamburger-Stouffer's	173.639	1	Each	23	18	39	410	0	0	0	0
55183	French Bread Pizza, Pepperoni-Stouffer's	159.465	1	Each	19	19	39	400	0	0	0	0
55185	French Bread Pizza, Sausage-Stouffer's	170.096	1	Each	20	21	40	430	0	0	0	0
55187	French Bread Pizza, Vegetable Deluxe-Stouffer's	180.727	1	Each	18	20	41	420	0	0	0	0
55761	French Onion Soup-Stouffer's	283.92	1	Cup	4.01	4.01	10.02	100.15	0	0	0	0
41337	Garden Potato Casserole-Healthy Choice	262.231	1	Each	12	4	23	180	0	0	20	2
55774	Garden Tomato Heat'n Serve Soup-Stouffer's	283.92	1	Cup	4.01	3	16.02	110.17	0	0	10.02	0
41273	Garden Vegetable Soup-Healthy Choice	212.62	1	Each	3	1	18	100	0	0	0	0
43399	Glazed Breast of Chicken, Top Shelf-Hormel	283.493	1	Each	19	2	19	170	0	0	35	1
55212	Glazed Chicken w/ Veg. Lean Cuisine-Stouffer's	240.969	1	Each	21	7	24	250	0	0	50	2
41307	Glazed Chicken-Healthy Choice	240.969	1	Each	21	3	27	220	0	0	45	1
55784	Glazed Chicken-Stouffer's	28.35	1	Ounce	2.9	1.1	1	26	0	0	9	0
55172	Green Bean Mushroom Casserole-Stouffer's	134.659	1	Each	5	10	13	160	0	0	0	0
55118	Green Pepper Steak w/ Rice-Stouffer's	297.668	1	Each	20	10	35	310	0	0	0	0

Monounsaturated Fat (gm)	Polyunsaturated Fat (gm)	Vitamin D (mg)	Vitamin K (mg)	Vitamin E (mg)	Vitamin A (re)	Vitamin C (mg)	Thiamin (mg)	Riboflavin (mg)	Niacin (mg)	Vitamin B6 (mg)	Folate (mg)	Vitamin B12 (mcg)	Calcium (mg)	Iron (mg)	Magnesium (mg)	Phosphorus (mg)	Potassium (mg)	Sodium (mg)	Zinc (mg)
8.23	1.99	0	0	0	3.45	6.1	0.16	0.05	2.6	0.3	37.95	0.14	18.4	1.55	37.95	152.95	818.8	187.45	0.6
9.11	2.84	0	0	0.22	3.45	6.1	0.16	0.05	2.6	0.3	37.95	0.14	18.4	1.55	37.95	152.95	818.8	187.45	0.6
0.84	0.7	0	0	0	24	0.96	0.22	0.12	2.88	0.55	19.2	0.12	50.4	1.13	43.2	132.01	705.67	544.85	0.77
7.72	0.94	0	0	0.24	5.76	10.94	0.16	0.03	2.15	0.33	15.84	0.03	14.4	0.96	31.68	138.24	534.24	580.32	0.43
3.66	3.5	0	0	0	45.76	0	0.39	0.46	5.9	0.33	40.48	2.06	183.04	5.05	40.48	401.28	344.96	1633.28	5.37
6.8	1.71	0	0	0	20.85	2.09	0.38	0.31	5.87	0.26	40.31	1.22	54.21	4.23	30.58	239.08	315.53	792.3	3.39
0.01	0.05	0	0	0	158.08	32.17	0.04	0.07	0.76	0.11	51.31	0	18.03	0.87	15.25	54.08	238.51	36.05	0.29
1.17	0.32	0	0	0	76.67	6.51	0.06	0.12	0.65	0.07	56.42	0.2	66.55	0.45	15.91	88.25	247.38	79.57	0.67
0.45	0.37	0	0	0	63.95	11.63	0.07	0.09	3.92	0.29	45.05	0.13	24.71	0.73	21.8	113.36	297.93	139.52	0.6
3.21	6.05	0	0	0	425.34	25.58	0.19	0.14	2.36	0.22	66.72	1.14	47.26	2.11	33.36	136.22	400.32	1048.05	1.11
0.55	0.32	0	0	0	51.92	6.14	0.08	0.11	0.77	0.09	58.21	2.52	39.33	0.6	25.17	106.99	269.04	325.68	0.85
2.09	0.1	0	0	0	6.96	0	0.03	0.14	0	0.01	6.72	0.07	3.12	0.34	5.28	48.72	48.96	153.12	0.18
3	0.11	0	0	0	6.24	0	0.04	0.16	0	0.01	8.22	0.03	14.46	0.51	6.8	59.54	31.75	250.05	0.21
3.67	2.3	0	0	0	30.8	3.78	0.28	0.25	5.01	0.25	61.6	1.08	63	3.54	33.6	204.4	359.8	547.4	3.11
8.23	2.28	0	0	0	79.8	12.31	1	0.8	5.49	0.14	54.72	1.09	189.24	2.51	68.4	287.28	394.44	1650.72	2.58
1.84	2.61	0	0	0	49.68	5.62	0.41	0.41	5.96	0.32	45.36	1.81	41.04	2.81	66.96	192.24	330.48	844.56	4.38
13.4	7.3	0	0	0	40.96	3.58	0.46	0.33	11.34	0.23	56.32	1.61	74.24	2.64	79.36	220.16	335.36	1292.8	1.87
3.03	1.01	0.31	0	0.9	68.2	3.41	0.06	0.29	0.95	0.05	12.4	0.6	189.1	0.22	27.9	217	317.75	195.3	0.82
2.33	0.81	0.47	0	0.66	56.88	2.37	0.06	0.3	1.07	0.13	9.48	0.65	206.98	0.58	33.18	227.52	395	181.7	0.95
2.66	1.02	0.46	0	0.78	58.14	1.99	0.06	0.28	0.9	0.08	18.36	0.64	160.65	0.32	24.48	154.53	270.81	91.8	0.66
10.11	1.48	0	0	0	226.18	3.42	0.24	0.68	4.94	0.37	36.82	1.6	339.27	3.71	107.83	312.97	728.51	1233.47	6.05
3.44	1.17	0	0	0	51.48	2.38	0.07	0.24	1.64	0.15	26.4	0.42	128.04	1.52	34.32	95.04	277.2	508.2	1.8
3.03	1.02	0	0	0	142.68	2.26	0.1	0.33	1.69	0.35	41.76	0.49	163.56	1.77	34.8	102.66	261	589.86	2.19
0.92	0.33	0	0	0	23.53	0.4	0.01	0.06	0.22	0.03	11.91	0.11	45.93	0.18	7.94	25.23	70.59	86.75	0.44
3.05	0.75	0	0	0	84.96	1.3	0.1	0.33	1.32	0.16	74.88	0.69	210.24	1.89	59.04	116.64	403.2	542.88	1.9
3.51	0.6	0	0	0	173.25	4.05	0.09	0.5	2.86	0.25	96.75	1.13	189	2.45	67.5	173.25	490.5	870.75	3.17
3.34	0.97	0	0	0	96.17	2.61	0.1	0.55	3.15	0.23	14.67	1.17	216.79	2.87	63.57	179.3	572.13	896.5	3.68
0	0	0	0	0	60	1.2	0	0	0	0	0	0	300	1.5	0	0	510	540	0
0	0	0	0	0	0	0	0.3	0.43	1.52	0	0	0	200	0.8	0	0	270	570	0
0	0	0	0	0	0	0	0.15	0.26	0.95	0	0	0	120	0.4	0	0	100	400	0
0	0	0	0	0	400	18	0.3	0.43	1.52	0	0	0	240	0.8	0	0	400	510	0
0	0	0	0	0	0	0	0	0.01	0	0	0	0	2.72	0	0	0	340.51	1812.72	0
0	2	0	0	0	150	0	0.45	0.51	3.8	0	0	0	120	1.5	0	310	450	480	0
0	0	0	0	0	450	42	0	0	0	0	0	0	72	1.5	0	0	490	480	0
0	0	0	0	0	0	6.01	0	0	0.19	0	0	0	2.4	1	0	0	430.64	711.07	0
0	1	0	0	0	20	27	0.15	0.34	1.9	0	0	0	120	0.4	0	0	800	490	0
0	2	0	0	0	500	1.2	0.15	0.34	1.9	0	0	0	120	0.4	0	0	780	590	0
0	0	0	0	0	60	3.6	0.45	0.34	2.85	0	0	0	200	1.5	0	0	300	630	0
0	1	0	0	0	80	0	0.45	0.34	3.8	0	0	0	200	2.5	0	280	350	500	0
0	0	0	0	0	100	6	0.45	0.43	3.8	0	0	0	160	1.5	0	0	350	950	0
0	0	0	0	0	40	6	0.45	0.51	3.8	0	0	0	360	1.5	0	0	320	850	0
0	0	0	0	0	60	6	0.38	0.34	3.8	0	0	0	160	1.5	0	0	340	650	0
0	0	0	0	0	100	6	0.53	0.43	3.8	0	0	0	160	1.5	0	0	300	880	0
0	0	0	0	0	80	6	0.6	0.43	3.8	0	0	0	160	1.5	0	0	340	840	0
0	0	0	0	0	250	3.6	0.45	0.43	3.8	0	0	0	280	1.5	0	0	230	830	0
0	0	0	0	0	0	0	0.02	0.02	0	0	0	0	240.36	0	0	0	170.26	2073.11	0
0	0	0	0	0	0	0	0	0	0	0	0	0	0	0	0	0	600	360	0
0	0	0	0	0	0	0	0	0	0.19	0	0	0	240.36	0.3	0	0	430.64	1051.58	0
0	0	0	0	0	350	9	0.09	0.07	0.76	0	0	0	16	0.4	0	0	230	560	0
1	1	0	0	0.76	400	3.6	0.06	0.17	7.6	0	0	0	32	0.4	35	0	804	780	1.05
0	4	0	0	0	20	3.6	0.15	0.17	7.6	0	0	0	16	0.2	0	0	580	590	0
0	1	0	0	0	0	1.2	0.15	0.14	6.65	0	0	0	0	0.6	0	240	370	510	0
0	0	0	0	0	0	0	0	0	0.23	0	0	0	24	0.01	0	0	45	105	0
0	0	0	0	0	40	2.4	0.06	0.17	0.38	0	0	0	64	0.2	0	0	200	550	0
0	0	0	0	0	40	6	0.15	0.17	3.8	0	0	0	16	1	0	0	410	700	0

USDA ID Code	Food Name	Weight in Grams*	Quantity of Units	Unit of Measure	Protein (gm)	Fat (gm)	Carbohydrates (gm)	Kcalories	Caffeine (gm)	Fiber (gm)	Cholesterol (mg)	Saturated Fat (gm)
55780	Green Pepper Steak-Stouffer's	28.35	1	Ounce	2.6	1.4	1.3	28	0	0	7	0
62617	Grilled Salisbury Steak-Weight Watchers	240.975	1	Each	19	9	24	250	0	4	30	3
55159	Ham and Asparagus Bake-Stouffer's	269.319	1	Each	18	35	32	520	0	0	0	0
62683	Hamburger Helper, Beef Noodle	220	1	Cup	4	10.5	23	260	0	1	5	4
62682	Hamburger Helper, Cheesy Italian	220	1	Cup	5	21	30	330	0	1	5	2
62681	Hamburger Helper, Chili Mac	220	1	Cup	3	16	30	290	0	1	4	4
55809	Heartland Medley-Stouffer's	28.35	1	Ounce	1.4	0.4	1.8	17	0	0	3	0
41279	Hearty Beef Soup-Healthy Choice	212.62	1	Each	9	1	17	120	0	0	20	0
41280	Hearty Chicken Soup-Healthy Choice	212.62	1	Each	7	2	17	110	0	0	25	0
41258	Herb Roasted Chicken-Healthy Choice	347.279	1	Each	22	5	50	300	0	0	40	2
41311	Homestyle Turkey w/ Vegetables-Healthy Choice	269.319	1	Each	26	2	34	260	0	0	30	0
55214	Honey Mustard Chicken, Lean Cuisine-Stouffer's	212.62	1	Each	18	4	30	230	0	0	40	1
41312	Honey Mustard Chicken-Healthy Choice	269.319	1	Each	26	4	41	310	0	0	45	1
43371	Hot Chili no Beans-Hormel	212.62	1	Each	16	27	14	360	0	0	60	11
43410	Hot Chili w/ Beans, Micro Cup-Hormel	209.076	1	Each	15	11	24	250	0	0	49	4
43372	Hot Chili w/ Beans-Hormel	212.62	1	Each	15	15	27	300	0	0	55	5
62622	Italian Cheese Lasagna-Weight Watchers	311.85	1	Each	29	8	28	300	0	7	25	3
43395	Italian Lasagna, Top Shelf-Hormel	283.493	1	Each	23	16	30	350	0	0	60	8
55798	Italian Style Vegetables-Stouffer's	28.35	1	Ounce	0.3	0.3	1.6	10	0	0	0	0
62613	Lasagna Florentine-Weight Watchers	283.5	1	Each	13	2	37	210	0	5	10	0.5
55215	Lasagna w/ Meat Sauce, Lean Cuisine-Stouffer's	290.581	1	Each	20	6	36	280	0	0	25	3
41308	Lasagna w/ Meat Sauce-Healthy Choice	283.493	1	Each	18	5	37	260	0	0	20	2
62623	Lasagna with Meat Sauce-Weight Watchers	290.59	1	Each	24	7	34	290	0	7	15	2.5
43403	Lasagna, Micro Cup-Hormel	212.62	1	Each	8	13	25	250	0	0	23	6
55134	Lasagna-Stouffer's	283.493	1	Each	18	12	40	340	0	0	0	0
41259	Lemon Pepper Fish-Healthy Choice	304.755	1	Each	13	5	52	300	0	0	40	1
41274	Lentil Soup-Healthy Choice	212.62	1	Each	8	1	23	140	0	0	0	0
55216	Linguini w/ Clam Sauce, Lean Cuisine-Stouffer's	272.862	1	Each	17	8	36	280	0	0	30	2
	Macaroni & Cheese, Deluxe Light, Kraft	90	1	Serving	14	4.5	48	290	0	0	15	2.5
	Macaroni & Cheese, Kraft	70	1	Serving	12	18.5	50	420	0	0	15	5
55217	Macaroni and Beef in Sauce, Lean Cuisine-Stouffer's	283.493	1	Each	14	6	35	250	0	0	25	1
55137	Macaroni and Beef w/ Tomatoes-Stouffer's	326.017	1	Each	21	12	38	340	0	0	0	0
41338	Macaroni and Beef-Healthy Choice	240.969	1	Each	12	3	32	200	0	0	15	1
62533	Macaroni and Cheese	111.912	1	Cup	1	12.99	43.97	359.72	0	15.99	39.97	7.99
57808	Macaroni and Cheese Pot Pie-Swanson	198.445	1	Each	7	8	24	200	0	0	0	0
55218	Macaroni and Cheese, Lean Cuisine-Stouffer's	255.144	1	Each	15	9	37	290	0	0	30	4
43406	Macaroni and Cheese, Micro Cup-Hormel	212.62	1	Each	12	11	28	260	0	0	45	6
41339	Macaroni and Cheese-Healthy Choice	255.144	1	Each	12	6	45	280	0	0	20	3
55155	Macaroni and Cheese-Stouffer's	170.096	1	Each	11	13	23	250	0	0	0	0
62624	Macaroni and Cheese-Weight Watchers	255.15	1	Each	11	7	49	300	0	7	20	2
41309	Mandarin Chicken-Healthy Choice	311.843	1	Each	23	2	39	260	0	0	50	0
55830	Marinara Sauce-Stouffer's	283.92	1	Cup	3	11.02	18.03	180.27	0	0	0	0
55219	Meatloaf w/ Mac. and Cheese, Lean Cuisine-Stouffer's	265.775	1	Each	26	8	26	280	0	0	55	3
41260	Meatloaf-Healthy Choice	340.192	1	Each	17	8	48	340	0	0	40	3
55779	Meatloaf-Stouffer's	28.35	1	Ounce	4.4	3.4	2.1	57	0	0	15	0
55812	Mexicali Chicken-Stouffer's	28.35	1	Ounce	1.4	0.8	1.8	20	0	0	5	0
55770	Minestrone Heat'n Serve Soup-Stouffer's	283.92	1	Cup	5.01	4.01	18.03	130.2	0	0	0	0
41281	Minestrone Soup-Healthy Choice	212.62	1	Each	6	1	30	160	0	0	0	0
55760	Minestrone Soup-Stouffer's	283.92	1	Cup	6.01	3	20.03	140.21	0	0	10.02	0
41313	Mushroom Gravy over Beef Sirloin Tips-Healthy Choice	269.319	1	Each	22	5	43	310	0	0	35	2
62619	Nacho Grande Chicken Enchiladas-Weight Watchers	255.15	1	Each	15	8	42	290	0	4	20	2.5
41340	Nacho Macaroni and Cheese-Healthy Choice	255.144	1	Each	13	5	44	280	0	0	20	3
55754	Navy Bean w/ Ham Soup-Stouffer's	283.92	1	Cup	11.02	8.01	31.05	240.36	0	0	20.03	0
55757	New England Clam Chowder Soup-Stouffer's	283.92	1	Cup	14.02	23.03	21.03	340.51	0	0	40.06	0
55829	Newburg Sauce Supreme-Stouffer's	283.92	1	Cup	7.01	41.06	20.03	480.72	0	0	120.18	0

Monounsaturated Fat (gm)	Polyunsaturated Fat (gm)	Vitamin D (mg)	Vitamin K (mg)	Vitamin E (mg)	Vitamin A (re)	Vitamin C (mg)	Thiamin (mg)	Riboflavin (mg)	Niacin (mg)	Vitamin B6 (mg)	Folate (mg)	Vitamin B12 (mcg)	Calcium (mg)	Iron (mg)	Magnesium (mg)	Phosphorus (mg)	Potassium (mg)	Sodium (mg)	Zinc (mg)
0	0	0	0	0	0	3.6	0	0	0.1	0	0	0	48	0.02	0	0	51	164	0
0	0	0	0	0	60	0	0	0	0	0	0	0	120	1.5	0	0	450	590	0
0	0	0	0	0	60	36	0.53	0.51	2.85	0	0	0	160	0.8	0	0	360	1100	0
0	0	0	0	0	60	0	0.23	0.17	3.8	0	0	0	24	1	0	0	240	900	0
0	0	0	0	0	60	0	0.3	0.34	3.8	0	0	0	120	1.5	0	0	400	900	0
0	0	0	0	0	200	0	0.3	0.26	4.75	0	0	0	24	1.5	0	0	0	900	0
0	0	0	0	0	0	0.6	0	0	0.06	0	0	0	40	0.02	0	0	60	85	0
0	0	0	0	0	150	9	0.06	0.1	1.9	0	0	0	32	0.4	0	90	280	540	0
0	0	0	0	0	200	2.4	0.09	0.17	1.9	0	0	0	32	0.4	0	90	190	520	0
0	1	0	0	0	250	24	0.15	0.14	7.6	0	0	0	32	0.8	0	280	370	560	0
0	0	0	0	0	100	4.8	0.03	0.07	0	0	0	0	32	0	0	0	100	550	0
0	1	0	0	0	200	2.4	0.15	0.17	3.8	0	0	0	16	0.4	0	0	340	540	0
0	0	0	0	0	100	3.6	0.15	0.03	1.52	0	0	0	16	0.8	0	0	110	520	0
13	1	0	0	10.56	330	0	0.05	0.22	2.47	0	0	0	40	1.4	35	0	497	860	2.7
4	0	0	0	1.95	190	0	0.14	0.15	1.71	0	0	0	48	1.9	45.5	0	677	977	2.7
6	1	0	0	0	210	0	0.09	0.17	1.71	0	0	0	48	1.8	49	0	777	1030	2.25
0	0	0	0	0	350	15	0	0	0	0	0	0	780	1.5	0	0	720	560	0
5	1	0	0	0.7	100	2.4	0.3	0.51	3.8	0	0	0	240	1.5	49	0	728	840	3.15
0	0	0	0	0	0	1.8	0	0	0.02	0	0	0	72	0.01	0	0	62	147	0
0	0	0	0	0	300	15	0	0	0	0	0	0	300	1.5	0	0	440	420	0
0	0	0	0	0	100	6	0.15	0.26	2.85	0	0	0	120	1	0	0	700	560	0
0	1	0	0	0	150	2.4	0.3	0.26	1.9	0	0	0	80	1.5	0	210	500	420	0
0	0	0	0	0	250	12	0	0	0	0	0	0	480	1.5	0	0	720	580	0
4	2	0	0	0	100	1.8	0.12	0.2	1.9	0	0	0	40	0.8	24.5	0	331	949	1.05
0	0	0	0	0	150	6	0.15	0.34	6.65	0	0	0	200	1	0	0	570	840	0
0	2	0	0	0	80	48	0.23	0.14	1.14	0	0	0	32	0.6	0	180	410	370	0
0	0	0	0	0	60	2.4	0.06	0.03	0.38	0	0	0	0	0.6	0	0	160	480	0
0	2	0	0	0	0	0	0.3	0.17	1.9	0	0	0	32	1.5	0	0	90	560	0
0	0	0	0	0	0	0	0	0	0	0	0	0	160	1.5	0	0	0	810	0
0	0	0	0	0	0	0	0	0	0	0	0	0	120	1.5	0	0	0	760	0
0	1	0	0	0	100	3.6	0.15	0.17	2.85	0	0	0	48	1.5	0	0	450	540	0
0	0	0	0	0	60	6	0.06	0.1	1.9	0	0	0	32	0.8	0	0	300	1440	0
0	0	0	0	0	200	15	0.3	0.26	0	0	0	0	32	1	0	0	530	420	0
0	0	0	0	0	99.92	0	0	0	0	0	0	0	239.81	1.5	0	0	0	1029.19	0
0	0	0	0	0	80	0	0.09	0.17	0.76	0	0	0	120	0.6	0	0	0	740	0
0	0	0	0	0	0	0	0.3	0.43	1.52	0	0	0	200	0.8	0	0	160	550	0
3	1	0	0	0	80	6	0.09	0.26	1.14	0	0	0	80	0.6	24.5	0	209	650	1.05
0	1	0	0	0	0	0	0.3	0.26	1.14	0	0	0	120	1	0	230	220	520	0
0	0	0	0	0	20	0	0.15	0.26	0.38	0	0	0	160	0.4	0	0	140	640	0
0	0	0	0	0	100	0	0	0	0	0	0	0	300	1	0	0	410	570	0
0	0	0	0	0	250	9	0.15	0.17	4.75	0	0	0	16	1	0	200	400	400	0
0	0	0	0	0	0	66.1	0	0	0.38	0	0	0	0	0.2	0	0	681.02	1221.83	0
0	1	0	0	0	60	9	0.23	0.43	3.8	0	0	0	120	2	0	0	550	540	0
0	1	0	0	0	0	0	0	0	0	0	0	0	0	0	0	240	690	560	0
0	0	0	0	0	0	0	0	0	0.13	0	0	0	48	0.06	0	0	4.4	193	0
0	0	0	0	0	0	4.2	0	0	0.11	0	0	0	88	0.02	0	0	68	48	0
0	0	0	0	0	0	0	0	0	0	0	0	0	0	0.2	0	0	310.46	1191.79	0
0	0	0	0	0	60	15	0.12	0.14	1.52	0	0	0	32	0.6	0	130	440	520	0
0	0	0	0	0	0	0	0	0	0.19	0	0	0	0	0.2	0	0	370.56	1281.92	0
0	0	0	0	0	60	2.4	0	0.03	0.38	0	0	0	0	0.2	0	0	80	500	0
0	0	0	0	0	300	12	0	0	0	0	0	0	360	0.6	0	0	600	560	0
0	0	0	0	0	0	0	0.6	0.51	0	0	0	0	160	0.8	0	0	420	560	0
0	0	0	0	0	0	0	0	0	0.19	0	0	0	70.11	3	0	0	570.86	1251.88	0
0	0	0	0	0	0	0	0	0.01	0.19	0	0	0	2.48	0.1	0	0	570.86	961.44	0
0	0	0	0	0	0	0	0	0.01	0	0	0	0	1.84	0	0	0	370.56	1051.58	0

USDA ID Code	Food Name	Weight in Grams*	Quantity of Units	Unit of Measure	Protein (gm)	Fat (gm)	Carbohydrates (gm)	Kcalories	Caffeine (gm)	Fiber (gm)	Cholesterol (mg)	Saturated Fat (gm)
43407	Noodles and Chicken, Micro Cup-Hormel	212.62	1	Each	7	7	19	174	0	0	29	2
55804	Noodles Romanoff-Stouffer's	283.92	1	Cup	17.03	25.04	36.05	440.66	0	0	40.06	0
41282	Old Fashioned Chicken Noodle Soup-Healthy Choice	212.62	1	Each	5	2	11	90	0	0	20	0
55806	Old-Fashion Stuff'n-Stouffer's	283.92	0.5	Cup	11.02	37.06	61.09	620.93	0	0	10.02	0
55220	Oriental Beef w/ Veg., Lean Cuisine-Stouffer's	244.513	1	Each	20	9	31	290	0	0	40	2
41314	Oriental Chicken w/ Spicy Peanut Sauce-Healthy Choice	269.319	1	Each	33	5	40	340	0	0	45	1
55221	Oven Baked Chicken, Lean Cuisine-Stouffer's	226.795	1	Each	17	5	21	200	0	0	35	2
	Pasta Accents - Primavera	175	1	Serving	9	10	27	230	0	0	0	0
55800	Pasta Florentine-Stouffer's	283.92	0.5	Cup	16.02	21.03	32.05	380.57	0	0	50.07	0
41294	Pasta Italiano-Healthy Choice	340.192	1	Each	16	5	59	350	0	0	30	2
55810	Pasta Roma-Stouffer's	283.92	0.5	Cup	16.02	7.01	31.05	260.39	0	0	30.04	0
41292	Pasta Shells w/ Tomato Sauce-Healthy Choice	340.192	1	Each	24	3	53	330	0	0	35	2
55142	Pasta Shells, Cheese w/ Sauce-Stouffer's	262.231	1	Each	17	13	28	300	0	0	0	0
41287	Pasta w/ Cacciatore Chicken-Healthy Choice	354.367	1	Each	26	3	47	310	0	0	35	0
41293	Pasta w/ Teriyaki Chicken-Healthy Choice	357.91	1	Each	24	3	58	350	0	0	45	1
41333	Pepperoni French Bread Pizza-Healthy Choice	170.096	1	Each	20	7	38	310	0	0	30	3
62625	Pepperoni Pizza-Weight Watchers	157.626	1	Each	23	12	46	390	0	4	45	4
55827	Pesto Sauce-Stouffer's	283.92	0.25	Cup	35.05	61.09	21.03	771.16	0	0	70.11	0
	Pizza, DiGiorno, 3 Meat	154	1	Slice	19	16	40	380	0	3.11	40	8
	Pizza, DiGiorno, 4 Cheese	139	1	Slice	16	11	39	320	0	3.11	25.1	6.1
	Pizza, Red Baron, Pepperoni	154	1	Slice	19	24	40	450	0	2	35	9
	Pizza, Red Baron, Special Deluxe	129	1	Slice	13	18	32	340	0	2	25	7
	Pizza, Tombstone, Sausage & Pepperoni	132	1	Slice	19	19	25	340	0	2	45	9
	Pizza, Tony's, Supreme, Sausage & Pepperoni	122	1	Slice	13	20	28	340	0	2	25	7
	Pizza, Totino's, Microwave for One Cheese	104	1	Each	10	11	25	240	0	1	15	3.5
	Pizza, Totino's, Microwave for One Pepperoni	104	1	Each	10	16	25	280	0	1	15	3.5
	Pizza, Totino's, Party Cheese	277	1	Slice	15	5	33	320	0	2	20	5
	Pizza, Totino's, Party Pepperoni	289	1	Slice	14	21	33	380	0	2	20	5
	Pizza, Totino's, Party Supreme	309	1	Slice	15	20	34	380	0	2	20	4.5
55174	Potatoes Au Gratin-Stouffer's	163.008	1	Each	5	9	17	170	0	0	0	0
62536	Ravioli, Beef	243.935	1	Cup	9	5	35.99	229.94	0	4	19.99	2.5
62537	Ravioli, Cheese	243.935	1	Cup	9	3	37.99	219.94	0	4	15	1.5
62662	Rice-a-Roni Wild Rice	56	1	Cup	5	1	43	240	0	1	0	0
55222	Rigatoni Bake, Lean Cuisine-Stouffer's	276.406	1	Each	18	8	27	250	0	0	25	3
41341	Rigatoni in Meat Sauce-Healthy Choice	269.319	1	Each	16	6	34	260	0	0	30	2
55782	Rigatoni w/ Meat Sauce-Stouffer's	283.92	0.5	Cup	16.02	11.02	31.05	290.44	0	0	30.04	0
62614	Roast Turkey Medallions-Weight Watchers	240.975	1	Each	10	2	34	190	0	4	20	0.5
41310	Roasted Turkey and Mushrooms in Gravy-Healthy Choice	240.969	1	Each	18	3	26	200	0	0	40	1
41290	Salisbury Steak w/ Mushroom Gravy-Healthy Choice	311.843	1	Each	21	6	35	280	0	0	55	3
43402	Salisbury Steak, Top Shelf-Hormel	283.493	1	Each	25	15	22	320	0	0	70	7
41262	Salsa Chicken-Healthy Choice	318.93	1	Each	20	2	36	240	0	0	50	1
43412	Scalloped Potatoes and Ham, Micro Cup-Hormel	212.62	1	Each	8	16	21	260	0	0	33	6
55175	Scalloped Potatoes-Stouffer's	163.008	1	Each	4	6	16	130	0	0	0	0
41263	Shrimp Marinara-Healthy Choice	297.668	1	Each	10	1	51	260	0	0	60	0
62615	Shrimp Marinara-Weight Watchers	255.15	1	Each	9	2	35	190	0	4	40	0.5
55143	Single Serving Stuffed Pepper-Stouffer's	283.493	1	Each	10	8	28	220	0	0	0	0
41264	Sirloin Beef w/ Barbecue Sauce-Healthy Choice	311.843	1	Each	17	4	44	280	0	0	25	2
41291	Sliced Turkey Breast w/ Gravy and Dressing-Healthy Choice	283.493	1	Each	27	4	30	270	0	0	50	2
41296	Sliced Turkey Breast w/ Gravy-Healthy Choice	340.192	1	Each	19	3	46	290	0	0	20	1
55225	Sliced Turkey w/ Dressing, Lean Cuisine-Stouffer's	223.251	1	Each	16	5	23	200	0	0	25	1
41265	Southwestern Style Chicken-Healthy Choice	354.367	1	Each	25	5	51	340	0	0	60	2
43404	Spaghetti and Meatballs, Micro Cup-Hormel	212.62	1	Each	10	7	27	210	0	0	20	3
55226	Spaghetti w/ Meat Sauce, Lean Cuisine-Stouffer's	326.017	1	Each	15	6	45	290	0	0	20	2
43396	Spaghetti w/ Meat Sauce, Top Shelf-Hormel	283.493	1	Each	14	6	37	260	0	0	20	2
41342	Spaghetti w/ Meat Sauce-Healthy Choice	283.493	1	Each	14	6	42	280	0	0	20	2

Monounsaturated Fat (gm)	Polyunsaturated Fat (gm)	Vitamin D (mg)	Vitamin K (mg)	Vitamin E (mg)	Vitamin A (re)	Vitamin C (mg)	Thiamin (mg)	Riboflavin (mg)	Niacin (mg)	Vitamin B6 (mg)	Folate (mg)	Vitamin B12 (mcg)	Calcium (mg)	Iron (mg)	Magnesium (mg)	Phosphorus (mg)	Potassium (mg)	Sodium (mg)	Zinc (mg)
3	2	0	0	0	270	8.4	0.08	0.12	1.71	0	0	0	32	0.7	21	0	254	1009	0.75
0	0	0	0	0	0	0	0	0.01	0.19	0	0	0	1.6	0.2	0	0	260.39	1992.99	0
0	0	0	0	0	80	12	0.03	0.1	1.9	0	0	0	16	0.2	0	60	130	540	0
0	0	0	0	0	0	0.84	0.01	0.01	0.74	0	0	0	0	0.33	0	0	200.3	1121.68	0
0	0	0	0	0	150	1.2	0.09	0.17	2.85	0	0	0	16	1	0	0	400	590	0
0	1	0	0	0	0	2.4	0	0	0.38	0	0	0	0	0.2	0	0	50	470	0
0	0	0	0	0	350	6	0.15	0.17	7.6	0	0	0	16	0.8	0	0	550	480	0
0	0	0	0	0	0	20	0	0	0	0	0	0	160	1.2	0	0	0	450	0
0	0	0	0	0	0	0.54	0	0.01	0.19	0	0	0	3.45	0.1	0	0	400.6	891.34	0
0	3	0	0	0	60	0	0.53	0.51	2.85	0	0	0	48	2	0	180	540	530	0
0	0	0	0	0	0	6.01	0.11	0.01	0.95	0	0	0	1.04	0.3	0	0	600.9	781.17	0
0	0	0	0	0	100	21	0.53	0.43	2.85	0	0	0	320	1.5	0	240	640	470	0
0	0	0	0	0	150	9	0.12	0.26	1.9	0	0	0	280	1	0	0	480	820	0
0	1	0	0	0	100	6	0.45	0.43	6.65	0	0	0	32	1.5	0	250	660	430	0
0	2	0	0	0	100	6	0.3	0.34	3.8	0	0	0	48	1.5	0	200	390	370	0
0	1	0	0	0	150	0	0.53	0.34	3.8	0	0	0	160	2.5	0	240	350	470	0
0	0	0	0	0	80	4.8	0	0	0	0	0	0	540	1	0	0	320	650	0
0	0	0	0	0	0	12.02	0	0.02	0.38	0	0	0	5.69	0.3	0	0	620.93	1362.04	0
0	1	0	0	0	138.3	0	0.5	0.3	3	0	0	0	330	1	0	200	330	1100	0
0	1	0	0	0	138.3	0	0.5	0.3	3	0	0	0	350	0.9	0	200	330	870	0
0	1	0	0	0	90	0	0	0	0	0	0	0	330	1.9	0	200	330	920	0
0	1	0	0	0	78	0	0	0	0	0	0	0	220	2.7	0	200	330	690	0
0	1	0	0	0	150	0	0	0	0	0	0	0	350	0.9	0	200	330	820	0
0	1	0	0	0	40	2.4	0	0	0	0	0	0	200	1.5	0	200	330	610	0
0	1	0	0	0	0	0	0	0	0	0	0	0	220	1.5	0	180	290	530	0
0	1	0	0	0	0	0	0	0	0	0	0	0	200	1.5	0	180	290	710	0
0	1	0	0	0	0	0	0	0	0	0	0	0	300	1.5	0	200	330	630	0
0	1	0	0	0	0	0	0	0	0	0	0	0	280	1.5	0	200	330	920	0
0	1	0	0	0	0	0	0	0	0	0	0	0	280	1.5	0	200	330	890	0
0	0	0	0	0	20	3.6	0	0.1	0.76	0	0	0	48	0.8	0	0	260	670	0
0	0	0	0	0	149.96	2.4	0	0	0	0	0	0	0	1.5	0	0	0	1149.69	0
0	0	0	0	0	59.98	1.2	0	0	0	0	0	0	23.99	1.5	0	0	0	1279.66	0
0	0	0	0	0	80	6	0.15	0.1	1.52	0	0	0	48	0.8	0	0	0	1110	0
0	1	0	0	0	200	6	0.23	0.34	3.8	0	0	0	160	1.5	0	0	620	430	0
0	0	0	0	0	200	2.4	0.3	0.26	2.85	0	0	0	120	1.5	0	200	700	540	0
0	0	0	0	0	0	48.07	0	0.01	0.76	0	0	0	2.08	0.3	0	0	620.93	851.28	0
0	0	0	0	0	100	4.8	0	0	0	0	0	0	24	1	0	0	220	530	0
0	1	0	0	0	200	0	0.12	0.14	2.85	0	0	0	16	0.8	0	150	260	380	0
0	0	0	0	0	0	0	0	0	0	0	0	0	0	0	0	260	630	500	0
8	1	0	0	0.03	0	3.6	0.03	0.26	4.75	0	0	0	16	1.5	35	0	801	910	5.7
0	0	0	0	0	200	66	0.23	0.17	3.8	0	0	0	64	0.6	0	200	540	450	0
8	2	0	0	0.39	0	11.4	0.09	0.1	2.09	0	0	0	32	0.4	21	0	425	768	0.9
0	0	0	0	0	0	2.4	0.03	0.14	0.76	0	0	0	80	0.2	0	0	375	610	0
0	0	0	0	0	100	114	0.23	0.14	1.14	0	0	0	48	1.5	0	130	390	320	0
0	0	0	0	0	150	6	0	0	0	0	0	0	120	1	0	0	440	400	0
0	0	0	0	0	20	6	0.23	0.17	2.85	0	0	0	32	1	0	0	400	1010	0
0	1	0	0	0	0	0	0	0	0	0	0	0	0	0	0	190	630	240	0
0	1	0	0	0	150	0	0.3	0.34	7.6	0	0	0	48	1	0	310	590	530	0
0	1	0	0	0	150	27	0.15	0.1	1.52	0	0	0	16	0.6	0	0	360	520	0
0	2	0	0	0	500	6	0.23	0.26	4.75	0	0	0	32	0.8	0	0	400	590	0
0	2	0	0	0	0	0	0	0	0	0	0	0	0	0	0	260	560	550	0
3	1	0	0	0	140	3.6	0.12	0.26	2.28	0	0	0	32	1.1	24.5	0	341	930	1.05
0	2	0	0	0	100	6	0.3	0.34	3.8	0	0	0	48	2	0	0	500	500	0
2	1	0	0	0.11	100	2.4	0.23	0.26	3.8	0	0	0	48	1.5	45.5	0	879	980	2.4
0	2	0	0	0	250	4.8	0.38	0.26	1.9	0	0	0	48	2	0	160	540	480	0

USDA ID Code	Food Name	Weight in Grams*	Quantity of Units	Unit of Measure	Protein (gm)	Fat (gm)	Carbohydrates (gm)	Kcalories	Caffeine (gm)	Fiber (gm)	Cholesterol (mg)	Saturated Fat (gm)
55247	Spaghetti w/ Meat Sauce-Stouffer's	364.998	1	Each	16	12	38	320	0	0	0	0
55150	Spaghetti w/ Meatballs, -Stouffer's	276.406	1	Each	14	9	37	290	0	0	0	0
55176	Spinach Souffle-Stouffer's	170.096	1	Each	9	15	11	220	0	0	0	0
41283	Split Pea and Ham Soup-Healthy Choice	212.62	1	Each	10	3	25	170	0	0	10	1
55766	Split Pea Soup w/ Ham-Stouffer's	283.92	1	Cup	15.02	3	35.05	220.33	0	0	10.02	0
55781	Stuffed Cabbage no Sauce-Stouffer's	28.35	1	Ounce	2	2.1	3.1	39	0	0	5	0
55228	Stuffed Cabbage w/ Meat, Lean Cuisine-Stouffer's	269.319	1	Each	13	6	26	210	0	0	30	2
55778	Stuffed Cabbage-Stouffer's	28.35	1	Ounce	1.4	1.4	2.7	29	0	0	4	0
55157	Stuffed Green Peppers-Stouffer's	219.707	1	Each	9	8	22	200	0	0	0	0
55229	Swedish Meatballs w/ Pasta, Lean Cuisine-Stouffer's	258.688	1	Each	23	8	31	290	0	0	55	3
55148	Swedish Meatballs w/ Pasta-Stouffer's	262.231	1	Each	24	21	32	420	0	0	0	0
41266	Sweet and Sour Chicken-Healthy Choice	326.017	1	Each	20	2	52	280	0	0	35	0
43438	Taco Shells, Chi-Chi's-Hormel	20	1	Each	1.41	4.94	11.99	98.77	0	0	0	0
43401	Tender Beef Roast, Top Shelf-Hormel	283.493	1	Each	28	6	19	240	0	0	60	2
41267	Teriyaki Chicken-Healthy Choice	347.279	1	Each	24	4	39	290	0	0	55	1
55811	Three Bean Chili-Stouffer's	283.92	1	Cup	10.02	5.01	32.05	210.32	0	0	20.03	0
41284	Tomato Garden Soup-Healthy Choice	212.62	1	Each	4	3	22	130	0	0	5	1
62538	Tortellini, Beef	257.894	1	Cup	5	1	45.98	229.91	0	9	14.99	0
55160	Tortellini-Cheese in Alfredo Sauce-Stouffer's	251.6	1	Each	26	37	35	580	0	0	0	0
55161	Tortellini-Cheese w/ Tomato Sauce-Stouffer's	262.231	1	Each	18	15	39	360	0	0	0	0
55162	Tuna Noodle Casserole-Stouffer's	283.493	1	Each	17	15	33	280	0	0	0	0
55814	Turkey and Gravy-Stouffer's	255	1	Each	11.99	2.47	2.12	77.6	0	0	23.28	0
55232	Turkey Dijon, Lean Cuisine-Stouffer's	269.319	1	Each	20	6	20	210	0	0	45	2
55791	Turkey Dijonnaise-Stouffer's	260	1	Each	8.47	5.29	7.05	112.88	0	0	28.22	0
55163	Turkey Pie-Stouffer's	283.493	1	Each	16	24	33	410	0	0	0	0
57809	Turkey Pot Pie-Swanson	198	1	Each	5.54	10.58	18.14	191.49	0	0	0	0
41243	Turkey Sausage Omelet on English Muffin-Healthy Choice	134.659	1	Each	16	4	30	210	0	0	20	2
41268	Turkey Tetrazzini-Healthy Choice	357.91	1	Each	23	6	49	340	0	0	40	3
55164	Turkey Tetrazzini-Stouffer's	283.493	1	Each	22	23	26	400	0	0	0	0
41275	Turkey Vegetable Soup-Healthy Choice	212.62	1	Each	4	3	17	110	0	0	15	1
41285	Vegetable Beef Soup-Healthy Choice	212.62	1	Each	8	1	21	130	0	0	15	0
55759	Vegetable Beef w/ Barley Soup-Stouffer's	283.92	1	Cup	4.01	13.02	15.02	190.29	0	0	10.02	0
55797	Vegetable Chow Mein-Stouffer's	28.35	1	Ounce	0.3	0.7	1.6	14	0	0	0	0
55166	Vegetable Lasagna-Stouffer's	274.042	1	Each	23	20	33	400	0	0	0	0
41343	Vegetable Pasta Italiano-Healthy Choice	283.493	1	Each	7	1	46	220	0	0	0	0
55758	Vegetarian Vegetable Soup-Stouffer's	283.92	1	Cup	6.01	2	20.03	120.18	0	0	0	0
55828	Veloute Sauce Supreme-Stouffer's	307.58	1	Cup	8.68	49.91	20.61	564.18	0	0	97.65	0
55167	Welsh Rarebit-Stouffer's	141.746	1	Each	13	20	9	270	0	0	0	0
41244	Western Style Omelet on English Muffin-Healthy Choice	134.659	1	Each	16	3	29	200	0	0	15	2
55826	Whipped Sweet Potatoes-Stouffer's	283.92	0.5	Cup	3	18.03	60.09	410.61	0	0	60.09	0
41269	Yankee Pot Roast-Healthy Choice	311.843	1	Each	19	4	36	260	0	0	55	2
55233	Zucchini Lasagna, Lean Cuisine-Stouffer's	311.843	1	Each	17	6	34	260	0	0	20	2
41344	Zucchini Lasagna-Healthy Choice	326.017	1	Each	14	3	41	250	0	0	15	2
32391	Arby's-Beef'N Cheddar Sandwich	194	1	Each	35.27	19.84	29.76	443.11	0	1.21	84.88	9.92
32433	Arby's-Boston Clam Chowder	226.795	1	Each	10	11	18	207	0	1.4	28	4
32400	Arby's-Chicken Breast Fillet Sandwich	204	1	Each	25.5	27.72	53.22	546.59	0	1.77	100.89	5.65
	Arby's-Chicken Cordon Bleu	240	1	Each	38	33	46	623	0	5	77	5.65
	Arby's-Chicken Fingers	102	1	Each	16	16	20	290	0	0.5	32	2
32434	Arby's-Cream of Broccoli Soup	226.795	1	Each	9	8	19	180	0	1.8	3	5
32413	Arby's-Curly Fries	99.223	1	Each	4.2	17.7	43.2	337	0	0	0	7.4
32405	Arby's-Fish Fillet Sandwich	221	1	Each	23	27	50	526	0	0	43.8	7
32411	Arby's-French Fries	70.873	1	Each	2.1	13.2	29.8	246	0	0	0	3
	Arby's-Grilled Chicken BBQ	201	1	Each	23	13	47	388	0	2	43	3
	Arby's-Grilled Chicken Delux	230	1	Each	23	20	47	430	0	3	61	4
32406	Arby's-Ham'N Cheese Sandwich	170.096	1	Each	24.47	18.64	38.45	411.26	0	1.17	67.57	7.46

Monounsaturated Fat (gm)	Polyunsaturated Fat (gm)	Vitamin D (mg)	Vitamin K (mg)	Vitamin E (mg)	Vitamin A (re)	Vitamin C (mg)	Thiamin (mg)	Riboflavin (mg)	Niacin (mg)	Vitamin B6 (mg)	Folate (mg)	Vitamin B12 (mcg)	Calcium (mg)	Iron (mg)	Magnesium (mg)	Phosphorus (mg)	Potassium (mg)	Sodium (mg)	Zinc (mg)
0	12	0	0	0	150	6	0.15	0.17	3.8	0	0	0	80	1.5	0	0	800	560	0
0	0	0	0	0	100	6	0.3	0.26	3.8	0	0	0	64	1.5	0	0	550	790	0
0	0	0	0	0	200	6	0.12	0.34	0.38	0	0	0	120	0.4	0	0	345	820	0
0	0	0	0	0	100	6	0.15	0.14	1.9	0	0	0	16	0.6	0	190	450	460	0
0	0	0	0	0	0	0	0.01	0	0.38	0	0	0	240.36	0.2	0	0	570.86	1191.79	0
0	0	0	0	0	0	0.6	0	0	0.08	0	0	0	72	0.04	0	0	48	150	0
0	1	0	0	0	80	6	0.12	0.17	3.8	0	0	0	64	1.5	0	0	600	560	0
0	0	0	0	0	0	3	0	0	0.06	0	0	0	48	0.02	0	0	51	145	0
0	0	0	0	0	60	6	0.12	0.14	2.85	0	0	0	32	0.8	0	0	380	650	0
0	1	0	0	0	20	0	0.23	0.34	3.8	0	0	0	48	1.5	0	0	450	550	0
0	0	0	0	0	20	1.2	0.15	0.26	2.85	0	0	0	48	1.5	0	0	350	740	0
0	0	0	0	0	250	30	0.15	0.17	8.55	0	0	0	32	1	0	220	480	320	0
0	0	0	0	0.09	0	0	0.06	0.07	0.54	0	0	0	0	0.14	0	0	0	3.53	0
2	1	0	0	0	400	2.4	0.75	0.43	5.7	0	0	0	16	1.5	42	0	933	880	4.5
0	2	0	0	0	20	6	0.09	0.1	7.6	0	0	0	32	0.8	0	250	520	560	0
0	0	0	0	0	0	6.01	0	0.01	0.57	0	0	0	1.2	0.4	0	0	891.34	861.29	0
0	0	0	0	0	100	6	0.06	0.1	1.14	0	0	0	32	0.4	0	70	440	510	0
0	0	0	0	0	149.94	3.6	0	0	0	0	0	0	95.96	1.5	0	0	0	769.68	0
0	0	0	0	0	40	3.6	0.3	0.51	1.9	0	0	0	320	0.8	0	0	270	830	0
0	0	0	0	0	150	6	0.23	0.34	1.9	0	0	0	240	1	0	0	420	720	0
0	0	0	0	0	20	0	0.15	0.34	3.8	0	0	0	120	0.6	0	0	380	1090	0
0	0	0	0	0	0	0.42	0	0	0.87	0	0	0	84.66	0.03	0	0	405.65	296.3	0
0	0	0	0	0	400	2.4	0.23	0.34	4.75	0	0	0	120	0.4	0	0	640	590	0
0	0	0	0	0	0	0.63	0	0	0.27	0	0	0	0	0.07	0	0	176.37	356.27	0
0	0	0	0	0	250	0	0.3	0.43	3.8	0	0	0	80	1	0	0	290	750	0
0	0	0	0	0	176.37	0	0.11	0.09	1.44	0	0	0	8.06	0.5	0	0	0	362.82	0
0	1	0	0	0	60	0	0.38	0.51	2.85	0	0	0	160	2	0	250	590	470	0
0	2	0	0	0	0	72	0.23	0.34	3.8	0	0	0	80	1	0	250	510	490	0
0	0	0	0	0	20	0	0.15	0.43	2.85	0	0	0	80	0.8	0	0	300	960	0
0	1	0	0	0	150	4.8	0.03	0.03	0.38	0	0	0	16	0.2	0	0	140	540	0
0	0	0	0	0	150	15	0.09	0.1	1.9	0	0	0	32	0.4	0	120	360	530	0
0	0	0	0	0	0	0	0	0	0.19	0	0	0	240.36	0.1	0	0	340.51	1251.88	0
0	0	0	0	0	0	0.6	0	0	0.02	0	0	0	24	0.01	0	0	26	156	0
0	0	0	0	0	250	0	0.12	0.43	0.76	0	0	0	160	0.6	0	0	350	760	0
0	0	0	0	0	250	0	0.45	0.26	1.52	0	0	0	32	2.5	0	0	380	330	0
0	0	0	0	0	0	0	0	0	0.19	0	0	0	0	0.1	0	0	400.6	911.37	0
0	0	0	0	0	0	0	0	0.01	0	0	0	0	2.26	0	0	0	368.89	1410.45	0
0	0	0	0	0	40	0	0.03	0.34	0	0	0	0	280	0.2	0	0	140	460	0
0	0	0	0	0	100	3.6	0.45	0.51	1.9	0	0	0	160	2	0	240	220	480	0
0	0	0	0	0	0	0	0	0	0.19	0	0	0	0	0.1	0	0	400.6	1111.67	0
0	0	0	0	0	100	9	0.15	0.17	1.52	0	0	0	32	1	0	150	350	400	0
0	0	0	0	0	150	6	0.15	0.26	1.9	0	0	0	200	0.8	0	0	650	520	0
0	0	0	0	0	350	6	0.38	0.26	1.9	0	0	0	200	1.5	0	250	830	400	0
4.08	3.86	0	0	0.44	63.93	1.32	0.42	0.51	6.5	0.37	45.19	2.26	201.72	5.62	44.09	442.01	380.28	1801.11	5.95
5	2	0	0	0.1	100	4	0.06	0.22	0.9	0.12	9	9.38	170	1.4	20	143	319	1157	0.7
10.64	11.42	0	0	2.88	16.63	0	0.5	0.43	16.41	0.72	35.48	0.38	123.07	3.88	51	321.52	365.87	1129.76	1.88
10.64	11.42	0	0	2.88	16.63	0	0.5	0.43	16.41	0.72	35.48	0.38	123.07	3.88	51	321.52	365.87	1594	1.88
4	4.1	0	0	1.4	2.6	0	0	0	0	0.09	17	0.19	92	1.9	22	140	190	677	0.3
2	1	0	0	1.4	50	9	0.11	0.42	0.8	0.18	46	0.59	237	0.8	55	193	455	1113	0.7
7.6	1.5	0	0	0	0	0	0.06	0.07	1.9	0	0	0	16	0.8	0	0	724	167	0
9.2	10.6	0	0	0	0	1.2	0.35	0.31	5.32	0	0	0	72	2.1	0	0	450	872	0
5.5	4.7	0	0	0	0	3.6	0.06	0	1.9	0	0	0	0	0.6	0	0	240	114	0
2	1	0	0	0	16.63	0	0.5	0.43	16.41	0.72	35.48	0.38	123.07	3.88	51	321.52	365.87	1002	1.88
2	1	0	0	0	16.63	0	0.5	0.43	16.41	0.72	35.48	0.38	123.07	3.88	51	321.52	365.87	848	1.88
7.81	1.63	0	0	1.28	111.84	3.5	0.36	0.57	3.15	0.23	82.72	0.63	151.46	3.84	18.64	177.09	337.86	899.41	1.63

USDA ID Code	Food Name	Weight in Grams*	Quantity of Units	Unit of Measure	Protein (gm)	Fat (gm)	Carbohydrates (gm)	Kcalories	Caffeine (gm)	Fiber (gm)	Cholesterol (mg)	Saturated Fat (gm)
32390	Arby's-Regular Roast Beef	155.921	1	Each	24.68	15.7	38.14	388.12	0	1.12	58.33	4.04
	Arby's-Roast Chicken Delux	195	1	Each	20	6	33	276	0	4	33	2
32393	Arby's-Super Roast Beef	240.969	1	Each	25.74	22.66	51.49	515.92	0	1.65	41.19	8.75
32410	Arby's-Turkey Sub	277	1	Each	32.86	28.17	53.99	598.6	0	0	82.16	6.22
32438	Arby's-Wisconsin Cheese Soup	226.795	1	Each	9	19	19	287	0	1.8	31	8
34858	Burger King Bacon Double Cheeseburger	218	1	Each	44	39	28	640	0	1	145	18
	Burger King Barbecue Dipping Sauce	28	1	Each	0	0	9	35	0	0	0	0
	Burger King Biscuit With Bacon, Egg and Cheese	171	1	Each	19	31	39	280	0	1	225	10
	Burger King Biscuit with Sausage	151	1	Each	16	40	41	360	0	1	45	13
	Burger King BK Big Fish sandwich	255	1	Each	26	41	56	700	0	3	90	6
	Burger King BK Broiler- chicken sandwich	248	1	Each	30	29	41	550	0	2	80	6
	Burger King Broiled Chicken Salad	302	1	Each	21	10	7	90	0	3	60	4
34856	Burger King Cheeseburger	138	1	Each	23	16	28	380	0	1	65	9
	Burger King Chicken Sandwich	229	1	Each	26	43	54	710	0	2	60	9
	Burger King Chicken Tenders - 8 piece	117	1	Each	21	17	19	310	0	3	50	4
	Burger King Chocolate Shake - Medium	397	1	Each	12	10	75	440	0	4	30	6
	Burger King Coated French Fries, medium, salted	102	1	Each	3	17	43	340	0	3	0	5
	Burger King Coca Cola Classic - medium	360	1	Each	0	0	70	280	3.08	0	0	0
	Burger King Croissan'Wich, w/ sausage, egg and cheese	176	1	Each	22	46	25	600	0	1	260	16
	Burger King Diet Coke - medium	360	1	Each	0	0	0	1	3.08	0	0	0
34857	Burger King Double Cheeseburger	210	1	Each	41	36	28	600	0	1	135	17
	Burger King Double Whopper	351	1	Each	33	46	46	730	0	3	115	16
	Burger King Double Whopper w/ cheese	375	1	Each	52	63	46	960	0	3	195	24
	Burger King Dutch Apple Pie	113	1	Each	3	15	39	300	0	2	0	3
	Burger King French Dressing	30	1	Each	0	10	11	140	0	0	0	2
	Burger King French Fries, medium, salted	116	1	Each	5	20	43	180	0	3	0	5
	Burger King French Toast Sticks	141	1	Each	4	27	60	500	0	1	0	27
	Burger King Garden Salad	255	1	Each	6	5	8	100	0	4	15	3
	Burger King Grape Jam	12	1	Each	0	0	8	30	0	0	0	0
34855	Burger King Hamburger	126	1	Each	20	15	28	330	0	1	55	6
	Burger King Hash Browns	71	1	Each	2	12	25	110	0	2	0	3
	Burger King Honey Dipping Sauce	28	1	Each	0	0	21	80	0	0	0	0
	Burger King Ketchup	14	1	Each	0	0	4	15	0	0	0	0
	Burger King Onion Rings	124	1	Each	4	14	41	310	0	6	0	2
	Burger King Ranch Dressing	30	1	Each	0	19	2	180	0	0	10	4
	Burger King Reduced Calorie light Italian Dressing	30	1	Each	0	0.5	3	15	0	0	0	0
34843	Burger King Salad w/ 1000 Island	176	1	Each	2	12	9	145	0	0	17	0
34842	Burger King Salad w/ Bleu Cheese	176	1	Each	3	16	7	184	0	0	22	0
34844	Burger King Salad w/ French	176	1	Each	2	11	13	152	0	0	0	0
34845	Burger King Salad w/ Golden Italian	176	1	Each	2	14	7	162	0	0	0	0
34841	Burger King Salad w/ House Dressing	176	1	Each	3	13	8	159	0	0	11	0
34846	Burger King Salad w/ Reduced-Calorie Italian	176	1	Each	2	1	7	42	0	0	0	0
	Burger King Side Salad	133	1	Each	3	3	4	60	0	2	5	2
	Burger King Strawberry Jam	12	1	Each	0	0	8	30	0	0	0	0
	Burger King Sweet & Sour Dipping Sauce	28	1	Each	0	0	11	45	0	0	0	0
	Burger King Thousand Island Dressing	30	1	Each	0	12	7	140	0	0	15	3
	Burger King Vanilla Shake - medium	397	1	Each	13	9	73	430	0	2	30	5
34859	Burger King Whopper	270	1	Each	27	39	45	640	0	3	90	11
	Burger King Whopper Jr.	164	1	Each	21	24	29	420	0	2	60	8
	Burger King Whopper Jr. with cheese	177	1	Each	23	28	29	460	0	2	75	10
37167	Dunkin' Donuts-Almond Croissant	105	1	Each	8	27	38	420	0	3	0	0
37146	Dunkin' Donuts-Apple Filled w/ Cinnamon Sugar	79	1	Each	5	11	33	250	0	1	0	0
37160	Dunkin' Donuts-Apple 'n Spice Muffin	100	1	Each	6	8	52	300	0	2	25	0
37159	Dunkin' Donuts-Banana Nut Muffin	103	1	Each	7	10	49	310	0	3	30	0
37147	Dunkin' Donuts-Bavarian Filled /w Chocolate	79	1	Each	5	11	32	240	0	2	0	0

Monounsaturated Fat (gm)	Polyunsaturated Fat (gm)	Vitamin D (mg)	Vitamin K (mg)	Vitamin E (mg)	Vitamin A (re)	Vitamin C (mg)	Thiamin (mg)	Riboflavin (mg)	Niacin (mg)	Vitamin B6 (mg)	Folate (mg)	Vitamin B12 (mcg)	Calcium (mg)	Iron (mg)	Magnesium (mg)	Phosphorus (mg)	Potassium (mg)	Sodium (mg)	Zinc (mg)
7.63	1.91	0	0	0.22	70.67	2.24	0.43	0.35	6.62	0.3	44.87	1.37	60.57	4.71	34.77	268.09	354.47	888.41	3.81
2	1	0	0	0	16.63	0	0.5	0.43	16.41	0.72	35.48	0.38	123.07	3.88	51	321.52	365.87	777	1.88
8.44	5.56	0	0	0.41	0	0	0.65	0.62	9.68	0.49	42.22	4.42	118.42	6.59	59.73	413.97	517.98	821.77	11.02
7.04	8.22	0	0	0	0	0	0.53	0.4	9.39	0	0	0	93.9	3.17	0	0	0	1431.95	0
8	3	0	0	0.4	90	2	0.03	0.24	0.7	0.05	7	0	252	1.3	7	241	441	1129	1.1
14.5	6.22	0	0	1.55	73.54	8.29	0.31	0.4	8.39	0.38	32.11	3.36	161.59	4.14	39.36	386.37	479.59	1240	6.63
0	0	0	0	0	0	0	0	0	0	0	0	0	0	0	0	0	0	400	0
0	0	0	0	0	0	0	0	0	0	0	0	0	0	0	0	0	0	1530	0
0	0	0	0	0	0	0	0	0	0	0	0	0	0	0	0	0	0	1390	0
0	0	0	0	0	0	0	0	0	0	0	0	0	0	0	0	0	0	980	0
0	0	0	0	0	0	0	0	0	0	0	0	0	0	0	0	0	0	4803	0
0	0	0	0	0	0	0	0	0	0	0	0	0	0	0	0	0	0	110	0
0	0	0	0	0	0	0	0	0	0	0	0	0	0	0	0	0	0	770	0
0	0	0	0	0	0	0	0	0	0	0	0	0	0	0	0	0	0	1400	0
0	0	0	0	0	0	0	0	0	0	0	0	0	0	0	0	0	0	710	0
0	0	0	0	0	0	0	0	0	0	0	0	0	0	0	0	0	0	330	0
0	0	0	0	0	0	0	0	0	0	0	0	0	0	0	0	0	0	680	0
0	0	0	0	0	0	0	0	0	0	0	0	0	0	0	0	0	0	0	0
0	0	0	0	0	0	0	0	0	0	0	0	0	0	0	0	0	0	1140	0
0	0	0	0	0	0	0	0	0	0	0	0	0	0	0	0	0	0	0	0
12.24	2.23	0	0	2	111.25	6.68	0.24	0.34	5.45	0.27	34.49	2.01	210.27	3.34	34.49	339.33	382.72	1060	4.45
0	0	0	0	0	0	0	0	0	0	0	0	0	0	0	0	0	0	1350	0
0	0	0	0	0	0	0	0	0	0	0	0	0	0	0	0	0	0	1420	0
0	0	0	0	0	0	0	0	0	0	0	0	0	0	0	0	0	0	230	0
0	0	0	0	0	0	0	0	0	0	0	0	0	0	0	0	0	0	190	0
0	0	0	0	0	0	0	0	0	0	0	0	0	0	0	0	0	0	240	0
0	0	0	0	0	0	0	0	0	0	0	0	0	0	0	0	0	0	490	0
0	0	0	0	0	0	0	0	0	0	0	0	0	0	0	0	0	0	115	0
0	0	0	0	0	0	0	0	0	0	0	0	0	0	0	0	0	0	0	0
0	0	0	0	0	0	0	0	0	0	0	0	0	0	0	0	0	0	530	0
0	0	0	0	0	0	0	0	0	0	0	0	0	0	0	0	0	0	320	0
0	0	0	0	0	0	0	0	0	0	0	0	0	0	0	0	0	0	20	0
0	0	0	0	0	0	0	0	0	0	0	0	0	0	0	0	0	0	180	0
0	0	0	0	0	0	0	0	0	0	0	0	0	0	0	0	0	0	810	0
0	0	0	0	0	0	0	0	0	0	0	0	0	0	0	0	0	0	170	0
0	0	0	0	0	0	0	0	0	0	0	0	0	0	0	0	0	0	50	0
0	0	0	0	0	0	25.8	0	0	0.19	0	0	0	336	0.14	98	528	405	251	0.08
0	0	0	0	0	0	25.2	0	0	0.19	0	0	0	528	0.13	101.5	664	382	333	0.09
0	0	0	0	0	0	25.8	0	0	0.19	0	0	0	320	0.14	98	480	410	330	0.07
0	0	0	0	0	0	25.2	0	0	0.19	0	0	0	320	0.13	98	480	389	292	0.06
0	0	0	0	0	0	25.2	0	0	0.19	0	0	0	352	0.13	94.5	592	402	293	0.08
0	0	0	0	0	0	25.2	0	0	0.19	0	0	0	320	0.14	105	472	390	430	0.06
0	0	0	0	0	0	0	0	0	0	0	0	0	0	0	0	0	0	55	0
0	0	0	0	0	0	0	0	0	0	0	0	0	0	0	0	0	0	5	0
0	0	0	0	0	0	0	0	0	0	0	0	0	0	0	0	0	0	50	0
0	0	0	0	0	0	0	0	0	0	0	0	0	0	0	0	0	0	190	0
0	0	0	0	0	0	0	0	0	0	0	0	0	0	0	0	0	0	330	0
14.99	2.39	0	0	4.24	208.55	14.12	0.02	0.03	5.65	0.34	33.67	3.05	112.96	6.52	54.31	338.89	564.81	870	5.76
0	0	0	0	0	0	0	0	0	0	0	0	0	0	0	0	0	0	530	0
0	0	0	0	0	0	0	0	0	0	0	0	0	0	0	0	0	0	770	0
0	0	0	0	0	0	0	0	0	0	0	0	0	0	0	0	0	0	280	0
0	0	0	0	0	0	0	0	0	0	0	0	0	0	0	0	0	0	280	0
0	0	0	0	0	0	0	0	0	0	0	0	0	0	0	0	0	0	360	0
0	0	0	0	0	0	0	0	0	0	0	0	0	0	0	0	0	0	410	0
0	0	0	0	0	0	0	0	0	0	0	0	0	0	0	0	0	0	260	0

USDA ID Code	Food Name	Weight in Grams*	Quantity of Units	Unit of Measure	Protein (gm)	Fat (gm)	Carbohydrates (gm)	Kcalories	Caffeine (gm)	Fiber (gm)	Cholesterol (mg)	Saturated Fat (gm)
37149	Dunkin' Donuts-Blueberry Filled	67	1	Each	4	8	29	210	0	2	0	0
37156	Dunkin' Donuts-Blueberry Muffin	101	1	Each	6	8	46	280	0	2	30	0
37157	Dunkin' Donuts-Bran Muffin w/ Raisins	104	1	Each	6	9	51	310	0	4	15	0
37151	Dunkin' Donuts-Cake Ring, Plain	62	1	Each	4	17	25	270	0	1	0	0
37163	Dunkin' Donuts-Chocolate Chunk Cookie	43	1	Each	3	10	25	200	0	1	30	0
37164	Dunkin' Donuts-Chocolate Chunk Cookie w/ Nuts	43	1	Each	3	11	23	210	0	2	30	0
37168	Dunkin' Donuts-Chocolate Croissant	94	1	Each	7	29	38	440	0	3	0	0
37145	Dunkin' Donuts-Chocolate Frosted Yeast Ring	55	1	Each	4	10	25	200	0	1	0	0
37158	Dunkin' Donuts-Corn Muffin	96	1	Each	7	12	51	340	0	1	40	0
37161	Dunkin' Donuts-Cranberry Nut Muffin	98	1	Each	6	9	44	290	0	2	25	0
37166	Dunkin' Donuts-Croissant, Plain	72	1	Each	7	19	27	310	0	2	0	0
37153	Dunkin' Donuts-Glazed Buttermilk Ring	74	1	Each	4	14	37	290	0	1	10	0
37152	Dunkin' Donuts-Glazed Chocolate Rings	71	1	Each	3.5	21	34	324	0	1.9	0	0
37144	Dunkin' Donuts-Glazed Coffee Roll	81	1	Each	5	12	37	280	0	2	0	0
37155	Dunkin' Donuts-Glazed French Cruller	38	1	Each	2	8	16	140	0	0	30	0
37143	Dunkin' Donuts-Glazed Yeast Ring	55	1	Each	4	9	26	200	0	1	0	0
37150	Dunkin' Donuts-Jelly Filled	67	1	Each	4	9	31	220	0	1	0	0
37148	Dunkin' Donuts-Lemon Filled	79	1	Each	4	12	33	260	0	1	0	0
37162	Dunkin' Donuts-Oat Bran Muffin	100	1	Each	7	11	50	330	0	3	0	0
37165	Dunkin' Donuts-Oatmeal Pecan Raisin Cookie	46	1	Each	3	9	28	200	0	1	25	0
40349	Hardee's-Big Cheese	141.75	1	Each	30	30	28	495	0	0	0	0
40350	Hardee's-Big Deluxe	248.1	1	Each	31	41	46	675	0	0	0	0
40356	Hardee's-Big Fish Sandwich	191.358	1	Each	20	26	49	514	0	0	0	0
40353	Hardee's-Big Roast Beef	163.008	1	Each	21.9	13.38	38.93	364.94	0	1.09	54.74	6.08
40351	Hardee's-Big Twin	141.746	1	Each	18.84	20.48	27.86	368.7	0	1.39	45.06	9.01
40358	Hardee's-Biscuit	77.961	1	Each	5	13	35	275	0	0	0	0
40348	Hardee's-Cheeseburger	100.631	1	Each	17	17	29	335	0	0	0	0
40357	Hardee's-Chicken Fillet	191.358	1	Each	27	26	42	510	0	0	0	0
40347	Hardee's-Hamburger	100.063	1	Each	17	13	29	305	0	0	0	0
40354	Hardee's-Hot Dog	50	1	Each	11	22	26	346	0	0	0	0
40355	Hardee's-Hot Ham & Cheese	141.746	1	Each	23	15	37	376	0	0	0	0
40352	Hardee's-Roast Beef Sandwich	141.746	1	Each	18.65	11.19	38.54	323.28	0	0.99	43.52	4.97
44118	Jack In The Box-Bacon Cheeseburger	242	1	Each	35	45	41	705	0	0	113	14.9
44101	Jack In The Box-Breakfast Jack	126	1	Each	18.74	13.54	29.16	313.44	0	0	189.52	5.31
44141	Jack In The Box-Cheesecake	99	1	Each	8	18	29	309	0	0	63	9.4
44115	Jack In The Box-Jumbo Jack	222	1	Each	25.27	26.17	40.61	497.24	0	0	72.2	10.29
44116	Jack In The Box-Jumbo Jack w/ Cheese	242	1	Each	28.47	31.14	40.04	558.74	0	0	97.87	13.35
44136	Jack In The Box-Regular French Fries	109	1	Each	4	17	45	351	0	0	0	4
44135	Jack In The Box-Small French Fries	68	1	Each	3	11	28	219	0	0	0	2.5
47265	K.F.C.-Colonel's Chicken Sandwich	166	1	Each	20.8	27	39	482	0	1.4	47	6
47261	K.F.C.-French Fries	77	1	Each	3.2	12	31	244	0	0	2	3
47260	K.F.C.-Mashed Potatoes and Gravy	98	1	Each	2.4	2	12	71	0	0	0	1
47239	K.F.C.-Original Recipe Center Breast	103	1	Each	25.18	15.26	9.16	260.93	0	0.08	86.98	3.81
47240	K.F.C.-Original Recipe Drumstick	57	1	Each	11.57	11.57	4.96	168.52	0	0	58.65	2.48
47241	K.F.C.-Original Recipe Thigh	95	1	Each	15.97	23.95	11.18	324.12	0	0.08	102.98	6.39
47237	K.F.C.-Original Recipe Wing	53	1	Each	11.8	11	5	172	0	0	59	3
48215	McDonald's-Apple Danish	105	1	Each	5	16	51	360	0	1.6	25	4
	McDonald's-Arch Deluxe	239	1	Each	28	31	39	550	0	4	90	11
	McDonald's-Arch Deluxe w/Bacon	247	1	Each	32	34	39	590	0	4	100	12
48204	McDonald's-Bacon, Egg and Cheese Biscuit	153	1	Each	18	28	36	470	0	1	235	8.04
48174	McDonald's-Big Mac	215	1	Each	25	32	43	560	0	0	103	10.1
48205	McDonald's-Biscuit w/ Spread	75	1	Each	5	13	32	260	0	1	1	3
	McDonald's-Breakfast Burrito	117	1	Each	13	19	23	320	0	1	195	7
48170	McDonald's-Cheeseburger	116	1	Each	15	13	35	320	0	0	50	5
48181	McDonald's-Chicken McNuggets	18.5	1	Each	3.33	2.5	2.83	45	0	0	9.17	0.58

Monounsaturated Fat (gm)	Polyunsaturated Fat (gm)	Vitamin D (mg)	Vitamin K (mg)	Vitamin E (mg)	Vitamin A (re)	Vitamin C (mg)	Thiamin (mg)	Riboflavin (mg)	Niacin (mg)	Vitamin B6 (mg)	Folate (mg)	Vitamin B12 (mcg)	Calcium (mg)	Iron (mg)	Magnesium (mg)	Phosphorus (mg)	Potassium (mg)	Sodium (mg)	Zinc (mg)
0	0	0	0	0	0	0	0	0	0	0	0	0	0	0	0	0	0	240	0
0	0	0	0	0	0	0	0	0	0	0	0	0	0	0	0	0	0	340	0
0	0	0	0	0	0	0	0	0	0	0	0	0	0	0	0	0	0	560	0
0	0	0	0	0	0	0	0	0	0	0	0	0	0	0	0	0	0	330	0
0	0	0	0	0	0	0	0	0	0	0	0	0	0	0	0	0	0	110	0
0	0	0	0	0	0	0	0	0	0	0	0	0	0	0	0	0	0	100	0
0	0	0	0	0	0	0	0	0	0	0	0	0	0	0	0	0	0	220	0
0	0	0	0	0	0	0	0	0	0	0	0	0	0	0	0	0	0	190	0
0	0	0	0	0	0	0	0	0	0	0	0	0	0	0	0	0	0	560	0
0	0	0	0	0	0	0	0	0	0	0	0	0	0	0	0	0	0	360	0
0	0	0	0	0	0	0	0	0	0	0	0	0	0	0	0	0	0	240	0
0	0	0	0	0	0	0	0	0	0	0	0	0	0	0	0	0	0	370	0
0	0	0	0	0	0	0	0	0	0	0	0	0	0	0	0	0	0	383	0
0	0	0	0	0	0	0	0	0	0	0	0	0	0	0	0	0	0	310	0
0	0	0	0	0	0	0	0	0	0	0	0	0	0	0	0	0	0	130	0
0	0	0	0	0	0	0	0	0	0	0	0	0	0	0	0	0	0	230	0
0	0	0	0	0	0	0	0	0	0	0	0	0	0	0	0	0	0	230	0
0	0	0	0	0	0	0	0	0	0	0	0	0	0	0	0	0	0	280	0
0	0	0	0	0	0	0	0	0	0	0	0	0	0	0	0	0	0	450	0
0	0	0	0	0	0	0	0	0	0	0	0	0	0	0	0	0	0	100	0
0	0	0	0	0	0	0	0	0	0	0	0	0	0	0	0	0	0	1251	0
0	0	0	0	0	0	0	0	0	0	0	0	0	0	0	0	0	0	1063	0
0	0	0	0	0	0	0	0	0	0	0	0	0	0	0	0	0	0	314	0
6.08	2.43	0	0	0.24	0	0	0.36	0.41	6.57	0.34	29.2	2.98	80.29	4.5	40.14	279.79	389.27	1070.5	7.42
7.37	4.1	0	0	0.74	13.93	2.46	0.23	0.25	5.49	0.22	27.86	1.86	65.55	3.28	28.68	161.41	229.42	475.22	3.77
0	0	0	0	0	0	0	0	0	0	0	0	0	0	0	0	0	0	650	0
0	0	0	0	0	0	2	0.51	0.32	5.5	0	0	0	0	0	0	0	0	789	0
0	0	0	0	0	0	0	0	0	0	0	0	0	0	0	0	0	0	360	0
0	0	0	0	0	0	2	0.55	0.58	6.4	0	0	0	0	0	0	0	0	682	0
0	0	0	0	0	0	0	0	0	0	0	0	0	0	0	0	0	0	744	0
0	0	0	0	0	0	0	0	0	0	0	0	0	0	0	0	0	0	1067	0
4.97	2.49	0	0	0.25	0	0	0.32	0.36	5.72	0.3	24.87	2.6	69.63	3.85	34.81	243.7	323.28	907.67	6.47
15.7	8.7	0	0	0.6	70	7.8	0.24	0.48	8.36	0	0	0	200	2.8	0	0	0	1240	0
5.21	2.6	0	0	0.14	138.5	3.12	0.43	0.49	5.31	0.15	0	1.15	184.31	2.6	24.99	322.81	197.85	1079.85	1.87
7.4	1.6	0	0	0.32	0	0	0.05	0.24	1.9	0	0	0	88	0.3	0	0	0	208	0
11.37	2.17	0	0	0.18	66.78	3.61	0.42	0.31	10.47	0.27	0	2.42	120.93	4.06	39.71	235.54	444	1023.37	3.79
11.21	1.78	0	0	0.21	195.74	4.45	0.46	0.34	10.05	0.28	0	2.71	242.89	4.09	43.6	365.67	443.96	1482.25	4.27
7	0	0	0	5.31	0	25.8	0.18	0.03	3.61	0	0	0	0	0.7	0	0	0	194	0
7	0	0	0	10.36	0	16.2	0.11	0	2.28	0	0	0	0	0.4	0	0	0	121	0
3.9	9	0	0	2.3	14	0	0.39	0.27	10.64	0.59	29	0.31	100	3.1	41	261	297	1060	1.5
7	1	0	0	0	0	15.6	0.15	0.05	1.9	0	0	0	0	0.3	0	0	0	139	0
0	0	0	0	0	0	0	0	0.03	1.14	0	0	0	16	0.2	0	0	0	339	0
3.59	1.53	0	0	0.46	15.26	0	0.08	0.13	14.04	0.59	3.81	0.35	16.02	1.22	30.52	238.04	264.75	602.74	1.14
3.06	1.65	0	0	0.41	14.04	0	0.05	0.13	3.39	0.2	4.96	0.18	6.61	0.74	13.22	99.13	129.7	267.65	1.65
5.59	3.19	0	0	0.48	27.94	0	0.09	0.23	6.55	0.32	7.98	0.29	12.77	1.44	23.15	176.43	223.53	549.24	2.39
6	2	0	0	0	0	0	0.03	0.07	2.85	0	0	0	24	0.3	0	0	0	383	0
11	2	0	0	3.8	35	15	0.3	0.17	2.2	0.03	3	0	14	1.4	8	31	69	290	0.2
0	0	0	0	0	10	0	0	0	0	0	0	0	6	25	0	0	0	1010	0
0	0	0	0	0	10	0	0	0	0	0	0	0	6	6	0	0	0	1150	0
15.79	1.96	0	0	1.47	156.92	0	0.35	0.32	2.45	0.17	17.65	0.58	181.44	2.55	30.4	442.33	232.44	1250	1.67
20.1	1.5	0	0	0	106	2	0.48	0.41	6.8	0.27	21	1.8	256	4	38	314	237	950	4.7
9	1	0	0	1.8	0	0	0.23	0.1	1.52	0.03	6	0.1	75	1.3	14	168	100	730	0.7
0	0	0	0	0	10	15	0	0	0	0	0	0	8	10	0	0	0	600	0
7.7	1	0	0	0.5	118	2	0.29	0.21	3.9	0.12	18	0.94	199	2.3	21	177	223	750	2.1
1.67	0.25	0	0	0	0	0	0.02	0.02	1.27	0	0	0	0	0.1	0	0	0	96.67	0

USDA ID Code	Food Name	Weight in Grams*	Quantity of Units	Unit of Measure	Protein (gm)	Fat (gm)	Carbohydrates (gm)	Kcalories	Caffeine (gm)	Fiber (gm)	Cholesterol (mg)	Saturated Fat (gm)
48226	McDonald's-Chocolate Lowfat Milk Shake	294.124	1	Each	11.04	1.71	66.25	321.23	0	0	10.04	0.7
	McDonald's-Cinnamon Roll	95	1	Each	7	20	47	400	0	2	75	5
	McDonald's-Crispy Chicken Deluxe	223	1	Each	26	25	43	0	0	3	55	4
48198	McDonald's-Egg McMuffin	135	1	Each	17.61	10.76	27.39	283.7	0	1.37	221.09	3.72
48201	McDonald's-English Muffin w/ Spread	58	1	Each	5	4	26	170	0	1.6	9	2.4
48175	McDonald's-Fish Filet Deluxe	141	1	Each	27	28	54	560	0	1.09	49.65	5.16
48188	McDonald's-Garden Salad	189	1	Each	4	2	6	50	0	0	65	0.6
	McDonald's-Grilled Chicken Deluxe	223	1	Each	27	20	38	300	0	3	50	1
	McDonald's-Grilled Chicken Sld Deluxe	257	1	Each	21	1.5	7	120	0	0	45	0
48169	McDonald's-Hamburger	102	1	Each	13	9	34	260	0	0	30	3.5
48209	McDonald's-Hash Brown Potatoes	53	1	Each	1	7	15	130	0	0	0	1
48210	McDonald's-Hotcakes w/ Margarine and Syrup	174	1	Each	13	19	100	570	0	0	15	3
48216	McDonald's-Iced Cheese Danish	110	1	Each	7	22	47	410	0	0	47	6
48180	McDonald's-Large French Fries	122	1	Each	6	22	57	450	0	0	0	5
	McDonald's-Lowfat Apple Bran Muffin	114	1	Each	6	3	61	300	0	3	0	0.5
48223	McDonald's-McDonaldland Cookies	56.699	1	Each	3	5	32	180	0	0	0	1
48171	McDonald's-Quarter Pounder	166	1	Each	23	21	37	420	0	0	85	8
	McDonald's-Quarter Pounderw/Chse	200	1	Each	28	30	38	530	0	2	95	13
48207	McDonald's-Sausage Biscuit	118	1	Each	11	31	35	470	0	0	44	8
48203	McDonald's-Sausage Biscuit w/ Egg	175	1	Each	19	28	27	440	0	0	260	10
48199	McDonald's-Sausage McMuffin	135	1	Each	15	20	27	345	0	0	57	7
48200	McDonald's-Sausage McMuffin w/ Egg	159	1	Each	21	25	27	430	0	0	270	8
48208	McDonald's-Scrambled Eggs	100	1	Each	12	10	1	140	0	0	425	3
48178	McDonald's-Small French Fries	68	1	Each	3	12	26	220	0	0	0	2.5
48227	McDonald's-Strawberry Lowfat Milk Shake	294.124	1	Each	11	9	60	360	0	0	10	0.6
	McDonald's-Super Size Fries	176	1	Each	8	26	68	540	0	6	0	4.5
48225	McDonald's-Vanilla Lowfat Milk Shake	294.124	1	Each	11	9	60	360	0	0	10	0.6
	McDonald's-Vanilla RF Ice Crm Cone	90	1	Each	4	4.5	23	150	0	0	20	3
52366	Pizza Hut-Cheese Pizza, Hand Tossed	70	1	Slice	17	10	27.5	259	0	0	27.5	6.8
52359	Pizza Hut-Cheese Pizza, Pan	70	1	Slice	15	9	28.5	246	0	0	17	4.5
53322	Pizza Hut-Cheese Pizza, Thin'n Crispy	70	1	Slice	14	8.5	18.5	199	0	0	16.5	5.2
52370	Pizza Hut-Pepperoni Personal Pan Pizza	250	1	Each	37	29	76	675	0	0	53	12.5
52367	Pizza Hut-Pepperoni Pizza, Hand Tossed	70	1	Slice	14	11.5	25	250	0	0	25	6.45
52360	Pizza Hut-Pepperoni Pizza, Pan	70	1	Slice	14.5	11	31	270	0	0	21	4.5
52363	Pizza Hut-Pepperoni Pizza, Thin'n Crispy	70	1	Slice	13	10	18	206.5	0	0	23	5.3
52365	Pizza Hut-Super Sprm Pizza, Thin'n Crispy	70	1	Slice	14.5	10.5	22	231.5	0	0	28	5.15
52362	Pizza Hut-Super Supreme Pizza, Pan	70	1	Slice	16.5	13	26.5	281.5	0	0	27.5	6
52369	Pizza Hut-Super Supreme, Hand Tossed	70	1	Slice	16.5	12.5	27	278	0	0	27	6.5
52371	Pizza Hut-Supreme Personal Pan Pizza	250	1	Each	33	28	76	647	0	0	49	11.2
52368	Pizza Hut-Supreme Pizza, Hand Tossed	70	1	Slice	16	13	25	270	0	0	27.5	6.1
52361	Pizza Hut-Supreme Pizza, Pan	70	1	Slice	16	15	26.5	294.5	0	0	24	7
52364	Pizza Hut-Supreme Pizza, Thin'n Crispy	70	1	Slice	14	11	20.5	229.5	0	0	21	5.5
54494	Red Lobster-Atlantic Ocean Perch, Lunch	141.746	1	Each	24	4	1	130	0	0	75	1.1
54506	Red Lobster-Calamari, Brded and Fried, Lunch	141.746	1	Each	13	21	30	360	0	0	140	5.6
54486	Red Lobster-Catfish, Lunch Portion	141.746	1	Each	20	10	0	170	0	0	85	2.5
54514	Red Lobster-Chicken Breast, Skinless, Lunch	113.397	1	Each	26	3	0	140	0	0	70	1
54487	Red Lobster-Cod, Atlantic, Lunch Portion	141.746	1	Each	23	1	0	100	0	0	70	0.3
54510	Red Lobster-Deep Sea Scallops, Lnch Portion	141.746	1	Each	26	2	2	130	0	0	50	0.4
54488	Red Lobster-Flounder, Lunch Portion	141.746	1	Each	21	1	1	100	0	0	70	0.3
54489	Red Lobster-Grouper, Lunch Portion	141.746	1	Each	26	1	0	110	0	0	65	0.3
54490	Red Lobster-Haddock, Lunch Portion	141.746	1	Each	24	1	2	110	0	0	85	0.3
54491	Red Lobster-Halibut, Lunch Portion	141.746	1	Each	25	1	1	110	0	0	60	0.3
54513	Red Lobster-Hamburger, Lunch Portion	151.181	1	Each	37	28	0	410	0	0	130	11
54504	Red Lobster-King Crab Legs, Lunch Portion	453.59	1	Each	32	2	6	170	0	0	100	0.5
54507	Red Lobster-Langostino, Lunch Portion	141.746	1	Each	26	1	2	120	0	0	210	0.2

Monounsaturated Fat (gm)	Polyunsaturated Fat (gm)	Vitamin D (mg)	Vitamin K (mg)	Vitamin E (mg)	Vitamin A (re)	Vitamin C (mg)	Thiamin (mg)	Riboflavin (mg)	Niacin (mg)	Vitamin B6 (mg)	Folate (mg)	Vitamin B12 (mcg)	Calcium (mg)	Iron (mg)	Magnesium (mg)	Phosphorus (mg)	Potassium (mg)	Sodium (mg)	Zinc (mg)
0.9	0.1	0	0	0	92.35	0	0.13	0.5	0.4	0	0	0	333.27	0.8	0	0	0	240.92	0
0	0	0	0	0	10	0	0	0	0	0	0	0	8	8	0	0	0	340	0
0	0	0	0	0	6	8	0	0	0	0	0	0	6	15	0	0	0	1060	0
5.97	1.27	0	0	1.76	146.74	0.98	0.46	0.32	3.62	0.16	43.04	0.78	250.43	2.74	32.28	312.07	208.37	723.91	1.76
2	1	0	0	0.1	37	0	0.33	0.14	2.5	0.1	51	0	151	1.6	12	60	74	285	0.4
10.13	10.72	0	0	0	43.69	0	0.3	0.14	2.68	0.1	19.86	0.81	163.84	1.79	26.81	227.39	148.94	1060	0.89
1	0.4	0	0	0	900	21	0.09	0.1	0.38	0	0	0	32	0.8	0	0	0	70	0
0	0	0	0	0	6	8	0	0	0	0	0	0	6	15	0	0	0	930	0
0	0	0	0	0	120	40	0	0	0	0	0	0	4	8	0	0	0	240	0
5	1	0	0	0	40	4	0.3	0.17	3.8	0	0	0	15	1.5	0	0	0	580	0
4	2	0	0	0	0	1.2	0.06	0	0.76	0	0	0	0	0	0	0	0	330	0
5	5	0	0	0	40	0	0.3	0.34	2.85	0	0	0	80	1	0	0	0	750	0
13	2	0	0	0	40	0	0.3	0.26	1.9	0	0	0	32	0.8	0	0	0	420	0
15	2	0	0	0	0	15	0.23	0	2.85	0	0	0	0	0.6	0	0	0	290	0
0	0	0	0	0	0	0	0	0	0	0	0	0	10	8	0	0	0	380	0
7	1	0	0	0	0	0	0.23	0.17	1.9	0	0	0	0	1	0	0	0	190	0
11	1	0	0	0	40	3.6	0.38	0.26	6.65	0	0	0	120	2	0	0	0	645	0
0	0	0	0	0	10	4	0	0	0	0	0	0	15	25	0	0	0	1290	0
17	3	0	0	0	0	0	0.45	0.17	3.8	0	0	0	64	1	0	0	0	1080	0
20	3	0	0	0	60	0	0.45	0.34	3.8	0	0	0	80	2	0	0	0	1210	0
11	2	0	0	0	40	0	0.53	0.26	4.75	0	0	0	160	1.5	0	0	0	770	0
14	3	0	0	0	100	0	0.53	0.43	4.75	0	0	0	200	2	0	0	0	920	0
5	2	0	0	0	100	0	0.06	0.26	0	0	0	0	48	1	0	0	0	290	0
8	1	0	0	0	0	9	0.15	0	1.9	0	0	0	0	0.2	0	0	0	110	0
0.6	0.1	0	0	0	60	0	0.12	0.51	0.38	0	0	0	280	0	0	0	0	170	0
0	0	0	0	0	0	0	0	0	0	0	0	0	35	8	0	0	0	350	0
0.6	0.1	0	0	0	60	0	0.12	0.51	0	0	0	0	280	0	0	0	0	170	0
0	0	0	0	0	6	2	0	0	0	0	0	0	10	2	0	0	0	75	0
3.2	0	0	0	0	50	4.8	0.24	0.25	2.57	0	0	0.3	300	1.5	31.5	220	198	638	2.33
4.5	0	0	0	0	45	3.6	0.28	0.3	2.47	0	0	0.3	252	1.5	26.25	188	160	470	2.03
3.3	0	0	0	0	35	2.4	0.2	0.2	2.28	0	0	0.25	264	0.9	21	188	130.5	433.5	1.8
16.5	0	0	0	0	120	10.2	0.56	0.66	7.79	0	0	0.44	584	3.2	52.5	360	408	1335	3.75
5.05	0	0	0	0	50	3.6	0.27	0.26	2.66	0	0	0.33	176	1.4	26.25	156	207.5	633.5	1.88
6.5	0	0	0	0	50	4.2	0.32	0.25	2.57	0	0	0.3	208	1.75	24.5	176	202.5	563.5	2.1
4.7	0	0	0	0	35	3	0.21	0.21	2.47	0	0	0.25	180	0.9	19.25	148	143.5	493	1.73
5.35	0	0	0	0	50	4.2	0.29	0.22	2.57	0	0	0.35	184	1.35	26.25	168	231.5	668	2.25
7	0	0	0	0	60	5.4	0.38	0.33	3.04	0	0	0.4	216	1.85	31.5	188	266	723.5	2.7
6	0	0	0	0	55	6	0.35	0.29	3.52	0	0	0.41	176	1.9	33.25	168	258	824	2.4
16.8	0	0	0	0	120	10.8	0.59	0.66	7.6	0	0	0.46	416	3.7	52.5	320	487	1313	3.75
6.9	0	0	0	0	55	6	0.35	0.26	3.42	0	0	0.4	192	2.25	35	184	289	735	2.85
8	0	0	0	0	60	4.8	0.41	0.4	2.85	0	0	0.38	200	1.4	33.25	184	290	831.5	2.78
5.5	0	0	0	0	50	4.8	0.3	0.25	2.57	0	0	0.3	172	1.65	29.75	160	272	664	2.33
0	1.2	0	0	0	0	0	0.06	0.1	1.52	0	0	0.3	0	0	21	160	0	190	0.3
0	1.5	0	0	0	0	0	0.23	0.14	1.52	0	0	2	0	0.6	21	360	0	1150	0.9
0	1.9	0	0	0	0	0	0.3	0.14	1.9	0	0	0.04	0	0	21	160	0	50	0.3
0	1	0	0	0	0	0	0.06	0.1	11.4	0	0	0.08	0	0.4	21	160	0	60	0.9
0	0.6	0	0	0	0	0	0.03	0.07	0.76	0	0	0.6	0	0	28	200	0	200	0.3
0	1.5	0	0	0	0	0	0	0.1	1.9	0	0	0.4	0	0	52.5	240	0	260	1.5
0	0.7	0	0	0	0	0	0.03	0	1.52	0	0	0.3	16	0	21	48	0	95	0.3
0	0.5	0	0	0	0	0	0.06	0.03	1.52	0	0	0.08	32	0	28	200	0	70	0.3
0	1.1	0	0	0	0	0	0.03	0.07	2.85	0	0	0.2	0	0	21	160	0	180	0.3
0	0.7	0	0	0	0	0	0.15	0	2.85	0	0	0.3	0	0	28	240	0	105	0
0	1	0	0	0	0	0	0.06	0.34	7.6	0	0	1.2	0	1.5	28	200	0	115	7.5
0	1.6	0	0	0	0	0	0.09	0.17	1.9	0	0	1.6	48	0	70	320	0	900	6
0	0.6	0	0	0	0	0	0.12	0	1.14	0	0	2	16	0.8	35	160	0	410	1.5

USDA ID Code	Food Name	Weight in Grams*	Quantity of Units	Unit of Measure	Protein (gm)	Fat (gm)	Carbohydrates (gm)	Kcalories	Caffeine (gm)	Fiber (gm)	Cholesterol (mg)	Saturated Fat (gm)
54500	Red Lobster-Lemon Sole, Lunch Portion	141.746	1	Each	27	1	1	120	0	0	65	0.3
54524	Red Lobster-Live Maine Lobster	510.288	1	Each	36	8	5	240	0	0	310	1.9
54492	Red Lobster-Mackerel, Lunch Portion	141.746	1	Each	20	12	1	190	0	0	100	3.6
54493	Red Lobster-Monkfish, Lunch Portion	141.746	1	Each	24	1	0	110	0	0	80	0.2
54498	Red Lobster-Norwegian Salmon, Lunch	141.746	1	Each	27	12	3	230	0	0	80	2.7
54495	Red Lobster-Pollock, Lunch Portion	141.746	1	Each	28	1	1	120	0	0	90	0.3
54502	Red Lobster-Rainbow Trout, Lunch Portion	141.746	1	Each	23	9	0	170	0	0	90	2.5
54496	Red Lobster-Red Rockfish, Lunch Portion	141.746	1	Each	21	1	0	90	0	0	85	0.3
54497	Red Lobster-Red Snapper, Lunch Portion	141.746	1	Each	25	1	0	110	0	0	70	0.4
54509	Red Lobster-Rock Lobster, Lunch Portion	368.541	1	Each	49	3	2	230	0	0	200	0.7
54511	Red Lobster-Shrimp, Lunch Portion	198.445	1	Each	25	2	0	120	0	0	230	0.5
54505	Red Lobster-Snow Crab Legs, Lunch Portion	453.59	1	Each	33	2	1	150	0	0	130	0.6
54499	Red Lobster-Sockeye Salmon, Lunch Portion	141.746	1	Each	28	4	3	160	0	0	50	1.1
54512	Red Lobster-Strip Steak, Lunch Portion	255.144	1	Each	47	40	0	560	0	0	150	17
54501	Red Lobster-Swordfish, Lunch Portion	141.746	1	Each	17	4	0	100	0	0	100	1.2
54503	Red Lobster-Yellow Fin Tuna, Lunch Portion	141.746	1	Each	32	2	6	180	0	0	70	0.5
	Subway B.L.T. - 6" white	191	1	Each	14	10	38	311	0	3	16	3
	Subway BMT - 6" Italian	213	1	Each	44	55	83	982	0	5	133	20
	Subway BMT - 6" Wheat	253	1	Each	21	22	45	460	0	3	56	7
	Subway Bologna - Deli Sandwich	171	1	Each	10	12	38	292	0	2	20	4
	Subway Chicken Taco Sub - 6" white	286	1	Each	24	16	43	421	0	3	52	5
	Subway Classic Italian B.M.T. - 6" white	246	1	Each	21	21	39	445	0	3	56	8
	Subway Club - 6" white	246	1	Each	21	5	40	297	0	3	26	1
	Subway Club Salad	331	1	Each	14	3	12	126	0	1	26	1
	Subway Club Sandwich - 12" Italian	213	1	Each	46	22	83	693	0	5	84	7
	Subway Club Sandwich - 12" Wheat	220	1	Each	47	23	89	722	0	6	84	7
	Subway Cold Cut Combo - 12" Italian	184	1	Each	46	40	83	853	0	5	166	12
	Subway Cold Cut Combo - 12" Wheat	184	1	Each	48	41	88	853	0	6	166	12
	Subway Cold Cut Trio - 6" white	246	1	Each	19	13	39	362	0	3	64	4
	Subway Cold Cut Trio Salad	330	1	Each	13	11	11	191	0	1	64	3
	Subway Ham - 6" white	232	1	Each	18	5	39	287	0	3	28	1
	Subway Ham - Deli Sandwich	171	1	Each	11	4	37	234	0	2	14	1
	Subway Ham and Cheese - 12" Italian	184	1	Each	38	18	81	643	0	5	73	7
	Subway Ham and Cheese - 12" Italian	239	1	Each	19	5	45	302	0	3	28	1
	Subway Meat Ball Sandwich - 12" Italian	215	1	Each	42	44	96	918	0	3	88	17
	Subway Meat Ball Sandwich - 12" Wheat	224	1	Each	44	45	101	947	0	0	88	17
	Subway Meatballs - 6" white	260	1	Each	18	16	44	404	0	3	33	6
	Subway Melt - 6" white	251	1	Each	22	12	40	366	0	3	42	5
	Subway Pizza Sub - 6" white	250	1	Each	19	22	41	448	0	3	50	9
	Subway Roast Beef - 12" Italian	184	1	Each	42	23	84	689	0	5	83	8
	Subway Roast Beef - 12" Wheat	189	1	Each	41	24	89	717	0	6	75	8
	Subway Roast Beef - 6" white	232	1	Each	19	5	39	288	0	3	20	1
	Subway Roast Beef - Deli Sandwich	180	1	Each	13	4	38	245	0	2	13	1
	Subway Roast Beef Salad	316	1	Each	12	3	11	117	0	1	20	1
	Subway Roasted Chicken Breast - 6" hot	246	1	Each	26	6	41	332	0	3	48	1
	Subway Seafood - 12" Italian	210	1	Each	29	57	94	986	0	0	56	11
	Subway Seafood - 12" Wheat	219	1	Each	31	58	100	1015	0	2.5	56	11
	Subway Seafood & Crab - 6" white	246	1	Each	19	19	38	415	0	3	34	3
	Subway Seafood & Crab Salad	331	1	Each	13	17	10	244	0	2	34	3
	Subway Spicy Italian - 12" Italian	213	1	Each	42	63	83	1043	0	5	137	23
	Subway Spicy Italian - 6" white	232	1	Each	20	24	38	467	0	3	57	9
	Subway Steak & Cheese - 6" white	257	1	Each	29	10	41	383	0	3	70	6
	Subway Steak and Cheese - 12" Italian	213	1	Each	43	32	83	765	0	6	82	12
	Subway Tuna - 6" white	246	1	Each	18	32	38	527	0	3	36	5
	Subway Tuna - Deli Sandwich, lite mayo	178	1	Each	11	9	38	279	0	2	16	2

Monounsaturated Fat (gm)	Polyunsaturated Fat (gm)	Vitamin D (mg)	Vitamin K (mg)	Vitamin E (mg)	Vitamin A (re)	Vitamin C (mg)	Thiamin (mg)	Riboflavin (mg)	Niacin (mg)	Vitamin B6 (mg)	Folate (mg)	Vitamin B12 (mcg)	Calcium (mg)	Iron (mg)	Magnesium (mg)	Phosphorus (mg)	Potassium (mg)	Sodium (mg)	Zinc (mg)
0	0.4	0	0	0	0	0	0.06	0.1	0.38	0	0	0.4	0	0	21	64	0	90	0.3
0	4.1	0	0	0	0	0	0.15	0.17	2.85	0	0	2	320	0.8	52.5	320	0	550	6.75
0	5.4	0	0	0	0	0	0.15	0.43	5.7	0	0	0.8	16	0.8	21	200	0	250	1.2
0	0.7	0	0	0	40	0	0.06	0.14	0.76	0	0	0.2	0	1	14	64	0	95	0.3
0	4.6	0	0	0	0	0	0.23	0.07	6.65	0	0	0.2	16	0	35	240	0	60	0.3
0	1	0	0	0	0	0	0.06	0.17	0.38	0	0	1	0	0	28	160	0	90	0.3
0	4	0	0	0	0	0	0.12	0.17	2.85	0	0	1	80	0	21	200	0	90	0.9
0	0.5	0	0	0	0	0	0.09	0.1	0.76	0	0	0.6	0	0	21	120	0	95	0.3
0	0.6	0	0	0	0	0	0.06	0.03	4.75	0	0	0.3	0	0	21	120	0	140	0.3
0	1.4	0	0	0	0	0	0	0.07	3.8	0	0	0.5	48	0	87.5	400	0	1090	6
0	1.1	0	0	0	0	0	0	0.03	1.9	0	0	0.5	32	0	35	120	0	110	1.5
0	1.8	0	0	0	0	0	0.03	0.1	1.9	0	0	1.6	80	0.2	70	200	0	1630	6
0	1.8	0	0	0	0	0	0.38	0.14	7.6	0	0	2	0	0	35	280	0	60	0.3
0	2	0	0	0	0	0	0.15	0.34	7.6	0	0	1.2	0	2	35	280	0	115	9
0	1	0	0	0	20	0	0.06	0.07	3.8	0	0	0.3	0	0	28	80	0	140	0.6
0	1.6	0	0	0	0	0	0.06	0.03	13.3	0	0	1.6	0	0.6	35	240	0	70	0.3
0	0	0	0	0	601	15	0	0	0	0	0	0	27	3	0	0	0	945	0
24	7	0	0	5.1	67	5	0.27	0.34	5.1	0.48	63	2.33	64	4.3	66	308	917	3139	6.1
25	7	0	0	0	753	15	0	0	0	0	0	0	44	4	0	0	1002	3199	0
0	0	0	0	0	565	14	0	0	0	0	0	0	39	3	0	0	0	744	0
0	0	0	0	0	1044	18	0	0	0	0	0	0	118	4	0	0	0	1264	0
0	0	0	0	0	753	15	0	0	0	0	0	0	44	4	0	0	0	1652	0
0	0	0	0	0	601	15	0	0	0	0	0	0	29	4	0	0	0	1341	0
0	0	0	0	0	1363	32	0	0	0	0	0	0	26	2	0	0	0	1067	0
8	4	0	0	1.3	74	20	0.48	0.33	12.5	0.58	47	0.95	58	3.1	66	384	971	2717	2.5
9	4	0	0	4.2	83	15	0.49	0.35	9.3	0.46	43	0.44	96	3.2	40	247	1055	2777	1.4
15	10	0	0	0.9	87	17	0.36	0.33	3.8	0.2	39	1.23	227	2.9	28	315	876	2218	2.7
15	10	0	0	0.9	90	18	0.37	0.35	3.9	0.21	41	1.28	235	3	29	327	1010	2278	2.8
0	0	0	0	0	649	16	0	0	0	0	0	0	49	4	0	0	0	1401	0
0	0	0	0	0	1412	33	0	0	0	0	0	0	46	2	0	0	0	1127	0
0	0	0	0	0	601	15	0	0	0	0	0	0	28	3	0	0	0	1308	0
0	0	0	0	0	565	14	0	0	0	0	0	0	24	3	0	0	0	773	0
8	4	0	0	3.8	174	17	0.53	0.39	3.6	0.34	45	0.76	304	2.2	50	527	834	1710	2.8
8	4	0	0	0	0	0	0	0	0	0	0	0	35	3	0	0	918	1319	0
17	4	0	0	1	72	19	0.33	0.39	9.4	0.4	35	3.21	78	5	47	263	1210	2022	6.2
18	4	0	0	0	0	0	0	0	0	0	0	0	0	0	0	0	1498	2082	0
0	0	0	0	0	712	16	0	0	0	0	0	0	32	4	0	0	0	1035	0
0	0	0	0	0	777	15	0	0	0	0	0	0	93	4	0	0	0	1735	0
0	0	0	0	0	1190	16	0	0	0	0	0	0	103	4	0	0	0	1609	0
9	4	0	0	4.4	58	5	0.23	0.29	4.4	0.42	54	2.01	55	3.7	57	266	910	2288	5.3
9	4	0	0	4.5	59	5	0.24	0.3	4.5	0.43	56	2.07	56	3.8	59	273	994	2348	5.4
0	0	0	0	0	601	15	0	0	0	0	0	0	25	4	0	0	0	928	0
0	0	0	0	0	565	14	0	0	0	0	0	0	23	3	0	0	0	638	0
0	0	0	0	0	1363	32	0	0	0	0	0	0	23	2	0	0	0	654	0
0	0	0	0	0	617	15	0	0	0	0	0	0	35	3	0	0	0	967	0
15	28	0	0	2.5	107	5	0.51	0.38	7	0.26	91	6.54	230	4.4	32	336	641	2027	5.3
16	28	0	0	0	0	0	0	0	0	0	0	0	0	0	0	0	557	1967	0
0	0	0	0	0	604	15	0	0	0	0	0	0	28	3	0	0	0	849	0
0	0	0	0	0	1366	32	0	0	0	0	0	0	25	2	0	0	0	575	0
28	7	0	0	0	0	0	0	0	0	0	0	0	0	0	0	0	880	2282	0
0	0	0	0	0	845	15	0	0	0	0	0	0	40	4	0	0	0	1592	0
0	0	0	0	0	877	18	0	0	0	0	0	0	88	5	0	0	0	1106	0
12	4	0	0	0.8	119	6	0.33	0.46	5.1	0.38	36	2.54	231	4.2	43	456	909	1556	6.8
0	0	0	0	0	627	15	0	0	0	0	0	0	32	3	0	0	0	875	0
0	0	0	0	0	628	14	0	0	0	0	0	0	26	3	0	0	0	583	0

USDA ID Code	Food Name	Weight in Grams*	Quantity of Units	Unit of Measure	Protein (gm)	Fat (gm)	Carbohydrates (gm)	Kcalories	Caffeine (gm)	Fiber (gm)	Cholesterol (mg)	Saturated Fat (gm)
	Subway Turkey Breast - 12" Wheat	192	1	Each	42	20	88	674	0	7	67	6
	Subway Turkey Breast - 6" white	232	1	Each	17	4	40	273	0	3	19	1
	Subway Turkey Breast - Deli sandwich	180	1	Each	12	4	38	235	0	2	12	1
	Subway Turkey Breast & Ham - 6" white	232	1	Each	18	5	39	280	0	3	24	1
	Subway Turkey Breast Salad	316	1	Each	11	2	12	316	0	1	19	1
	Subway Veggie Delight - 6" white	175	1	Each	9	3	38	222	0	3	0	0
	Subway Veggie Delite - 6" wheat	182	1	Each	9	3	44	237	0	3	0	0
	Subway Veggie Delite Salad	260	1	Each	2	1	10	51	0	1	0	0
58318	Taco Bell-Bean Burrito	206	1	Each	15	14	63	387	0	3	9	4
58319	Taco Bell-Beef Burrito	206	1	Each	25	21	48	431	0	2	57	8
58321	Taco Bell-Burrito Supreme	198	1	Each	20	22	55	440	0	3	33	8
62585	Taco Bell-Light 7-Layer Burrito	276	1	Each	19	9	67	440	0	0	5	0
62583	Taco Bell-Light Bean Burrito	198	1	Each	14	6	55	330	0	0	5	0
62586	Taco Bell-Light Burrito Supreme	248	1	Each	20	8	50	350	0	0	25	0
62584	Taco Bell-Light Chicken Burrito	170	1	Each	12	6	45	290	0	0	30	0
62587	Taco Bell-Light Chicken Burrito Supreme	248	1	Each	18	10	62	410	0	0	65	0
62582	Taco Bell-Light Chicken Soft Taco	120	1	Each	9	5	26	180	0	0	30	0
62575	Taco Bell-Light Soft Taco	99	1	Each	13	5	19	180	0	2	25	4
62581	Taco Bell-Light Soft Taco Supreme	128	1	Each	14	5	23	200	0	0	25	0
62574	Taco Bell-Light Taco	78	1	Each	11	5	11	140	0	1	20	4
62588	Taco Bell-Light Taco Salad	464	1	Each	30	9	35	330	0	0	50	0
62580	Taco Bell-Light Taco Supreme	106	1	Each	14	5	23	160	0	0	20	0
58328	Taco Bell-Mexican Pizza	223	1	Each	21	37	40	575	0	3	52	11
58325	Taco Bell-Nachos	106	1	Each	7	18	37	346	0	1	9	6
58323	Taco Bell-Nachos Bell Grande	287	1	Each	22	35	61	649	0	4	36	12
58329	Taco Bell-Pintos 'N Cheese	128	1	Each	9	9	19	190	0	2	16	4
58337	Taco Bell-Salsa	10	1	Each	1	0	4	18	0	0.4	0	0
58314	Taco Bell-Soft Taco	92	1	Each	12	12	18	225	0	2	32	5
58313	Taco Bell-Taco	78	1	Each	10	11	11	183	0	1	32	5
58332	Taco Bell-Taco Salad	575	1	Each	34	61	55	905	0	4	80	19
58333	Taco Bell-Taco Salad w/o Shell	520	1	Each	28	31	22	484	0	3	80	14
58316	Taco Bell-Tostada	156	1	Each	9	11	27	243	0	2	16	4
	Wendy's Big Bacon Classic	285	1	Each	34	30	46	580	0	3	100	12
61273	Wendy's Big Classic	251	1	Each	27	23	44	480	0	0	75	7
62322	Wendy's Bkd Potato w/ Bacon and Cheese	380	1	Each	17	17	75	510	0	0	15	4
61287	Wendy's Bkd Potato w/ Broccoli and Cheese	411	1	Each	9	14	77	450	0	0	0	2
62524	Wendy's Bkd Potato w/ Cheese	383	1	Each	14	24	74	550	0	0	30	8
	Wendy's Breaded Chicken Sandwich	208	1	Each	28	18	44	440	0	2	60	3.5
	Wendy's Cheesburger, Kids' Meal	123	1	Each	17	13	33	320	0	2	45	6
61281	Wendy's Chicken Club Sandwich	216	1	Each	31	20	44	470	0	2	70	4
61292	Wendy's Chili, Large	340	1	Each	28	9	31	290	0	0	60	4
61291	Wendy's Chili, Small	227	1	Each	19	6	21	190	0	0	40	2
61285	Wendy's French Fries, Biggie	170	1	Each	7	23	61	450	0	0	0	5
61284	Wendy's French Fries, Medium	136	1	Each	5	17	50	360	0	0	0	4
61283	Wendy's French Fries, Small	91	1	Each	3	12	33	240	0	0	0	2
61302	Wendy's Frosty Dairy Dessert, Large	402.22	1	Each	15	17	91	570	0	0	70	9
61301	Wendy's Frosty Dairy Dessert, Medium	321.776	1	Each	12	13	76	460	0	0	55	7
61300	Wendy's Frosty Dairy Dessert, Small	241.332	1	Each	9	10	57	340	0	0	40	5
	Wendy's Grilled Chicken Sandwich	189	1	Each	27	8	35	310	0	2	65	1.5
	Wendy's Hamburger, Kids' Meal	111	1	Each	15	10	33	270	0	2	30	3.5
	Wendy's Jr. Bacon Cheesburger	166	1	Each	20	19	34	380	0	2	60	7
	Wendy's Jr. Cheeseburger	130	1	Each	17	13	34	320	0	2	45	6
	Wendy's Jr. Cheesburger Deluxe	180	1	Each	18	17	36	360	0	3	50	6
	Wendy's Jr. Hamburger	118	1	Each	15	10	34	270	0	2	30	3.5
61271	Wendy's Plain Single	133	1	Each	24	16	31	360	0	2	65	6

Monounsaturated Fat (gm)	Polyunsaturated Fat (gm)	Vitamin D (mg)	Vitamin K (mg)	Vitamin E (mg)	Vitamin A (re)	Vitamin C (mg)	Thiamin (mg)	Riboflavin (mg)	Niacin (mg)	Vitamin B6 (mg)	Folate (mg)	Vitamin B12 (mcg)	Calcium (mg)	Iron (mg)	Magnesium (mg)	Phosphorus (mg)	Potassium (mg)	Sodium (mg)	Zinc (mg)
7	7	0	0	0	0	0	0	0	0	0	0	0	0	0	0	0	605	2520	0
0	0	0	0	0	601	15	0	0	0	0	0	0	30	4	0	0	0	1391	0
0	0	0	0	0	565	14	0	0	0	0	0	0	26	3	0	0	0	944	0
0	0	0	0	0	601	15	0	0	0	0	0	0	29	3	0	0	0	1350	0
0	0	0	0	0	1363	32	0	0	0	0	0	0	28	2	0	0	0	1117	0
0	0	0	0	0	601	15	0	0	0	0	0	0	25	0	0	0	0	3	0
0	0	0	0	0	601	15	0	0	0	0	0	0	32	3	0	0	0	593	0
0	0	0	0	0	1363	32	0	0	0	0	0	0	23	1	0	0	0	308	0
0	2	0	0	0	0	53	0.4	2	2.8	0	0	0	190	4	0	0	495	1148	0
0	2	0	0	0	0	2	0.4	0.3	3.2	0	0	0	150	3	0	0	380	1311	0
0	2	0	0	0	0	26	0.4	2.1	3.6	0	0	0	190	4	0	0	501	1181	0
0	0	0	0	0	350	4.8	0	0	0	0	0	0	300	2.5	0	0	0	1130	0
0	0	0	0	0	300	2.4	0	0	0	0	0	0	120	2	0	0	0	1340	0
0	0	0	0	0	600	9	0	0	0	0	0	0	96	1.5	0	0	0	1160	0
0	0	0	0	0	200	3.6	0	0	0	0	0	0	72	1.5	0	0	0	900	0
0	0	0	0	0	250	4.8	0	0	0	0	0	0	72	1.5	0	0	0	1190	0
0	0	0	0	0	150	4.8	0	0	0	0	0	0	48	0.8	0	0	0	570	0
0	1	0	0	0	40	0	0.4	0.2	2.8	0	0	0	48	0.6	0	0	196	554	0
0	0	0	0	0	100	2.4	0	0	0	0	0	0	48	0.6	0	0	0	610	0
0	1	0	0	0	40	0	0.1	0.1	1.2	0	0	0	0	0	0	0	159	276	0
0	0	0	0	0	1200	27	0	0	0	0	0	0	120	1.5	0	0	0	1610	0
0	0	0	0	0	100	2.4	0	0	0	0	0	0	0	0	0	0	0	340	0
0	10	0	0	0	0	31	0.3	0.3	3	0	0	0	257	4	0	0	408	1031	0
0	2	0	0	0	0	2	0	0.2	0.6	0	0	0	191	1	0	0	159	399	0
0	3	0	0	0	0	58	0.1	0.3	2.2	0	0	0	297	3	0	0	674	997	0
0	1	0	0	0	0	52	0.1	0.2	0.4	0	0	0	156	1	0	0	384	642	0
0	0	0	0	0	0	0	0	0.1	0	0	0	0	36	1	0	0	376	376	0
0	1	0	0	0	0	1	0.4	0.2	2.8	0	0	0	116	2	0	0	196	554	0
0	1	0	0	0	0	1	0.1	0.1	1.2	0	0	0	84	1	0	0	159	276	0
0	12	0	0	0	0	75	0.5	0.6	4.8	0	0	0	320	6	0	0	673	910	0
0	2	0	0	0	0	74	0.2	0.4	3.2	0	0	0	290	4	0	0	612	680	0
0	1	0	0	0	0	45	0.1	0.2	0.6	0	0	0	180	2	0	0	401	596	0
0	0	0	0	0	15	25	0	0	0	0	0	0	25	30	0	0	0	1460	0
8	7	0	0	0	60	12	0.45	0.26	6.65	0	0	0	120	3.5	0	0	500	850	0
3	8	0	0	0	100	36	0.45	0.17	6.65	0	0	0	80	2.5	0	0	1370	1170	0
3	7	0	0	0	200	60	0.3	0.14	4.75	0	0	0	80	2.5	0	0	1310	450	0
6	7	0	0	0	150	36	0.3	0.17	3.8	0	0	0	240	2	0	0	1210	640	0
0	0	0	0	0	4	10	0	0	0	0	0	0	10	16	0	0	0	840	0
0	0	0	0	0	6	0	0	0	0	0	0	0	17	18	0	0	0	830	0
7	9	0	0	0	20	9	0.6	0.43	15.2	0	0	0	80	8	0	0	470	970	0
2	1	0	0	0	150	12	0.15	0.17	2.85	0	0	0	80	4.5	0	0	660	1000	0
1	1	0	0	0	100	6	0.09	0.14	1.9	0	0	0	64	3	0	0	440	670	0
15	1	0	0	0	0	12	0.3	0.07	3.8	0	0	0	16	0.8	0	0	950	280	0
12	1	0	0	0	0	9	0.23	0.03	2.85	0	0	0	16	0.6	0	0	760	220	0
8	1	0	0	0	0	6	0.15	0.03	1.9	0	0	0	0	0.4	0	0	510	150	0
4	1	0	0	0	100	0	0.23	1.36	0.76	0	0	0	400	1	0	0	1040	330	0
3	1	0	0	0	100	0	0.15	1.02	0.76	0	0	0	320	0.8	0	0	830	260	0
3	0	0	0	0	80	0	0.12	0.77	0.38	0	0	0	240	0.6	0	0	630	200	0
0	0	0	0	0	4	10	0	0	0	0	0	0	10	15	0	0	0	790	0
0	0	0	0	0	2	0	0	0	0	0	0	0	11	17	0	0	0	610	0
0	0	0	0	0	8	10	0	0	0	0	0	0	17	19	0	0	0	850	0
0	0	0	0	0	6	2	0	0	0	0	0	0	17	18	0	0	0	830	0
0	0	0	0	0	10	10	0	0	0	0	0	0	18	19	0	0	0	890	0
0	0	0	0	0	2	2	0	0	0	0	0	0	11	17	0	0	0	610	0
7	2	0	0	0	0	0	0.38	0.17	5.7	0	0	0	80	3	0	0	280	580	0

USDA ID Code	Food Name	Weight in Grams*	Quantity of Units	Unit of Measure	Protein (gm)	Fat (gm)	Carbohydrates (gm)	Kcalories	Caffeine (gm)	Fiber (gm)	Cholesterol (mg)	Saturated Fat (gm)
61272	Wendy's Single w/ everything	219	1	Each	25	20	37	420	0	3	70	6
	Wendy's Spicy Chicken Sandwich	213	1	Each	28	15	43	410	0	2	65	2.5
62477	White Castle-Cheeseburger Sandwich	64.8	1	Each	7.8	11.2	15.53	199.58	0	2.7	0	0
62481	White Castle-Chicken Sandwich	63.786	1	Each	7.99	7.45	20.49	185.75	0	1.73	0	0
62478	White Castle-Fish Sandwich, w/o Tartar	59.333	1	Each	5.78	4.98	20.87	155.44	0	1.41	0	0
62483	White Castle-French Fries	96.83	1	Each	2.49	14.7	37.73	301.14	0	4.64	0	0
62476	White Castle-Hamburger Sandwich	58.5	1	Each	5.88	7.94	15.38	161.27	0	2.13	0	0
62485	White Castle-Onion Chips	92.135	1	Each	3.72	16.55	38.83	328.66	0	3.52	0	0
62484	White Castle-Onion Rings	60.17	1	Each	2.91	13.38	26.62	245.49	0	2.61	0	0
62479	White Castle-Sausage and Egg Sandwich	96.25	1	Each	12.55	22.02	16.05	322.37	0	3.03	0	0
62480	White Castle-Sausage Sandwich	48.667	1	Each	6.67	12.29	13.3	196.1	0	1.95	0	0
15002	Anchovy, European, Cnd In Oil	28.35	3	Ounce	8.19	2.75	0	59.54	0	0	24.1	0.62
15187	Bass, Freshwater, Ckd, Dry Heat	28.35	3	Ounce	6.86	1.34	0	41.39	0	0	24.66	0.28
15188	Bass, Striped, Ckd, Dry Heat	28.35	3	Ounce	6.44	0.85	0	35.15	0	0	29.2	0.18
15189	Bluefish, Ckd, Dry Heat	28.35	3	Ounce	7.28	1.54	0	45.08	0	0	21.55	0.33
15235	Catfish, Channel, Farmed, Ckd, Dry Heat	28.35	3	Ounce	5.31	2.27	0	43.09	0	0	18.14	0.51
15233	Catfish, Channel, Wild, Ckd, Dry Heat	28.35	3	Ounce	5.24	0.81	0	29.77	0	0	20.41	0.21
15011	Catfish, Fried	28.35	3	Ounce	5.13	3.78	2.28	64.92	0	0	22.96	0.93
15012	Caviar, Black and Red, Granular	16	1	Tbsp.	3.94	2.86	0.64	40.32	0	0	94.08	0.65
15158	Clam, Ckd, Breaded and Fried	28.35	3	Ounce	4.04	3.16	2.93	57.27	0	0	17.29	0.76
15159	Clam, Ckd, Moist Heat	28.35	3	Ounce	7.24	0.55	1.45	41.96	0	0	18.99	0.05
15160	Clam, Cnd, Drained Solids	28.35	3	Ounce	7.24	0.55	1.45	41.96	0	0	18.99	0.05
15016	Cod, Atlantic, Ckd, Dry Heat	28.35	3	Ounce	6.47	0.24	0	29.77	0	0	15.59	0.05
15017	Cod, Atlantic, Cnd	28.35	3	Ounce	6.45	0.24	0	29.77	0	0	15.59	0.05
15137	Crab, Alaska King, Ckd, Moist Heat	28.35	3	Ounce	5.49	0.44	0	27.5	0	0	15.03	0.04
15138	Crab, Alaska King, Imitation	28.35	3	Ounce	3.41	0.37	2.9	28.92	0	0	5.67	0.07
15140	Crab, Blue, Ckd, Moist Heat	28.35	3	Ounce	5.73	0.5	0	28.92	0	0	28.35	0.06
15141	Crab, Blue, Cnd	28.35	3	Ounce	5.82	0.35	0	28.07	0	0	25.23	0.07
15142	Crab, Blue, Crab Cakes	28.35	3	Ounce	5.73	2.13	0.14	43.94	0	0	42.53	0.42
15226	Crab, Dungeness, Ckd, Moist Heat	28.35	3	Ounce	6.33	0.35	0.27	31.19	0	0	21.55	0.05
15227	Crab, Queen, Ckd, Moist Heat	28.35	3	Ounce	6.72	0.43	0	32.6	0	0	20.13	0.05
15243	Crayfish, Farmed, Ckd, Moist Heat	28.35	3	Ounce	4.97	0.37	0	24.66	0	0	38.84	0.06
15146	Crayfish, Wild, Ckd, Moist Heat	28.35	3	Ounce	4.75	0.34	0	24.95	0	0	37.71	0.05
15027	Fish Fillets and Sticks, Fried	28.35	3	Ounce	4.44	3.47	6.73	77.11	0	0	31.75	0.89
15029	Flounder, Ckd, Dry Heat	28.35	3	Ounce	6.85	0.43	0	33.17	0	0	19.28	0.1
15032	Grouper, Ckd, Dry Heat	28.35	3	Ounce	7.04	0.37	0	33.45	0	0	13.32	0.08
15034	Haddock, Ckd, Dry Heat	28.35	3	Ounce	6.87	0.26	0	31.75	0	0	20.98	0.05
15035	Haddock, Smoked	28.35	3	Ounce	7.15	0.27	0	32.89	0	0	21.83	0.05
15037	Halibut, Ckd, Dry Heat	28.35	3	Ounce	7.57	0.83	0	39.69	0	0	11.62	0.12
15196	Halibut, Greenland, Ckd, Dry Heat	28.35	3	Ounce	5.22	5.03	0	67.76	0	0	16.73	0.88
15040	Herring, Ckd, Dry Heat	28.35	3	Ounce	6.53	3.29	0	57.55	0	0	21.83	0.74
15042	Herring, Kippered	28.35	3	Ounce	6.97	3.51	0	61.52	0	0	23.25	0.79
15197	Herring, Pacific, Ckd, Dry Heat	28.35	3	Ounce	5.96	5.04	0	70.88	0	0	28.07	1.18
15041	Herring, Pickled	28.35	3	Ounce	4.02	5.1	2.73	74.28	0	0	3.69	0.68
15148	Lobster, Northern, Ckd, Moist Heat	28.35	3	Ounce	5.81	0.17	0.36	27.78	0	0	20.41	0.03
15228	Lobster, Spiny, Ckd, Moist Heat	28.35	3	Ounce	7.49	0.55	0.88	40.54	0	0	25.52	0.09
15056	Mullet, Striped, Ckd, Dry Heat	28.35	3	Ounce	7.03	1.38	0	42.53	0	0	17.86	0.41
15165	Mussel, Blue, Ckd, Moist Heat	28.35	3	Ounce	6.75	1.27	2.1	48.76	0	0	15.88	0.24
15168	Oyster, Eastern, Breaded and Fried	28.35	3	Ounce	2.49	3.57	3.29	55.85	0	0	22.96	0.91
15170	Oyster, Eastern, Cnd	28.35	3	Ounce	2	0.7	1.11	19.56	0	0	15.59	0.18
15245	Oysters, Raw	28.35	3	Ounce	1.48	0.44	1.57	16.73	0	0	7.09	0.13
15058	Perch, Atlantic, Ckd, Dry Heat	28.35	3	Ounce	6.77	0.59	0	34.3	0	0	15.31	0.09
15061	Perch, Ckd, Dry Heat	28.35	3	Ounce	7.05	0.33	0	33.17	0	0	32.6	0.07
15063	Pike, Northern, Ckd, Dry Heat	28.35	3	Ounce	7	0.25	0	32.04	0	0	14.18	0.04
15204	Pike, Walleye, Ckd, Dry Heat	28.35	3	Ounce	6.96	0.44	0	33.74	0	0	31.19	0.09

Monounsaturated Fat (gm)	Polyunsaturated Fat (gm)	Vitamin D (mg)	Vitamin K (mg)	Vitamin E (mg)	Vitamin A (re)	Vitamin C (mg)	Thiamin (mg)	Riboflavin (mg)	Niacin (mg)	Vitamin B6 (mg)	Folate (mg)	Vitamin B12 (mcg)	Calcium (mg)	Iron (mg)	Magnesium (mg)	Phosphorus (mg)	Potassium (mg)	Sodium (mg)	Zinc (mg)
7	7	0	0	0	60	9	0.38	0.17	6.65	0	0	0	80	3	0	0	430	920	0
0	0	0	0	0	4	10	0	0	0	0	0	0	11	15	0	0	0	1280	0
0	0	0	0	0	0	0	0	0	0	0	0	0	0	0	0	0	0	361	0
0	0	0	0	0	0	0	0	0	0	0	0	0	0	0	0	0	0	497	0
0	0	0	0	0	0	0	0	0	0	0	0	0	0	0	0	0	0	201	0
0	0	0	0	0	0	0	0	0	0	0	0	0	0	0	0	0	0	193	0
0	0	0	0	0	0	0	0	0	0	0	0	0	0	0	0	0	0	266	0
0	0	0	0	0	0	0	0	0	0	0	0	0	0	0	0	0	0	823	0
0	0	0	0	0	0	0	0	0	0	0	0	0	0	0	0	0	0	566	0
0	0	0	0	0	0	0	0	0	0	0	0	0	0	0	0	0	0	698	0
0	0	0	0	0	0	0	0	0	0	0	0	0	0	0	0	0	0	488	
1.07	0.73	0	0	1.42	5.95	0	0.02	0.1	5.64	0.06	3.54	0.25	65.77	1.31	19.56	71.44	154.22	1039.88	0.69
0.52	0.39	0	0	0	9.92	0.6	0.02	0.03	0.43	0.04	4.82	0.65	29.2	0.54	10.77	72.58	129.28	25.52	0.24
0.24	0.28	0	0	0	8.79	0	0.03	0.01	0.73	0.1	2.84	1.25	5.39	0.31	14.46	72.01	92.99	24.95	0.14
0.65	0.38	0	0	0	39.12	0	0.02	0.03	2.05	0.13	0.57	1.76	2.55	0.18	11.91	82.5	135.23	21.83	0.29
1.18	0.39	0	0	0	4.25	0.23	0.12	0.02	0.71	0.05	1.98	0.79	2.55	0.23	7.37	69.46	91	22.68	0.3
0.31	0.18	0	0	0	4.25	0.23	0.06	0.02	0.68	0.03	2.84	0.82	3.12	0.1	7.94	86.18	118.79	14.18	0.17
1.59	0.94	0	0	0	2.27	0	0.02	0.04	0.65	0.05	4.68	0.54	12.47	0.41	7.65	61.24	96.39	79.38	0.24
0.74	1.19	0.93	0	1.12	89.6	0	0.03	0.1	0.02	0.05	8	3.2	44	1.9	48	56.96	28.96	240	0.15
1.29	0.81	0	0	0	25.52	2.84	0.03	0.07	0.59	0.02	5.16	11.42	17.86	3.94	3.97	53.3	92.42	103.19	0.41
0.05	0.16	0	0	0	48.48	6.27	0.04	0.12	0.95	0.03	8.16	28.03	26.08	7.93	5.1	95.82	178.04	31.75	0.77
0.05	0.16	0	0	0.28	48.48	6.27	0.04	0.12	0.95	0.03	8.16	28.03	26.08	7.93	5.1	95.82	178.04	31.75	0.77
0.04	0.08	0	0	0.09	3.97	0.28	0.02	0.02	0.71	0.08	2.3	0.3	3.97	0.14	11.91	39.12	69.17	22.11	0.16
0.04	0.08	0.6	0	0.06	3.97	0.28	0.02	0.02	0.71	0.08	2.3	0.3	5.95	0.14	11.62	73.71	149.69	61.8	0.16
0.05	0.15	0	0	0	2.55	2.15	0.02	0.02	0.38	0.05	14.46	3.26	16.73	0.22	17.86	79.38	74.28	303.91	2.16
0.06	0.19	0	0	0	5.67	0	0.01	0.01	0.05	0.01	0.45	0.45	3.69	0.11	12.19	79.95	25.52	238.42	0.09
0.08	0.19	0	0	0.28	0.57	0.94	0.03	0.01	0.94	0.05	14.4	2.07	29.48	0.26	9.36	58.4	91.85	79.1	1.2
0.06	0.12	0	0	0.28	0.57	0.77	0.02	0.02	0.39	0.04	12.05	0.13	28.63	0.24	11.06	73.71	106.03	94.41	1.14
0.8	0.64	0	0	0	22.96	0.79	0.03	0.02	0.82	0.05	11.77	1.68	29.77	0.31	9.36	60.39	91.85	93.56	1.16
0.06	0.12	0	0	0	8.79	1.02	0.02	0.06	1.03	0.05	11.91	2.94	16.73	0.12	16.44	49.61	115.67	107.16	1.55
0.09	0.15	0	0	0	14.74	2.04	0.03	0.07	0.82	0.05	11.91	2.94	9.36	0.82	17.86	36.29	56.7	195.9	1.02
0.07	0.12	0	0	0	4.25	0.14	0.01	0.02	0.47	0.04	3.12	0.88	14.46	0.31	9.36	68.32	67.47	27.5	0.42
0.07	0.1	0	0	0.43	4.25	0.26	0.01	0.02	0.65	0.02	12.47	0.61	17.01	0.24	9.36	76.55	83.92	26.65	0.5
1.44	0.9	0	0	0	8.79	0	0.04	0.05	0.6	0.02	5.16	0.51	5.67	0.21	7.09	51.31	73.99	165	0.19
0.09	0.12	0	0	0	3.12	0	0.02	0.03	0.62	0.07	2.61	0.71	5.1	0.1	16.44	81.93	97.52	29.77	0.18
0.08	0.11	0	0	0	14.18	0	0.02	0	0.11	0.1	2.89	0.2	5.95	0.32	10.49	40.54	134.66	15.03	0.14
0.04	0.09	0	0	0	5.39	0	0.01	0.01	1.31	0.1	3.77	0.39	11.91	0.38	14.18	68.32	113.12	24.66	0.14
0.04	0.09	0	0	0.11	6.24	0	0.01	0.01	1.44	0.11	4.34	0.45	13.89	0.4	15.31	71.16	117.65	216.31	0.14
0.27	0.27	0	0	0	15.31	0	0.02	0.03	2.02	0.11	3.91	0.39	17.01	0.3	30.33	80.8	163.3	19.56	0.15
3.05	0.5	0	0	0	5.1	0	0.02	0.03	0.55	0.14	0.28	0.27	1.13	0.24	9.36	59.54	97.52	29.2	0.14
1.36	0.78	0	0	0.38	8.79	0.2	0.03	0.08	1.17	0.1	3.26	3.73	20.98	0.4	11.62	85.9	118.79	32.6	0.36
1.45	0.83	0.85	0	0.28	11.06	0.28	0.04	0.09	1.25	0.12	3.88	5.3	23.81	0.43	13.04	92.14	126.72	260.25	0.39
2.5	0.88	0	0	0	9.92	0	0.02	0.07	0.8	0.15	1.7	2.73	30.05	0.41	11.62	82.78	153.66	26.93	0.19
3.39	0.48	4.82	0	0.28	73.14	0	0.01	0.04	0.94	0.05	0.68	1.21	21.83	0.35	2.27	25.23	19.56	246.65	0.15
0.05	0.03	0	0	0.28	7.37	0	0	0.02	0.3	0.02	3.15	0.88	17.29	0.11	9.92	52.45	99.79	107.73	0.83
0.1	0.21	0	0	0	1.7	0.6	0	0.02	1.39	0.05	0.28	1.15	17.86	0.4	14.46	64.92	58.97	64.35	2.06
0.39	0.26	0	0	0	11.91	0.34	0.03	0.03	1.79	0.14	2.78	0.07	8.79	0.4	9.36	69.17	129.84	20.13	0.25
0.29	0.34	0	0	0.24	25.8	3.86	0.09	0.12	0.85	0.03	21.43	6.8	9.36	1.91	10.49	80.8	75.98	104.61	0.76
1.33	0.94	0	0	0	25.52	1.08	0.04	0.06	0.47	0.02	3.86	4.43	17.58	1.97	16.44	45.08	69.17	118.22	24.7
0.07	0.21	0	0	0.24	25.52	1.42	0.04	0.05	0.35	0.03	2.52	5.42	12.76	1.9	15.31	39.41	64.92	31.75	25.78
0.04	0.17	0	0	0	2.27	1.33	0.03	0.02	0.36	0.02	5.1	4.59	0	1.64	9.36	26.37	35.15	50.46	10.75
0.23	0.16	0	0	0	3.97	0.23	0.04	0.04	0.69	0.08	2.95	0.33	38.84	0.33	11.06	78.53	99.23	27.22	0.17
0.06	0.13	0	0	0	2.84	0.48	0.02	0.03	0.54	0.04	1.64	0.62	28.92	0.33	10.77	72.86	97.52	22.4	0.41
0.06	0.07	0	0	0	6.8	1.08	0.02	0.02	0.79	0.04	4.9	0.65	20.7	0.2	11.34	79.95	93.84	13.89	0.24
0.11	0.16	0	0	0	6.8	0	0.09	0.06	0.79	0.04	4.82	0.65	39.97	0.47	10.77	76.26	141.47	18.43	0.22

USDA ID Code	Food Name	Weight in Grams*	Quantity of Units	Unit of Measure	Protein (gm)	Fat (gm)	Carbohydrates (gm)	Kcalories	Caffeine (gm)	Fiber (gm)	Cholesterol (mg)	Saturated Fat (gm)
15205	Pollock, Atlantic, Ckd, Dry Heat	28.35	3	Ounce	7.06	0.36	0	33.45	0	0	25.8	0.05
15069	Pompano, Florida, Ckd, Dry Heat	28.35	3	Ounce	6.72	3.44	0	59.82	0	0	18.14	1.28
15071	Rockfish, Pacific, Ckd, Dry Heat	28.35	3	Ounce	6.82	0.57	0	34.3	0	0	12.47	0.13
15232	Roughy, Orange, Ckd, Dry Heat	28.35	3	Ounce	5.34	0.26	0	25.23	0	0	7.37	0.01
15209	Salmon, Atlantic, Wild, Ckd, Dry Heat	28.35	3	Ounce	7.21	2.3	0	51.6	0	0	20.13	0.36
15210	Salmon, Chinook, Ckd, Dry Heat	28.35	3	Ounce	7.29	3.79	0	65.49	0	0	24.1	0.91
15211	Salmon, Chum, Ckd, Dry Heat	28.35	3	Ounce	7.32	1.37	0	43.66	0	0	26.93	0.31
15087	Salmon, Cnd.	28.35	3	Ounce	5.8	2.07	0	43.38	0	0	12.47	0.47
15239	Salmon, Coho, Farmed, Ckd, Dry Heat	28.35	3	Ounce	6.89	2.33	0	50.46	0	0	17.86	0.55
15247	Salmon, Coho, Wild, Ckd, Dry Heat	28.35	3	Ounce	6.65	1.22	0	39.41	0	0	15.59	0.3
15082	Salmon, Coho, Wild, Ckd, Moist Heat	28.35	3	Ounce	7.76	2.13	0	52.16	0	0	16.16	0.45
15212	Salmon, Pink, Ckd, Dry Heat	28.35	3	Ounce	7.25	1.25	0	42.24	0	0	18.99	0.2
15088	Sardine, Atlantic, Cnd In Oil	28.35	3	Ounce	6.98	3.25	0	58.97	0	0	40.26	0.43
15173	Scallop, Breaded and Fried	28.35	3	Ounce	5.12	3.1	2.87	60.95	0	0	17.29	0.76
15174	Scallop, Imitation	28.35	3	Ounce	3.62	0.12	3.01	28.07	0	0	6.24	0.02
62652	Scallops, Sauteed	28.35	3	Ounce	9.67	0.33	0.67	50	0	0	20	0
15092	Sea Bass, Ckd, Dry Heat	28.35	3	Ounce	6.7	0.73	0	35.15	0	0	15.03	0.19
15096	Shark, Ckd, Batter-dipped and Fried	28.35	3	Ounce	5.28	3.92	1.81	64.64	0	0	16.73	0.91
15150	Shrimp, Ckd, Breaded and Fried	28.35	3	Ounce	6.06	3.48	3.25	68.61	0	0	50.18	0.59
15151	Shrimp, Ckd, Moist Heat	28.35	3	Ounce	5.93	0.31	0	28.07	0	0	55.28	0.08
15152	Shrimp, Cnd	28.35	3	Ounce	6.54	0.56	0.29	34.02	0	0	49.05	0.11
15149	Shrimp, Fresh	28.35	3	Ounce	5.76	0.49	0.26	30.05	0	0	43.09	0.09
15153	Shrimp, Imitation	28.35	3	Ounce	3.51	0.42	2.59	28.63	0	0	10.21	0.08
15100	Smelt, Rainbow, Ckd, Dry Heat	28.35	3	Ounce	6.41	0.88	0	35.15	0	0	25.52	0.16
15102	Snapper, Ckd, Dry Heat	28.35	3	Ounce	7.46	0.49	0	36.29	0	0	13.32	0.1
15176	Squid, Fried	28.35	3	Ounce	5.09	2.12	2.21	49.61	0	0	73.71	0.53
15218	Sunfish, Ckd, Dry Heat	28.35	3	Ounce	7.05	0.26	0	32.32	0	0	24.38	0.05
15111	Swordfish, Ckd, Dry Heat	28.35	3	Ounce	7.2	1.46	0	43.94	0	0	14.18	0.4
15219	Trout, Ckd, Dry Heat	28.35	3	Ounce	7.55	2.4	0	53.87	0	0	20.98	0.42
15241	Trout, Rainbow, Farmed, Ckd, Dry Heat	28.35	3	Ounce	6.88	2.04	0	47.91	0	0	19.28	0.6
15116	Trout, Rainbow, Wild, Ckd, Dry Heat	28.35	3	Ounce	6.5	1.65	0	42.53	0	0	19.56	0.46
15128	Tuna Salad	28.35	3	Ounce	4.55	2.63	2.67	53.01	0	0	3.69	0.44
15183	Tuna, Light Meat, Cnd In Oil	28.35	3	Ounce	8.26	2.33	0	56.13	0	0	5.1	0.43
15184	Tuna, Light Meat, Cnd In Water	28.35	3	Ounce	8.39	0.14	0	37.14	0	0	5.1	0.05
15121	Tuna, Light, Cnd In Water	28.35	3	Ounce	7.23	0.23	0	32.89	0	0	8.51	0.07
15220	Tuna, Skipjack, Ckd, Dry Heat	28.35	3	Ounce	8	0.37	0	37.42	0	0	17.01	0.12
15185	Tuna, White Meat, Cnd In Oil	28.35	3	Ounce	7.52	2.29	0	52.73	0	0	8.79	0.47
15186	Tuna, White Meat, Cnd In Water	28.35	3	Ounce	7.56	0.7	0	38.56	0	0	11.91	0.19
15221	Tuna, Yellowfin, Ckd, Dry Heat	28.35	3	Ounce	8.5	0.35	0	39.41	0	0	16.44	0.09
15223	Whitefish, Ckd, Dry Heat	28.35	3	Ounce	6.94	2.13	0	48.76	0	0	21.83	0.33
15131	Whitefish, Smoked	28.35	3	Ounce	6.63	0.26	0	30.62	0	0	9.36	0.06
15225	Yellowtail, Ckd, Dry Heat	28.35	3	Ounce	8.41	1.91	0	53.01	0	0	20.13	0
15135	Yellowtail, Fresh	28.35	3	Ounce	6.56	1.49	0	41.39	0	0	15.59	0.36
19065	Almond Joy Candy Bar	50	1	Bar	2.35	13.85	29.2	232	0	0	1	8.31
19066	Alpine White Bar w/ Almonds	35	1	Bar	3.5	12.92	17.64	197.4	0	1.89	4.2	6.67
62631	Bagel Chips	28.35	1	Ounce	4	6	20	150	0	1	0	1
19400	Banana Chips	28.35	1	Ounce	0.65	9.53	16.56	147.14	0	2.18	0	8.21
19002	Beef Jerky, Chopped and Formed	28.35	3	Ounce	11.25	3.69	4.11	95.82	0	0.03	32.04	1.66
18151	Brownies	56	1	Each	2.69	9.13	35.78	226.8	0	1.34	9.52	2.42
18155	Butter Cookies	5	1	Each	0.31	0.94	3.45	23.35	0	0.12	4.35	0.54
19069	Butterfinger Bar	61	1	Bar	4.7	11.29	40.5	266.57	2.44	1.65	0.61	5.17
19070	Butterscotch Candy	6	1	Piece	0.01	0.21	5.72	23.7	0	0	0.54	0.07
19074	Caramels	8	1	Piece	0.37	0.65	6.16	30.56	0	0.1	0.56	0.53
	Carefree Bubble Gum	3	1	Each	0	0	2	10	0	0	0	0
	Carefree Gum	3	1	Each	0	0	2	8	0	0	0	0

Monounsaturated Fat (gm)	Polyunsaturated Fat (gm)	Vitamin D (mg)	Vitamin K (mg)	Vitamin E (mg)	Vitamin A (re)	Vitamin C (mg)	Thiamin (mg)	Riboflavin (mg)	Niacin (mg)	Vitamin B6 (mg)	Folate (mg)	Vitamin B12 (mcg)	Calcium (mg)	Iron (mg)	Magnesium (mg)	Phosphorus (mg)	Potassium (mg)	Sodium (mg)	Zinc (mg)
0.04	0.18	0	0	0	3.4	0	0.02	0.06	1.13	0.09	0.85	1.04	21.83	0.17	24.38	80.23	129.28	31.19	0.17
0.94	0.41	0	0	0	10.21	0	0.19	0.04	1.08	0.07	4.9	0.34	12.19	0.19	8.79	96.67	180.31	21.55	0.2
0.13	0.17	0	0	0	18.71	0	0.01	0.02	1.11	0.08	2.95	0.34	3.4	0.15	9.64	64.64	147.42	21.83	0.15
0.17	0	0	0	0	6.8	0	0.03	0.05	1.04	0.1	2.27	0.65	10.77	0.07	10.77	72.58	109.15	22.96	0.27
0.76	0.92	0	0	0	3.69	0	0.08	0.14	2.86	0.27	8.22	0.86	4.25	0.29	10.49	72.58	178.04	15.88	0.23
1.63	0.75	0	0	0	42.24	1.16	0.01	0.04	2.85	0.13	9.92	0.81	7.94	0.26	34.59	105.18	143.17	17.01	0.16
0.56	0.33	0	0	0	9.64	0	0.03	0.06	2.42	0.13	1.42	0.98	3.97	0.2	7.94	102.91	155.93	18.14	0.17
0.79	0.65	0	0	0.45	15.03	0	0	0.05	1.55	0.09	2.78	0.09	67.76	0.3	8.22	92.42	106.88	152.52	0.29
1.03	0.56	0	0	0	16.73	0.43	0.03	0.03	2.1	0.16	3.97	0.9	3.4	0.11	9.64	94.12	130.41	14.74	0.13
0.45	0.36	0	0	0	11.06	0.4	0.02	0.04	2.25	0.16	3.69	1.42	0	0.17	9.36	91.29	123.04	16.44	0.16
0.77	0.71	0	0	0	9.07	0.28	0.03	0.05	2.21	0.16	2.55	1.27	13.04	0.2	9.92	84.48	128.99	15.03	0.15
0.34	0.49	0	0	0	11.62	0	0.06	0.02	2.42	0.07	1.42	0.98	4.82	0.28	9.36	83.63	117.37	24.38	0.2
1.1	1.46	1.93	0	0.09	18.99	0	0.02	0.06	1.49	0.05	3.35	2.53	108.3	0.83	11.06	138.92	112.55	143.17	0.37
1.28	0.81	0	0	0	6.24	0.65	0.01	0.03	0.43	0.04	5.16	0.37	11.91	0.23	16.73	66.91	94.41	131.54	0.3
0.02	0.06	0	0	0	5.67	0	0	0	0.09	0.01	0.45	0.45	2.27	0.09	12.19	79.95	29.2	225.38	0.09
0	0	0	0	0	0	0.6	0	0	0	0	0	0	8	0	0	0	0	91.67	0
0.15	0.27	0	0	0	18.14	0	0.04	0.04	0.54	0.13	1.64	0.09	3.69	0.1	15.03	70.31	92.99	24.66	0.15
1.68	1.05	0	0	0	15.31	0	0.02	0.03	0.79	0.09	1.47	0.34	14.18	0.31	12.19	55	43.94	34.59	0.14
1.08	1.44	0	0	0	15.88	0.43	0.04	0.04	0.87	0.03	2.3	0.53	18.99	0.36	11.34	61.8	63.79	97.52	0.39
0.06	0.12	0	0	1.03	18.71	0.62	0.01	0.01	0.73	0.04	0.99	0.42	11.06	0.88	9.64	38.84	51.6	63.5	0.44
0.08	0.21	0	0	0.71	5.1	0.65	0.01	0.01	0.78	0.03	0.51	0.32	16.73	0.78	11.62	66.06	59.54	47.91	0.36
0.07	0.19	1.08	0	0.81	15.31	0.57	0.01	0.01	0.72	0.03	0.85	0.33	14.74	0.68	10.49	58.12	52.45	41.96	0.31
0.06	0.21	0	0	0	5.67	0	0.01	0.01	0.05	0.01	0.45	0.45	5.39	0.17	12.19	79.95	25.23	199.87	0.09
0.23	0.32	0	0	0	4.82	0	0	0.04	0.5	0.05	1.3	1.13	21.83	0.33	10.77	83.63	105.46	21.83	0.6
0.09	0.17	0	0	0	9.92	0.45	0.02	0	0.1	0.13	1.64	0.99	11.34	0.07	10.49	56.98	147.99	16.16	0.12
0.78	0.61	0	0	0	3.12	1.19	0.02	0.13	0.74	0.02	1.5	0.35	11.06	0.29	10.77	71.16	79.1	86.75	0.49
0.04	0.09	0	0	0	4.82	0.28	0.03	0.02	0.41	0.04	4.82	0.65	29.2	0.44	10.77	65.49	127.29	29.2	0.56
0.56	0.34	0	0	0	11.62	0.31	0.01	0.03	3.34	0.11	0.65	0.57	1.7	0.29	9.64	95.54	104.61	32.6	0.42
1.18	0.54	0	0	0	5.39	0.14	0.12	0.12	1.64	0.07	4.25	2.12	15.59	0.54	7.94	89.02	131.26	18.99	0.24
0.59	0.66	0	0	0	24.38	0.94	0.07	0.02	2.49	0.11	6.8	1.41	0	0.09	9.07	75.41	125.02	11.91	0.14
0.49	0.52	0	0	0	4.25	0.57	0.04	0.03	1.64	0.1	5.39	1.79	0	0.11	8.79	76.26	127.01	15.88	0.14
0.82	1.17	0	0	0	7.65	0.62	0.01	0.02	1.9	0.02	2.07	0.34	4.82	0.28	5.39	50.46	50.46	113.97	0.16
0.84	0.82	0	0	0.34	6.52	0	0.01	0.03	3.52	0.03	1.5	0.62	3.69	0.39	8.79	88.17	58.68	14.18	0.26
0.04	0.04	0	0	0.15	6.52	0	0.01	0.03	3.52	0.11	1.33	0.62	3.4	0.91	8.22	52.73	89.02	14.18	0.12
0.05	0.1	0	0	0.15	4.82	0	0.01	0.02	3.76	0.1	1.13	0.85	3.12	0.43	7.65	46.21	67.19	95.82	0.22
0.07	0.11	0	0	0	5.1	0.28	0.01	0.03	5.32	0.28	2.84	0.62	10.49	0.45	12.47	80.8	147.99	13.32	0.3
0.7	0.96	0	0	0	6.8	0	0.02	0	3.32	0.12	1.3	0.62	1.13	0.18	9.64	75.69	94.41	14.18	0.13
0.18	0.26	0	0	0	6.8	0	0	0.01	1.64	0.12	1.16	0.62	1.13	0.17	9.64	75.69	80.23	14.18	0.13
0.06	0.1	0	0	0	5.67	0.28	0.14	0.02	3.38	0.29	0.57	0.17	5.95	0.27	18.14	69.46	161.31	13.32	0.19
0.73	0.78	0	0	0	11.06	0	0.05	0.04	1.09	0.1	4.82	0.27	9.36	0.13	11.91	98.09	115.1	18.43	0.36
0.08	0.08	0	0	0.06	16.16	0	0.01	0.03	0.68	0.11	2.07	0.92	5.1	0.14	6.52	37.42	119.92	288.89	0.14
0	0	0	0	0	8.79	0.82	0.05	0.01	2.47	0.05	1.13	0.35	8.22	0.18	10.77	56.98	152.52	14.18	0.19
0.56	0.4	0	0	0	8.22	0.79	0.04	0.01	1.93	0.05	1.05	0.37	6.52	0.14	8.51	44.51	119.07	11.06	0.15
2.63	1.19	0	0	0	2	0.1	0.02	0.08	0.24	0.03	4	0.06	39.5	0.6	33	70	185.5	67	0.4
4.81	0.88	0	0	0	8.75	0.14	0.03	0.15	0.03	0.03	4.55	0.3	80.85	0.2	13.3	81.55	146.3	25.55	0.4
3	2	0	0	0	0	0	0	0	0	0	0	0	0	0.4	0	0	0	190	0
0.55	0.18	0	0	1.53	2.27	1.79	0.02	0	0.2	0.07	3.97	0	5.1	0.35	21.55	15.88	151.96	1.7	0.21
1.51	0.16	0	0	0.04	0	0	0.03	0.26	2.61	0.13	4.82	1.13	3.12	1.56	14.46	107.73	169.25	815.06	2.3
4.73	1.44	0	0	0	11.2	0.06	0.14	0.12	0.96	0.02	6.72	0.08	16.24	1.26	17.36	56.56	83.44	174.72	0.4
0.26	0.05	0	0	0	7.55	0	0.02	0.02	0.16	0	0.3	0.01	1.45	0.11	0.6	5.1	5.55	17.55	0.02
3.82	1.81	0	0	0.81	11.59	1.71	0.09	0.03	2.01	0.04	18.91	0.09	14.64	0.64	27.45	57.95	129.32	82.96	0.45
0.03	0	0	0	0	2.04	0	0	0	0	0	0	0	0.18	0	0.06	0.18	0.24	2.58	0
0.07	0.01	0	0	0.04	0.64	0.04	0	0.01	0.02	0	0.4	0	11.04	0.01	1.36	9.12	17.12	19.6	0.04
0	0	0	0	0	0	0	0	0	0	0	0	0	0	0	0	0	0	0	0
0	0	0	0	0	0	0	0	0	0	0	0	0	0	0	0	0	0	0	0

USDA ID Code	Food Name	Weight in Grams*	Quantity of Units	Unit of Measure	Protein (gm)	Fat (gm)	Carbohydrates (gm)	Kcalories	Caffeine (gm)	Fiber (gm)	Cholesterol (mg)	Saturated Fat (gm)
19163	Chewing Gum	3	1	Stick	0	0.01	2.9	10.23	0	0	0	0
	Chewing Gum - Cinnamon	3	1	Each	0	0	2	10	0	0	0	0
	Chewing Gum - Mint Flavors	3	1	Each	0	0	2	10	0	0	0	0
62672	Chewing Gum, Sugar-Free	1.7	1	Stick	0	0	1	5	0	0	0	0
19033	Chex Mix	42.525	1	Cup	4.68	7.36	27.68	180.73	0	0	0	0
18198	Chocolate Chip Cookies, Dietary	7	1	Each	0.27	1.18	5.14	31.5	0	0	0	0.57
18159	Chocolate Chip Cookies, Higher Fat, Enr	10	1	Each	0.54	2.26	6.68	48.1	0	0.25	0	0.78
18158	Chocolate Chip Cookies, Lower Fat	10	1	Each	0.58	1.54	7.33	45.3	0	0	0	0.45
18160	Chocolate Chip Cookies, Soft-type	15	1	Each	0.53	3.65	8.87	68.7	0	0.48	0	1.12
18157	Chocolate Wafers	6	1	Each	0.4	0.85	4.34	25.98	0	0	0.12	0.22
19119	Chunky Bar	35	1	Bar	3.15	10.22	19.99	173.25	10.15	1.68	3.85	8.13
19219	Coconut Cream Pudding	280	1	Cup	8.68	7	49.84	291.2	0	0	19.6	5.04
19049	Combos Snacks Cheddar Pretzel	28.35	1	Ounce	2.78	5.53	18.43	135.51	0	0	2.55	0
62589	Cookie Cakes, Devils Food, Fat Free-SnackWell	16	1	Each	1	0	13	50	0	0.5	0	0
62591	Cookie Cakes, Double Fudge, Fat Free-SnackWell	16	1	Each	1	0	12	50	0	0.5	0	0
62656	Corn Chips	2.231	13	Chips	0.15	0.85	1.15	12.31	0	0.08	0	0.12
19401	Cornnuts, Barbecue-flavor	28.35	1	Ounce	2.55	4.05	20.33	123.61	0	2.38	0	0.73
19402	Cornnuts, Nacho-flavor	28.35	1	Ounce	2.66	4.03	20.3	124.17	0	2.27	0.57	0.73
19009	Cornnuts, Plain	28.35	1	Ounce	2.41	4	20.78	124.46	0	1.96	0	0.72
18150	Crackers, Animal	2.5	1	Each	0.17	0.35	1.85	11.15	0	0	0	0.09
19032	Doo Dads Snack Mix, Original Flavor	56.7	1	Cup	5.84	10.49	36.46	258.55	0	3.86	0.57	0
	Doritos - Cool Ranch	28	1	Ounce	2	7	18	140	0	0	0	1
	Doritos - Nacho Cheese	28	1	Ounce	2	7	17	140	0	0	0	1
62686	Doughnut Holes	15	1	Each	0.78	3.44	7.62	63.9	0	0	4.8	0.8
19168	Egg Custards	282	1	Cup	14.38	13.25	30.17	296.1	0	0	245.34	6.63
19098	Fifth Avenue Bar	60	1	Bar	4.74	12.72	40.8	279.6	0	0	2.4	0
18170	Fig Bars	16	1	Each	0.59	1.17	11.34	55.68	0	0.74	0	0.21
	Fig Newton - Fat Free	29	2	Each	1	0	22	100	0	0	0	0
	Fritos	28	1	Ounce	2	10	15	160	0	0	0	1.5
	Fritos-Barbecue	28	1	Ounce	2	9	16	160	0	0	0	1.5
62638	Frosted Pop Tart, Fruit	52	1	Each	2	5	38	200	0	1	0	1.5
19226	Frostings, Chocolate, Creamy	28.35	1	Ounce	0.31	4.99	17.92	112.55	0	0	0	1.57
19713	Frostings, Cream Cheese-flavor	28.35	1	Ounce	0.03	4.9	18.91	117.09	0	0	0	1.43
19229	Frostings, Sour Cream-flavor	28.35	1	Ounce	0.03	4.88	19.16	116.8	0	0	0	1.42
19230	Frostings, Vanilla, Creamy	28.35	1	Ounce	0.03	4.76	19.67	118.79	0	0	0	1.39
41319	Frozen Dessert, Bordeaux Cherry-Healthy Choice	132.969	1	Cup	6	4	46	240	0	0	10	0
41320	Frozen Dessert, Butter Pecan Crunch-Healthy Choice	132.969	1	Cup	6	4	52	280	0	0	10	0
41321	Frozen Dessert, Chocolate Chip-Healthy Choice	132.969	1	Cup	6	4	48	260	0	0	10	0
41322	Frozen Dessert, Coffee Toffee-Healthy Choice	132.969	1	Cup	6	4	50	260	0	0	10	0
41323	Frozen Dessert, Cookies 'n Cream-Healthy Choice	132.969	1	Cup	8	4	48	260	0	0	10	0
41324	Frozen Dessert, Double Fudge Swirl-Healthy Choice	132.969	1	Cup	6	4	48	260	0	0	10	0
41325	Frozen Dessert, Fudge Brownie-Healthy Choice	132.969	1	Cup	6	4	54	280	0	0	10	0
41326	Frozen Dessert, Mint Chocolate Chip-Healthy Choice	132.969	1	Cup	6	4	50	280	0	0	10	0
41327	Frozen Dessert, Neapolitan-Healthy Choice	132.969	1	Cup	6	4	44	240	0	0	10	0
41328	Frozen Dessert, Praline and Caramel-Healthy Choice	132.969	1	Cup	6	4	52	260	0	0	10	0
41329	Frozen Dessert, Rocky Road-Healthy Choice	132.969	1	Cup	6	4	64	320	0	0	10	0
41330	Frozen Dessert, Vanilla-Healthy Choice	132.969	1	Cup	8	4	42	240	0	0	10	0
	Frozen Yogurt - low fat	72	0-Jan	Cup	3	3	22	120	0	0	10	2
19263	Fruit and Juice Bars	77	1	Bar	0.92	0.08	15.55	63.14	0	0	0	0
19381	Fudge, Brown Sugar w/ Nuts	14	1	Piece	0.41	1.41	10.86	55.44	0	0	0.84	0.25
19100	Fudge, Chocolate	17	1	Piece	0.29	1.45	13.52	64.77	0	0.14	2.38	0.88
19101	Fudge, Chocolate w/ Nuts	19	1	Piece	0.65	3.06	13.83	80.94	0	0.25	2.66	1.07
19102	Fudge, Peanut Butter	16	1	Piece	0.59	1.04	12.53	59.36	0	0	0.64	0.24
19103	Fudge, Vanilla	16	1	Piece	0.18	0.86	13.17	59.04	0	0	2.56	0.54
19104	Fudge, Vanilla w/ Nuts	15	1	Piece	0.44	2	11.28	62.25	0	0.09	2.1	0.56

Monounsaturated Fat (gm)	Polyunsaturated Fat (gm)	Vitamin D (mg)	Vitamin K (mg)	Vitamin E (mg)	Vitamin A (re)	Vitamin C (mg)	Thiamin (mg)	Riboflavin (mg)	Niacin (mg)	Vitamin B6 (mg)	Folate (mg)	Vitamin B12 (mcg)	Calcium (mg)	Iron (mg)	Magnesium (mg)	Phosphorus (mg)	Potassium (mg)	Sodium (mg)	Zinc (mg)
0	0	0	0	0	0	0	0	0	0	0	0	0	0	0	0	0	0.12	0.18	0
0	0	0	0	0	0	0	0	0	0	0	0	0	0	0	0	0	0	0	0
0	0	0	0	0	0	0	0	0	0	0	0	0	0	0	0	0	0	0	0
0	0	0	0	0	0	0	0	0	0	0	0	0	0	0	0	0	0	0	0
0	0	0	0	0	5.95	20.2	0.66	0.21	7.16	0.66	0	5.27	14.88	10.5	26.79	79.52	114.39	432.48	0.89
0.47	0.07	0	0	0	0	0	0.02	0.01	0.18	0	0.42	0	2.31	0.24	1.75	6.23	13.93	0.77	0.04
1.15	0.22	0	0	0	0	0	0.02	0.03	0.27	0.01	0.9	0	2.5	0.28	3.1	10.8	13.5	31.5	0.06
0.79	0.17	0	0	0	0	0.03	0.03	0.03	0.28	0.03	0.6	0	1.9	0.31	2.8	8.4	12.3	37.7	0.07
1.95	0.4	0	0	0	0.15	0	0.02	0.03	0.24	0.02	0.75	0	2.25	0.36	5.25	7.5	13.95	48.9	0.07
0.45	0.1	0	0	0	0.12	0	0.01	0.02	0.17	0	0.66	0	1.86	0.24	3.18	7.92	12.6	34.8	0.07
0.11	1.54	0	0	0	3.85	0.11	0.03	0.14	0.67	0.04	7.7	0.13	50.05	0.44	25.55	72.8	186.9	18.55	0.64
1.46	0.2	0	0	0	140	1.96	0.09	0.41	0.25	0.41	11.2	0.73	316.4	0.56	44.8	249.2	445.2	456.4	1.04
0	0	0	0	0	1.98	0	0.03	0.16	0.9	0.01	2.27	0.03	54.15	0.86	6.24	40.54	36.86	316.67	0.21
0	0	0	0	0	0	0	0	0	0	0	0	0	0	0	0	0	0	25	0
0	0	0	0	0	0	0	0	0	0	0	0	0	0	0.2	0	0	0	70	0
0	0	0	0	0	0	0	0	0	0	0	0	0	5.54	0.02	0	0	0	15.38	0
2.09	0.91	0	0	0	9.64	0.11	0.1	0.04	0.43	0.05	0	0	4.82	0.48	30.9	80.23	81.08	276.7	0.53
2.07	0.91	0	0	0	1.13	4.39	0.1	0.02	0.34	0.06	4.25	0	9.92	0.48	30.9	87.6	88.17	179.74	0.51
2.06	0.9	0	0	0.29	0	0	0.01	0.04	0.48	0.06	0	0	2.55	0.47	32.04	77.96	78.81	155.64	0.5
0.19	0.05	0	0	0	0	0	0.01	0.01	0.09	0	0.35	0	1.08	0.07	0.45	2.85	2.5	9.83	0.02
0	0	0	0	0	24.38	0.06	0.2	0.15	3.04	0.12	22.68	0.01	41.96	1.42	34.02	167.83	157.06	720.66	1.28
0	0	0	0	0	0	0	0	0	0	0	0	0	32	0.2	0	0	0	170	0
0	0	0	0	0	0	0	0	0	0	0	0	0	32	0.2	0	0	0	200	0
1.79	0.39	0	0	0	0.45	0.02	0.03	0.03	0.23	0	1.8	0.03	9	0.16	2.55	17.55	15.3	60.3	0.07
4.26	0.99	0	0	0	169.2	1.41	0.09	0.64	0.24	0.14	28.2	0.87	315.84	0.85	39.48	318.66	431.46	217.14	1.49
0	0	0	0	0	4.8	0	0.01	0.13	1.96	0.06	33	0.11	42	0.6	37.8	90	196.8	111.6	0.65
0.64	0.2	0	0	0	0.64	0.03	0.03	0.03	0.3	0.01	1.6	0	10.24	0.46	4.32	9.92	33.12	56	0.06
0	0	0	0	0	0	0	0	0	0	0	0	0	0	0	0	0	0	115	0
0	0	0	0	0	0	0	0	0	0	0	0	0	0	0	0	0	0	160	0
0	0	0	0	0	0	0	0	0	0	0	0	0	0	0	0	0	0	310	0
0	0	0	0	0	100	0	0.15	0.17	1.9	0.2	20	0	0	1	0	16	0	170	0
2.56	0.6	0	0	0	56.13	0	0	0	0.03	0	0	0	2.27	0.4	5.95	22.4	55.57	51.88	0.08
2.56	0.67	0	0	0	0	0	0	0	0	0	0	0	0.85	0.05	0.57	0.85	9.92	11.06	0
2.55	0.66	0	0	0	34.59	0	0	0.01	0.19	0	0.28	0	0.57	0.02	0.57	1.13	55	57.83	0
2.49	0.65	0	0	0	64.07	0	0	0	0	0	0	0	0.85	0.03	0.28	11.06	10.49	25.52	0
0	2	0	0	0	0	0	0.06	0.34	0	0	0	0	160	0	0	200	300	100	0
0	2	0	0	0	0	2.4	0.12	0.34	0	0	0	0	160	0	0	160	300	160	0
0	2	0	0	0	0	2.4	0.12	0.27	0	0	0	0	160	0.4	0	160	320	140	0
0	2	0	0	0	0	2.4	0.12	0.34	0	0	0	0	160	0	0	160	320	160	0
0	2	0	0	0	0	0	0.06	0.34	0	0	0	0	240	0	0	200	360	160	0
0	2	0	0	0	0	0	0.12	0.27	0	0	0	0	160	0.8	0	200	420	140	0
0	2	0	0	0	0	0	0.06	0.27	0	0	0	0	160	0.4	0	160	380	140	0
0	4	0	0	0	0	0	0.12	0.27	0	0	0	0	160	0.4	0	0	340	160	0
0	2	0	0	0	0	0	0.06	0.34	0	0	0	0	160	0	0	200	320	120	0
0	2	0	0	0	0	0	0.06	0.34	0	0	0	0	160	0	0	200	320	140	0
0	2	0	0	0	0	0	0.06	0.34	0	0	0	0	160	0	0	200	380	140	0
0	2	0	0	0	0	0	0.12	0.51	0	0	0	0	240	0	0	200	360	120	0
0	0	0	0	0	0	0	0	0	0	0	0	0	64	0	0	0	0	55	0
0	0	0	0	0	2.31	7.32	0.01	0.01	0.12	0.02	4.62	0	3.85	0.15	3.08	4.62	40.81	3.08	0.04
0.34	0.76	0	0	0	2.38	0.08	0.01	0.01	0.03	0.01	1.54	0	15.54	0.25	6.86	12.04	52.36	13.72	0.09
0.44	0.05	0	0	0.02	7.82	0.03	0	0.01	0.02	0	0.34	0.01	7.14	0.08	4.25	9.86	17.51	10.54	0.07
0.82	1.03	0	0	0.08	8.93	0.11	0.01	0.02	0.04	0.02	1.9	0.01	9.5	0.14	8.55	17.67	30.02	11.4	0.14
0.48	0.27	0	0	0	1.6	0.03	0	0.01	0.24	0.01	1.76	0.01	6.72	0.04	3.52	10.4	20.96	11.68	0.07
0.25	0.03	0	0	0.03	8	0.03	0	0.01	0	0	0.16	0.01	6.24	0.01	0.8	5.12	8	10.72	0.02
0.5	0.83	0	0	0.07	6.9	0.09	0.01	0.01	0.03	0.01	1.5	0.01	7.05	0.06	4.05	10.65	16.95	9.15	0.08

USDA ID Code	Food Name	Weight in Grams*	Quantity of Units	Unit of Measure	Protein (gm)	Fat (gm)	Carbohydrates (gm)	Kcalories	Caffeine (gm)	Fiber (gm)	Cholesterol (mg)	Saturated Fat (gm)
19215	Gelatin Pops	44	1	Each	0.53	0.04	7.35	30.8	0	0	0	0
18172	Gingersnaps	7	1	Each	0.39	0.69	5.38	29.12	0	0.15	0	0.12
19105	Goobers	1	1	Piece	0.14	0.34	0.49	5.13	0.22	0	0.09	0.12
62684	Granola Bar, Low-Fat	28	1	Each	2	2	21	110	0	1	0	0
19016	Granola Bars, Hard, Almond	28.35	1	Each	2.18	7.23	17.58	140.33	0	0	0	3.55
19017	Granola Bars, Hard, Chocolate Chip	28.35	1	Each	2.07	4.62	20.44	124.17	0	1.25	0	3.23
19019	Granola Bars, Hard, Peanut	28.35	1	Each	3.12	6.07	18.06	135.8	0	0	0	0.71
19420	Granola Bars, Hard, Peanut Butter	28.35	1	Each	2.78	6.75	17.66	136.93	0	0	0	0.91
19015	Granola Bars, Hard, Plain	28.35	1	Each	2.86	5.61	18.26	133.53	0	1.5	0	0.67
19404	Granola Bars, Soft, Chocolate Chip	28.35	1	Each	2.07	4.71	19.59	119.07	0	1.36	0.28	2.89
19406	Granola Bars, Soft, Nut and Raisin	28.35	1	Each	2.27	5.78	18.03	128.71	0	1.59	0.28	2.7
19021	Granola Bars, Soft, Peanut Butter	28.35	1	Each	2.98	4.48	18.26	120.77	0	1.22	0.28	1.03
19027	Granola Bars, Soft, Peanut Butter and Choc Chip	28.35	1	Each	2.78	5.67	17.63	122.47	0	1.19	0.28	1.58
19020	Granola Bars, Soft, Plain	28.35	1	Each	2.1	4.88	19.08	125.59	0	1.3	0.28	2.05
19022	Granola Bars, Soft, Raisin	28.35	1	Each	2.15	5.05	18.82	127.01	0	1.19	0.28	2.71
19106	Gumdrops	3.5	1	Each	0	0	3.46	13.51	0	0	0	0
	Ice Cream - fat free	72	0.5	Cup	4	0	23	100	0	0	0	0
	Ice Cream - Haagen Dazs - Low Fat	92	0.5	Cup	7	2.5	29	170	0	0	0	0
	Ice Cream - light	67	0.5	Cup	3	4.5	18	130	0	0	35	2.5
	Ice Cream - Starbucks	99	0.5	Cup	4	13	30	250	0	0	60	8
	Ice Cream - Starbucks - Low Fat	99	0.5	Cup	5	3	31	170	0	0	10	1.5
18271	Ice Cream Cones, Cake or Wafer-type	4	1.5	Each	0.32	0.28	3.16	16.68	0	0.16	0	0.04
18272	Ice Cream Cones, Sugar, Rolled-type	10	1.5	Each	0.79	0.38	8.41	40.2	0	0.46	0	0.06
62640	Ice Cream Sandwich	63	1	Each	3	6	27	170	0	1	10	3
19270	Ice Cream, Chocolate	91	0.5	Cup	4.2	14.9	20.2	232	1.5	0	0	0
19090	Ice Cream, French Vanilla, Soft-serve	88	0.5	Cup	4.3	11.2	19.2	185	0	0	78	6.4
19271	Ice Cream, Strawberry	90	0.5	Cup	4.22	11.09	36.43	253.44	0	0	38.28	0
19095	Ice Cream, Vanilla	90	0.5	Cup	4.62	14.52	31.15	265.32	0	0	58.08	8.96
19089	Ice Cream, Vanilla, Rich	90	0.5	Cup	4.65	21.54	29.79	320.46	0	0	81.11	13.26
19088	Ice Milk, Vanilla	66	0.5	Cup	2.5	2.8	15	92	0	0	9	1.7
19096	Ice Milk, Vanilla, Soft Serve	88	0.5	Cup	4.3	2.3	19.2	111	0	0	11	1.4
19283	Ice Pops	52	1	Bar	0	0	9.83	37.44	0	0	0	0
19717	Ice Pops, w/ Added Ascorbic Acid	52	1	Bar	0	0	9.83	37.44	0	0	0	0
19173	Jello	140	0.5	Cup	1.7	0	19.6	83	0	0	0	0
19108	Jellybeans	1.1	1	Each	0	0.01	1.02	4.04	0	0	0	0
19109	Kit Kat Wafer Bar	46	1	Bar	3.08	13.11	28.47	234.6	5.06	0.41	11.5	7.67
19110	Krackel Chocolate Bar	47	1	Bar	2.91	13.07	29.09	235.94	8.46	0	8.93	5.55
19107	Lollipop	6	1	Each	0	0	5.89	22.38	0	0	0	0
19140	M&M's Peanut	49	1	Pkg	5.24	13.18	28.91	242.55	0	1.57	6.37	0
19141	M&M's Plain	48	1	Pkg	3.02	10.66	32.74	228.48	0	1.49	7.2	0
62667	M&M's, Almond	42	1	Pkg	4	13	25	230	0	2	5	4
19116	Marshmallows	46	1	Cup	0.83	0.09	37.4	146.28	0	0.05	0	0
19120	Milk Chocolate	44	1	Bar	3.04	13.46	26.09	225.72	11	1.54	9.68	8.09
19126	Milk Chocolate Coated Peanuts	28.35	1	Ounce	3.71	9.5	14	147.14	6.24	1.19	2.55	4.14
19127	Milk Chocolate Coated Raisins	28.35	1	Ounce	1.16	4.2	19.36	110.57	7.09	1.19	0.85	2.49
19132	Milk Chocolate w/ Almonds	41	1	Bar	3.69	14.1	21.81	215.66	9.02	2.54	7.79	6.96
19135	Milky Way Bar	60	1	Bar	2.7	9.12	43.5	251.4	0	0.96	12	4.73
18177	Molasses Cookies	15	1	Each	0.84	1.92	11.07	64.5	0	0	0	0.35
19142	Mounds Candy Bar	20	1	Bar	0.72	4.32	11.58	72.2	0	0.64	0	2.3
19143	Mr. Goodbar Chocolate Bar	50	1	Bar	6.3	16.15	25.65	257	5	2.15	10	9.03
19145	Nestle Crunch	40	1	Bar	2.48	10.4	25.68	197.6	9.6	1.04	7.6	5.74
18200	Oatmeal Cookies, Dietary	7	1	Each	0.34	1.26	4.89	31.43	0	0	0	0.56
18178	Oatmeal Cookies, Regular	18	1	Each	1.12	3.26	12.37	81	0	0.56	0	0.6
18179	Oatmeal Cookies, Soft-type	15	1	Each	0.92	2.21	9.86	61.35	0	0.41	1.35	0.43
18199	Oreos, Dietary	10	1	Each	0.45	2.21	6.77	46.1	0	0	0	1.04

Monounsaturated Fat (gm)	Polyunsaturated Fat (gm)	Vitamin D (mg)	Vitamin K (mg)	Vitamin E (mg)	Vitamin A (re)	Vitamin C (mg)	Thiamin (mg)	Riboflavin (mg)	Niacin (mg)	Vitamin B6 (mg)	Folate (mg)	Vitamin B12 (mcg)	Calcium (mg)	Iron (mg)	Magnesium (mg)	Phosphorus (mg)	Potassium (mg)	Sodium (mg)	Zinc (mg)
0	0	0	0	0	0	0	0	0	0	0	0	0	0.88	0.01	0.44	0	0.88	20.24	0.01
0.39	0.1	0	0	0	0	0	0.01	0.02	0.23	0.01	0.42	0	5.39	0.45	3.43	5.81	24.22	45.78	0.04
0.15	0.05	0	0	0	0	0	0	0	0.05	0	0.08	0	1.27	0.01	1.19	2.96	5.02	0.41	0.02
0	0	0	0	0	0	0	0	0	0	0	0	0	0	0.2	0	0	0	70	0
2.19	1.07	0	0	0	1.13	0	0.08	0.02	0.17	0.01	3.4	0	9.07	0.71	22.96	64.64	77.4	72.58	0.45
0.75	0.36	0	0	0	1.13	0.03	0.05	0.03	0.16	0.02	3.69	0	21.83	0.86	20.41	57.83	71.16	97.52	0.55
1.63	3.37	0	0	0	0.85	0	0.05	0.02	0.41	0.02	6.52	0	11.06	0.71	31.19	85.05	86.47	78.81	0.59
1.98	3.42	0	0	0	0.57	0.06	0.06	0.03	0.56	0.03	5.1	0	11.62	0.68	15.59	39.41	82.5	80.23	0.35
1.24	3.42	0	0	0	4.25	0.26	0.07	0.03	0.45	0.02	6.52	0	17.29	0.84	27.5	78.53	95.26	83.35	0.58
1	0.56	0	0	0	1.42	0	0.06	0.04	0.27	0.03	6.24	0.05	26.37	0.72	22.11	65.21	96.39	77.11	0.43
1.2	1.56	0	0	0	1.13	0	0.05	0.05	0.74	0.03	8.51	0.07	23.81	0.62	25.8	68.32	111.13	72.01	0.45
1.87	1.21	0	0	0	0.57	0	0.06	0.04	0.89	0.03	9.07	0.06	25.8	0.6	24.38	70.88	82.5	115.95	0.53
2.37	1.31	0	0	0	0.57	0	0.03	0.03	0.89	0.03	9.36	0.13	22.68	0.55	24.95	74.28	106.88	92.99	0.48
1.08	1.51	0	0	0	0	0	0.08	0.05	0.15	0.03	6.8	0.11	29.77	0.73	20.98	65.21	92.14	78.81	0.43
0.81	0.91	0	0	0	0	0	0.07	0.05	0.31	0.03	5.95	0.05	28.63	0.69	20.41	62.37	102.63	79.95	0.37
0	0	0	0	0	0	0	0	0	0	0	0	0	0.11	0.01	0.04	0.04	0.18	1.54	0
0	0	0	0	0	0	0	0	0	0	0	0	0	120	0	0	0	0	65	0
0	0	0	0	0	0	0	0	0	0	0	0	0	160	0	0	0	0	50	0
0	0	0	0	0	0	0	0	0	0	0	0	0	80	0	0	0	0	50	0
0	0	0	0	0	0	0	0	0	0	0	0	0	120	0	0	0	0	15	0
0	0	0	0	0	0	0	0	0	0	0	0	0	80	0	0	0	0	65	0
0.11	0.1	0	0	0	0	0	0.01	0.01	0.18	0	0.2	0	1	0.14	1.04	3.88	4.48	5.72	0.03
0.15	0.15	0	0	0	0	0	0.05	0.04	0.51	0.01	0.5	0	4.4	0.44	3.1	10.3	14.5	32	0.08
0	0	0	0	0	20	0	0	0	0	0	0	0	48	0.4	0	0	0	140	0
0	0	0	0	0	0	0	0.01	0.19	0	0.6	0	0	84	0.46	0	96	200	45	0
3	0.4	0	0	0	132	1	0.04	0.16	0.1	0.06	8	0.43	113	0.19	10	100	152	52	0.45
0	0	0	0	0	102.96	10.16	0.06	0.34	0.22	0.07	15.84	0.4	158.4	0.28	18.48	132	248.16	79.2	0.45
4.18	0.54	0	0	0	154.44	0.79	0.05	0.32	0.15	0.06	6.6	0.51	168.96	0.12	18.48	138.6	262.68	105.6	0.91
6.2	0.8	0	0	0	244.66	0.93	0.05	0.22	0.11	0.05	6.65	0.48	155.57	0.07	14.63	126.32	211.42	74.46	0.53
0.8	0.1	0	0	0	31	1	0.04	0.17	0.1	0.04	4	0.44	92	0.07	10	72	139	56	0.29
0.7	0.1	0	0	0	26	1	0.07	0.17	0.1	0.04	5	0.44	138	0.05	12	106	194	62	0.47
0	0	0	0	0	0	0	0	0	0	0	0	0	0	0	0.52	0	2.08	6.24	0.01
0	0	0	0	0	0	5.56	0	0	0	0	0	0	0	0	0.52	0	2.08	6.24	0.01
0	0	0	0	0	0	0	0	0	0	0	0	0	3	0.04	1	31	1	59	0.04
0	0	0	0	0	0	0	0	0	0	0	0	0	0.03	0.01	0.02	0.04	0.41	0.28	0
3.58	0.22	0	0	0.36	13.8	0.83	0.03	0.12	0.19	0.02	0	0.32	82.8	0.39	20.24	80.04	141.68	46.46	0.46
3.3	2.6	0	0	0	5.64	0.19	0.02	0.14	0.21	0.02	3.76	0.27	84.13	0.38	25.85	103.87	160.74	63.92	0.57
0	0	0	0	0	0	0	0	0	0	0	0	0	0.18	0.02	0.18	0.18	0.3	2.28	0
0	0	0	0	2.72	4.41	0	0.03	0.1	1.56	0.09	27.44	0.17	65.17	0.73	40.18	134.26	191.1	45.57	0.74
0	0	0	0	0.6	12.48	0	0.03	0.12	0.26	0.03	3.84	0.2	81.12	0.73	32.16	93.6	187.68	48.96	0.61
0	0	0	0	0	0	0	0	0	0	0	0	0	72	0.4	0	0	0	20	0
0	0	0	0	0	0	0	0	0	0.04	0	0.46	0	1.38	0.11	0.92	3.68	2.3	21.62	0.02
4.39	0.4	0	0	0.55	21.12	0.18	0.03	0.13	0.14	0.02	3.08	0.17	84.04	0.61	26.4	95.04	169.4	36.08	0.61
3.66	1.23	0	0	0.72	0	0	0.03	0.05	1.2	0.06	2.27	0.13	29.48	0.37	25.52	60.1	142.32	11.62	0.53
1.34	0.14	0	0	0.27	1.98	0.06	0.02	0.05	0.11	0.03	1.42	0.06	24.38	0.48	12.76	40.54	145.72	10.21	0.22
5.53	0.93	0	0	5.18	5.74	0.08	0.02	0.18	0.3	0.02	4.51	0.22	91.84	0.67	36.9	108.24	182.04	30.34	0.55
3.28	0.32	0	0	0.39	28.2	0.54	0.02	0.13	0.21	0.03	5.4	0.31	78	0.46	20.4	98.4	144.6	144	0.43
1.11	0.27	0	0	0	0	0	0.05	0.04	0.45	0.04	1.05	0	11.1	0.96	7.8	14.25	51.9	68.85	0.07
1.33	0.15	0	0	0.38	0.2	0.02	0	0.01	0.01	0.01	0.6	0	4.6	0.75	13.6	24	42	25	0.21
5.65	0.76	0	0	0.62	5	0	0.03	0.14	2.36	0.06	36	0.23	55.5	0.6	47.5	140	225	17	0.9
3.81	0.4	0	0	0	6	0.12	0.02	0.11	0.2	0.03	3.6	0.15	67.6	0.26	18.4	71.2	137.6	59.2	0.44
0.53	0.11	0	0	0	0.14	0.04	0.02	0.01	0.14	0	0.56	0	3.22	0.23	2.24	10.08	12.25	0.63	0.05
1.87	0.49	0	0	0	0.36	0.07	0.05	0.04	0.4	0.01	1.26	0	6.66	0.46	5.94	24.84	25.56	68.94	0.14
1.22	0.35	0	0	0	0.6	0.05	0.03	0.03	0.27	0.01	1.2	0	13.5	0.42	4.5	31.35	20.25	52.35	0.07
0.91	0.15	0	0	0	0.1	0	0.04	0.03	0.31	0	1	0.01	5.8	0.52	6.6	17.7	29.5	24.3	0.11

USDA ID Code	Food Name	Weight in Grams*	Quantity of Units	Unit of Measure	Protein (gm)	Fat (gm)	Carbohydrates (gm)	Kcalories	Caffeine (gm)	Fiber (gm)	Cholesterol (mg)	Saturated Fat (gm)
18166	Oreos, Regular	10	1	Each	0.47	2.06	7.03	47.2	0	0.3	0	0.41
18168	Oreos, w/ Extra Creme Filling	13	1	Each	0.47	3.28	8.85	65	0	0	0	0.63
19031	Oriental Mix, Rice-based	28.35	1	Ounce	5.67	11.54	9.38	154.51	0	3.74	0	5.04
19147	Peanut Bar	40	1	Bar	6.2	13.48	18.96	208.8	0	1.32	2.8	1.72
19148	Peanut Brittle	28.35	1	Ounce	2.13	5.41	19.65	128.43	0	0.57	3.69	1.42
18185	Peanut Butter Cookies, Regular	15	1	Each	1.44	3.54	8.84	71.55	0	0	0.15	0.8
18186	Peanut Butter Cookies, Soft-type	15	1	Each	0.8	3.66	8.66	68.55	0	0.26	0	0.81
18201	Peanut Butter Sandwich Cookies, Dietary	10	1	Each	1	3.4	5.08	53.5	0	0	0	1.18
18190	Peanut Butter Sandwich Cookies, Regular	14	1	Each	1.23	2.95	9.18	66.92	0	0	0	0.63
19034	Popcorn, Air-popped	8	1	Cup	0.96	0.34	6.23	30.56	0	1.21	0	0.05
19806	Popcorn, Air-popped, White Popcorn	8	1	Cup	0.96	0.34	6.23	30.56	0	0	0	0.05
19036	Popcorn, Cakes	10	1	Cake	0.97	0.31	8.01	38.4	0	0.29	0	0.05
19038	Popcorn, Caramel-coated, w/ Peanuts	35.182	1	Cup	2.25	2.74	28.39	140.73	0	1.34	0	0.37
19039	Popcorn, Caramel-coated, w/o Peanuts	35.2	1	Cup	1.34	4.51	27.84	151.71	0	1.83	1.76	1.27
19040	Popcorn, Cheese-flavor	6	1	Cup	1.02	3.65	5.68	57.86	0	1.09	1.21	0.71
62649	Popcorn, Microwave	14	4	Cup	0.75	3	4.25	42.5	0	0.75	0	0.75
62650	Popcorn, Microwave, Low-Fat	14	4	Cup	0.67	1	3.67	23.33	0	0.5	0	0.17
	Popcorn, Microwave-Pop Secret-94% Fat Free	5	1	Serving	1	0	4	20	0	0	0	0
19035	Popcorn, Oil-popped	11	1	Cup	0.99	3.09	6.29	55	0	1.1	0	0.54
19807	Popcorn, Oil-popped, White Popcorn	11	1	Cup	0.99	3.09	6.29	55	0	0	0	0.54
62602	Popsicles	56	1	Each	0	0	11	40	0	0	0	0
19408	Pork Skins, Barbecue-flavor	28.35	1	Ounce	16.41	9.02	0.45	152.52	0	0	32.6	3.28
19041	Pork Skins, Plain	28.35	1	Ounce	17.38	8.87	0	154.51	0	0	26.93	3.22
	Potato Chips - Baked Lays	28	1	Ounce	2	1.5	23	110	0	0	0	0
	Potato Chips - Barbeque	28	1	Ounce	2	10	15	160	0	0	0	1.5
19042	Potato Chips, Barbecue-flavor	28.35	1	Ounce	2.18	9.19	14.97	139.2	0	1.25	0	2.28
19421	Potato Chips, Cheese-flavor	28.35	1	Ounce	2.41	7.71	16.36	140.62	0	0	1.13	2.44
19422	Potato Chips, Light	28.35	1	Ounce	2.01	5.9	18.97	133.53	0	0	0	1.18
19411	Potato Chips, Plain, Salted	28.35	1	Ounce	1.98	9.81	15	151.96	0	1.28	0	3.11
19811	Potato Chips, Plain, Unsalted	28.35	1	Ounce	1.98	9.81	15	151.96	0	0	0	3.11
19412	Potato Chips, Pringles, Cheese-flavor	28.35	1	Ounce	1.98	10.49	14.35	156.21	0	0	1.13	2.71
19045	Potato Chips, Pringles, Light	28.35	1	Ounce	1.59	7.29	18.4	142.03	0	1.02	0	1.45
19410	Potato Chips, Pringles, Plain	28.35	1	Ounce	1.67	10.89	14.46	158.19	0	1.02	0	2.68
19046	Potato Chips, Pringles, Sour-cream&onion-flavor	28.35	1	Ounce	1.87	10.49	14.54	155.07	0	0	0.85	2.68
19043	Potato Chips, Sour-cream-and-onion-flavor	28.35	1	Ounce	2.3	9.61	14.6	150.54	0	1.47	1.98	2.52
11920	Potato Chips, w/o Salt Added	28.35	1	Ounce	1.82	10.03	14.7	148.27	0	1.36	0	2.57
19415	Potato Sticks	28.35	1	Ounce	1.9	9.75	15.11	147.99	0	0.96	0	2.52
62693	Power Bar	65	1	Each	10	2.5	45	230	0	3	0	0.5
19216	Praline	39	1	Piece	1.09	9.48	24.18	177.06	0	0	0	0.73
19047	Pretzels, Hard, Plain, Salted	28.35	1	Ounce	2.58	0.99	22.45	108.01	0	0.91	0	0.21
19814	Pretzels, Hard, Plain, Unsalted	28.35	1	Ounce	2.58	0.99	22.45	108.01	0	0.79	0	0.21
19050	Pretzels, Hard, Whole-wheat	28.35	1	Ounce	3.15	0.74	23.02	102.63	0	0	0	0.16
19072	Pudding Pops, Chocolate	47	1	Each	1.88	2.21	11.94	71.91	0	0.19	0.94	0
19073	Pudding Pops, Vanilla	47	1	Each	1.88	2.07	12.6	74.73	0	0	0.94	0
19311	Pudding, Banana	298.116	1	Cup	7.15	10.73	63.2	378.61	0	0	0	1.67
19167	Pudding, Bread	252	1	Cup	13.1	14.87	61.99	423.36	0	0	166.32	5.77
19183	Pudding, Chocolate	298.116	1	Cup	8.05	11.92	67.97	396.49	14.91	2.98	8.94	2.12
19380	Pudding, Lemon	298.116	1	Cup	0.3	8.94	74.53	372.65	0	0	0	1.34
19193	Pudding, Rice	298.116	1	Cup	5.96	22.36	65.59	485.93	0	0	2.98	3.49
19218	Pudding, Tapioca	298.116	1	Cup	5.96	11.03	57.83	354.76	0	0.3	2.98	1.79
19201	Pudding, Vanilla	298.116	1	Cup	6.86	10.73	65.29	387.55	0	0.3	20.87	1.7
18191	Raisin Cookies, Soft-type	15	1	Each	0.62	2.04	10.2	60.15	0	0	0.3	0.53
19149	Raisinets	1	10	Piece	0.05	0.16	0.71	4.12	0.25	0	0.04	0.07
62607	Reduced Fat Chocolate Chip Cookies	0.448	2	Each	1	1.25	10.5	50	0	0.02	0	0.02
62595	Reduced Fat Chocolate Sandwich Cookies-SnackWell	12.5	2	Each	0.5	1.25	10.5	50	0	0.5	0	0.25

Monounsaturated Fat (gm)	Polyunsaturated Fat (gm)	Vitamin D (mg)	Vitamin K (mg)	Vitamin E (mg)	Vitamin A (re)	Vitamin C (mg)	Thiamin (mg)	Riboflavin (mg)	Niacin (mg)	Vitamin B6 (mg)	Folate (mg)	Vitamin B12 (mcg)	Calcium (mg)	Iron (mg)	Magnesium (mg)	Phosphorus (mg)	Potassium (mg)	Sodium (mg)	Zinc (mg)
1.18	0.27	0	0	0	0	0	0.01	0.02	0.21	0	0.5	0	2.6	0.39	4.5	9.8	17.5	60.4	0.08
1.91	0.43	0	0	0	0	0	0.01	0.02	0.2	0	0.52	0	3.12	0.37	4.42	11.83	15.86	64.09	0.08
2.96	2.66	0	0	0	1.42	0.23	0.08	0.04	2.98	0.05	24.66	0	21.83	0.78	39.69	111.98	146.57	235.02	1.3
6.71	4.27	0	0	0.39	20.4	0	0.04	0.06	3.17	0.04	24	0.01	31.2	0.39	29.6	61.2	162.8	96.4	0.55
2.4	1.33	0	0	0.46	13.32	0	0.05	0.01	0.99	0.03	19.85	0	8.51	0.39	14.18	31.47	58.97	128.14	0.27
1.32	1.22	0	0	0	1.35	0	0.03	0.03	0.64	0.01	4.8	0.01	5.25	0.38	6.75	12.9	25.05	62.25	0.08
1.99	0.66	0	0	0	0	0	0.04	0.02	0.32	0.01	0.75	0	1.8	0.13	4.8	13.05	16.05	50.4	0.08
1.53	0.51	0	0	0	0	0	0.02	0.01	0.5	0.01	3.3	0	5.4	0.23	5	18.8	29.4	41.2	0.18
1.54	0.58	0	0	0	0.14	0.01	0.05	0.04	0.52	0.01	2.1	0.01	7.42	0.36	6.86	26.32	26.88	51.52	0.15
0.09	0.15	0	0	0.01	1.6	0	0.02	0.02	0.16	0.02	1.84	0	0.8	0.21	10.48	24	24.08	0.32	0.28
0.09	0.15	0	0	0	0.24	0	0.02	0.02	0.16	0.02	1.84	0	0.8	0.21	10.48	24	24.08	0.32	0.28
0.09	0.14	0	0	0.01	0.7	0	0.01	0.02	0.6	0.02	1.8	0	0.9	0.19	15.9	27.7	32.7	28.8	0.4
0.96	1.15	0	0	0.53	2.11	0	0.02	0.04	0.7	0.07	5.63	0	23.22	1.38	28.15	44.68	124.9	103.79	0.44
1.01	1.58	0	0	0.42	3.52	0	0.02	0.02	0.77	0.01	0.7	0	15.14	0.61	12.32	29.22	38.37	72.51	0.2
1.07	1.69	0	0	0.01	4.84	0.06	0.01	0.03	0.16	0.03	1.21	0.06	12.43	0.25	10.01	39.71	28.71	97.79	0.22
0	0	0	0	0	0	0	0	0	0	0	0	0	0	0.05	0	0	0	72.5	0
0	0	0	0	0	0	0	0	0	0	0	0	0	0	0.07	0	0	0	55	0
0	0	0	0	0	0	0	0	0	0	0	0	0	0	0	0	0	0	40	0
0.9	1.48	0	0	0.01	1.65	0.03	0.01	0.01	0.17	0.02	1.87	0	1.1	0.31	11.88	27.5	24.75	97.24	0.29
0.9	1.48	0	0	0	0.22	0.03	0.01	0.01	0.17	0.02	1.87	0	1.1	0.31	11.88	27.5	24.75	97.24	0.29
0	0	0	0	0	0	1.2	0	0	0	0	0	0	0	0	0	0	0	10	0
4.26	0.98	0	0	0	51.6	0.43	0.02	0.12	0.95	0.04	8.79	0.04	12.19	0.29	0	62.37	51.03	756.09	0.2
4.19	1.03	0	0	0	11.06	0.14	0.03	0.08	0.44	0.01	0	0.18	8.51	0.25	3.12	24.1	36	521.07	0.16
0	0	0	0	0	0	0	0	0	0	0	0	0	48	0.4	0	0	0	150	0
0	0	0	0	0	0	6.4	0	0	0	0	0	0	0	0.2	0	0	0	300	0
1.85	4.64	0	0	1.42	6.24	9.61	0.06	0.06	1.33	0.18	23.53	0	14.18	0.55	21.26	52.73	357.49	212.63	0.27
2.19	2.71	0	0	0	2.27	15.34	0.04	0.04	1.42	0.1	0	0	20.41	0.52	21.26	84.77	433.19	224.82	0.26
1.36	3.1	0	0	0	0	7.29	0.06	0.08	1.98	0.19	7.65	0	5.95	0.38	25.23	54.72	494.42	139.48	0.02
2.79	3.45	0	0	1.38	0	8.82	0.05	0.06	1.08	0.19	12.76	0	6.8	0.46	18.99	46.78	361.46	168.4	0.31
2.79	3.45	0	0	0	0	8.82	0.05	0.06	1.08	0.19	12.76	0	6.8	0.46	18.99	46.78	361.46	168.4	0.31
2.02	5.29	0	0	0	0	2.41	0.05	0.03	0.74	0.15	5.1	0	31.19	0.45	15.03	46.21	108.01	214.04	0.18
1.68	3.82	0	0	1.42	0	3.4	0.05	0.02	1.19	0.22	6.52	0	9.64	0.43	17.86	43.66	284.92	121.34	0.17
2.06	5.66	0	0	1.38	0	2.32	0.06	0.03	0.89	0.04	1.98	0	6.8	0.43	16.44	44.51	285.77	185.98	0.17
2.02	5.32	0	0	0	27.78	2.69	0.05	0.03	0.71	0.13	6.52	0	18.14	0.4	15.59	47.91	140.62	204.12	0.2
1.74	4.94	0	0	0	5.95	10.57	0.05	0.06	1.14	0.19	17.58	0.28	20.41	0.45	20.98	49.9	377.34	177.19	0.28
1.77	5.15	0	0	2.23	0	11.79	0.04	0.01	1.19	0.14	12.81	0	6.8	0.34	16.73	43.38	367.98	2.27	0.3
1.75	5.07	0	0	1.38	0	13.41	0.03	0.03	1.36	0.09	11.34	0	5.1	0.64	18.14	48.76	350.69	70.88	0.28
1.5	0.5	0	0	0	0	0	1.5	1.7	19	2	200	2	360	3.5	122.5	280	0	90	5.25
5.92	2.35	0	0	0	1.95	0.27	0.12	0.02	0.13	0.03	5.46	0	12.09	0.46	20.28	42.51	82.29	24.18	0.79
0.39	0.35	0	0	0.06	0	0	0.13	0.18	1.49	0.03	23.53	0	10.21	1.22	9.92	32.04	41.39	486.2	0.24
0.39	0.35	0	0	0.06	0	0	0.13	0.18	1.49	0.03	23.53	0	10.21	1.22	9.92	32.04	41.39	81.93	0.24
0.29	0.24	0	0	0	0	0.28	0.12	0.08	1.85	0.08	15.31	0	7.94	0.76	8.51	35.44	121.91	57.55	0.18
0	0	0	0	0.01	15.51	0.19	0.02	0.08	0.06	0.01	1.41	0.25	66.27	0.22	9.87	52.64	105.28	77.55	0.17
0	0	0	0	0.01	24.44	0.14	0.02	0.09	0.02	0.02	2.35	0.17	60.63	0.03	5.17	47.47	64.86	49.82	0.16
4.56	3.96	0	0	0	89.43	1.49	0.06	0.44	0.49	0.06	5.96	0.54	253.4	0.39	23.85	205.7	327.93	584.31	0.83
5.42	2.39	0	0	0	163.8	2.02	0.23	0.56	1.58	0.19	32.76	0	287.28	2.77	47.88	274.68	564.48	582.12	1.31
5.07	4.26	0	0	0.37	32.79	5.37	0.08	0.46	1.03	0.08	8.94	0	268.3	1.52	62.6	238.49	536.61	384.57	1.25
3.88	3.4	0	0	0	0	0.3	0	0.01	0.01	0	0	0	5.96	0.21	2.98	14.91	2.98	417.36	0.09
9.57	8.32	0	0	0	104.34	1.49	0.05	0.21	0.48	0.09	8.94	0.63	155.02	0.89	23.85	202.72	178.87	253.4	1.46
4.71	4.05	0	0	0.27	0	2.09	0.07	0.29	0.93	0.29	11.92	0.33	250.42	0.69	23.85	235.51	310.04	351.78	0.8
4.59	3.99	0	0	0.37	17.89	0	0.07	0.41	0.75	0.03	0	0.3	262.34	0.39	23.85	202.72	336.87	402.46	0.75
1.12	0.27	0	0	0	1.8	0.05	0.03	0.03	0.3	0.01	1.35	0.02	6.9	0.34	3.15	12.45	21	50.7	0.05
0.06	0.02	0	0	0	0.09	0	0	0	0	0	0.05	0	1.08	0.01	0.45	1.44	5.14	0.36	0.01
0.02	0	0	0	0	0	0	0	0	0	0	0	0	0	0.01	0	0	0	2.63	0
0.25	0	0	0	0	0	0	0	0	0	0	0	0	0	0.2	0	0	0	95	0

USDA ID Code	Food Name	Weight in Grams*	Quantity of Units	Unit of Measure	Protein (gm)	Fat (gm)	Carbohydrates (gm)	Kcalories	Caffeine (gm)	Fiber (gm)	Cholesterol (mg)	Saturated Fat (gm)
62593	Reduced Fat Classic Golden Crackers-SnackWell	2.33	6	Each	0.17	0.17	1.83	9.99	0	0	0	0
62594	Reduced Fat Creme Sandwich Cookies-SnackWell	13	2	Each	0.5	1.25	10.5	55	0	0.5	0	0.25
62597	Reduced Fat French Onion Snack Crackers-SnackWell	0.938	32	Each	0.06	0.06	0.72	3.75	0	0.03	0.72	0
62598	Reduced Fat Oatmeal Raisin Cookies-SnackWell	13.5	2	Each	1	1.25	10	55	0	0.5	0	0
62525	Reduced Fat Zesty Cheese Snack Crackers-SnackWell	0.938	32	Each	0.09	0.06	0.72	3.75	0	0.03	0.16	0.02
19150	Reese's Peanut Butter Cups	7	1	Each	0.77	2.18	3.35	33.95	0.77	0.29	1.05	1.61
19151	Reese's Pieces Candy	55	1	Pkg	7.21	11.39	34.16	257.95	0	2.26	2.2	0
19052	Rice Cakes, Brown Rice, Buckwheat	9	1	Cake	0.81	0.32	7.21	34.2	0	0.34	0	0.06
19817	Rice Cakes, Brown Rice, Buckwheat, Unsalted	9	1	Cake	0.81	0.32	7.21	34.2	0	0	0	0.06
19413	Rice Cakes, Brown Rice, Corn	9	1	Cake	0.76	0.29	7.31	34.65	0	0.26	0	0.06
19414	Rice Cakes, Brown Rice, Multigrain	9	1	Cake	0.77	0.32	7.21	34.83	0	0.27	0	0.05
19818	Rice Cakes, Brown Rice, Multigrain, Unsalted	9	1	Cake	0.77	0.32	7.21	34.83	0	0	0	0.05
19051	Rice Cakes, Brown Rice, Plain	9	1	Cake	0.74	0.25	7.34	34.83	0	0.38	0	0.05
19816	Rice Cakes, Brown Rice, Plain, Unsalted	9	1	Cake	0.74	0.25	7.34	34.83	0	0.38	0	0.05
19416	Rice Cakes, Brown Rice, Rye	9	1	Cake	0.73	0.34	7.19	34.74	0	0.36	0	0.05
62669	Rice Krispie Treats	40	1	Cup	1.33	2	33.33	160	0	0	0	0
	Ruffles - Reduced Fat	28	1	Ounce	2	6.7	18	140	0	0	0	1
19418	Sesame Sticks, Wheat-based, Salted	28.35	1	Ounce	3.09	10.4	13.18	153.37	0	0.79	0	1.84
19820	Sesame Sticks, Wheat-based, Unsalted	28.35	1	Ounce	3.09	10.4	13.18	153.37	0	0	0	1.84
19097	Sherbet, All Flavors	192	1	Cup	2.11	3.84	58.37	264.96	0	0	9.6	2.23
18193	Shortbread Cookies, Pecan	14	1	Each	0.69	4.55	8.16	75.88	0	0.25	4.62	0.99
18192	Shortbread Cookies, Plain	8	1	Each	0.49	1.93	5.16	40.16	0	0	1.6	0.49
19370	Skittles Bite Size Candies	65	1	Pkg	0.2	1.95	62.4	254.8	0	0	0	0
19407	Slim Jims, Smoked	28.35	1	Ounce	6.1	14.06	1.53	155.93	0	0	37.71	5.9
19155	Snickers Bar	61	1	Bar	5.86	13.6	36.78	277.55	0	1.83	7.32	7.29
	Sorbet - Ben & Jerry's	110	0.5	Cup	0	0	32	130	0	0	0	0
62599	Sorbet, All Flavors	180.053	0.5	Cup	0	0	50.01	200.06	0	2	0	0
19164	Special Dark Sweet Chocolate Bar	79	1	Bar	3.71	23.86	48.66	376.04	60.04	4.35	0	0
18203	Sugar Cookies, Dietary	7	1	Each	0.81	0.91	4.85	30.17	0	0	0	0.16
18204	Sugar Cookies, Regular (includes Vanilla)	15	1	Each	0.77	3.17	10.19	71.7	0	0	7.65	0.81
	Sun Chips - original	28	1	Ounce	1	6	20	140	0	0	0	1
19093	Symphony Milk Chocolate Bar	68	1	Bar	5.3	22.03	38.62	354.96	0	0	19.04	0
19113	Syrup, Pancake, w/ Butter	20	1	Tbsp.	0	0.32	14.82	59.2	0	0	0.8	0.2
19382	Taffy	15	1	Piece	0.02	0.5	13.71	56.4	0	0	1.35	0.31
19524	Taro Chips	28.35	1	Ounce	0.65	7.06	19.31	141.18	0	2.04	0	1.82
19159	Three Musketeers Bar	60	1	Bar	1.92	7.74	46.08	249.6	0	0.96	6.6	3.9
18361	Toaster Pastries, Brown-sugar-cinn.	52	1	Each	2.65	7.38	35.41	214.24	0	0	0	1.87
18362	Toaster Pastries, Fruit	52	1	Each	2.44	5.3	36.97	204.36	0	0	0	0.8
19383	Toffee	12	1	Piece	0.13	3.94	7.72	65.04	0	0	12.6	2.45
62655	Tortilla Chips, Low-Fat, Baked	2.181	13	Chips	0.23	0.08	1.85	8.46	0	0.15	0	0
19057	Tortilla Chips, Nacho-flavor	28.35	1	Ounce	2.21	7.26	17.69	141.18	0	1.5	0.85	1.39
19424	Tortilla Chips, Nacho-flavor, Light	28.35	1	Ounce	2.47	4.31	20.3	126.16	0	0	0.85	0.82
19056	Tortilla Chips, Plain	28.35	1	Ounce	1.98	7.43	17.83	142.03	0	1.87	0	1.42
19058	Tortilla Chips, Ranch-flavor	28.35	1	Ounce	2.15	6.75	18.31	138.92	0	0	0.28	1.29
19063	Tortilla Chips, Taco-flavor	28.35	1	Ounce	2.24	6.86	17.89	136.08	0	0	1.42	1.32
	Tostitos - Baked	28	1	Ounce	2	1	24	110	0	0	0	0
	Tostitos - Baked, salsa & sour cream	28	1	Ounce	2	3	21	120	0	0	0	0.5
19059	Trail Mix, Regular	150	1	Cup	20.7	44.1	67.35	693	0	0	0	8.33
19821	Trail Mix, Regular, Unsalted	150	1	Cup	20.7	44.1	67.35	693	0	0	0	8.33
19062	Trail Mix, Regular, w/ Chocolate Chips	146	1	Cup	20.73	46.57	65.55	706.64	0	0	5.84	8.91
19061	Trail Mix, Tropical	140	1	Cup	8.82	23.94	91.84	569.8	0	0	0	11.87
62673	Triscuits	4.429	7	Each	0.43	0.71	3	20	0	0.57	0	0.14
62674	Triscuits, Low-Fat	4	8	Each	0.38	0.38	3	16.25	0	0.5	0	0.06
19138	Truffles	12	1	Piece	0.68	4.12	5.4	58.56	0	0	6.24	2.58
19160	Twix	57	1	Each	3.08	13.4	37.45	272.46	1.71	0.97	5.13	0

Monounsaturated Fat (gm)	Polyunsaturated Fat (gm)	Vitamin D (mg)	Vitamin K (mg)	Vitamin E (mg)	Vitamin A (re)	Vitamin C (mg)	Thiamin (mg)	Riboflavin (mg)	Niacin (mg)	Vitamin B6 (mg)	Folate (mg)	Vitamin B12 (mcg)	Calcium (mg)	Iron (mg)	Magnesium (mg)	Phosphorus (mg)	Potassium (mg)	Sodium (mg)	Zinc (mg)
0	0	0	0	0	0	0	0	0	0	0	0	0	3.99	0.07	0	0	0	23.3	0
0.5	0	0	0	0	0	0	0	0	0	0	0	0	12	0.1	0	0	0	47.5	0
0.02	0	0	0	0	0	0	0	0	0	0	0	0	1.5	0.02	0	0	0	9.06	0
0.25	0.25	0	0	0	0	0	0	0	0	0	0	0	12	0.2	0	0	0	67.5	0
0.02	0	0	0	0	0	0	0	0	0	0	0	0	1.5	0.02	0	0	0	10.94	0
0.15	0.15	0	0	0.09	1.33	0	0	0.01	0.28	0.01	1.96	0.03	5.46	0.08	5.95	16.8	28	20.3	0.1
0	0	0	0	0.73	2.2	0.28	0.03	0.13	3.14	0.07	30.8	0.18	73.15	0.83	44.55	126.5	242	82.5	0.61
0.1	0.1	0	0	0	0	0	0.01	0.01	0.73	0.01	1.89	0	0.99	0.1	13.59	34.2	26.91	10.44	0.23
0.1	0.1	0	0	0	0	0	0.01	0.01	0.73	0.01	1.89	0	0.99	0.1	13.59	34.2	26.91	0.36	0.23
0.1	0.1	0	0	0	0	0	0.01	0.01	0.58	0.01	1.71	0	0.81	0.11	10.26	28.8	24.75	26.19	0.2
0.1	0.13	0	0	0	0	0	0.01	0.02	0.59	0.01	1.8	0	1.89	0.18	12.33	33.3	26.46	22.68	0.23
0.1	0.13	0	0	0	0	0	0.01	0.02	0.59	0.01	1.8	0	1.89	0.18	12.33	33.3	26.46	0.36	0.23
0.09	0.09	0	0	0.06	0.45	0	0.01	0.01	0.7	0.01	1.89	0	0.99	0.13	11.79	32.4	26.1	29.34	0.27
0.09	0.09	0	0	0.01	0.45	0	0.01	0.01	0.7	0.01	1.89	0	0.99	0.13	11.79	32.4	26.1	2.34	0.27
0.12	0.14	0	0	0	0	0	0.01	0.01	0.63	0.01	0.45	0	1.89	0.16	12.96	34.2	27.99	9.9	0.27
1.33	0	0.67	0	0	200	20	0.5	0.57	6.33	0.67	0	0.67	0	1.33	0	21.33	26.67	226.67	0
0	0	0	0	0	0	0	0	0	0	0	0	0	0	0.2	0	0	0	130	0
3.09	4.94	0	0	1.11	2.55	0	0.03	0.02	0.44	0.02	6.24	0	48.2	0.21	12.76	39.12	50.18	421.85	0.33
3.09	4.94	0	0	0	2.55	0	0.03	0.02	0.44	0.02	6.24	0	48.2	0.21	12.76	39.12	50.18	8.22	0.33
1.02	0.15	0	0	0	26.88	8.26	0.05	0.13	0.18	0.07	7.68	0.25	103.68	0.27	15.36	76.8	184.32	88.32	0.92
2.65	0.68	0	0	0	0.28	0.03	0.04	0.03	0.35	0	1.12	0	4.2	0.34	2.52	11.9	10.22	39.34	0.08
1.08	0.25	0	0	0	0.96	0	0.03	0.03	0.27	0	0.72	0.01	2.8	0.22	1.36	8.64	8	36.4	0.04
0	0	0	0	0	0	0	0	0	0	0	0	0	1.95	0.07	0.65	1.95	14.95	29.9	0.01
5.8	1.25	0	0	0	47.91	1.93	0.04	0.12	1.29	0.06	0	0.28	19.28	0.96	5.95	51.03	72.86	419.58	0.69
4.11	0.52	0	0	3.39	18.91	0.18	0.03	0.11	1.82	0.11	24.4	0.25	70.15	0.48	36.6	128.71	198.86	163.48	0.7
0	0	0	0	0	0	0	0	0	0	0	0	0	80	0	0	0	0	10	0
0	0	0	0	0	0	24.01	0	0	0	0	0	0	0	0	0	0	0	20.01	0
0	0	0	0	0.8	1.58	0	0.02	0.19	0.53	0.04	3.16	0	15.01	1.66	90.85	126.4	268.6	7.9	1.19
0.53	0.13	0	0	0	0	0	0.03	0.01	0.22	0	0.49	0	2.1	0.27	0.63	5.67	7.28	0.21	0.02
1.76	0.4	0	0	0	4.05	0.02	0.03	0.03	0.4	0.01	1.65	0.02	3.15	0.32	1.8	12	9.45	53.55	0.06
0	0	0	0	0	0	1.2	0	0	0	0	0	0	0	0	0	0	0	115	0
0	0	0	0	0	8.84	0.27	0.06	0.26	0.22	0.03	4.76	0.27	159.8	0.68	37.4	170	261.8	58.48	0.77
0.09	0.01	0	0	0	3	0	0	0	0	0	0	0	0.4	0.02	0.4	2	0.6	19.6	0.01
0.14	0.02	0	0	0	4.95	0	0	0	0	0	0	0	0.45	0.01	0.15	0.45	0.6	13.35	0
1.26	3.65	0	0	1.39	0	1.42	0.05	0.01	0.15	0.12	5.67	0	17.01	0.34	23.81	37.14	214.04	96.96	0.11
2.57	0.27	0	0	0.28	15.6	0.24	0.02	0.08	0.14	0.01	0	0.13	50.4	0.44	17.4	54.6	79.8	116.4	0.33
4.15	0.96	0	0	0	116.48	0.1	0.19	0.3	2.38	0.22	41.6	0.06	17.68	2.1	12.48	69.16	59.28	220.48	0.33
2.14	2.01	0	0	0	55.12	0.16	0.15	0.19	2.05	0.2	41.6	0.03	13.52	1.81	9.36	57.72	58.24	217.88	0.34
1.14	0.15	0	0	0	38.16	0.02	0	0.01	0	0	0.24	0.01	4.08	0.01	0.48	3.96	6	22.44	0.02
0	0	0	0	0	0	0	0	0	0	0	0	0	3.69	0	0	0	0	10.77	0
4.28	1	0	0	0	11.62	0.51	0.04	0.05	0.41	0.08	3.97	0.01	41.67	0.41	23.25	69.17	61.24	200.72	0.34
2.54	0.6	0	0	0	11.91	0.06	0.06	0.08	0.12	0.07	7.37	0	45.08	0.46	27.5	90.15	77.11	284.35	0
4.38	1.03	0	0	0.39	5.67	0	0.02	0.05	0.36	0.08	3.12	0	43.66	0.43	24.95	58.12	55.85	149.69	0.43
3.98	0.94	0	0	0	7.65	0.26	0.03	0.07	0.41	0.06	4.82	0	39.97	0.41	25.23	67.76	69.17	173.5	0.35
4.05	0.95	0	0	0	25.8	0.26	0.07	0.06	0.57	0.08	5.95	0	43.94	0.57	24.95	67.76	61.52	223.11	0.36
0	0	0	0	0	0	0	0	0	0	0	0	0	32	0.2	0	0	0	200	0
0	0	0	0	0	0	0	0	0	0	0	0	0	32	0.2	0	0	0	190	0
18.8	14.48	0	0	0	3	2.1	0.69	0.3	7.07	0.45	106.5	0	117	4.58	237	517.5	1027.5	343.5	4.83
18.8	14.48	0	0	0	3	2.1	0.69	0.3	7.07	0.45	106.5	0	117	4.58	237	517.5	1027.5	15	4.83
19.77	16.48	0	0	0	7.3	1.9	0.6	0.33	6.43	0.38	94.9	0	159.14	4.95	235.06	565.02	946.08	176.66	4.58
3.49	7.22	0	0	0	7	10.64	0.63	0.16	2.07	0.46	58.8	0	79.8	3.7	134.4	260.4	992.6	14	1.64
0.07	0.21	0	0	0	0	0	0	0	0	0	0	0	0	0.11	0	11.43	0	24.29	0
0	0.13	0	0	0	0	0	0	0	0	0	0	0	0	0.13	0	15	0	22.5	0
1.22	0.13	0	0	0	17.16	0.05	0.01	0.03	0.03	0	0.12	0.04	18.6	0.12	5.64	21.24	36.6	8.52	0.13
0	0	0	0	0.4	18.24	0.11	0.03	0.11	0.21	0.02	3.99	0.22	67.26	0.38	16.53	76.38	117.42	114.57	0.39

USDA ID Code	Food Name	Weight in Grams*	Quantity of Units	Unit of Measure	Protein (gm)	Fat (gm)	Carbohydrates (gm)	Kcalories	Caffeine (gm)	Fiber (gm)	Cholesterol (mg)	Saturated Fat (gm)
19112	Twizzlers Strawberry Candy	71	1	Pkg	2.34	1.14	65.82	262.7	0	0	0	0
18210	Vanilla Sandwich Cookies w/ Creme Filling	10	1	Each	0.45	2	7.21	48.3	0	0.15	0	0.36
18213	Vanilla Wafers, Higher Fat	6	1	Each	0.26	1.16	4.27	28.38	0	0	0	0.3
18212	Vanilla Wafers, Lower Fat	4	1	Each	0.2	0.61	2.94	17.64	0	0	2.32	0.14
62675	Wheat Thins	1.813	16	Each	0.13	0.38	1.19	8.75	0	0.13	0	0.06
62676	Wheat Thins, Low-Fat	1.611	18	Each	0.11	0.22	1.17	6.67	0	0.11	0	0.03
19393	Yogurt, Soft-serve, Chocolate	144.089	1	Cup	5.76	8.65	35.88	230.54	0	0	7.2	5.23
19293	Yogurt, Soft-serve, Vanilla	144.089	1	Cup	5.76	8.07	34.87	229.1	0	0	2.88	4.93
	York Peppermint Pattie (large)	42	1	Lg Patty	0.92	2.98	33.64	165.06	0	0.84	0.42	1.81
19091	York Peppermint Pattie (small)	17	1	Sm Patty	0.37	1.2	13.61	66.81	0	0.34	0.17	0.73
6474	Soup, Bean w/ Bacon	253	1	Cup	7.9	5.9	22.8	172	0	8.6	3	1.5
6007	Soup, Bean w/ Ham	256	1	Cup	12.61	8.51	27.12	230.85	0	11.18	21.87	3.33
6406	Soup, Bean w/ Hot Dogs	256	1	Cup	9.97	6.97	22	187.5	0	0	12.5	2.12
6404	Soup, Bean w/ Pork	253	1	Cup	7.89	5.95	22.8	172.04	0	8.6	2.53	1.52
6008	Soup, Beef Broth or Bouillon	240	1	Cup	3	0.53	1	30	0	0	0	0.5
6547	Soup, Beef Mushroom	244	1	Cup	5.8	3	6.3	73	0	0	7	1.5
6409	Soup, Beef Noodle	244	1	Cup	4.83	3.07	8.98	82.96	0	0.73	4.88	1.15
6070	Soup, Beef, Chunky	230	1	Cup	11.74	5.14	19.56	170.4	0	1.44	14.4	2.54
6402	Soup, Black Bean	247	1	Cup	5.63	1.51	19.81	116.09	0	4.45	0	0.4
6478	Soup, Cauliflower	253	1	Cup	2.89	1.72	10.73	69.15	0	0	0	0.26
6411	Soup, Cheese	247	1	Cup	5.41	10.47	10.52	155.61	0	0	29.64	6.67
6480	Soup, Chicken Broth or Bouillon	244	1	Cup	1.34	1.1	1.44	21.96	0	0	0	0.27
6417	Soup, Chicken Gumbo	244	1	Cup	2.64	1.44	8.37	56.12	0	1.95	4.88	0.32
6549	Soup, Chicken Mushroom	244	1	Cup	4.39	9.15	9.27	131.76	0	0	9.76	2.39
6419	Soup, Chicken Noodle	241	1	Cup	4.05	2.46	9.35	74.71	0	0.72	7.23	0.65
6018	Soup, Chicken Noodle, Chunky	240	1	Cup	12.72	6	17.04	175.2	0	3.84	19.2	1.39
6485	Soup, Chicken Rice	241	1	Cup	2.45	1.44	9.25	60.67	0	0.76	2.53	0.33
6022	Soup, Chicken Rice, Chunky	243	1	Cup	12.26	3.19	12.98	127.2	0	0.96	12	0.96
6425	Soup, Chicken Vegetable	241	1	Cup	3.62	2.84	8.58	74.71	0	0.96	9.64	0.84
6024	Soup, Chicken Vegetable, Chunky	240	1	Cup	12.31	4.82	18.89	165.6	0	0	16.8	1.44
6412	Soup, Chicken w/ Dumplings	241	1	Cup	5.62	5.52	6.05	96.4	0	0.72	33.74	1.3
6423	Soup, Chicken w/ Rice	241	1	Cup	3.54	1.9	7.16	60.25	0	0.72	7.23	0.46
6015	Soup, Chicken, Chunky	251	1	Cup	12.7	6.63	17.27	178.21	0	1.51	30.12	1.98
6426	Soup, Chili Beef	250	1	Cup	6.7	6.6	21.45	170	0	9.5	12.5	3.35
6027	Soup, Clam Chowder, Manhattan Style	244	1	Cup	2.2	2.2	12.2	78	0	1.5	2	0.4
6230	Soup, Clam Chowder, New England	248	1	Cup	4.8	2.9	12.4	95	0	1.5	5	0.4
6034	Soup, Crab	240	1	Cup	5.49	1.51	10.3	75.64	0	0.73	9.76	0.39
6201	Soup, Cream Of Asparagus	248	1	Cup	6.32	8.18	16.39	161.2	0	0.74	22.32	3.32
6210	Soup, Cream Of Celery	248	1	Cup	5.68	9.7	14.53	163.68	0	0.74	32.24	3.94
6216	Soup, Cream Of Chicken	248	1	Cup	7.46	11.46	14.98	190.96	0	0.25	27.28	4.64
6243	Soup, Cream Of Mushroom	248	1	Cup	6.05	13.59	15	203.36	0	0.5	19.84	5.13
6246	Soup, Cream Of Onion	248	1	Cup	6.8	9.37	18.35	186	0	0.74	32.24	4.04
6253	Soup, Cream Of Potato	248	1	Cup	5.78	6.45	17.16	148.8	0	0.5	22.32	3.77
6256	Soup, Cream Of Shrimp	248	1	Cup	6.82	9.3	13.91	163.68	0	0.25	34.72	5.78
6501	Soup, Cream Of Vegetable	260.1	1	Cup	1.9	5.7	12.3	106.64	0	0.52	0	1.43
6036	Soup, Gazpacho	244	1	Cup	8.69	2.24	0.78	56.12	0	3.66	0	0.29
	Soup, Hot and Sour	244	1	Cup	15	8	5	162	0	0.5	34	3
	Soup, Instant	240	1	Cup	3	1	7	50	0	0.7	2	0.001
6037	Soup, Lentil w/ ham	248	1	Cup	9.28	2.78	20.24	138.88	0	0	7.44	1.12
6440	Soup, Minestrone	241	1	Cup	4.27	2.51	11.23	81.94	0	0.96	2.41	0.55
6039	Soup, Minestrone, Chunky	240	1	Cup	5.11	2.81	20.74	127.2	0	1.92	4.8	1.49
6493	Soup, Mushroom	253	1	Cup	2.23	4.86	11.13	96.14	0	0.76	0	0.81
6445	Soup, Onion	241	1	Cup	3.76	1.74	8.17	57.84	0	0.96	0	0.27
6249	Soup, Pea, Green	254	1	Cup	12.62	7.04	32.23	238.76	0	2.79	17.78	4.01
6451	Soup, Pea, Split w/ Ham	253	1	Cup	10.32	4.4	27.96	189.75	0	0	7.59	1.77

Monounsaturated Fat (gm)	Polyunsaturated Fat (gm)	Vitamin D (mg)	Vitamin K (mg)	Vitamin E (mg)	Vitamin A (re)	Vitamin C (mg)	Thiamin (mg)	Riboflavin (mg)	Niacin (mg)	Vitamin B6 (mg)	Folate (mcg)	Vitamin B12 (mcg)	Calcium (mg)	Iron (mg)	Magnesium (mg)	Phosphorus (mg)	Potassium (mg)	Sodium (mg)	Zinc (mg)
0	0	0	0	0	0	0	0.01	0.03	0.07	0.01	0	0	24.85	0.36	4.26	220.1	45.44	196.67	0.11
1.18	0.28	0	0	0	0	0	0.03	0.02	0.27	0	0.4	0	2.7	0.22	1.4	7.5	9.1	34.9	0.04
0.66	0.15	0	0	0	0	0	0.02	0.01	0.18	0	0.48	0	1.5	0.13	0.72	3.84	6.42	18.36	0.02
0.24	0.15	0	0	0	0.72	0	0.01	0.01	0.12	0	0.36	0	1.92	0.1	0.56	4.16	3.88	12.48	0.01
0.03	0.16	0	0	0	0	0	0	0	0	0	0	0	1.5	0.03	0	0	0	10.63	0
0	0.08	0	0	0	0	0	0	0	0	0	0	0	1.33	0.02	0	4.44	0	12.22	0
2.52	0.32	0	0	0	61.96	0.43	0.05	0.3	0.44	0.11	15.85	0.42	211.81	1.8	38.9	200.28	376.07	141.21	0.71
2.29	0.3	0	0	0.07	82.13	1.15	0.05	0.32	0.41	0.12	8.65	0.42	206.05	0.43	20.17	185.88	304.03	125.36	0.61
1.05	0.084	0	0	0	0	0	0	0	0	0	0	0	6.3	0.42	0	0	54.18	10.08	0
0.43	0.034	0	0	0	0.11	0	0	0.01	0.09	0	0.44	0	2.55	0.17	0	0	21.93	4.08	0
2.2	1.8	0	0	0.26	89	2	0.09	0.03	0.6	0.04	32	0.05	81	2.05	46	132	402	951	1.03
3.84	0.95	0	0	0.07	396.09	4.37	0.15	0.15	1.7	0.12	29.16	0.07	77.76	3.23	46.17	143.37	425.25	972	1.07
2.72	1.65	0	0	0	87.5	1	0.11	0.06	1.03	0.13	30	0.07	87.5	2.35	47.5	165	477.5	1092.5	1.18
2.18	1.82	0	0	0.08	88.55	1.52	0.09	0.03	0.57	0.04	31.88	0.05	80.96	2.05	45.54	131.56	402.27	951.28	1.03
0.44	0.04	0	0	0	0	0	0	0.1	3.74	0.04	9.6	0.34	40	0.8	9.6	62	260	1800	0
1.2	0.1	0	0	0	0	5	0.04	0.06	1	0.05	10	0.2	5	0.88	10	34	154	942	1.46
1.24	0.49	0	0	0	63.44	0.24	0.07	0.06	1.07	0.04	4.39	0.2	14.64	1.1	4.88	46.36	100.04	951.6	1.54
2.14	0.22	0	0	0.17	261.6	6.96	0.06	0.15	2.7	0.13	13.44	0.62	31.2	2.33	4.8	120	336	866.4	2.64
0.54	0.47	0	0	0.07	49.4	0.74	0.08	0.05	0.53	0.09	24.7	0.02	44.46	2.15	41.99	106.21	274.17	1197.95	1.41
0.74	0.64	0	0	0	0	2.56	0.08	0.08	0.51	0.03	2.56	0.18	10.24	0.51	2.56	51.22	105	842.57	0.26
2.96	0.3	0	0	0	108.68	0	0.02	0.14	0.4	0.02	4.94	0	140.79	0.74	4.94	135.85	153.14	958.36	0.64
0.41	0.37	0	0	0.02	12.2	0	0.01	0.03	0.2	0	2.44	0.02	14.64	0.07	4.88	12.2	24.4	1483.52	0.01
0.66	0.34	0	0	0.04	14.64	4.88	0.02	0.05	0.66	0.06	4.88	0.02	24.4	0.9	4.88	24.4	75.64	954.04	0.38
4.03	2.32	0	0	0	112.24	0	0.02	0.11	1.63	0.05	0.24	0.05	29.28	0.88	9.76	26.84	153.72	941.84	0.98
1.11	0.55	0	0	0.07	72.3	0.24	0.05	0.06	1.39	0.03	2.17	0.14	16.87	0.77	4.82	36.15	55.43	1106.19	0.4
2.66	1.51	0	0	0.79	122.4	0	0.07	0.17	4.32	0.05	4.8	0.31	24	1.44	9.6	72	108	849.6	0.96
0.63	0.43	0	0	0.04	0	0	0	0	0.36	0.03	0.51	0.08	7.58	0	0	10.11	10.11	980.86	0.13
1.44	0.67	0	0	0.09	585.6	3.84	0.02	0.1	4.1	0.05	3.84	0.31	33.6	1.87	9.6	72	108	888	0.96
1.28	0.6	0	0	0.08	265.1	0.96	0.04	0.06	1.23	0.05	4.82	0.12	16.87	0.87	7.23	40.97	154.24	944.72	0.37
2.16	1.01	0	0	0	600	5.52	0.04	0.17	3.29	0.1	12	0.24	26.4	1.46	9.6	105.6	367.2	1068	2.16
2.53	1.3	0	0	0.14	53.02	0	0.02	0.07	1.75	0.04	2.41	0.17	14.46	0.63	4.82	60.25	115.68	860.37	0.37
0.92	0.41	0	0	0.05	65.07	0.24	0.02	0.02	1.13	0.02	0.96	0.14	16.87	0.75	0	21.69	101.22	814.58	0.26
2.96	1.38	0	0	0.18	130.52	1.26	0.09	0.17	4.42	0.05	4.52	0.25	25.1	1.73	7.53	112.95	175.7	888.54	1
2.8	0.27	0	0	0.17	150	4	0.06	0.07	1.07	0.16	17.5	0.32	42.5	2.12	30	147.5	525	1035	1.4
0.4	1.3	0	0	0.1	98	4	0.03	0.04	0.8	0.1	10	4.05	27	1.63	12	41	188	578	0.98
1.2	1.1	0	0	0.15	0	2	0.02	0.04	1	0.08	4	8	44	1.49	7	54	146	915	0.75
0.68	0.39	0	0	0.1	51.24	0	0.2	0.07	1.34	0.12	14.64	0.2	65.88	1.22	14.64	87.84	326.96	1234.64	1.46
2.08	2.23	0	0	0.84	84.32	3.97	0.1	0.28	0.88	0.06	29.76	0.5	173.6	0.87	19.84	153.76	359.6	1041.6	0.93
2.46	2.65	0	0	0.97	66.96	1.49	0.07	0.25	0.44	0.06	8.43	0.5	186	0.69	22.32	151.28	310	1009.36	0.2
4.46	1.64	0	0	0.24	94.24	1.24	0.07	0.26	0.92	0.07	7.69	0.55	181.04	0.67	17.36	151.28	272.8	1046.56	0.67
2.98	4.61	0	0	1.34	37.2	2.23	0.08	0.28	0.91	0.06	9.92	0.5	178.56	0.6	19.84	156.24	270.32	1076.32	0.64
3.27	1.59	0	0	0.07	66.96	2.48	0.1	0.27	0.61	0.07	12.4	0.5	178.56	0.69	22.32	153.76	310	1004.4	0.62
1.74	0.57	0	0	0.1	66.96	1.24	0.08	0.24	0.64	0.09	9.18	0.5	166.16	0.55	17.36	161.2	322.4	1061.44	0.67
2.68	0.35	0	0	0.87	54.56	1.24	0.06	0.23	0.53	0.45	9.92	1.04	163.68	0.6	22.32	146.32	248	1036.64	0.8
2.55	1.48	0	0	1.24	2.6	3.9	1.22	0.11	0.52	0.03	7.8	0.13	31.21	0.52	10.4	54.62	96.24	1170.45	0.26
0.54	1.32	0	0	0.46	19.52	3.17	0.05	0.02	0.93	0.15	9.76	0	24.4	0.98	7.32	36.6	224.48	1183.4	0.24
0.3	0.68	0	0	0.3	0.03	0.6	0	0	0	0	0	0	32	1.65	0	0	0	1011	0
0	0	0	0	0	0.03	0.03	0	0	0	0	0	0	27	0.45	0	0	0	1222	0
1.29	0.32	0	0	0	34.72	4.22	0.17	0.11	1.35	0.22	49.6	0.3	42.16	2.65	22.32	183.52	357.12	1319.36	0.74
0.7	1.11	0	0	0.07	233.77	1.21	0.05	0.04	0.94	0.1	16.15	0	33.74	0.92	7.23	55.43	313.3	910.98	0.74
0.91	0.26	0	0	0.72	434.4	4.8	0.06	0.12	1.18	0.24	31.2	0	60	1.78	14.4	110.4	612	864	1.44
2.25	1.54	0	0	0.63	0	1.01	0.28	0.11	0.5	0.03	5.06	0.25	65.78	0.51	5.06	75.9	199.87	1019.59	0.09
0.75	0.65	0	0	0.29	0	1.21	0.03	0.02	0.6	0.05	15.18	0	26.51	0.67	2.41	12.05	67.48	1053.17	0.61
2.18	0.53	0	0	0.18	58.42	2.79	0.15	0.27	1.34	0.1	7.87	0.43	172.72	2.01	55.88	238.76	375.92	1046.48	1.76
1.8	0.63	0	0	0	45.54	1.52	0.15	0.08	1.47	0.07	2.53	0.25	22.77	2.28	48.07	212.52	399.74	1006.94	1.32

USDA ID Code	Food Name	Weight in Grams*	Quantity of Units	Unit of Measure	Protein (gm)	Fat (gm)	Carbohydrates (gm)	Kcalories	Caffeine (gm)	Fiber (gm)	Cholesterol (mg)	Saturated Fat (gm)
6050	Soup, Pea, Split w/ Ham, Chunky	240	1	Cup	11.09	3.98	26.81	184.8	0	4.08	7.2	1.58
	Soup, Sweet & Sour	244	1	Cup	3	1	14	72	0	1.6	5	0.001
6359	Soup, Tomato	248	1	Cup	6.1	6	22.3	161.2	0	0.5	17.36	2.9
6461	Soup, Tomato Beef w/ noodle	244	1	Cup	4.47	4.29	21.15	139.08	0	1.46	4.88	1.59
6463	Soup, Tomato Rice	247	1	Cup	2.1	2.72	21.93	118.56	0	1.48	2.47	0.52
6499	Soup, Tomato Vegetable	253	1	Cup	2	0.86	10.22	55.66	0	0.51	0	0.38
6465	Soup, Turkey Noodle	244	1	Cup	3.9	2	8.64	68.32	0	0.73	4.88	0.56
6466	Soup, Turkey Vegetable	241	1	Cup	3.08	3.04	8.63	72.3	0	0.48	2.41	0.89
6064	Soup, Turkey, Chunky	236	1	Cup	10.22	4.41	14.07	134.52	0	0	9.44	1.23
6500	Soup, Vegetable Beef	253.1	1	Cup	2.94	1.11	8.02	53.15	0	0.51	0	0.56
6067	Soup, Vegetable, Chunky	240	1	Cup	3.5	3.7	19.01	122.4	0	1.2	0	0.55
6468	Soup, Vegetarian Vegetable	241	1	Cup	2.1	1.93	11.98	72.3	0	0.48	0	0.29
	Soup, Won-Ton	241	1	Cup	14	7	14	182	0	0.9	53	2
19294	Apple Butter	18	1	Tbsp.	0.02	0.05	8.59	33.12	0	0.23	0	0
9020	Applesauce, Sweetened	255	1	Cup	0.46	0.46	50.77	193.8	0	3.06	0	0.08
9019	Applesauce, Unsweetened	244	1	Cup	0.41	0.12	27.55	104.92	0	2.93	0	0.02
62678	Bean Dip	15	2	Tbsp.	0.5	0	2	10	0	0.5	0	0
11935	Catsup	15	1	Tbsp.	0.23	0.05	4.09	15.6	0	0.19	0	0.01
11949	Catsup, Low Sodium	15	1	Tbsp.	0.23	0.05	4.09	15.6	0	0.24	0	0.01
18242	Croutons, Plain	30	0.5	Cup	3.57	1.98	22.05	122.1	0	1.53	0	0.47
18243	Croutons, Seasoned	40	0.5	Cup	4.32	7.32	25.4	186	0	2	1.2	2.01
62677	French Onion Dip	15	2	Tbsp.	0.5	2.5	1	30	0	0	7.5	1.5
6114	Gravy, Au Jus, Cnd	149	0.25	Cup	2.86	0.48	5.96	38.14	0	0	0	0.24
6116	Gravy, Beef, Cnd	234	0.25	Cup	8.8	5.6	11.2	124	0	1	8	2.3
6119	Gravy, Chicken, Cnd	238	0.25	Cup	4.6	13.61	12.92	188.34	0	0.95	4.77	3.36
6121	Gravy, Mushroom, Cnd	298	0.25	Cup	3	6.46	13.04	119.2	0	0.95	0	0.95
6125	Gravy, Turkey, Cnd	298	0.25	Cup	6.2	5.01	12.16	121.58	0	0.95	4.77	1.48
6527	Gravy, Unspecified Type	298	0.25	Cup	3.22	1.99	14.38	86.26	0	0	4.77	0.71
19296	Honey	21	1	Tbsp.	0.06	0	17.3	63.84	0	0.04	0	0
19297	Jams and Preserves	20	1	Tbsp.	0.14	0.04	12.88	48.4	0	0.22	0	0
19300	Jellies	19	1	Tbsp.	0.08	0.02	13.45	51.49	0	0.19	0	0
19303	Marmalade, Orange	20	1	Tbsp.	0.06	0	13.26	49.2	0	0.04	0	0
62646	Mustard	5	1	Tbsp.	0	0	0	0	0	0	0	0
62679	Nacho Cheese Dip	16.5	2	Tbsp.	0	1.25	2	20	0	0	0	0.25
11958	Pickle Relish, Hamburger	15	1	Tbsp.	0.09	0.08	5.17	19.35	0	0.48	0	0.01
11944	Pickle Relish, Hot Dog	15	1	Tbsp.	0.22	0.07	3.5	13.65	0	0	0	0.01
11945	Pickle Relish, Sweet	15	1	Tbsp.	0.06	0.07	5.26	19.5	0	0	0	0.01
62651	Salt Substitute	4.8	0.25	Tsp.	0	0	0	0	0	0	0	0
2047	Salt, Table	6	1	Tsp.	0	0	0	0	0	0	0	0
	Sauce, A-1 Steak	31.3	2	Tbsp.	0.003	0.005	5	19	0	0.5	0	0.002
6150	Sauce, Barbecue	250	0.5	Cup	4.5	4.5	32	187.5	0	3	0	0.67
	Sauce, Chinese Mustard	15	1	Tbsp.	1	1	1	11	0	0.4	0	0.002
11256	Sauce, Marinara	250	0.5	Cup	4	8.37	25.45	170	0	0	0	1.2
6134	Sauce, Soy (Tamari)	18	1	Tbsp.	0.93	0.01	1.53	9.54	0	0	0	0
11455	Sauce, Spaghetti	249	0.5	Cup	4.53	11.88	39.67	271.41	0	8.47	0	1.7
6112	Sauce, Teriyaki	18	1	Tbsp.	1.07	0	2.87	15.12	0	0.02	0	0
6313	Sauce, White	263.8	0.5	Cup	10.21	13.45	21.39	240.06	0	0	34.29	6.41
	Sauce, Worcestershire	34	2	Tbsp.	0	0	6	23	0	0	0	0
62666	Spaghetti Sauce w/garlic and herbs, Healthy Choice	113	1	Cup	2	0.59	9	40			0	
62665	Spaghetti Sauce, Prego	146	1	Cup	3.56	4.15	26.11	154.31		3.56	0	1.19
62664	Spaghetti Sauce, Ragu	146	1	Cup	3.56	4.75	20.18	130.57	0	3.56	0	1.78
19334	Sugar, Brown	5	1	Tsp.	0	0	4.87	18.8	0	0	0	0
19335	Sugar, Granulated	4	1	Tsp.	0	0	4	15.48	0	0	0	0
19336	Sugar, Powdered	8	1	Tbsp.	0	0.01	7.96	31.12	0	0	0	0
19349	Syrup, Corn, Dark	20	1	Tbsp.	0	0	15.32	56.4	0	0	0	0

Monounsaturated Fat (gm)	Polyunsaturated Fat (gm)	Vitamin D (mg)	Vitamin K (mg)	Vitamin E (mg)	Vitamin A (re)	Vitamin C (mg)	Thiamin (mg)	Riboflavin (mg)	Niacin (mg)	Vitamin B6 (mg)	Folate (mg)	Vitamin B12 (mcg)	Calcium (mg)	Iron (mg)	Magnesium (mg)	Phosphorus (mg)	Potassium (mg)	Sodium (mg)	Zinc (mg)
1.63	0.58	0	0	0.14	487.2	6.96	0.12	0.09	2.52	0.22	4.56	0.24	33.6	2.14	38.4	177.6	304.8	964.8	3.12
0	0	0	0	0	30	16.8	0	0	0	0	0	0	27	0.45	0	0	0	1292	0
1.61	1.12	0	0	2.6	109.12	67.7	0.13	0.25	1.52	0.16	20.83	0.45	158.72	1.81	22.32	148.8	448.88	932.48	0.29
1.73	0.68	0	0	0.78	53.68	0	0.08	0.09	1.87	0.09	7.32	0.2	17.08	1.12	7.32	56.12	219.6	917.44	0.75
0.59	1.36	0	0	0.79	76.57	14.82	0.06	0.05	1.05	0.08	13.58	0	22.23	0.79	4.94	34.58	330.98	815.1	0.51
0.3	0.08	0	0	0.81	20.24	6.07	0.06	0.05	0.79	0.05	10.12	0	7.59	0.63	20.24	30.36	103.73	1146.09	0.17
0.81	0.49	0	0	0.06	29.28	0.24	0.07	0.06	1.4	0.04	2.2	0.15	12.2	0.95	4.88	48.8	75.64	814.96	0.58
1.33	0.67	0	0	0.14	243.41	0	0.03	0.04	1	0.05	4.82	0.17	16.87	0.77	4.82	40.97	175.93	906.16	0.61
1.77	1.09	0	0	0	715.08	6.37	0.04	0.11	3.59	0.31	11.09	2.12	49.56	1.91	23.6	103.84	361.08	922.76	2.12
0.46	0.05	0	0	0.03	22.78	1.27	0.03	0.04	0.46	0.05	7.59	0.25	12.65	0.86	22.78	35.43	75.93	1002.28	0.27
1.58	1.39	0	0	0.6	588	6	0.07	0.06	1.2	0.19	16.56	0	55.2	1.63	7.2	72	396	1010.4	3.12
0.82	0.72	0	0	0.8	301.25	1.45	0.05	0.05	0.92	0.06	10.6	0	21.69	1.08	7.23	33.74	209.67	821.81	0.46
0.001	0.003	0	0	0	100	3.6	0	0	0	0	0	0	29	1.5	0	0	0	543	0
0	0	0	0	0	0	0.32	0	0	0.01	0.01	0	0	0.9	0.02	0.54	1.08	16.38	0	0.01
0.02	0.14	0	0	0.13	2.55	4.34	0.03	0.07	0.48	0.07	1.53	0	10.2	0.89	7.65	17.85	155.55	7.65	0.1
0	0.03	0	0	0.12	7.32	2.93	0.03	0.06	0.46	0.06	1.46	0	7.32	0.29	7.32	17.08	183	4.88	0.07
0	0	0	0	0	0	0	0	0	0	0	0	0	0	0.1	0	0	0	75	0
0.01	0.02	0	0	0.22	15.3	2.26	0.01	0.01	0.21	0.03	2.25	0	2.85	0.1	3.3	5.85	72.15	177.9	0.03
0.01	0.02	0	0	0.22	15.3	2.26	0.01	0.01	0.21	0.03	2.25	0	2.85	0.1	3.3	5.85	72.15	3	0.03
1.01	0.32	0	0	0	0		0.19	0.08	1.63	0.01	6.6	0	22.8	1.22	9.3	34.5	37.2	209.4	0.27
3.82	1	0	0	0	2	0	0.2	0.17	1.86	0.03	16	0.03	38.4	1.13	16.8	56	72.4	495.2	0.38
0	0	0	0	0	20	0.6	0	0	0	0	0	0	12	0	0	0	0	52.5	0
0.19	0.02	0	0	0	0	2.38	0.05	0.14	2.15	0.02	4.77	0.24	9.54	1.43	4.77	71.52	193.1	119.2	2.38
2.2	0.2	0	0	0.3	0	0	0.08	0.08	1.6	0.02	4	0.24	14	1.64	4	70	190	1330	2.34
6.08	3.58	0	0	0.37	264.62	0	0.04	0.1	1.06	0.02	4.77	0.24	47.68	1.12	4.77	69.14	259.86	1375.57	1.91
2.79	2.43	0	0	0.15	0	0	0.08	0.15	1.6	0.05	28.61	0	16.69	1.57	4.77	35.76	252.7	1358.88	1.67
2.15	1.17	0	0	0.14	0	0	0.05	0.19	3.1	0.02	4.77	0.24	9.54	1.67	4.77	69.14	259.86	1375.57	1.91
0.78	0.39	0	0	0	0	1.83	0.05	0.11	0.78	0.03	3.4	0.18	36.6	0.26	10.46	49.67	65.35	1422.02	0.26
0	0	0	0	0	0	0.11	0	0.01	0.03	0.01	0.42	0	1.26	0.09	0.42	0.84	10.92	0.84	0.05
0.02	0	0	0	0	0.2	1.76	0	0	0.01	0	6.6	0	4	0.1	0.8	2.2	15.4	8	0.01
0	0	0	0	0	0.38	0.17	0	0	0.01	0	0.19	0	1.52	0.04	1.14	0.95	12.16	6.84	0.01
0	0	0	0	0	1	0.96	0	0	0.01	0	7.2	0	7.6	0.03	0.4	1.2	7.4	11.2	0.01
0	0	0	0	0	0	0	0	0	0	0	0	0	0	0	0	0	0	75	0
0	0	0	0	0	0	0	0	0	0	0	0	0	12	0	0	0	0	100	0
0.04	0.02	0	0	0	4.05	0.34	0	0.01	0.09	0	0.15	0	0.6	0.17	1.05	2.55	11.4	164.4	0.02
0.03	0.02	0	0	0	2.55	0.15	0.01	0.01	0.07	0	0.15	0	0.75	0.19	2.85	6	11.7	163.65	0.03
0.03	0.02	0	0	0	2.4	0.15	0	0	0.03	0	0.15	0	0.45	0.13	0.75	2.1	3.75	121.65	0.02
0	0	0	0	0	0	0	0	0	0	0	0	0	0	0	0	0	2440	0	0
0	0	0	0	0	0	0	0	0	0	0	0	0	2.7	0.01	0.12	0	0.48	2325.48	0
0	0	0	0	0	32	4.8	0	0	0	0	0	0	12	0.3	0	0	0	454	0
1.92	1.7	0	0	2.77	217.5	17.5	0.07	0.05	2.25	0.19	10	0	47.5	2.25	45	50	435	2037.5	0.5
0	0	0	0	0	0	0	0	0	0	0	0	0	12	0.3	0	0	0	188	0
4.28	2.29	0	0	0	240	32	0.11	0.15	3.97	0.62	33.75	0	45	2	60	87.5	1060	1572.5	0.67
0	0.01	0	0	0	0	0	0.01	0.02	0.6	0.03	2.79	0	3.06	0.36	6.12	19.8	32.4	1028.7	0.07
6.07	3.25	0	0	6.22	306.27	27.89	0.14	0.15	3.75	0.88	53.78	0	69.72	1.62	59.76	89.64	956.16	1235.04	0.52
0	0	0	0	0	0	0	0.01	0.01	0.23	0.02	3.6	0	4.5	0.31	10.98	27.72	40.5	689.94	0.02
4.7	1.69	0	0	0	92.33	2.64	0.08	0.45	0.53	0.07	15.83	1.06	424.72	0.26	263.8	255.89	443.18	796.68	0.55
0	0	0	0	0	0.003	4.2	0	0	0	0	0	0	43	1.5	0	0	0	333	0
0	0	0	0	0	56	18	0	0	0	0	0	0	24	0.8	0	0	0	390	0
0	0	0	0	0	356.1	21.37	0	0	0	0	0	0	85.46	0.71	0	0	0	724.07	0
0	0	0	0	0	178.05	1.42	0	0	0	0	0	0	56.98	0.71	0	0	0	652.85	0
0	0	0	0	0	0	0	0	0	0	0	0.05	0	4.25	0.1	1.45	1.1	17.3	1.95	0.01
0	0	0	0	0	0	0	0	0	0	0	0	0	0.04	0	0	0.08	0.08	0.04	0
0	0	0	0	0	0	0	0	0	0	0	0	0	0.08	0	0	0.16	0.16	0.08	0
0	0	0	0	0	0	0	0	0	0	0	0	0	3.6	0.07	1.6	2.2	8.8	31	0.01

USDA ID Code	Food Name	Weight in Grams*	Quantity of Units	Unit of Measure	Protein (gm)	Fat (gm)	Carbohydrates (gm)	Kcalories	Caffeine (gm)	Fiber (gm)	Cholesterol (mg)	Saturated Fat (gm)
19351	Syrup, Corn, High-fructose	19	1	Tbsp.	0	0	14.44	53.39	0	0	0	0
19350	Syrup, Corn, Light	20	1	Tbsp.	0	0	15.32	56.4	0	0	0	0
19352	Syrup, Malt	24	1	Tbsp.	1.49	0	17.11	76.32	0	0	0	0
19353	Syrup, Maple	20	1	Tbsp.	0	0.04	13.44	52.4	0	0	0	0
19128	Syrup, Pancake, Lo Cal	19.98	1	Tbsp.	0	0	8.85	32.77	0	0	0	0
19360	Syrup, Pancake, w/ 2% Maple	20	1	Tbsp.	0	0.02	13.92	53	0	0	0	0
19364	Toppings, Butterscotch or Caramel	20.513	1	Tbsp.	0.31	0.02	13.52	51.69	0	0	0.21	0.02
62550	Toppings, Caramel	16.68	1	Tbsp.	0.27	0	13.01	51.71	0	0	0	0
19348	Toppings, Chocolate	21	1	Tbsp.	0.92	2.81	12.37	72.66	1.89	0.25	2.52	1.18
62549	Toppings, Hot Fudge	19.018	1	Tbsp.	1	2	11.01	70.07	0	0	0	0.5
19365	Toppings, Marshmallow Cream	20.513	1	Tbsp.	0.35	0.04	16.31	63.59	0	0	0	0
19367	Toppings, Nuts in Syrup	20.513	1	Tbsp.	0.92	4.51	10.95	83.69	0	0.33	0	0.4
19366	Toppings, Pineapple	21.268	1	Tbsp.	0.02	0.02	14.12	53.81	0	0.21	0	0
19137	Toppings, Strawberry	21.268	1	Tbsp.	0.04	0.02	14.1	54.02	0	0.21	0	0

Monounsaturated Fat (gm)	Polyunsaturated Fat (gm)	Vitamin D (mg)	Vitamin K (mg)	Vitamin E (mg)	Vitamin A (re)	Vitamin C (mg)	Thiamin (mg)	Riboflavin (mg)	Niacin (mg)	Vitamin B6 (mg)	Folate (mg)	Vitamin B12 (mcg)	Calcium (mg)	Iron (mg)	Magnesium (mg)	Phosphorus (mg)	Potassium (mg)	Sodium (mg)	Zinc (mg)
0	0	0	0	0	0	0	0	0	0	0	0	0	0	0.01	0	0	0	0.38	0
0	0	0	0	0	0	0	0	0	0	0	0	0	0.6	0.01	0.4	0.4	0.8	24.2	0
0	0	0	0	0	0	0	0	0.09	1.95	0.12	2.88	0	14.64	0.23	17.28	56.64	76.8	8.4	0.03
0	0	0	0	0	0	0	0	0	0.01	0	0	0	13.4	0.24	2.8	0.4	40.8	1.8	0.83
0	0	0	0	0	0	0	0	0	0	0	0	0	0.2	0	0	8.59	0.6	39.96	0
0	0	0	0	0	0	0	0	0	0	0	0	0	0	0.01	0.4	2	1.2	12.2	0.05
0	0	0	0	0	5.54	0.06	0	0.02	0.01	0	0.41	0.02	10.87	0.04	1.44	9.64	17.23	71.59	0.04
0	0	0	0	0	0	0	0	0	0	0	0	0	2.34	0	0	4.67	5.67	11.01	0.03
0.77	0.68	0	0	0	4.62	0.11	0.01	0.05	0.04	0.01	0.84	0.06	21	0.25	10.08	35.7	45.15	27.3	0.17
0	0	0	0	0	0	0	0	0	0	0	0	0	36.03	0.2	0	0	0	35.03	0
0	0	0	0	0	0	0	0	0	0.02	0	0.21	0	0.62	0.05	0.41	1.64	1.03	9.44	0.01
1.02	2.82	0	0	0.18	0.82	0.23	0.04	0.02	0.08	0.04	4.31	0	8.21	0.22	12.92	22.77	42.87	8.62	0.21
0	0	0	0	0	0.43	12.46	0.01	0	0.02	0	0.64	0	4.68	0.1	0.43	1.7	67.42	13.4	0.1
0	0	0	0	0.03	0.43	5.3	0	0	0.05	0	0.43	0	5.1	0.21	0.85	2.76	15.53	4.47	0.1

Appendix B Amino Acid Content of Foods, 100 g, Edible Portion

Protein content and nitrogen conversion factor	Trypto-phan (g)	Threo-nine (g)	Iso-leucine (g)	Leucine (g)	Lysine (g)	Methi-onine (g)	Cystine (g)	Phenyl-alanine (g)	Tyro-sine (g)	Valine (g)	Argi-nine (g)	Histi-dine (g)
Milk, milk products												
Milk (protein, N × 6.38)												
Cow												
Fluid, whole and nonfat (3.5% protein)	0.049	0.161	0.223	0.344	0.272	0.086	0.031	0.170	0.178	0.240	0.128	0.092
Canned												
Evaporated, unsweetened (7.0% protein)	0.099	0.323	0.447	0.688	0.545	0.171	0.063	0.340	0.357	0.481	0.256	0.185
Condensed, sweetened (8.1% protein)	0.114	0.374	0.518	0.796	0.631	0.198	0.072	0.393	0.413	0.557	0.296	0.214
Dried												
Whole (25.8% protein)	0.364	1.191	1.648	2.535	2.009	0.632	0.231	1.251	1.316	1.774	0.944	0.680
Nonfat (35.6% protein)	0.502	1.641	2.271	3.493	2.768	0.870	0.318	1.724	1.814	2.444	1.300	0.937
Goat (3.3% protein)	0.039	0.217	0.087	0.278	0.312	0.065	—	0.121	—	0.139	0.174	0.068
Human (1.4% protein)	0.023	0.062	0.075	0.124	0.090	0.028	0.027	0.060	0.071	0.086	0.055	0.030
Milk products												
Buttermilk (3.5% protein, N × 6.38)	0.038	0.165	0.219	0.346	0.291	0.082	0.032	0.186	0.137	0.262	0.168	0.099
Casein (100% protein, N × 6.29)	1.335	4.277	6.550	10.048	8.013	3.084	0.382	5.389	5.819	7.393	4.070	3.021
Cheese (protein, N × 6.38)												
Blue mold (21.5% protein)	0.293	0.799	1.449	2.096	1.577	0.559	0.121	1.153	1.028	1.543	0.785	0.701
Camembert (17.5% protein)	0.239	0.650	1.179	1.706	1.284	0.455	0.099	0.938	0.837	1.256	0.639	0.571
Cheddar processed (23.2% protein)	0.316	0.862	1.563	2.262	1.702	0.604	0.131	1.244	1.109	1.665	0.847	0.756
Cheese foods, Cheddar (20.5% protein)	0.280	0.761	1.382	1.998	1.504	0.533	0.116	1.099	0.980	1.472	0.749	0.668
Cottage (17.0% protein)	0.179	0.794	0.989	1.826	1.428	0.469	0.147	0.917	0.917	0.978	0.802	0.549
Cream cheese (9.0% protein)	0.080	0.408	0.519	0.923	0.721	0.229	0.085	0.547	0.408	0.538	0.313	0.278
Limburger (21.2% protein)	0.289	0.788	1.429	2.067	1.555	0.552	0.120	1.136	1.014	1.522	0.774	0.691
Parmesan (36.0% protein)	0.491	1.337	2.426	3.510	2.641	0.937	0.203	1.930	1.721	2.584	1.315	1.174
Swiss (27.5% protein)	0.375	1.021	1.853	2.681	2.017	0.715	0.155	1.474	1.315	1.974	1.004	0.896
Swiss processed (26.4% protein)	0.360	0.981	1.779	2.574	1.937	0.687	0.149	1.415	1.262	1.895	0.964	0.861
Eggs, chicken (protein, N × 6.25)												
Fresh or stored												
Whole (12.8% protein)	0.211	0.637	0.850	1.126	0.819	0.401	0.299	0.739	0.551	0.950	0.840	0.307
Whites (10.8% protein)	0.164	0.477	0.698	0.950	0.648	0.420	0.263	0.689	0.449	0.842	0.634	0.233
Yolks (16.3% protein)	0.235	0.827	0.996	1.372	1.074	0.417	0.274	0.717	0.756	1.121	1.132	0.368

Protein content and nitrogen conversion factor	Trypto-phan (g)	Threo-nine (g)	Iso-leucine (g)	Leucine (g)	Lysine (g)	Methi-onine (g)	Cystine (g)	Phenyl-alanine (g)	Tyro-sine (g)	Valine (g)	Argi-nine (g)	Histi-dine (g)
Dried												
Whole (46.8% protein)	0.771	2.329	3.108	4.118	2.995	1.468	1.093	2.703	2.014	3.474	3.070	1.123
Whites (85.9% protein)	1.306	3.793	5.553	7.559	5.154	3.340	3.089	5.484	3.573	6.693	5.044	1.855
Yolks (31.2% protein)	0.449	1.582	1.907	2.626	2.057	0.799	0.524	1.373	1.448	2.147	2.167	0.704

Meat, poultry, fish, and shellfish (their products)

Protein content and nitrogen conversion factor	Trypto-phan (g)	Threo-nine (g)	Iso-leucine (g)	Leucine (g)	Lysine (g)	Methi-onine (g)	Cystine (g)	Phenyl-alanine (g)	Tyro-sine (g)	Valine (g)	Argi-nine (g)	Histi-dine (g)
Meat (protein, N × 6.25)												
Beef cuts, medium fat												
Chuck (18.6% protein)	0.217	0.821	0.973	1.524	1.625	0.461	0.235	0.765	0.631	1.033	1.199	0.646
Flank (19.9% protein)	0.232	0.879	1.041	1.630	1.738	0.494	0.252	0.818	0.675	1.105	1.283	0.691
Hamburger (16.0% protein)	0.187	0.707	0.837	1.311	1.398	0.397	0.202	0.658	0.543	0.888	1.032	0.556
Porterhouse (16.4% protein)	0.192	0.724	0.858	1.343	1.433	0.407	0.207	0.674	0.556	0.911	1.057	0.569
Rib roast (17.4%)	0.203	0.768	0.910	1.425	1.520	0.432	0.220	0.715	0.590	0.966	1.122	0.604
Round (19.5% protein)	0.228	0.861	1.020	1.597	1.704	0.484	0.246	0.802	0.661	1.083	1.257	0.677
Rump (16.2% protein)	0.189	0.715	0.848	1.327	1.415	0.402	0.205	0.666	0.550	0.899	1.045	0.562
Sirloin (17.3% protein)	0.202	0.764	0.905	1.417	1.511	0.429	0.219	0.711	0.587	0.960	1.116	0.601
Beef, canned (25.0% protein)	0.292	1.104	1.308	2.048	2.184	0.620	0.316	1.028	0.848	1.388	1.612	0.868
Beef, dried or chipped (34.3% protein)	0.401	1.515	1.795	2.810	2.996	0.851	0.434	1.410	1.163	1.904	2.212	1.191
Lamb cuts, medium fat												
Leg (18.0% protein)	0.233	0.824	0.933	1.394	1.457	0.432	0.236	0.732	0.625	0.887	1.172	0.501
Rib (14.9% protein)	0.193	0.682	0.772	1.154	1.206	0.358	0.195	0.606	0.517	0.734	0.970	0.415
Shoulder (15.6% protein)	0.202	0.714	0.809	1.208	1.263	0.374	0.205	0.634	0.542	0.769	1.016	0.434
Pork cuts, medium fat, fresh												
Ham (15.2% protein)	0.197	0.705	0.781	1.119	1.248	0.379	0.178	0.598	0.542	0.790	0.931	0.525
Loin (16.4% protein)	0.213	0.761	0.842	1.207	1.346	0.409	0.192	0.646	0.585	0.853	1.005	0.567
Miscellaneous lean cuts (14.5% protein)	0.188	0.673	0.745	1.067	1.190	0.362	0.169	0.571	0.517	0.754	0.889	0.501
Pork, cured												
Bacon, medium fat (9.1% protein)	0.095	0.306	0.399	0.728	0.587	0.141	0.106	0.434	0.234	0.434	0.622	0.246
Fat back or salt pork (3.9% protein)	0.006	0.141	0.110	0.367	0.317	0.055	0.043	0.157	0.052	0.168	0.379	0.035
Ham (16.9% protein)	0.162	0.692	0.841	1.306	1.420	0.411	0.273	0.646	0.652	0.879	1.068	0.544
Luncheon meat												
Boiled ham (22.8% protein)	0.219	0.934	1.135	1.762	1.915	0.554	0.368	0.872	0.879	1.186	1.441	0.733
Canned, spiced (14.9% protein)	0.143	0.610	0.741	1.161	1.252	0.362	0.241	0.570	0.575	0.775	0.942	0.479
Rabbit, domesticated, flesh only (21.9% protein)	—	1.021	1.082	1.636	1.818	0.541	—	0.793	—	1.021	1.176	0.474
Veal cuts, medium fat												
Round (19.5% protein)	0.256	0.846	1.030	1.429	1.629	0.446	0.231	0.792	0.702	1.008	1.270	0.627
Shoulder (19.4% protein)	0.255	0.841	1.024	1.422	1.620	0.444	0.230	0.788	0.698	1.003	1.263	0.624
Stew meat (18.3% protein)	0.240	0.793	0.966	1.341	1.528	0.419	0.217	0.744	0.659	0.946	1.192	0.589
Poultry (protein, N × 6.25)												
Chicken, fresh only												
Broilers or fryers (20.6% protein)	0.250	0.877	1.088	1.490	1.810	0.537	0.277	0.811	0.725	1.012	1.302	0.593
Hens (21.3% protein)	0.259	0.907	1.125	1.540	1.871	0.556	0.286	0.838	0.750	1.046	1.346	0.613
Ducks, domesticated, flesh only (21.4% protein)	—	0.935	1.109	1.657	1.842	0.531	—	0.842	—	1.027	1.301	0.486
Turkey, flesh only (24.0% protein)	—	1.014	1.260	1.836	2.173	0.664	0.330	0.960	—	1.187	1.513	0.649
Fish and shellfish (protein, N × 6.25)												
Bluefish (20.5% protein)	0.203	0.889	1.040	1.548	1.797	0.597	0.276	0.761	0.554	1.092	1.155	—
Cod												
Fresh (16.5% protein)	0.164	0.715	0.837	1.246	1.447	0.480	0.222	0.612	0.446	0.879	0.929	—
Dried (81.8% protein)	0.811	3.547	4.149	6.178	7.172	2.382	1.099	3.036	2.212	4.358	4.607	—

Continued

Protein content and nitrogen conversion factor	Trypto-phan (g)	Threo-nine (g)	Iso-leucine (g)	Leucine (g)	Lysine (g)	Methi-onine (g)	Cystine (g)	Phenyl-alanine (g)	Tyro-sine (g)	Valine (g)	Argi-nine (g)	Histi-dine (g)
Croaker (17.8% protein)	0.177	0.772	0.903	1.344	1.561	0.518	0.239	0.661	0.481	0.948	1.002	—
Eel (18.6% protein)	0.185	0.806	0.943	1.405	1.631	0.542	0.250	0.690	0.503	0.991	1.048	—
Flounder (14.9% protein)	0.148	0.646	0.756	1.125	1.306	0.434	0.200	0.553	0.403	0.794	0.839	—
Haddock (18.2% protein)	0.181	0.789	0.923	1.374	1.596	0.530	0.245	0.676	0.492	0.970	1.025	—
Halibut (18.6% protein)	0.185	0.806	0.943	1.405	1.631	0.542	0.250	0.690	0.503	0.991	1.048	—
Herring												
Atlantic (18.3% protein)	0.182	0.793	0.928	1.382	1.605	0.533	0.246	0.679	0.495	0.975	1.031	—
Mackerel, canned, solids and liquid												
Pacific (21.1% protein)	0.209	0.915	1.070	1.593	1.850	0.614	0.284	0.783	0.571	1.124	1.188	—
Salmon												
Raw, Pacific (Chinook or King) (17.4% protein)	0.173	0.754	0.883	1.314	1.526	0.507	0.234	0.646	0.470	0.927	0.980	—
Canned, solids and liquid (sockeye or red) (20.2% protein)	0.200	0.876	1.025	1.526	1.771	0.588	0.271	0.750	0.546	1.076	1.138	—
Sardines, canned, solids and liquid												
Atlantic type (21.1% protein)	0.209	0.915	1.070	1.593	1.850	0.614	0.284	0.783	0.571	1.124	1.188	—
Shrimp, canned, solids and liquid (18.7% protein)	0.186	0.811	0.948	1.412	1.640	0.545	0.251	0.694	0.506	0.996	1.053	—
Products from meat, poultry, and fish (protein, N × 6.25)												
Brains (10.4% protein)	0.138	0.494	0.504	0.845	0.760	0.220	0.145	0.506	0.433	0.536	0.614	0.278
Chitterlings (8.6% protein)	0.094	0.398	0.308	0.457	0.670	0.193	0.109	0.359	0.228	0.462	1.406	0.169
Gizzard, chicken (23.1% protein)	0.207	1.072	1.094	1.689	1.567	0.554	0.218	0.968	0.680	1.116	1.741	0.480
Heart												
Beef or pork (16.9% protein)	0.219	0.776	0.857	1.509	1.387	0.403	0.168	0.765	0.627	0.973	1.068	0.433
Kidney												
Beef (15.0% protein)	0.221	0.665	0.730	1.301	1.087	0.307	0.182	0.706	0.557	0.876	0.934	0.377
Liver												
Beef or pork (19.7% protein)	0.296	0.936	1.031	1.819	1.475	0.463	0.243	0.993	0.738	1.239	1.201	0.523
Calf (19.0% protein)	0.286	0.903	0.994	1.754	1.423	0.447	0.234	0.958	0.711	1.195	1.158	0.505
Chicken (22.1% protein)	0.332	1.050	1.156	2.040	1.655	0.520	0.272	1.114	0.827	1.390	1.347	0.587
Sausage												
Bologna (14.8% protein)	0.126	0.606	0.718	1.061	1.191	0.313	0.185	0.540	0.481	0.744	1.028	0.398
Braunschweiger (15.4% protein)	0.172	0.668	0.754	1.291	1.200	0.320	0.187	0.700	0.471	0.956	0.954	0.458
Frankfurters (14.2% protein)	0.120	0.582	0.688	1.018	1.143	0.300	0.177	0.518	0.461	0.713	0.986	0.382
Head cheese (15.0% protein)	0.079	0.418	0.509	0.946	0.907	0.250	0.209	0.569	0.569	0.617	1.075	0.278
Liverwurst (16.7% protein)	0.187	0.724	0.818	1.400	1.301	0.347	0.203	0.759	0.510	1.037	1.034	0.497
Pork, links or bulk, raw (10.8% protein)	0.092	0.442	0.524	0.774	0.869	0.228	0.135	0.394	0.351	0.543	0.750	0.290
Salami (23.9% protein)	0.023	0.979	1.159	1.713	1.923	0.505	0.298	0.872	0.776	1.201	1.660	0.642
Vienna sausage, canned (15.8% protein)	0.134	0.647	0.766	1.133	1.272	0.334	0.197	0.576	0.513	0.794	1.097	0.425
Tongue												
Beef (16.4% protein)	0.197	0.708	0.792	1.286	1.364	0.357	0.207	0.661	0.548	0.840	1.065	0.412
Pork (16.8% protein)	0.202	0.726	0.812	1.317	1.398	0.366	0.212	0.677	0.562	0.860	1.091	0.422
Veal and pork loaf, canned (17.2% protein)	0.198	0.627	0.859	1.236	1.258	0.418	0.209	0.619	0.468	0.958	0.916	0.388

Legumes (dry seed), common nuts, other nuts, and dry seeds (their products)

Legume seeds and their products												
Beans (*Phaseolus vulgaris*) (N × 6.25)												
Pinto and red Mexican (23.0% protein)	0.213	0.997	1.306	1.976	1.708	0.232	0.228	1.270	0.887	1.395	1.384	0.655

Protein content and nitrogen conversion factor	Trypto-phan (g)	Threo-nine (g)	Iso-leucine (g)	Leucine (g)	Lysine (g)	Methi-onine (g)	Cystine (g)	Phenyl-alanine (g)	Tyro-sine (g)	Valine (g)	Argi-nine (g)	Histi-dine (g)
Red kidney												
Raw (23.1% protein)	0.214	1.002	1.312	1.985	1.715	0.233	0.229	1.275	0.891	1.401	1.390	0.658
Canned, solids and liquid (5.7% protein)	0.053	0.247	0.324	0.490	0.423	0.057	0.057	0.315	0.220	0.346	0.343	0.162
Other common beans, including navy, peabean, white marrow												
Raw (21.4% protein)	0.199	0.928	1.216	1.839	1.589	0.216	0.212	1.181	0.825	1.298	1.287	0.609
Baked with pork, canned (5.8% protein)	0.057	0.274	0.291	0.486	0.354	0.059	0.018	0.333	0.165	0.312	0.251	0.186
Broadbeans, raw (25.4% protein, N × 6.25)	0.236	0.829	1.593	2.211	1.426	0.106	0.179	1.057	0.687	1.276	1.780	0.748
Chickpeas (20.8% protein, N × 6.25)	0.170	0.739	1.195	1.538	1.434	0.276	0.296	1.012	0.692	1.025	1.551	0.559
Cowpeas (22.9% protein, N × 6.25)	0.220	0.901	1.110	1.715	1.491	0.352	0.297	1.198	0.678	1.293	1.473	0.692
Lentils, whole (25.0% protein, N × 6.25)	0.216	0.896	1.316	1.760	1.528	0.180	0.294	1.104	0.664	1.360	1.908	0.548
Lima beans (20.7% protein, N × 6.25)	0.195	0.980	1.199	1.722	1.378	0.331	0.311	1.222	0.543	1.298	1.315	0.669
Lupine (32.3% protein, N × 6.25)	—	1.101	1.618	1.964	1.447	0.114	—	1.271	—	1.328	2.718	0.811
Mung beans (24.4% protein, N × 6.25)	0.180	0.765	1.351	2.202	1.667	0.265	0.152	1.167	0.390	1.444	1.370	0.543
Peas (*Pisum sativum*) (N × 6.25)												
Entire seeds (23.8% protein)	0.251	0.918	1.340	1.969	1.744	0.286	0.308	1.200	0.960	1.333	2.102	0.651
Split (24.5% protein)	0.259	0.945	1.380	2.027	1.795	0.294	0.318	1.235	0.988	1.372	2.164	0.670
Soybeans, whole (34.9% protein, N × 5.71)	0.526	1.504	2.054	2.946	2.414	0.513	0.678	1.889	1.216	2.005	2.763	0.911
Soybean flour, flakes, and grits (protein, N × 5.71)												
Low fat (44.7% protein)	0.673	1.926	2.630	3.773	3.092	0.658	0.869	2.419	1.558	2.568	3.538	1.166
Medium fat (42.5% protein)	0.640	1.831	2.501	3.588	2.940	0.625	0.826	2.300	1.481	2.441	3.364	1.109
Full fat (35.9% protein)	0.541	1.547	2.112	3.030	2.483	0.528	0.698	1.943	1.251	2.062	2.842	0.937
Soybean curd (7.0% protein, N × 5.71)	—	—	—	—	—	0.081	0.091	—	—	—	—	—
Soybean milk (3.4% protein, N × 5.71)	0.051	0.176	0.175	0.305	0.269	0.054	0.071	0.195	0.193	0.186	0.302	0.121
Common nuts and their products												
Almonds (18.6% protein, N × 5.18)	0.176	0.610	0.873	1.454	0.582	0.259	0.377	1.146	0.618	1.124	2.729	0.517
Brazil nuts (14.4% protein, N × 5.46)	0.187	0.422	0.593	1.129	0.443	0.941	0.504	0.617	0.483	0.823	2.247	0.367
Cashews (18.5% protein, N × 5.30)	0.471	0.737	1.222	1.522	0.792	0.353	0.527	0.946	0.712	1.592	2.098	0.415
Coconut (3.4% protein, N × 5.30)	0.033	0.129	0.180	0.269	0.152	0.071	0.062	0.174	0.101	0.212	0.486	0.069
Coconut meal (20.3% protein, N × 5.30)	0.199	0.770	1.076	1.605	0.908	0.421	0.372	1.038	0.605	1.268	2.899	0.414
Filberts (12.7% protein, N × 5.30)	0.211	0.415	0.853	0.939	0.417	0.139	0.165	0.537	0.434	0.934	2.171	0.288
Peanuts (26.9% protein, N × 5.46)	0.340	0.828	1.266	1.872	1.099	0.271	0.463	1.557	1.104	1.532	3.296	0.749
Pecans (9.4% protein, N × 5.30)	0.138	0.389	0.553	0.773	0.435	0.153	0.216	0.564	0.316	0.525	1.185	0.273
Walnuts (15.0% protein, N × 5.30)	0.175	0.589	0.767	1.228	0.441	0.306	0.320	0.767	0.583	0.974	2.287	0.405

Continued

Protein content and nitrogen conversion factor	Trypto-phan (g)	Threo-nine (g)	Iso-leucine (g)	Leucine (g)	Lysine (g)	Methi-onine (g)	Cystine (g)	Phenyl-alanine (g)	Tyro-sine (g)	Valine (g)	Argi-nine (g)	Histi-dine (g)
Other nuts and seeds and their products (protein N × 5.30)												
Acorns (10.4% protein)	0.126	0.434	0.561	0.808	0.636	0.139	0.184	0.473	—	0.718	0.722	0.251
Amaranth (14.6% protein)	0.149	0.832	0.882	1.209	1.074	0.372	0.521	1.141	—	0.849	1.747	0.441
Cottonseed flour and meal (42.3% protein)	0.591	1.764	1.884	2.945	2.139	0.686	0.814	2.610	1.365	2.458	5.603	1.325
Pumpkin seed (30.9% protein)	0.560	0.933	1.737	2.437	1.411	0.577	—	1.749	—	1.679	4.810	0.711
Safflower seed meal (42.1% protein)	0.675	1.462	1.914	2.740	1.525	0.731	—	2.605	—	2.446	4.623	0.985
Sesame Seed (19.3% protein)	0.331	0.707	0.951	1.679	0.583	0.637	0.495	1.457	0.951	0.885	1.992	0.441
Sunflower Kernel (23.0% protein)	0.343	0.911	1.276	1.736	0.868	0.443	0.464	1.220	0.647	1.354	2.370	0.586
Grains and their products												
Barley (12.8% protein, N × 5.83)	0.160	0.433	0.545	0.889	0.433	0.184	0.257	0.661	0.466	0.643	0.659	0.239
Bread, white (4% nonfat dry milk, flour basis) (8.5% protein, N × 5.70)	0.091	0.282	0.429	0.668	0.225	0.142	0.200	0.465	0.243	0.435	0.340	0.192
Buckwheat flour Dark (11.7% protein, N × 6.25)	0.165	0.461	0.440	0.683	0.687	0.206	0.228	0.442	0.240	0.607	0.930	0.256
Cereal combinations Corn and soy grits (18.0% protein, N × 6.25)	0.161	0.792	0.841	1.656	0.772	0.271	0.311	0.832	0.562	1.054	0.982	0.472
Infants food, precooked, mixed cereals with nonfat dry milk and yeast (19.4% protein, N × 6.25)	0.118	—	—	—	0.273	0.310	0.137	0.543	0.447	—	0.447	0.233
Oat-corn-rye mixture, puffed (14.5% protein, N × 5.83)	0.172	0.545	0.841	1.368	0.343	0.388	0.234	0.933	0.622	0.900	0.776	0.326
Corn, field (10.0% protein, N × 6.25)	0.061	0.398	0.462	1.296	0.288	0.186	0.130	0.454	0.611	0.510	0.352	0.206
Cornmeal Whole ground (9.2% protein, N × 6.25)	0.056	0.367	0.425	1.192	0.265	0.171	0.119	0.418	0.562	0.470	0.324	0.190
Degermed (7.9% protein, N × 6.25)	0.048	0.315	0.365	1.024	0.228	0.147	0.102	0.359	0.483	0.403	0.278	0.163
Corn products Flakes (8.1% protein, N × 6.25)	0.052	0.275	0.306	1.047	0.154	0.135	0.152	0.354	0.283	0.386	0.231	0.226
Germ (14.5% protein, N × 6.25)	0.144	0.622	0.578	1.030	0.791	0.232	0.130	0.483	0.343	0.789	1.134	0.464
Gluten (10.0% protein, N × 6.25)	0.059	0.344	0.443	1.563	0.179	0.282	0.141	0.558	0.582	0.512	0.322	0.200
Grits (8.7% protein, N × 6.25)	0.053	0.347	0.402	1.128	0.251	0.161	0.113	0.395	0.532	0.444	0.306	0.180
Hominy (8.7% protein, N × 6.25)	0.084	0.316	0.349	0.810	0.358	0.099	—	0.333	0.331	0.398	0.444	0.203
Masa (2.8% protein, N × 6.25)	0.010	—	—	—	0.103	0.108	0.030	—	—	—	—	—
Pozole (5.9% protein, N × 6.25)	0.042	0.336	0.304	0.591	0.234	0.087	—	0.254	—	0.267	0.197	0.122
Tortilla (5.8% protein, N × 6.25)	0.031	0.235	0.345	0.939	0.145	0.111	—	0.252	—	0.304	0.223	0.128
Zein (16.1% protein, N × 6.25)	0.010	0.495	0.822	3.184	—	0.281	0.162	1.664	0.981	0.654	0.286	0.216

Protein content and nitrogen conversion factor	Trypto-phan (g)	Threo-nine (g)	Iso-leucine (g)	Leucine (g)	Lysine (g)	Methi-onine (g)	Cystine (g)	Phenyl-alanine (g)	Tyro-sine (g)	Valine (g)	Argi-nine (g)	Histi-dine (g)
Millet												
Pearl millet (11.4% protein, N × 5.83)	0.248	0.456	0.635	1.746	0.383	0.270	0.152	0.506	—	0.682	0.524	0.240
Ragimillet (6.2% protein, N × 5.83)	0.085	0.270	0.398	0.620	0.202	0.270	0.187	0.263	—	0.473	0.100	0.079
Oatmeal and rolled oats (14.2% protein, N × 5.83)	0.183	0.470	0.733	1.065	0.521	0.209	0.309	0.758	0.524	0.845	0.935	0.261
Quinoa (11.0% protein, N × 6.25)	0.120	0.523	0.722	0.781	0.729	0.278	0.107	0.394	0.253	0.447	0.820	0.297
Rice												
Brown (7.5% protein, N × 5.95)	0.081	0.294	0.352	0.646	0.296	0.135	0.102	0.377	0.343	0.524	0.432	0.126
White and converted (7.6% protein, N × 5.95)	0.082	0.298	0.356	0.655	0.300	0.137	0.103	0.382	0.347	0.531	0.438	0.128
Rice products												
Flakes or puffed (5.9% protein, N × 5.95)	0.046	—	—	—	0.056	—	0.044	0.286	0.124	—	0.137	0.137
Germ (14.2% protein, N × 5.95)	0.270	2.177	0.630	0.838	1.707	0.420	0.169	0.750	0.929	0.938	1.559	0.430
Rye (12.1% protein, N × 5.83)	0.137	0.448	0.515	0.813	0.494	0.191	0.241	0.571	0.390	0.631	0.591	0.276
Rye flour, medium (11.4% protein, N × 5.83)	0.129	0.422	0.485	0.766	0.465	0.180	0.227	0.538	0.368	0.594	0.557	0.260
Sorghum (11.0% protein, N × 6.25)	0.123	0.394	0.598	1.767	0.299	0.190	0.183	0.547	0.303	0.628	0.417	0.211
Teosinte (22.0% protein, N × 6.25)	0.049	—	—	—	0.348	0.496	—	—	—	—	—	—
Wheat flour												
Whole grain (13.3% protein, N × 5.83)	0.164	0.383	0.577	0.892	0.365	0.203	0.292	0.657	0.497	0.616	0.636	0.271
White (10.5% protein, N × 5.70)	0.129	0.302	0.483	0.809	0.239	0.138	0.210	0.577	0.539	0.453	0.466	0.210
Wheat products												
Bran (12.0% protein, N × 6.31)	0.196	0.342	0.485	0.717	0.491	0.145	0.270	0.434	0.259	0.552	0.742	0.280
Bulgur (12.4% protein, N × 5.83)	0.070	—	—	—	0.430	0.300	0.319	—	—	—	—	—
Farina (10.9% protein, N × 5.70)	0.124	—	—	—	0.199	0.143	0.184	0.579	0.447	—	0.424	0.268
Flakes (10.8% protein, N × 5.70)	0.121	0.356	0.496	0.891	0.360	0.127	0.191	0.478	0.311	0.572	0.559	0.231
Germ (25.2% protein, N × 5.80)	0.265	1.343	1.177	1.708	1.534	0.404	0.287	0.908	0.882	1.364	1.825	0.687
Macaroni or spaghetti (12.8% protein, N × 5.70)	0.150	0.499	0.642	0.849	0.413	0.193	0.243	0.669	0.422	0.728	0.582	0.303
Noodles, containing egg solids (12.6% protein, N × 5.70)	0.133	0.533	0.621	0.834	0.411	0.212	0.245	0.610	0.312	0.745	0.621	0.301
Shredded Wheat (10.1% protein, N × 5.83)	0.085	0.405	0.449	0.684	0.331	0.139	0.204	0.481	0.236	0.577	0.523	0.236
Whole wheat with added germ (12.8% protein, N × 5.83)	0.136	—	—	—	0.466	—	0.246	0.755	0.481	—	0.742	0.371

Note: Fruits are not a significant source of amino acids.

Continued

Protein content and nitrogen conversion factor	Trypto-phan (g)	Threo-nine (g)	Iso-leucine (g)	Leucine (g)	Lysine (g)	Methi-onine (g)	Cystine (g)	Phenyl-alanine (g)	Tyro-sine (g)	Valine (g)	Argi-nine (g)	Histi-dine (g)
Vegetables												
Immature seeds (protein, N × 6.25)												
Corn, sweet, white or yellow												
Raw (3.7% protein)	0.023	0.151	0.137	0.407	0.137	0.072	0.062	0.207	0.124	0.231	0.174	0.095
Canned, solids and liquid (2.0% protein)	0.012	0.082	0.074	0.220	0.074	0.039	0.033	0.112	0.067	0.125	0.094	0.052
Cowpeas (9.4% protein)	0.099	0.353	0.465	0.653	0.617	0.131	—	0.523	—	0.513	0.615	0.310
Lima beans												
Raw (7.5% protein)	0.097	0.338	0.460	0.605	0.474	0.080	0.083	0.389	0.259	0.485	0.454	0.247
Canned, solids and liquid (3.8% protein)	0.049	0.171	0.233	0.306	0.240	0.041	0.042	0.197	0.131	0.246	0.230	0.125
Peas												
Raw (6.7% protein)	0.056	0.245	0.308	0.418	0.316	0.054	0.073	0.257	0.163	0.274	0.595	0.109
Canned, solids and liquid (3.4% protein)	0.028	0.125	0.156	0.212	0.160	0.027	0.037	0.131	0.083	0.139	0.302	0.055
Leafy vegetables, raw (protein, N × 6.25)												
Amaranth (3.5% protein)	0.038	0.056	0.164	0.206	0.141	0.025	0.024	0.096	0.105	0.136	0.134	0.069
Beet greens (2.0% protein)	0.024	0.076	0.084	0.129	0.108	0.034	—	0.116	—	0.101	0.083	0.026
Brussels sprouts (4.4% protein)	0.044	0.153	0.186	0.194	0.197	0.046	—	0.148	—	0.193	0.279	0.106
Cabbage (1.4% protein)	0.011	0.039	0.040	0.057	0.066	0.013	0.028	0.030	0.030	0.043	0.105	0.025
Chard (1.4% protein)	0.014	0.058	0.060	0.076	0.055	0.004	—	0.046	—	0.055	0.035	0.018
Chicory (1.6% protein)	0.024	—	—	—	0.052	0.016	0.006	—	0.040	—	—	0.024
Collards (3.9% protein)	0.055	0.114	0.121	0.218	0.202	0.046	0.059	0.124	0.151	0.195	0.258	0.087
Kale (3.9% protein)	0.042	0.139	0.133	0.252	0.121	0.035	0.036	0.158	—	0.184	0.202	0.062
Lettuce (1.2% protein)	0.012	—	—	—	0.070	0.004	—	—	—	—	—	—
Mustard greens (2.3% protein)	0.037	0.060	0.075	0.062	0.111	0.024	0.035	0.074	0.121	0.108	0.167	0.041
Parsley, curly garden (2.5% protein)	0.050	—	—	—	0.160	0.012	—	—	—	—	—	—
Spinach (2.3% protein)	0.037	0.102	0.107	0.176	0.142	0.039	0.046	0.099	0.073	0.126	0.116	0.049
Turnip greens (2.9% protein)	0.045	0.125	0.107	0.207	0.129	0.052	0.045	0.146	0.105	0.149	0.167	0.051
Watercress (1.7% protein)	0.028	0.084	0.076	0.131	0.091	0.010	—	0.062	0.036	0.084	0.053	0.034
Starchy roots and tubers (protein, N × 6.25)												
Cassava												
Flour (1.6% protein)	0.021	0.044	0.045	0.066	0.066	0.010	0.018	0.045	0.030	0.049	0.159	0.025
Root (1.1% protein)	0.014	0.030	0.031	0.045	0.045	0.007	0.012	0.031	0.021	0.033	0.110	0.017
Potatoes												
Raw (2.0% protein)	0.021	0.079	0.088	0.100	0.107	0.025	0.019	0.088	0.036	0.107	0.099	0.029
Canned, solids and liquid (1.7% protein)	0.018	0.067	0.075	0.085	0.091	0.021	0.016	0.075	0.030	0.091	0.084	0.024
Sweet potatoes (*Ipomoea batatas*), raw (1.8% protein)	0.031	0.085	0.087	0.103	0.085	0.033	0.029	0.100	0.081	0.135	0.094	0.036
Taro (1.9% protein)	0.035	0.089	0.099	0.169	0.110	0.021	—	0.099	—	0.114	0.118	0.032
Yam (*Dioscorea* spp.) (2.1% protein)	0.035	—	—	—	0.110	0.034	—	—	—	—	—	—
Other vegetables (protein, N × 6.25)												
Asparagus												
Raw (2.2% protein)	0.027	0.066	0.080	0.096	0.103	0.032	—	0.069	—	0.106	0.123	0.036
Canned, solids and liquid (1.9% protein)	0.023	0.057	0.069	0.083	0.089	0.027	—	0.060	—	0.092	0.106	0.031
Beans, snap												
Raw (2.4% protein)	0.033	0.091	0.109	0.139	0.126	0.035	0.024	0.057	0.050	0.115	0.101	0.045
Canned, solids and liquid (1.0% protein)	0.014	0.038	0.045	0.058	0.052	0.014	0.010	0.024	0.021	0.048	0.042	0.019

Protein content and nitrogen conversion factor	Tryptophan (g)	Threonine (g)	Isoleucine (g)	Leucine (g)	Lysine (g)	Methionine (g)	Cystine (g)	Phenylalanine (g)	Tyrosine (g)	Valine (g)	Arginine (g)	Histidine (g)
Beets												
Raw (1.6% protein)	0.014	0.034	0.051	0.055	0.086	0.006	—	0.027	—	0.049	0.028	0.022
Canned, solids and liquid (0.9% protein)	0.0008	0.019	0.029	0.031	0.048	0.003	—	0.015	—	0.028	0.016	0.012
Broccoli (3.3% protein)	0.037	0.122	0.126	0.163	0.147	0.050	—	0.119	—	0.170	0.192	0.063
Carrots												
Raw (1.2% protein)	0.010	0.043	0.046	0.065	0.052	0.010	0.029	0.042	0.020	0.056	0.041	0.017
Canned, solids and liquid (0.5% protein)	0.004	0.018	0.019	0.027	0.022	0.004	0.012	0.018	0.008	0.023	0.017	0.007
Cauliflower (2.4% protein)	0.033	0.102	0.104	0.162	0.134	0.047	—	0.075	0.034	0.144	0.110	0.048
Celery (1.3% protein)	0.012	—	—	—	0.021	0.015	0.006	—	0.016	—	—	—
Chayote (0.6% protein)	0.008	—	—	—	0.038	0.001	—	—	—	—	—	—
Cowpeas, yardlong, immature pod (3.4% protein)	0.034	—	—	—	0.203	0.021	—	—	—	—	—	—
Cucumbers (0.7% protein)	0.005	0.019	0.022	0.030	0.031	0.007	—	0.016	—	0.024	0.053	0.001
Cushaw (1.5% protein)	0.014	—	—	—	0.044	0.008	—	—	—	—	—	—
Eggplant (1.1% protein)	0.010	0.038	0.056	0.068	0.030	0.006	—	0.048	—	0.065	0.037	0.019
Mallow (3.7% protein)	0.144	0.155	—	0.259	0.155	0.030	—	0.166	—	0.181	0.189	0.063
Mushrooms												
*Agaricus campestris**	0.006	—	0.532	0.281	—	0.167	—	—	—	0.378	0.235	—
Lactarius spp.†	0.006	0.156	0.201	0.139	0.088	0.021	—	0.018	—	0.116	0.021	0.027
Okra (1.8% protein)	0.018	0.066	0.069	0.101	0.076	0.022	0.017	0.065	0.079	0.091	0.093	0.030
Onions, mature (1.4% protein)	0.021	0.022	0.021	0.037	0.064	0.013	—	0.039	0.046	0.031	0.180	0.014
Peppers (1.2% protein)	0.009	0.050	0.046	0.046	0.051	0.016	—	0.055	—	0.033	0.024	0.014
Prickly pears (1.1% protein)	0.009	0.053	0.044	0.057	0.044	0.008	—	0.059	—	0.041	0.032	0.016
Pumpkin (1.2% protein)	0.016	0.028	0.044	0.063	0.058	0.011	—	0.032	0.016	0.045	0.043	0.019
Radishes (1.2% protein)	0.005	0.059	—	—	0.034	0.002	—	—	—	0.030	—	—
Soybean sprouts (6.2% protein)	—	0.159	0.225	0.265	0.211	0.045	—	0.186	—	0.225	0.225	0.133
Squash, summer (0.6% protein)	0.005	0.014	0.019	0.027	0.023	0.008	—	0.016	—	0.022	0.027	0.009
Tomatoes and cherry tomatoes (1.0% protein)	0.009	0.033	0.029	0.041	0.042	0.007	—	0.028	0.014	0.028	0.029	0.015
Turnips (1.1% protein)	—	—	0.020	—	0.057	0.012	—	0.020	0.029	—	—	—
Miscellaneous food items												
Vegetable patty or steak (principally wheat protein) (15% protein, N × 5.70)	0.142	0.411	0.884	1.079	0.321	0.253	—	0.811	—	0.705	0.597	0.321
Yeast												
Baker's, compressed (N × 6.25)	0.122	0.655	0.655	1.151	0.914	0.248	0.120	0.607	0.580	0.840	0.536	0.353
Brewer's dried (N × 6.25)	0.710	2.353	2.398	3.226	3.300	0.836	0.548	1.902	1.902	2.723	2.250	1.251

*Total nitrogen is 0.58%. This is equivalent to 2.4% protein on the basis that two thirds of the nitrogen is protein nitrogen. If total nitrogen is used for the calculation, the protein content is 3.6%.

†Total nitrogen is 0.69%. This is equivalent to 2.9% protein on the basis that two thirds of the nitrogen is protein nitrogen. If total nitrogen is used for the calculation, the protein content is 4.3%.

Appendix C   Fatty Acid Content of Common Vegetable Oils

Vegetable oil	Polyunsaturated (%)	Monounsaturated (%)	Saturated (%)
Safflower	74	12	9
Walnut	66	15	11
Sunflower	64	21	10
Wheat germ	61	16	17
Corn	58	25	13
Soybean (unhydrogenated)	58	23	15
Cottonseed	51	19	26
Sesame seed	40	40	15
Soybean (partially hydrogenated)	40	47	13
Peanut	30	46	19
Olive	9	72	14
Palm	9	38	48
Coconut	2	6	86

Modified from Brown HB: Current focus on fat in the diet, ADA White Paper, *J Am Diet Assoc* 68:25, 1977. Other substances in the oils that make up total composition (100%) include such materials as sterols, vitamins, phospholipids, and water.

Relative Ratios of Polyunsaturated Fat and Saturated Fat (P/S Ratio) in Representative Foods

P/S ratio	Foods	P/S ratio	Foods
High >2.5:12	Almonds Corn oil Cottonseed oil Mayonnaise (made with oils in this group) Safflower oil Sesame oil Soft margarines Soybean oil Sunflower oil Walnuts	Low 0.1-0.5:1	Chicken liver Lamb Lard Olive oil Palm oil Pork Veal
Medium high 2:1	Chicken Fish Peanut oil Semisolid margarines	Very low < 0.1:1	Beef Butter, cream Coconut oil Egg yolk Whole milk, milk products
Medium 1:1	Beef heart, liver Hydrogenated or hardened vegetable oils (shortenings, special products) Peanuts, peanut butter Pecans Solid margarines		

Appendix E Caffeine Content of Common Beverages and Drugs

Source	Caffeine (mg)
Beverages (180 ml cup)	
Brewed coffee	80-140
Instant coffee	60-100
Decaffeinated coffee	1-6
Leaf tea	30-80
Tea bags	25-75
Instant tea	30-60
Cocoa	10-50
Cola drinks (8 oz)	15-50
Candy bar, chocolate (1 oz)	20
Caffeine-containing analgesics	
General	30 (per unit)
Excedrine	60 (per unit)
Cafergot	100 (per unit)

Food	Amount	Weight (g)	Total dietary fiber (g)	Noncellulose polysaccharides (g)	Cellulose (g)	Lignin
Apple	1 med					
Flesh		138	1.96	1.29	0.66	0.01
Skin		100	3.71	2.21	1.01	0.49
Banana	1 small	119	2.08	1.33	0.44	0.31
Beans						
Baked	1 cup	255	18.53	14.45	3.59	0.48
Green, cooked	1 cup	125	4.19	2.31	1.61	0.26
Bread						
White	1 slice	25	0.68	0.50	0.18	Trace
Whole meal	1 slice	25	2.13	1.49	0.33	0.31
Broccoli, cooked	1 cup	155	6.36	4.53	1.78	0.05
Brussels sprouts, cooked	1 cup	155	4.43	3.08	1.24	0.11
Cabbage, cooked	1 cup	145	4.10	2.55	1.00	0.55
Carrots, cooked	1 cup	155	5.74	3.44	2.29	Trace
Cauliflower, cooked	1 cup	125	2.25	0.84	1.41	Trace
Cereals						
All-Bran	1 oz	30	8.01	5.35	1.80	0.86
Corn Flakes	1 cup	25	2.75	1.82	0.61	0.33
Grapenuts	¼ cup	30	2.10	1.54	0.38	0.17
Puffed Wheat	1 cup	15	2.31	1.55	0.39	0.37
Rice Krispies	1 cup	30	1.34	1.04	0.23	0.07
Shredded Wheat	1 biscuit	25	3.07	2.20	0.66	0.21
Special K	1 cup	30	1.64	1.10	0.22	0.32
Cherries	10 cherries	68	0.84	0.63	0.17	0.05
Cookies						
Ginger	4 snaps	28	0.56	0.41	0.08	0.07
Oatmeal	4 cookies	52	2.08	1.64	0.21	0.22
Plain	4 cookies	48	0.80	0.68	0.05	0.06
Corn	1 cup	165	7.82	7.11	0.51	0.20
Canned	1 cup	165	9.39	8.20	1.06	0.13
Flour						
Bran	1 cup	100	44.00	32.70	8.05	3.23
White	1 cup	115	3.62	2.90	0.69	0.03
Whole meal	1 cup	120	11.41	7.50	2.95	0.96
Grapefruit	½ cup	100	0.44	0.34	0.04	0.06
Jam, strawberry	1 tbsp	20	0.22	0.17	0.02	0.03
Lettuce	⅙ head	100	1.53	0.47	1.06	Trace
Marmalade, orange	1 tbsp	20	0.14	0.13	0.01	Trace
Onions, raw, sliced	1 cup	100	2.10	1.55	0.55	Trace

Continued

Food	Amount	Weight (g)	Total dietary fiber (g)	Noncellulose polysaccharides (g)	Cellulose (g)	Lignin
Orange	1 cup	200	0.58	0.44	0.08	0.06
Parsnips, raw, diced	1 cup	100	4.90	3.77	1.13	Trace
Peach, flesh and skin	1 med	100	2.28	1.46	0.20	0.62
Peanuts	1 oz	30	2.79	1.92	0.51	0.36
Peanut butter	1 tbsp	16	1.21	0.90	0.31	Trace
Pear	1 med					
Flesh		164	4.00	2.16	1.10	0.74
Skin		100	8.59	3.72	2.18	2.67
Peas, canned	1 cup	170	13.35	8.84	3.91	0.60
Peas, raw or frozen	1 cup	100	7.75	5.48	2.09	0.18
Plums	1 plum	66	1.00	0.65	0.15	0.20
Potato, raw	1 med	135	4.73	3.36	1.38	Trace
Raisins	1 oz	30	1.32	0.72	0.25	0.35
Strawberries	1 cup	149	2.65	1.39	1.04	0.22
Tomato						
Raw	1 med	135	1.89	0.88	0.61	0.41
Canned, drained	1 cup	240	2.04	1.08	0.89	0.07
Turnips, raw	1 med	100	2.20	1.50	0.70	Trace

Modified from Southgate DAT et al: A guide to calculating intakes of dietary fiber, *J Hum Nutr* 30:303, 1976.

Appendix G

Sodium Content of Popular Condiments, Fats, and Oils

Product	Portion size	Sodium (mg)	Product	Portion size	Sodium (mg)
Salt	1 tsp	1938	Pickle, sweet	1 pickle	128
Garlic salt	1 tsp	1850	Relish (sweet)	1 tbsp	124
Meat tenderizer (regular)	1 tsp	1750	Italian dressing (bottled, store bought)	1 tbsp	116
Onion salt	1 tsp	1620	Butter (regular)	1 tbsp	116
Soy sauce	1 tbsp	1029	Thousand Island dressing (regular)	1 tbsp	109
Dill pickle	1 pickle	928	Pickles, bread-and-butter	2 slices	101
Baking soda	1 tsp	821	Mission olives, ripe	3 olives	96
Teriyaki sauce	1 tbsp	690	French dressing (home recipe)	1 tbsp	92
Monosodium glutamate (MSG)	1 tsp	492	Mayonnaise	1 tbsp	78
Baking powder	1 tsp	339	Butter (whipped)	1 tbsp	74
Green olives	4 olives	323	Mustard (prepared)	1 tsp	65
A-1 Steak Sauce	1 tbsp	275	Chili powder	1 tsp	26
French dressing (dry mix, prepared)	1 tbsp	253	Tabasco sauce	1 tsp	24
Chili sauce (regular)	1 tbsp	227	Chili sauce (low sodium)	1 tbsp	11
French dressing (bottled, store bought)	1 tbsp	214	Parsley, dried	1 tbsp	6
Worcestershire sauce	1 tbsp	206	Catsup (low sodium)	1 tbsp	3
Horseradish (prepared)	1 tbsp	198	French dressing (low sodium)	1 tbsp	3
Tartar sauce	1 tbsp	182	Butter (unsalted)	1 tbsp	2
Italian dressing (dry mix, prepared)	1 tbsp	172	Meat tenderizer (low sodium)	1 tsp	1
Catsup (regular)	1 tbsp	156	Onion powder	1 tsp	1
Thousand Island dressing (low kcalorie)	1 tbsp	153	Black pepper	1 tsp	1
Blue cheese dressing	1 tbsp	153	Vinegar	1/2 cup	1
Margarine (regular)	1 tbsp	140	Margarine (unsalted)	1 tbsp	1
Russian dressing	1 tbsp	133	Oil, vegetable (corn, olive, soybean)	1 tbsp	0
Barbecue sauce	1 tbsp	130			

Modified from *The sodium content of your food*, Home and Garden Bulletin No 233, US Department of Agriculture, Washington, DC, Aug 1980, US Government Printing Office.

Appendix **H** Salt-Free Seasoning Guide

Fish

Breaded, battered fillets
  Dry mustard, onion;
  oregano, basil, garlic;
  thyme
Broiled steaks or fillets
  Chili or curry powder;
  tarragon
Fillets in butter sauce
  Thyme, chervil; dill; fennel
Fish soup
  Italian seasoning; bay leaf,
  thyme, tarragon
Fish cakes
  Tarragon, savory; dry mus-
  tard, white pepper; red
  pepper, oregano

Beef

Swiss steak
  Rosemary, black pepper; bay
  leaf, thyme; clove
Roast beef
  Basil, oregano; bay leaf; nut-
  meg; tarragon, marjoram
Beef stew
  Chili powder; bay leaf, tar-
  ragon; caraway; marjoram
Meatballs
  Garlic, thyme; basil,
  oregano, onion; thyme,
  garlic; black pepper, dry
  mustard
Beef stroganoff
  Red pepper, onion, garlic;
  nutmeg, onion; curry
  powder

Poultry and veal

Fried chicken
  Basil, oregano, garlic; onion,
  dill; sesame seed, nutmeg
Roast chicken or turkey
  Ginger, garlic; onion, thyme,
  tarragon
Chicken croquettes
  Dill; curry; chili, cumin;
  tarragon, oregano
Veal patties
  Italian seasoning; tarragon;
  dill, onion, sesame seed
Barbecue chicken
  Garlic, dry mustard; clove,
  allspice, dry mustard; basil,
  garlic, and oregano

Gravies and sauces

Barbecue
  Bay leaf, thyme, red pepper;
  cinnamon, ginger, allspice,
  dry mustard, red pepper;
  chili powder
Brown
  Chervil, onion; onion, bay
  leaf, thyme; onion, nutmeg;
  tarragon
Chicken
  Dry mustard; ginger, garlic;
  marjoram, thyme, bay leaf
Cream
  White pepper, dry mustard;
  curry powder; dill, onion,
  paprika; tarragon, thyme

Soups

Chicken
  Thyme, savory; ginger;|
  clove, white pepper,
  allspice
Clam chowder
  Basil, oregano; nutmeg,
  white pepper; thyme,
  garlic powder
Mushroom
  Ginger; oregano; thyme,
  tarragon; bay leaf, black
  pepper; chili powder
Onion
  Curry, caraway; marjoram,
  garlic; cloves
Tomato
  Bay leaf, thyme; Italian
  seasoning; oregano, onion;
  nutmeg
Vegetable
  Italian seasoning; paprika,
  caraway; rosemary, thyme;
  fennel, thyme

Salads

Chicken
  Curry or chili powder;
  Italian seasoning; thyme,
  tarragon
Coleslaw
  Dill; caraway; poppy; dry
  mustard, ginger
Fish or seafood
  Dill; tarragon, ginger, dry
  mustard, red pepper;
  ginger, onion, garlic
Macaroni
  Dill; basil, thyme, oregano;
  dry mustard, garlic
Potato
  Chili powder; curry; dry
  mustard, onion

Pasta, beans, and rice

Baked beans
  Dry mustard; chili powder;
  clove, onion; ginger, dry
  mustard
Rice and vegetables
  Curry; thyme, onion,
  paprika; rosemary, garlic;
  ginger, onion, garlic
Spanish rice
  Cumin, oregano, basil;
  Italian seasoning
Spaghetti
  Italian seasoning, nutmeg;
  oregano, basil, nutmeg;
  red pepper, tarragon
Rice pilaf
  Dill; thyme; savory, black
  pepper

Vegetables

Asparagus
  Ginger; sesame seed; basil,
  onion
Broccoli
  Italian seasoning; marjoram,
  basil; nutmeg, onion;
  sesame seed
Cabbage
  Caraway; onion, nutmeg;
  allspice, clove
Carrots
  Ginger; nutmeg; onion, dill
Cauliflower
  Dry mustard; basil; paprika,
  onion
Tomatoes
  Oregano; chili powder; dill,
  onion
Spinach
  Savory, thyme; nutmeg;
  garlic, onion

654

Appendix | Physical Growth NCHS Percentiles

GIRLS: BIRTH TO 36 MONTHS
PHYSICAL GROWTH
NCHS PERCENTILES*

NAME_____   RECORD #_____

Ross
Growth &
Development
Program

DATE	AGE	LENGTH	WEIGHT	HEAD CIRC.	COMMENT
	BIRTH				

MOTHER'S STATURE _____   GESTATIONAL
FATHER'S STATURE _____   AGE _____ WEEKS

BOYS: BIRTH TO 36 MONTHS
PHYSICAL GROWTH
NCHS PERCENTILES*

NAME _____   RECORD # _____

*Adapted from: Hamill PVV, Drizd TA, Johnson CL, Reed RB, Roche AF, Moore WM: Physical growth: National Center for Health Statistics percentiles. AM J CLIN NUTR 32:607-629, 1979. Data from the Fels Research Institute, Wright State University School of Medicine, Yellow Springs, Ohio.

© 1982 ROSS LABORATORIES

Ross
Growth &
Development
Program

GIRLS: BIRTH TO 36 MONTHS
PHYSICAL GROWTH
NCHS PERCENTILES*

NAME_____ RECORD #_____

*Adapted from: Hamill PVV, Drizd TA, Johnson CL, Reed RB Roche AF, Moore WM. Physical growth: National Center for Health Statistics percentiles. AM J CLIN NUTR 32:607-629, 1979. Data from the Fels Research Institute, Wright State University School of Medicine, Yellow Springs, Ohio.

© 1982 ROSS LABORATORIES

DATE	AGE	LENGTH	WEIGHT	HEAD CIRC.	COMMENT

Recommend the formulation you prefer
with the name you trust

SIMILAC®
SIMILAC® WITH IRON
SIMILAC® WITH WHEY
Infant Formulas

The **ISOMIL®** System of
Soy Protein Formulas

ADVANCE®
Nutritional Beverage

ROSS LABORATORIES
COLUMBUS, OHIO 43216
Division of Abbott Laboratories, USA

G106/JUNE 1983   LITHO IN USA

BOYS: BIRTH TO 36 MONTHS
PHYSICAL GROWTH
NCHS PERCENTILES*

NAME_____ RECORD #_____

*Adapted from: Hamill PVV, Drizd TA, Johnson CL, Reed RB, Roche AF, Moore WM: Physical growth: National Center for Health Statistics percentiles. AM J CLIN NUTR 32:607-629, 1979. Data from the Fels Research Institute, Wright State University School of Medicine, Yellow Springs, Ohio.
© 1982 ROSS LABORATORIES

DATE	AGE	LENGTH	WEIGHT	HEAD CIRC.	COMMENT

Recommend the formulation you prefer
with the name you trust

SIMILAC®
SIMILAC® WITH IRON
SIMILAC® WITH WHEY
Infant Formulas

The **ISOMIL®** System of
Soy Protein Formulas

ADVANCE®
Nutritional Beverage

ROSS LABORATORIES
COLUMBUS, OHIO 43216
Division of Abbott Laboratories, USA

G105/JUNE 1983   LITHO IN USA

GIRLS: 2 TO 18 YEARS
PHYSICAL GROWTH
NCHS PERCENTILES*

NAME_____   RECORD #_____

*Adapted from: Hamill PVV, Drizd T.A, Johnson CL, Reed RB, Roche AF, Moore WM: Physical growth: National Center for Health Statistics percentiles. AM J CLIN NUTR 32:607-629, 1979. Data from the National Center for Health Statistics (NCHS) Hyattsville, Maryland.

Ross Growth & Development Program

© 1982 ROSS LABORATORIES

BOYS: 2 TO 18 YEARS
PHYSICAL GROWTH
NCHS PERCENTILES*

NAME _____ RECORD # _____

Ross
Growth &
Development
Program

GIRLS: PREPUBESCENT
PHYSICAL GROWTH
NCHS PERCENTILES*

NAME_____ RECORD #_____

* Adapted from: Hamill PVV, Drizd TA, Johnson CL, Reed RB, Roche AF, Moore WM: Physical growth. National Center for Health Statistics percentiles. AM J CLIN NUTR 32:607-629, 1979. Data from the National Center for Health Statistics (NCHS) Hyattsville, Maryland.

© 1982 ROSS LABORATORIES

Recommend the formulation you prefer with the name you trust
SIMILAC®
SIMILAC® WITH IRON
SIMILAC® WITH WHEY
Infant Formulas

The **ISOMIL®** System of **ADVANCE®**
Soy Protein Formulas   **Nutritional Beverage**

ROSS LABORATORIES
COLUMBUS, OHIO 43216
Division of Abbott Laboratories, USA

G108/JUNE 1983   LITHO IN USA

BOYS: PREPUBESCENT
PHYSICAL GROWTH
NCHS PERCENTILES*

NAME _____ RECORD # _____

DATE	AGE	STATURE	WEIGHT	COMMENT

*Adapted from: Hamill PVV, Drizd TA, Johnson CL, Reed RB, Roche AF, Moore WM: Physical growth: National Center for Health Statistics percentiles. AM J CLIN NUTR 32:607-629, 1979. Data from the National Center for Health Statistics (NCHS) Hyattsville, Maryland.

© 1982 ROSS LABORATORIES

STATURE

cm 85 90 95 100 105 110 115 120 125 130 135 140 145

in 34 35 36 37 38 39 40 41 42 43 44 45 46 47 48 49 50 51 52 53 54 55 56 57 58

Recommend the formulation you prefer with the name you trust

SIMILAC®
SIMILAC® WITH IRON
SIMILAC® WITH WHEY
Infant Formulas

The ISOMIL® System of
Soy Protein Formulas

ADVANCE®
Nutritional Beverage

ROSS LABORATORIES
COLUMBUS, OHIO 43216
Division of Abbott Laboratories, USA

G107/JUNE 1983   LITHO IN USA

Appendix J Assessment of Nutritional Status: Percentiles

Mid-upper-arm circumference percentiles (cm)

Age (yr)	Female percentiles					Male percentiles				
	5th	25th	50th	75th	95th	5th	25th	50th	75th	95th
1	13.8	14.8	15.6	16.4	17.7	14.2	15.0	15.9	17.0	18.3
2	14.2	15.2	16.0	16.7	18.4	14.1	15.3	16.2	17.0	18.5
3	14.3	15.8	16.7	17.5	18.9	15.0	16.0	16.7	17.5	19.0
4	14.9	16.0	16.9	17.7	19.1	14.9	16.2	17.1	18.0	19.2
5	15.3	16.5	17.5	18.5	21.1	15.3	16.7	17.5	18.5	20.4
6	15.6	17.0	17.6	18.7	21.1	15.5	16.7	17.9	18.8	22.8
7	16.4	17.4	18.3	19.9	23.1	16.2	17.7	18.7	20.1	23.0
8	16.8	18.3	19.5	21.4	26.1	16.2	17.7	19.0	20.2	24.5
9	17.8	19.4	21.1	22.4	26.0	17.5	18.7	20.0	21.7	25.7
10	17.4	19.3	21.0	22.8	26.5	18.1	19.6	21.0	23.1	27.4
11	18.5	20.8	22.4	24.8	30.3	18.6	20.2	22.3	24.4	28.0
12	19.4	21.6	23.7	25.6	29.4	19.3	21.4	23.2	25.4	30.3
13	20.2	22.3	24.3	27.1	33.8	19.4	22.8	24.7	26.3	30.1
14	21.4	23.7	25.2	27.2	32.2	22.0	23.7	25.3	28.3	32.3
15	20.8	23.9	25.4	27.9	32.2	22.2	24.4	26.4	28.4	32.0
16	21.8	24.1	25.8	28.3	32.4	24.4	26.2	27.8	30.3	34.3
17	22.0	24.1	26.4	29.5	35.0	24.6	26.7	28.5	30.8	34.7
18	22.2	24.1	25.8	28.1	32.5	24.5	27.6	29.7	32.1	37.9
19-25	21.1	24.7	26.5	29.0	34.5	26.2	28.8	30.8	33.1	37.2
25-35	23.3	25.6	27.7	30.4	36.8	27.1	30.0	31.9	34.2	37.5
35-45	24.1	26.7	29.0	31.7	37.8	27.8	30.5	32.6	34.5	37.4
45-55	24.2	27.4	29.9	32.8	38.4	26.7	30.1	32.2	34.2	37.6
55-65	24.3	28.0	30.3	33.5	38.5	25.8	29.6	31.7	33.6	36.9
65-75	24.0	27.4	29.9	32.6	37.3	24.8	28.5	30.7	32.5	35.5

Data derived from the Health and Nutrition Examination Survey data of 1971-1974, using same population samples as those of the National Center for Health Statistics (NCHS) growth percentiles for children. Modified from Frisancho AR: New norms of upper limb fat and muscle areas for assessment of nutritional status, *Am J Clin Nutr* 34:2540, 1981.

Triceps skinfold percentiles (mm)

Age (yr)	Female percentiles					Male percentiles				
	5th	25th	50th	75th	95th	5th	25th	50th	75th	95th
1	6	8	10	12	16	6	8	10	12	16
2	6	9	10	12	16	6	8	10	12	15
3	7	9	11	12	15	6	8	10	11	15
4	7	8	10	12	16	6	8	9	11	14
5	6	8	10	12	18	6	8	9	11	15
6	6	8	10	12	16	5	7	8	10	16
7	6	9	11	13	18	5	7	9	12	17
8	6	9	12	15	24	5	7	8	10	16
9	8	10	13	16	22	6	7	10	13	18
10	7	10	12	17	27	6	8	10	14	21
11	7	10	13	18	28	6	8	11	16	24
12	8	11	14	18	27	6	8	11	14	28
13	8	12	15	21	30	5	7	10	14	26
14	9	13	16	21	28	4	7	9	14	24
15	8	12	17	21	32	4	6	8	11	24
16	10	15	18	22	31	4	6	8	12	22
17	10	13	19	24	37	5	6	8	12	19
18	10	15	18	22	30	4	6	9	13	24
19-25	10	14	18	24	34	4	7	10	15	22
25-35	10	16	21	27	37	5	8	12	16	24
35-45	12	18	23	29	38	5	8	12	16	23
45-55	12	20	25	30	40	6	8	12	15	25
55-65	12	20	25	31	38	5	8	11	14	22
65-75	12	18	24	29	36	4	8	11	15	22

Mid-upper-arm muscle circumference percentiles (cm)

Age (yr)	Female percentiles					Male percentiles				
	5th	25th	50th	75th	95th	5th	25th	50th	75th	95th
1	10.5	11.7	12.4	13.9	14.3	11.0	11.9	12.7	13.5	14.7
2	11.1	11.9	12.6	13.3	14.7	11.1	12.2	13.0	14.0	15.0
3	11.3	12.4	13.2	14.0	15.2	11.7	13.1	13.7	14.3	15.3
4	11.5	12.8	13.8	14.4	15.7	12.3	13.3	14.1	14.8	15.9
5	12.5	13.4	14.2	15.1	16.5	12.8	14.0	14.7	15.4	16.9
6	13.0	13.8	14.5	15.4	17.1	13.1	14.2	15.1	16.1	17.7
7	12.9	14.2	15.1	16.0	17.6	13.7	15.1	16.0	16.8	19.0
8	13.8	15.1	16.0	17.1	19.4	14.0	15.4	16.2	17.0	18.7
9	14.7	15.8	16.7	18.0	19.8	15.1	16.1	17.0	18.3	20.2
10	14.8	15.9	17.0	18.0	19.7	15.6	16.6	18.0	19.1	22.1
11	15.0	17.1	18.1	19.6	22.3	15.9	17.3	18.3	19.5	23.0
12	16.2	18.0	19.1	20.1	22.0	16.7	18.2	19.5	21.0	24.1
13	16.9	18.3	19.8	21.1	24.0	17.2	19.6	21.1	22.6	24.5
14	17.4	19.0	20.1	21.6	24.7	18.9	21.2	22.3	24.0	26.4
15	17.5	18.9	20.2	21.5	24.4	19.9	21.8	23.7	25.4	27.2
16	17.0	19.0	20.2	21.6	24.9	21.3	23.4	24.9	26.9	29.6
17	17.5	19.4	20.5	22.1	25.7	22.4	24.5	25.8	27.3	31.2
18	17.4	19.1	20.2	21.5	24.5	22.6	25.2	26.4	28.3	32.4
19-25	17.9	19.5	20.7	22.1	24.9	23.8	25.7	27.3	28.9	32.1
25-35	18.3	19.9	21.2	22.8	26.4	24.3	26.4	27.9	29.8	32.6
35-45	18.6	20.5	21.8	23.6	27.2	24.7	26.9	28.6	30.2	32.7
45-55	18.7	20.6	22.0	23.8	27.4	23.9	26.5	28.1	30.0	32.6
55-65	18.7	20.9	22.5	24.4	28.0	23.6	26.0	27.8	29.5	32.0
65-75	18.5	20.8	22.5	24.4	27.9	22.3	25.1	26.8	28.4	30.6

Values derived by formula calculation. Data derived from the Health and Nutrition Examination Survey data of 1971-1974, using same population samples as those of the National Center for Health Statistics (NCHS) growth percentiles for children. Modified from Frisancho AR: New norms of upper limb fat and muscle areas for assessment of nutritional status, *Am J Clin Nutr* 34:2540, 1981.

IS YOUR WEIGHT HEALTHY?

Moderately to severely overweight range

Healthy weight range

Normal Constituents of Blood and Urine in Adults

Normal Constituents of Blood in the Adult

Physical measurements

Specific gravity		1.025-1.029
Viscosity (water as unity)		4.5
Bleeding time (capillary)	Minutes	1-3
Prothrombin time (plasma) (Quick)	Seconds	10-20
Sedimentation rate (Wintrobe method)		
Men	mm/hr	0-9
Women	mm/hr	0-20

Hemologic studies

Cell volume	%	39-50
Red blood cells	Million per mm^3	4.25-5.25
White blood cells	Per mm^3	5000-9000
Lymphocytes	%	25-30
Neutrophils	%	60-65
Monocytes	%	4-8
Eosinophils	%	0.5-4
Basophils	%	0-1.5
Platelets	Per mm^3	125,000-300,000

Proteins

Total protein (serum)	g/dl	6.5-7.5
Albumin (serum)	g/dl	4.5-5.5
Globulin (serum)	g/dl	1.5-2.5
Albumin:globulin ratio		1.8-2.5
Fibrinogen (plasma)	g/dl	0.2-0.5
Hemoglobin		
Males	g/dl	14-17
Females	g/dl	13-16

Nitrogen constituents

Nonprotein N (serum)	mg/dl	20-36
(whole blood)	mg/dl	25-40
Urea (whole blood)	mg/dl	18-38
Urea N (whole blood)	mg/dl	8-18
Creatinine (whole blood)	mg/dl	1-2
Uric acid (whole blood)	mg/dl	2.5-5.0
Amino acid N (whole blood)	mg/dl	3-6

Carbohydrates and lipids

Glucose (whole blood)	mg/dl	70-90
Ketones—as acetone (whole blood)	mg/dl	1.5-2
Fats (total lipids) (serum)	mg/dl	570-820
Cholesterol (serum)	mg/dl	100-230
Bilirubin (serum)	mg/dl	0.1-0.25
Icteric index (serum)	units	4-6

Blood gases

CO_2 content (serum)	vol %	55-75
	mmol/L	(24.5-33.5)
CO_2 content (whole blood)	vol %	40-60
	mmol/L	(18.0-27.0)
Oxygen capacity (whole blood)		
Males	vol %	18.7-22.7
Females	vol %	17.0-21.0
Oxygen saturation		
Arterial blood	%	94-96
Venous blood	%	60-85

Abbreviations and conversion factors:

dl	=	deciliter
ml	=	milliliter
µg	=	microgram

$$mEq/L = \frac{mg/L}{\text{Equivalent weight}}$$

$$\text{Equivalent weight} = \frac{\text{Atomic weight}}{\text{Valence of element}}$$

g	=	gram
mm^3	=	cubic millimeter
mEq	=	milliequivalent

$$mmol \text{ (millimole)}/L = \frac{mg/L}{\text{Molecular weight}}$$

vol % (volumes percent) = mmol/L x 2.24

Normal Constituents of Blood in the Adult—cont'd

Acid-base constituents

Base, total fixed (serum)	mEq/L	142-150	Lactic acid (venous blood)	mg/dl	10-20
Sodium (serum)	mg/dl	320-335		mEq/L	(1.1-2.2)
	mEq/L	(139-146)	Serum protein base binding power	mEq/L	(15.5-18.0)
Potassium (serum)	mg/dl	16-22			
	mEq/L	(4.1-5.6)	Base bicarbonate HCO_3 (serum)	mEq/L	(19-30)
Calcium (serum)	mg/dl	9.0-11.5			
	mEq/L	(4.5-5.8)	pH (blood or plasma at 38° C)		7.3-7.45
Magnesium (serum)	mg/dl	1.0-3.0			
	mEq/L	(1.0-2.5)	**Miscellaneous**		
Phosphorus, inorganic (serum)	mg/dl	3.0-5.0	Phosphatase (serum)	Bodansky units per deciliter	5
	mEq/L	(1.0-1.6)			
Chlorides, expressed as Cl (serum)	mg/dl	352-383	Iron (whole blood)	mg/dl	46-55
	mEq/L	(99-108)	Ascorbic acid (whole blood)	mg/dl	0.75-1.50
As NaCl (serum)	mg/dl	580-630			
	mEq/L	(99-108)	Carotene (serum)	μg/dl	75-125
Sulfates, inorganic as SO_4 (serum)	mg/dl	2.5-5.0			
	mEq/L	(0.5-1.0)			

Normal Constituents of Urine in the Adult

Urine constituents	g/24 hr
Total solids	55-70
Nitrogenous constituents	
Total nitrogen	10-17
Ammonia	0.5-1.0
Amino acid N	0.4-1
Creatine	None
Creatinine	1-1.5
Protein	None
Purine bases	0.016-0.060
Urea	20-35
Uric acid	0.5-0.7
Acetone bodies	0.003-0.015
Bile	None
Calcium	0.2-0.4
Chloride (as NaCl)	10-15
Glucose	None
Indican	0-0.030
Iron	0.001-0.005
Magnesium (as MgO)	0.15-0.30
Phosphate, total (as phosphoric acid)	2.5-3.5
Potassium (as K_2O)	2.0-3.0
Sodium (as Na_2O)	4.0-5.0
Sulfates, total (as sulfuric acid)	1.5-3.0

Physical measurements

Specific gravity	1.010-1.025
Reaction (pH)	5.5-8.0
Volume (ml/24 hr)	800-1600

Exchange Lists for Meal Planning

Starch exchange list

(One exchange = 15 g carbohydrate, 3 g protein, 0-1 g fat, 80 kcal)

Bread

Bagel	½ (1 oz)
Bread, reduced-calorie	2 slices (1½ oz)
Bread, white, whole wheat, pumpernickel, rye	1 slice (1 oz)
Bread sticks, crisp, 4 inches long × ½ inch	2 (⅔ oz)
English muffin	½
Hot dog or hamburger bun	½ (1 oz)
Pita, 6 inches across	½
Roll, plain, small	1 (1 oz)
Raisin bread, unfrosted	1 slice (1 oz)
Tortilla, corn, 6 inches across	1
Tortilla, flour, 7-8 inches across	1
Waffle, 4½ inches square, reduced-fat	1

Cereals and grains

Bran cereals	½ cup
Bulgur	½ cup
Cereals	½ cup
Cereals, unsweetened, ready-to-eat	¾ cup
Cornmeal (dry)	3 tbsp
Couscous	⅓ cup
Flour (dry)	3 tbsp
Granola, low-fat	¼ cup
Grape-Nuts	¼ cup
Grits	½ cup
Kasha	½ cup
Millet	¼ cup
Muesli	¼ cup
Oats	½ cup
Pasta	½ cup
Puffed cereal	1½ cups
Rice milk	½ cup
Rice, white or brown	⅓ cup
Shredded Wheat	½ cup
Sugar-frosted cereal	½ cup
Wheat germ	3 tbsp

Starchy vegetables

Baked beans	⅓ cup
Corn	½ cup
Corn on cob, medium	1 (5 oz)
Mixed vegetables with corn, peas, or pasta	1 cup
Peas, green	½ cup
Plantain	½ cup
Potato, baked or boiled	1 small (3 oz)
Potato, mashed	½ cup
Squash, winter (acorn, butternut)	1 cup
Yam, sweet potato, plain	½ cup

Crackers and snacks

Animal crackers	8
Graham crackers, 2½ inches square	3
Matzoh	¾ oz
Melba toast	4 slices
Oyster crackers	24
Popcorn (popped, no fat added or low-fat microwave)	3 cups
Pretzels	¾ oz
Rice cakes, 4 inches across	2
Saltine-type crackers	6
Snack chips, fat-free (tortilla, potato)	15-20 (¾ oz)
Whole-wheat crackers, no fat added	2-5 (¾ oz)

Dried beans, peas, and lentils

(Count as 1 starch exchange, plus 1 very lean meat exchange)

Beans and peas (garbanzo, pinto, kidney, white, split, black-eyed)	½ cup
Lima beans	⅔ cup
Lentils	½ cup
Miso	3 tbsp

Starchy foods prepared with fat

(Count as 1 starch exchange, plus 1 fat exchange)

Biscuit, 2½ inches across	1
Chow mein noodles	½ cup
Corn bread, 2-inch cube	1 (2 oz)
Crackers, round butter type	6
Croutons	1 cup
French-fried potatoes	16-25 (3 oz)
Granola	¼ cup
Muffin, small	1 (1½ oz)
Pancake, 4 inches across	2
Popcorn, microwave	3 cups

Starchy foods prepared with fat—cont'd

Sandwich crackers, cheese or peanut butter filling	3
Stuffing, bread (prepared)	1/3 cup
Taco shell, 6 inches across	2
Waffle, 4 1/2 inches square	1
Whole-wheat crackers, fat added	4-6 (1 oz)

Fruit exchange list

(One exchange = 15 g carbohydrate, 60 kcal; weight includes skin, core, seeds, and rind)

Fruit

Apple, unpeeled, small	1 (4 oz)
Applesauce, unsweetened	1/2 cup
Apples, dried	4 rings
Apricots, fresh	4 whole (5 1/2 oz)
Apricots, dried	8 halves
Apricots, canned	1/2 cup
Banana, small	1 (4 oz)
Blackberries	3/4 cup
Blueberries	3/4 cup
Cantaloupe, small	1/3 melon (11 oz) or 1 cup cubes
Cherries, sweet, fresh	12 (3 oz)
Cherries, sweet, canned	1/2 cup
Dates	3
Figs, fresh	1 1/2 large or 2 medium (3 1/2 oz)
Figs, dried	1 1/2
Fruit cocktail	1/2 cup
Grapefruit, large	1/2 (11 oz)
Grapefruit sections, canned	3/4 cup
Grapes, small	17 (3 oz)
Honeydew melon	1 slice (10 oz) or 1 cup cubes
Kiwi	1 (3 1/2 oz)
Mandarin oranges, canned	3/4 cup
Mango, small	1/2 fruit (5 1/2 oz) or 1/2 cup
Nectarine, small	1 (5 oz)
Orange, small	1 (6 1/2 oz)
Papaya	1/2 fruit (8 oz) or 1 cup cubes
Peach, medium, fresh	1 (6 oz)
Peaches, canned	1/2 cup
Pear, large, fresh	1/2 (4 oz)
Pears, canned	1/2 cup
Pineapple, fresh	3/4 cup

Pineapple, canned	1/2 cup
Plums, small	2 (5 oz)
Plums, canned	1/2 cup
Prunes, dried	3
Raisins	2 tbsp
Raspberries	1 cup
Strawberries	1 1/4 cup whole berries
Tangerines, small	2 (8 oz)
Watermelon	1 slice (13 1/2 oz) or 1 1/4 cup cubes

Fruit juice

Apple juice/cider	1/2 cup
Cranberry juice cocktail	1/3 cup
Cranberry juice cocktail, reduced-calorie	1 cup
Fruit juice blends, 100% juice	1/3 cup
Grape juice	1/3 cup
Grapefruit juice	1/2 cup
Orange juice	1/2 cup
Pineapple juice	1/2 cup
Prune juice	1/3 cup

Milk exchange list

(One exchange = 12 g carbohydrate, 8 g protein)

Skim and very low-fat milk

(0-3 g fat per serving)

Skim milk	1 cup
1/2% milk	1 cup
1% milk	1 cup
Nonfat or low-fat buttermilk	1 cup
Evaporated skim milk	1/2 cup
Nonfat dry milk	1/3 cup dry
Plain nonfat yogurt	3/4 cup
Nonfat or low-fat fruit-flavored yogurt sweetened with aspartame or with a nonnutritive sweetener	1 cup

Low-fat milk

(5 g fat per serving)

2% milk	1 cup
Plain low-fat yogurt	3/4 cup
Sweet acidophilus milk	1 cup

Whole milk

(8 g fat per serving)

Whole milk	1 cup
Evaporated whole milk	1/2 cup
Goat's milk	1 cup
Kefir	1 cup

Other carbohydrates list

(One exchange = 15 g carbohydrate, or 1 starch, 1 fruit, or 1 milk)

Food	*Serving size*	*Exchanges per serving*
Angel food cake, unfrosted	1/12 cake	2 carbohydrates
Brownie, small, unfrosted	2 inches square	1 carbohydrate, 1 fat
Cake, unfrosted	2 inches square	1 carbohydrate, 1 fat
Cake, frosted	2 inches square	2 carbohydrates, 1 fat

Other carbohydrates list—cont'd

Food	Serving size	Exchanges per serving
Cookie, fat-free	2 small	1 carbohydrate
Cookie or sandwich cookie with creme filling	2 small	1 carbohydrate, 1 fat
Cupcake, frosted	1 small	2 carbohydrates, 1 fat
Cranberry sauce, jellied	1/4 cup	2 carbohydrates
Doughnut, plain cake	1 medium (1 1/2 oz)	1 1/2 carbohydrates, 2 fats
Doughnut, glazed	3 3/4 inches across (2 oz)	2 carbohydrates, 2 fats
Fruit juice bars, frozen, 100% juice	1 bar (3 oz)	1 carbohydrate
Fruit snacks, chewy (pureed fruit concentrate)	1 roll (3/4 oz)	1 carbohydrate
Fruit spreads, 100% fruit	1 tbsp	1 carbohydrate
Gelatin, regular	1/2 cup	1 carbohydrate
Gingersnaps	3	1 carbohydrate
Granola bar	1 bar	1 carbohydrate, 1 fat
Granola bar, fat free	1 bar	2 carbohydrates
Hummus	1/3 cup	1 carbohydrate, 1 fat
Ice cream	1/2 cup	1 carbohydrate, 2 fats
Ice cream, light	1/2 cup	1 carbohydrate, 1 fat
Ice cream, fat-free, no sugar added	1/2 cup	1 carbohydrate
Jam or jelly, regular	1 tbsp	1 carbohydrate
Milk, chocolate, whole	1 cup	2 carbohydrates, 1 fat
Pie, fruit, 2 crusts	1/6 pie	3 carbohydrates, 2 fats
Pie, pumpkin or custard	1/8 pie	1 carbohydrate, 2 fats
Potato chips	12-18 (1 oz)	1 carbohydrate, 2 fats
Pudding, regular (made with low-fat milk)	1/2 cup	2 carbohydrates
Pudding, sugar-free (made with low-fat milk)	1/2 cup	1 carbohydrate
Salad dressing, fat-free	1/4 cup	1 carbohydrate
Sherbet, sorbet	1/2 cup	2 carbohydrates
Spaghetti or pasta sauce, canned	1/2 cup	1 carbohydrate, 1 fat
Sweet roll or Danish	1 (2 1/2 oz)	2 1/2 carbohydrates, 2 fats
Syrup, light	2 tbsp	1 carbohydrate
Syrup, regular	1 tbsp	1 carbohydrate
Syrup, regular	1/4 cup	4 carbohydrates
Tortilla chips	6-12 (1 oz)	1 carbohydrate, 2 fats
Vanilla wafers	5	1 carbohydrate, 1 fat
Yogurt, frozen, low fat, fat-free	1/3 cup	1 carbohydrate, 0-1 fat
Yogurt, frozen, fat-free, no sugar added	1/2 cup	1 carbohydrate
Yogurt, low fat with fruit	1 cup	3 carbohydrates, 0-1 fat

Vegetable exchange list

(One exchange = 5 g carbohydrate, 2 g protein, 0 g fat, 25 kcal)

One exchange equals 1/2 cup of cooked vegetables or vegetable juice, or 1 cup of raw vegetables.

Artichoke
Artichoke hearts
Asparagus
Beans (green, wax, Italian)
Bean sprouts
Beets
Broccoli
Brussels sprouts
Cabbage
Carrots
Cauliflower
Celery
Cucumber
Eggplant
Green onions or scallions
Greens (collard, kale, mustard, turnip)
Kohlrabi
Leeks
Mixed vegetables (without corn, peas, or pasta)
Mushrooms
Okra
Onions
Pea pods
Radishes
Salad greens
Sauerkraut
Spinach
Summer squash
Tomato
Tomatoes, canned
Tomato sauce
Tomato/vegetable juice
Turnips
Water chestnuts
Watercress
Zucchini

Meat exchange list

Very lean meat and substitutes

(One exchange = 0 g carbohydrate, 7 g protein, 0-1 g fat, 35 kcal)

Poultry: Chicken or turkey (white meat, no skin), Cornish hen (no skin)	1 oz
Fish: Fresh or frozen cod, flounder, haddock, trout; tuna fresh or canned in water	1 oz
Shellfish: Clams, crab, lobster, scallops, shrimp, imitation shellfish	1 oz
Game: Duck or pheasant (no skin), venison, buffalo, ostrich	1 oz
Cheese with 1 g or less fat per ounce:	
Nonfat or low-fat cottage cheese	¼ cup
Fat-free cheese	1 oz
Other:	
Processed sandwich meats with 1 g or less fat per ounce, such as deli thin, shaved meats, chipped beef, turkey ham	1 oz
Egg whites	2
Egg substitutes, plain	¼ cup
Hot dogs with 1 g or less fat per ounce	1 oz
Kidney (high in cholesterol)	1 oz
Sausage with 1 g or less fat per ounce	1 oz
Count as one very lean meat and one starch exchange:	
Dried beans, peas, lentils (cooked)	½ cup

Lean meat and substitutes

(One exchange = 0 g carbohydrate, 7 g protein, 3 g fat, 55 kcal)

Beef: USDA Select or Choice grades of lean beef trimmed of fat, such as round, sirloin, and flank steak; tenderloin; roast (rib, chuck, rump); steak (T-bone, porterhouse, cubed); ground round	1 oz
Pork: Lean pork, such as fresh ham; canned, cured, or boiled ham; Canadian bacon, tenderloin, center loin chop	
Lamb: Roast, chop, leg	1 oz
Veal: Lean chop, roast	
Poultry: Chicken, turkey (dark meat, no skin), chicken white meat (with skin), domestic duck or goose (well-drained of fat, no skin)	1 oz
Fish: Herring (uncreamed or smoked)	1 oz
Oysters	6 medium
Salmon (fresh or canned), catfish	1 oz
Sardines (canned)	2 medium
Tuna (canned in oil, drained)	1 oz
Game: Goose (no skin), rabbit	1 oz
Cheese: 4.5% fat cottage cheese	¼ cup
Grated parmesan	2 tbsp
Cheeses with 3 g or less fat per ounce	1 oz
Other: Hot dogs with 3 g or less fat per ounce	1½ oz
Processed sandwich meat with 3 g or less fat per ounce, such as turkey pastrami or kielbasa	1 oz
Liver, heart (high in cholesterol)	1 oz

Medium-fat meat and substitutes

(One exchange = 0 g carbohydrate, 7 g protein, 5 g fat, 75 kcal)

Beef: Most beef products fall into this category (ground beef, meat loaf, corned beef, short ribs, prime grades of meat trimmed of fat, such as prime rib)	1 oz
Pork: Top loin, chop, Boston butt, cutlet	1 oz
Lamb: Rib roast, ground	1 oz
Veal: Cutlet (ground or cubed, unbreaded)	1 oz
Poultry: Chicken dark meat (with skin), ground turkey or ground chicken, fried chicken (with skin)	1 oz
Fish: Any fried fish product	1 oz
Cheese: With 5 g or less fat per ounce	
Feta	1 oz
Mozzarella	1 oz
Ricotta	¼ cup (2 oz)
Other: Egg (high in cholesterol, limit to 3 per week)	1

Medium-fat meat and substitutes—cont'd

Sausage with 5 g or less fat per ounce	1 oz
Soy milk	1 cup
Tempeh	¼ cup
Tofu	4 oz or ½ cup

High-fat meat and substitutes

(One exchange = 0 g carbohydrate, 7 g protein, 8 g fat, 100 kcal)

These items are high in saturated fat, cholesterol, and calories and may raise blood cholesterol levels if eaten on a regular basis.

Pork: Spareribs, ground pork, pork sausage	1 oz
Cheese: All regular cheeses, such as American, cheddar, Monterey Jack, Swiss	1 oz
Other: Processed sandwich meats with 8 g or less fat per ounce, such as bologna, pimento loaf, salami	1 oz
Sausage, such as bratwurst, Italian, knockwurst, Polish, smoked	1 oz
Hot dog (turkey or chicken)	1 (10 per lb)
Bacon	3 slices (20 slices per lb)
Count as 1 high-fat meat plus 1 fat exchange:	
Hot dog (beef, pork, or combination)	1 (10 per lb)
Peanut butter (contains unsaturated fat)	2 tbsp

Fat Exchange List

(One exchange = 5 g fat, 45 kcal)

Monounsaturated fats

Avocado, medium	⅛ (1 oz)
Oil (canola, olive, peanut)	1 tsp
Olives: ripe (black)	8 large
Green, stuffed	10 large
Nuts: almonds, cashews	6 nuts
Mixed (50% peanuts)	6 nuts
Peanuts	10 nuts
Pecans	4 halves
Peanut butter, smooth or crunchy	2 tsp
Sesame seeds	1 tbsp
Tahini paste	2 tsp

Polyunsaturated fats

Margarine: stick, tub, or squeeze	1 tsp
Margarine: lower-fat (30% to 50% vegetable oil)	1 tbsp
Mayonnaise: regular	1 tsp
Mayonnaise: reduced-fat	1 tbsp
Nuts: walnuts, English	4 halves
Oil (corn, safflower, soybean)	1 tsp
Salad dressing: regular	1 tbsp
Salad dressing: reduced-fat	2 tbsp
Miracle Whip salad dressing: regular	2 tsp
Miracle Whip salad dressing: reduced-fat	1 tbsp
Seeds: pumpkin, sunflower	1 tbsp

Saturated fats

Bacon, cooked	1 slice (20 slices per lb)
Bacon, grease	1 tsp
Butter, stick	2 tsp
Butter, whipped	2 tsp
Butter, reduced-fat	1 tbsp
Chitterlings, boiled	2 tbsp (½ oz)
Coconut, sweetened, shredded	2 tbsp
Cream, half and half	2 tbsp
Cream cheese, regular	1 tbsp (½ oz)
Cream cheese, reduced-fat	2 tbsp (1 oz)
Shortening or lard	1 tsp
Sour cream, regular	2 tbsp
Sour cream, reduced-fat	3 tbsp

Free foods

A free food is any food or drink that contains less than 20 kcal or less than 5 g carbohydrate per serving. You can eat as much as you want of those items that have no serving size specified. You may eat two or three servings per day of those items that have a specific serving size. Be sure to spread them out through the day.

Fat-free or reduced-fat foods

Cream cheese, fat-free	1 tbsp
Creamers, nondairy, liquid	1 tbsp
Creamers, nondairy, powdered	2 tsp
Mayonnaise, fat-free	1 tbsp
Mayonnaise, reduced-fat	1 tsp
Margarine, fat-free	4 tbsp
Margarine, reduced-fat	1 tsp
Miracle Whip, nonfat	1 tbsp
Miracle Whip, reduced-fat	1 tsp
Nonstick cooking spray	
Salad dressing, fat-free	1 tbsp
Salad dressing, fat-free, Italian	2 tbsp
Salsa	¼ cup
Sour cream, fat-free, reduced-fat	1 tbsp
Whipped topping, regular or light	2 tbsp

Sugar-free or low-sugar foods

Candy, hard, sugar-free	1 candy
Gelatin dessert, sugar-free	
Gelatin, unflavored	
Gum, sugar-free	
Jam or jelly, low-sugar or light	2 tsp
Syrup, sugar-free	2 tbsp

Sugar substitutes, alternatives, or replacements that are approved by the Food and Drug Administration (FDA) are safe to use. Common brand names include:

Equal (aspartame)

Sugar-free or low-sugar foods—cont'd

Sprinkle Sweet (saccharin)
Sweet One (acesulfame K)
Sweet-10 (saccharin)
Sugar Twin (saccharin)
Sweet 'n Low (saccharin)

Drinks

Bouillon, broth, consomme
Bouillon or broth, low-sodium
Carbonated or mineral water
Cocoa powder, unsweetened   1 tbsp
Coffee
Club soda
Diet soft drinks, sugar-free
Drink mixes, sugar-free
Tea
Tonic water, sugar-free

Condiments

Catsup   1 tbsp
Horseradish

Lemon juice
Lime juice
Mustard
Pickles, dill   1½ large
Soy sauce, regular or light
Taco sauce   1 tbsp
Vinegar

Seasonings

Be careful with seasonings that contain sodium or are salts, such as garlic or celery salt, and lemon pepper.
Flavoring extracts
Garlic
Herbs, fresh or dried
Pimento
Spices
Tabasco or hot pepper sauce
Wine, used in cooking
Worcestershire sauce

Combination food lists

Many combination foods do not fit into any one exchange list. This is a list of exchanges for some typical combination foods.

Entrees

Food	Serving size	Exchanges per serving
Tuna noodle casserole, lasagna, spaghetti with meatballs, chili with beans, macaroni and cheese	1 cup (8 oz)	2 carbohydrates, 2 medium-fat meats
Chow mein (without noodles or rice)	1 cup (16 oz)	1 carbohydrate, 2 lean meats
Pizza, cheese, thin crust	¼ of 10 inch (5 oz)	2 carbohydrates, 2 medium-fat meats, 1 fat
Pizza, meat topping, thin crust	¼ of 10 inch (5 oz)	2 carbohydrates, 2 medium-fat meats, 2 fats
Pot pie	1 (7 oz)	2 carbohydrates, 1 medium-fat meat, 4 fats

Frozen entrees

Food	Serving size	Exchanges per serving
Salisbury steak with gravy, mashed potato	1 (11 oz)	2 carbohydrates, 3 medium-fat meats, 3-4 fats
Turkey with gravy, mashed potato, dressing	1 (11 oz)	2 carbohydrates, 2 medium-fat meats, 2 fats
Entree with less than 300 calories	1 (8 oz)	2 carbohydrates, 3 lean meats

Soups

Food	Serving size	Exchanges per serving
Bean	1 cup	1 carbohydrate, 1 very lean meat
Cream (made with water)	1 cup (8 oz)	1 carbohydrate, 1 fat
Split pea (made with water)	½ cup (4 oz)	1 carbohydrate
Tomato (made with water)	1 cup (8 oz)	1 carbohydrate
Vegetable beef, chicken noodle, or other broth-type	1 cup (8 oz)	1 carbohydrate

Fast foods

Food	Serving size	Exchanges per serving
Burritos with beef	2	4 carbohydrates, 2 medium-fat meats, 2 fats
Chicken nuggets	6	1 carbohydrate, 2 medium-fat meats, 1 fat
Chicken breast and wing, breaded and fried	1 each	1 carbohydrate, 4 medium-fat meats, 2 fats
Fish sandwich with tartar sauce	1	3 carbohydrates, 1 medium-fat meat, 3 fats
French fries, thin	20-25	2 carbohydrates, 2 fats
Hamburger, regular	1	2 carbohydrates, 2 medium-fat meats
Hamburger, large	1	2 carbohydrates, 3 medium-fat meats, 1 fat
Hot dog with bun	1	1 carbohydrate, 1 high-fat meat, 1 fat
Individual pan pizza	1	5 carbohydrates, 3 medium-fat meats, 3 fats
Soft-serve cone	1 medium	2 carbohydrates, 1 fat
Submarine sandwich	1 sub (6 inch)	3 carbohydrates, 1 vegetable, 2 medium-fat meats, 1 fat
Taco, hard shell	1 (6 oz)	2 carbohydrates, 2 medium-fat meats, 2 fats
Taco, soft shell	1 (3 oz)	1 carbohydrate, 1 medium-fat meat, 1 fat

From American Dietetic Association and American Diabetes Association: *Exchange lists for meal planning*, Chicago, IL, 1995, ADA/ADA.

Appendix M Dietary Guidelines for Americans

EAT A VARIETY OF FOODS

About 40 different known nutrients, and probably more as yet unknown factors, are needed to maintain health. No single food can supply all the essential nutrients in the amounts needed to maintain health. Thus the greater the variety of foods used, the less likely a person is to develop either a deficiency or an excess of any single nutrient. One way to ensure a varied balanced diet is to select foods each day from all the major food groups.

MAINTAIN HEALTHY WEIGHT

Excessive fatness is associated with some chronic disorders such as hypertension and diabetes, which in turn relate to heart disease. The healthy body weight, however, must be determined individually because many factors are involved, such as body composition (muscle/fat ratio), body metabolism, genetics, and physical activity.

CHOOSE A DIET LOW IN FAT, SATURATED FAT, AND CHOLESTEROL

Americans have traditionally consumed a high-fat diet. In some persons, excess fat leads to high levels of blood fats and cholesterol. Elevated blood levels of these fats and cholesterol are associated with a higher risk of coronary heart disease. Thus it is wise to reduce intake of fats in general, using them only in moderation.

CHOOSE A DIET WITH PLENTY OF VEGETABLES, FRUITS, AND GRAIN PRODUCTS

Increasing use of these foods will help supply more of the needed starches (complex carbohydrates) for energy, many essential nutrients, and necessary dietary fiber. Research indicates that certain types of dietary fiber may help control chronic bowel diseases, contribute to improved blood glucose management for persons with diabetes mellitus, and bind dietary cholesterol.

USE SUGARS IN MODERATION

The major health hazard from eating too much sugar is tooth decay (dental caries). Contrary to popular opinion, however, too much sugar does not in itself cause diabetes. It can only contribute to poor control of diabetes in persons who have inherited the disease. Most Americans consume a relatively large amount of sugar, over 100 pounds per person per year, much of it in processed food products. Again, moderation is the key.

USE SALT AND SODIUM IN MODERATION

Our main source of dietary sodium is in ordinary table salt. Excessive salt is not healthy for anyone and certainly not for persons with hypertension. Many processed food products contain considerable amounts of salt and other sodium compounds, and many Americans use more salt in foods than they need. Thus it is wise to limit salt use in food preparation or at the table and to reduce the use of "salty" food products. This approach will lower individual salt tastes, which are learned habits and not biologic necessities. There is ample sodium as a natural mineral in foods to meet usual needs.

DRINK ALCOHOLIC BEVERAGES IN MODERATION

Alcoholic beverages tend to be high in kcalories and low in other nutrients. Limited food intake may accompany excessive alcohol intake. Heavy drinking also contributes to chronic liver disease and some neurologic disorders, as well as some throat and neck cancers. Moreover, it is a major factor in highway deaths. Thus if alcohol is used at all, moderation is the key, and persons should *never* drink and drive

Guidelines for Nutritional Assessment and Care of Cystic Fibrosis

STEP ONE: CALCULATION OF BASAL METABOLIC RATE (BMR)

In cystic fibrosis care, if a patient fails to grow adequately while receiving kcalorie intake based on Recommended Daily Allowances (RDAs), use this table to calculate BMR daily energy requirement.

World Health Organization equations for calculating BMR (kcal) from body weight (kg)

Age (years)	BMR (kcal)	
	Females	Males
0-3	$61.0 \times (wt\ kg) - 51$	$60.9 \times (wt\ kg) - 54$
3-10	$22.5 \times (wt\ kg) + 499$	$22.7 \times (wt\ kg) + 495$
10-18	$12.2 \times (wt\ kg) + 746$	$17.5 \times (wt\ kg) + 651$
18-30	$14.7 \times (wt\ kg) + 496$	$15.3 \times (wt\ kg) + 679$
30-60	$8.7 \times (wt\ kg) + 829$	$11.6 \times (wt\ kg) + 879$

Adapted from World Health Organization *Energy and protein requirements*, WHO Technical Report Series, Volume 924, No 724, 1985; Ramsey, BW et al: Nutritional assessment and management in cystic fibrosis, *Am J Clin Nutr* 55:108, 1992, and Cystic Fibrosis Foundation guidelines.

STEP TWO: CALCULATION OF DAILY ENERGY EXPENDITURE (DEE) IN THERAPY

$$DEE = BMR \times (AC + DC)$$

Abbreviations

DEE	=	daily energy expenditure (kcal)
BMR	=	basal metabolic rate (kcal)
AC	=	activity coefficient
DC	=	disease coefficient

GUIDELINES FOR AC AND DC VALUES

Use the following tables to establish the appropriate activity coefficient and disease coefficient values.

Activity Coefficients (AC)

Activity level of patient	AC value
Confined to bed	1.3
Sedentary	1.5
Active	1.7

Disease Coefficients (DC)

Lung functioning level in cystic fibrosis	Forced air expiration volume in 1 second ($FEV_{1.0}$) (100% = normal FEV)	DC value
Close to normal lung function	>80%	0.0
Moderate lung disease	40%-79%	0.2
Severe lung disease	<40%	0.3
Very severe lung disease	<40%	0.5

Modified from Ramsey BW et al: Nutritional assessment and management in cystic fibrosis, *Am J Clin Nutr* 55:108, 1992, and Cystic Fibrosis Foundation guidelines.

DEE CALCULATION

Determine the DEE for a school-age child with cystic fibrosis who is attending school, is relatively sedentary, and has a measured $FEV_{1.0}$ of 50% of predicted normal value.

$$DEE = BMR \times (AC + DC)$$
$$= BMR \times (1.5 + 0.2)$$
$$= BMR \times 1.7$$

STEP THREE: CALCULATION OF DAILY ENERGY REQUIREMENT (DER) FROM DAILY ENERGY EXPENDITURE (DEE)

CALCULATION METHOD

1. Calculate the coefficient of fat absorption (CFA):

$$CFA = \frac{\text{Fat absorption (FA)}}{\text{Fat intake (FI)}} = \text{Fat absorption } \%*$$

2. Use one of the following guideline formulas for DER:

If CFA > 0.93, then DER = DEE

or

If CFA = 0.93, then $DER = DEE \times \dfrac{0.93}{CFA}$

Abbreviations

CFA = coefficient of fat absorption
FA = fat absorption (kcal)
FI = fat intake (kcal)
DEE = daily energy expenditure (kcal)
DER = daily energy requirement (kcal)

DER CALCULATION EXAMPLE

The fat absorption of a cystic fibrosis patient on enzyme therapy has been determined by laboratory analysis to be 78% of normal. Therefore the CFA for this patient is 0.78. The DEE for this same patient is calculated to be 2000 kcal. Therefore the DER for this patient is:

$$DER = DEE \times \frac{0.93}{CFA}$$

$$DER = 2000 \text{ kcal} \times \frac{0.93}{0.78}$$

$$DER = 2384 \text{ kcal/day}$$

---

*NOTE 1: The fat absorption % (CFA) is usually calculated in a clinical setting by medical laboratory analysis from a patient stool sample.

NOTE 2: If no laboratory analysis report is available, then use CFA = 0.85 as an approximation value in the DER calculation. Modified from Ramsey BW et al: Nutritional assessment and management in cystic fibrosis, *Am J Clin Nutr* 55:108, 1992, and Cystic Fibrosis Foundation guidelines.

Low-calcium diet (approximately 400 mg calcium)

	Foods allowed	Foods not allowed
Beverage*	Carbonated beverage, coffee, tea	Chocolate-flavored drinks, milk, milk drinks
Bread	White, light rye bread, crackers	
Cereals	Refined cereals	Oatmeal, whole-grain cereals
Desserts	Cake, cookies, gelatin desserts, pastries, pudding, sherbets, all made without chocolate, milk, or nuts; if egg yolk is used, it must be from one egg allowance	
Fat	Butter, cream, 2 tbsp/day; French dressing, margarine, salad oil, shortening	Cream (except in amount allowed), mayonnaise
Fruits	Canned, cooked, or fresh fruits or juice except rhubarb	Dried fruit, rhubarb
Meat, eggs	224 g (8 oz) daily of any meat, fowl, fish except clams, oysters, shrimp; not more than one egg daily, including those used in cooking	Clams, oysters, shrimp, cheese
Potato or substitute	Potato, hominy, macaroni, noodles, refined rice, spaghetti	Whole-grain rice
Soup	Broth, vegetable soup made from vegetables allowed	Bean or pea soup, cream or milk soup
Sweets	Honey, jam, jelly, sugar	
Vegetables	Any canned, cooked, fresh vegetables or juice except those listed	Dried beans, broccoli, green cabbage, celery, chard, collards, endive, greens, lettuce, lentils, okra, parsley, parsnips, dried peas, rutabagas
Miscellaneous	Herbs, pickles, popcorn, relishes, salt, spices, vinegar	Chocolate, cocoa, milk gravy, nuts, olives, white sauce

*Depending on calcium content of local water supply. In instances of high calcium content, distilled water may be indicated.

Appendix O-2

Low-phosphorus diet (approximately 1 g phosphorous and 40 g protein)

	Foods allowed	Foods not allowed
Milk	Not more than 1 cup daily; whole, skim, buttermilk or 3 tbsp powdered, including the amount used in cooking	
Beverages	Fruit juices, tea, coffee, carbonated drinks, Postum	Milk and milk drinks except as allowed
Bread	White only; enriched commercial, French, hard rolls, soda crackers, rusk	Rye and whole-grain breads, cornbread, biscuits, muffins, waffles
Cereals	Refined cereals, such as Cream of Wheat, Cream of Rice, rice, cornmeal, dry cereals, cornflakes, spaghetti, noodles	All whole-grain cereals
Desserts	Berry or fruit pies, cookies, cakes in average amounts; Jell-O, gelatin, angel food cake, sherbet, meringues made with egg whites, puddings if made with one egg or milk allowance	Desserts with milk and eggs, unless made with the daily allowance
Eggs	Not more than one egg daily, including those used in cooking; extra egg whites may be used	
Fats	Butter, margarine, oils, shortening	
Fruits	Fresh, frozen, canned, as desired	Dried fruits such as raisins, prunes, dates, figs, apricots
Meat	One large serving or two small servings daily of beef, lamb, veal, pork, rabbit, chicken, turkey	Fish, shellfish (crab, oyster, shrimp, lobster), dried and cured meats (bacon, ham, chipped beef), liver, kidney, sweetbreads, brains
Cheese	None	Avoid all cheeses and cheese spreads
Vegetables	Potatoes as desired; at least two servings per day of any of the following: asparagus, carrots, beets, green beans, squash, lettuce, rutabagas, tomatoes, celery, peas, onions, cucumber, corn; no more than 1 serving daily of either cabbage, spinach, broccoli, cauliflower, brussels sprouts, artichokes	Dried vegetables such as peas, mushrooms, lima beans
Miscellaneous	Sugar, jams, jellies, syrups, salt, spices, seasonings; condiments in moderation	Chocolate, nuts, nut products such as peanut butter, cream sauces

Sample menu pattern

Breakfast	Lunch	Dinner
Fruit juice	Meat, 56 g (2 oz)	Meat, 56 g
Refined cereal	Potato	Potato
Egg	Vegetable	Vegetable
White toast	Salad	Salad
Butter	Bread, white	Bread, white
1/2 cup milk	Butter	Butter
Coffee or tea	1/2 cup milk	Dessert
	Dessert	Coffee or tea
	Coffee or tea	

Appendix O-3

Low-calcium test diet (200 mg calcium)

	Grams	Calcium (mg)
Breakfast		
Orange juice, fresh	100	19.00
Bread (toast), white	25	19.57
Butter	15	3.00
Rice Krispies	15	3.70
Cream, 20% butterfat	35	33.95
Sugar	7	0.00
Jam	20	2.00
Distilled water, coffee, or tea*		0.00
TOTAL		81.22
Lunch		
Beef steak, cooked	100	10.00
Potato	100	11.00
Tomatoes	100	11.00
Bread	25	19.57
Butter	15	3.00
Honey	20	1.00
Applesauce	20	1.00
Distilled water, coffee, or tea		0.00
TOTAL		56.57
Dinner		
Lamb chop, cooked	90	10.00
Potato	100	11.00
Frozen green peas	80	10.32
Bread	25	19.57
Butter	15	3.00
Jam	20	2.00
Peach sauce	100	5.00
Distilled water, coffee, or tea		0.00
TOTAL		60.89
TOTAL MILLIGRAMS CALCIUM		198.68

*Use distilled water only for cooking and for beverages.

Appendix O-4

Acid ash diet

The purpose of this diet is to furnish a well-balanced diet in which the total acid ash is greater than the total alkaline ash each day. It lists (1) unrestricted foods, (2) restricted foods, (3) foods not allowed, and (4) sample of a day's diet.

Unrestricted foods

Eat as much as desired of the following foods:
- Bread: any, preferably whole grain; crackers, rolls
- Cereals: any, preferably whole grain
- Desserts: angel food or sunshine cake; cookies made without baking powder or baking soda; cornstarch pudding, cranberry desserts, custards, gelatin desserts, ice cream, sherbet, plum or prune desserts; rice or tapioca pudding
- Fats: any, as butter, margarine, salad dressings, shortening, lard, salad oils, olive oil
- Fruits: cranberries, plums, prunes
- Meat, eggs, cheese; any meat, fish, or fowl, two servings daily; at least one egg daily
- Potato substitutes: corn, hominy, lentils, macaroni, noodles, rice, spaghetti, vermicelli
- Soup: broth as desired; other soups from foods allowed
- Sweets: cranberry or plum jelly; sugar, plain sugar candy
- Miscellaneous: cream sauce, gravy, peanut butter, peanuts, popcorn, salt, spices, vinegar, walnuts

Restricted foods

Do not eat any more than the amount allowed each day.
- Milk: 2 cups daily (may be used in other ways than as beverage)
- Cream: 1/3 cup or less daily
- Fruits: one serving of fruit daily (in addition to prunes, plums, cranberries); certain fruits listed under "Sample menu" are not allowed at any time
- Vegetables including potato: two servings daily; certain vegetables listed under "Foods not allowed" are not allowed at any time

Foods not allowed

- Carbonated beverages, such as ginger ale, cola, root beer
- Cakes or cookies made with baking powder or soda
- Fruits: dried apricots, bananas, dates, figs, raisins, rhubarb
- Vegetables: dried beans, beet greens, dandelion greens, carrots, chard, lima beans
- Sweets: chocolate or candies other than those under "Unrestricted foods"; syrups
- Miscellaneous: other nuts, olives, pickles

Sample menu

Breakfast	Lunch	Dinner
Grapefruit	Creamed chicken	Broth
Wheatena	Steamed rice	Roast beef, gravy
Scrambled eggs	Green beans	Buttered noodles
Toast, butter, plum jam	Stewed prunes	Sliced tomato
	Bread, butter	Mayonnaise
Coffee, cream, sugar	Milk	Vanilla ice cream
		Bread, butter

Appendix O-5

Low-purine diet (approximately 125 mg purine)

General directions
- During acute stages use only list 1.
- After acute stage subsides and for chronic conditions, use the following schedule:
  Two days a week, not consecutive, use list 1 entirely.
  The remaining days add foods from list 2 and 3, as indicated.
  Avoid list 4 entirely.
- Keep diet moderately low in fat.

Typical meal pattern

Breakfast	Lunch	Dinner
Fruit	Egg or cheese dish	Egg or cheese dish
Refined cereal and/or egg	Vegetables, as allowed (cooked or salad)	Cream of vegetable soup, if desired
White toast	Potato or substitute	Starch (potato or substitute)
Butter, 1 tsp	White bread	Colored vegetable, as allowed
Sugar	Butter, 1 tsp	White bread, butter, 1 tsp, if desired
Coffee	Fruit or simple dessert	Salad, as allowed
Milk, if desired	Milk	Fruit or simple dessert
		Milk

Food list 1: may be used as desired; foods that contain an insignificant amount of purine bodies

Beverages	Cheese of all kinds*	Celery
Carbonated	Eggs	Corn
Chocolate	Fats of all kinds* (moderation)	Cucumber
Cocoa	Fruits of all kinds	Eggplant
Coffee	Gelatin, Jell-O	Endive
Fruit juices	Milk: buttermilk, evaporated, malted, sweet	Kohlrabi
Postum	Nuts of all kinds,* peanut butter*	Lettuce
Tea	Pies* (except mincemeat)	Okra
Butter*	Sugar and sweets	Parsnips
Bread: white and crackers, cornbread	Vegetables	Potato, white and sweet
Cereals and cereal products	Artichokes	Pumpkin
Corn	Beets	Rutabagas
Rice	Beet greens	Sauerkraut
Tapioca	Broccoli	String beans
Refined wheat	Brussels sprouts	Summer squash
Macaroni	Cabbage	Swiss chard
Noodles	Carrots	Tomato
		Turnips

*High in fat.

Appendix O-5

Low-purine diet (approximately 125 mg purine)—cont'd

Food list 2: one item four times a week; foods that contain a moderate amount (up to 75 mg) of purine bodies in 100 g serving

Asparagus	Finnan haddie	Mushrooms	Salmon
Bluefish	Ham	Mutton	Shad
Bouillon	Herring	Navy beans	Spinach
Cauliflower	Kidney beans	Oatmeal	Tripe
Chicken	Lima beans	Oysters	Tuna fish
Crab	Lobster	Peas	Whitefish

Food list 3: one item once a week; foods that contain a large amount (75-150 mg) of purine bodies in 100 g serving

Bacon	Duck	Perch	Sheep
Beef	Goose	Pheasant	Shellfish
Calf tongue	Halibut	Pigeon	Squab
Carp	Lentils	Pike	Trout
Chicken soup	Liver sausage	Pork	Turkey
Codfish	Meat soups	Quail	Veal
	Partridge	Rabbit	Venison

Food list 4: avoid entirely; foods that contain large amounts (150-1000 mg) of purine bodies in 100 g serving

Sweetbreads	825 mg	Liver (calf, beef)	233 mg	Meat extracts	160-400 mg
Anchovies	363 mg	Kidneys (beef)	200 mg	Gravies	Variable
Sardines (in oil)	295 mg	Brains	195 mg		

Appendix O-6

Low-methionine diet

	Foods allowed	Foods not allowed
Soup	Any soup made without meat stock or addition of milk	Rich meat soups, broths, canned soups made with meat broth
Meat or meat substitute	Peanut butter sandwich; spaghetti, or macaroni dish made without addition of meat, cheese, or milk; one serving per day: chicken, lamb, veal, beef, pork, crab, or bacon (3)	Fish and those not listed above
Beverages	Soy milk, tea, coffee	Milk in any form
Vegetables	Asparagus, artichoke, beans, beets, carrots, chicory, cucumber, eggplant, escarole, lettuce, onions, parsnips, potatoes, pumpkin, rhubarb, tomatoes, turnips	Those not listed as allowed
Fruits	Apples, apricots, bananas, berries, cherries, fruit cocktail, grapefruit, grapes, lemon juice, nectarines, oranges, peaches, pears, pineapple, plums, tangerines, watermelon, cantaloupe	Those not listed as allowed
Salads	Raw or cooked vegetable or fruit salad	
Cereals	Macaroni, spaghetti, noodles	
Bread	Whole wheat, rye, white	
Nuts	Peanuts	
Desserts	Fresh or cooked fruit, ices, fruit pies	
Eggs		In any form
Cheese		All varieties
Concentrated sweets	Sugar, jams, jellies, syrup, honey, hard candy	
Concentrated fats	Butter, margarine, cream	
Miscellaneous	Pepper, mustard, vinegar, garlic, oil, herbs, spices	

Meal pattern

Breakfast	Lunch	Dinner
1 cup fruit juice	1 serving soup	56 g (2 oz) meat
1/2 cup fruit	1 serving sandwich	1 med starch
1 slice toast	1 cup fruit	1/2 cup vegetable
1 1/2 pats butter	240 ml (8 oz) soy milk*	1 serving salad
2 tsp jelly	3 tsp sugar	1 tbsp dressing
1 tbsp sugar	1 tbsp cream	1 slice bread
Beverage	Beverage	1 serving dessert
1 tbsp cream		1 tbsp sugar
		1 tbsp cream
		1 1/2 pats butter
		Beverage

Sample menu

Breakfast	Lunch	Dinner
Orange juice	Vegetable soup, vegetarian	Chicken, roast
Applesauce	Peanut butter sandwich	Baked potato
Whole-wheat toast	Canned peaches	Artichoke
Butter	Soy milk*	Sliced tomatoes
Jelly	Sugar	French dressing
Sugar	Cream	Whole-wheat bread
Coffee	Coffee or tea	Fruit ice
Cream		Sugar
		Cream
		Butter
		Coffee or tea

Modified from Smith DR, Kolb FO, and Harper HA: The management of cystinuria and cystine-stone disease, *J Urol* 81:61, 1959.
*Optional: use in children to include protein intake. Omit if urine calcium level is elevated in adults.

Calculation Aids and Conversion Tables

More than 185 years ago a group of French scientists set up the metric system of weights and measures. Today, with refinements over years of use, it is called the "Systeme International" (SI). In 1975 the United States Congress passed the Metric Conversion Act, which provides for conversion of our customary British/American system to the simpler metric system used by the rest of the world. We are now in the midst of this conversion, as evidenced by distance signs along highways and labels on many packaged foods in supermarkets. Here are a few conversion factors to help you make these transitions in your necessary calculations.

Metric System of Measurement

Like our money system, this is a simple decimal system based on units of 10. It is uniform and used internationally.

Weight units: 1 kilogram (kg) = 1000 grams (gm or g)
1 g = 1000 milligrams (mg)
1 mg = 1000 micrograms (mcg or µg)

Length units: 1 meter (m) = 100 centimeters (cm)
1000 meters = 1 kilometer

Volume units: 1 liter (L) = 1000 milliliters (ml)
1 milliliter = 1 cubic centimeter (cc)

Temperature units: Celsius (C) scale, based on 100 equal units between 0° C (freezing point of water) and 100° C (boiling point of water); this scale is used in all scientific work.

Energy units: Kilocalorie (kcal) = Amount of energy required to raise 1 kg water 1° C
Kilojoule (kJ) = Amount of energy required to move 1 kg mass 1 m by a force of 1 newton
1 kcal = 4.184 kJ

In 1970 the American Institute of Nutrition's Committee on Nomenclature recommended that the term *Kilojoule* (kJ) replace the kilocalorie (kcal). This change is gradually coming about.

British/American System of Measurement

This system is a confusion of units with no uniform relationships. It is not a decimal system, but rather a jumbled collection of different units collected in usage and language over time. It is used mainly in America

Weight units: 1 pound (lb) = 16 ounces (oz)

Length units: 1 foot (ft) = 12 inches (in)
1 yard (yd) = 3 feet (ft)

Volume units: 3 teaspoons (tsp) = 1 tablespoon (tbsp)
16 tbsp = 1 cup
1 cup = 8 fluid ounces (fl oz)
4 cups = 1 quart (qt)
5 cups = 1 imperial quart (qt), Canada

Temperature units: Fahrenheit (F) scale, based on 180 equal units between 32° F (freezing point of water) and 212° F (boiling point of water) at standard atmospheric pressure

Conversions Between Measurement Systems

Weight: 1 oz = 28.35 g (usually used as 28 or 30 g)
2.2 lb = 1 kg

Length: 1 in = 2.54 cm
1 ft = 30.48 cm
39.37 in = 1 m

Volume: 1.06 qt = 1 L
                         0.85 imperial qt = 1 L (Canada)

Temperature: Boiling point of   100° C   212° F
               water
               Body temperature   37° C   98.6° F
               Freezing point of   0° C   32° F
               water

Interconversion formulas:
  Fahrenheit temperature (°F) = $\frac{9}{5}$ (°C + 32)
  Celsius temperature (°C) = $\frac{5}{9}$ (°F − 32)

RETINOL EQUIVALENTS

The following internationally agreed on definitions and equivalences provide a basis for calculating retinol equivalent conversions.

Definitions

International units (IU) and retinol equivalents (RE) are defined as follows:

  1 IU = 0.3 μg retinol (0.0003 mg)
  1 IU = 0.6 μg beta-carotene (0.0006 mg)
  1 RE = 6 μg retinol
  1 RE = 6 μg beta-carotene
  1 RE = 12 μg other provitamin A carotenoids
  1 RE = 3.33 IU retinol
  1 RE = 10 IU beta-carotene

Conversion formulas

On the basis of weight, beta-carotene is $\frac{1}{2}$ as active as retinol; on the basis of structure the other provitamin carotenoids are $\frac{1}{4}$ as active as retinol. In addition, retinol is more completely absorbed in the intestine, whereas the provitamin carotenoids are much less well utilized, with an average absorption of about $\frac{1}{3}$. Therefore in overall activity, beta-carotene is $\frac{1}{6}$ as active as retinol and the other carotenoids are $\frac{1}{12}$ as active. These differences in utilization provide the basis for the 1:6:12 relationship shown in the equivalences given and in the following formulas for calculating retinol equivalents from values of vitamin A, beta-carotene, and other active carotenoids, expressed either as international units or micrograms:

If retinol and beta-carotene are given in micrograms:

Micrograms of retinol +
            (Micrograms of beta-carotene ÷ 6) = RE

            If both are given as IU:

(International units of retinol ÷ 3.33) +
        (International units of beta-carotene ÷ 10) = RE

If beta-carotene and other carotenoids are given in micrograms:

(Micrograms of beta-carotene ÷ 6) +
        (Micrograms of other carotenoids ÷ 12) = RE

Appendix P

Approximate metric conversions

When you know	Multiply by	To find
Weight		
Ounces	28	Grams
Pounds	0.45	Kilograms
Length		
Inches	2.5	Centimeters
Feet	30	Centimeters
Yards	0.9	Meters
Miles	1.6	Kilometers
Volume		
Teaspoons	5	Millimeters
Tablespoons	15	Millimeters
Fluid ounces	30	Millimeters
Cups	0.24	Liters
Pints	0.47	Liters
Quarts	0.95	Liters
Temperature		
Fahrenheit temperature	5/9 (after subtracting 32)	Celsius temperature

Cultural group	Bread, cereal, rice, pasta group	Vegetable group
Native American	Blue corn flour (ground dried blue corn kernels) used to make cornbread, mush dumplings; fruit dumplings (walakshi); fry bread (biscuit dough deep fried); ground sweet acorn; tortillas; wheat or rye used to make cornmeal and flours	Cabbage, carrots, cassava, dandelion greens, eggplant, milkweed, onions, pumpkin, squash (all varieties), sweet and white potatoes, turnips, wild tullies (a tuber), yellow corn
African-American	Biscuits; cornbread as spoon bread; corn-pone or hush puppies; grits	Leafy greens, including dandelion greens, kale, mustard greens, collard greens, turnips
Japanese	Rice and rice products, rice flour (mochiko), noodles (comen/soba); seaweed around rice with or without fish (sushi)	Bamboo shoots (takenoko), burdock (gobo), cabbage (nappa), dried mushrooms (shiitake), eggplant, horseradish (wasabi), Japanese parsley (seri), lotus root (renkon), mustard greens, pickled cabbage (kimchee), pickled vegetables, seaweed (laver, nori, wakame, kombu), vegetable soup (mizutaki), white radish (daikon)
Chinese	Rice and related products (flour, cakes, and noodles); noodles made from barley, corn, and millet; wheat and related products (breads, noodles, spaghetti, stuffed noodles [won ton] and filled buns [bow])	Bamboo shoots; cabbage (napa); Chinese celery; Chinese parsley (coriander); Chinese turnips (lo bok); dried day lilies; dry fungus (Black Juda's ear); leafy green vegetables, including kale, Chinese cress, Chinese mustard greens (gai choy), Chinese chard (bok choy), amaranth greens (yin choy), wolfberry leaves (gou gay), and Chinese broccoli (gai lan); lotus tubers; okra; snow peas; stir-fried vegetables (chow yuk); taro roots, white radish (daikon)
Filipino	Noodles, rice, rice flour (mochiko), stuffed noodles (won ton), white bread (pan de sal)	Bamboo shoots, dark green leafy vegetables (malunggay and salvyot), eggplant, sweet potatoes (camotes), okra, palm, peppers, turnips, root crop (gabi)

Modified from Grodner et al: *Foundations and clinical applications of nutrition, a nursing approach*, St Louis, 1996, Mosby.

*Only foods that are specifically associated with these cultural groups are noted. Individuals may also consume typical American foods; assumptions of dietary patterns cannot be made, but knowledge of these unique foods provides a common understanding of the range of possible food choices.

†The foods reflect both religious and cultural customs of Jewish people. Adherence to religious dietary patterns by followers of the different forms of Judaism (Orthodox, Conservative, Reform, and Reconstructionist) vary. Generally, Orthodox Jews and many Conservative Jews follow kosher dietary rules both at home and when eating out. Others may only observe these rules when in their own homes.

Fruit group	Milk, yogurt, cheese group	Meat, poultry, fish, dry beans, eggs, nut group	Fats, oils, sweets
Dried wild cherries and grapes; wild banana, berries, and yucca	None	Duck eggs, fish eggs (roe), geese, groundhog, kidney beans, lentils, peanuts, pinenuts, pinto beans, all nuts, venison, wild rabbit	None
None	Buttermilk	Pork and pork products, scrapple (cornmeal and pork), chitterlings (pork intestines), bacon, pig's feet, pig ears, souse, pork neck bones; fried meats and poultry; organ meats (kidney, liver, tongue, tripe); venison; rabbit; catfish, buffalo fish, mackerel; legumes (black-eyed peas, kidney, navy, chickpeas)	Lard
Pear-like apple (nasi), persimmons	None	Fish and shellfish, including dried fish with bones, raw fish (sashimi), and fish cake (kamaboko); soybeans as soybean curd (tofu), fermented soy bean paste (miso), and sprouts; red beans (azuki)	Soy and rice oil
Kumquat	None	Fish and seafood (all kinds, dried and fresh), hen, legumes, nuts, organ meats, pigeon eggs, pork and pork products, soybean curd (tofu), steamed stuffed dumplings (dim sum)	Peanut, soy, sesame and rice oil, lard
Avocado, bitter melon (ampalaya), guavas, jackfruit, limes, mangoes, papaya, pod fruit (tamarind), pomelos, tangelo (naranghita)	Custards	Fish in all forms; dried fish (dilis); egg roll (lumpia); fish sauce (alamang and bagoong); legumes such as mung beans, bean sprouts, chickpeas, organ meats (liver, heart intestines); pork with chicken in soy sauce (adobo); pork sausage; soybean curd (tofu)	None

Cultural group	Bread, cereal, rice, pasta group	Vegetable group
Southeastern Asians (Laos, Cambodia, Thailand, Viet Nam, the Hmong and the Mien)	Rice (long and short grain) and related products such as noodles; Hmong cornbread or cake	Bamboo shoots, broccoli, Chinese parsley (coriander), mustard greens, pickled vegetables, water chestnuts, Thai chili peppers
Mexican	Corn and related products; taco shells (fried corn tortillas); tortillas (corn and flour); white bread	Cactus (nopoles), chili peppers, salsa, tomatoes, yambean root (jicama), yucca root (cassava or manioc)
Puerto Rican and Cuban	Rice; starchy green bananas, usually fried (plantain)	Beets; eggplant; tubers (yucca); white yams (boniato)
Jewish†	Bagel, buckwheat groats (kasha), dumplings made with matzoh meal (matzoh balls or knaidelach), egg bread (challah), noodle or potato pudding (kugel), a crepe filled with farmer cheese and/or fruit (blintz), unleavened bread or large cracker made with wheat flour and water (matzoh)	Potato pancakes (latkes); a vegetable stew made with sweet potatoes, carrots, prunes, and sometimes brisket (tzimmes); beet soup (borscht)

Continued

Fruit group	Milk, yogurt, cheese group	Meat, poultry, fish, dry beans, eggs, nut group	Fats, oils, sweets
Apple pear (Asian pear), bitter melon, coconut cream and milk, guava, jack fruit, mango	Sweetened condensed milk	Beef; chicken; deer; eggs; fish and shellfish (all kinds freshwater and saltwater); legumes, including black-eyed peas, peanuts, kidney beans, and soybeans; organ meats (liver, stomach); pork; rabbit; soybean curd (tofu)	Lard, peanut oil
Avocado; guacamole (mashed avocado, onion, cilantro [coriander], and chilis); papaya	Cheese, flan, sour cream	Black or pinto beans (reijoles); refried beans (frijoles refritos); flour tortilla stuffed with beef, chicken, eggs, or beans (burrito); corn tortilla stuffed with chicken, cheese, or beef topped with chili sauce (enchilada); Mexican sausage (chorizo)	Bacon fat, lard (manteca), salt pork
Coconuts, guava, mango, oranges (sweet and sour), prune and mango paste	Flan, hard cheese (queso de mano)	Chicken, fish (all kinds and preparations, including smoked, salted, canned, and fresh), legumes (all kinds, especially black beans), pork (fried), sausage (chorizo)	Olive and peanut oil, lard
None	None	A mixture of fish formed into balls and poached (gefilte fish); smoked salmon (lox)	Chicken fat

Appendix R

The Prudent Diet as Compared with the Usual American Diet

	Prudent diet	Usual American diet
Total kcalories	Sufficient to maintain ideal body weight	Often excessive for need
Cholesterol	300 mg	600-800 mg
Total fats (% of kcalories)	30%-35%	40%-45%
Saturated	10% or less	15%-20%
Monounsaturated	15%	15%-20%
Polyunsaturated	10%	5%-6%
P/S ratio (polyunsaturated/saturated fat in the diet)	1-1.5%	0.3:1
Carbohydrates (% of kcalories)	50%-55%	40%-45%
Starch (complex CHO)	30%-35%	20%-25%
Simple sugars	10%	15%-20%
Proteins (% of total kcalories)	12%-20%	12%-15%
Sodium	130 mEq	200-250 mEq

From American Heart Association Nutrition Committee: Rational for the diet-heart statement of the American Heart Association, *Arterioscler Thromb* 4:177, 1982.

Appendix S

American Heart Association Revised Prudent Diet Guidelines for Lowering Elevated Blood Lipid Levels	Step 1 % total kcalories	Step 2 % total kcalories
Total fat	<30	<30
Saturated	<10	<7
Monounsaturated	10-15	10-15
Polyunsaturated	10	10
Carbohydrates	50-60	50-60
Protein	15-20	15-20
Cholesterol	<300 mg/day	<200 mg/day

From Repka FJ, Leighton RF: Step management of hypercholesterolemia, *Am Fam Physician* 36:238, 1987.

Glossary

achlasia (Gr *a-*, negative, without; *cholasis*, relaxation) Failure to relax the smooth muscle fibers of the gastrointestinal tract at any point of juncture of its parts; especially failure of the esophagogastric sphincter to relax when swallowing, caused by degeneration of ganglion cells in the wall of the organ. The lower esophagus also loses its normal peristaltic activity. Also called cardiospasm.

actin (Gr *aktis*, a radiating activating substance) Myofibril protein whose synchronized meshing action in conjunction with **myosin** causes muscles to contract and relax.

adenosine triphosphate (ATP) The high-energy compound formed in the cell, called the "energy currency " of the cell because of the binding of energy in its high-energy phosphate bonds for release for cell work as these bonds are split. A compound of adenosine (a nucleotide containing adenine and ribose) that has three phosphoric acid groups, ATP is a high-energy phosphate compound important in energy exchange for cellular activity. The splitting off of the terminal phosphate bond (PO_4) of ATP to produce adenosine diphosphate (ADP) releases bound energy and transfers it to free energy available for body work. The reforming of ATP in cell oxidation again stores energy in high-energy phosphate bonds for use as needed. They may be charged and discharged according to conditions in the cell.

adipocyte (L *adipis*, fat; Gr *kytos*, hollow vessel) A fat cell. All cell names end in the suffix *-cyte*, with the type of cell indicated by the root word to which it is added.

adipose (L *adeps*, fat; *adiposus*, fatty) Fat present in cells of adipose (fatty) tissue.

admixture (L *admixtus*, admixture) A mixture resulting from adding or mingling another ingredient; a combination of two or more substances that are not chemically united or that exist in no fixed proportion to each other.

aerobic capacity (Gr *aer*, air or gas) Milliliters of oxygen consumed per kilogram of body weight per minute; influenced by body composition.

aldosterone Potent hormone of the cortex of the adrenal glands, which acts on the distal renal tubule to cause reabsorption of sodium in an ion exchange with potassium. The aldosterone mechanism is essentially a sodium-conserving mechanism but indirectly also conserves water, since water absorption follows the sodium reabsorption.

alpha-fetoprotein A fetal antigen in amniotic fluid that provides an early pregnancy test for fetal malformations such as neural tube defect.

amine An organic compound containing nitrogen. Many different amine organic compounds are found.

amino acid (*amino*, the monovalent chemical group—NH_2) An acid containing the essential element nitrogen (in the chemical group—NH_2). Amino acids are the structural units of protein and the basic building blocks of the body.

aminopeptidase (Chemistry: *amino*, nitrogen-containing; Gr *pepsis*, digestion) Protein-splitting enzyme that cuts the peptide bond (linkage) at the amino end of amino acids, splitting off the amino group—NH_2.

amnionic fluid (Gr *amnion*, bowl) The watery fluid within the membrane enveloping the fetus, in which the fetus is suspended.

amphoteric (Gr *amphoteros*, both) Having opposite characteristics; capable of acting either as an acid or a base, combining with both acids and bases.

ampullae (L *ampulla*, a jug) A general term for flask-like wider portions of a tubular structure; spaces under the nipple of the breast for storing milk.

amyloid (Gr *amylon*, starch; *-oid, eidos*, form, shape) A glycoprotein substance having a relation to starchlike structure but more a protein compound; an abnormal complex material forming characteristic brain deposits of fibrillary tangles always found in postmortem examinations of patients with Alzheimer's disease, the only means of definitive diagnosis; found in various body tissues that can form lesions that destroy functional cells and injure the organ.

amyotrophic lateral sclerosis (Gr *a-*, negative; *mys*, muscle; *trophē*, nourishment; L *lateralis*, to the side;

sklērōsis, hardness) A progressive neuromuscular disease characterized by the degeneration of the neurons of the spinal cord and the motor cells of the brain stem, causing a deficit of upper and lower motor neurons; death usually occurs in 2 to 3 years.

anabolism (Gr *anabole,* a building up) Metabolic process by which body tissues are built.

anemia (Gr *an-,* negative prefix; *haima,* blood) Blood condition characterized by decreased number of circulating red blood cells, hemoglobin, or both.

anergy (Gr *an-,* negative prefix, *ergon,* work) Diminished immunologic reactivity to specific antigens.

anorexia nervosa (Gr "want of appetite") Extreme psychophysiologic aversion to food, resulting in life-threatening weight loss; a psychiatric eating disorder caused by a morbid fear of fatness, in which the person's distorted body image is reflected as fat when the body is actually malnourished and extremely thin from self-starvation.

anthropometry (Gr *anthropos,* man; *metron,* measure) The science of measuring the size, weight, and proportions of the human body.

antibody Any of numerous protein molecules produced by B cells as a primary immune defense for attaching to specific related **antigens;** animal protein made up of a specific sequence of amino acids that is designed to interact with its specific antigen during an allergic response or to prevent infection.

antigen (antibody + Gr *gennan,* to produce) Any foreign or "non-self" substances, such as toxins, viruses, bacteria, and foreign proteins, that stimulate the production of **antibodies** specifically designed to interact with them.

antimetabolite A substance bearing a close structural resemblance to one required for normal physiologic functioning and exerting its effect by interfering with the utilization of the essential metabolite.

antioxidant (Gr *anti,* against; *oxys* keen) A substance that inhibits oxidation of polyunsaturated fatty acids and formation of free radicals in the cells.

apoprotein (Gr *apo,* from, separation or derivation from; *prōtos, f*irst, protein compound) A separate protein compound that attaches to its specific receptor site on a particular lipoprotein and activates certain functions, such as synthesis of a related enzyme. An example is apoprotein C II, an apoprotein of HDL and VLDL that functions to activate the enzyme lipoprotein lipase.

areola (L *areola,* area, space) A defined space; a circular area of different color surrounding a central point, such as the darkened pigmented ring surrounding the nipple of the breast.

ariboflavinosis Group of clinical manifestations of riboflavin deficiency.

arteriosclerosis (Gr *arteria,* from *aēr,* air, and *tērein,* to keep, because of the ancient belief that the arteries contained vital air; *sklēros,* hard) Blood vessel disease characterized by thickening and hardening of artery walls, with loss of functional elasticity, mainly affecting the intima (inner lining) of the arteries.

arthroplasty (Gr *arthron,* joint; *plassein,* to form) Surgical procedure for replacing degenerated joints such as the hip with a mechanical joint of metal or special plastic; formation of movable joint replacement, developed by team of biomedical engineers and orthopedists.

asterixis (Gr *a,* negative prefix; *sterixis,* a fixed position) Neuromotor disturbance marked by an inability to hold outstretched hands in a steady position, resulting in an intermittent flapping of the hands, characteristic of hepatic coma.

atheroma (Gr *athērē,* gruel; *-oma,* a mass or body of tissue) A mass of fatty plaque formed in inner arterial walls in atherosclerosis.

atherosclerosis (Gr *athere,* gruel; *skleros,* hard) Common form of arteriosclerosis, characterized by the gradual formation,—beginning in childhood in genetically predisposed individuals,—of yellow cheese like streaks of cholesterol and fatty material that develop into hardened plaques in the intima or inner lining of major blood vessels, such as coronary arteries, eventually in adulthood cutting off blood supply to the tissue served by the vessels; the underlying pathology of coronary heart disease.

atrium (L *atrion,* hall) An anatomical chamber; usually used alone to designate one of the pair of smaller upper chambers of the heart, with thin muscular walls, which receives blood from the body's inflowing circulation via the superior and inferior vena cava and delivers it to the thicker walled ventricles.

autonomy (Gr *autos,* self; *nomos,* law) The state of functioning independently, without extraneous influence.

azotemia (Gr *a,* negative; *zoe,* life; *azote,* nitrogen; haima, blood) An excess of urea or other nitrogenous substances in the blood.

basal metabolic rate (BMR) Amount of energy required to maintain the resting body's internal activities after an overnight fast. See also **resting metabolic rate (RMR).**

benign (L *benignus,* kind, generous) Not malignant or recurrent; favorable for recovery.

beriberi (Singhalese "I cannot, I cannot") A disease of the peripheral nerves caused by a deficiency of thiamin (vitamin B_1). It is characterized by pain (neuritis) and paralysis of the extremities, cardiovascular changes, and edema. Beriberi is common in the Orient, where diets consist largely of milled rice with little protein.

bile (L *bilis,* bile) A fluid secreted by the liver and transported to the gallbladder for concentration and storage. It is released into the duodenum upon entry of fat to facilitate enzymatic fat digestion by acting as an emulsifying agent.

bilirubin (L *bilis,* bile; *ruber,* red) A reddish bile pigment resulting from the degradation of heme by reticuloedothelial cells in the liver; a high level in the blood produces the yellow skin symptomatic of jaundice.

bioavailability Amount of a nutrient ingested in food that is absorbed and thus available to the body for metabolic use.

blood urea nitrogen (BUN) The nitrogen component of urea in the blood; a measure of kidney function; elevated levels of BUN indicate a disorder of kidney function.

body composition The relative sizes of the four basic body compartments that make up the total body: lean body mass (muscle mass), fat, water, and bone.

bolus (Gr *bolos,* lump) Rounded mass of food formed in the mouth and ready to be swallowed.

buffer Mixture of acidic and alkaline components that, when added to a solution, is able to protect the solution against wide variations in its pH, even when strong acids and bases are added to it. If an acid is added, the alkaline partner reacts to counteract the acidic effect. If a base is added, the acid partner reacts to counteract the alkalizing effect. A solution to which a buffer has been added is called a buffered solution.

bulimia nervosa (L *bous,* ox; *limos,* hunger) A psychiatric eating disorder related to the person's fear of fatness, in which cycles of gorging on large quantities of food are followed by self-induced vomiting and use of diuretics and laxatives to maintain a "normal" body weight.

cachexia (Gr *kakos,* bad; *hexis,* habit) A specific profound effect caused by malnutrition and a disturbance in glucose metabolism usually seen in patients with terminal cancer or heart failure; general poor health and malnutrition indicated by an emaciated appearance.

calcitonin (L *calx,* lime, calcium; *tonus,* balance) A polypeptide hormone secreted by the thyroid gland in response to hypercalcemia, which acts to lower both calcium and phosphate in the blood.

calcitriol Activated hormone form of vitamin D $(1,25[OH]_2D_3)$-1,25-dihydroxycholecalciferol.

callus (L *callositis,* callus, bone) Unorganized meshwork of newly grown, woven bone developed on pattern of original fibrin clot (formed after fracture or surgery) and normally replaced in the healing process by hard adult bone.

calorie (L *calor,* heat) A unit of heat energy. The calorie used in the study of metabolism is the large calorie, or *kilocalorie,* defined as the amount of heat required to raise the temperature of 1 kg of water 1° Celsius (centigrade).

calorimetry (L *calor,* heat; Gr *metron,* measure) Measurement of amounts of heat absorbed or given out. *Direct method:* measurement of amount of heat produced by a subject enclosed in a small chamber. *Indirect method:* measurement of amount of heat produced by a subject by the quantity of nitrogen and carbon dioxide eliminated.

cancer (L *cancer,* crab) A malignant cellular tumor with properties of tissue invasion and spread to other parts of the body.

candidiasis (L *candidus,* glowing white) Infection with the fungus of the genus *Candida,* generally caused by *C. albicans,* so-named for the whitish appearance of its small lesions; usually a superficial infection in moist areas of the skin or inner mucous membranes.

capillary fluid shift mechanism Process that controls the movement of water and small molecules in solution (electrolytes, nutrients) between the blood in the capillary and the surrounding interstitial area. Filtration of water and solutes out of the capillary at the arteriole end and reabsorption at the venule end are accomplished by shifts in balance between the intracapillary hydrostatic blood pressure and the colloidal osmotic pressure exerted by the plasma proteins.

carbohydrate Compound of carbon, hydrogen, and oxygen; starches, sugars, cellulose, and gums made and stored in plants; major energy source in the human diet.

carboxyl (COOH) The monovalent radical,—COOH occurring in those organic acids termed carboxylic acids.

carboxypeptidase (L *carbo-,* carbon; *oxy,* oxygen) A protein enzyme that splits off the chemical group *carboxyl* (—COOH) at the end of peptide chains, acting on the peptide bond of the terminal amino acid having a free-end carboxyl group.

carcinoma (Gr *karkinos,* crab; *onkoma,* a swelling) A malignant new growth made up of epithelial cells, infiltrating the surrounding tissue and spreading to other parts of the body.

cardiac output (Gr *kardia,* heart) Total volume of blood propelled from the heart with each contraction; equal to the stroke output multiplied by the number of beats per the time unit used in the calculation.

carnitine A naturally occurring amino acid $(C_{17}H_{15}NO_3)$ formed from methionine and lysine, required for transport of long-chain fatty acids across the mitochondrial membrane, where they are oxidized as fuel substrate for metabolic energy.

casein hydrolysate formula (L *caseus,* cheese) Infant formula with base of hydrolyzed casein, major milk protein, produced by partially breaking down the casein into smaller peptide fragments, making a product that is more easily digested.

catabolism (Gr *katabole,* a throwing down) The breaking-down phase of metabolism, the opposite of anabolism. Catabolism includes all the processes in which complex substances are progressively broken down into simpler ones. Catabolism usually involves the release of energy. Together, anabolism and catabolism constitute metabolism, which is the coordinated operation of anabolic and catabolic processes into a dynamic balance of energy and substance.

chemical bonding Process of linking the radicals, chemical elements, or groups of a chemical compound.

cholecalciferol Chemical name for vitamin D in its inactive dietary form (D_3). When the inactive cholecalciferol is consumed or its counterpart cholesterol compound is developed in the skin, its first stage of acti-vation occurs in the liver and then is completed in the kidney to the active vitamin D hormone form *calcitriol* (1,25-dihydroxycholecalciferol, or shorter form 1,25 $[OH]_2D_3$).

cholecystectomy (Gr *cholē,* bile; *kystis,* bladder; *ektomē,* a cutting out) Surgical removal of the gallbladder.

cholecystokinin (CCK) (Gr *chole,* bile or gall; *kystis,* bladder, *kinein,* to move) A peptide hormone secreted by the duodenal mucosa in the presence of fat. The cholecystokinin causes the gallbladder to contract. This contraction propels bile into the duodenum, where it is needed to emulsify the fat. The fat is thus prepared for digestion and absorption.

cholesterol A fat-related compound, a sterol ($C_{27}H_{45}OH$). It is a normal constituent of bile and a principal constituent of gallstones. In body metabolism cholesterol is important as a precursor of various steroid hormones, such as sex hormones and adrenal corticoids. Cholesterol is synthesized by the liver. It is widely distributed in nature, especially in animal tissue such as glandular meats and egg yolk.

chorea (L *choreia,* dance) A wide variety of ceaseless involuntary movements that are rapid, complex, and jerky, yet appear to be well coordinated; characteristic movements of Huntington's disease.

chronic dieting syndrome (Gr *chronos,* time, persisting over a long period of time; *diaita,* way of living, customary allowance of food and drink; *syndrome,* concurrence, a set of symptoms that occur together) A compulsive eating disorder, commonly referred to as **compulsive overeating.** It includes binge eating episodes, but without the purging behavior of persons with bulimia nervosa. This is an emotional, reactive eating pattern occurring in response to stress or anxiety and used to soothe painful feelings.

chylomicrons (L *chylus,* juice, milky fluid taken up by lacteals of the intestinal villi; Gr *mikros,* small) Initial lipoproteins, carrying a large fat load, formed in the intestinal wall after a meal for absorption of the food fats into circulation.

chyme (Gr *chymos,* juice) Semifluid food mass in gastrointestinal tract following gastric digestion.

chymotrypsin (Gr *chymos,* chyme, creamy gruel-like material produced by gastric digestion of food) One of the protein-splitting and milk-curdling pancreatic enzymes, activated in the intestine from precursor chymotrypsinogen. It breaks peptide linkages of the amino acids phenylalanine and tyrosine.

cirrhosis (Gr *kirrhos,* orange-yellow) Chronic liver disease, characterized by loss of functional cells, with fibrous and nodular regeneration.

cisterni chyli Cistern or receptacle of the chyle is a dilated sac at the origin of the thoracic duct, which is the common truck that receives all the lymphatic vessels. The cisterna chyli lies in the abdomen between the second lumbar vertebra and the aorta. It receives the lymph from the intestinal trunk, the right and left lumbar lymphatic trunks, and two descending lymphatic trunks. The chyle, after passing through the cisterna chyli, is carried upward into the chest through the thoracic duct and empties into the venous blood at the point where the left subclavian vein joins the left internal jugular vein.

clinical nutrition specialist Specialty practice of a registered dietitian with an advanced degree in nutritional science and training in clinical nutrition.

coenzyme factors A major metabolic role of the micronutrients, vitamins and minerals, as essential partners with cell enzymes in a variety of reactions in both energy and protein metabolism.

cognitive (L *cognoscere,* to know) Pertaining to the mental processes of perceptions, memory, judgment, and reasoning, as contrasted with emotional and volitional processes.

collagen (Gr *kolla,* glue; *gennan,* to produce) The protein substance of the white fibers (collagenous fibers) of skin, tendon, bone, cartilage, and all other connective tissue; it is converted into gelatin by boiling.

collagen disease (Gr *kolla,* glue; *gennan,* to produce) Diseases attacking collagen tissues, the protein substance of the white fibers (collagenous fibers) of skin, tendon, bone, cartilage, and other connective tissue; any of a group of diseases that are clinically distinct but have in common widespread pathologic changes in the connective tissue, such as rheumatoid arthritis, lupus erythematosus, scleroderma, and rheumatic fever.

colloid (Gr *kollōdēs,* glutinous) Glutinous, gluelike; a dispersion of matter throughout a liquid.

colloidal osmotic pressure (COP) Pressure produced by the protein molecules in the plasma and in the cell. Because proteins are large molecules, they do not pass through the separating membranes of the capillary cells. Thus they remain in their respective compartments, exerting a constant osmotic pull that protects vital plasma and cell fluid volumes in these compartments.

colon (Gr *kolon,* colon) The part of the large intestine extending from the cecum to the rectum.

colostrum (L *colostrum,* premilk) Thin yellow fluid first secreted by the mammary gland a few days before and after childbirth, preceding the mature breast milk. It contains up to 20% protein including a large amount of lactalbumin, more minerals and less lactose and fat than does milk, and immunoglobulins representing the antibodies found in maternal blood.

compartment The collective quantity of material of a given type in the body. The four body compartments are lean body mass (muscle), bone, fat, and water.

complement (L *complere,* to fill) A complex series of enzymatic proteins occurring in normal serum that interact to combine with and augment (fill out, complete) the antigen-antibody complex of the body's immune system, producing lysis when the antigen is an intact cell; composed of 11 discrete proteins or functioning components, activated by the immunoglobulin factors IgG and IgM.

corticotropin-releasing factor (CRF) (L *cortex,* shell or rind, external layer; Gr *tropikos,* turning, *-tropic,* suffix indicating turning toward or changing) Hypothalamus factor stimulating release of anterior pituitary hormone ACTH (adrenocorticotropic hormone).

creatinine (Gr *kreas,* flesh) End product of the breakdown of body tissue; found in muscles and blood and excreted in urine. High levels indicate abnormally high catabolism of body proteins and possibly inadequate intake of carbohydrate and fat, which have a protein-sparing effect.

cretinism (F *cretinisine*) A congenital disease resulting from absence or deficiency of normal thyroid secretion, characterized by physical deformity, dwarfism, & mental retardation, and often goiters.

cruciferous (L *cruces,* cross; *forma,* form) Bearing a cross; botanical term for plants belonging to the botanical family *Cruciferae* or *Brassicaceae,* the mustard family, so called because of crosslike, four-petaled flowers; name given to certain vegetables of this family, such as broccoli, cabbage, brussels sprouts, and cauliflower.

cyclosporine An immunosuppressant drug widely used following organ transplants to control the immune system and prevent rejection of the new tissue.

cytokines (Gr *kytos,* hollow vessel, cell; *kinētos,* movable, changing) Substances produced in tissues that can cause inflammatory changes in tissue cells, e.g., tumor necrosis factor and interleukin-1.

deamination Removal of amino group (NH_2) from amino acid.

decubitus ulcer (L *decubitus,* lying down; *ulcus,* ulcer) Pressure sores in long-term bed-bound or immobile patients at points of bony protuberances, where prolonged pressure of body weight in one position cuts off adequate blood circulation to that area, causing tissue death and ulceration.

dehiscence (L *dehiscere,* to gape) A splitting open; the separation of the layers of a surgical wound, either (1) partial or superficial or (2) complete, with total disruption requiring resuturing.

dehydrocholesterol A precursor cholesterol compound in the skin that is irratiated by sunlight to produce an initial stage in the process of forming activated vitamin D hormone.

demographic (Gr *demos,* people; *graphein,* to write) The statistical data of a population, especially those showing average age, income, education, births, deaths, and so on.

diabetes insipidus (Gr *dia,* through; *bainein,* to go; *diabetes,* siphon; L *insipidus,* tasteless, not sweet, as compared to diabetes *mellitus,* L honey) A condition of the pituitary gland and insufficiency of one of its hormones, vasopressin or antidiuretic hormone; characterized by a copious output of a nonsweet urine, great thirst, and sometimes a large appetite. In diabetes insipidus these symptoms result from a specific injury to the pituitary gland, not a collection of metabolic disorders as in diabetes mellitus. The injured pituitary gland produces less vasopressin, a hormone that normally helps the kidneys reabsorb adequate water.

dialysis (Gr *dia,* through; *lysis,* dissolution) Process of separating crystalloids and colloids in solution by the difference in their rates of diffusion through a semipermeable membrane; crystalloids pass through readily and colloids very slowly or not at all.

dideoxynucleosides (chemistry *di-,* two; *de-,* removal; *oxy-,* oxygen; *nucleoside,* basic type of chemical compound involved) A class of drugs used treat HIV-infected persons; a nucleoside is a combination of a sugar (a pentose) with a purine or pyrimidine (two types of compounds that provide the cross-linking "ladders" of the double strands of DNA) base.

dietary fiber Nondigestible form of carbohydrate that is of nutritional importance in gastrointestinal disease such as diverticulosis and in reducing serum lipid and glucose levels related to chronic conditions such as heart disease and diabetes.

dietetics Management of diet and the use of food; the science concerned with the nutritional planning and preparation of foods.

disability Mental or physical impairment that prevents an individual from performing one or more gainful activities; not synonymous with **handicap,** which implies serious disadvantage.

disaccharides (Gr *di,* two; *saccharide,* sugar) Class of compound sugars composed of two molecules of monosaccharide. The three most common are sucrose, lactose, and maltose.

disulfiram White to off-white crystalline antioxidant; inhibits oxidation of the acetaldehyde metabolized from alcohol. It is used in the treatment of alcoholism, producing extremely uncomfortable symptoms when alcohol is ingested following oral administration of the drug.

diverticulitis (L *divertere,* to turn aside) Inflammation of pockets of tissue (diverticuli) in the lining of the mucous membrane of the colon.

dysentery (Gr *dys,* painful, bad; *enteron,* intestine) A general term given to a number of disorders marked by inflammation of the intestines, especially of the colon, and attended by abdominal pain and frequent stools containing blood and mucus. The causative agent may be chemical irritants, bacteria, protozoa, or parasites.

dyspnea (Gr *dysnoia,* difficulty of breathing) Labored, difficult breathing.

eclampsia (Gr *eklampein,* to shine forth) Advanced pregnancy-induced hypertension (PIH), manifested by convulsions.

ecology (Gr *oikos,* house) Relations between organisms and their environments.

eicosanoids (Gr *eikosa,* twenty) Long chain fatty acids composed of 20 carbon atoms.

electrolytes (Gr *electron,* amber [which emits electricity when rubbed]; *lytos,* soluble) A chemical element or compound that in solution dissociates as ions carrying a positive or negative charge (for example, H^+, Na^+, K^+, Ca^{++}, Mg^{++}, and Cl^-, HCO_3-, HPO_4-, SO_4-. Electrolytes constitute a major force controlling fluid balances within the body through their concentrations and shifts from one place to another to restore and maintain balance—*homeostasis.*

elemental formula A nutrition support formula composed of simple elemental nutrient components that require no further digestive breakdown and are thus readily absorbed; infant formula produced with elemental ready-to-be-absorbed components of free amino acids and carbohydrate as simple sugars.

emulsifier An agent that breaks down large fat globules to smaller, uniformly distributed particles. This action is accomplished in the intestine chiefly by the bile acids, which lower surface tension of the fat particles. Emulsification greatly increases the surface area of fat, facilitating contact with fat-digesting enzymes.

encephalopathy (Gr *enkephalos,* brain; *pathos,* disease) Any degenerative disease of the brain.

endemic (Gr *endemos,* dwelling in a place) Characterizing a disease of low morbidity that remains constantly in a human community but is clinically recognizable in only a few.

endocarditis (Gr *endon,* within; *kardia,* heart) Inflammation of the endocardium, the serous membrane that lines the cavities of the heart.

endothelium (Gr *endo-,* within; *thēlē,* nipple) Layer of epithelial cells that line the cavities of the heart, the blood and lymph vessels, and the serous cavities of the body, originating from the mesoderm.

energy (Gr *en,* in, with; *ergon,* work) The capacity of a system for doing work; available power. Energy is manifest in various forms—motion, position, light, heat, and sound. Energy is interchangeable among these various forms and is constantly being transformed and transferred among them.

enteral (Gr *enteron,* intestine) A mode of feeding that uses the gastrointestinal tract, oral or tube feeding.

enterogastrone (Gr *enteron,* intestine; *gaster,* stomach; -*one,* suffix for hormones) A duodenal peptide hormone that inhibits gastric hydrochloric acid secretion and motility.

enzyme (Gr *en,* in; *zyme,* leaven) Various complex proteins produced by living cells that act independently of these cells. Enzymes are capable of producing certain chemical changes in other substances without themselves being changed in the process. Their action is therefore that of a catalyst. Digestive enzymes of the gastrointestinal secretions act on food substances to break them down into simpler compounds and greatly accelerate the speed of these chemical reactions. An enzyme is usually named according to the substance (substrate) on which it acts, with the common suffix -ase; for example, sucrase is the specific enzyme for sucrose and breaks it down to glucose and fructose.

epidemiology (Gr *epidemois,* prevalent; -*ology,* study) The study of factors determining the frequency, distribution, and strength of diseases in population groups.

ergogenic (Gr *ergo,* work; *gennan,* to produce) Tendency to increase work output; various substances that increase work or exercise capacity and output.

erythema (Gr *erythros,* red; *erythema,* flush upon the skin) Redness of the skin produced by coagulation of the capillaries; results from a variety of causes, e.g., radiant heat or burns.

essential amino acid Any one of nine amino acids that the body cannot synthesize at all or in sufficient amounts to meet body needs, so it must be supplied by the diet, and is hence a *dietary* essential. These nine specific amino acids are histidine, isoleucine, leucine, lysine, methionine, phenylalanine, threonine, tryptophan, and valine.

essential fatty acid (L *essentialis,* necessary or inherent) A fatty acid required in the diet because the body cannot synthesize it.

essential hypertension An inherent form of hypertension with no specific discoverable cause and considered to be familial; also called primary hypertension.

ester A compound produced by the reaction between an acid and an alcohol with elimination of a molecule of water. This process is called *esterification*. For example, a triglyceride is a glycerol ester. Cholesterol esters are formed in the mucosal cells by combination with fatty acids, largely linoleic acid.

exudate (L *exsudare,* to sweat out) Various materials such as cells, cellular debris, and fluids, usually resulting from inflammation, that have escaped from blood vessels and are deposited in or on surface tissues; has a high protein content.

fasciculi (L *fascis,* bundle) A general term for a small bundle or cluster of muscle, tendon, or nerve fibers.

fatty acid The structural components of fats.

ferritin Protein-iron compound in which iron is stored in tissues; the storage form of iron in the body.

fetor hepaticus (L *fetor,* stench, offensive odor; *hepaticus,* liver) The peculiar odor of the breath that is characteristic of advanced liver disease.

fetus (L *fetus,* unborn offspring) The unborn offspring in the postembryonic period, after major structures have been outlined; in humans the growing offspring from 7 to 8 weeks after fertilization until birth.

filtration (L *filtrum,* felt used to strain liquids) Passage of a fluid through a semipermeable membrane (a membrane that permits passage of water and small solutes but not large molecules) as a result of a difference in pressures on the two sides of the membrane. For example, the net filtration pressure in the capillaries is the difference between the outward-pushing hydrostatic force of the blood pressure and the opposing inward-pulling force of the colloidal osmotic pressure exerted by the plasma proteins retained in capillary.

fistula (L *fistula,* pipe) Abnormal passageway, usually between two internal organs, or leading from an internal organ to the surface of the body.

flushing reaction Short-term reaction resulting in redness of neck and face.

fuel factor The kilocalorie value (energy potential) of food nutrients; that is, the number of kilocalories that 1 g of the nutrient yields when oxidized. The kilocalorie fuel factor for carbohydrate is 4; for protein, 4; and for fat, 9. The basic figures are used in computing diets and energy values of foods. (For example, 10 g of fat yields 90 kcal.)

fulminant (L *fulminare,* to flare up) Sudden, severe; occurring suddenly with great intensity.

gastrectomy (Gr *gaster,* stomach; *ektome,* excision) Surgical removal of the whole (total gastrectomy) or part (partial gastrectomy) of the stomach.

gastrin Hormone secreted by mucosal cells in the antrum of the stomach that stimulates the parietal cells to produce hydrochloric acid. Gastrin is released in response to stimulants, especially coffee, alcohol, and meat extractives, into the stomach. When the gastric pH reaches 2.0 to 3.0, a feedback mechanism cuts off gastrin secretion and prevents excess acid formation.

gastritis (Gr *gaster,* stomach) Inflammation of the stomach.

geriatrics (Gr *geras,* old age; *iatrike,* surgery, medicine) Branch of medicine specializing in medical problems associated with old age.

gerontology (Gr *geronto,* old man; *logy,* work, reason, study) Study of the aging process and its remarkable progressive events.

gestation (L *gestatio,* from; *gestare,* to bear) The period of embryonic and fetal development from fertilization to birth; pregnancy.

glomerulosclerosis (L *glomus,* ball, cluster; *sklerosis,* hardness) Intercapillary degeneration of the nephron glomerulus, a cluster of capillary loops cupped at the head of each nephron, resulting in the degeneration of the entire nephron; a diabetic complication, with symptoms of albuminuria, nephrotic edema, hypertension, and renal insufficiency.

glossitis (Gr *glossa,* tongue + *itis*) Swollen, reddened tongue; riboflavin deficiency symptom.

glucagon (Gr *glykys,* sweet; *gone,* seed) A polypeptide hormone secreted by the A cells of the pancreatic islets of Langerhans in response to hypoglycemia; has an opposite balancing effect to that of insulin, raising the blood sugar, thus is used as a quick-acting antidote for the hypoglycemic reaction of insulin. It stimulates the breakdown of glycogen (glycogenolysis) in the liver by activating the liver enzyme phosphorylase and thus raises blood sugar levels during fasting states to ensure adequate levels for normal nerve and brain function.

gluconeogenesis (Gr *gleukos,* sweetness; *neos,* new; *genesis,* production, generation) Production of glucose from keto-acid carbon skeleton from deaminated amino acids and the glycerol portion of fatty acids.

glucose tolerance factor (GTF) A biologically active complex of chromium and nicotinic acid that facilitates the reaction of insulin with receptor sites on tissues.

glyceride Group name for fats; any of a group of esters obtained from glycerol by the replacement of one, two, or three hydroxyl (OH) groups with a fatty acid. Monoglycerides contain one fatty acid; diglycerides contain two fatty acids; triglycerides contain three fatty acids. Glycerides are the principal constituent of adipose tissue and are found in animal and vegetable fats and oils.

glycerol A colorless, odorless, syrupy, sweet liquid; a constituent of fats usually obtained by the hydrolysis of fats. Chemically glycerol is an alcohol; it is esterified with fatty acids to produce fats.

glycogen (Gr *glykys,* sweet; *genes,* born, produced) A polysaccharide, that is, a large compound of many saccharide (i.e., sugar) units. It is the main body storage form of carbohydrate, largely stored (with relatively rapid turnover) in the liver, with lesser amounts stored in muscle tissue.

glycogenolysis (*glycogen* + Gr *lysis,* dissolution) Specific term for conversion of glycogen into glucose in the liver; chemical process of enzymatic hydrolysis or breakdown by which this conversion is accomplished.

glycolysis Initial energy production enzyme pathway outside the mitochondria, by which 6-carbon glucose is changed to active 3-carbon fragments of acetyl CoA, the fuel ready for final energy production in the mitochondria to the high-energy phosphate bond compound adenosine triphosphate (ATP).

goiter (L *guttur,* throat) Enlargement of the thyroid gland caused by lack of sufficient available iodine to produce the thyroid hormone, thyroxine.

gravida (L *gravida,* heavy, loaded) A pregnant woman.

growth acceleration (L *celerare,* to quicken) Period of increased speed of growth at different points of childhood development.

growth channel The progressive regular growth pattern of children, guided along individual genetically controlled channels, influenced by nutritional and health status.

growth chart grids Grids comparing stature (length), weight, and age of children by percentile; used for nutritional assessment to determine how their growth is progressing. The most commonly used grids are those of the National Center for Health Statistics (NCHS), by the Fels Research Institute.

growth deceleration (L *de,* from; *celerare,* to quicken) Period of decreased speed of growth at different points of childhood development.

growth velocity (L *velocitas,* speed) Rapidity of motion or movement; rate of childhood growth over normal periods of development, as compared with a population standard.

handicap Mental or physical defect that may or may not be congenital that prevents the individual from participating in normal life activities; implies disadvantage.

Heimlich maneuver A first-aid maneuver to relieve a person who is choking from blockage of the breathing passageway by a swallowed foreign object or food particle. Standing behind the person, clasp the victim around the waist, placing one fist just under the sternum (breastbone) and grasping the fist with the other hand. Then make a quick, hard, thrusting movement inward and upward to dislodge the object.

hematuria (Gr *haima,* blood; *ouron,* urine) The abnormal presence of blood in the urine.

heme iron Dietary iron from animal sources, from the heme portion of hemoglobin in red blood cells. Heme iron is more easily absorbed and transported in the body than nonheme iron from plant sources, but it supplies the smaller portion of the body's total dietary iron intake.

hemodialysis (Gr *haima,* blood; *dia,* through; *lysis,* dissolution) Removal of certain elements from the blood according to their rates of diffusion through a semipermeable membrane, e.g., by a hemodialysis machine.

hemoglobin (Gr *haima, blood; L globus,* a ball) Oxygen-carrying pigment in red blood cells; a conjugated protein containing four heme groups combined with iron and four long polypeptide chains forming the protein globin, named for its ball-like form; made by the developing red blood cells in bone marrow. Hemoglobin carries oxygen in the blood to body cells.

hemolytic anemia (Gr *haima,* blood; *lysis,* dissolution) An anemia (reduced number of red blood cells) caused by breakdown of red blood cells and loss of their hemoglobin.

hemophilia (Gr *hemo-,* blood; *philein,* to love) A heredity hemorrhagic disease caused by deficiency of blood coagulation factor VIII; characterized by spontaneous or traumatic bleeding; transmitted as an X-linked (maternal) recessive trait to male children. This X chromosome–linked deficiency of factor VIII has played a major role in the history of royal families of Europe.

hemosiderin (Gr *haima,* blood; *sideros,* iron) Insoluble iron oxide–protein compound in which iron is stored in the liver if the amount of iron in the blood exceeds the storage capacity of ferritin, for example, during rapid destruction of red blood cells (malaria, hemolytic anemia).

herpes zoster (Gr *herpēs,* herpes; *zoster,* a girdle or encircling structure or pattern) An acute self-limiting viral inflammatory disease of posterior nerve roots causing skin eruptions in a lateral pattern across the back of the torso served by these nerves, accompanied by neuralgic pain; caused by the virus of chickenpox and commonly called *shingles.*

homeostasis (Gr *homoios,* like, unchanging; *stasis,* standing, stable) State of relative dynamic equilibrium within the body's internal environment; a balance achieved through the operation of various interrelated physiologic mechanisms.

hormones Various internally secreted substances from the endocrine organs, which are conveyed by the blood to another organ or tissue on which they act to stimulate increased functional activity or secretion. This tissue or substance is called its target organ or substance.

hydrogenation Process of hardening liquid vegetable oils by injecting hydrogen gas to produce margarines and shortenings.

hydrolysis (Gr *hydro,* water; *lysis,* dissolution) Process by which a chemical compound is split into other simpler compounds by taking up the elements of water, as in the manufacture of infant formulas to produce easier-to-digest derivatives of the main protein casein in the cow's milk base. This process occurs naturally in digestion.

25-hydroxycholecalciferol (25, [OH]D$_3$) Initial product formed in the liver in the process of developing the active vitamin D hormone.

hygroscopic (Gr *hygros,* moist) Taking up and retaining moisture readily.

hypercapnia (Gr *hyper,* above; *kapnos,* smoke) Excess carbon dioxide in the blood.

hyperemesis gravidarum (Gr *hyper,* above, excessive; *emesis,* vomiting; L *gravida,* heavy loaded) Severe vomiting during pregnancy that is potentially fatal.

hyperlipoproteinemia (Gr *hyper,* above; *lipoprotein,* fat-protein compound; *-emia,* suffix referring to *haima,* blood) Elevated level of lipoproteins in the blood.

hypernatremia (Gr *hyper,* above; L *natron,* sodium; *haima,* blood) Excessive levels of sodium in the blood.

hyperparathyroidism (Gr *hyper,* above; *para,* alongside; *thyroidism,* thyroid gland function and, by extension, parathyroid gland function) Abnormally increased activity of the parathyroid gland, resulting in excessive secretion of parathyroid hormone, which normally helps regulate serum calcium levels in balance with vitamin D hormone; excess secretion occurs when the serum calcium level falls below normal, as in chronic renal disease or in vitamin D deficiency.

hypovolemia (Gr *hypo,* under; *haima,* blood) Abnormally decreased volume of circulating blood in the body.

hypoxemia (Gr *hypo,* under; *-ox-,* oxygen; *emia (haima),* blood) Deficient oxygenation of the blood, resulting in *hypoxia,* reduced oxygen supply to tissue.

iatrogenic (Gr *iatros,* healer; *genesis,* origin or source) Describing a medical disorder caused by physician diagnosis, manner, or treatment.

icterus (Gr *ikteros,* jaundice) Alternate term for jaundice: **nonicteric** indicates absence of jaundice; **pre-icteric** indicates a state prior to development of icterus, or jaundice.

immunocompetence (L *immunis,* free, exempt) The ability or capacity to develop an immune response—that is, antibody production and/or cell-mediated immunity—following exposure to antigen.

incomplete protein food A protein food having a ratio of amino acids different from that of the average body protein and therefore less valuable for nutrition than complete protein food.

indole A compound produced in the intestines by the decomposition of tryptophan; also found in the oil of jasmine and clove.

infarct (L *infarcire,* to stuff in) An area of tissue necrosis caused by local ischemia, resulting from obstruction of blood circulation to that area.

insulin (L *insula,* island) Hormone formed in the B cells of the islets of Langerhans in the pancreas. Insulin is secreted when blood glucose and amino acid levels rise and assists their entry into body cells. It also promotes glycogenesis and conversion of glucose into fat and inhibits lipolysis and gluconeogenesis (protein breakdown). Commercial insulin is manufactured from pigs and cows; new "artificial" human insulin products have recently been made available.

interferon (L *inter,* between; *ferire,* to strike) One of a class of small soluble proteins produced and released by cells invaded by a virus, which induces in noninfected cells the formation of an antiviral protein that interferes with viral multiplication.

intermittent claudication (L *claudicatio,* limping or lameness) A symptomatic pattern of peripheral vascular disease, characterized by absence of pain or discomfort in a limb, usually the legs, when at rest, which is followed by pain and weakness when walking, intensifying until walking becomes impossible, and then disappearing again after a rest period; seen in occlusive arterial disease.

interstitial fluid (L *inter,* between; *sistere,* to set) The fluid situated between parts or in the interspaces of a tissue.

intima (L *intima,* inner area) General term indicating an innermost part of a structure or vessel; inner layer of the blood vessel wall.

intramural nerve plexus (L *intra,* within; *murus,* wall; plexus, plait or network) Network of nerves in the walls of the intestine that make up the enteric nervous system controlling muscle action and secretions for digestion and absorption.

ischemia (Gr *ischein,* to suppress; *haima,* blood) Deficiency of blood to a particular tissue, caused by functional blood vessel constriction or actual obstruction.

jaundice (Fr *jaune,* yellow) A syndrome characterized by hyperbilirubinemia and deposits of bile pigment in the skin, mucous membranes, and sclera, giving a yellow appearance to the patient.

joule (James Prescott Joule, 1818-1889, English physicist) The international (SI) unit of energy and heat, defined as the work done by the force of 1 newton acting over the distance of 1 meter. A newton (named for Sir Isaac Newton, 1643-1727, English mathematician, physicist, and astronomer) is the international unit of force, defined as the amount of force that, when applied in a vacuum to a body having a mass of 1 kg, accelerates it at the rate of 1 meter per second. These are examples of the exactness with which terms and values used by the world's scientific community must be defined, as illustrated in the *Système International d'Unitēs (SI).*

keratinization The process of creating the protein *keratin,* which is the principal constituent of skin, hair, nails, horny tissues, and the organizing matrix of the enamel of the teeth. It is a very insoluble protein.

keto acid   Amino acid residue after deamination. The glycogenic keto acids are used to form carbohydrates. The ketogenic keto acids are used to form fats.

kilocalorie   (Fr *chilioi*, thousand; L *calor*, heat) The general term *calorie* refers to a unit of heat measure and is used alone to designate the *small calorie*. The calorie used in nutritional science and the study of metabolism is the *large calorie*, 1000 calories, or kilocalori (kcalorie), to be more accurate and avoid use of very large numbers in calculations.

kinetic   (Gr *kinetikos*, moving) Energy released from body fuels by cell metabolism and now active in moving muscles and energizing all body activities.

kyphosis   (Gr *hyphos*, a hump) Increased, abnormal convexity of the upper part of the spine; hunchback.

lactase   Enzyme that splits the disaccharide lactose into its two monosaccharides, glucose and galactose.

lactated Ringer's solution   Sterile solution of calcium chloride, potassium chloride, sodium chloride, and sodium lactate in water given to replenish fluid and electrolytes; developed by English physiologist Sydney Ringer (1835-1910).

lactiferous ducts   (L *lac*, milk; *ferre*, to bear) Branching channels in the mammary gland that carry breast milk to holding spaces near the nipple, ready for the infant's feeding.

limiting amino acid   The amino acid in foods occurring in the smallest amount, thus limiting its availability for tissue structure.

linoleic acid   The ultimate essential fatty acid for humans.

lipase   (Gr *lipos*, fat; *-ase*, enzyme) Group of fat enzymes that cut the ester linkages between the fatty acids and glycerol of triglycerides (fats).

lipids   (Gr *lipos*, fat) Chemical group name for fats and fat-related compounds such as cholesterol, lipoproteins, and phospholipids; general group name for organic substances of a fatty nature, including fats, oils, waxes, and related compounds.

lipoprotein   Noncovalent complexes of fat with protein. The lipoproteins function as major carriers of lipids in the plasma, since most of the plasma fat is associated with them. Such a combination makes possible the transport of fatty substances in a water medium such as plasma.

lumen   (L *lumen*, light) The cavity or channel within a tube or tubular organ, such as the intestines.

lymphocytes   (L *lympho-*, water; Gr *kytos*, hollow vessel, suffix for a cell type of the root to which it is designated or attached) Special white cells from lymphoid tissue that participate in humeral and cell-mediated immunity.

lymphoma   (L *lympha*, water; Gr *sōma*, body) General term applied to any neoplastic disorder (cancer) of the lymphoid tissue.

macrocytic anemia   (Gr *makros*, large; *cyte*, hollow vessel, cell) An anemia (deficiency of normal red cells) characterized by abnormally large red cells.

macronutrients   (Gr *makros*, large; L *nutriens*, nourishment) The three large energy-yielding nutrients: carbohydrates, fats, and proteins.

malignant   (L *malignare*, to act suspiciously) An abnormal condition such as a tumor that tends to become progressively worse and results in death.

malignant melanoma   (L *malignans*, acting maliciously; Gr *melos*, black) A tumor tending to become progressively worse, composed of melanin, the dark pigment of the skin and other body tissues, usually arising from the skin and aggravated by excessive sun exposure.

maltase   Enzyme that breaks down the disaccharide maltose into two units of glucose, a monosaccharide.

median   (L *medianus*, middle, midpoint) In statistics, the middle number in a sequence of numbers.

medical foods   Specially formulated nutrient mixtures for use under medical supervision to treat various metabolic diseases.

medulla   (L *medulla*, marrow, center) General term for the inner or central portion of an organ or structure. The renal medulla is the inner part of the kidney, holding the lower parts (loop of Henle and collecting tubule) of the nephron, which are organized grossly into pyramids with glomerular heads of the nephrons in the outer portion (cortex) of the kidney.

megaloblastic anemia   (Gr *mega*, great size; *blastos*, embryo, germ) Anemia resulting from faulty production of abnormally large immature red blood cells, caused by a deficiency of vitamin B_{12} and folate.

menadione   The parent compound of vitamin K in the body; called also *vitamin K_3*.

menaquinone   Form of vitamin K synthesized by intestinal bacteria; called also *vitamin K_2*.

menarche   (Gr *men*, month; *arche*, beginning) The beginning of first menstruation with the onset of puberty.

meningitis   (Gr *meninx*, membrane) Inflammation of the *meninges*, the three membranes that envelop the brain and spinal cord, caused by a bacterial or viral infection and characterized by high fever, severe headache, and stiff neck or back muscles.

metabolism   (Gr *metaballein*, to change, alter) Sum of all the various biochemical and physiologic processes by which the body grows and maintains itself (**anabolism**) and breaks down and reshapes tissue (**catabolism**), transforming energy to do its work. Products of these various reactions are called **metabolites.**

metabolite   Any substance produced by metabolism or by a metabolic process.

micellar bile-fat complex   (L *mica*, crumb, particle) A combination of bile and fat in which the bile emulsifies fat into very minute globules or particles that can be absorbed easily into the small intestine wall in preparation for the final stage of absorption into circulation to the cells.

microaneurysm (Gr *mikros,* small; *aneurysma,* a widening) A small sac formed by the widening of the wall of small blood vessels; diabetic aneurysms may form in the basement membrane of capillaries throughout vascular beds, as in the eye.

micronutrients (Gr *mikros,* small; L *nutriens,* nourishment) The two classes of small non-energy-yielding elements and compounds—minerals and vitamins—essential in very small amounts for regulation and control functions in cell metabolism and building certain body structures.

microvilli (Gr *mikros,* small; L *villus,* tuft of hair) Minute vascular structures protruding from the surface of villi covering the inner surface of the small intestine, forming a "brush border" that facilitates absorption of nutrients.

monosaccharide (Gr *mono,* single; *sakcharon,* sugar) Simple single sugar; a carbohydrate containing a single saccharide (sugar) unit.

motivation Forces that affect individual goal-directed behavior toward satisfying needs or achieving personal goals.

mucosa (L *mucus*) The mucous membrane comprising the inner surface layer of gastrointestinal tract tissues, providing extensive nutrient absorption and transport functions.

mucus Viscid fluid secreted by mucous membranes and glands, consisting mainly of mucin (a glycoprotein), inorganic salts, and water. Mucus serves to lubricate and protect the gastrointestinal mucosa and to help move the food mass along the digestive tract.

myasthenia gravis (Gr *mys,* muscle; *asthenia,* weakness; L *gravis,* heavy, weighty, grave) A progressive neuromuscular disease caused by faulty nerve conduction resulting from the presence of antibodies to acetylcholine receptors at the neuromuscular junction.

myelin (Gr *myelos,* marrow) High lipid-to-protein substance forming a fatty sheath to insulate and protect neuron axons and facilitate their neuromuscular impulses.

myelin sheath (Gr *myelos,* marrow; *thēkē,* sheath) Covering of myelin, a lipid-protein substance with a high fat proportion to protein, surrounding nerve axons; serves as electrical insulator and speeds the conduction of nerve impulses; interrupted at intervals along the length of the axon by gaps known as Ranvier's nodes.

myofibril (Gr mys, muscle; L *fibrilla,* very small fiber) Slender thread of muscle; runs parallel to the muscle fiber's long axis.

myofilaments (Gr *mys,* muscle; L *filare,* to wind thread, spin) Threadlike filaments of actin or myosin, which are components of myofibrils.

myosin (Gr *mys,* muscle) Myofibril protein whose synchronized meshing action in conjunction with **actin** causes muscles to contract and relax.

necrosis (Gr *nekrosis,* deadness) Cell death caused by progressive enzyme breakdown.

neoplasm (Gr *neos,* new; *plasma,* formation) Any new or abnormal cellular growth, specifically one that is uncontrolled and progressive.

nephron (Gr *nephros,* kidney) Microscopic anatomic and functional unit of the kidney that selectively filters and reabsorbs essential blood factors, secretes hydrogen ions as needed for maintaining acid-base balance, then reabsorbs water to protect body fluids, and forms and excretes a concentrated urine for elimination of wastes. The nephron includes the renal corpuscle (glomerulus), the proximal convoluted tubule, the loop of Henle, the distal convoluted tubule, and the collecting tubule, which empties the urine into the renal medulla. The urine passes into the papilla and then to the pelvis of the kidney. Urine is formed by filtration of blood in the glomerulus and by the selective reabsorption and secretion of solutes by cells that comprise the walls of the renal tubules. There are approximately 1 million nephrons in each kidney.

nephropathy (Gr *nephros,* kidney; *pathos,* disease) Disease of the kidneys; in diabetes, renal damage associated with functional and pathologic changes in the nephrons, which can lead to glomerulosclerosis and chronic renal failure.

nephrosis (Gr *nephros,* kidney) Nephrotic syndrome caused by degenerative epithelial lesions of the renal tubules of the nephrons, especially the *mesangium,* the thin basement membrane that helps support the capillary loops in a renal glomerulus; marked by edema, albuminuria, and decreased serum albumin.

neuropathy (Gr *neuron,* nerve; *pathos,* disease) General term for functional and pathologic changes in the peripheral nervous system; in diabetes, a chronic sensory condition affecting mainly the nerves of the legs, marked by numbness from sensory impairment, loss of tendon reflexes, severe pain, weakness, and wasting of muscles involved.

niacin equivalent (NE) A measure of the total dietary sources of niacin equivalent to 1 mg of niacin. Thus an NE is 1 mg of niacin or 60 mg of tryptophan.

night blindness Inability to see well at night in diminished light, resulting from lack of required vitamin A.

nitrogen balance The metabolic balance between nitrogen intake in dietary protein and output in urinary nitrogen compounds such as urea and creatinine. For every 6.25 g dietary protein consumed, 1 g nitrogen is excreted.

nonheme iron The larger portion of dietary iron, including all the plant food sources and 60% of the animal food sources, which lacks the more easily absorbed and bioavailable heme iron in the remaining 40% of the animal food sources that contain hemoglobin residues of iron-containing heme.

norepinephrine (*nor-,* prefix, normal or parent form of a compound; Gr *epi-,* on, upon, or over; *nephros,* kidney) One of the catecholamines; a neurohormone, principal neurotransmitter of adrenergic nerves; secreted by inner part of the adrenal glands, which lie on top of the kidneys.

nulligravida (L *nullus,* none; *gravida,* pregnant) A woman who has never been pregnant.

nutrients (L *nutriens,* nourishment) Substances in food that are essential for energy, growth, normal functioning of the body, and maintenance of life.

nutrition (L *nutritio,* nourishment) The sum of the processes involved in taking in food nutrients, assimilating and using them to maintain body tissue and provide energy; a foundation for life and health.

nutritional science The body of scientific knowledge, developed through controlled research, that relates to the processes involved in nutrition\Mnational, international, community, and clinical.

obesity (L *obesus,* excessively fat) Fatness; an excessive accumulation of fat in the body.

occult bleeding (L *occultus,* concealed) Obscure, difficult to detect, concealed from observation; such a small blood loss that it can be detected only by a microscope or chemical test.

oligosaccharides (Gr *oligos,* little; *saccharide,* sugar) Intermediate products of polysaccharide carbohydrate breakdown that contain a small number (from 4 to 10) of single sugar units of the monosaccharide glucose.

oliguria (Gr *oligos,* little; *ouron,* urine) Secretion of a very small amount of urine in relation to fluid intake.

oncogene (Gr *onkos,* mass; *genesis,* generation, production) Any of various genes that, when activated as by radiation or a virus, may cause a normal cell to become cancerous; viral genetic material carrying the potential of cancer and passed from parent to offspring.

organic (Gr *organikos,* organ) Carbon-based chemical compounds.

orthotopic (Gr *ortho,* straight, normal, correct; *topos,* place) Occurring at the normal place in the body; placement of a transplanted organ in the position formerly occupied by tissue of the same kind.

osmolality (Gr *osmos,* impulse, osmotic force) Property of a solution that depends on the concentration of the solute per unit of the solvent.

osteodystrophy (Gr *osteon,* bone) Defective bone formation.

osteoporosis (Gr *osteon,* bone; *poros,* passage, pore) Abnormal thinning of bone, producing a porous, fragile, latticelike bone tissue of enlarged spaces that is prone to fracture or deformity.

palliative (L *palliatus,* cloaked) Care affording relief but not cure; useful for comfort when cure is still unknown or obscured.

palmar grasp (L *palma,* palm) Early grasp of the young infant, clasping an object in the palm and wrapping the whole hand around it.

pancreatic enzyme preparations Commercial preparations of pancreatic enzymes—protease, lipase, and amylase—that have the same action as do the human enzymes from the pancreas; used in the treatment of pancreatic insufficiency.

pandemic (Gr *pan,* all; *dēmos,* people) A widespread epidemic, distributed through a region, continent, or the world.

pantothenic acid (Gr *pantothen,* "from all sides" or "in every corner") A B vitamin found widely distributed in nature and occurring throughout the body tissues. Pantothenic acid is an essential constituent of coenzyme A, which has extensive metabolic responsibility as an activating agent of a number of compounds in many tissues.

paradigm (Gr *para,* side-by-side; *deiknynai,* to show) A pattern or model serving as an example; a standard or ideal for practice or behavior based on a fundamental value or theme.

parasite (Gr *para,* along side; *sitos,* food, grain; *parasitos,* one who eats at another's table; in ancient Greece, a term for a person who received free meals in return for amusing or flattering conversation) An organism that lives on or in an organism of another species, known as the host, from whom all life-cycle nourishment is obtained.

parenchymal cells (Gr *parenchyma,* "anything poured in beside") Functional cells of an organ, as distinguished from the cells comprising its structure or framework.

parenteral (Gr *para,* along side, beyond, accessory; *enteron,* intestine) A mode of feeding that does not use the gastrointestinal tract but instead provides nutrition by intravenous delivery of nutrient solutions.

paresthesia (Gr *para,* beyond; *aisthesis,* perception) Abnormal sensations such as prickling, burning, and "crawling" of skin.

parity (L *parere,* to bring forth, produce) The condition of a woman with respect to having borne viable offspring.

pepsin The main gastric enzyme specific for proteins. Pepsin begins breaking large protein molecules into shorter chain polypeptides, proteoses, and peptones. Gastric hydrochloric acid is necessary to activate pepsin.

peptide bond The characteristic joining of amino acids to form proteins. Such a chain of amino acids is termed a peptide. Depending on its size, it may be a dipeptide fragment of protein digestion or a large polypeptide.

percentile (L *per,* throughout, in space or time; *centrum,* a hundred) One of 100 equal parts of a measured series of values; rate or proportion per hundred.

peristalsis (Gr *peri,* around; *stalsis,* contraction) A wavelike progression of alternate contraction and relaxation of the muscle fibers of the gastrointestinal tract.

peritoneal dialysis Dialysis through the peritoneum into and out of the peritoneal cavity.

peritoneum (Gr *per,* around; *teinein,* to stretch) A strong smooth surface, a serous membrane, lining the abdominal/pelvic walls and the undersurface of the diaphragm, forming a sac enclosing the body's vital visceral organs within the peritoneal cavity.

pernicious anemia A chronic macrocytic anemia occurring most commonly after age 40. It is caused by absence of the intrinsic factor normally present in the gastric juices and necessary for the absorption of cobalamin vitamin B_{12} and controlled by intramuscular injections of vitamin B_{12}.

phagocytes (Gr *phagein,* to eat; *kytos,* hollow vessel, cell) Cells that ingest microorganisms, other cells, or foreign particles; macrophages.

phospholipid Any of a class of fat-related substances that contain phosphorus, fatty acids, and a nitrogenous base. The phospholipids are essential elements in every cell.

photosynthesis (Gr *photos,* light; *synthesis,* putting together) Process by which plants containing chlorophyll are able to manufacture carbohydrate by combining CO_2 from air and water from soil. Sunlight is used as energy; chlorophyll is a catalyst. $6\ CO_2 + 6\ H_2O + Energy \rightarrow$ Chlorophyll $\rightarrow C_6H_{12}O_6 + 6\ O_2$

phylloquinone A fat-soluble vitamin of the K group, $C_3,H_{46}O_2$, found in green plants or prepared synthetically.

physiologic age (Gr *physis,* nature; *logikos,* or speech or reason) Rate of biologic maturation in individual adolescents that varies widely and accounts more for wide and changing differences in their metabolic rates, nutritional needs, and food requirements than does chronologic age.

pincer grasp Later digital grasp of the older infant, usually picking up smaller objects with a precise grip between thumb and forefinger.

placenta (L *placenta,* a flat cake) Special organ developed in early pregnancy that provides nutrients to the fetus and removes metabolic waste.

plaque (Fr *plaque,* patch or flat area) Thickened deposits of fatty material, largely cholesterol, within the arterial wall that eventually may fill the lumen and cut off blood supply to the tissue served by the damaged vessel.

polysaccharides (Gr *poly,* many; *saccharide,* sugar) Class of complex carbohydrates composed of many monosaccharide units. Common members are starch, dextrins, dietary fiber, and glycogen.

portal An entryway, usually referring to the portal circulation of blood through the liver. Blood is brought into the liver by the portal vein and out by the hepatic vein.

postprandial (L *post* after; *prandium,* breakfast, a meal) Occurring after a meal.

potential (L *potentia,* power) Energy existing in stored fuels and ready for action, but not yet released and active.

prealbumin (PAB) Plasma protein with short life used as a biochemical measure for assessing current nutritional status.

precursor (L *praecursor,* a forerunner) Something that precedes; in biology, a substance from which another substance is derived.

primigravida (L *prima,* first; *gravida,* pregnant) A woman pregnant for the first time.

proctocolectomy (Gr *prōktos,* anus; *-col-,* colon; *ektomē,* excision) Surgical removal of the rectum and colon.

proenzyme An inactive precursor converted to the active enzyme by the action of an acid, another enzyme, or other means; also called zymogen.

prostaglandins (Gr *prostates,* standing before; L *glans,* acorn; hence, male prostate gland) Group of naturally occurring substances, first discovered in semen, derived from long-chain fatty acids that have multiple local hormonelike actions, including regulation of gastric acid secretion, platelet aggregation, body temperature, and tissue inflammation.

protein balance (Gr *protos,* first) Body tissue protein balance between building up tissue (**anabolism**) and breaking down tissue (**catabolism**) to maintain healthy body growth and maintenance.

proteinuria (Gr *protos,* first, protein; *ouron,* urine) The presence of an excess of serum proteins, such as albumin in the urine.

prothrombin (Gr *pro,* before; *thrombos,* clot) Blood-clotting factor (number II) synthesized in the liver from glutamic acid and carbon dioxide, catalyzed by vitamin K.

P/S ratio Ratio of polyunsaturated to saturated fats in the diet.

public health nutritionist A professional nutritionist, accredited by academic degree course of university and special graduate study (MPH, DrPH) in schools of public health accredited by the American Association of Public Health, responsible for nutrition components of public health programs in varied community settings—county, state, national, international.

pulmonary edema Accumulation of fluid in tissues of the lung.

pyrosis (Gr *pyro,* fire, burning) Heartburn.

raffinose (Fr *raffin,* to refine) A colorless crystalline trisaccharide component of legumes, composed of galactose and sucrose connected by bonds that human enzymes cannot break, thus it remains whole in the intestines and produces gas as bacteria attack it.

receptor (L *receptor,* receiver) Any one of various specific protein molecules in surface membranes of cells and cell organelles, to which complementary molecules (such as hormones, neurotransmitters, drugs, viruses, or other antigens or antibodies) may become bound.

Recommended Dietary Allowances (RDAs) Recommended daily allowances of nutrients and energy intake for population groups according to age and sex, with defined weight and height. The RDAs are established and reviewed periodically by a representative group of nutritional scientists in response to current research. These standards vary very little among the developed countries.

Registered Dietitian (RD) A professional dietitian, accredited by academic degree course of university and graduate study (MS, PhD), clinical and administration training, and passing required registration examinations administered by the American Dietetic Association.

renal solute load (L *ren,* kidney) Collective number and concentration of solute particles in a solution, carried by the blood to the kidney nephrons for excretion in the urine. These particles are usually nitrogenous products from protein metabolism and the electrolytes Na^+, K^+, Cl^-, and $HPO_4=$.

renin-angiotensin-aldosterone mechanism Three-stage system of sodium conservation, hence control of water loss, in response to diminished filtration pressure in the kidney nephrons: (1) pressure loss causes kidney to secrete the enzyme renin, which combines with and activates angiotensinogen from the liver; (2) active angiotensin stimulates of the adjacent adrenal gland to release the hormone aldosterone; (3) the hormone causes reabsorption of sodium from the kidney nephrons and water follows.

replicate (L *replicare,* to fold back) To make an exact copy; to repeat, duplicate, or reproduce. In genetics, replication is the process by which double-stranded DNA makes copies of itself, each separating strand synthesizing a complementary strand. Cell replication is the process by which living cells, under gene control, make exact copies of themselves a programmed number of times during the life span of the organism. The process can be reproduced in the laboratory with cultured cell lines for special studies in cell biology.

resting metabolic rate (RMR) Amount of energy required to maintain the resting body's internal activities when in a normal environment temperature. Because of small differences in measuring techniques, RMR may be slightly different from the same person's **basal metabolic rate (BMR).** In practice, however, RMR and BMR measurments may be used interchangeably.

retinal Organic compound that is the aldehyde form of **retinol,** derived by the enzymatic splitting of absorbed carotene. It performs vitamin A activity. In the retina of the eye, retinal combines with opsins to form visual pigments. In the rods it combines with scotopsin to form rhodopsin (visual purple). In the cones it combines with photopsin to form the three pigments responsible for color vision.

retinol Chemical name for vitamin A, derived from its function relating to the retina of the eye and light-dark adaptation. Daily RDA standards are stated in retinol equivalents (RE) to account for sources of the preformed vitamin A and its precursor provitamin A, beta-carotene.

retinol Equivalent (RE) Unit of measure for dietary sources of vitamin A, both preformed vitamin, retinol, and the precursor provitamin, beta-carotene. 1 RE = 1 μg retinol or 6 μg beta-carotene.

retinopathy (L *rete,* net, network; *retina,* innermost layer covering the eyeball; *pathos,* disease) Noninflammatory disease of the retina, visual tissue of the eye, characterized by microaneurysms, intraretinal hemorrhages, waxy yellow exudates, "cotton wool" patches, and macular edema; a complication of diabetes that may lead to proliferation of fibrous tissue, retinal detachment, and blindness.

retrovirus (L *retro-,* backward) Any of a family of single-strand RNA viruses having an envelope and containing a reverse coding enzyme that allows for a reversal of genetic transcription from RNA to DNA rather than the usual DNA to RNA, the newly transcribed viral DNA then being incorporated into the host cell's DNA strand for the production of new RNA retroviruses.

rooting reflex A reflex in a newborn in which stimulation of the side of the cheek or the upper or lower lip causes the infant to turn its mouth and face to the stimulus.

sarcoma (Gr *sarkos,* flesh; *onkoma,* a swelling) Tumors, usually malignant, arising from connective tissue.

saturated (L *saturare,* to fill) To cause to unite with the greatest possible amount of another substance through solution, chemical combination, or the like. A saturated fat, for example, is one in which the component fatty acids are filled with hydrogen atoms. A fatty acid is said to be saturated if all available chemical bonds of its carbon chain are filled with hydrogen. If one bond remains unfilled, it is a monounsaturated fatty acid. If two or more bonds remain unfilled, it is a polyunsaturated fatty acid.

Fats of animal sources are more saturated. Fats of plant sources are unsaturated.

scurvy A hemorrhagic disease caused by lack of vitamin C. Diffuse tissue bleeding occurs, limbs and joints are painful and swollen, bones thicken as a result of subperiosteal hemorrhage, ecchymoses (large irregular discolored skin areas caused by tissue hemorrhages) form, bones fracture easily, wounds do not heal well, gums are swollen and bleeding, and teeth loosen.

sebaceous (L *sebum,* suet) Secreting the fatty lubricating substance *sebum.*

secretin Hormone produced in the mucous membrane of the duodenum in response to the entrance of the acid contents of the stomach into the duodenum. Secretin in turn stimulates the flow of pancreatic juice, providing needed enzymes and the proper alkalinity for their action.

senescence (L *senescere,* to grow old) The process of growing old; a consequence of advancing age or of premature aging process from disease.

sepsis (Gr *sēpsis,* decay) Presence in the blood or other tissues of pathogenic microorganisms or their toxins; conditions associated with such pathogens.

serosa Outer surface layer of the intestines interfacing with the blood vessels of the portal system going to the liver.

serotonin A neurotransmitter in the brain that effectively suppresses appetite and heavy eating.

solutes (Gr *solvere,* to solve) Particles of a substance in solution; a solution consists of solutes and a dissolving medium (solvent), usually a liquid.

somatostatin (Gr *soma,* body; *stasis,* standing still, maintaining a constant level) A hormone formed in the D cells of the pancreatic islets of Langerhans and the hypothalamus. It is a balancing factor in maintaining normal blood glucose levels by inhibiting insulin and glucagon production in the pancreas as needed.

spina bifida (L *spina,* spine; *bifidus,* cleft into two parts or branches) Congenital defect in the fetal closing of the neural tube to form a portion of the lower spine, leaving the spine unclosed and the spinal cord open in various degrees of exposure and damage.

sprue Alternate term for adult celiac disease, a malabsorption syndrome.

steroids (Gr *stereos,* solid; L *-ol, oleum,* oil) Group name for lipid-based sterols, including hormones, bile acids, and cholesterol.

stoma (Gr *stoma,* mouth, opening) The opening established in the abdominal wall, connecting with the ileum or colon, for elimination of intestinal wastes after surgical removal of diseased portions of the intestinal tract.

stomatitis (Gr *stoma,* mouth; *-itis,* inflammation) Inflammation of the oral mucosa, especially the buccal tissue lining the inside of the cheeks, but also possibly the tongue, palate, floor of the mouth, and gums.

stroke volume (Gr *streich,* to strike or stretch) The amount of blood pumped from a ventricle (chamber of the heart releasing blood to body circulations) with each beat of the heart.

substrate (L *sub,* under; *stratum,* layer) The specific organic substance on which a particular enzyme acts to produce new metabolic products.

sucrase Enzyme splitting the disaccharide sucrose into its two monosaccharides of glucose and fructose.

synergism (Gr *syn,* with or together; *ergon,* work) The joint action of separate agents in which the total effect of their combined action is greater than the sum of their separate actions. (Adjective: **synergistic.**)

synosheath (Gr syno-, with, together; *thēkē,* sheath) Protective pliable connective tissue surrounding the bony-collagen meshwork and fluid that come together in the synovial area between major bone heads in joints, allows normal padded and lubricated joint movement and motion.

tachycardia (Gr *tachys,* swift; *kardia,* heart) Excessively rapid action of the heart; usually applied to a heart rate above 100 beats per minute.

tactile (L *tactus,* touch) Pertaining to the sense of touch.

taurine A sulfur-containing amino acid, $NH_2(CH_2)_2$ SO_2OH, formed from the essential amino acid methionine. It is found in various body tissues, such as lungs and muscles, and in bile and breast milk.

thermic effect of food (Gr *therme,* heat, of or pertaining to heat) Body heat produced by food; amount of energy required to digest and absorb food and transport nutrients to the cells. This basic preparatory work accounts for about 10% of the day's total energy (kcalories) requirement.

thiamin pyrophosphate (TPP) Activating coenzyme form of thiamin that plays a key role in carbohydrate metabolism.

tocopherol (Gr *tokos,* childbirth; *pherein,* to carry) Chemical name for vitamin E. It was so named by early investigators because their initial work with rats indicated a reproductive function, which did not turn out to be the case with humans. In humans it functions as a strong antioxidant to preserve structural membranes, such as cell walls.

transmural (L *trans-,* through; *murrus,* wall) Through the wall of an organ; extending through or affecting the entire thickness of the wall of an organ or cavity.

triglyceride (Gr *tri,* three) Chemical name for fat, indicating structure: attachment of three fatty acids to a glycerol base; a neutral fat, synthesized from carbohydrate and stored in adipose tissue. It releases free fatty acids into the blood when hydrolyzed by enzymes.

trypsin   (Gr *trypein,* to rub; *pepsis,* digestion) A protein-splitting enzyme formed in the intestine by action of enterokinase on the inactive precursor trypsinogen.

vagotomy   (L *vagus,* wandering; Gr *tomē,* a cutting) A cutting of the vagus nerve (tenth cranial nerve), which regulates muscular and secretory actions of the stomach.

valence   (L *valens,* powerful) Power of an element or a radical to combine with or to replace other elements or radicals. Atoms of various elements combine in definite proportions. The valence number of an element is the number of atoms of hydrogen with which one atom of the element can combine.

varices   (plural form) (L *varix* [singular], enlarged vein) Varicose veins; enlarged and tortuous veins, full of twists, turns, curves, or windings.

vasoactive   (L *vas,* vessel) Having an effect on the diameter of blood vessels.

ventricle   (L *venter,* belly, abdomen; *ventriculus,* diminutive form indicating relation to front aspect of the body) A small cavity; one of the pair of lower chambers of the heart, with thick muscular walls, that make up the bulk of the heart. The ventricles receive blood from the atria and in turn force blood out into body circulation to the lungs for oxygenation and then into systemic body circulation to service the cells.

villi   (L *villus,* "tuft of hair") Small protrusions from the surface of a membrane; fingerlike projections covering the mucosal surfaces of the small intestine.

virus   (L *virus,* poison; *virion,* individual virus particle) Minute infectious agent characterized by lack of independent metabolism and by the ability to reproduce with genetic continuity only within living host cells. Viruses range in decreasing size from about 200 nanometers (nm) down to only 15 nanometers (nm). (A nanometer is a linear measure equal to one-billionth of a meter; it is also called a millimicron.) Each particle (virion) consists basically of nucleic acids (genetic material) and a protein shell that protects and contains the genetic material and any enzymes present.

viscous (viscid)   (L *viscidus,* glutinous or sticky) Physical property of a substance dependent on the friction of its component molecules as they slide by one another; viscosity.

VO_2max   Maximum uptake volume of oxygen during exercise; used to measure the intensity and duration of exercise a person can perform.

xanthoma   (Gr *xanthos,* yellow; *-oma,* mass or body of material) A plaque of yellow lipid deposits in the skin; fatty streaks or nodules.

Zollinger-Ellison syndrome   An intractable, sometimes fulminating atypical peptic ulcer disease, characterized by extreme gastric hyperacidity.

Index

Page numbers in *italics* indicate figures and boxed items. Page numbers followed by a *t* indicate tables.

Median Height and Weight and Recommended Energy Intake, 10th edition RDAs

Category	Age (years) or condition	Weight (kg)	Weight (lb)	Height (cm)	Height (in)	REE* (kcal/day)	Multiples of REE	Per kg	Per day†
Infants	0-0.5	6	13	60	24	320		108	650
	0.5-1	9	20	71	28	500		98	850
Children	1-3	13	29	90	56	740		102	1300
	4-6	20	44	112	44	950		90	1800
	7-10	28	62	132	52	1130		70	2000
Men	11-14	45	99	157	62	1440	1.70	55	2500
	15-18	66	145	176	69	1760	1.67	45	3000
	19-24	72	160	177	70	1780	1.67	40	2900
	25-50	79	174	176	70	1800	1.60	37	2900
	51+	77	170	173	68	1530	1.50	30	2300
Women	11-14	46	101	157	62	1310	1.67	47	2200
	15-18	55	120	163	64	1370	1.60	40	2200
	19-24	58	128	164	65	1350	1.60	38	2200
	25-50	63	138	163	64	1380	1.55	36	2200
	51+	65	143	160	63	1280	1.50	30	1900
Pregnant	1st trimester								+0
	2nd trimester								+300
	3rd trimester								+300
Lactating	1st 6 months								+500
	2nd 6 months								+500

*Resting energy expenditure (REE); calculation based on FAQ equations and then rounded. This is the same as RMR (resting metabolic rate).
†Figure is rounded.

1983 Metropolitan Life Insurance Company Height-Weight Table*†

Height Ft	Height In	Women Frame* Small	Women Frame* Medium	Women Frame* Large	Height Ft	Height In	Men Frame* Small	Men Frame* Medium	Men Frame* Large
4	10	102-111	109-121	118-131	5	2	128-134	131-141	138-150
4	11	103-113	111-123	120-134	5	3	130-136	133-143	140-153
5	0	104-115	113-126	122-137	5	4	132-138	135-145	142-156
5	1	106-118	115-129	125-140	5	5	134-140	137-148	144-160
5	2	108-121	118-132	128-143	5	6	136-142	139-151	146-164
5	3	111-124	121-135	131-147	5	7	138-145	142-154	149-168
5	4	114-127	124-138	134-151	5	8	140-148	145-157	152-172
5	5	117-130	127-141	137-155	5	9	142-151	148-160	155-176
5	6	120-133	130-144	140-159	5	10	144-154	151-163	158-180
5	7	113-136	133-147	143-163	5	11	146-157	154-166	161-184
5	8	126-139	136-150	146-167	6	0	149-160	157-170	164-188
5	9	129-142	139-153	149-170	6	1	152-164	160-174	168-192
5	10	132-145	142-156	152-173	6	2	155-168	164-178	172-197
5	11	135-148	146-159	155-176	6	3	158-172	167-182	176-202
6	0	138-151	148-162	158-179	6	4	162-176	171-187	181-207

*Based on a weight-height mortality study conducted by the Society of Actuaries and the Association of Life Insurance Medical Directors of American, Metropolitan Life Insurance Medical Directors of America, Metropolitan Life Insurance Company, revised 1983.
†Weights at ages 25 to 59 based on lowest mortality. Height includes 1-in heel. Weight for women includes 3 lb. for indoor clothing. Weight for men includes 5 lb. for indoor clothing.